THEORY AND PRACTICE OF HISTOLOGICAL TECHNIQUES

Commissioning Editor: Michael Houston
Development Editor: Sheila Black
Editorial Assistant: Liz MacSween
Project Manager: Alan Nicholson
Designer: Sarah Russell
Illustration Manager: Bruce Hogarth
Marketing Managers: John Canelon (UK); Kathleen Neely (USA)

THEORY AND PRACTICE OF HISTOLOGICAL TECHNIQUES

Sixth Edition

John D. Bancroft

Formerly Pathology Directorate Manager and Business Manager
Queen's Medical Centre
Nottingham, UK
Email: jcbancroft550@hotmail.com

Marilyn Gamble

Formerly Quality Assurance Coordinator
Cellular Pathology Services
Kaiser Permanente
Regional Reference Laboratories
North Hollywood, CA, USA

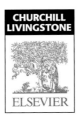

CHURCHILL
LIVINGSTONE

ELSEVIER

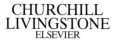

CHURCHILL LIVINGSTONE
An imprint of Elsevier Limited
© 2008, Elsevier Limited All rights reserved.

The author of chapter 17 is a US Federal employee. Its contents are therefore in the public domain.

First edition 1977
Second edition 1982
Third edition 1990
Fourth edition 1996
Fifth edition 2002
Sixth edition 2008

The right of J.D. Bancroft and M. Gamble to be identified as authors of this work has been asserted by them in accordance with the Copyright, Designs and Patents Act 1988

ISBN: 978-0-443-10279-0

British Library Cataloguing in Publication Data
A catalogue record for this book is available from the British Library

Library of Congress Cataloging in Publication Data
A catalog record for this book is available from the Library of Congress

Notice
Medical knowledge is constantly changing. Standard safety precautions must be followed, but as new research and clinical experience broaden our knowledge, changes in treatment and drug therapy may become necessary or appropriate. Readers are advised to check the most current product information provided by the manufacturer of each drug to be administered to verify the recommended dose, the method and duration of administration, and contraindications. It is the responsibility of the practitioner, relying on experience and knowledge of the patient, to determine dosages and the best treatment for each individual patient. Neither the Publisher nor the author assume any liability for any injury and/or damage to persons or property arising from this publication.

The Publisher

Printed in China
Last digit is the print number: 9 8 7 6 5 4 3 2 1

Contents

v

List of contributors

Caroline Astbury PhD
Clinical Cytogeneticist
Genetic Testing Laboratory
Southern California Permanente Medical Group
Los Angeles, CA, USA

John D. Bancroft
Formerly Pathology Directorate Manager
and Business Manager
Queen's Medical Centre
Nottingham, UK

Iain Banks FIBMS
Laboratory Manager
Department of Histopathology and Molecular
Pathology
Leeds Teaching Hospitals NHS Trust
Leeds, UK

Jeanine H. Bartlett BS HT(ASCP) QIHC
Histotechnologist
Centers for Disease Control and Prevention
National Center for Zoonotic, Vector-Borne, and
Enteric Diseases
Division of Viral and Rickettsial Diseases
Infectious Diseases Pathology Branch
Atlanta, GA, USA

Paul E. Billings Jr
Laboratory Manager
Tissue Procurement
University of Alabama at Birmingham
Birmingham, AL, USA

David Blythe FIBMS
Chief Biomedical Scientist
Haematological Malignancy Diagnostic Service
Laboratory
Leeds Teaching Hospitals NHS Trust
Leeds, UK

Gayle M. Callis BS MT HT HTL(ASCP)
Histopathology Supervisor
Veterinary Molecular Biology
Montana State University
Bozeman, MT, USA

Charles J. Churukian BA HTL(ASCP)
Senior Technical Associate and Supervisor
Histochemistry Laboratory
Department of Pathology and Laboratory Medicine
University of Rochester Medical Center
Rochester, NY, USA

Richard W. Dapson PhD
Consultant
Dapson & Dapson, LLC
Richland, MI, USA

Alton D. Floyd PhD
Consultant, ImagePath Systems Inc.
Edwardsburg, MI, USA
and Adjunct Associate Professor
Department of Pathology and Laboratory Medicine
University of Rochester School of Medicine
Rochester, NY, USA

Jerry L. Fredenburgh PhD
President and Chief Operating Officer
Surgipath Medical Industries, Inc.
Richmond, IL, USA

Marilyn Gamble HT(ASCP) HTL
Formerly Quality Assurance Coordinator
Cellular Pathology Services
Kaiser Permanente
Regional Reference Laboratories
North Hollywood, CA, USA

William E. Grizzle MD PhD
Professor of Pathology
Department of Pathology
University of Alabama at Birmingham
Birmingham, AL, USA

Neil M. Hand MPhil CSci FIBMS
Chief Biomedical Scientist
Department of Histopathology
Queen's Medical Centre Campus
Nottingham University Hospitals NHS Trust
Nottingham, UK

Christa L. Hladik HT(ASCP) QIHC
Laboratory Manager, Immunohistochemistry and
Neuropathology
Department of Pathology
University of Texas Southwestern Medical School
Dallas, TX, USA

Richard W. Horobin BSc PhD
Senior Research Fellow
Division of Neuroscience and Biomedical Systems
Institute of Biomedical and Life Sciences
University of Glasgow
Glasgow, UK

Peter Jackson MPhil CSci FIBMS
Chief Biomedical Scientist
Department of Histopathology and Molecular
Pathology
The General Infirmary at Leeds
Leeds Teaching Hospitals NHS Trust
Leeds, UK

M. Lamar Jones BS HT(ASCP)
Manager, Anatomic Pathology
Pathology Department
Wake Forest University Baptist Medical Center
Winston-Salem, NC, USA

Wanda G. Jones HT(ASCP)
Field Service Specialist
Vision BioSystems
Boston, MA, USA

Janet I. Minshew HT(ASCP) HTL
Marketing Manager, Pathology Diagnostics
Leica Microsystems, Inc.
Bannockburn, IL, USA

Russell B. Myers PhD
Vice President of Immunohistochemistry and
Molecular Biology
Surgipath Medical Industries, Inc.
Richmond, IL, USA

Scott L. Nestor DO FASCP FCAP
Clinical Assistant Professor
Department of Pathology
Wheeling Hospital
Wheeling, WV, USA

Lena T. Spencer MA HT HTL(ASCP) QIHC
Senior Histotechnologist
Anatomic Pathology Department
Norton Healthcare
Louisville, KY, USA

Diane L. Sterchi MS HTL(ASCP)
Associate Senior Biologist
Department of Integrative Biology
Eli Lilly and Company
Greenfield, IN, USA

John W. Stirling BSc(Hons) MLett AFRCPA MAIMS
Principal Medical Scientist
Electron Microscope Unit
Department of Anatomical Pathology
SouthPath, Flinders Medical Centre
Bedford Park, SA, Australia

Geoffrey H. Vowles BSc FIBMS CSci
Quality Manager
Cellular Pathology Division
Royal London Hospital
London, UK

Charles L. White, III MD
Professor of Pathology
Director, Neuropathology and Immunohistochemistry
Department of Pathology
University of Texas Southwestern Medical School
Dallas, TX, USA

Anthony E. Woods BA BSc(Hons) PhD MAIMS
Associate Professor
School of Pharmacy and Medical Sciences
University of South Australia
Adelaide, SA, Australia

Preface to the sixth edition

In the 30 years since the first edition of this book, histotechnology has continued to develop into a highly complex branch of laboratory medicine. Immunohistochemistry, in situ hybridization, molecular pathology, genetic testing and laser capture are all techniques currently in use to establish a diagnosis or to assess the changes occurring in tissues and cells in the disease process. Far more information can be obtained from these techniques than from many of the empirical methods used previously, but knowledge of the old and new is required by trained and trainee histotechnologists as well as the pathologist. The successful training of laboratory staff of all grades requires a thorough grounding in all aspects of histological techniques.

In producing this edition, we continued to be faced with the problem of achieving a balance between the new and old technology. To help achieve this some chapters from the last edition have been amalgamated to allow the introduction of the new material.

There are a number of new chapters and contributors for this edition. The new chapters include The gross room/surgical cutup by Paul Billings and William Grizzle, Tissue microarray by Wanda Grace-Jones, Genetic testing by Caroline Astbury, Laser microdissection by Diane Sterchi, and Jan Minshew has written Ergonomics.

New contributors are William Grizzle, Jerry Fredenburgh and Russell Myers who between them rewrote Fixation of tissues, Carbohydrates, and Proteins and nucleic acids. Lena Spencer updated Tissue processing and Microtomy. William Grizzle also updated the Neuroendocrine chapter, Jeanie Bartlett Microorganisms, and Scott Nestor Neuropathology and Enzyme histochemistry. Peter Jackson and David Blythe rewrote the Practical immunohistochemical chapter and Charles White its Applications in pathology. Christa Hladik with Charles White rewrote Quality control in immunohistochemistry and immunofluorescent techniques. Diane Sterchi has updated Molecular pathology. William Grizzle, Jerry Fredenburgh and Russell Myers have updated the Appendices.

As with the last edition we have had to remove some more of the less commonly used histological methods, which is unfortunate but a necessity, otherwise the book would have been impossibly large. The chapters on Cytology have not been included in this edition, as it has developed into specialized subject with numerous excellent textbooks devoted to it. Microwave methods have been assimilated into appropriate chapters.

Where relevant, we have continued the policy of outlining the uses of histological techniques in solving specific diagnostic problems.

John D. Bancroft **Marilyn Gamble**
Nottingham, UK   Morgantown, West Virginia, USA
2007

Preface to the first edition

In recent years histological techniques have become increasingly sophisticated, incorporating a whole variety of specialities, and there has been a corresponding dramatic rise in the level and breadth of knowledge demanded by the examiner of trainees in histology and histopathology technology.

We believe that the time has arrived when no single author can produce a comprehensive book on histology technique sufficiently authoritative in the many differing fields of knowledge with which the technologist must be familiar. Many books exist which are solely devoted to one particular facet such as electron microscopy or autoradiography, and the dedicated technologist will, of course, read these in the process of self-education. Nevertheless the need has arisen for a book which covers the entire spectrum of histology technology, from the principles of tissue fixation and the production of paraffin sections, the more esoteric level of the principles of scanning electron microscopy. It has been our aim then, to produce a book which the trainee technologist can purchase at the beginning of his career and which will remain valuable to him as he rises on the ladder of experience and seniority.

The book has been designed as a comprehensive reference work for those preparing for examinations in histopathology, both in Britain and elsewhere. Although the content is particularly suitable for students working towards the Special Examination in Histopathology of the Institute of Medical Laboratory Sciences, the level is such that more advanced students, along with research workers, histologists, and pathologists, will find the book beneficial. To achieve this we have gathered a team of expert contributors, many of whom have written specialised books or articles on their own subject; most are intimately involved in the teaching of histology and some are examiners in the HNC and Special Examination in Histopathology. The medically qualified contributors are also involved in technician education.

All contributors have taken care to give, where applicable, the theoretical basis of the techniques, for we believe that the standard of their education has risen so remarkably in recent years that the time is surely coming when medical laboratory technicians will be renamed 'medical laboratory scientists'; we hope that the increase in 'scientific' content in parts of this book will assist in this essential transformation.

John D. Bancroft
Alan Stevens
Nottingham, 1977

General acknowledgments

Many Laboratory Scientists and Pathologists have contributed in different ways to the six editions of this text and to acknowledge their individual advice and assistance is impossible. We express our thanks to everyone who has contributed since 1977. We owe Harry Cook special thanks for his advice and contributions to the earlier editions. Our thanks are also due to the colleagues we worked with in Nottingham and Los Angeles during the lifetime of this book.

We would like to thank all of our current authors, and those contributors whose previous work remains in some of the chapters in this new edition. Special thanks go to Richard Horobin who has contributed to all of the editions, and Bob Francis and David Hopwood who contributed to the first five.

Our thanks go to those who assisted in the preparation of the manuscripts and the production of the illustrations. We are grateful to Carol Bancroft for her considerable help with the editing and proof-reading.

Finally, we wish to thank the staff of our publishers for their unfailing help and courtesy.

John D. Bancroft   **Marilyn Gamble**
Nottingham, UK   Morgantown, West Virginia, USA
2007

Acknowledgment to Alan Stevens

I have known Alan since he joined the Pathology Department at the University of Nottingham some thirty years ago. We had many discussions in those early years over whether the time had arrived for a multi-authored text on histological technique. It was apparent at that time that the subject was becoming too diverse for any single or two authors to cover in the depth that was required in the laboratories or the colleges where histotechnologists received their academic education.

In 1977 the first edition of this text was published and was due in no small part to Alan's vision and diligent work in editing and even rewriting some of the chapters. His contributions to the succeeding editions were just as important and his medical knowledge was a significant factor in the development of the book. It has been a great pleasure working with him and I have greatly missed his contribution to the editing of this new edition, although much of his writing in the various chapters remains. The success over the years of Bancroft and Stevens owes a great deal to Alan Stevens. I wish to thank him and wish him well in his current and future medical education publications.

John D. Bancroft
Nottingham, UK
2001

1

Managing the Laboratory

Marilyn Gamble, Iain Banks and John D. Bancroft

INTRODUCTION

Management is an important aspect of the day-to-day life of the histopathology laboratory particularly since the emergence of accreditation. The accreditation standards include management as part of the evaluation and it is necessary that the laboratory worker is familiar with the processes involved. There are excellent books available which cover management issues in depth, and it is not the objective of this chapter to be a comprehensive guide to the subject. It discusses and concentrates on specific areas which have an impact on the operation of the laboratory; these are:

- Risk management
- Quality management and establishing a quality system.

RISK MANAGEMENT

Every laboratory has to have an effective risk management policy, because, as in most aspects of life, 'if it can go wrong, it will go wrong'. In the laboratory, it is important that the chance of something going wrong is either negated or minimized. The risk management process involves:

- Identifying all risks that exist within your environment
- Assessing risks for likelihood and severity
- Eliminating those risks that can be removed
- Reducing the effect of risks that cannot be eliminated.

Medicine itself is a risky business, which requires careful clinical management. Histopathology is a significant aspect of the medical risk management process. The surgical biopsy is sent for histopathological assessment to corroborate or dispute the clinical diagnosis by providing confirmation of data provided from other diagnostic tests. It gives the clinician valuable information on how to proceed with the treatment of the disease. Major resections are referred to the laboratory to confirm the diagnosis, and in the case of malignant tumors to ensure that there are adequate resection margins, to determine the extent of lymphatic involvement and/or direct spread, and to stage and classify the disease. Autopsies provide definitive data for medical audit, and can be used to determine where medical procedures have been ineffective and also to give additional data for the future treatment of other patients with similar medical conditions. Cervical cytological smears are used as a screening process to assist in the early diagnosis of disease prior to the development of symptoms and thereby enable effective treatment. This is accomplished by using non-invasive or minimally invasive techniques, which have a low risk of complications to the patient.

These clinical diagnostic aspects are not the only types of risk that apply to the laboratory. To function effectively and safely all of its procedures and activities are subjected to the risk management process. The risks in the laboratory are similar worldwide with a variation due to local circumstances. Health and safety and quality assurance incorporate a major aspect of risk management. All aspects of our working life incorporate a degree of risk and the risk management process allows us to prioritize, evaluate, and handle the risk appropriately. It is not possible to avoid or eliminate all risks, and in reality this may not be practical or possible. It is important to identify and understand the risks that are involved in your working practices. An individual's perception of risk is dependent upon that individual's role within the organization. The chief executive, for example, will be concerned mainly with risks associated with strategic issues affecting the organization as a whole and would only include histopathology within the risk assessment if it had a direct impact on these issues. Matters concerning the day-to-day running of the laboratory would not be of direct interest unless, of course, there was a significant reason for involvement such as political or major financial concerns.

The laboratory manager or supervisor deals with the risks associated with ensuring that adequate resources are available to deliver the service and guaranteeing that the laboratory provides a service that is safe. Staffing levels and competence, budgetary management, consumable and equipment supplies, and maintenance are some of the areas of concern, but also included would be ensuring that risk management procedures are in place for the laboratory.

The laboratory manager must ensure that day-to-day errors do not arise as a result of inadequacies in laboratory procedures and that quality control checks are in place to eradicate human errors such as transcription or misreading. Standard operating procedures (SOPs) should be detailed to include Control of Substances Hazardous to Health (COSHH) risk assessments and also to include other health and safety information relevant to the procedure.

The histotechnologists and biomedical scientists at the bench face risks that involve equipment malfunction due to poor maintenance or design; poor-quality reagents produce poor processing of tissues or inaccurate staining results. The routine use of laboratory equipment, e.g. in microtomy, can result in one of the most common accidents that occur in the laboratory, cutting a finger or hand on microtome knives or blades. It is the responsibility of each laboratory worker to reduce the risks associated with their day-to-day work by using safety guards where available, checking the quality of reagents, and carrying out checks with diligence.

The risk management process

Risk management is a continual process and not a single step evaluation. Figure 1.1 shows the complete process.

Risk identification

A group of individuals with different roles in the laboratory best identifies risks. This ensures that the broadest

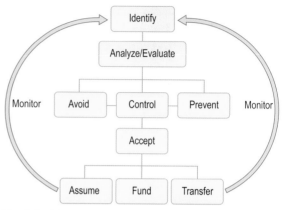

Fig. 1.1   The risk management process.

possible spectrum of viewpoints is considered. During this process it is also useful to divide the risks into different categories such as 'political', 'organizational', 'financial', 'clinical', 'physical', 'chemical', 'infectious', etc. This helps to ensure that all aspects of the laboratory's operation are included. Different professions and grades of staff will be best placed to ensure the identification of all risks in the above categories.

Risk analysis/evaluation

Analysis and evaluation of potential risks is an essential part of the process, and one that is used to identify both the likelihood and severity of these risks. By scoring the risks for likelihood and severity, it is then possible to use the matrix (Figure 1.2) as a tool that will put a value on specific risks, which helps in prioritizing them for further action.

The risk manager should put a system in place whereby all incidents and accidents are reported no matter how small. It is only by recording data that the full picture can be obtained and analyzed.

Severity and likelihood values

Incidents may be scored on a scale of 1–5 for severity.

1 *No injury*, potential for individual claim up to $10,000:
   - Breach of guidance
   - Minimal loss of reputation
   - No/minimal disruption to normal services.
2 *Minor injury*, potential for multiple or individual claims $10,000–50,000:

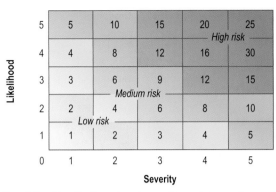

Fig. 1.2 The likelihood and severity matrix can be used as a tool to put a value on specific risks, prioritizing them for further action.

- Breach of legal requirement or authoritative guidance
- Loss of reputation
- Disruption to normal services.

3 *Moderate* potential for multiple or individual claims $50,000–200,000:
  - Breach of significant legal requirement or authoritative guidance
  - Significant loss of reputation
  - Significant disruption to normal services.

4 *Moderately severe injury*, potential for multiple or individual claims $200,000–2.5 million:
  - Breach of significant legal requirement with likely enforcement action
  - Serious loss of reputation
  - Serious disruption to normal services.

5 *Serious injury*, potential for multiple claims or individual claim exceeding $2.5 million:
  - Breach of significant legal requirement with imminent action
  - Serious loss of reputation
  - Serious disruption to normal services.

Incidents may also be scored 1–5 for likelihood:

1. Incident unlikely to occur.
2. Incident likely to occur once in a 5-year period.
3. Incident likely to occur yearly.
4. Incident likely to occur once in a 6-month period.
5. Incident likely to occur once every 4 weeks or more frequently.

Risks should also be evaluated against the standards of one's peers to ascertain whether or not the risk is accept-able, as there could be more than one reason for obtaining poor results. A surgeon who has a record of poor results could either be a bad surgeon, or could be operating mainly on high-risk cases. The results may be poor in general comparison with other surgeons, but may be exceptionally good when compared to other surgeons operating on similar cases. It is for these reasons that laboratories should participate in benchmarking, and as laboratories deal with variable types of work the benchmarking should be compared to other similar operations, i.e. teaching hospital laboratories should only be compared to other teaching hospital laboratories. Benchmarking results are an effective aid to risk management and let you know how you are performing compared to your peers.

Risk control

The objective of the whole risk management process is to control risks. It may be possible in certain circumstances to avoid a risk or even prevent it completely. This would be possible, for example, by looking for alternatives to high-risk, harmful chemicals used in the laboratory. Prior to the 1970's, it was common practice to use mercuric chloride as a constituent of fixatives and, although this gave excellent quality fixation, it was extremely harmful to the environment and also to laboratory staff. Its use was subsequently stopped and alternative fixatives replaced it.

Despite efforts to eliminate risks it is not possible to remove them totally. Efforts should be made to reduce the effect or the possibility of the risk happening, but some risk may remain. Ways of controlling risk are numerous, but frequently there will be expert guidance or regulations issued by professional bodies or government that the risk manager should ensure are implemented. Where there is residual risk it must be funded as part of the control mechanism.

Risk funding

Risk management is not only about insurance, although this is an important option. All medical staff carry medical liability insurance, which covers them in the event of any negligence claims. Similarly, professional indemnity insurance is commonly available today for non-medical laboratory staff who are much more at risk in today's litigation-conscious society. The decision whether or not to insure should be based on the risk assessment and the severity and likelihood of the risk. Some risks will not be appropriate for insurance cover for whatever reason, and in these instances the risk must be accepted by the organization.

Risk monitoring

Monitoring risk is an ongoing process and diligent documentation of all incidents and accidents is necessary for the process to be successful. The records are analyzed to identify whether or not the control measures implemented are effective. Each incident should be investigated, and where possible additional measures taken to ensure a repeat is avoided. It is important to realize that when an effective monitoring system is utilized the likelihood is that the number of reported incidents will increase due to the higher profile that risk management has with the staff. If not handled correctly this can have a detrimental effect on staff morale, as the initial perception will be that incidents have increased in number.

Risk management and quality control

Powers (2005) maintained that the laboratory quality control requirements should be based on risk management principles and answer the real question that the laboratory must answer, 'What are the appropriate laboratory controls to minimize patient risk?' He refers to the ISO 14971 risk management process as a systematic way to answer that question and recommends that standards be developed for clinical laboratories. In the interest of patient safety, determining the appropriate amount of quality control (QC) may require going beyond the current regulatory and accreditation requirements.

QUALITY MANAGEMENT

Accreditation/certification/regulatory agencies' standards, with some variation, utilize the components listed in the ISO section (see page 6). In conjunction with 'quality assurance' and 'continuing quality improvement', 'quality control' is an integral component of a required 'quality system'. A good QC system provides information for quality assurance activities.

Quality control (QC)

This system checks that the work process is functioning properly. It includes processes utilized in the laboratory to recognize and eliminate errors. It ensures that the quality of work produced by the laboratory conforms to specified requirements prior to its release for diagnoses. Errors and/or deviations from expected results must be documented and include the corrective action taken. It is not the intention of this chapter to give step-by-step guidelines for performing quality control. In the laboratory, quality control has long been a component of accreditation requirements and is ingrained in histotechnologists as a daily practice. Most laboratories have experienced technologists who have the responsibility of performing routine quality control checks prior to the release of slides for diagnoses. This QC evaluation will include, but is not limited to: accurate patient identification, fixation, adequate processing, appropriate embedding techniques, acceptable microtomy, unacceptable artefacts, and inspection of controls to determine correctness of special staining and immunohistochemistry methods. Criteria should be established that would trigger a repeat if the QC findings were qualitatively or quantitatively discordant with expected findings. Despite having a conscientious QC system in the laboratory, pathologists with a higher level of expertise perform the final QC examination as they 'read' the slide. It is their responsibility to determine that the section/slide is adequate for diagnostic interpretation. Errors/problems reported by pathologists and others should be included as part of the laboratory QC data collection.

Quality assurance (QA)

This is a shift from a focus on the end product or service to a focus on the process. Subsequent statistical analysis of good QC documentation provides the data for quality assurance activities where correlation of errors, complaints, failures or other unexpected results are evaluated against the laboratory expectations. This monitoring program evaluates errors and problems and addresses resolution. Reviewing the data allows identification of declining quality in specific areas and should trigger appropriate corrective action. A high number of 'repeats', for example, would indicate that a system check be done to identify the problem and implement corrective action. Participation in external programs/schemes also contributes valuable information for a quality assurance program.

Continuing quality improvement (CQI)

This is the system used proactively to approach, evaluate, and identify opportunities to improve quality before problems occur through evaluation of all systems/processes in the laboratory. The goal is to improve patient care and safety through recognition of potential problems/errors before they can occur. Good managers now realize that many failures, errors, and/or problems that occur are usually due to the system process and not the fault of the employee(s).

Quality system

This is the 'high level' organizational structure, responsibilities, procedures, processes, and resources needed to implement quality management. It should be noted that all processes, equipment, and procedures must be evaluated, validated, and written in a format that is easy to read, easy to follow, and readily available to the staff. Employees must meet personnel requirements, be adequately informed, well trained and tested for competency prior to performing methods on patient samples, and competency re-evaluated on a regular basis. Documentation, of all, must be available to inspectors for verification.

Quality assurance systems and schemes/surveys

In addition to local data collection and monitoring for a quality assurance program, external programs provide valuable information regarding quality and peer comparisons. In the UK, quality assurance of laboratory techniques is organized on a national basis. It is a system of peer review and registration with appropriate schemes. The non-profit-making organization NEQAS (National External Quality Assurance Scheme) organizes a program for immunohistochemistry and tinctorial staining.

In the USA, the National Society of Histotechnology (NSH) in partnership with the College of American Pathologists (CAP) (2006) created the His-

tology Quality Improvement Program (HistoQIP). Additionally, CAP establishes national surveys for immunohistochemistry.

UK quality assurance schemes were started by members of the profession to establish quality standards within histopathology. The process was subsequently developed to include preparations for immunohistochemistry and tinctorial staining techniques organized on a national basis, and registration with the schemes is now a requirement for accreditation.

The quality assurance process is based on peer review of the stained sections submitted by participating laboratories. There are also medical quality assurance schemes for many of the sub-specialties of histopathology. There are two distinct systems that can be used to deliver quality assurance; some schemes are organized on a mixture of both systems.

> Selective system—stained preparations from departmental archival records are used to assess the quality of staining.
> Distributive system—participating laboratories are asked to stain sections that have been submitted by the scheme organizer.

The quality assurance schemes currently used in the UK are coordinated under the auspices of UK NEQAS and within this organization there are two individual schemes for histopathology, the NEQAS for immunohistochemistry and the NEQAS for cellular pathology technique.

The immunohistochemistry scheme gives participants the option to be assessed on general antibody panels, or more specialist laboratories may choose to participate only in the lymphoma or breast specialist areas. The cellular pathology scheme is subdivided into general, veterinary and neuropathology.

The assessment process
USA, NSH/CAP HistoQIP

The HistoQIP program is designed as an educational program to improve the preparation of histological slides. Twice each year, participating laboratories submit one stained and coverslipped glass slide from five different cases (two hematoxylin and eosin (H&E), two special, and one immunohistochemistry stain). All submitted slides are recuts of specific surgical tissue types or positive control tissue that vary from one challenge to the next. Submitted slides are evaluated for histological technique by an expert panel of histotechnologists, biomedical scientists, and pathologists using uniform grading criteria. The following areas are evaluated: fixation, tissue processing and embedding, microtomy, staining, and coverslipping.

For each set of slides submitted, participants receive an evaluation specific to their laboratory, an educational critique, and a participant summary report that includes peer comparison data, performance benchmarking data, and information regarding best-performing procedures and techniques.

USA, CAP immunohistochemistry

Surveys are designed for laboratories performing immuno-histochemistry procedures. Slides are mailed to participants. They are asked to stain slides with antibodies to suggested 'markers', using the remaining slides for an H&E stain and appropriate negative controls, and provide interpretation. The survey consists of four cases in each of the two shipments for a total of eight case challenges per year. At least one breast carcinoma is offered during the year with HER2 as the specified antibody. Additional immunohistochemistry surveys are available for immunohistochemistry tissue microarrays. Participants receive a summary report with peer comparison data and educational information.

UK NEQAS for immunohistochemistry

Participating laboratories are assessed on four runs per year. All slides are anonymized by the scheme organizer and are assessed collectively by a panel of four assessors (usually a mixture of medical and non-medical laboratory staff) who mark each slide out of five points using lists of predefined assessment criteria. Accreditation standards demand that action be taken by poor performers to improve the quality of their preparations. The scheme offers expert assistance and advice to laboratories that fall below the acceptable score.

UK NEQAS for cellular pathology

This scheme currently has six runs per year. Again slides are anonymized and assessed collectively by a panel of assessors. Slides are assessed using lists of predefined assessment criteria. The result for each of the criteria is computerized and a final score calculated. The participating laboratory receives an accumulated score for each slide submitted. A histogram of all participants is included which indicates individual performance compared to all other participants nationally. A regional coordinator monitors poor performance, and assistance in improving performance is available. A poor performance trigger mechanism is activated when participants have accrued a designated number of low marks in an assessment period. Scoring excessive low marks in a row can result in the laboratory being referred to NEQAP (National External Quality Assurance Panel), who may take further action which could ultimately mean referral to the Department of Health and potential closure of the laboratory.

Establishing a quality system

International standards

ISO

The development of international standards (in most fields except electrotechnical) is the purview of the International Organization for Standardization (ISO). ISO is a network of the national standards institutes of 148 countries, one member per country, with the Central Secretariat in Geneva, Switzerland, which coordinates the system. ISO standards are developed by technical committees composed of experts that participate as national delegates, chosen by the ISO national member body for the country concerned.

ISO 9000

ISO 9000 (Harrington & Mathers 1997) is a family name for a set of standards that are concerned with the management of quality systems, and includes at least the following standards: ISO 9000:2000, ISO 9001:2000 (Paradis & Trubiano 2001), and ISO 9004:2000. In more recent years, ISO 9000 standards migrated into the healthcare setting (DOH 1994). Standards are developed and maintained by ISO Technical Committee 176, which includes representatives from its member countries. They periodically review and update standards and documents. The ISO Technical Management Board (TMB) established ISO Technical Committee (ISO/TC) 212 in 1995, to provide a focus for coordination of international standardization in the clinical laboratory-testing field. The current standard, ISO 15189:2003, *Medical laboratories—particular requirements for quality and competence* (2006), is quickly becoming accepted as the certification standard for clinical laboratories. This standard does not replace national regulations, but in the future could be adopted as the accepted standard by accreditation agencies worldwide.

CLSI (formerly NCCLS)

The National Committee for Clinical Laboratory Science (NCCLS) changed its name in 2005 and is now known as The Clinical and Laboratory Standards Institute (CLSI), Wayne, Pennsylvania, USA (CLSI 2006). Its core business is the development of globally applicable voluntary consensus documents for healthcare testing. It manages two distinct processes:

- The CLSI consensus process for developing globally applicable standards and guidelines; and
- The International Organization for Standardization or ISO process, for developing international standards as the Secretariat for ISO/TC 212, clinical laboratory testing and in vitro diagnostic test systems.

The CLSI is a global, non-profit, membership-based organization dedicated to developing standards and guidelines for the healthcare and medical testing community. The organization continues to provide NCCLS standards and guidelines (NCCLS 2002a, 2002b, 2004) and to produce new CLSI guidelines under the same global consensus process.

Description of ISO 9000

Basically, the ISO 9000 quality system is a series of standards and guidelines which require an organization to be sure that it is doing the correct thing, at the right time; documenting what it is doing, and doing what is documented. Documents must conform to the requirements of the standard, operations must conform to the documents, and records must show past conformance to documents.

To become successfully ISO 9000 registered the quality system is developed to meet the quality requirements specified by the standards selected. This is done while utilizing the ISO's guidelines. After the quality system is developed and implemented, internal audits are conducted as preparation for the ISO audit. An accredited external auditor (registrar) is invited to evaluate the effectiveness of the quality system. If all ISO requirements are met, the organization is recorded in the registry. The registrar generally maintains a long-term contract with the organization with periodic interim assessments to ensure that the quality system is main-

tained and improved. While the process sounds simplistic, the estimated time for project completion is 12 to 24 months. Management must make the commitment, and take an active role in achieving certification, through strategic planning. Responsibility and authority must be defined, a timeline established, a project team formed, and the project leader identified. Once a conformance model is selected, the team is responsible for the certification process, which includes assessment of the current system and gap analysis, to determine if there are gaps between the existing quality system and the ISO requirements. Corrective action is taken to resolve differences and close those gaps between organizational operations and documents.

Description of ISO 15189:2003

The ISO 15189 standard is a quality system standard for medical laboratories which contains two major parts: management requirements for quality management systems (Table 1.1) and technical requirements for activities carried out by technical laboratories (Table 1.2). The tables contain condensed information to give a brief content description. The standard should be reviewed in its entirety to gain full understanding. If you choose to follow NCCLS guidelines, you will find that the NCCLS document organizes the standards into 'Quality System Essentials (QSEs)' and provides specific 'how to' information on compliance (Berte 2004).

ADVANTAGES OF A QUALITY SYSTEM

Establishing an internationally recognized quality system in the medical laboratory goes beyond quality assurance monitors. A quality system contains universal quality elements for each laboratory operation, and includes criteria to meet regulations and accreditation requirements. Compliance with the standards improves documentation and record keeping, and requires that the management team provide greater awareness of responsibility and quality for the laboratory staff. Once the quality elements are in place the laboratory has the basis for establishing a quality system that provides the foundation for true continuous improvement and total quality management. In this age of globalization of services, successful implementation and registration demonstrates achieved standards of quality that are recognized and respected throughout the world.

Table 1.1   ISO 15189:2003

4. Management	
4.1 Organization and management	Introduces management requirements and responsibilities in meeting legal and accreditation requirements; definition of responsibilities and authorities of all personnel; definition and implementation of policies and organizational structure.
4.2 Quality management system	Implementation of a quality system which includes a defined quality manual, internal quality control, inter-laboratory comparisons, monitoring program, and preventive maintenance.
4.3 Document control	A document control system must be in place for the all documents that form its quality documentation. This includes the creation and approval of documents, reviews, removal, and storage.
4.4 Review of contracts	Establish and maintain procedures for review of contracts to ensure that they meet the requirements of the customers.
4.5 Examination by referral laboratories	Evaluating and selecting referral laboratories and/or consultants. Must monitor quality and competency.
4.6 External services and supply	Includes selection and use of purchased services, equipment and consumable supplies and includes documentation criteria for inspection, acceptance, rejection, and storage of materials.
4.7 Advisory services	Documented professional and clinical staff meetings to provide advice on use of services, including repeat frequency and required type of sample.
4.8 Resolution of complaints	Includes documentation of feedback (good and bad), complaints, resolutions, and corrective actions.
4.9 Identification and control of nonconformities	All process deviations or unexpected outcomes are investigated, analyzed, and corrective actions taken. This includes errors, accidents, and customer complaints.
4.10 Corrective action	Corrective action procedures include an investigation process to determine underlying cause(s) in order to implement preventive action where appropriate.
4.11 Preventive action	Analysis of nonconformities and development and implementation of preventive action plans to prevent occurrences.
4.12 Continual improvement	Regular review to identify potential sources of nonconformance or other opportunities for improvement.
4.13 Quality and technical records	Quality and technical records maintenance, indexing, ready access, storage time, and safe disposal.
4.14 Internal audits	Identification and measurement of quality indicators and measuring effectiveness to verify that operations (management and technical) continue to comply with the quality management system.
4.15 Management review	Laboratory management must conduct an annual review to ensure continuing suitability and effectiveness in support of patient care and to introduce changes or improvements. Review results are part of a plan that includes goals, objectives, and action plans for the coming year.

Table 1.2 ISO 15189:2003

5. Technical requirements	
5.1 Personnel	Evaluation of personnel competence, training requirements and records, job descriptions, personnel files, evaluations, continuing education, confidentiality and protection of patient data.
5.2 Accommodation and environmental conditions	Adequate space allocations, efficient design. Comfort and safety of personnel. Monitoring, control, and recording environmental conditions required by specifications or where they may influence the quality of results.
5.3 Laboratory equipment	Selection and monitoring of instruments, reference materials, consumables, reagents, computer software, and analytical systems.
5.4 Pre-examination procedures	Identification of the patient and authorized requester. Defining criteria for request forms, collection, identification, handling, transportation, and receipt of patient samples. Requires a manual for collection of samples; procedures and acceptance and rejection criteria.
5.5 Examination procedures	Control of the analytical process including validation, reference and critical intervals, and documented procedures. Defines required reviews of methods and procedures, approvals, and required documentation.
5.6 Assuring quality of examination procedures	Quality control procedures. Internal quality control systems to verify that intended quality of results is achieved. Calibration program requirements; participation in inter-laboratory comparison programs and external quality assessment programs; documentation of actions taken upon results from comparisons.
5.7 Post-examination process	Definition of criteria for storage and safe disposal of samples; review and release of results.
5.8 Reporting of results	Requirements for reports formatting, transmitting and alteration; communication of delays, retention period of results, etc.

REFERENCES

Berte L.M. (2004) Managing laboratory quality—a systematic approach. Chicago, IL: Laboratory Medicine (September), ASCP.

Clinical and Laboratory Standards Institute (2006) Press release: From NCCLS to CLSI: One year. Online. Available at: www.clsi.org.

College of American Pathologists (2006) NSH/CAP Histo-QIP program. Online. Available at: www.cap.org.

DOH (1994) Risk management in the NHS: D026/RISK/3M. London: Department of Health.

Harrington H.J., Mathers D.D. (1997) ISO 9000 and beyond. New York: McGraw-Hill, 59–67.

ISO 14971:2000 (2006) Medical devices—application of risk management to medical devices. Geneva, Switzerland: International Organization for Standardization.

ISO 15189:2003 (2006) Medical laboratories—particular requirements for quality and competence. Geneva, Switzerland: International Organization for Standardization.

ISO 9001 (1996) Quality systems-model for quality assurance in design, development, production, installation and servicing. ISO Standards Compendium, 6th edn. Geneva, Switzerland: International Organization for Standardization.

NCCLS (2002a) Application of a quality management system model for laboratory services; approved guideline GP26-A3. Wayne, PA: NCCLS.

NCCLS (2002b) Clinical technical procedures manuals. Approved guideline GP2-A2. Wayne, PA: NCCLS.

NCCLS (2004) A quality management system model for health care. NCCLS approved guideline HS1-A2. Wayne, PA: NCCLS.

Paradis G.W., Trubiano J.D. (2001) Demystifiying ISO 9001:2000: Information Mapping's Guide to the ISO 9001 Standard, 2nd edn. Upper Saddle River, NJ: Prentice Hall.

Powers Donald M. (2005) Laboratory quality control requirements should be based on risk management principles. LABMEDICINE, October, 2005.

WEBSITES

CLSI, Clinical and Laboratory Standards Institute, website: About CLSI: www.clsi.org.

CLSI, Clinical and Laboratory Standards Institute, website: Standards Development: www.clsi.org.

College of American Pathologists Immunohistochemistry survey (2006): www.cap.org.

2

Safety in the Laboratory

Richard W. Dapson

Most textbooks in the field of histotechnology have contained little if any information on health, safety, and environmental issues. This has been less a deliberate omission on the part of the authors than a direct reflection upon the state of histology laboratories around the world. Until recently, these facilities usually were relegated to the darkest recesses of a building, lacking ventilation and windows. A few decades ago, some were retrofitted with ventilation that merely redistributed the odd odors and toxic fumes elsewhere in the facility. Worker safety was rarely considered, in great part because no one understood the dangers of histological chemicals.

Curiously, as the rest of society became aware of workplace hazards, the sector that treated the illnesses emanating from them became one of the last to remedy its own conditions. Even today, there are laboratories where nobody should work. Many countries have now passed regulations designed to improve workplace conditions; there are even some directed specifically at laboratories. While these vary from country to country, an underlying theme is becoming essentially universal. Risk management pertains not just to personal health and safety in the conventional sense, but also to environmental health and safety. Healthcare and research facilities have seen significant improvements in workplace conditions, but they remain one of the worst contributors to environmental pollution.

The goal of this chapter is to lay out a risk management plan that is applicable worldwide. While general in scope to encompass a variety of regulations, it will be specific regarding the hazards unique to histology. Most of the information is from Dapson and Dapson (2005), which contains detail and pertinent references for these and many other related topics. Other references which

should be in every laboratory include Montgomery (1995), the Prudent Practices Series (National Research Council 1989, 1995), aids for preparing chemical hygiene plans (Stricoff & Walters 1990), as well as guidelines from the Clinical and Laboratory Standards Institute concerning laboratory safety (2004), biohazards (2005) and waste management (2002). Indispensable publications from the Centers for Disease Control (USA) include guidelines for safety (1988), HIV and tuberculosis (1990, 1994).

RISK MANAGEMENT

Identify and evaluate hazards

The first step in risk management is to identify all hazards in and emanating from the workplace. If this has never been done, it may be a formidable task, especially if there are old reagents or chemicals in poorly labeled containers. Anything that is unidentifiable or questionable should be set aside for disposal. Identification of hazards goes beyond making a chemical inventory, although that is a significant part of the effort. Electrical, mechanical and biological hazards are also included. In this initial identification stage, include the nature of the hazard(s) with the name, its location and the procedure(s) involved with its use. If no current use is found, then dispose of the item.

For hazardous chemicals, data sheets are available in most countries, and today should be obtainable anywhere from databases on the internet. A file of data sheets should be kept in a secure location, and employees must be given reasonable access to it. It is also advisable to keep a duplicate file readily accessible in the laboratory in case of emergencies. Some reagents found in storage areas may be obsolete; sheets will be impossible to find for these. This creates a problem with no simple solution, because legitimate disposal may require having a data sheet, yet keeping the chemical also dictates that a sheet be on file (a data sheet will have to be created, or a qualified firm hired to do so).

Evaluate the severity of each of the hazards. What is the volume or magnitude of the hazardous item? How much is used per day (or some other meaningful unit of time)? Now put that information together with the data sheet. These are written for industrial-scale exposures, and must be weighed against the scale of use in the laboratory. This evaluation must include risks associated with spillage and disposal as well as normal use. The hazards of a 5-gallon container of formalin emptying onto the floor of a laboratory are quite different from spilling a 30 ml (1oz) specimen container in a dermatologist's office. Likewise, emptying hundreds of small formalin-filled specimen containers into a disposal drum or sink might present a far greater exposure risk than handling each one during grossing. Do not underestimate risk, but keep the assessment proportional to scale and scope of operations.

Plan to minimize risk

Once the hazards have been listed and evaluated, decide how to reduce risk. Each item should be scrutinized, not just those offering the greatest dangers. Prioritize later. The goal is to reduce risks to acceptable levels, preferably through a cascading series of options that become progressively more burdensome and expensive. Work practice controls are the best way to tackle the problem; when pursued aggressively and with commitment at all levels of the institution, they usually are the only changes needed. Work practice controls involve eliminating, reducing, and recycling everything possible. If they do not succeed, engineering controls should be implemented. These involve ventilation systems, fire protection devices, and other expensive alterations to the facility. If all of these measures fail or are impossible to accomplish, personal protective equipment (PPE) must be used as a last resort. PPE should never be the first choice, although it may seem the most obvious way to protect workers.

There are several ways to reduce risk, the first of which should be to eliminate the hazard altogether. The list of obsolete chemicals in some of our labs is growing

rapidly; how many does your lab still use? Remember using benzene and dioxane? No? Then do not be surprised in another few years to have histotechnologists and biomedical scientists who never used xylene, toluene, chloroform, methacrylate, picric acid, uranyl nitrate, and formaldehyde. A surprising number of laboratories are free of one or more of these highly dangerous substances and a few have eliminated all of them.

Practically every seriously hazardous chemical can be replaced today with a safer and technically superior substitute. The question is not whether it can be done, but if it might be done; the obstacle is rarely technical feasibility; most likely, it is human obstinacy. The notion that substitutes are not as good has been debased so often in everyday life that it is a wonder that it persists so strongly in the medical profession. Antifreeze, correction fluid, nail polish, hard surface cleaners, cosmetics, contact lens solutions, and gasoline are just a few of the thousands of common materials in our lives that have undergone radical reformulation. In all cases, the products are safer, many work better, and some are less expensive. In no case is quality degraded: such products simply do not survive the competitive marketplace.

If elimination of a hazard is out of the question, consider reduction. This will involve procedural changes, so be sure to weigh all implications before pushing ahead. A common idea for reduction is to use smaller specimen containers for fixation. Unfortunately, many labs already use less volume of fixative than is necessary for good fixation; so further reduction here will only exacerbate problems with specimen quality that are rampant in surgical pathology today. Recycling is a final option for risk minimization. The volume in use at any given time might not be reduced, but the amount involved in storage and disposal will be cut drastically.

The plan must include justification to managers. Rationale for change should not rely solely upon improving safety. If worker health and safety had been high priorities within a facility, then making a new plan would not have to be done now, as it would have been accomplished years ago when authorities around the world recognized the risks. Financial considerations weigh heavily in any business, and could be the strongest argument for change. While many changes will cost more money initially, the long-term benefits are usually easy to calculate. For example, formalin substitutes are more expensive than formalin, but their use creates significant savings later. Workplaces and personnel do not need to be monitored for hazardous vapors, and disposal costs are usually reduced to zero. Less tangible, but nonetheless real, are the cost benefits of a healthier workforce.

Implement the plan

Having a plan, even a written one, will do no good unless it is implemented. Prioritize the changes described in the plan. While easy changes should be tackled immediately, do not put off the challenging items that carry high health or environmental risk. Achieving financial gain quickly will help the cause, so be sure to include something at the outset that will have an immediate, positive economic impact.

Design standard operating procedures for working with hazards

Nearly all laboratories operate under a set of written, standardized procedures (SOPs) mandated by a variety of accreditory or regulatory agencies. Detailed procedures for handling hazardous substances certainly should be central in these procedures, but other topics ought to be addressed as well. Personal hygiene practices should be a subconscious part of every worker's behavior, but must be spelled out in the SOPs. Define the criteria for invoking the use of specific control measures, such as the use of protective equipment. Describe how to assure that fume hoods and other pieces of protective equipment are functioning properly. Make provisions for employee training, medical consultations, and medical examinations. Detail spill procedures; define the kinds of spills that should be handled by lab workers and those too serious for anyone except trained hazmat responders. Establish a qualified officer or committee of qualified people to develop and administer these safety procedures.

Train personnel

Safety training is mandated by a variety of governmental regulations in several countries, and should be part of every department's personnel practices. Trained people work more safely, efficiently, and economically. In addition, the threat of employee litigation against the department is reduced. Regulations rarely address the issue of who should provide the training. In the past, it was common for one of the technical staff (usually the super-

visor) to do this—that person obtaining the information as best he/she could. It is preferable, however, to have the trainer specially educated and experienced in health and safety matters.

Training must include general practices and may deal with very specific topics such as respirator use, handling select carcinogens, and working with formaldehyde. Each employee should sign a form verifying that training was received, a copy of which becomes part of the employee's permanent record. The employee's name, date, and subject of training should be included on the certification form. Yearly retraining should be mandatory and documented. New employees, or employees assigned new hazardous tasks, must be adequately trained before beginning work.

Periodic reviews

On at least a yearly basis, all SOPs, risk assessments, and training programs should be reviewed and updated as needed. Each written document should bear the date of creation and latest revision. Continue to minimize risks. Address any new risks that occur when different hazardous materials are brought into the workplace. Revise risk assessments and protocols to accommodate increased use of hazardous substances, especially as workloads increase.

Record keeping

Government regulations often prescribe what records must be kept and for how long. Consider that a minimum requirement. It is prudent to record everything that pertains to regulatory compliance, risk assessment, causes and prevention of occupational illness or injury, employee health and safety training, exposure monitoring, occupational medical records, personal protective equipment, and hazardous waste disposal practices. Records should be kept indefinitely, although 30 years past the duration of a worker's employment is often prescribed by regulatory agencies. If in doubt, consider this: for how long would you want your estate to have access to health and safety records relating to your employment?

Occupational exposure limits

Most chemicals are hazardous to some degree; the question really is how hazardous are they? In other words, what would a safe level of exposure be? From many years of actual industrial experience, various agencies have developed standards for exposure to widely used chemicals. Generically, these are called occupational exposure limits, but each agency refers to its own values by unique names. OSHA's Permissible Exposure Limits (PELs) are based upon scientifically based recommendations from the National Institute of Occupational Safety and Health, or NIOSH (2005), but are also influenced by special interest groups and Congressional actions. OSHA limits therefore typically are more lenient. Another source of exposure limits, called Threshold Limit Values (TLVs®), is ACGIH® (American Conference of Governmental Industrial Hygienists 2007). These limits are more widely used around the world for occupational standards.

An exposure limit is the maximum allowable airborne concentration of a chemical (vapor, fume, or dust) to which a worker may be exposed. Presumably, it represents the concentration at or below which it is safe for most people to work, but there will be individuals who react adversely below the limits because of hypersensitivity.

It is important to realize that exposure limits are properties of the worker and the workplace combined. They are not simply the maximum limits of vapor, fume, or dust in the workplace; they are the maximum limits of exposure. This is especially important to consider when monitoring exposure levels. Monitor employees, not the workplace. Monitoring devices should be positioned as close as possible to the worker's face in order to capture actual breathable quantities of hazardous material. For example, airborne levels of formaldehyde vapor a few inches above a grossing station's cutting board may be much higher than concentrations at nose level, especially with well-designed ventilation.

Kinds of exposure limit based upon the duration of exposure

TWA (or TWAEV). The time-weighted average (time-weighted average exposure value) is the employee's average exposure over an 8-hour work shift. Shorter exposures may exceed this value as long as the average exposure does not. There may be some short exposure that is too high for safety; that is covered below. When additional exposure is likely through the skin, that may be noted after the TWA. This is especially true for chemicals such as phenol and methanol that pass quickly through skin.

STEL (or STEV). The short-term exposure limit (or value) is the highest permissible time-weighted average exposure for any 15-minute period during the work shift. It should be measured during the worst 15-minute period. The STEL is always higher than the TWA.

CL (or CEV). The Ceiling Limit (Ceiling Exposure Value) is the maximum permissible instantaneous exposure during any part of the work shift. Few chemicals are given both a STEL and a CL; the CL is usually reserved for highly dangerous substances.

For chemicals lacking either a STEL or CL, prudent values may be determined by multiplying the TWA by 3 for the STEL or by 5 for the CL, as is suggested by the Ontario (Canada) Ministry of Labor (1991). When more than one harmful substance is present, complex formulas must be used to determine combined occupational exposure limits. These formulas are prescribed by various governments and vary from country to country.

IDLH. This airborne concentration is immediately dangerous to life and health. Chemicals with low IDLH should be considered very dangerous when spilled or when significant volumes are being dispensed. A single inhalation at or above this limit could have serious, if not lethal, consequences.

Biological exposure indices

Can a worker determine if significant exposure has occurred? Can the chemical in question be detected in the worker by a clinical test? In a few instances, the answer is 'yes'. ACGIH® has established Biological Exposure Indices (BEIs®) as maximum values of analytes determined from clinical tests on exhaled air, urine, or blood for a variety of hazardous chemicals, but only four are pertinent to histology: N,N-dimethylformamide, methanol, phenol, and xylenes. Consult the latest booklet issued yearly by ACGIH® for details on the first three chemicals.

Because xylene is used so pervasively in histology, and so many histologists are concerned with its effects, further information is presented here on this chemical. The isomers of xylene are metabolized to methylhippuric acids, which can be measured in exposed workers' urine. The BEI® for xylenes is 1.5 g methylhippuric acids per g creatinine. Samples are collected immediately at the end of a work shift.

BEIs® are not intended to be used in diagnosing occupational illness. They are not maximum safe permissible values. Rather, they are to be used as indicators that workers may be exposed to significant concentrations of harmful substances, particularly if an individual worker or a group of co-workers repeatedly show values of the analyte at or above the BEI®. For xylene in a well-ventilated histology lab, high methylhippuric acids in urine would probably indicate significant skin exposure.

Types of hazard

Systems of classifying the hazardous nature of chemicals range from simple pictographs with numerical ratings to comprehensive lists of formally defined terms. Even within a single country, government agencies may differ in how hazards are defined. While no single system will suffice worldwide, the following terms do have nearly universal meaning and should serve on a practical basis for describing the hazards encountered in histology. For convenience, hazards are first divided into two broad categories, health and physical. The latter certainly have ramifications for health, but present more immediate problems for storage, handling, and building codes.

Biohazards can be infectious agents themselves or items (solutions, specimens, or objects) contaminated with them. Anything that can cause disease in humans, regardless of its source, is considered biohazardous, even if the disease primarily occurs in animals. In many countries, biohazardous materials are specially labeled and disposal is generally strictly controlled.

Irritants are chemicals that cause reversible inflammatory effects at the site of contact with living tissue. Most often, eyes, skin and respiratory passages are affected. Nearly all chemicals can be irritating given sufficient exposure to tissue, so general hygiene practices dictate that direct contact be avoided as much as possible.

Corrosive chemicals present both physical and health hazards. When exposed to living tissue, destruction or irreversible alteration occurs. In contact with certain inanimate surfaces (generally metal), corrosives destroy the material. Interestingly, a chemical may be corrosive to tissue but not to steel, or vice versa; few are corrosive to both.

Sensitizers cause allergic reactions in a substantial proportion of exposed subjects. Nearly any chemical may cause an allergic reaction in hypersensitive individu-

als, so the key here is the prevalence of the reaction in the exposed population. True sensitizers are very serious hazards, because sensitization lasts for life and only gets worse with subsequent exposure. Sensitization may occur at work because of the high exposure level, but chances are the chemicals will also be found outside the workplace in lower concentrations that aggravate the allergy. Formaldehyde is a prime example here. Its vapors come off permanent press clothing, draperies, upholstery, wall coverings, plywood, and many other building materials. Affected persons can never get away from it.

Carcinogens: While many substances induce tumors in experimental animals exposed to unrealistically high dosages, officially recognized carcinogens must present a special risk to humans. Criteria for the carcinogenic designation differ slightly among agencies, but in the end any carcinogenic chemical used in histology is universally recognized as such. Examples include chloroform, chromic acid, dioxane, formaldehyde, nickel chloride, and potassium dichromate. Additionally, a number of dyes are carcinogens: auramine O (CI 41000), basic fuchsin (pararosaniline hydrochloride, CI 42500), ponceau 2R (ponceau de xylidine, CI 16150) and any dye derived from benzidine (including Congo red, CI 22120; diaminobenzidine and chlorazol black E, CI 30235).

Toxic materials are capable of causing death by ingestion, skin contact or inhalation at certain specified concentrations. These concentrations vary slightly according to the agency making the designation, but differences are insignificant to the histologist. Some countries use the term *poison* when referring to this category. Toxic chemicals pose an immediate risk greater than the previously covered hazards, and some are so dangerous that they are given the designation *highly toxic*. Methanol is toxic; chromic acid, osmium tetroxide, and uranyl nitrate are highly toxic. Use extreme caution when handling toxic substances; avoid highly toxic ones if possible.

Chemicals causing specific harm to select anatomical or physiological systems are said to have *target organ effects*. These are particularly dangerous substances because their effects are not immediately evident but are cumulative and frequently irreversible. There are numerous histologically relevant examples: xylene and toluene are neurotoxins and benzene affects the blood. Reproductive toxins are especially prevalent (chloroform, methanol, methyl methacrylate, mercuric chloride, xylene, and toluene, to name a few) and may warrant special consideration under occupational safety regulations of some countries.

The remaining hazard classes pertain to physical risks. *Combustibles* have flash points at or above a specified temperature. Flash point is the temperature at which vapors will ignite in the presence of an ignition source under carefully defined conditions using specified test equipment. It is a guide to the likelihood of which vapors might ignite under real workplace conditions. Flash point is not the temperature at which a substance will ignite spontaneously. Different countries and various agencies within those countries have their own unique values for the specified temperature. In the USA, OSHA defines it as 100°F (38°C), while the Department of Transportation uses 141°F (60.5°C). Combustible liquids pose little risk of fire under routine laboratory conditions, but they will burn readily during a fire. It is better to choose a combustible product over a flammable one if all other considerations are equal. Clearing agents offer this choice.

Flammable materials have flash points below the specified temperature discussed above, and thus are of greater concern. Vapors should be controlled carefully to prevent build up around electrical devices that spark. Special provisions for storage are usually mandated by national regulations, but local codes may impose even stricter measures. Storage rooms, cabinets, and containers may have to be specially designed for flammable liquids; volumes stored therein may also be limited. Original manufacturers' containers should be used whenever possible, and preferably should not exceed 1 gallon (4–5 liters).

Explosive chemicals are rare in histology, the primary example being picric acid. Certain silver solutions may become explosive upon aging, which is why they should never be stored after use. In both cases, explosions may occur simply by shaking. Picric acid also forms dangerous salts with certain metals, which, unlike the parent compound, are potentially explosive even when wet. The best defense against explosive reagents is to avoid them altogether; this is certainly feasible today with picric acid.

Oxidizers initiate or promote combustion in other materials. Harmless by themselves, they may present a serious fire risk when in contact with suitable substances. Sodium iodate is a mild oxidizer that poses little risk under routine laboratory conditions. Mercuric oxide and chromic acid are oxidants that are more serious.

Organic peroxides are particularly dangerous oxidizers sometimes used to polymerize plastic resins. Limit their volume on hand to extremely small quantities. *Pyrophoric, unstable (reactive)* and *water-reactive* substances are not generally found in histology. All involve fire or excessive heat.

CONTROL OF CHEMICALS HAZARDOUS TO HEALTH AND THE ENVIRONMENT

Personal hygiene practices

There must be no eating, drinking or smoking in the lab. Application of cosmetics other than hand lotion likewise has no place within the laboratory setting. Wash hands frequently, but keep skin supple and hydrated with a good lotion. If hazardous powders have been handled, wash around your nose and mouth so that adherent particles are not ingested or inhaled. Solutions must never be pipetted by mouth.

Labeling

Every chemical should be labeled with certain basic information; indeed, proper labeling of all containers of chemicals is mandated in some countries. Most reagents purchased recently will have most of the following already on the label, but older inventories may lack certain critical hazard warnings. Remember that solutions created in your lab must be fully labeled. Minimum information includes:

- chemical name and, if a mixture, names of all ingredients
- manufacturer's name and address if purchased commercially, or person making the reagent
- date purchased or made
- expiration date, if known
- hazard warnings and safety precautions.

When putting a reagent's name (or names of ingredients) on the label, use terminology that will be useful to those needing the information. In histology, we have many reagent names that are unfamiliar to chemically knowledgeable people who might be involved in an emergency. This is why it is so important to list ingredients, using names with widespread acceptance in the general field of chemistry; for example, use formaldehyde for formalin, acid fuchsin and picric acid for Van Gieson's, and mercuric chloride, sodium acetate, and formaldehyde for B-5.

Commercial products in their original containers will have the name and address of the manufacturer or supplier. If the material is put into another container, even 'temporarily', include this information on the new label. Chemicals in 'temporary' storage conditions have a bad habit of remaining there for years after lab personnel have moved on.

If the reagent is made in the lab, indicate who made it and when. Traceability could be critical if other information is lacking, as in the case of a Coplin jar of 'silver stain' left in a refrigerator. Is the solution one of those that is potentially explosive? Does anyone know which silver solution it is?

Many laboratories use small self-adhesive labels that say 'Received:____'. These are dated and affixed to each incoming container. Similarly, an expiration date should also be included for those chemicals that do not have an indefinite shelf life. Most inorganic compounds and many non-perishable organic chemicals are good for many years, but mixtures frequently deteriorate in a briefer time. Information on shelf life is hard to come by, and the best source is experience since each lab has different conditions and perhaps slightly varied formulations. Kiernan (1999) has included shelf life data from his own extensive experience, which should serve as a good first approximation for use.

Hazard warnings at a minimum should include the designations listed in the preceding section. This is the simplest and least ambiguous system. Pictographs (flames, corroding objects, etc.) are not universally recognized; some are obscure as to meaning. Hazard diamonds are popular but carry risks of misinterpretation, especially since there are several systems in use. When there is an emergency, people may not think clearly or have time to figure something out. They need immediate access to the nature of the danger, and nothing provides that so effectively as the printed word. Briefly worded safety precautions may be appended to the hazard warning: for example irritant, avoid contact with skin and eyes.

A multicultural workforce, not all of whom may have the same native language, staffs many labs. It is prudent to accommodate their needs by providing multilingual hazard warnings. Again, in an emergency there should be no impediments to prompt and correct action.

Warning signs

Various countries have established different guidelines or mandatory regulations involving signage, so specific recommendations cannot be given here.

Protective equipment

General guidelines for clothing suitable for laboratory work should be considered before protective equipment. Secure, close-toed footwear should be mandated; open-toed shoes and sandals offer no protection against spills or dropped items. While nearly all fabric today is resistant to destruction by histological solvents, such was not always the case. Certain early acrylic and acetate fibers dissolved almost instantly when in contact with xylene or toluene, creating a great deal of embarrassment when tiny drops of solvent hit the cloth. The possibility that such fabric still exists is real enough to take heed.

Aprons, goggles, gloves, and respirators are the personal protective equipment (PPE) most likely to be used in the histology laboratory. In some countries, laws for certain hazardous situations require specified PPE. The following set of recommendations should be a routine part of general laboratory hygiene and will satisfy the most stringent regulations. When very specific requirements exist for certain chemicals, such information will be included below in the section detailing common histological reagents. Aprons should be made of material impervious to the chemicals being used. Simple disposable plastic aprons are usually quite satisfactory, although heavy rubber aprons may be warranted when handling concentrated acids. Cloth laboratory coats are suitable only for protection against powders or very small quantities of hazardous liquids. Do not use them for protection against formaldehyde.

Goggles should be chosen specifically for each worker to accommodate the diversity of facial shapes and prescription glasses. Goggles not only come in a variety of sizes and shapes, they are also made for different functions. Choose only vented splash-proof goggles for routine work in histology. These allow for ventilation, which reduces bothersome fogging of the lenses, but the vent holes are baffled so that splashing liquids are not likely to reach the eyes. Never cut holes in goggles to improve ventilation, as this defeats the protective function of the equipment. For severe conditions of exposure, wear a face shield over splash-proof goggles; never use a face shield without the goggles. Finally, safety glasses are no substitute for goggles when handling hazardous liquids.

The issue of contact lenses arises frequently in discussions about eye protection (American College of Occupational and Environmental Medicine 2003). If liquids with no irritating fumes are being handled, contact lenses may be used safely in conjunction with appropriate goggles. However, conventional goggles offer no protection against harmful vapors, which can become trapped beneath the lenses, causing greater corneal damage. Stinging or watering eyes indicate that the inhalation exposure is almost certainly beyond permissible or prudent limits: regardless of whether contact lenses are being worn or not, work under those conditions, even for brief periods, should not be undetaken.

Gloves are the most controversial PPE, and misinformation abounds. It is vitally important to understand how gloves work, so that informed decisions can be made about glove selection. Glove material is rarely completely impermeable; it delays penetration of harmful material for a time sufficient to provide adequate protection. Chemical resistance refers to how well material holds up in the presence of solvents, but says nothing about how readily substances move through the material. In most cases, liquids rarely penetrate intact glove material. The vapors are the problem, both because they penetrate more efficiently through gloves and skin, and because the worker usually cannot detect them. Reputable manufacturers of gloves evaluate their products in somewhat standardized tests, measuring the time it takes for detectable amounts of a particular chemical to appear on the far side of the material. This is called the breakthrough time, and it increases non-linearly with glove thickness. A glove twice as thick as another made from the same material will not have a breakthrough time double that of the thinner glove. Schwope et al (1987) present the most comprehensive listing of data on this subject.

Latex is one of the most permeable of all glove materials. Thick (8 mil) rubber gloves have a breakthrough time of 12 minutes with formaldehyde solutions. Latex surgical gloves are so thin (1.0–1.5 mil) that they offer *no* effective protection against formaldehyde or histological solvents. These gloves are suitable only for protection from biohazards. Keep in mind the startling increase in the incidence of latex sensitization, which has accompanied the widespread use of these gloves since the beginning of the AIDS epidemic.

Nitrile gloves are the best option for histological use. They are available in surgical-type thinness for brief intermittent exposures where fine dexterity is necessary. Exposures that are more serious can be safely tolerated with 8 mil nitrile gloves. Remember, however, that no glove material is effective against all classes of chemicals, and nitrile is no exception. Some chemicals in wide histological usage (xylene, toluene, chloroform) will permeate nitrile in seconds.

Respiratory protection against chemical vapors should rarely if ever be needed except in emergencies. Regulatory agencies stress that respirators are the protective equipment of last resort. No one in histology should be in a workplace whose vapor levels are even transiently higher than the PELs. Wearing respirators is uncomfortable, expensive, and fraught with compliance hassles. Leave them to the people specially trained not only in respiratory use but also in dealing with such dangerous environments.

In the following discussion, the word 'should' is used, but substitute 'must' in countries having stringent respiratory protection standards. Workers should receive special training for wearing respirators because of the complexities of proper usage. Each worker needing this level of protection should be individually fitted with a respirator that exactly fits the contours of the face. The efficacy of the fit is then assured through a series of complicated tests that should be documented and repeated on a periodic basis. Workers should undergo medical evaluations and respiratory function tests to determine if they are physically qualified to wear respirators. Cartridges for respirators must be chosen carefully for the chemical environment. Both the type of chemical and the vapor concentration are vitally important considerations. Respiratory protection from airborne infectious materials is another matter altogether. Surgical masks are unacceptable because they fit poorly and have too large a pore size to filter out aerosols. HEPA (high-efficiency particulate air) filters are suitable. Workers wearing HEPA masks may have to comply with applicable provisions of respiratory protection standards.

Ventilation

Ventilation is the foremost engineering control; ensuring proper airflow through a laboratory is the first critical step in improving working conditions. While much of the design of a ventilating system is beyond the scope of this discussion, every laboratory scientist should be aware of the following basic principles. For further details on hood design and placement, see Dapson and Dapson (2005) and Saunders (1993). Laboratories should have two separate systems of ventilation, one for general air circulation (often combined with heating and air conditioning and called HVAC), the other for local removal of hazardous fumes. They must work in concert to be effective, and must not merely shift the noxious vapors to another part of the facility.

General ventilation is for the physical comfort of the occupants of the room. Each hour, the entire volume of room air should be exchanged 4–12 times. That air should not contain significant quantities of hazardous vapors. If such vapors are originating somewhere in the room (from a grossing area, for instance), they should be dealt with at their source with an independent system of local ventilation.

Properly designed chemical fume hoods enclose the emission area, isolating it structurally and functionally from the rest of the room. A motor somewhere in the ductwork (preferably far from the hood) moves air directly to the outside. A sliding door (sash) usually fronts the system, and is an integral part of the way it works by controlling the face velocity of air entering the enclosure. It is a common misconception that high face velocities are good. In fact, strong airflow may create such turbulence inside the hood that contaminated air spills back out into the room. For vapor levels usually encountered in histology labs, a face velocity of 80–120 linear feet per minute is ideal; this is controlled by adjusting the height of the sash. As lifting the sash enlarges the opening, face velocity declines. A vanometer, built into the hood or obtained as an inexpensive handheld device, measures face velocity. Always keep the sash at least partially open (unless the hood is designed to admit room air from another port) to prevent overtaxing the motor.

Improperly designed hoods will not be able to achieve optimal face velocity with the sash opened to a comfortable working height. Avoid these, literally at all costs, as the facility's money will only be wasted and give the staff a dangerously false sense of security. There are important dimensional considerations that determine a hood's effectiveness: the hood will develop dangerous eddies if too shallow and may not be able to move the full volume of air if too expansive.

There are other, external factors that influence how a hood works, and all center on the air supplied to the face of the hood. It should be obvious that a device removing air from a workplace must have a supply to draw upon. This is in addition to the amount required by the general ventilating system to exchange 4–12 room air changes per hour. Heating and air conditioning must also be balanced to account for the removal of air through the hood. Location of a hood is critical. Airflow into the face should be smooth and unimpeded. Surprisingly strong crosscurrents are generated by doors opening and closing, or by people walking by. Even the draft from general HVAC ducts can adversely affect hood performance. Any of these disturbances can draw harmful vapors out of the enclosure into the room, even against a net inward flow of air. Locate the hood, and by inference the hazardous work area, out of main traffic patterns and away from HVAC ducts.

Do not use fume hoods as storage or disposal devices. Objects within a hood disrupt airflow, and may block important air passages. Containers that emit vapors should not be placed within a hood except as a temporary safety measure. Remove the offending substance as soon as possible and put it into a secure container. Finally, do not put a waste chemical into a hood for evaporating it away unless there is no alternative in an emergency. Doing so is probably a violation of environmental regulations, and it may exceed the capacity of the hood to carry fumes away safely.

Ventilation devices other than fume hoods are used in histology labs; few are suitable unless vapor levels are already low. A non-enclosed system, such as a duct located above or behind the work area, may be powerful enough to draw contaminated air away from the worker as long as no crosscurrents are generated, but that is an unrealistic assumption. Workers must move about, and that usually destroys the effectiveness of unenclosed devices. Hoods that return air to the room after passing it through a filter may be suitable for localized workstations generating modest vapor emissions. Filters must be chosen with care. Vapor levels will dictate the size needed. Formaldehyde is not effectively captured by the filtration media used for solvent vapors. Filters become loaded and must be replaced, but how often this occurs is usually a mystery until odors are noticed out in the room. Since most workers in histology labs have impaired senses of smell, dangerous vapor levels may accumulate before anyone detects them. If filtration devices must be used, figure out how to determine effective life of the filters and establish a strict replacement regimen.

Air purification systems based upon ozone should be not be used. They generate a chemical that is more hazardous than most of the fumes found in histology labs: ozone has a Ceiling Limit of 0.1 ppm according to ACGIH®. Further, ozone from these purifiers does not seem to be effective in destroying formaldehyde vapors (Esswein & Boeniger 1994).

First aid

With laboratory chemicals, the most common accidents requiring first aid are ingestion, eye contact, and extensive skin contact. All healthcare professionals should have basic training in dealing with these situations at least and preferably with all aspects of first aid. Yearly safety training should include preparedness exercises on the most likely chemical accidents. Ingestion is encountered with patients and other non-laboratory staff, and frequently involves formalin. This is a tragic consequence of administrative neglect of basic safety issues. Laboratory chemicals should never be accessible to unattended patients, particularly those who because of age or illness are unable to think clearly about their actions. Improperly labeled containers are another cause of accidental ingestion. Patients should not be allowed to take fixed surgical specimens home; they present such a large risk from poisoning that no argument to the contrary is sufficient. If a body part needs to be specially cared for as part of a religious purpose, it should be given only to a responsible adult who can assure that it will never be accessible to unattended children.

First aid for ingestion of hazardous chemicals is not a simple matter. Some reagents will cause more damage if vomited and subsequently aspirated into respiratory passages; others are so toxic that the risk of aspiration is outweighed by the necessity to get the offending substance out of the body quickly. To solve this dilemma, some countries have established sophisticated networks of emergency response teams, which are admirably qualified to provide the best advice. If you have access to a Poison Control Center, or something similar, post the telephone number on each telephone in your laboratory. Time is of the essence in such emergencies, and preparedness may save a life. If enough people are available, get the victim to the emergency room while someone else contacts a Poison Control Center. If outside help is not possible, give a conscious victim a large quantity of water.

Splashing of dangerous chemicals into eyes is a common accident among those who fail to wear suitable goggles. Except for concentrated mineral acids, routine histological chemicals, including formaldehyde, are not likely to cause serious harm to eyes as long as proper treatment immediately follows an accident. All labs should be equipped with emergency eyewash stations, as either freestanding devices or small appliances affixed to sink faucets (the latter must be tested frequently to assure free flow of water). Current recommendations are to have such devices no more than 10 seconds or 100 feet from hazardous work areas. Ideally, the water temperature should be controlled to a range of 15–35°C. Portable eyewash bottles are not recommended and may be deemed unacceptable by regulatory agencies. These containers hold little liquid and may become contaminated with microorganisms.

Rinse the affected eye for 15–30 minutes, pulling the lids away from the eyeball. This is a seemingly interminable period, but do not shorten it. Emergency healthcare should be sought only after this treatment.

Treatment of skin contact with hazardous chemicals is simple: wash with water for 15–30 minutes. A quick rinse will not be sufficient for the more dangerous chemicals. Emergency showers should be as accessible as eyewash stations. If the substance is not readily water-soluble, use soap with the water wash. Immediately remove contaminated clothing, including wet shoes. Launder before wearing again, or discard the article. Formaldehyde-soaked leather will be difficult to salvage.

Radiation

The advantages of using radioactive chemicals are rarely sufficient to justify their risks to health and the environment. Exceptions may pertain to therapeutic radio-isotopes used as tracers. These emit very low levels of poorly penetrating radiation, and have half-lives measured in hours.

If radioactive substances are handled, a qualified radiation safety officer must oversee all aspects of the project, including waste disposal. Participating staff must be specially trained in radiation safety. This will allay fears as much as create a responsible workforce. The work area should be monitored periodically with a radiation detector. Workers should wear dosimeters.

Storage of hazardous chemicals

Most laboratory chemicals can be safely stored in conventional cupboards. Dangerous liquids are best stored below countertop height to minimize the risk of bodily exposure in case a bottle is dropped and broken. Buy dangerous reagents in plastic or plastic-coated glass bottles whenever possible. Special storage provisions are warranted for acids, flammables, radioactive isotopes, controlled substances, and hazardous chemicals in bulk containers.

Specialized acid cabinets are designed to contain the fumes emanating from most containers of strong mineral acids. They should be vented to the outside, using acid-resistant ductwork. Curiously, many of these storage devices contain some mild steel parts, which soon rust. Choose this equipment carefully for that reason. Paper labels on acid bottles should be checked periodically for corrosion that could lead to illegibility. Other special storage cabinets are usually mandated for all but the smallest quantities of flammable materials. These are designed to contain a fire within the cabinet. If they are vented, provisions must be made in the ductwork to prevent the spread of fire from the cabinet.

Certain flammable liquids present unusual fire and explosion risks because of their highly volatile nature and very low flash point. Isopentane and diethyl ether ('ether') are common examples. Opened containers cannot be resealed reliably. Never store these in a refrigerator or freezer unless these appliances are certified as suitable for an explosive atmosphere (mistakenly referred to as 'explosion-proof'). The best advice is to avoid using these chemicals altogether. If that is not possible, buy only the quantity immediately needed, use it up if possible and do not try to store any leftovers.

Radioactive chemicals and controlled substances must be stored separately from other reagents. Cabinets should be locked. Access should be limited to a few specially qualified people.

Large containers present other risks. Even 5 gallon (20 liter) quantities can be too heavy for people to handle, especially for pouring operations. Equip these containers with spigots and keep the spigot above fluid level when not in use, if that is possible. Larger drums up to 55 gallons (208 liters) require special handling equipment for moving and dispensing. Be sure any pumping device is completely compatible with the chemical. Avoid mild steel parts for fixatives and most plastics for xylene and toluene.

Transporting hazardous materials from storage to work areas can be risky. Carry glass containers with both hands, one hand beneath the jar or bottle. Special rubber buckets should be used to carry highly dangerous materials such as glass containers of mineral acids.

Spills and containment

Preparedness for spills begins with laboratory design. The goal is to prevent hazardous materials from reaching the outside environment. There should be no open floor drains unless they lead to special containment equipment that can be pumped out or drained by a hazardous waste hauler. Floor drains for showers can be built with a low dike that prevents liquids on the floor from entering and keeps most of the water from the shower from getting out onto the floor.

How laboratory personnel respond to a spill will depend upon the nature of the hazard, the volume of the spill, and the qualifications of the staff. Each chemical should be evaluated with these factors in mind. A gallon of alcohol spilled onto the floor presents a risk of fire but little health hazard, while the same quantity of formalin could be life threatening (20 ppm is imminently hazardous to life). Small spills are defined as those that can be safely handled by the immediate staff. Large spills present risks that surpass the qualifications of the same people to deal safely with the emergency and require specially trained hazmat or emergency response teams. Each lab must draw the line between small and large spills based on its unique merits. Keep in mind that, in some cases, emergency responders by law receive special training and medical evaluation.

Develop plans for dealing with each family of hazardous material (acids, bases, flammables, etc.). Detail exactly what protective equipment is needed, and how each type of spill will be handled. Establish who will be called in the event the spill requires outside help, then contact them so they will be prepared. They may want an on-site visit to familiarize themselves with the facility's layout, and certainly will want to discuss the types and magnitudes of hazards. Finally, train the laboratory staff on spill procedures, and practice doing it with harmless material. Not having had the time to do this will prove to be a sorry excuse when the accident occurs.

If the amount of spilled material is limited to a few grams or milliliters, it should simply be wiped up with towel or sponge. Protect the hands with suitable gloves. Dispose of the towel or sponge appropriately; do not put it into the general trash, and protect the room from its vapors by sealing it within an impermeable plastic bag or other container.

In contrast to such very small incidents, an entirely different approach should be used for any other spills of dangerous materials. All personnel should evacuate the room or immediate vicinity and assemble in a designated spot. Check everyone is there and, on the way out, watch for co-workers and assist anyone needing help. Provide first aid if anyone has been splashed or is feeling the effects of vapors. Calmly discuss the magnitude of the spill and determine if it is large or small. There should be no mention of cause or blame here: it is immaterial to the immediate problem. If the spill is large, call an emergency response team and seal off the area; if small, decide how to handle the spill based on pre-arranged plans.

Spill neutralizing and containment kits should be available immediately outside the hazardous work area. These may be commercially purchased or assembled from common materials, and should include protective equipment and cleanup aids. Nitrile gloves similar in thickness to dishwashing gloves are adequate for most spills likely in histology; several sizes are available. Splash-proof goggles and a faceshield are important. Provide disposable plastic aprons for chemical spills and disposable gowns for biohazards. If the staff is qualified and trained, equip the kit with respirators appropriate for the type of spill (do not forget a HEPA respirator for biohazards).

A good basic kit would also include cleanup items such as a dustpan and brush for powders, sponges, towels, and mops for liquids, adsorbent material (vermiculite, kitty litter or a commercial sorbent), bleach (sodium hypochlorite) for biohazards, baking soda for acids, vinegar (5% acetic acid) for alkalis, and a commercial formalin neutralizing product. Have a sealable plastic bucket and heavy plastic bags for containment of the salvaged waste. Kits that are more sophisticated would contain instantaneous vapor monitoring devices so that the contaminated area can be checked before cleanup operations begin. Remember: the level of expertise of the staff will dictate how far to go with this.

Recycling

One very effective way to control hazardous chemicals is through recycling, as this reduces the quantities purchased, stored, and discarded. Many clearing agents, alcohol, and formalin can be recycled very satisfactorily with proper equipment. Because these are the highest volume chemicals in histology, the cost savings can be impressive despite an initial outlay of capital funds. Buy wisely, however, because there are inexpensive units on the market that will not yield a recycled product of acceptable purity.

Formalin is a mixture of volatile formaldehyde and nonvolatile salts in a solvent of water or water and alcohol (the small amount of stabilizing methanol can be ignored). Used solutions also contain solubilized and particulate components from the specimens. Through the process of simple distillation, water and formaldehyde are separated from all the other constituents. While that leaves the undesirable parts behind, the recycled product now lacks its salts and may not be at the proper concentration. Formaldehyde content can be assayed with a simple kit and adjusted as necessary. Fresh salts are readily restored to the solution.

Solvents should be fractionally distilled, as some of the contaminants in the waste are also volatile. Simple distillation will not separate these, and the resultant product may contain unacceptable amounts of water. Poorly described devices with inordinately high or fast throughput that are priced thousands of dollars below fractional distillation equipment are likely to cause great trouble. They have certainly given distillation a bad name, which is unfortunate because recycling does work and saves money when done correctly.

The most common problem with good distillation equipment is a foul amine odor detectable in the recycled product. It comes from deamination of protein in the waste during the distillation process. The freed amines evaporate readily and pass over with the other volatile components. Keeping the distillation chamber scrupulously clean is usually the key to avoiding the problem altogether. Formalin that has been heavily enriched with blood protein (as from fixing placentas) may require diluting with less bloody waste formalin. Pre-filter solutions containing many tissue fragments or coagulated protein.

Hazardous chemical waste disposal

Healthcare facilities are in business to prevent and treat illness, yet they are significant contributors to environmental harm especially in countries that have seen significant improvements in industrial pollution. On the other hand, there should be little waste to deal with if an effective pollution prevention program has been put into effect. Reducing toxics use by substitution and minimization, coupled with recycling, could lead to amazingly low quantities of waste to be hauled away. The three highest volume reagents, formalin, alcohol, and clearant, can all be recycled. Formalin can be replaced with an effective glyoxal-based fixative that is drain disposable in nearly all communities because of its ready biodegradability and low aquatic toxicity.

Options for disposal of hazardous chemical waste depend heavily upon national and local regulations, but the following recommendations should be valid any-where. First, keep waste streams separated; do not mix different chemicals together unless told to do so by a qualified waste official. Second, know the hazard(s) of the waste. Is it flammable? Water-soluble? Toxic? Each of these factors affects the choice of disposal method. The best option for disposal is to pour the waste down the sanitary drain, from which it can be treated before enter-ing the environment. Such waste, however, must not harm the biological processes that waste treatment facil-ities depend upon, nor must it pass through the system untreated. An example of the former would be formalde-hyde in sufficient strength and quantity to kill off the bacteria driving the treatment process. Xylene typifies the latter, because its rate of biodegradation is too slow to be affected by the 1–3-day residence time in the waste-water treatment plant.

Formaldehyde is readily biodegradable. Nearly all organisms have an enzyme, formaldehyde dehydroge-nase, that decomposes this chemical. The trick is to feed it into the system slowly enough so that it is diluted below toxic concentrations by the normal flow of water. Never dilute toxic material before pouring it down the drain, or follow disposal by 'flushing with copious amounts of water'. It is illegal to do so in some countries (including the USA). Furthermore, the practice increases the volume passing through the treatment plant, which shortens the residence time and may impair biodegradation.

Work with your wastewater authorities. You may be very surprised at what they allow. Inform them of the nature of the waste (chemical composition and hazard-ous characteristics), and offer material data sheets. Propose a plan for disposal which includes the volume of waste, the time period over which it will be dumped, and the frequency of disposal. For example, you may wish to dispose of 2 gallons (7.6 liters) of waste formalin con-taining 3.7% or 37,000 ppm formaldehyde over a 1-hour period each working day. This could be accomplished by trickling the waste into a sink from a carboy equipped with bottom spigot adjusted so that it takes an hour to become empty. There would be no risk to the treatment

plant at this flow rate of 2 ml/second. Dumping a large volume of waste all at once is not good because it tends to travel in a slug and may fail to become sufficiently diluted to protect the treatment plant.

Some waste can be rendered more acceptable for drain disposal. Acids and bases can be neutralized and formalin can be detoxified with commercial products. Be sure the pretreatment process is safe, effective, and acceptable. Never attempt to detoxify formalin by mixing with bleach (sodium hypochlorite) or ammonia. Both reactions are exothermic and could quickly get out of control, spewing vapors and hot fluid all over the lab. Know what the reaction products are, and be certain that they are indeed suitably low in toxicity. Water-insoluble solvents are never drain disposable, even if purportedly biodegradable. If they are combustible with sufficiently high caloric value, they may be eligible to be mixed with the fuel in an oil-fired heating system in certain countries. Good candidates for this option are any of the clearing agents except the halogenated sol-vents chloroform, trichloroethane, and their relatives. Note that this method is not burning the waste in an incinerator. The difference is subtle but important. An incinerator exists for the sole purpose of destroying waste, while a furnace provides heat.

If you cannot get rid of a waste by drain disposal or combustion in a furnace, you must resort to a waste hauler. This is the option of last resort. Despite strict regulations and the best of intentions, the hazardous waste disposal industry has a poor record of accomplish-ment. In some countries, the waste generator (your facil-ity) bears the ultimate responsibility and liability for the waste that someone else takes away and supposedly deals with properly. If you are generating waste that must be removed from the premises for burial or incin-eration, you should do everything possible to eliminate that chemical from your lab. There is no better advice, however you want to view it, whether from a financial, health, or environmental perspective.

CONTROL OF BIOLOGICAL SUBSTANCES HAZARDOUS TO HEALTH AND THE ENVIRONMENT

Preparation

An exposure control plan for biohazards should be written. It may be part of the chemical hygiene plan or an independent document, but definitely should be part of your SOPs. As with chemical hazards, workers should be trained initially, refreshed at least yearly, and immediately introduced to any new procedures that present additional risks.

Handling

People who work in histology laboratories may not be exposed to quite the level of risk that many healthcare workers are, but they face hazards that may be more subtle. Keep in mind that there are three potential routes of exposure: inhalation of aerosols, contact with non-intact skin, and contact with mucous membranes (eyes, nose, and mouth). Knowing how infectious agents can reach you is the foundation of protecting yourself and your co-workers. Practice universal precautions: handle every specimen as if it were infectious.

Fresh specimens of human origin must always be considered potentially infectious. Most animal tissue does not carry that risk, but there are important exceptions. Species known to be capable of transmitting disease to humans, and animals intentionally infected or known to be naturally infected with transmissible diseases, must be handled with the same precautions as would be used for human tissue.

The first and most obvious source of biological risk is with fresh tissue and body fluids; grossing carries the highest risk of all histological activities. Fixed specimens have a much-reduced risk because nearly all infectious agents are readily deactivated by histological fixation. Specimens must be thoroughly fixed for this to happen, however. Certain tissues such as liver, spleen, placenta, and lung do not fix well unless grossed thinly, and may remain raw (unfixed) in the center after days of exposure to the fixative. Those centers are potentially infectious. Also, realize that some fixatives require more time than that available in rushed pathology labs, so tissues in the first several stations of a tissue processor may remain biohazardous. Complete penetration by alcohol will kill all infectious agents except prions, so it is safe to say that properly processed specimens are free from microbial risk and can be handled without special precautions.

Prions, the agents of spongiform encephalopathies such as Creutzfeldt–Jakob disease, scrapie, chronic wasting disease, and mad cow disease present a more difficult challenge. Even normal steam sterilization fails to inactivate these particles, and common effective chemical treatments such as sodium hypochlorite and phenol create artifacts in tissue. Histological specimens can be decontaminated by immersion in formalin for 48 hours, followed by treatment for 1 hour in concentrated formic acid and additional formalin fixation for another 48 hours. Rank (1999) reviewed the risks and decontamination protocols for histology labs.

Cryotomy presents special risks because tissue is usually fresh. Small dust-like particles generated from sectioning may become airborne, a risk vastly magnified with the use of cryogenic sprays. Never use these; they are dangerous to you and anyone nearby in the room. Do not clean the cabinet with a vacuum unless the device is equipped with a HEPA filter. Sterilize surfaces with chlorine bleach or a suitable commercial disinfectant; avoid formaldehyde solutions as these present a chemical risk to the person doing the cleaning. Good quality latex or nitrile surgical gloves are perfectly acceptable protective devices for biohazards. Goggles should be worn during grossing anyway to protect against chemical splashes, and will do double duty against infectious agents. A face shield may be warranted in some cases. Aprons or lab coats will keep clothes clean, but do not wear these used protective articles outside the lab (especially to the cafeteria!).

Disposal of biohazardous waste

Biohazardous waste should be incinerated on-site or hauled away. Either way, potentially infectious waste ought to be segregated from chemical and non-regulated waste, which may be barred from incinerators designed for biohazardous materials. Fixed wet specimens and their fluid are chemically hazardous and may be infectious. Together they pose a difficult problem. Haulers of biohazardous waste may not be equipped to handle chemical waste, and chemical waste haulers may balk at disposing of biohazardous materials. Clarification may come soon as regulators become more aware of this dilemma.

CONTROL OF PHYSICAL HAZARDS

Equipment may present risks from electrical and mechanical factors, which can be minimized by proper installation, care, and personnel training. Keep a log for each piece of equipment listing installation date, person and firm performing the installation, and initial diagnostic test results to insure the item is working properly.

Also, include a schedule for preventive maintenance and a complete service record. Such record keeping may be mandatory in some countries, and it certainly is good laboratory practice anywhere.

Electrical shock most often arises from improperly grounded devices. Have a qualified person verify that all outlets are properly polarized and grounded. Plug equipment into outlets, not into extension cords. Limit purchases of equipment to those that have met the standards of one of the internationally recognized testing agencies.

Electrical equipment also poses a risk of igniting flammable vapors. Nearly all switches may spark, including those associated with doors. Devices sold as 'explosion-proof' have their switches sealed to prevent contact with flammable vapors. Refrigerators and freezers must never be used to store highly flammable chemicals such as ether and isopentane unless they are rated as suitable for flammable environments. Likewise, household microwave ovens should not be used to heat flammables because the door interlock switch may spark (this switch stops the magnetron when the door is opened). Some laboratory microwave appliances vent the chamber sufficiently to prevent potentially explosive vapor concentrations from building.

Today, mechanical dangers from histological equipment are generally confined to burns from hot surfaces. Most modern devices have adequate safety features that have eliminated some of the more common hazards encountered decades ago. If your lab still uses older equipment be aware of its shortcomings. Many centrifuges have lockout devices that prevent the lid from being opened while the rotor is moving. Distillation equipment should be purchased only if it has safety features that include high temperature and low liquid volume cutoff switches. Specialized apparatus for electron microscopy should be used only by people specially trained in the inherent risks.

Devices that emit an open flame (such as Bunsen burners or alcohol lamps) must never be used in an environment where flammable solvents are present. Electrical appliances for heating or sterilizing are far safer and more convenient than a gas-fired or alcohol-fueled implement.

Broken glass articles and disposable microtome blades present special risks, particularly if they are contaminated with chemical or biological material. Special 'sharps' containers must be used for the disposal of such items. Microtomes and cryostats are particularly dangerous; be sure to remove blades before cleaning such equipment.

HAZARDS AND HANDLING OF COMMON HISTOLOGICAL CHEMICALS

Extracting succinct information from data sheets and reference books is a time-consuming task that has served as a major impediment to designing proper training programs and labels. The following compilation includes most of the chemicals commonly used in histology laboratories on a routine basis. Permissible exposure values are from OSHA unless otherwise indicated as being taken from ACGIH® (2007) or NIOSH (2005). All IDLH values are from NIOSH and Biological Exposure Indices (BEIs) are from ACGIH®. Many PELs have been revised downward since 2002. The listed hazards are applicable to the quantities normally handled on a laboratory scale and may be inappropriate for bulk quantities. Recommendations for glove material are from Schwope et al (1987). In reality, selection of glove material may have to balance chemical resistance against practicality for the tasks likely to be encountered. Some chemicals have been deemed essentially non-hazardous under normal laboratory conditions of use.

The intent of this section, and indeed this entire chapter, is to provide guidelines for a truly safe workplace for everyone. Most hazardous chemicals can be handled safely with a minimum of effort and equipment, but a few simply cannot. These have been identified clearly and should be eliminated or at least reduced to the smallest quantity possible. Suitable substitutes have been identified. Keep in mind that the toxicology of most chemicals is not well known, and new information, usually damaging, continues to become available. Realize also that the dangerous effects of exposure accumulate subtly, without the cognizance of the victim.

Acetic acid. TWA = 10 ppm; STEL = 15 ppm (ACGIH®); IDLH = 50 ppm. Irritating to respiratory system (target organ effects); concentrated solutions are severe skin and eye irritants, corrosive to most metals and combustible (flash point = 110°F). Avoid skin, eye, and respiratory contact. Use a chemical fume hood, nitrile gloves, goggles, and impermeable apron when dispensing concentrated acid. Do not use rubber (latex) gloves. Always add acid to water, never water to acid, to avoid severe splattering. Do not mix concentrated (glacial) acetic acid with chromic acid, nitric acid or sodium/potassium hydroxide. Dilute (1–10%) aqueous solutions are relatively benign.

Acetone. TWA = 1000 ppm (500 ppm ACGIH®, 250 ppm NIOSH); STEL = 750 ppm; BEI = 50 mg acetone/liter of urine at the end of the shift. Highly flammable (flash point = 4°F) and very volatile. Great risk of fire from heavy vapors traveling along counters or floors to a distant ignition source. Not a serious health hazard under most conditions of use but be aware that acetone can be narcotic in high concentration. Inhalation may cause dizziness, headache, and irritation to respiratory passages. Skin contact can cause excessive drying and dermatitis. Moderately toxic by ingestion. Protect skin with Neoprene gloves.

Aliphatic hydrocarbon clearing agents. TWA = 196 ppm (manufacturer's recommendation). Very low toxicity: non-irritating and non-sensitizing to normal human skin. Combustible (104°F) or flammable (flash point = 74°F). Limit skin exposure to minimize de-fatting effects. Neoprene or nitrile gloves are satisfactory. Recycle by fractional distillation, burn as a fuel supplement or use a licensed waste hauler for disposal.

Aluminum ammonium sulfate, aluminum potassium sulfate, and aluminum sulfate. Not dangerous in laboratory quantities except as eye irritants.

Ammonium hydroxide. TWA = 50 ppm OSHA (25 ppm ACGIH®), STEL = 35 ppm as ammonia gas; IDLH = 300 ppm. Severe irritant to skin, eyes, and respiratory tract. Target organ effects on respiratory system (fibrosis and edema). Wear rubber or nitrile gloves. Store away from acids. Do not mix with formaldehyde as this generates heat and toxic vapors. Spills of 500 ml or more may warrant evacuation of the room.

Aniline. TWA = 5 ppm (2 ppm ACGIH®) with additional exposure likely through the skin; IDLH = 100 ppm. A very dangerous reagent, which should not be used if possible. Moderate skin and severe eye irritant, sensitizer, toxic by skin absorption, carcinogen. Excessive exposure may cause drowsiness, headache, nausea, and blue discoloration of extremities.

Celloidin (stabilized nitrocellulose). Harmless as a health hazard but dangerously flammable as a solid. May deteriorate into a crumbly, potentially explosive substance requiring professional assistance for removal. Solutions usually contain highly flammable ether and alcohol.

Chloroform. CL = 50 ppm; STEL = 2 ppm (NIOSH); IDLH = 500 ppm. Toxic by ingestion and inhalation. Overexposure to vapors can cause disorientation, unconsciousness, and death. Target organ effects on liver, reproductive, fetal, central nervous, blood, and gastrointestinal systems. Carcinogenic. Practical glove materials are not available. This is one of the most dangerous and difficult chemicals in histology because workers in most laboratories simply cannot receive adequate protection from vapors and skin contact. Legitimate disposal may be very challenging. Do not burn. Do not evaporate solvent to the atmosphere. Avoid all use.

Chromic acid (chromium trioxide). TWA = 0.5 mg chromium/cubic meter (ACGIH®); CL = 0.1 (0.05 ACGIH®) mg chromium/cubic meter; IDLH = 15 mg chromium/cubic meter. Highly toxic with target organ effects on kidneys; corrosive to skin and mucous membranes; carcinogenic. Strong oxidizer. Avoid all skin contact. Nitrile, latex, and Neoprene gloves are not suitable except for limited contact; suitable protective material not readily available or practical for lab use. Chromium is a serious environmental toxin. Drain disposal is not a legitimate option for any solution containing chromium, including subsequent processing fluids following fixation or rinses following staining procedures involving chromium. Give this chemical high priority for complete elimination from your lab.

Diaminobenzidine (DAB). Human carcinogen. Solutions pose little health risk under normal conditions of use. Disposal of DAB and subsequent rinse solutions down the drain creates environmental problems. These wastes can be detoxified with acidified potassium permanganate according to the methods of Lunn and Sansone (1990); see Dapson and Dapson (2005: 183–184) for a simplified procedure. Do not use chlorine bleach as the reaction products remain mutagenic (Lunn & Sansone 1991).

Dimethylformamide (DMF). TWA = 10 ppm; additional exposure likely through skin contact; IDLH = 500 ppm. Eye, nose, and skin irritant. May cause nausea. May be a reproductive toxin. Facilitates transport of other harmful materials through skin and mucous membranes. Combustible liquid (flash point = 136°F). Avoid all skin and respiratory contact. Use DMF only in a fume hood with suitable gloves (butyl rubber). Common glove materials do not provide adequate protection. Dispose of DMF only through a licensed waste hauler.

Dioxane (1,4-dioxane). TWA = 100 pm (20 ppm ACGIH®); additional exposure likely through skin contact; CL 1 ppm (NIOSH); IDLH = 500 ppm. Skin and eye irritant: overexposure may cause corneal damage. Readily absorbed through skin and mucous membranes. Delayed target organ effects in central nervous system, liver, and kidneys. Only butyl or Teflon gloves are suitable. Flammable liquid that develops explosive properties (peroxides) after a year. Do not recycle as the risk of creating explosive peroxides increases greatly. Avoid all use of this chemical.

Dyes. There are thousands of dyes and many have been implicated in causing cancers in rats under highly unrealistic circumstances. All should be handled with due caution when in the powder state, but liquids pose little risk except through skin contact and ingestion. Dyes containing the benzidine nucleus are now considered known human carcinogens and must be treated accordingly in both handling and disposal. See the section on carcinogens earlier in this chapter for examples.

Ethanol. TWA = 1000 ppm. Skin and eye irritant. Toxic properties are not likely to be significant under intended conditions of use in a laboratory. Use butyl or nitrile gloves, not rubber or Neoprene. Flammable liquid. Recycle via distillation.

Ether (diethyl ether). TWA = 400 ppm. Mild to moderate skin and eye irritant. Over-exposure to vapors can produce disorientation, unconsciousness, or death. Target organ effects on nervous system following inhalation or skin absorption. Dangerously flammable liquid that forms explosive peroxides. It is extremely volatile and difficult to contain. Do not store in a refrigerator or freezer unless the appliance is rated for an explosive atmosphere. Use a licensed waste hauler. Because of the uncontrollable physical hazard, avoid use of this substance if possible.

Ethidium bromide. May be harmful by ingestion, inhalation, or absorption through the skin. Irritating to skin, eyes, mucous membranes, and upper respiratory tract. Chronic exposure may cause alteration of genetic material. Dispense powder under a fume hood and wear any type of gloves.

Ethylene glycol ethers (ethylene glycol monomethyl or monoethyl ether, Cellosolves). TWA = 200 ppm (5 ppm (ACGIH®); additional exposure likely through skin. Toxic by inhalation, skin contact, and ingestion, with target organ effects involving reproductive, fetal, urinary, and blood systems. Combustible liquids (flash point = 110–120°F). Avoid all use, substituting propylene-based glycol ethers. If substitution is not possible, wear butyl gloves and use a fume hood for all tasks involving these reagents.

Formaldehyde and paraformaldehyde. TWA = 0.75 ppm (0.016 ppm NIOSH), STEL = 2 ppm; CL = 0.3 ppm for 15 minutes ACGIH® (0.1 ppm NIOSH); IDLH = 20 ppm. Severe eye and skin irritant. Sensitizer by skin and respiratory contact (this is the most serious hazard for most laboratory workers). Toxic by ingestion and inhalation. Target organ effects on respiratory system. Carcinogen. Corrosive to most metals. All workers exposed to formaldehyde should be monitored for exposure levels on a periodic basis. Exposure of the skin during grossing is the greatest risk in a well-ventilated lab. Latex surgical gloves are nearly worthless as protective devices. Thin nitrile gloves are better but cannot be used safely for extended periods. Recycle as much waste as possible by distillation and have the remainder taken away by a licensed waste hauler or detoxified by a commercial product. Drain disposal of limited quantities of formaldehyde may be permitted in some communities. Satisfactory substitutes are now available worldwide and offer substantial technical advantages.

Formic acid. TWA = 5 ppm; STEL = 10 ppm (ACGIH®); IDLH = 30 ppm. Mild skin and severe eye irritant. Corrosive to metal. Avoid skin, eye, and respiratory contact; use a chemical fume hood. All common glove materials except latex are suitable. Always add acid to water, never water to acid, to avoid severe splattering.

Glutaraldehyde. CL = 0.2 ppm NIOSH (0.05 ppm ACGIH®). Severe skin and eye irritant; toxic by ingestion. Wear butyl or Neoprene gloves and use a hood.

Glycol methacrylate monomer. No established PELs. Sensitizer. Flammable liquid. Avoid all skin, eye, and respiratory contact. Common glove materials are probably not suitable, based on information concerning other methacrylates. To avoid a dangerous exothermic reaction, do not polymerize large quantities of this monomer. Polymerize small quantities for disposal.

Glyoxal. No established PELs. Glyoxal solutions have no vapor pressure (do not give off fumes) and thus pose no inhalation risk. Irritant to skin and eyes. Ingestion may produce adverse fixative effects on the gastrointestinal tract. Wear nitrile gloves and goggles.

Favorable ecotoxicity profile. An excellent substitute for formaldehyde-based fixatives.

Hydrochloric acid. CL = 5 ppm (2 ppm ACGIH®); IDLH = 50 ppm. Strong irritant to skin, eyes, and respiratory system. Target organ effects via inhalation on respiratory, reproductive, and fetal systems. Corrosive to most metals. Concentrated acid is particularly dangerous because it fumes. Use a fume hood, goggles, apron, and gloves made of any common material except butyl rubber. Always add acid to water, never water to acid, to avoid severe splattering.

Hydrogen peroxide. TWA = 1 ppm; IDLH = 75 ppm. Solutions less than 5% are essentially harmless. Concentrated solutions are very hazardous and should not be used.

Hydroquinone. TWA = 2 mg/cubic meter; CL = 2 mg/cubic meter for 15 minutes (NIOSH). Irritant capable of causing dermatitis and corneal ulceration. Toxic by ingestion and inhalation. May cause dizziness, sense of suffocation, vomiting, headache, cyanosis, delirium, and collapse. Urine may become green or brownish green. Lethal adult dose is 2 grams. All common glove materials are suitable except latex. Avoid contact with sodium hydroxide.

Iodine. CL = 0.1 ppm; IDLH = 2 ppm. Strong irritant and possibly corrosive to eyes, skin, and respiratory system. Dermal sensitizer. Toxic by ingestion and inhalation. Wear nitrile gloves and use a hood when handling iodine crystals. Histological solutions are essentially harmless except if ingested.

Isopentane. TWA = 1000 ppm (600 ppm ACGIH®, 120 ppm NIOSH); CL = 610 ppm for 15 minutes; IDLH = 1500 ppm. Excessive exposure to vapors causes irritation of respiratory tract, cough, mild depression, and irregular heartbeat. Ingestion causes vomiting, swelling of abdomen, headache, and depression. Chilled isopentane may freeze the skin but otherwise is harmless to it. Extremely flammable (flash point = −70°F) and highly volatile, making this a very dangerous chemical. Never store it in a refrigerator or freezer unless the appliance is rated for an explosive atmosphere. Protect hands from frostbite.

Isopropanol. TWA = 400 ppm (200 ppm ACGIH®); STEL = 400 ppm; IDLH = 2000 ppm. Mild skin and moderate eye irritant. Toxic by ingestion. Flammable liquid (flash point = 53°F). Practically harmless except for flammability under normal conditions of use. Recycle by fractional distillation.

Limonene. No PELs established. Generally regarded as safe as a food additive in minute quantities, but a dangerous sensitizer when handled as in histology. May cause respiratory distress if inhaled. Use a hood and gloves (butyl, Neoprene, or nitrile). Clearing agents containing limonene usually cannot be recycled back to the original product because they also include non-volatile antioxidants and diluents.

Mercuric chloride. TWA = 0.01 mg mercury/cubic meter; additional exposure likely through skin contact; IDLH = 10 mg mercury/cubic meter. Severe skin and eye irritant; target organ effects on reproductive, urogenital, respiratory, gastrointestinal, and fetal systems following ingestion and inhalation. Severe environmental hazard. Corrosive to metals. Avoid all use if possible because of the impossibility of preventing environmental contamination. Most processing solutions will become contaminated with mercury if any specimens have been fixed in B-5, Helly's, Zenker's, or similar fixatives. Reagents used to 'de-Zenkerize' sections release mercury. None of these must be allowed to go down the drain. Legitimate disposal of mercury-containing waste is difficult and very expensive, if not impossible, in some areas of the world. Replace mercuric fixatives with zinc formalin or glyoxal solutions.

Mercuric oxide. Strong oxidizer. See mercuric chloride for other information.

Methanol. TWA = 200 ppm; STEL = 250 ppm (ACGIH®); additional exposure likely through the skin; IDLH = 6000 ppm. Moderate skin and eye irritant. Toxic by ingestion and inhalation, with target organ effects on reproductive, fetal, respiratory, gastrointestinal, and nervous systems. May cause blindness or death. Flammable (flash point = 54°F) and rather volatile. Use butyl gloves; other common glove materials are ineffective. Recyclable.

Methenamine. No PELs established. Powder may cause irritation; solutions pose little risk under normal conditions of use.

Methyl methacrylate monomer. TWA = 100 ppm (50 ppm ACGIH®); STEL = 100 ppm (ACGIH®); IDLH = 1000 ppm. Target organ effects from inhalation include fetal, reproductive, and behavioral symptoms. Flammable liquid. May overheat dangerously if large quantities are mixed with polymerizing agents. Keep away from strong acids and bases. Common glove materials are not effective; use Teflon. Work in a hood. Polymerize small quantities for disposal.

Nickel chloride. TWA = 1.0 mg nickel/cubic meter (0.1 mg nickel/cubic meter ACGIH®, 0.015 mg nickel/cubic meter NIOSH); IDLH = 10 mg nickel/cubic meter. Carcinogenic to humans. Toxic by inhalation of dust. Solutions pose little risk to workers but are an environmental problem. Use gloves (any material) and hood when handling the powder. Do not use drain disposal for these solutions or for subsequent rinse fluids.

Nitric acid. TWA = 2 ppm; STEL = 4 ppm ACGIH®, NIOSH; IDLH = 25 ppm. Corrosive to skin, mucous membranes, and most metals. Toxic by inhalation. Target organ effects on reproductive and fetal systems after ingestion. Oxidizer. Concentrated acid is very hazardous. Use Neoprene gloves for extensive use; nitrile, butyl, and latex are not effective except to protect against minor splashes. Wear apron and goggles for handling any quantity. Always add acid to water, never water to acid, to avoid severe splattering. Explosive mixtures may be formed with hydrogen peroxide, diethyl ether, and anion exchange resins.

Nitrogen, liquid. No PELs established. Asphyxiant gas: excessive inhalation may cause dizziness, unconsciousness, or death. Use extreme caution to avoid thermal (cold) burns.

Osmium tetroxide (osmic acid). TWA = 0.0002 ppm osmium; STEL = 0.0006 ppm osmium (ACGIH®); IDLH = 0.1 ppm. Vapors are extremely dangerous. Corrosive to eyes and mucous membranes. Toxic by inhalation with target effects on reproductive, sensory, and respiratory systems. Avoid all contact with vapors. Do not open containers in air. In a hood, score vial and break under water or other solvent. Information on protective glove materials is not available.

Oxalic acid. TWA = 1 mg/cubic meter; STEL = 2 mg/cubic meter; IDLH = 500 mg/cubic meter. Corrosive solid; causes severe burns of the eyes, skin, and mucous membranes. Toxic by inhalation and ingestion, with target organ effects on kidneys and cardiovascular system. Repeated skin contact can cause dermatitis and slow-healing ulcers. Will corrode most metals. Risks are minimal with quantities usually encountered in histology.

Periodic acid. No PELs established. Mild oxidizer. Quantities used in histology pose little physical or health risk.

Phenol. TWA = 5 ppm; additional exposure likely through skin contact; CL = 15.6 ppm for 15 minutes; IDLH = 250 ppm. Toxic by ingestion, inhalation, and skin absorption. Readily absorbed through skin, causing increased heart rate, convulsions, and death. Will burn eyes and skin. Target organ effects on digestive, urinary, and nervous systems. Combustible liquid (flash point = 172°F). Avoid all contact if possible, or use extreme caution. Purchase the smallest quantity possible. Use only butyl rubber gloves and work only under a fume hood. Mixing concentrated formaldehyde and phenol may produce an uncontrollable reaction.

Phosphomolybdic and phosphotungstic acids. TWA = 1 mg/cubic meter ACGIH®; STEL = 3 mg/cubic meter ACGIH®, NIOSH; IDLH = 1000 mg/cubic meter. All PELs are expressed as the quantity of the metal molybdenum or tungsten. Oxidants. These reagents present minor risk under normal conditions of use in histology.

Picric acid. TWA = 0.1 mg/cubic meter; additional exposure likely through skin contact. Toxic by skin absorption. Explosive when dry or when complexed with metal and metallic salts. Do not move bottles containing dry picric acid; get professional help immediately. Do not allow any picric acid solutions, including yellow rinse fluids or processing solvents, to go down the drain, as these may form explosive picrates with metal pipes. Avoid all use if possible, substituting zinc formalin or glyoxal for Bouin's or similar fixatives, and tartrazine for a yellow counterstain. If you must have it, check containers monthly to keep the salts wet. Always wipe jar and cap threads with a damp towel to prevent material from drying within them.

Potassium dichromate. See chromic acid for information on chromium toxicity.

Potassium ferricyanide and potassium ferrocyanide. Low toxicity to humans and the environment in quantities likely to be encountered in histology.

Potassium hydroxide. CL = 2 mg/cubic meter as dust (NIOSH, ACGIH®). Corrosive to eyes and skin. Use care when dissolving solids in water, as the reaction may be violently exothermic and cause splattering.

Potassium permanganate. Skin and eye irritant. Ingestion will cause severe gastrointestinal distress. Strong oxidant: do not mix with ethylene glycol, ethanol, acetic acid, formaldehyde, glycerol, hydrochloric acid, sulfuric acid, hydrogen peroxide, or ammonium hydroxide. Use butyl gloves.

Propidium iodide. Mutagen, irritant, and suspected carcinogen. Material is irritating to mucous membranes and upper respiratory tract. All common glove materials except latex are suitable.

Propylene glycol ethers. TWA = 100 ppm; STEL = 150 ppm (ACGIH®). Used as a less toxic substitute for ethylene-based glycol ethers.

Pyridine. TWA = 5 ppm (1 ppm ACGIH®); IDLH = 1000 ppm. Toxic by ingestion, inhalation, and skin absorption. Overexposure causes nausea, headache, and increased urinary frequency. Target organ effects on liver and kidneys. Irritant to skin and eyes. Highly offensive odor. Flammable liquid (flash point = 68°F). Use only under a fume hood, with butyl gloves. Do not mix with chromic acid.

Silver salts and solutions. TWA = 0.01 mg silver/cubic meter; IDLH = 10 mg silver/cubic meter. Skin and eye irritants. Ingestion will cause violent gastrointestinal discomfort. Little risk to workers when fresh, but some aged solutions become explosive. Serious environmental hazard. Do not discard solutions or rinse fluids down the drain. Silver may be recoverable in special equipment or by metal reclaimers.

Sodium azide. CL = 0.3 mg/cubic meter for the powder (NIOSH, ACGIH®). Poison, very toxic. May be fatal if swallowed or absorbed through the skin. Evolves highly toxic gas when mixed with acids. When used as a preservative in biochemical solutions there is little risk to workers except by ingestion and skin absorption. Forms explosive compounds with metals. Do not discard waste down the drain.

Sodium bisulfite. TWA = 5 mg/cubic meter (NIOSH, ACGIH®). Irritant to skin, eyes, and mucous membranes. Strong reducing agent: keep from oxidants. Dilute solutions generally pose no risk.

Sodium hydroxide. See potassium hydroxide.

Sodium hypochlorite (liquid chlorine bleach). No PELs established. Eye irritant. May be toxic by ingestion unless diluted considerably. Strong oxidant, corrosive to most metals. All common glove materials provide suitable protection. Do not mix bleach with formaldehyde, aminoethylcarbazole (AEC), or diaminobenzidine (DAB).

Sodium iodate. Little risk likely with laboratory quantities. Use to replace mercuric oxide in Harris hematoxylin.

Sodium metabisulfite. See sodium bisulfite.

Sodium phosphate, monobasic and dibasic. Harmless to workers. May pose an environmental problem from eutrophication (over-enrichment of aquatic systems).

Sodium sulfite. See sodium bisulfite.

Sodium thiosulfate. Health risks are minimal under normal conditions of use in histology. Solutions used to 'de-Zenkerize' sections will contain significant amounts of mercury and must not be discarded down the drain.

Sulfuric acid. TWA = 1 mg/cubic meter (0.2 mg/cubic meter ACGIH®); IDLH = 15 mg/cubic meter. Strong irritant to skin, eyes, and respiratory system. Concentrated acid is especially dangerous because it fumes. Target organ effects from inhalation on respiratory, reproductive, and fetal systems. Dilute solutions pose little risk. Corrosive to most materials. Use a fume hood, apron, goggles, and gloves (any common material except butyl). Always add acid to water, never water to acid, to avoid severe splattering.

Tetrahydrofuran (THF). TWA = 200 ppm; STEL = 250 ppm; IDLH = 2000 ppm; BEI = 50 mg THF/liter urine at end of shift. Toxic by ingestion and inhalation. Vapors cause nausea, dizziness, headache, and anesthesia. Liquid can defat the skin. Eye and skin irritant. Flammable liquid. Dangerous fire hazard because of low flash point (5°F) and high evaporation rate. Only Teflon gloves are suitable. Avoid all use, as there is no practical way to protect against skin contact.

Toluene. TWA = 200 ppm (50 ppm ACGIH®); STEL = 150 ppm; IDLH = 500 ppm; BEI = 50 mg o-cresol/liter urine at end of shift. Skin and eye irritant. Toxic by ingestion, inhalation, and skin contact. Target organ effects on fetal, respiratory, and central nervous systems. Repeated exposure produces neurotoxic effects (impaired memory, poor coordination, mood swings, and permanent nerve damage). Flammable (flash point = 40°F). Avoid all use if possible or restrict use severely. No common glove material will provide adequate protection. Substitute one of the short-chain aliphatic hydrocarbon clearing agents except as a diluent in mounting media and for removing coverslips. Exposure may be monitored by measuring the amount of methylhippuric acids in urine (see page 14).

Trichloroethane. TWA = 350 ppm; STEL = 450 ppm. Irritant to skin and eyes. Target organ effects on gastrointestinal and central nervous systems. Noncombustible. No common glove material is suitable. Chlorinated solvents pose severe environmental risks and serious disposal problems. Avoid all use.

Uranyl nitrate. TWA = 0.05 mg uranium/cubic meter; STEL = 0.6 mg/cubic meter ACGIH®; IDLH = 10 mg/cubic meter. Corrosive to tissue and most metals. Highly toxic, with target organ effects on liver, urinary, circulatory, and respiratory systems. Radiation hazard from inhalation of fine particles; most substances block radioactivity, so handling solutions poses little risk. Any type of glove material except latex is satisfactory. Severe environmental toxin. Problems with transportation and disposal have made this chemical very difficult or impossible to obtain. Find alternate stains for most uses and employ immunohistochemistry for equivocal cases. This will eliminate both uranyl nitrate and silver from the lab.

Xylene. TWA = 100 ppm; STEL = 150 ppm; IDLH = 900 ppm; BEI = 1.6 g hippuric acid/g creatinine in urine at end of shift. See toluene for further information.

Zinc chloride. Corrosive to most metals, including stainless steel. All common glove materials except latex are satisfactory. Do not use zinc chloride solutions in tissue processors. Skin and eye irritant. Ingestion can cause intoxication and severe gastrointestinal upset.

Zinc formalin. A solution of zinc sulfate or zinc chloride and formaldehyde. See individual entries for those ingredients.

Zinc sulfate. Eye irritant, but otherwise not hazardous in quantities used in histology.

Acknowledgment

This chapter appeared in the second, third, and fourth editions written by George Coghill. Our acknowledgments are due to him for his earlier contribution.

REFERENCES

American College of Occupational and Environmental Medicine (2003) The use of contact lenses in an industrial environment. Online. Available at: www.acoem.org/guidelines/article.asp?ID=58.

American Conference of Governmental Industrial Hygienists (2007) TLVs® and BEIs®. Cincinnati: ACGIH®.

Centers for Disease Control (1988) Guidelines for protecting the safety and health of health care workers, CDC Publication No. 88–119. Washington, DC: US Government Printing Office.

Centers for Disease Control (1990) Guidelines for preventing the transmission of tuberculosis in health-care settings, with special focus on HIV-related issues. Morbidity and Mortality Weekly Report 39:1–29.

Centers for Disease Control (1994) Guidelines for preventing the transmission of *Mycobacterium tuberculosis* in health-care facilities. Morbidity and Mortality Weekly Report 43:1–132.

Clinical and Laboratory Standards Institute (2002) Clinical laboratory waste management: approved guideline, 2nd edn. Document GP05-A2. Wayne, PA: CLSI.

Clinical and Laboratory Standards Institute (2004) Clinical laboratory safety: approved guideline, 2nd edn. Document GP17-A2. Wayne, PA: CLSI.

Clinical and Laboratory Standards Institute (2005) Protection of laboratory workers from occupationally acquired infections: approved guideline, 3rd edn. Document M29-A3. Wayne, PA: CLSI.

Dapson J.C., Dapson R.W. (2005) Hazardous materials in the histopathology laboratory: regulations, risks, handling and disposal, 4th edn. Battle Creek, MI: Anatech Ltd.

Esswein E.J., Boeniger M.F. (1994) Effect of an ozone-generating air-purifying device on reducing concentrations of formaldehyde in air. Applied Occupational Environmental Hygiene 9:139–146.

Kiernan J.A. (1999) Histological and histochemical methods: theory and practice, 3rd edn. Boston: Butterworth Heinemann.

Lunn G., Sansone E.B. (1990) Destruction of hazardous chemicals in the laboratory. New York: Wiley.

Lunn G., Sansone E.B. (1991) The safe disposal of diaminobenzidine. Applied Occupational and Environmental Hygiene 6:49–53.

Montgomery L. (1995) Health and safety guidelines for the laboratory. Chicago: American Society of Clinical Pathologists.

National Institute for Occupational Safety and Health (2005) NIOSH pocket guide to chemical hazards. DHHS (NIOSH) Publication No. 2005-149.

National Research Council (1989) Prudent practices for the handling and disposal of infectious materials. Washington, DC: National Academy Press.

National Research Council (1995) Prudent practices in the laboratory: handling and disposal. Washington, DC: National Academy Press.

Ontario (Canada) Ministry of Labor (1991) Regulation respecting control of exposure to biological or chemical agents made under the Occupational Health and Safety Act. Toronto: Ontario Government Publications.

Rank J.P. (1999) How can histotechnologists protect themselves from Creutzfeldt–Jakob disease? Laboratory Medicine 30:305–306.

Saunders G.T. (1993) Laboratory fume hoods: a user's manual. Cincinnati, OH: American Conference of Governmental Industrial Hygienists.

Schwope A.D., Costas P.P., Jackson J.O., Stull J.O., Weitzman D.J. (1987) Guidelines for the selection of chemical protective clothing. Cincinnati, OH: American Conference of Governmental Industrial Hygienists.

Stricoff R.S., Walters B.D. (1990) Laboratory health and safety handbook: a guide for the preparation of a chemical hygiene plan. New York: Wiley.

3

Light Microscopy

John D. Bancroft and Alton D. Floyd

LIGHT AND ITS PROPERTIES

Visible light occupies a very narrow portion of the electromagnetic spectrum. The electromagnetic spectrum extends from what we perceive as heat, all the way to gamma rays. Electromagnetic energy is complex, having properties that are both wave-like and particle-like. A discussion of these topics is well beyond the scope of this chapter. Suffice it to say that visible light is that portion of the electromagnetic spectrum that can be detected by the human eye. In physics texts, this range is generally defined as wavelengths of light ranging from approximately 400 nm (deep violet) to 800 nm (far red). Practically speaking, most humans cannot see light of wavelengths much above about 700 nm (deep red).

It is common practice to illustrate the electromagnetic spectrum as a sine wave. This is a convenient representation as the distance from one sine peak to another (Fig. 3.1) represents the wavelength of light. Light that has a single wavelength is monochromatic, that is, a single color. The majority of sources of light provide a complex mixture of light of different wavelengths, and when this mixture approximates the mixture of light that derives from the sun, we perceive this as 'white' light. By definition, white light is a mixture of light that contains some percentage of wavelengths from all of the visible portions of the electromagnetic spectrum. It should be understood that almost all light sources provide a mixture of wavelengths of light (exceptions being devices such as lasers which generate monochromatic, coherent light). One measure of the mixture of light given off by a light source is *color temperature*. In practical terms, the higher the color temperature, the closer the light is to natural daylight derived from the sun. Natural daylight from the sun is generally stated to

have a color temperature of approximately 5200° kelvin. Incandescent light, from tungsten bulbs, has a color temperature of approximately 3200° kelvin. These values will be familiar to those using color film for photography, as film type must be chosen for the illumination source. As a general rule, the higher the color temperature, the more 'blue' or white the light appears to the eye. Lower color temperatures appear more red to yellow, and are regarded as 'warmer' in color.

Shorter wavelengths of light (toward the blue to violet end of the spectrum) have a higher energy content for a given brightness of light. As one goes to even shorter wavelengths of the electromagnetic spectrum, the energy content becomes even higher (X-rays and gamma rays). The energy content of light is generally expressed as an energy level, or amplitude based on the electron volts per photon (the particle representation of light). Visible light has an energy level of approximately one electron volt per photon, and the energy level increases as one moves toward the violet and ultraviolet range of the spectrum. As one approaches the soft X-ray portion of the spectrum, the energy level per photon ranges from 50 to 100 electron volts. It is this increased energy in shorter wavelengths of light (the ultraviolet and blue end of the spectrum) that is exploited to elicit fluorescence in some materials.

Light sources give off light in all directions, and most light sources supply a complex mixture of wavelengths. This mixture of wavelengths is what defines the color temperature of the light source. It should also be noted that the mixture of wavelengths is influenced by the type of material making up the source. Since the majority of light sources used in microscopy are either heated filaments or arcs of molten metal, each source will provide a specific set of wavelengths

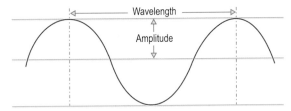

Fig. 3.1 Representation of a light ray showing wavelength and amplitude.

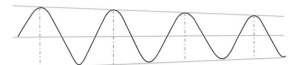

Fig. 3.2 The amplitude (i.e. brightness) diminishes as light gets further from the source because of absorption into the media through which it passes.

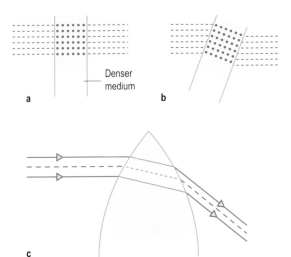

Fig. 3.3 (a) Rays passing from one medium to another, perpendicular to the interface, are slowed down at the same moment. (b) Rays passing at any other angle to the interface are slowed down in the order that they cross the interface and are deviated. (c) Rays passing through a curved lens exhibit both retardation and refraction.

related to the material being heated. This is referred to as the *emission spectrum*. Some sources provide relatively uniform mixtures of wavelengths, although of different amplitudes or intensities, such as tungsten filament lamps and xenon lamps. Others, such as mercury lamps, provide very discrete wavelengths scattered over a broad range, but with distinct gaps of no emission between these peaks.

Although light sources are inherently non-coherent (with the exception of lasers), standard diagrams of optics always draw light rays as straight lines. This is a simplification, and it should be remembered that the actual light consists of every possible angle of light rays from the source, not just the single ray illustrated in the diagram. Another property of light that is important for an understanding of microscope optics is absorption of some of the light by the medium through which the light passes (Fig. 3.2). This is seen as a reduction in the amplitude, or energy level, of the light. The medium through which light passes can also have an effect on the actual speed at which the light passes through the material, and this is referred to as *retardation*.

Retardation and refraction

Media through which light is able to pass will slow down or *retard* the speed of the light in proportion to the density of the medium. The higher the density, the greater the degree of *retardation*. Rays of light entering a sheet of glass at right angles are retarded in speed but their direction is unchanged (Fig. 3.3a). If the light enters the glass at any other angle, a deviation of direction will occur in addition to the retardation and this is called *refraction* (Fig. 3.3b). A curved lens will exhibit both retardation and refraction (Fig. 3.3c), the extent of which is governed by (a) the angle at which the light strikes the lens—the *angle of incidence*, (b) the density of the glass—its *refractive index*, and (c) the curvature of the lens.

The angle to which the rays are deviated within the glass or other transparent medium is called the *angle of refraction* and the ratio of the sine values of the angles of incidence (i) and refraction (r) gives a figure known as the *refractive index* (RI) of the medium (Fig. 3.4a). The greater the RI, the higher the density of the medium. The RI of most transparent substances is known and is of great value in the computation and design of lenses, microscope slides and coverslips, and mounting media. Air has a refractive index of 1.00, water 1.30, and glass a range of values depending on type but averaging 1.5.

As a general rule light passing from one medium into a more dense medium is refracted towards the normal, and when passing into a less dense medium is refracted away from the normal. The angle of incidence may

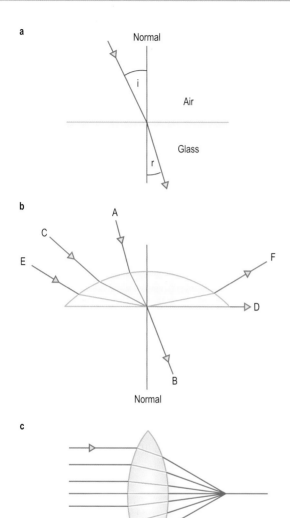

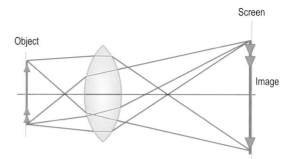

Fig. 3.5 A real image is formed by rays passing through the lens from the object, and can be focused on a screen.

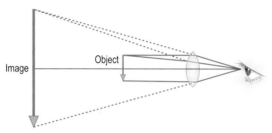

Fig. 3.6 A virtual image is viewed through the lens. It appears to be on the object side of the lens.

Fig. 3.4 (a) Angle of incidence (i) and refraction (r). (b) Ray C–D is lost through the edge of the lens. Ray E–F shows total internal reflection. (c) Parallel rays entering a curved lens are brought to a common focus.

increase to the point where the light emerges parallel to the surface of the lens. Beyond this angle of incidence, *total internal reflection* will occur, and no light will pass through (Fig. 3.4b).

Image formation

Parallel rays of light entering a simple lens are brought together by refraction to a single point, the 'principal focus' or *focal point*, where a clear image will be formed of an object (Fig. 3.4c). The distance between the optical center of the lens and the principal focus is the *focal length*. In addition to the principal focus, a lens also has other pairs of points, one either side of the lens, called *conjugate foci* such that an object placed at one will form a clear image on a screen placed at the other. The conjugate foci vary in position, and as the object is moved nearer the lens the image will be formed further away, at a greater magnification, and inverted. This is the '*real image*' and is that formed by the objective lens of the microscope (Fig. 3.5).

If the object is placed yet nearer the lens, within the principal focus, the image is formed on the same side as the object, is enlarged, the right way up, and cannot be projected onto a screen. This is the '*virtual image*' (Fig. 3.6) and is that formed by the eyepiece of the microscope of the real image projected from the objective. This appears to be at a distance of approximately 25 cm from the eye—around the object stage level. Figure 3.7 illustrates the formation of both images in the upright compound microscope, as is commonly used in histopathology.

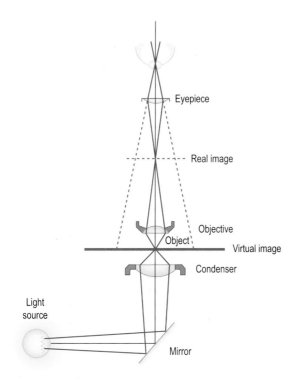

Fig. 3.7 Ray path through the microscope. The eye sees the magnified virtual image of the real image, produced by the objective.

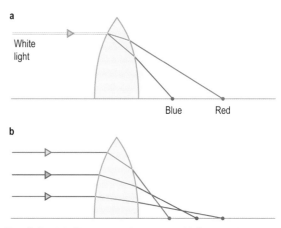

Fig. 3.8 (a) Chromatic aberration. (b) Spherical aberration.

IMAGE QUALITY

White light is composed of all the spectral colors and, on passing through a simple lens, each wavelength will be refracted to a different extent, with blue being brought to a shorter focus than red. This lens defect is *chromatic aberration* (Fig. 3.8a) and results in an unsharp image with colored fringes. It is possible to construct compound lenses of different glass elements to correct this fault. An *achromat* is corrected for two colors, blue and red, producing a secondary spectrum of yellow/green, which in turn can be corrected by adding more lens components—the more expensive *apochromat*.

Microscope objectives of both achromatic and apochromatic types (see p. 38, Fig. 3.11) are usually overcorrected for longitudinal chromatic aberration and must be combined with matched compensating eyepieces to form a good quality image. This restriction on changing lens combinations is overcome by using chromatic aberration-free (CF) optics, which correct for both longitudinal and lateral chromatic aberrations and remove all color fringes, being particularly useful for fluorescence and interference microscopes.

Other distortions in the image may be due to coma, astigmatism, curvature of field, and spherical aberration, and are due to lens shape and quality. *Spherical aberration* is caused when light rays entering a curved lens at its periphery are refracted more than those rays entering the center of the lens and are thus not brought to a common focus (Fig. 3.8b).

These faults are also corrected by making combinations of lens elements of different glass, e.g. fluorite, and of differing shapes.

THE COMPONENTS OF A MICROSCOPE

Light source

Light, of course, is an essential part of the system; at one time sunlight was the usual source. A progression of light sources has developed, from oil lamps to the low-voltage electric lamps of today. These operate via a transformer and can be adjusted to the intensity required. The larger instruments have their light sources built into them. Dispersal of heat, collection of the greatest amount of light, and direction and distance are all carefully calculated by the designer for greatest efficiency. To obtain a more balanced white light approximation, these light sources must often be operated at excessive brightness levels. The excess brightness is reduced to comfortable viewing levels through the use of *neutral density filters*.

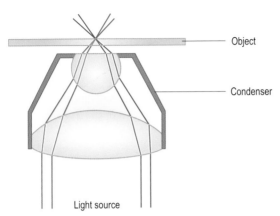

Fig. 3.9 The function of the condenser is to concentrate, or focus, the light rays at the plane of the object.

Condensers

Light from the lamp is directed into the first major optical component, the substage condenser, either directly or by a mirror or prism. The main purpose of the condenser is to focus or concentrate the available light into the plane of the object (Fig. 3.9). Within comfortable limits, the more light at the specimen, the better is the resolution of the image.

Many microscopes have condensers capable of vertical adjustment, in order to allow for varying heights or thickness of slides. Once the correct position of the condenser has been established, there is no reason to move it, as any alteration will change the light intensity and impair the resolution. In most cases condensers are provided with adjustment screws for centering the light path. Checking and, if necessary, adjusting the centration before using the instrument should be a routine procedure for every microscopist. All condensers have an aperture diaphragm with which the diameter of the light beam can be controlled.

Adjustment of this iris diaphragm will alter the size and volume of the cone of light focused on the object. If the diaphragm is closed too much, the image becomes too contrasty and refractile, whereas if the diaphragm is left wide open, the image will suffer from *glare* due to extraneous light interference. In both cases resolution of the image is poor. The correct setting for the diaphragm is when the numerical aperture of the condenser is matched to the numerical aperture of the objective in use (Fig. 3.10) and the necessary adjustment should be made when changing from one objective to another. This is achieved, approximately, by removing the eye-

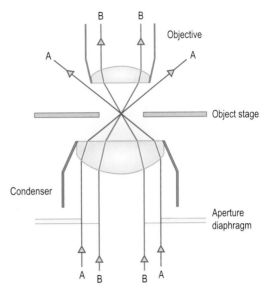

Fig. 3.10 Rays A illustrate the 'glare' position resulting in extraneous light and poor resolution. Rays B indicate the correct setting of the substage iris diaphragm.

piece, viewing the substage iris diaphragm in the back focal plane of the objective, and closing it down to two-thirds of the field of view.

With experience the correct setting can be estimated from the image quality. Under no circumstances should the iris diaphragm be closed to reduce the intensity of the light; use filters or the rheostat of the lamp transformer. Many condensers are fitted with a swing-out top lens. This is turned into the light path when the higher power objectives are in use. It focuses the light into a field more suited to the smaller diameter of the objective front lens. Swing it out of the path with the lower power objectives, or the field of view will only be illuminated at the center. When using apochromatic or fluorite objectives the substage condenser should also be of a suitable quality, such as an aplanatic or a highly corrected achromatic condenser.

Object stage

Above the condenser is the object stage, which is a rigid platform with an aperture through which the light may pass. The stage supports the glass slide bearing the specimen, and should therefore be sturdy and perpendicular to the optical path. In order to hold the slide firmly, and to allow the operator to move it easily and smoothly, a mechanical stage is either attached or built in. This allows controlled movement in two directions, and in most cases Vernier scales are incorporated to enable the operator to return to an exact location in the specimen at a later occasion.

Objectives

The next and most important piece of the microscope's equipment is the objective, the type and quality of the objective having the greatest influence on the performance of the microscope as a whole.

Within the objective there may be lenses and elements from 5 to 15 in number, depending on image ratio, type and quality (Fig. 3.11). The main task of the objective is to collect the maximum amount of light possible from the object, unite it, and form a high quality magnified real image, some distance above. Older microscopes used objectives computed for an optical tube length of 160 mm (DIN standard), or 170 mm (Leitz only), but these fixed tube length systems have now been largely replaced by *infinity corrected objectives* that can greatly extend this tube length (see also page 39) and permit the addition of other devices into the optical path.

Magnifying powers or, more correctly, object-to-image ratios of objectives are from 1:1 to 100:1 in normal biological instruments.

The ability of an objective to resolve detail is indicated by its *numerical aperture* and not by its magnifying power. The numerical aperture or NA is expressed as a value,

and will be found engraved on the body of the objective. The value expresses the product of two factors and can be calculated from the formula:

$$NA = n \times sin\,u$$

where n is the refractive index of the medium between the coverglass over the object and the front lens of the objective, for example air, water, or immersion oil, and u is the angle included between the optical axis of the lens and the outermost ray that can enter the front lens (Fig. 3.12).

In Figure 3.12 the point where the axis meets the specimen is regarded as a light source; rays radiate from this point in all directions. Some will escape to the outside, and some will be reflected back from the surface of the coverglass. Ray r is the outermost ray that can enter the front lens; the angle u between ray r and the axis gives us the *sin* value we require. In theory the greatest possible angle would be if the surface of the front lens coincided with the specimen, giving a value for u of 908. In the above formula, with air (RI = 1.00) as the medium, and a value for u of 908 ($sin\,u \times 1$), the resulting NA = 1.00. Of course this is impossible as there must always be some space between the surfaces and a value of 908 for u is unobtainable. In practice the maximum NA attainable with a dry objective is 0.95. Similar limitations apply to water and oil immersion objectives; theoretical maximum values for NA are 1.30 and 1.50 respectively. In practice values of 1.20 and 1.40 are the highest obtainable.

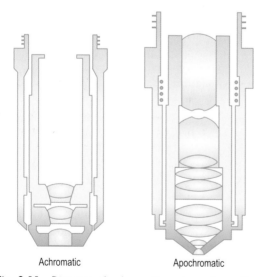

Achromatic   Apochromatic

Fig. 3.11 Diagram of achromatic and apochromatic objectives. Some examples of the latter may have as many as 15 separate lens elements.

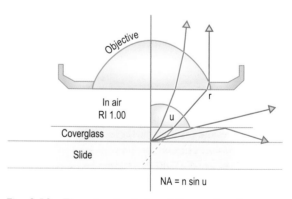

Fig. 3.12 The refractive index of the medium between the coverglass and the surface of the objective's front lens (in this case air, RI = 1.00), and the sine of the angle (u) between the optical axis and the outermost accepted ray (r), gives the numerical aperture (see text).

Resolution does not depend entirely on the NA of a lens but also on the wavelength of light used, with the following relationship:

$$\frac{\lambda \, resolution}{NA} = 0.61\lambda$$

where the resolution is the smallest distance between two dots or lines that can be seen as separate entities, and λ is the wavelength of light.

The *resolving power* of the objective is its ability to resolve the detail that can be measured. In summary, as the NA of an objective increases, the resolving power increases but working distance, flatness of field, and focal length decrease.

Objectives are available in varying quality and types (Fig. 3.11). The *achromatic* is the most widely used for routine purposes; the more highly corrected *apochromats*, often incorporating fluorite glass, are used for more critical work, while *plan-apochromats* (which have a field of view that is almost perfectly flat) are recommended for photomicrography. For cytology screening, flat-field objectives—often plan-achromats—are particularly useful. On modern microscopes, up to six objectives are mounted onto a revolving *nosepiece* to enable rapid change from one to another and, ideally, the focus and field location should require the minimum of adjustment. Such lenses are said to be *par-focal* and *par-central*.

Most objectives are designed for use with a coverglass protecting the object. If so, a value giving the correct coverglass thickness should be found engraved on the objective. Usually this is 0.17 mm. Some objectives, notably apochromats between 40:1 and 63:1, require coverslip thickness to be precise. Some are mounted in a correction mount and can be adjusted to suit the actual thickness of the coverglass used.

Body tube

Above the nosepiece is the body tube. Three main forms are available: monocular, binocular, and the combined photo-binocular. The last sometimes has a prism system allowing 100% of the light to go either to the observation eyepieces, or to the camera located on the vertical part, and sometimes has a beam-splitting prism dividing the light, 20% to the eyes and 80% to the camera. This facilitates continuous observation during photography. Provision is made in binocular tubes for the adjustment of the interpupillary distance, enabling each observer to adjust for the individual facial proportions. Alteration of this interpupillary distance may alter the mechanical tube length, and thus the length of the optical path. This can be corrected either by adjusting the individual eyepiece tubes, or by a compensating mechanism built into the body tube.

Modern design tends towards shortening the physical lengths of the components, and in consequence intermediate optics are sometimes included in the optical path to compensate. These lenses are mounted on a rotating turret and are designated by their magnification factor (see below). Additionally, a tube lens may be incorporated for objectives that are *infinity corrected*, as these objectives form only a virtual image of the object, which must be converted to a real image focused at the lower focal plane of the eyepiece.

Eyepiece

Eyepieces are the final stage in the optical path of the microscope. Their function is to magnify the image formed by the objective within the body tube, and present the eye with a virtual image, apparently in the plane of the object being observed; usually this is an optical distance of 250 mm from the eye.

Early types of eyepiece, like objectives, were subject to aberrations, especially of color. Compensating eyepieces were designed to overcome these problems and can be used with all modern objectives. The eyepiece design of Huyghens (1690) is still available, together with periplanatic (flat-field) and wide-field types, and eyepieces for holding measuring graticules and photographic formats. High focal point eyepieces are designed for spectacle wearers. For older fixed tube length microscopes, manufacturers often placed different amounts of the various corrections in the optical train in either the objective or the eyepiece. Therefore it is important to use eyepieces from the same manufacturer with objectives from that manufacturer. Eyepieces designed for infinity objectives must be used with the newer infinity-corrected systems.

MAGNIFICATION AND ILLUMINATION

Magnification values

Total magnification is the product of the magnification values of the objective and eyepiece, provided the system is standardized to an optical tube length of 160 mm. For variations of the latter the formula is:

$$\frac{\text{Optical tube length}}{\text{Focal length of objective}} \times \text{Magnification of the eyepiece}$$

Where additional tube lenses are included, simply multiply by the designated factor; for example, objective 40×, eyepiece 10×, and tube lens factor 1.25× gives a total magnification of 500×. Choosing the correct eyepiece magnification is important, as a total magnification may be reached without further resolution of the object; this is *empty magnification*. As a guide, total magnification should not exceed 1000 × NA of the objective. Therefore an objective designated 100/1.30 would allow a total magnification of 1300 (1000 × 1.3NA), so eyepieces in excess of 12.5× would serve no useful purpose. For accurate measurements, calibration of the optics with a stage micrometer is necessary.

Illumination

Critical illumination, often used with simple equipment and a separate light source, is when the light source is focused by the substage condenser in the same plane as the object, when the object is in focus (Fig. 3.13). At one time, ribbon filament lamps were available for microscope illumination. Modern filament lamps use a spring-like filament, and the image of the filament causes uneven illumination, which is unacceptable.

For photography and all the specialized forms of microscopy it is best to use *Köhler illumination*, where an image of the light source is focused by the lamp collector or field lens in the focal plane of the substage condenser (on the aperture diaphragm).

The image of the field or lamp diaphragm will now be focused in the object plane and the illumination is even. The image of the light source and the aperture diaphragm will in turn be focused at the back focal plane of the objective and can be examined with the eyepiece removed. Poor resolution will result unless the illumination is centered with respect to the optical axis of the microscope. Figure 3.13 shows the main differences between critical and Köhler systems.

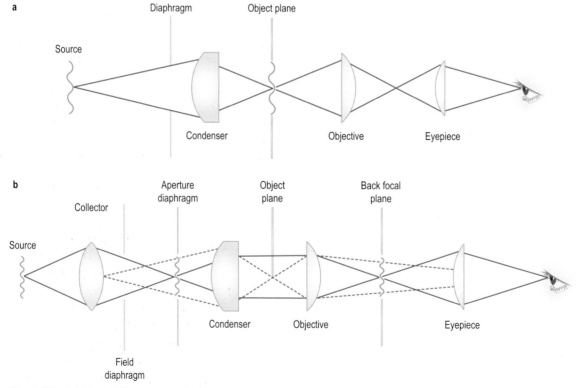

Fig. 3.13   (a) Critical illumination. (b) Köhler illumination.

Dark-field illumination

So far the microscope has been shown as suitable for the examination of stained preparations. Staining aids the formation of images by absorbing part of the light (some of the wavelengths) and producing an image of amplitude differences and color. Occasions arise when it is preferable, or essential, that unstained sections or living cells are examined. Such specimens and their components have refractive indices close to that of the medium in which they are suspended and are thus difficult to see by bright-field techniques, due to their lack of contrast. Dark-field microscopy overcomes these problems by preventing direct light from entering the front of the objective and the only light gathered is that reflected or diffracted by structures within the specimen (Fig. 3.14). This causes the specimen to appear as a bright image on a dark background, the contrast being reversed and increased. Dark-field permits the detection of particles smaller than the optical resolution that would be obtained in bright-field, due to the high contrast of the scattered light.

In the microscope, oblique light is achieved by using a modified or special condenser to form a hollow cone of direct light which will pass through the specimen but outside the objective (Fig. 3.14). Dark-field condensers may be for either dry, low-power objectives, or for oil

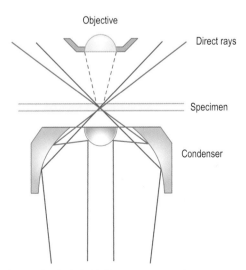

Fig. 3.14 In dark-field illumination no direct rays enter the objective. Only scattered rays from the edges of structures in the specimen form the image (dotted lines).

immersion high-power objectives. Whichever is used, the objective must have a lower numerical aperture than the condenser (in bright-field illumination, optimum efficiency is obtained when the NAs of both objective and condenser are matched). In order to obtain this condition it is sometimes necessary to use objectives with a built-in iris diaphragm or, more simply, by inserting a funnel stop into the objective. Perfect centering of the condenser is essential, and with the oil immersion systems it is necessary to put oil between the condenser and the object slide in addition to the oil between the slide and the objective. As only light diffracted by the specimen will enter the objective, a high-intensity light source is required.

Most bright-field microscopes can be converted for dark-field work by using simple patch stops, made of black paper, placed on top of the condenser lens or suspended in the filter holder. Alternatively the patch stops can be constructed from different colored filters (*Rheinberg illumination*) using a dark color for the center disc and a contrasting lighter color for the periphery. This system reduces the glare of conventional dark field and reveals the specimen in, say, red on a blue background.

Variable intensity dark-field is obtained by making the Rheinberg discs from polarizing filters, the center being oriented at right angles to the periphery. This allows good photomicrography. Dark-field illumination is particularly useful for spirochetes, flagellates, cell suspensions, flow cell techniques, parasites, and autoradiographic grain counting, and was once commonly used in fluorescence microscopy. Thin slides and coverglasses should be used and the preparation must be free of hairs, dirt, and bubbles. Many small structures are more easily visualized by dark-field techniques due to increased contrast, although resolution may be inferior to bright-field microscopy.

PHASE CONTRAST MICROSCOPY

Unstained and living biological specimens have little contrast with their surrounding medium, even though small differences of refractive index (RI) exist in their structures. To see them clearly involves either:

a. closing down the iris diaphragm of the condenser, which reduces its numerical aperture (NA) producing diffraction effects and destroying the resolving power of the objective, *or*

b. using dark-field illumination, which enhances contrast by reversal, but often fails to reveal internal detail.

Phase contrast overcomes these problems by a controlled illumination using the full aperture of the condenser and improving resolution. The higher the RI of a structure, the darker it will appear against a light background, i.e. with more contrast.

Optical principle

If a diffraction grating is examined under the microscope, diffraction spectra are formed in the back focal plane (BFP) of the objective due to interference between the direct and diffracted rays of light. The grating consists of alternate strips of material with slightly different RIs, through which light acquires small phase differences, and these form the image. Unstained cells are similar to diffraction gratings as their contents also differ very slightly in RI.

Two rays of light from the same source, having the same frequency, are said to be coherent, and when recombined will double in amplitude or brightness if they are in phase with each other (*constructive interference*). If however they are out of phase with each other, *destructive interference* will occur.

Figure 3.15a represents the waveform of a light ray. In Figure 3.15b the rays are identical but one is $\frac{1}{4}\lambda$ out of phase with the other and they interfere but with no increase in amplitude. Figure 3.15c shows one ray now $\frac{1}{2}\lambda$ out of phase with the other, and they cancel each other out. This is maximum destructive interference and no light is seen, resulting in maximum contrast. However, if one ray is brighter than the other (increased amplitude) and is still $\frac{1}{2}\lambda$ out of phase (Fig. 3.15d) then the difference in amplitude can be seen, while maintaining maximum interference. This last position is that which occurs in the phase contrast microscope.

The phase contrast microscope

To achieve phase contrast the microscope requires modified objectives and condenser, and relies on the specimen retarding light by between $\frac{1}{8}$ and $\frac{1}{4}\lambda$. An intense light source is required to be set up for Köhler illumination.

The microscope condenser usually carries a series of annular diaphragms made of opaque glass, with a clear narrow ring, to produce a controlled hollow cone of light. Each objective requires a different size of annulus, an image of which is formed by the condenser in the back

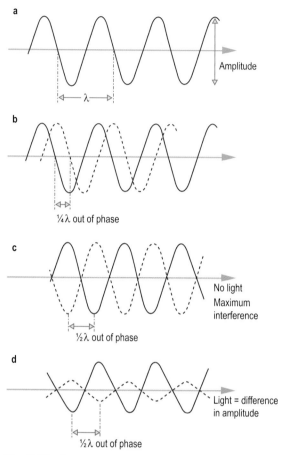

Fig. 3.15　Interference of light rays in phase contrast microscopy.

focal plane (BFP) of the objective as a bright ring of light (Fig. 3.16). The objective is modified by a phase plate which is placed at its BFP (Fig. 3.16). A positive phase plate consists of a clear glass disc with a circular trough etched in it, to half the depth of the disc. The light passing through the trough has a phase difference of $\frac{1}{4}\lambda$ compared to the rest of the plate. The trough also contains a neutral-density light-absorbing material to reduce the brightness of the direct rays, which would otherwise obscure the contrast obtained.

It is essential that the image of the bright annular ring from the condenser is centered and superimposed on the dull trough of the objective phase plate. This is achieved by using either a focusing telescope in place of the eyepiece or a Bertrand lens situated in the body tube of the microscope. Each combination of annulus and objective phase plate will require centration. When the hollow cone of direct light from the annulus enters the

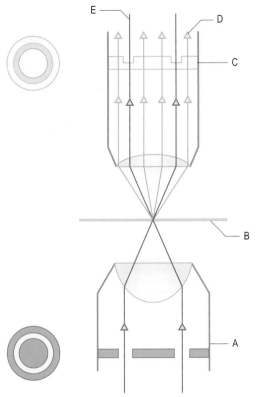

Fig. 3.16   A = annulus at focal plane of condenser;
B = object plane; C = phase plate at BFP of objective;
D = light rays diffracted and retarded by specimen,
total retardation $\frac{1}{2}\lambda$ compared with direct light;
E = direct light rays unaffected by specimen.

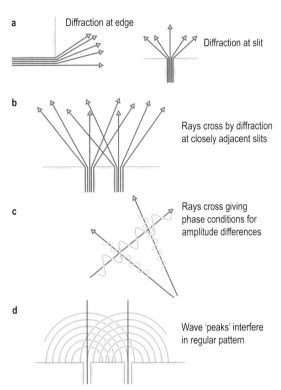

Fig. 3.17   Diffraction and interference of coherent rays
(see text).

specimen, some will pass through unaltered while some rays will be retarded (or diffracted) by approximately $\frac{1}{4}\lambda$. The direct light will mostly pass through the trough in the phase plate while the diffracted rays pass through the thicker clear glass and are further retarded.

The total retardation of the diffracted rays is now $\frac{1}{2}\lambda$ and interference will occur when they are recombined with the direct light. Thus an image of contrast is achieved revealing even small details within unstained cells. This is a quick and efficient way of examining unstained paraffin, resin, and frozen sections, as well as studying living cells and their behavior.

INTERFERENCE MICROSCOPY

In phase contrast microscopy, the specimen retards some light rays with respect to those which pass through the surrounding medium. The resulting interference of these rays provides image contrast but with an artifact called the 'phase halo'. In the interference microscope the retarded rays are entirely separated from the direct or reference rays, allowing improved image contrast, color graduation, and quantitative measurements of phase change (or 'optical path difference'), refractive index, dry mass of cells (optical weighing), and section thickness.

Whenever light passes across the edge of an opaque object the rays close to that edge are diffracted, or bent away from their normal path. If, instead of a single edge, the rays pass through a narrow slit, then the rays at the edge of the beam will fan out on either side to quite wide angles (Fig. 3.17a). Two slits closely side by side form two fans of rays which will cross (Fig. 3.17b) and, if coherent, will observably 'interfere'. If each ray is regarded as a wave it can be seen that phase conditions of increased amplitude and extinction are bound to occur at points where the waves cross and interfere (Figs 3.17c,d). The result of this in the microscope is a series of parallel bands, alternately bright and dark across the field of view. With white light, bands of the spectral colors are seen, because the wavelengths making up white light are diffracted at different angles. With monochromatic light the bands are alternately dark and light, and of a single color. The same effect can be shown if separate beams of coherent light are reunited. This phenomenon is known as 'interference'.

Early microscope models split a light beam into two parts, each traversing two sets of perfectly matched optics, one beam passing through the specimen (measuring beam) and the other acting as a reference beam. The beams were widely separated and suitable only for large specimens and interference fringe measurements. Later models used a double beam system, where the separation is produced by birefringent materials and is close enough to require only one objective (Fig. 3.18a).

If the two paths are equal and in the same phase, the interference bands can be seen running straight and parallel across the field. If into one beam path an object is introduced that causes some shift in the phase, this will be seen as a displacement in the interference bands (Fig. 3.18b). When using monochromatic light, each interval comprising one dark and one light band is one

wavelength wide, and thus the distance in nanometers is known. Displacement of the bands is measured with a micrometer eyepiece and with this information, coupled with either the RI or object thickness, the measurements referred to earlier can be determined.

Two types of double-beam system have been used. One involved focusing the reference beam below the object—the 'double focus' system—and the other involved a lateral displacement of the reference beam called 'shearing', where the separation of the beams is very small. Figures 3.19a,b illustrate this latter system

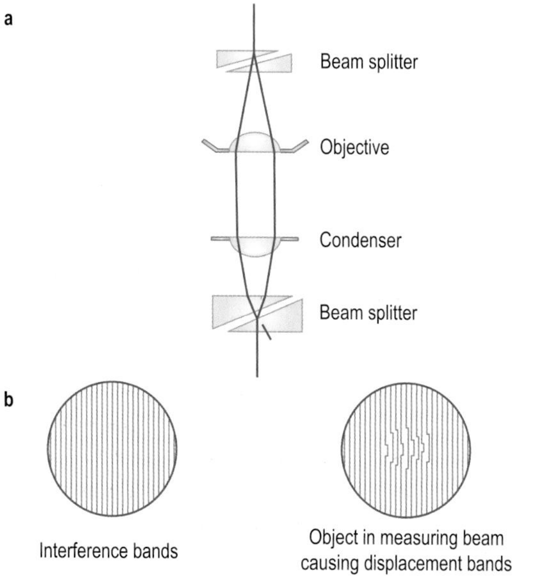

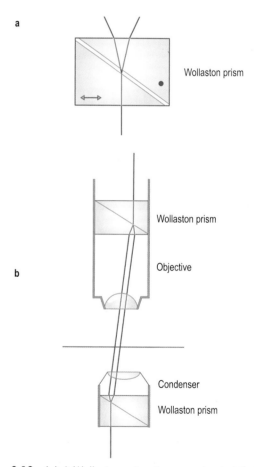

a

Fig. 3.18 (a) Ray path of an interference microscope using a single objective. The beams should be separated sufficiently for one to pass through an empty part of the preparation, otherwise the 'ghost' images formed can cause confusion. (b) Appearance of interference bands in the field of view.

a

Beam splitter

Objective

Condenser

Beam splitter

b

Interference bands

Object in measuring beam causing displacement bands

Fig. 3.19 (a) A Wollaston prism is so constructed that rays passing through the center are in phase. Those passing at other points have a phase difference. The arrows and dot represent the optic axes of the prisms, being at right angles to each other. (b) Ray path in the microscope. Each ray is polarized on separation and they vibrate at right angles to each other, producing interference colors when recombined.

using polarized light and Wollaston prisms. The first birefringent prism in the condenser separates the beams and after passing through the object they are recombined by the second identical prism at the back of the objective. A different pair of prisms is required for each magnification. This produces 'interference contrast' and together with rotation of the polarizers enhances the three-dimensional effect in the image. Nomarski in 1952 modified the Wollaston prisms, so that the lateral separation is less than the resolving power of the microscope, producing excellent 3D colored images from unstained specimens. This system is referred to as *differential interference contrast* or DIC. Additionally only one such prism is required at the objective level for all magnifications. This system permits enhanced visualization of immuno-histochemical preparations.

POLARIZED LIGHT MICROSCOPY

The use of polarized light in microscopy has many useful and diagnostic applications. Numerous crystals, fibrous structures (both natural and artificial), pigments, lipids, proteins, bone, and amyloid deposits exhibit birefringence. Every cellular pathology laboratory should have at least a simple system of polarizing microscopy.

Earlier in this chapter, light was described as a series of pulses of energy radiating away from a source, and shown diagrammatically as a sine curve, with wavelength and amplitude defined. Light can also be described as an electromagnetic vibration, which travels outwards from the source of its propagation, much in the same way as a vibration will travel along a rope when it is jerked in a direction at right angles to its length. The vibrations in the rope will be generated in the direction of the force that caused them, and this is called the *plane of vibration*, or *vibration direction* (Fig. 3.20). Natural light vibrates in many planes or vibration directions, whereas polarized light vibrates in only one plane, as in the rope, and can be produced for microscopy purpose by passing natural light through a polarizer, which is an optical component made from a substance that will allow vibrations of only one vibration direction to pass.

Substances or crystals capable of producing plane-polarized light are called *birefringent*. Light entering a birefringent crystal such as calcite is split into two light paths, each determined by a different refractive index (RI) and each vibrating in one direction only (i.e. polarized) but at right angles to each other (Fig. 3.21). The

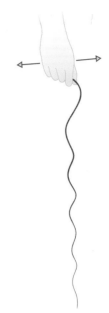

Fig. 3.20   Plane of vibration produced on a rope.

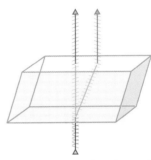

Fig. 3.21   A birefringent crystal such as calcite can split a ray of light into two light paths, each vibrating at right angles to the other.

higher the RI, the greater the retardation of the ray, so that each ray leaves the crystal at a different velocity. The high RI ray is called *slow* and the low RI ray is called *fast*. There is also a phase difference between the rays, so that, if they are recombined, interference occurs and various spectral colors are seen.

Originally, polarizers, made from calcite and known as Nicol prisms after their inventor, were cemented together with Canada balsam in such a way that the *slow* ray was reflected away from the optical path and into the mount of the prism, leaving only the polarized *fast* ray to pass through (Fig. 3.22).

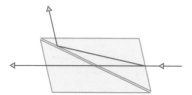

Fig. 3.22 A Nicol prism is constructed so that one part of the ray is allowed to pass whilst the other is directed away from the optical path and is lost.

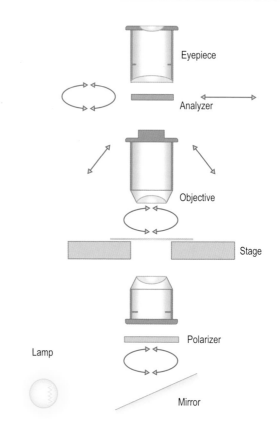

Fig. 3.23 A microscope equipped for polarized light.

There will be a direction within a birefringent crystal along which light may pass unaltered; this is called the optic axis (see Wollaston prism). Substances through which light can pass in any direction and at the same velocity are called *isotropic* and are not able to produce polarized light. A knowledge of RI and polarization measurements identifies many crystalline structures and is particularly useful to the materials scientist but is of limited use to the histologist.

Some substances and crystals can produce plane polarized light by differential absorption and give rise to the phenomenon of *dichroism*. Such crystals suspended in thin plastic films and oriented in one direction have replaced the bulky and expensive Nicol prisms. These thin films totally absorb the slow rays and are *pleochroic* (absorbing all colors equally), and are the most useful in microscopy as they occupy very little space and can be used with any microscope.

The dedicated polarizing microscope uses two polarizers (Fig. 3.23). One, always referred to as the *polarizer*, is placed beneath the substage condenser and held in a rotatable graduated mount, and can be removed from the light path when not required. The other, called the *analyzer*, is placed between the objective and the eyepiece and is also graduated for measurement to be taken. A circular rotating stage would also be present for rotation of the specimen.

The human eye is not able to distinguish any difference between polarized and natural light, although when looking through a single polarizer there is an obvious loss of intensity, some of which is due to the color of the filter, as well as the splitting and absorption of the rays. Polarizing spectacles used as sunglasses make full use of both properties, but their chief advantage is the elimination of glare and reflected light from such surfaces as water and glass, which act as polarizers, much of the reflected light being polarized at right angles to that which penetrates the surface. Looking through

two polarizers, if their vibration directions are parallel, results in a further slight loss of intensity (Fig. 3.24a), due to the increase of the thickness and subsequent absorption, but as one is rotated in relation to the other, intensity decreases to extinction when the vibration directions are crossed, and at right angles (Fig. 3.24b). The first polarizer only allows the passage of rays vibrating in its own vibration direction; if parallel, the second polarizer will allow those rays to pass; if crossed, passage of the rays is blocked.

Two phenomena detected in polarized light are interesting to the histologist; both are briefly discussed in Chapter 10. The first is birefringence. When a birefringent substance is rotated between two polarizers that are crossed, the image appears and disappears alternately at each 45° of rotation. In a complete revolution of 360° the image appears four times, and four times it is extinguished completely. In a thin section of rock composed of many types of crystal this phenomenon is very dramatic, especially when interference colors, due to

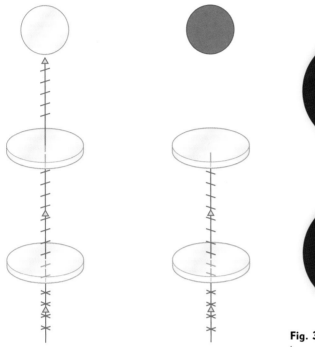

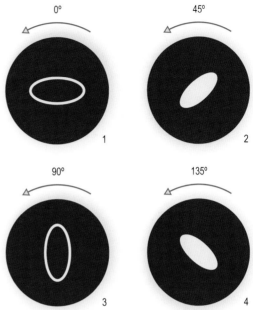

Fig. 3.24 (a) When polarizer and analyzer are parallel, rays vibrating in the parallel plane are able to pass. (b) When polarizer and analyzer are crossed, rays able to pass the polarizer are blocked by the analyzer. The condition when no light reaches the observer is known as *extinction*.

Fig. 3.25 When a birefringent substance is rotated between crossed polarizers, it is visible when it is in the diagonal position (i.e. when it is halfway (45°) between the vibration planes of the polarizers). Extinction occurs when one of its planes of vibration is parallel to either polarizer. Both conditions occur four times in a complete revolution of 360°.

varying thickness of crystal, are present. When one of the planes of vibration of the object is in a parallel plane to the polarizer, only one part ray can develop, and its further passage is blocked by the analyzer in the crossed position. At 45°, however, phase differences between the two rays which can develop are able to combine in the analyzer and form a visible image (Fig. 3.25).

Some birefringent substances are also dichroic, which is the second of the phenomena useful to the histologist. Only the polarizer is used and, if no rotating stage is available, the polarizer itself can be rotated. Changes in intensity and color are seen during rotation. The color changes in a rotation of 90°, and back to its original color in the next 90° (Fig. 3.26). This is due to differential absorption of light, depending upon the vibration direction of the two rays in a birefringent substance. Weak birefringence in biological specimens is enhanced by the addition of dyes or impregnating metals, in an orderly linear alignment, for example along amyloid

fibrils. Although only one polarizer is needed to detect the resulting dichroism, the use of the analyzer in addition can enhance the image.

Sign of birefringence

Reference was made earlier to the separated *slow* and *fast* rays in a birefringent substance. Additionally, if the *slow* ray (higher RI) is parallel to the length of the crystal or fiber, the birefringence is *positive*. If the *slow* ray is perpendicular to the long axis of the structure, the birefringence is *negative*. The *sign of birefringence* is diagnostically useful and is determined by the use of a compensator (birefringent plate of known retardation) either above the specimen or below the polarizer at 45° to the direction of polarized light. Rotate the compensator or the specimen until the *slow* direction of the compensator (indicated by arrows) is parallel to the long axis of the crystal or fiber. The field is now red and if the crystal is *blue* the birefringence is *positive*. If the crystal is *yellow*,

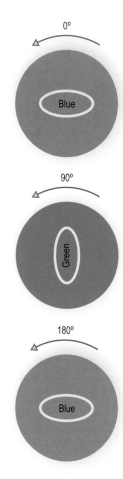

Fig. 3.26   A dichroic substance rotated in polarized light (i.e. using polarizer only). Changes of color and intensity can be seen after rotating 90°. The original color returns after a further 90° rotation. This is due to the differential absorption of the two rays in some birefringent substances, depending on the direction of the polarization.

the *slow* direction of the compensator is parallel to the *fast* direction of the crystal and the birefringence is *negative*. Quartz and collagen exhibit positive birefringence while polaroid discs, calcite, urates, and chromosomes are negative. Simple compensators can be made from mica or layers of sellotape.

FLUORESCENCE MICROSCOPY

Fluorescence is the property of some substances which, when illuminated by light of a certain wavelength, will re-emit the light at a longer wavelength. In fluorescence microscopy, the exciting radiation is usually in the ultraviolet wavelength (ca 360 nm) or blue region (ca 400 nm), although longer wavelengths can be used with some modern dyes.

A substance that possesses a 'fluorophore' will fluoresce naturally. This is known as *primary fluorescence* or *autofluorescence*. Ultraviolet excitation is required for optimum results with substances such as vitamin A, porphyrins, and chlorophyll. Dyes, chemicals, and antibiotics added to tissues produce *secondary fluorescence* of structures and are called 'fluorochromes'. This is the most common use of fluorescence microscopy and the majority of fluorochromes require only blue light excitation.

Induced fluorescence is a term applied to substances such as the catecholamines, which after treatment with formaldehyde vapor are converted to fluorescent quinoline compounds (see Chapter 16).

The applications of fluorescence microscopy are numerous in both qualitative and quantitative systems, and some of these are contained in other chapters of this book, e.g. Chapters 15 and 24.

Transmitted light fluorescence

Light sources

All light sources emit a wide range of wavelengths including the shorter ultraviolet and blue wavelengths which are of interest for fluorescence. Only a few sources are suitable in that they emit sufficient shortwave light for practical use.

Most commonly used are the high-pressure gas lamps such as the mercury vapor and xenon gas lamps. For some wavelength excitation, in the blue and green range for instance, halogen filament lamps produce enough light to be useful. The choice of a suitable source depends upon the type of work to be performed, and for routine observation purposes it is better to use the mercury vapor burners. These operate on alternating current and their starting equipment is not so costly. The xenon burners operate on direct current and require rectifiers to be included with the starter equipment, if they are to be used on normal mains supply. Xenon burners on a DC supply can be stabilized and are therefore suitable for fluorimetry or the measurement of fluorescence emission. The two types of lamp differ in their emission curves, that is to say, the mercury lamps at some wavelengths reach very high amplitudes whereas at other parts of the wavelength range the emission is low. The curve in general has a very spiky profile; xenon on the other hand has a smoother, more continuous curve. Fortunately the peaks in the mercury vapor emission coincide with the excitation wavelengths of some of the more widely used fluorochromes.

Because they contain gas at high pressure, these burners must be handled with great care, and housed in strong, protective lamphouses. Heat and infrared waves are filtered out before the light from the source begins its journey. At one time all fluorescence systems used the transmitted light route common to normal light microscopy; nowadays, the incident route is widely used (see page 50). High-pressure arc lamps also have specific lifetimes, and in the case of mercury lamps this is approximately 200 hours. Operation for longer times than this may result in explosive destruction of the lamp, with release of mercury vapor into the immediate vicinity.

In recent years, a new type of illumination source has been introduced. This is the LED source, which is a type of solid-state, semiconductor device. These LED sources have exceptionally long lifetimes, with little change in light output over that lifetime. Another characteristic is that these sources emit light of a single wavelength, with a very narrow peak width. Therefore these devices are finding increasing use in illuminators for microscopy. While they are not yet as bright as arc lamps, they do not require much optical filtering to select the wavelength of interest, and they do not suffer from the flicker and 'arc wandering' of the high-pressure lamps. They also do not pose the risk of explosion and they have essentially unlimited lifetimes. For different emission wavelengths, different LEDs are required, but there is no need to select a new set of emission filters as the LED itself provides a narrow band of excitation light.

Filters

Preparations for fluorescence may contain other fluorescing material in addition to that in which one is interested. It is necessary therefore to filter out all but the specific excitation wavelength to avoid confusion between the important and the unimportant fluorescence (Fig. 3.27).

A variety of filters are available for this purpose. 'Dyed in the glass' filters, with such designations as UG 1 and BG 12, are broadband filters and transmit a wide range of wavelengths, the width of the range depending upon the composition and thickness of the filter. Besides the

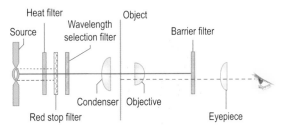

Fig. 3.27 Light path for transmitted fluorescence. Light of all wavelengths passes from the source through a heat-absorbing filter, into a second filter which removes red light, and then through an exciter filter, which allows only the desired wavelength(s) to pass. On passing through the specimen, the objective collects both exciting and fluorescent wavelengths. The former is removed by a barrier filter to protect the eye of the observer.

possibility of non-specific and auto-fluorescence, there may also be materials that are excited at more than one excitation wavelength, so it is better to employ filters of a narrower band transmission that have their transmission peaks closer to the excitation maximum of the fluorochrome, such as FITC. Narrow band filters are often of the 'interference' filter type, and are vacuum-coated layers of metals on a glass support. They have a mirror-like surface, and must be inserted in the beam with the reflective face towards the light source. The better quality filters are carefully selected for their transmission characteristics, and only a few are finally judged suitable. For this reason, they are expensive; careful handling to avoid corrosive fingermarks and scratches is essential. When used with high-intensity light sources, these filters may also degrade with time, and so should be checked with an accurate spectrophotometer at regular intervals.

Barrier or suppression filters are placed before the eyepiece to prevent short wavelength light from damaging the retina of the eye (Fig. 3.27). They must, however, allow the fluorescing color to pass, otherwise a negative result may be obtained. Barrier filters are colorless through yellow to dark orange and of specific wavelength transmission. For example a K.470 filter will block all wavelengths below 470 nm. Colored barrier filters may alter the final color rendering of the fluorescent specimen, and for this reason *all* filters used in the system must be recorded when reporting results.

Condensers for fluorescence microscopy

Bright-field condensers are able to illuminate the object, using all the available energy, but they also direct the rays beyond the object into the objective. Not only is this a potential hazard to the eyes of the observer, but it can set up disturbing autofluorescence in the cement and component layers in the objective itself. In consequence most systems employ a dark-field condenser which does not allow direct light into the objective, and in addition is more certain to give a dark contrasting background to the fluorescence. At the same time it should be realized that only about one-tenth of the available energy is used, limited by the design of the condenser.

Fluorescent light emission is in most cases very poor in relation to the amount of energy absorbed by fluorochromes or fluorophores, with an efficiency ratio somewhere between 1 : 1000 and 1 : 100 at best, and so any system that reduces the available energy to any extent should be well considered before being put into use.

Objectives

Objectives too must be carefully chosen. It has already been noted that autofluorescence is a hazard with bright-field illumination, and for that system only the simpler achromat objectives are practical. With dark-ground illumination the range of objectives is considerably widened, and more elaborate lenses with higher apertures and better 'light gathering power' are possible.

Incident light fluorescence

The trend today in fluorescence techniques is in incident illumination, or lighting from above and through the objective down to the object (Fig. 3.28). A number of advantages are gained over the transmitted route.

In principle the excitation beam, after passing the selection filters, is diverted through the objective on to the preparation where fluorescence is stimulated. This fluorescence travels back to the observer by the normal route (Fig. 3.28a). Dichroic mirrors have been produced to divide and divert the beam. These mirrors have the property of being able to transmit light of some wavelengths and reflect other wavelengths (Fig. 3.28b). By selection of the appropriate mirror, the wavelength desired is reflected to the object; the remainder passes through to be lost. At the same time, visible fluorescent light collected by the objective in the normal way can pass to the eyepiece, and any excitation rays bouncing

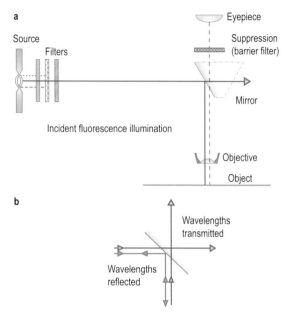

Fig. 3.28   (a) Diagram of incident fluorescence microscope layout. (b) Effect of dichroic mirror.

back (from slide and coverglass) are reflected back along their original path to the source, thus being prevented from reaching the observer. Since the objective in this system also acts as a condenser, the illumination and objective numerical apertures are one and the same, optically correct, and at their most efficient condition. Fluorescence is stimulated on the observer's side of the preparation, and is therefore more brilliant, not being masked by covering material or section thickness.

It is also possible to bring into use any type of objective, including sophisticated phase contrast and interference contrast objectives, for simultaneous transmitted illumination with normal tungsten lighting, and to demonstrate both the fluorescence and the morphology of the preparation. This is useful where normal stains cannot be used for fear of masking any fluorescent reactions.

The use of dichroic mirrors in these systems has made possible much brighter images, since up to 90% of the exciting energy can reach the preparation, and 90% of the resultant visible light can be presented to the eye. In addition, new objectives, of both oil and water immersion types, in low and high powers, have been developed. As immersion objectives they have higher numerical apertures, and can gather more light, avoiding much of the lost stray light reflected from coverslips. The use of low-magnification eyepieces is now more widely accepted, improving fluorescence techniques far beyond anything hitherto possible.

Due to the filters and light sources used in fluorescence microscopy, modern systems generally rely on digital image capture, and these images are monochrome (black and white) images. The highly colored fluorescence images appearing in publications are all the result of pseudocoloring composite images.

The confocal microscope

In fluorescence microscopy using conventional epi-fluorescence microscopes, the fluorochrome present in the field of view will be excited whether in or out of focus. The effect is that the out-of-focus fluorescence will reduce the contrast and resolution of the image. The confocal system uses a pinhole stop to observe the specimen in such a way as to exclude the out-of-focus portion of the image. In essence the axial resolution in the confocal system is greatly improved to $0.35\ \mu m$ (in reflection) with additional small but important gains in lateral resolution, and therefore the method lends itself to optical sectioning. With modern computer technology and Windows®-based software a series of optical sections can be recombined to create a 3D image of a cell or structure even with multiple labeling techniques.

Other techniques

A number of specialized techniques for use in fluorescence microscopy have appeared in recent years. One significant technique is *fluorescence resonance energy transfer* or FRET, in which the excitation of one fluorescence material is captured locally by a second material, causing fluorescence of the second material and quenching of the first. Many new techniques have been developed based on the availability of new fluorescence labels and dyes. Many of these new dyes have unique emission spectra, and may also be much more resistant to fading than earlier dyes. A promising new fluorescence label is quantum dots, a label composed on nanometer-sized particles of semiconductor metals. These quantum dots are excited over a wide range of wavelengths, and emit very narrow band light based on the size of the semiconductor particle. The advantage of quantum dots is that many different dots can be excited by the same excitation light, and each will emit a specific color based on the dot size.

The advent of powerful computers and sophisticated programs has led to many new approaches to microscopy. One specific technique that should be mentioned is *multispectral imaging*, in which a number of images are collected at narrow, specific wavelengths. Such images provide new information as individual components of the image can be easily enhanced, thus improving contrast or perceived resolution of specimen morphology.

USE OF THE MICROSCOPE

The microscope itself should receive some attention before it is used. Is the illumination correctly centered? Is the condenser centered and in its proper position? Make sure that the objectives are firmly screwed home, and that the eyepieces are indeed a pair. If the microscope is set aside exclusively for your personal use, these things will probably be in order, but if the instrument is in communal use then it is likely that someone has altered or readjusted something to suit their own purpose. Above all, make sure that the optical parts are clean, and free from dust. Greasy fingerprints and dust are enemies of the optical glass.

Often when an immersion objective has been used, the next objective is swung into position, straight into the oil drop on the slide. Sometimes oil is left on the front of an immersion lens, forgotten for some time, and by the time it is used it has gathered some dust and formed a translucent film. Use oil only for an oil immersion objective. Keep it away from everything else. After a session with immersion objectives, clean them. Gross amounts of oil can be wiped off with lens tissue. The use of xylene for washing the front lens is now frowned upon. Petroleum spirit is recommended by some manufacturers. Alcohol and acetone should be avoided as they may seep into the mount and dissolve the cements.

The front lenses of some objectives are difficult to clean because of their concave shape, and many people recommend the use of swabs of cotton wool or tissue to remove the dirt from the concavity. A better method is the use of a piece of expanded polystyrene such as is used in the packing of delicate equipment and lamp bulbs. A freshly broken surface will be dust free and contain no hard crystals; it cannot scratch the glass. By pressing the polystyrene on to the lens and rotating it in the optical axis, grease, moisture, and dust are quickly removed, even from the deepest of concave lenses. Do *not* use polystyrene if the lens is wet with xylene, or it will coat the glass with a layer of dissolved plastic and make matters worse.

Eyepieces become coated with a fine film of grease from eyelashes. They should be cleaned from time to time with a lens tissue. Tissues are better than cloths as they are usually stored in small numbers in a protective packet, and are discarded after use. Cloths are liable to lie around on the bench for some time, picking up dust and other harmful substances.

SETTING UP THE MICROSCOPE

Centering the lamp

This is possible on most modern microscopes (some have precentered bulbs and do not require attention), either by a pair of centering screws acting against a spring, or by loosening a screw collar and orienting the lamp holder. A ground glass or plastic disc with concentric circles engraved upon it is placed in the light path, usually on the dust protection glass in the foot of the microscope. By adjusting the lamp condenser, or by moving the lamp in its mounting, the filament can be imaged on the ground-glass disc. It is then a simple matter to adjust the bulb position until the image is in the center.

Adjusting the condenser

If the microscope has an adjustable condenser, this is also a simple procedure. First, select a low-power objective (10×) and, with a suitable preparation on the stage, focus the specimen (to establish the plane of the object). Most condensers have a top lens that is normally swung into the light path for the higher power objectives. This should be turned into position. Open the aperture diaphragm (in the condenser), close the field diaphragm (in the foot of the microscope) to a small aperture. An image of the field diaphragm should now be visible in the field of view. Adjust the height of the condenser until the image of the field diaphragm is sharply focused. This will be the correct position for slides of the same thickness. Now with the adjusting screws move the diaphragm image to the center. If the aperture is opened until it almost reaches the sides of the field of view, the centering

is more accurate. When the correct position has been reached, open the field diaphragm until it just disappears from view. Adjust the aperture (or substage) iris diaphragm, by closing it down, removing an eyepiece and, while looking down the tube, open the diaphragm until it occupies one third of the field of view. Replace the eyepiece. If the image is dark at the edge, open the aperture diaphragm a little more. This has now adjusted the numerical aperture of the condenser to approximately that of the objective in use and achieved the optimum resolution. The illumination should now be correctly adjusted and ready for use.

Inserting the slide

When changing slides it is always good practice to lower the stage before removing the slide. The risk of damaging the objective is reduced. When a new slide is placed on the stage and the objective lowered towards the focal plane, watch from the side and gently lower the objective (or rather, raise the stage) until it is almost in contact, then look into the eyepieces and complete the focusing by bringing the objective away from the preparation. If you look through the eyepiece as the objective approaches the slide, you stand a great chance of missing the focus plane and of crashing the objective through the slide with the possible destruction of both the objective and the specimen.

Make sure that the slide is the right way up. With the higher power objectives, the working distance is very short and you may never find the image.

Additional resources

Many additional resources for microscopy may be found on the internet. A site containing much information as well as graphical examples is the Molecular Expressions Microscopy Primer: http://micro.magnet.fsu.edu/primer.

Acknowledgments

This chapter was originally written by Roger Rose for the first edition; Ralph Nunn, John Bancroft, and Peter Frost have updated it through subsequent editions. Our acknowledgments are due to them for their contributions.

4

Fixation of Tissues

William E. Grizzle, Jerry L. Fredenburgh and Russell B. Myers

INTRODUCTION

The concept of fixation of biological tissues in order to understand biological function and structure has led to the development of many types of fixatives over the last century. The mechanisms and principles by which specific fixatives act to harden and preserve tissues and to prevent the loss of specific molecules fall into broad categories. These include the covalent addition of reactive groups and of cross-links, dehydration, and the effects of acids, salt formation, and heat, along with combinations of these actions. Compound fixatives may function via several of these mechanisms.

Each fixative has advantages and disadvantages. These include molecular loss from 'fixed' tissues, swelling or shrinkage of tissues during the process, variations in the quality of histochemical and immunohistochemical staining, the ability to perform biochemical analysis accurately, and varying capabilities to maintain the structures of cellular organelles. One of the major problems with fixation using formaldehyde has been the loss of antigen immunorecognition due to that type of fixation combined with processing the tissue to paraffin, (Eltoum et al 2001a, 2001b). Similarly the analysis of mRNA and DNA from formalin-fixed, paraffin-embedded tissue has been problematic (Grizzle et al 2001; Jewell et al 2002; Steg et al 2006). All widely used fixatives are selected by compromise; good aspects are balanced against less desirable features. This chapter discusses the basics of fixation, disadvantages and advantages of specific fixatives, and provides some of the formulas for specific fixatives currently used in pathology, histology, and anatomy.

The major objective of fixation in pathology has been to maintain clear and consistent morphological features,

(Eltoum et al 2001a, 2001b; Grizzle et al 2001). The development of specific fixatives usually has been empiric and much of the understanding of the mechanisms of fixation has been based upon information obtained from leather tanning and vaccine production. In order to visualize the microanatomy of tissues, stained sections of tissue must maintain the microscopic relationships among cells, cellular components (e.g. the cytoplasm and nuclei), and extracellular material with little disruption of the organization of the tissue, maintaining the tissue's local chemical composition. Many components of tissues are soluble in aqueous acid or other liquid environments and a reliable view of the microanatomy and microenvironment of these tissues requires that the soluble components are not lost during fixation and tissue processing. Minimizing the loss of cellular components, including proteins, peptides, mRNA, DNA, and lipids, prevents the destruction of macromolecular structures such as cytoplasmic membranes, smooth endoplasmic reticulum, rough endoplasmic reticulum, nuclear membranes, lysosomes, and mitochondria. Each fixative combined with the tissue processing protocol maintains some molecular and macromolecular aspects of the tissue better than other fixative processing combinations. For example, if soluble components are lost from the cytoplasm of cells, the color of the cytoplasm on hematoxylin and eosin (H&E) staining will be reduced or modified and aspects of the appearance of the microanatomy of the tissue, e.g. mitochondria, will be lost or damaged. Similarly, immunohistochemical evaluations of structure and function may be reduced or lost.

Almost any method of fixation induces shrinkage, swelling, and hardening of tissues and color variations in various histochemical stains (Sheehan & Hrapchak 1980; Horobin 1982; Fox et al 1985; Carson 1990;

53

Kiernan 1999; O'Leary & Mason 2004). Various methods of fixation always produce some artifacts in the appearance of tissue on staining; however, for diagnostic pathology it is important that artifacts are consistent.

The fixative acts to 'fix at a point in time' by minimizing the loss or enzymatic destruction of cellular and extracellular molecules, maintaining macromolecular structures and protecting tissues from destruction by microorganisms. This results in one view of a dynamically changing, viable tissue (Grizzle et al 2001). A fixative should also prevent the subsequent breakdown of the tissue or molecular features by enzymatic activity and/or by microorganisms during long-term storage, because diagnostic/therapeutic tissues removed from patients are an important resource which may be re-analyzed in the future.

A fixative not only interacts initially with the tissue in its aqueous environment but subsequently the unreacted fixative and the chemical modifications induced by the fixative continue to react. Fixation interacts with all phases of processing and staining from dehydration to staining of tissue sections using histochemical, enzymatic or immunohistochemical stains (Eltoum et al 2001b; Rait et al 2004). A stained tissue section produced after specific fixation combined with tissue processing produces a compromise in the picture of one or more features representing the original living tissue. To date a universal or ideal fixative has not been identified. Fixatives are therefore selected based on their ability to produce a final product needed to demonstrate a specific feature of a specific tissue (Grizzle et al 2001). In diagnostic pathology, the fixative of choice of most pathologists has been 10% neutral buffered formalin (Grizzle et al 2001).

The most important characteristic of a fixative is to support high quality and consistent staining with hematoxylin and eosin (H&E) both initially and after storage of the paraffin blocks for at least a decade. The fixative must have the ability to prevent short- and long-term destruction of the micro-architecture of the tissue by stopping the activity of catabolic enzymes and hence autolysis, minimizing the diffusion of soluble molecules from their original locations. Another important characteristics of a good fixative is the destruction of infectious agents, which helps maintain tissue and cellular integrity. It is important to have good toxicological and flammability profiles that permit the safe use of the fixative (Grizzle & Fredenburgh 2005). The advent of new biological methods, increased understanding of the human genome, and the need to evaluate rapidly the biology of disease processes, means that fixatives should also permit the recovery of macromolecules including proteins, mRNA, and DNA without extensive biochemical modifications from fixed and paraffin-embedded tissues.

Other important characteristics of an ideal fixative include being useful for a wide variety of tissues including fatty, lymphoid, and neural tissues. It should preserve small and large specimens and support histochemical, immunohistochemical, in situ hybridization and other specialized procedures. It should penetrate and fix tissues rapidly, have a shelf life of at least one year, and be compatible with automated tissue processors. The fixative should be readily disposable or recyclable and support long-term tissue storage giving excellent microtomy of paraffin blocks, and should be cost effective (Dapson 1993).

Hopwood in the last edition of this text, Horobin (1982), Eltoum et al (2001a, 2001b), and Rait et al (2004, 2005) have reviewed theoretical aspects of fixation.

TYPES OF FIXATION

Fixation of tissues can be accomplished by physical and/or chemical methods. Physical methods such as heating, microwaving, and freeze-drying are independent processes and not used commonly in the routine practice of medical or veterinary pathology, anatomy, and histology except for the use of dry heat fixation of microorganisms prior to Gram staining. Most methods of fixation used in processing of tissue for histopathological diagnoses rely on chemical fixation carried out by liquid fixatives. The requirement of fixatives used for diagnostic pathology is reproducibility over time of the microscopic appearances of tissues on H&E staining. Methods of fixation used in research protocols may be more varied including fixation using vapors and fixation of whole animals by perfusing the animal's vascular system with a fixative (Eltoum et al 2001a, 2001b).

Several chemicals or combinations of chemicals can act as good fixatives and accomplish many of the stated goals of fixation. Some fixatives add covalent reactive groups which may induce cross-links between proteins, individual protein moieties, within nucleic acids, and between nucleic acids and proteins (Horobin 1982; Eltoum et al 2001a, 2001b; Rait et al 2004, 2005). The best examples of such 'cross-linking fixatives' are formaldehyde and glutaraldehyde. Another approach to fixation is the use of agents that remove free water from tissues and hence precipitate and coagulate proteins; examples of these dehydrants include ethanol, methanol, and acetone. Other fixatives such as acetic acid, trichloroacetic acid, mercuric chloride, and zinc acetate rely on denaturing proteins and nucleic acids through changes in pH or via salt formation. Some fixatives are mixtures of reagents and are referred to as compound fixatives, e.g. alcoholic formalin acts to fix tissues by adding covalent hydroxymethyl groups and cross-links as well as by coagulation and dehydration.

PHYSICAL METHODS OF FIXATION

Heat fixation

The simplest form of fixation is heat. Boiling or poaching an egg precipitates the proteins and, on cutting, the yolk and egg white can be identified separately. Each component is less soluble in water after heat fixation than the same component of a fresh egg. Picking up a frozen section on a warm microscope slide both attaches the section to the slide and partially fixes it by heat and dehydration. Even though adequate morphology could be obtained by boiling tissue in normal saline, in histopathology, heat is primarily used to accelerate other forms of fixation as well as the steps of tissue processing.

Microwave fixation

Microwave heating speeds fixation and can reduce times for fixation of some gross specimens and histological sections from more than 12 hours to less than 20 minutes (Anonymous 2001; Kok & Boon 2003; Leong 2005). Microwaving tissue in formalin results in the production of large amounts of dangerous vapors so in the absence of a hood for fixation, or a microwave processing system designed to handle these vapors, this may cause safety problems. Recently, commercial glyoxal-based fixatives which do not form vapors when heated at 55°C have been introduced as an efficient method of microwave fixation.

Freeze-drying and freeze substitution

Freeze-drying is a useful technique in studying soluble materials and small molecules; tissues are cut into thin sections, immersed in liquid nitrogen, and the water is removed in a vacuum chamber at −40°C. The tissue can be post-fixed with formaldehyde vapor. In substitution, specimens are immersed in cold (−40°C) fixatives, such as acetone or alcohol, which slowly remove water through dissolution of ice crystals, and the proteins are not denatured; bringing the temperature gradually to 4°C will complete the fixation process (Pearse 1980). The advantages and drawbacks of these two techniques are discussed in more detail in Chapter 7.

CHEMICAL FIXATION

Chemical fixation utilizes organic or non-organic solutions to maintain adequate morphological preservation. Chemical fixatives can be considered as members of three major categories: coagulant, cross-linking, and compound fixatives.

Coagulant fixatives

Both organic and non-organic solutions may coagulate proteins making them insoluble. Cellular architecture is maintained primarily by lipoproteins and by fibrous proteins such as collagen; coagulating such proteins maintains tissue histomorphology at the light microscopic level. Unfortunately, because coagulant fixatives result in cytoplasmic flocculation as well as poor preservation of mitochondria and secretory granules, such fixatives are not useful in ultrastructural analysis.

Dehydrant coagulant fixatives

The most commonly used coagulating fixatives are alcohols (e.g. ethanol, methanol) and acetone. Methanol is closer to the structure of water than ethanol. Ethanol therefore competes more strongly than methanol in the interaction with hydrophobic areas of molecules; thus, coagulant fixation begins at a concentration of 50–60% for ethanol but requires a concentration of 80% or more for methanol (Lillie & Fullmer 1976). Removal and replacement of free water from tissue by any of these agents has several potential effects on proteins within the tissue. Water molecules surround hydrophobic areas of proteins and, by repulsion, force hydrophobic chemical groups into closer contact with each other and hence stabilize hydrophobic bonding. By removing water, the opposite principle weakens hydrophobic bonding. Similarly, molecules of water participate in hydrogen bonding in hydrophilic areas of proteins, so removal of water destabilizes this hydrogen bonding. Together, these changes act to disrupt the tertiary structure of proteins. In addition, with the water removed, the structure of the protein may become partially reversed, with hydrophobic groups moving to the outside surface of the protein. Once the tertiary structure of a soluble protein has been modified, the rate of reversal to a more ordered soluble state is slow and most proteins after coagulation remain insoluble even if returned to an aqueous environment.

Disruption of the tertiary structure of proteins, i.e. denaturation, changes their physical properties, potentially causing insolubility and loss of function. Even though most proteins become less soluble in organic environments, up to 13% of protein may be lost, e.g. with acetone fixation (Horobin 1982). Factors that influence the solubility of macromolecules include:

1   Temperature, pressure, and pH.
2   Ionic strength of the solute.
3   The salting-in constant, which expresses the contribution of the electrostatic interactions.
4   The salting-in and salting-out interactions.
5   The type(s) of denaturing reagent(s) (Herskovits et al 1970; Horobin 1982; Papanikolau & Kokkinidis 1997; Bhakuni 1998).

Alcohol denatures protein differently depending on the choice and concentration of alcohol, the presence of organic and non-organic substances, and the pH and temperature of fixation. For example, ethanol denatures proteins > phenols > water and polyhydric alcohols > monocarboxylic acids > dicarboxylic acids (Bhakuni 1998).

Other types of coagulant fixative

Acidic coagulants such as picric acid and trichloroacetic acid change the charges on the ionizable side chains, e.g. $(—NH_2 \rightarrow NH_3^+)$ and $(COO \rightarrow COOH)$, of proteins and disrupt electrostatic and hydrogen bonding. These acids also may insert a lipophilic anion into a hydrophilic region and hence disrupt tertiary structures of proteins (Horobin 1982). Acetic acid coagulates nucleic acids but does not fix or precipitate proteins; it is therefore added to other fixatives to prevent the loss of nucleic acids. Trichloroacetic acid (Cl_3CCOOH) can penetrate hydrophobic domains of proteins and the anion produced $(—C—COO^-)$ reacts with charged amine groups. This interaction precipitates proteins and extracts nucleic

acids. Picric acid or trinitrophenol slightly dissolves in water to form a weak acid solution (pH 2.0). In reactions, it forms salts with basic groups of proteins, causing the proteins to coagulate. If the solution is neutralized, precipitated protein may redissolve. Picric acid fixation produces brighter staining, but the low pH solutions of picric acid may cause hydrolysis and loss of nucleic acids

Non-coagulant cross-linking fixatives

Several chemicals were selected as fixatives secondary to their potential actions of forming cross-links within and between proteins and nucleic acids as well as between nucleic acids and proteins. Cross-linking may not be a major mechanism at current short times of fixation, and therefore 'covalent additive fixatives' may be a better name for this group. Examples include formaldehyde, glutaraldehyde, and other aldehydes, e.g. chloral hydrate and glyoxal, metal salts such as mercuric and zinc chloride, and other metallic compounds such as osmium tetroxide. Aldehyde groups (i.e. $-C\begin{smallmatrix}H\\\\O\end{smallmatrix}$) are chemically and biologically reactive and are responsible for many histochemical reactions, e.g. free aldehyde groups may be responsible for argentaffin reactions (Papanikolau & Kokkinidis 1997).

Formaldehyde fixation

Formaldehyde in its 10% neutral buffered form (NBF) is the most common fixative used in diagnostic pathology. Pure formaldehyde is a vapor that when completely dissolved in water forms a solution containing 37–40% formaldehyde; this aqueous solution is known as 'formalin'. The usual '10% formalin' used in fixation of tissues is a 10% solution of formalin, i.e. it contains about 4% weight to volume of formaldehyde. The reactions of formaldehyde with macromolecules are numerous and complex. Fraenkel-Conrat and his colleagues, using simple chemistry, meticulously identified most of the reactions of formaldehyde with amino acids and proteins (French & Edsall 1945; Fraenkel-Conrat & Olcott 1948a, 1948b; Fraenkel-Conrat & Mecham 1949). In an aqueous solution formaldehyde forms methylene hydrate, a methylene glycol as the first step in fixation (Singer 1962).

$$H_2C{=}O + H_2O \rightarrow HOCH_2OH$$

Methylene hydrate reacts with several side chains of proteins to form reactive hydroxymethyl side groups

($-CH_2-OH$). With relatively short times of fixation with 10% neutral buffered formalin (hours to days), the formation of hydroxymethyl side chains is probably the primary and characteristic reaction. The formation of actual cross-links may be relatively rare at the currently used relatively short times of fixation.

Formaldehyde also reacts with nuclear proteins and nucleic acids (Kok & Boon 2003; Leong 2005). It penetrates between nucleic acids and proteins and stabilizes the nucleic acid–protein shell, and it also modifies nucleotides by reacting with free amino groups of nucleotides as in proteins. In naked and free DNA, the cross-linking reactions are believed to start at adenine–thymidine (AT)-rich regions and cross-linking increases with increasing temperature (McGhee & von Hippel 1975a, 1975b, 1977a, 1977b). Formaldehyde reacts with $C=C$ and $-SH$ bonds in unsaturated lipids but does not interact with carbohydrates (French & Edsall 1945; Hayat 1981).

The side chains of peptides or proteins that are most reactive with methylene hydrate and hence have the highest affinity for formaldehyde include lysine, cysteine, histidine, arginine, tyrosine, and reactive hydroxyl groups of serine and threonine (see Table 4.1) (Means & Feeney 1995).

Table 4.1 Side chains of peptides or proteins and their bound hydroxymethyl group

Side chains of peptides/proteins:	Bound hydroxymethyl group:
Arginine side chain	
N-terminal amino acids such as lysine	
The thiol (sulfydryl) group of cysteine	

Gustavson (1956) reported that one of the most important cross-links in 'over-fixation', i.e. in tanning, is that between lysine and the amide group of the protein backbone. Due to the shorter times of fixation of current diagnostic pathology and biological applications, cross-linking reactions with the protein backbone are unlikely (French & Edsall 1945; Fraenkel-Conrat et al 1945, 1947; Fraenkel-Conrat & Olcott 1948a, 1948b; Fraenkel-Conrat & Mecham 1949; Gustavson 1956).

Reversibility of formaldehyde— macromolecular reactions

The reactive groups may combine with hydrogen groups or with each other forming methylene bridges. If the formalin is washed away, reactive groups may rapidly return to their original states, but any bridging that has already occurred may remain.

$$—(CH_2)_4—NH—CH_2OH\ +\ H_2O \xrightarrow[\text{washing}]{\text{Extensive}}$$

Lysine hydroxymethyl

$$—(CH_2)_4—NH_2\ +\ \begin{array}{c}\text{Formaldehyde is}\\ \text{washed away}\end{array}$$

Lysine $(HO—CH_2—OH)$

Washing for 24 hours removes 50% of reactive groups and 4 weeks of washing removes up to 90% (Helander 1994). This suggests that actual cross-linking is a relatively slow process, so, in the rapid fixation used in diagnostic pathology, most 'fixation' with formaldehyde prior to tissue processing stops with the formation of reactive hydroxymethyl groups.

On long-term storage in formalin, the reactive groups may be oxidized to the more stable groups (e.g. acids —NH—COOH) which are not easily removed by washing in water or alcohol. Thus, following fixation, returning the specimen to water or alcohol reduces further fixation of the specimen because the reactive groups induced by the initial reaction with formalin may reverse and may be removed. Although it was initially thought that cross-linking was most important for fixation of tissue for biological uses (based on the limited number of cross-links over short periods of fixation), it is likely that formation of these hydroxymethyl groups actually denatures macromolecules and renders them insoluble. As these washing experiments have not been reproduced, the actual mechanisms and their importance to fixation from formaldehyde are uncertain. As well as simple washing under running water, over-fixation of tissue may be partially corrected by soaking the tissue in concentrated ammonia plus 20% chloral hydrate (Lhotka & Ferreira 1949). Fraenkel-Conrat and his colleagues frequently noted that the addition and condensation reactions of formaldehyde with amino acids and proteins were unstable and could be reversed easily by dilution or dialysis (Fraenkel-Conrat et al 1945, 1947; Fraenkel-Conrat & Olcott 1948a, 1948b; Fraenkel-Conrat & Mecham 1949).

The principal type of cross-link in short-term fixation is thought to be between the hydroxymethyl group on lysine side chains and arginine (through secondary amino groups), aspargine, glutamine (through secondary amide groups), or tyrosine (through hydroxyl group) (Tome et al 1990). For example, a lysine methyl hydroxyl amine group can react with an arginine group to form a lysine—CH_2—arginine cross-link; similarly a tyrosine methyl hydroxyl amine group can bind with a cysteine group to form a tyrosine—CH_2—cysteine cross-link. Each of these cross-links between macromolecules has varying degrees of stability, which can be modified by the temperature, pH, and type of environment surrounding and permeating the tissue (Eltoum et al 2001b). The time to saturation of human and animal tissues with active groups by formalin is about 24 hours, but cross-linking may continue for many weeks (Helander 1994).

When formaldehyde dissolves in an unbuffered aqueous solution, it forms an acid solution (pH 5.0–5.5) because a 5–10% component of commercially available formaldehyde is formic acid. Acid formalin may react more slowly with proteins than NBF because amine groups become charged (e.g. —N^+H_3). In solution, this requires a much lower pH than 5.5; however, the requirement for a lower pH to produce —N^+H_3 groups may not be equivalent to that required in peptides. Acid formalin also preserves immunorecognition much better than NBF (Arnold et al 1996). The disadvantage of using acid formalin for fixation is the formation of a brown–black pigment with degraded hemoglobulin. This heme-related pigment which forms in tissue is usually not a great problem unless patients have a blood abnormality (e.g. sickle cell disease, malaria).

Formaldehyde primarily preserves peptide–protein bonds and the general structure of cellular organelles; it can interact with nucleic acids but has little effect on carbohydrates and preserves lipids if the solutions contain calcium (Bayliss High & Lake 1996).

Glutaraldehyde fixation

Less is known about glutaraldehyde's biological reactions and effects compared to formaldehyde, as it has not been used as widely in biological applications. Glutaraldehyde is a bifunctional aldehyde that probably combines with the same reactive groups as does formaldehyde. In aqueous solutions glutaraldehyde polymerizes forming cyclic and oligomeric compounds (Hopwood 1985) and is also oxidized to glutaric acid. To aid in stability, it requires storage at 4°C and pH around 5 (Hopwood 1969).

$$\underset{O}{\overset{H}{\diagdown}}C-(CH_2)_3-C\underset{H}{\overset{O}{\diagup}}$$

Unlike formaldehyde, glutaraldehyde has an aldehyde group on both ends of the molecule. With each reaction, an unreacted aldehyde group may be introduced into the protein and these aldehyde groups can act to further cross-link the protein. Alternatively, the aldehyde groups may react with the wide range of histochemical reagents including antibodies, enzymes, or proteins. The reaction of glutaraldehyde with an isolated protein such as bovine serum albumin is maximal at pH 6–7, is faster (Habeeb 1966), and results in more cross-linking than formaldehyde (Habeeb 1966; Hopwood 1969). Cross-linking is irreversible and withstands acids, urea, semicarbazide, and heat (Hayat 1981). Like formaldehyde, reactions with lysine are the most important in cross-linking.

Extensive cross-linking by glutaraldehyde results in better preservation of ultrastructure, but this method of fixation negatively affects immunohistochemical methods and slows the penetration by the fixative. Thus, any tissue fixed in glutaraldehyde must be small (0.5 mm maximum) and, unless the aldehyde groups are blocked, increased background staining will result if several histochemical methods are used (Grizzle 1996a). Glutaraldehyde does not react with carbohydrates or lipids unless they contain free amino groups as are found in some phospholipids (Hayat 1981). At room temperature glutaraldehyde does not cross-link nucleic acids in the absence of nucleohistones but it may react with nucleic acids at or above 45°C (Hayat 1981).

Osmium tetroxide fixation

Osmium tetroxide (OsO_4), a toxic solid, is soluble in water as well as non-polar solvents and can react with hydrophilic and hydrophobic sites including the side chains of proteins, potentially causing cross-linking (Hopwood et al 1990). The reactive sites include sulfydryl, disulfide, phenolic, hydroxyl, carboxyl, amide, and heterocyclic groups. Osmium tetroxide is known to interact with nucleic acids, specifically with the 2,3-glycol moiety in terminal ribose groups and the 5,6 double bonds of thymine residues. Nuclei fixed in OsO_4 and dehydrated with alcohol may show prominent clumping of DNA. This unacceptable artifact can be prevented by pre-fixation with potassium permanganate ($KMnO_4$), post-fixation with uranyl acetate, or by adding calcium ions and tryptophan during fixation (Hayat 1981). The reaction of OsO_4 with carbohydrates is uncertain (Hayat 1981). Large proportions of proteins and carbohydrates are lost from tissues during osmium fixation; some of this may be due to the superficial limited penetration of OsO_4 (i.e. <1 mm) into tissues or its slow rates of reaction. In electron microscopy, this loss is minimized by initial fixation of tissue in glutaraldehyde (see Chapter 30). The most characterized reaction with osmium is its reaction with unsaturated bonds within lipids and phospholipids:

$$\begin{array}{l} H-\overset{|}{C} \\ \parallel \\ H-\overset{|}{C} \end{array} + OsO_4 \longrightarrow \begin{array}{l} H-\overset{|}{C}-O \\ \quad\quad\quad\diagdown Os \diagup\diagdown O \\ H-\overset{|}{C}-O \diagup \quad \diagdown O \end{array}$$

In this reaction, osmium in its +8 valence state converts to a +6 valence state, which is colorless. If two unsaturated bonds are close together there may be cross-linking by osmium tetroxide:

$$\begin{array}{ll} H-\overset{|}{C} & O\diagdown \quad \diagup O \\ \parallel & \quad Os \quad + \\ H-\overset{|}{C} & O\diagup \quad \diagdown O \end{array} + \begin{array}{l} \overset{|}{C}-H \\ \parallel \\ \overset{|}{C}-H \end{array} \longrightarrow$$

$$\begin{array}{ll} H\overset{|}{C}-O\diagdown & \diagup O-\overset{|}{C}-H \\ \quad\quad\quad Os \\ H\overset{|}{C}-O\diagup & \diagdown O-\overset{|}{C}-H \end{array}$$

Although the complex is colorless at this point, the typical black staining of membranes expected from fixation with osmium requires the production of osmium dioxide ($OsO_2 \cdot 2H_2O$). Osmium dioxide is black, electron dense, and insoluble in aqueous solution; it precipitates as the above unstable compounds break down and becomes deposited on cellular membranes. The breakdown of osmium +6 valence complexes to osmium dioxide (+4 valence state) is facilitated by a reaction with solutions of ethanol:

$$-\overset{|}{\underset{|}{C}}-O \diagdown \hspace{-0.3em} \underset{O \diagup}{\overset{\diagup O}{Os}} \diagdown \hspace{-0.3em} \diagup O \; + \; C_2H_5OH \; + 2H_2O \longrightarrow$$

$$-\overset{|}{\underset{|}{C}}-OH$$
$$-\overset{|}{\underset{|}{C}}-OH \quad + \; OsO_2 \cdot 2H_2O\downarrow + \; CH_3CHO$$

In addition to its use as a secondary fixative for electron microscopic examinations, osmium tetroxide can also be used to stain lipids in frozen sections. Osmium tetroxide fixation causes tissue swelling which is reversed during dehydration steps. Swelling can also be minimized by adding calcium or sodium chloride to osmium-containing fixatives (Hayat 1981).

Cross-linking fixatives for electron microscopy

Cell organelles such as cytoplasmic and nuclear membranes, mitochondria, membrane-bound secretory granules, and smooth and rough endoplasmic reticulum need to be preserved carefully for electron microscopy. The lipids in these structures are extracted by many fixatives with dehydrants (e.g. alcohols) and therefore for ultrastructural examination it is important to use a fixative that does not solubilize lipids. The preferred fixatives are a strong cross-linking fixative such as glutaraldehyde, a combination of glutaraldehyde and formaldehyde, or Carson's modified Millonig's, followed by post-fixation in an agent that further stabilizes as well as emphasizes membranes such as osmium tetroxide (see Chapter 30 for more detail).

Mercuric chloride

The chemistry of fixation using mercuric chloride is not understood well. It is, however, known that mercuric chloride reacts with ammonium salts, amines, amides, amino acids, and sulfydryl groups, and hardens tissues. It is especially reactive with cysteine forming a dimercaptide (Hopwood 2002) and acidifying the solution:

$$\text{sulfydryl} \quad -2(R-S-H) + HgCl_2 \rightleftharpoons$$
$$(R-S)_2-Hg + 2H^+ + 2Cl^-$$

If only one cysteine is present, a reactive group of $R-S-Hg-Cl$ is likely.

Mercury-based fixatives are toxic and should be handled with care. They should not be allowed to come into contact with metal, and should be dissolved in distilled water to prevent the precipitation of mercury salts. Mercury-containing chemicals are an environmental disposal problem. These fixatives penetrate slowly so specimens must be thin, and mercury and acid formaldehyde hematein pigments may deposit in tissue after fixation. Mercury fixatives (Hopwood 1973) are no longer used routinely except by some laboratories for fixing hematopoietic tissues (especially B5). A potential replacement for mercuric chloride is zinc sulfate. Special formulations of zinc sulfate in formaldehyde replacing mercuric chloride in B5 may give better nuclear detail than formaldehyde alone and improve tissue penetration (Carson 1990).

SPECIAL FIXATIVES

Dichromate and chromic acid fixation

Chromium trioxide $\overset{O}{\underset{O}{\diagup\diagdown}} Cr^{+6}{=}O$ dissolves in water to produce an acid solution, chromic acid, with a pH of 0.85. Chromic acid is a powerful oxidizing agent which produces aldehyde from the 1,2-diglycol residues of polysaccharides. These aldehydes can react in histochemical stains (PAS and argentaffin/argyrophil) and should increase the background of immunohistochemical staining (Grizzle 1996a).

$$CrO_3 + H_2O \rightleftharpoons H^+ + HCrO_4^- \text{ (red)}$$
$$2HCrO_4 \rightleftharpoons Cr_2O_7^{-2} \text{ (orange)} + H_2O$$

Actual chromic salts (i.e. chromium ions in +3 valence state) may destroy animal tissues (Kiernan 1999) but chromium ions in their +6 state coagulate proteins and nucleic acids. The fixation and hardening reactions are not understood completely but probably involve oxidation of proteins, which varies in strength depending upon the pH of the fixative, plus interaction of the reduced chromate ions directly in cross-linking proteins (Pearse & Stoward 1980). Chromium ions specifically interact with carboxyl and hydroxyl side chains of proteins. Chromic acid also interacts with disulfide bridges and attacks lipophilic residues such as tyrosine and methionine (Horobin 1982). Fixatives containing chromate at a pH of 3.5–5.0 are good fixatives which make proteins insoluble without coagulation. Chromate is reported to make unsaturated but not saturated lipids insoluble upon prolonged (>48 hours) fixation and hence mitochondria are well preserved by dichromate fixatives.

Dichromate-containing fixatives have been used primarily to prepare tissue for staining of endocrine tissues, especially normal adrenal medulla and its tumors. Many of these stains, such as the chromaffin reaction used to identify chromaffin granules, are not used frequently. They are unreliable and require controls (adrenal medulla fixed appropriately) which are seldom available. These stains have therefore largely been replaced by immunohistochemical stains such as neuron-specific enolase, chromagranin A, and synaptophysin (Grizzle 1996a, 1996b).

Metallic ions as a fixative supplement

Multiple metallic ions have been used as aids in fixation including Hg^{2+}, Pb^{2+}, Co^{2+}, Cu^{2+}, Cd^{2+}, $[UO_2]^{2+}$, $[PtCl_6]^{2-}$, and Zn^{2+}. Mercury, lead, and zinc are used most commonly in current fixatives, e.g. zinc-containing formaldehyde is suggested as a better fixative for immunohistochemistry than formaldehyde alone. This does however depend upon the pH of the formaldehyde as well as the zinc formaldehyde (Arnold et al 1996; Eltoum et al 2001a).

COMPOUND FIXATIVES

Pathologists use formaldehyde-based fixatives to produce reproducible histomorphometric patterns. Other agents may be added to formaldehyde to produce specific effects not possible with formaldehyde alone. The dehydrant ethanol, for example, can be added to formaldehyde to produce alcoholic formalin. This combination preserves molecules such as glycogen and results in less shrinkage and hardening than pure dehydrants.

Compound fixatives are useful for specific tissues, e.g. alcoholic formalin for fixation of fatty tissues such as breast in which preservation of the lipid is not important. In addition, fixation of gross specimens in alcoholic formalin may aid in identifying lymph nodes embedded in fat. Some combined fixatives including alcoholic formalin are good in preserving antigen immunorecognition, but non-specific staining or increased background staining in immunohistochemical procedures can be increased. Unreacted aldehyde groups in glutaraldehyde–formaldehyde fixation for example may increase background staining, and alcoholic formalin may cause non-specific staining of myelinated nerves (Grizzle et al 1995, 1997, 1998a,b; Arnold et al 1996; Grizzle 1996b).

FACTORS AFFECTING THE QUALITY OF FIXATION

Buffers and pH

The effect of pH on fixation with formaldehyde may be profound depending upon the applications to which the tissues will be exposed. In a strongly acid environment, the primary amine target groups ($—NH_2$) attract hydrogen ions ($—NH^+_3$) and become unreactive to the hydrated formaldehyde (methylene hydrate or methylene glycol), and carboxyl groups (COO^-) lose their charges ($—COOH$); this may affect the structure of proteins. Similarly the hydroxyl groups of alcohols ($—OH$) including serine and threonine may become less reactive in a strongly acid environment. The extent of formation of reactive hydroxymethyl groups and cross-linking is reduced in unbuffered 4% formaldehyde (Means & Feeney 1995), which is slightly acidic (French & Edsall 1945), because the major methylene cross-links are between lysine and the free amino group on side chains. The decrease in the effectiveness of formaldehyde fixation and hence cross-linking in the slightly acid environment supports the observation that unbuffered formalin is a better fixative than NBF with respect to immunorecognition of many antigens (Arnold et al 1996; Eltoum et al 2001b). The changes in amines and carboxyl groups require a strong acid environment and should be minimal at this slightly acidic pH of acid formalin unless the environment of the peptide has an effect.

At the acidic pH of unbuffered formaldehyde, hemoglobin metabolic products are chemically modified to form a brown–black insoluble crystalline birefringent pigment. The pigment forms at a pH of less than 5.7, and the extent of pigment formation increases in the pH range of 3.0 to 5.0. Formalin pigment is recognized easily and should not affect diagnoses except in patients with large amounts of hemoglobin breakdown products secondary to hematopoietic diseases. The pigment is removed easily with an alcoholic solution of picric acid. To avoid the formation of formalin pigment, neutral buffered formalin is used as the preferred formaldehyde-based fixative.

Acetic acids and other acids work mainly through lowering pH and disrupting the tertiary structure of proteins. Buffers are used to maintain pH at an optimum. The choice of specific buffer depends on the type of fixative and analyte. Commonly used buffers are phosphate, cacodylate, bicarbonate, Tris, and acetate. It is necessary to use low salt-buffered formalin in the new complex tissue processors in order to keep the machine 'clean', and reduce problems in its operation.

Duration of fixation and size of specimens

The factors that govern diffusion of a fixative into tissue were investigated by Medawar (1941). He found that the depth (d) reached by a fixative is directly proportional to the square root of duration of fixation (t) and expressed this relation as:

$$d = k\sqrt{t}$$

The constant (k) is the coefficient of diffusability, which is specific for each fixative. The coefficient of diffusability is 0.79 for 10% formaldehyde, 1.0 for 100% ethanol, and 1.33 for 3% potassium dichromate (Hopwood 1969). Thus, for most fixatives, the time of fixation is approximately equal to the square of the distance the fixative must penetrate. Most fixatives, such as NBF, will penetrate tissue to the depth of approximately 1 mm in one hour, e.g. for a 10-mm sphere, the fixative will not penetrate to the center of the sphere until after $(5)^2$ or 25 hours of fixation. It is important to note that the components of a compound fixative penetrate at different rates, so that these aspects of the fixative will be best manifest in thin specimens.

Gross specimens should not rest on the bottom of a container of fixative: they should be separated from the bottom by wadded fixative-soaked paper or cloth allowing penetration of fixative or processing fluids in all directions. In addition, unfixed gross specimens which are to be cut and stored in fixative prior to processing should not be thicker than 0.5 cm. When surgical specimens are to be processed to paraffin blocks, the time of penetration by fixative is more critical. Specific issues related to the processing of tissues have been reviewed separately (Grizzle et al 2001; Jones et al 2001; and Chapter 6).

Fixation proceeds slowly and the period between the formation of reactive hydroxymethyl groups and the formation of a significant number of cross-links is unknown. Ninety percent of reactive groups can be removed by 4 weeks of washing (Helander 1994), confirming that cross-linking is not a rapid process and may require weeks for completion of potential bonds.

Proteins inactivate fixatives, especially those in blood or bloody fluids. Bloody gross specimens should therefore be washed with saline prior to being put into fixative. The fixative volume should be at least ten times the volume of the tissue specimen for optimal, rapid fixation. Currently, thin specimens may be fixed in NBF for only 5–6 hours including the short time of fixation in tissue processors. The extent of formation of cross-links during such rapid NBF 'fixation' is uncertain, so most aspects of formaldehyde fixation may be due to formation of hydroxymethyl groups. Rapid fixation is acceptable as long as histochemical staining continues to be adequate; in fact, immunohistochemistry and other molecular techniques are likely to be improved by shorter times of fixation using an aldehyde (e.g. formaldehyde)-based fixation.

Temperature of fixation

The diffusion of molecules increases with rising temperature due to their more rapid movement and vibration, i.e. the rate of penetration of a tissue by formaldehyde is faster at higher temperatures. Microwaves therefore have been used to speed formaldehyde fixation by both increasing the temperature and molecular movements. Increased vapors, however, are a safety problem (Grizzle & Fredenburgh 2001, 2005). Most chemical reactions also occur more rapidly at higher temperatures and therefore formaldehyde reacts more rapidly with proteins (Hopwood 1985). Closed tissue processors have their processing retort directly above the paraffin holding stations which are held at 60–65°C, making the retort slightly warmer than room temperature.

Concentration of fixative

Effectiveness and solubility primarily determine the appropriate concentration of fixatives. Concentrations of formalin above 10% tend to cause increased hardening and shrinkage (Fox et al 1985); ethanol concentrations below 70% do not remove free water from tissues efficiently.

Osmolality of fixatives and ionic composition

The osmolality of buffer and fixative is important; hypertonic and hypotonic solutions lead to shrinkage and swelling respectively. The best results are obtained with solutions that are slightly hypertonic (400–450 mOsm), however; the osmolality for 10% NBF is about 1500 mOsm. Similarly, various ions (Na^+, K^+, Ca^{2+}, Mg^{2+}) can affect cell shape and structure regardless of the osmotic effect. The ionic composition of fluids should be as isotonic as possible to the tissues.

Additives

The addition of electrolytes and non-electrolytes to fixatives improves the morphology of the fixed tissue. These additives include calcium chloride, potassium thiocyanate, ammonium sulfate, and potassium dihydrogen phosphate. The electrolytes may react either directly with proteins causing denaturation, or independently with the fixatives and cellular constituents (Hayat 1981). The choice of electrolytes to be added to fixatives used on a tissue processor may vary. Fixatives buffered with electrolytes such as phosphates may cause problems with some processors due to precipitation of the salts. The addition of non-electrolyte substances such as sucrose, dextran, and detergent has also been reported to improve fixation (Hayat 1981).

Selecting or avoiding specific fixatives

We have emphasized that the choice of a fixative is a compromise balancing between beneficial and detrimental effects. Kiernan (1999) originally produced a table of the actions of fixatives; this was later modified and published by Eltoum et al (2001b), and Table 4.2 is a further modification of the latter.

Specific fixatives are, however, unsuitable for most uses and should be avoided. The main problem with fixatives used in histological staining is the loss by solution/extraction of molecules that are targets of specific histochemical methods. Typically, some molecules are soluble in aqueous fixatives (e.g. glycogen), while others are soluble in organic-based fixatives (e.g. lipids). Some fixatives may chemically modify targets of histochemical staining and thus affect the quality of special stains (e.g. glutaraldehyde for silver stains); this includes modification of staining secondary to changes in pH induced by fixation. A good discussion of the effects of fixation on histochemistry is by Sheehan and Hrapchak (1980).

We previously modified (Eltoum et al 2001b) the table of Sheehan and Hrapchak (1980) so that harmful methods of fixation could be identified rapidly. Table 4.3 of this chapter is a further modification of the table.

Fixation for selected individual tissues

Eyes

The globe must be firmly fixed in order to cut good sections for embedding. Eyes may be fixed in NBF, usually for about 48 hours; to speed fixation one or two small windows can be cut into the globe (avoid the retina and iris) after 24 hours. After gross description, the anterior (iris) and posterior (e.g. optic nerve) are removed with a new, sharp razor blade and the components of the globe are fixed for an additional 48 hours or more in buffered formaldehyde before being processed. Embedding may be in celloidin or paraffin. Perfusion fixation of the eye is recommended for studies of the canal of Schlemm and/or the aqueous outflow pathways.

Brain

The problem of fixing a whole brain is to render it firm enough to investigate the neuroanatomy and to produce sections to show histopathology and to respond to immunochemistry if required. Conventionally this fixation takes at least 2 weeks. Adickes et al (1997) proposed a perfusion technique which allows all of the above to be accomplished and the report issued in 5–6 days. This method depends on the perfusion of the brain via the middle cerebral arteries. Fixatives may also be enhanced by the use of microwave technology (Anonymous 2001; Kok & Boon 2003; Leong 2005). Alcoholic formalin should not be used for fixation if immunohistochemistry is to be performed using biotin–avidin (strepavidin) methods (Grizzle et al, unpublished data). See also Chapter 19.

Lungs

Lung biopsies are typically fixed in NBF. The lungs from autopsies may be inflate-fixed in NBF via the trachea or

Table 4.2 Action of major single or combination fixatives

Category of fixative	Dehydrants	Aldehyde cross-linkers	Combination mercuric chloride with formaldehyde or acetic acid	Osmium tetroxide	Picric acid plus formalin and acetic acid	Combination alcohols plus formalin
Examples of category	Ethanol Methanol Acetone	Formaldehyde Glutaraldehyde	Zenker's B5	Post-fixation after glutaraldehyde	Bouin's	Alcoholic formalin
Effect on proteins	Precipitates without chemical addition	Cross-linkers: adds active hydroxy-methyl groups to amines, amides, reactive alcohols, and sulfydryl groups; cross-links amine/amide or sulfydryl side chains of proteins	Additive plus coagulation	Additive cross-links; some extraction; some destruction	Additive and non-additive coagulant; some extraction	Additive plus precipitation
mRNA/DNA	Slight	Slowly cross-links; slightly extracts	Coagulation	Slight extraction	No action	Slight
Lipids	Extensive extraction	No action	No action	Made insoluble by cross-links with double bonds	No action	Extensive extraction
Carbohydrates	No action	None on pure carbohydrates; cross-linking of glycoproteins	No action	Slight oxidation	No action	No action
Quality of H&E staining	Satisfactory	Good	Good	Poor	Good	Good

Effect on ultrastructure (organelles)	Destroys ultrastructure including mitochondria, proteins, coagulates	Good (NBF) to excellent preservation with glutaraldehyde; adequate to good in Carson–Millonig's	Poor preservation	Used for visualization of membranes	Poor—tends to destroy membranes	Poor
Usual formulation	70–100% solution or in combination with other types of fixative	Formaldehyde (37%) – 10% V/V aqueous solution buffered with phosphates to 7.2–7.4. Glutaraldehyde – 2% buffered to 7.4	Mercuric chloride combined either with acetic acid plus dichromate or with formaldehyde plus acetate	1% solution buffered to 7.4	Aqueous picric acid, formalin, glacial acetic acid	10% formaldehyde (37%) with 90% ethanol
Important variables/issues	Time, specimen thickness – should be used only for small or thin specimens	Time, temperature, pH, concentration/ specimen thickness	Toxic	Extremely toxic	Mitochondria and integrity of nuclear membrane destroyed; not appropriate for some stains; mordant	Time, specimen dimensions. Note good fixative for renal tissues
Special uses	Preserves small non-lipid molecules such as glycogen; preserves enzymatic activity	General all-round fixative; best for ultrastructure if used with osmium tetroxide post-fixation	Excellent for hematopoietic tissues	Ultrastructural visualization of membranes; lipids on frozen sections	Mordant for connective tissue stains (trichrome)	Good general fixative; good for specific immunohistochemical reactions and good to detect lymph nodes in fatty tissue; removes fats from tissue

Table 4.3 Incompatible stains and fixatives

Target of special stain	Type of special stain	Do not use this fixative	Required or best fixative
Amebas	Best's carmine	Aqueous fixative	Alcohol or alcoholic formalin
Cholesterol and cholesterol esters	Schultz's method	Bouin's; Zenker's	10% NBF (frozen section)
	Digitonin	Bouin's; Zenker's	10% NBF (frozen section)
Chromaffin granules	Ferric ferricyanide reduction test		Orth's; Möller's
	Gomori–Burtner methenamine silver Periodic acid–Schiff (PAS)		Orth's; Möller's
	Mallory's aniline blue collagen stain	Dichromate and alcohol bases	10% NBF; Bouin's; Heiden Hain's mercuric chloride
Connective tissue	Wilder's reticulum Masson's trichrome	No picric acid fixatives NBF tissues must be post-fixed with (Bouin's)	10% NBF; Zenker's; Helly's Bouin's
	Mallory's analine blue collagen stain	All except required/best	Zenker's
Copper	Mallory's stain	Formalin	Alcohol-based fixatives
Degenerating myelin	Marchi's method	All except required/best	Orth's for 48 hours; 10% NBF
DNA/RNA	Feulgen	Bouiv's, strong acids	Ethanol
Elastic fibers	Gomori's aldehyde fuchsin	No chromates	10% NBF
Fats/lipids	Nile blue sulfate	All except required/best	Formal calcium
	Osmic acid (frozen section)	All except required best	10% NBF
	Oil red O (frozen section)	Zenker's; Helly's	10% NBF
	Sudan black B (frozen section)	Zenker's; Helly's	10% NBF
Fibrin	Mallory's phosphotungstic acid hematoxylin	Bouin's	Zenker's
	Weigert's stain for fibrin	Bouin's	Absolute ethanol; Carnoy's; alcoholic formalin
Glycogen	Bauer–Feulgen	Aqueous fixative	Carnoy's or Gendre's
	PAS	Aqueous fixative	Acid alcoholic formalin
	Best's carmine	Aqueous fixative	Absolute alcohol; Carnoy's
Glycoproteins	Müller–Mowry colloidal iron	Chromates	Alcoholic formalin Carnoy's
Hemoglobin	Lepehne's (frozen section)	Zenker's	Short time in 10% NBF
	Dunn–Thompson	Bouin's, Zenker's, Helly's	10% NBF

Table 4.3 *(continued)*			
Target of special stain	Type of special stain	Do not use this fixative	Required or best fixative
Hepatitis B surface antigen	Orcein	No chromates	
	Aldehyde fuchsin	No chromates	
Iron	Mallory's stain	Formalin	Alcohol-based fixatives
Juxtaglomerular cells of kidney	Bowie's stain	All except required/best	Helly's
Melanin pigments	DOPA oxidase	All except required/best	See procedure
Mitochondria		Dehydrants, ethanol, methanol, acetone	Carson–Millonig's
Mucoproteins	PAS	Glutaraldehyde	
Neuroendocrine granules	Rapid argyrophil Fontana–Masson	Ethanol, methanol, acetone	10% NBF
Pancreas α, β, & δ cells	Trichrome–PAS	Zenker's, Bouin's Alcohol based	10% NBF or Helly's
Paneth cell granules	Phloxine tartrazine	Acid	10% NBF
Peripheral nerve elements	Bielschowski's for neurofibrils and axis cylinders	All except required/best	3–6 weeks in 10% NBF
	Bodian's for myelinated and non-myelinated nerve fibers	All except required/best	9 parts ethanol 1 part formalin
	Nonidez's for neurofibrils and axis cylinders	All except required/best	100 ml 50% ethanol plus 25 g chloral hydrate
	Rio–Hortega for neutrofibrils	All except required/best	10% NBF
	Immunohistochemistry biotin–streptavidin	Alcoholic formalin	Zn acid 10% formalin
Phospholipids	Smith–Dietrich (frozen section)	All except required/best	Formal calcium
	Baker's acid hematin (frozen section)	All except required/best	10% NBF
Pituitary β cells	Congo red for β cells		10% NBF
	Gomori's aldehyde Fuchsin for β cells	NBF requires mordant	Bouin's
Silver stains	Fontana–Masson–Grimelius	Glutaraldehyde	
Spirochetes	Giemsa	Bouin's; Zenker's	
	Gram's technique	Bouin's; Zenker's	
	Levaditi	Bouin's; Zenker's	
	Warthin–Starry	All except required/best	10% NBF
Uric acid crystals	Gomori's methenamine, silver for urate	All except required/best	Absolute thanol
	Gomori's chrome alum hematoxylin–phloxine	Avoid chromates	Bouin's

major bronchi, and in our experience these lungs can be cut within 2 hours. Gross sections are fixed overnight and sections to be processed and cut the next day.

Lymphoid tissue

Special care should be taken with all lymphoid tissue as many organisms (e.g. *Mycobacterium tuberculosis* and viruses) may sequester themselves in the lymphoid reticular system. The lymphoid tissue is usually split and a representative sample of fresh tissue is sent for special studies (e.g. fluorescent flow cytometry). The rest of the lymph node is fixed in NBF, though some laboratories fix part of the tissue in B5 or zinc.

Testis

Biopsies of the testes are fixed routinely in NBF.

Muscle biopsies

Biopsies of muscle are received fresh. A portion is separated for enzyme histochemistry (see Chapters 7 and 20). The tissue for routine histology is fixed in NBF and embedded so the fibers of the specimens are viewed in cross-section and longitudinally. After processing this is stained with H&E, a trichrome stain, and Congo red if amyloid is suspected.

Renal biopsies

Renal core biopsies should be subdivided as they are obtained into three components, each of which should contain adequate numbers of glomeruli. Each portion is then fixed depending upon the method to be used for analysis:

- NBF or Carson's modified Millonig's for routine histology
- Carson's modified Millonig's fixative or 2% buffered glutaraldehyde (pH 7.3) for ultrastructural analysis
- Commercial transfer solutions, e.g. Zeus®, for immunofluorescence examination.

USEFUL FORMULAS FOR FIXATIVES

Gray (1954) lists over 600 formulations for various fixatives. The following is a list of the fixatives and formulas most commonly used by histotechnologists/anatomists. Many of these formulas are based on those presented in standard textbooks of histochemistry (Sheehan & Hrapchak 1980; Carson 1990; Kiernan 1999). The formulas

vary slightly from text to text, but these variations are unlikely to cause problems.

For routine histology, 10% neutral buffered formalin (NBF) is frequently used for initial fixation and for the first station on tissue processors. NBF is composed of a 10% solution of phosphate buffered formaldehyde. Formaldehyde is commercially supplied as a 37–40% solution and in the following formulas is referred to as 37% formaldehyde.

Neutral buffered 10% formalin

Tap water	900 ml
Formalin (37% formaldehyde solution)	100 ml
Sodium phosphate, monobasic, monohydrate	4 g
Sodium phosphate, dibasic, anhydrous	6.5 g

The pH should be 7.2–7.4

There are other formulations of NBF and related fixatives. NBF purchased from commercial companies may vary widely in its aldehyde content, and commercial companies may add material such as methanol (Fox et al 1985) or other agents to stabilize NBF preparations (Grizzle et al unpublished).

Carson's modified Millonig's phosphate buffered formalin

Formaldehyde (37–40%)	10 ml
Tap water	90 ml
Sodium phosphate, monobasic	1.86 g
Sodium hydroxide	0.42 g

Deionized water can be used if tap water is hard and/or contains solids. The pH should be 7.2–7.4. This formula is reported to be better for ultrastructural preservation than NBF.

Sometimes the term 'formal' is used to refer to 10% formalin or 3.7% formaldehyde.

Formal (10% formalin), calcium acetate

Tap water	900 ml
Formaldehyde (37%)	100 ml
Calcium acetate	20 g

This is a good fixative for preservation of lipids.

Formal (10% formalin), saline

Tap water	900 ml
Formaldehyde (37%)	100 ml
Sodium chloride	9 g

Formal (10% formalin), zinc, unbuffered

Tap water	900 ml
Formaldehyde (37%)	100 ml
Sodium chloride	4.5 g
Zinc chloride or (zinc sulfate)	1.6 g (or 3.6 g)

Zinc formalin is reported to be an excellent fixative for immunohistochemistry.

Formalin, buffered saline

Tap water	900 ml
Formaldehyde (37%)	100 ml
Sodium chloride	9 g
Sodium phosphate, dibasic	12 g

Formalin, buffered zinc

10% neutral buffered formalin	1000 ml
Zinc chloride	1.6 g

Mercuric fixatives

A problem with fixation in mercury solutions is that several types of pigment may combine with the mercury. These pigments are removed from sections by using iodine treatment followed by sodium thiosulfate.

Zenker's solution

Distilled water	250 ml
Mercuric chloride	12.5 g
Potassium dichromate	6.3 g
Sodium sulfate	2.5 g

Just before use add 5 ml of glacial acidic acid to 95 ml of above solution. This is a good fixative for bloody (congested) specimens and trichrome stains.

Helly's solution

Distilled water	250 ml
Mercuric chloride	12.5 g
Potassium dichromate	6.3 g
Sodium sulfate	2.5 g

Just before use add 5 ml of 37% formaldehyde to 95 ml of above solution. It is excellent for bone marrow extramedullary hematopoiesis and intercalated discs.

Schaudinn's solution

Distilled water	50 ml
Mercuric chloride	3.5 g
Absolute ethanol	25 ml

Ohlmacher's solution

Absolute ethanol	32 ml
Chloroform	6 ml
Glacial acetic acid	2 ml
Mercuric chloride	8 g

This fixative penetrates rapidly.

Carnoy–Lebrun solution

Absolute ethanol	15 ml
Chloroform	15 ml
Glacial acetic acid	15 ml
Mercuric chloride	8 g

This fixative penetrates rapidly.

B5 fixative

Stock solution:

Mercuric chloride	12 g
Sodium acetate	2.5 g
Distilled water	200 ml

Add 2 ml of formaldehyde (37%) to 20 ml of stock solution just before use.

Frequently used for bone marrow, lymph nodes, spleen, and other hematopoietic tissues.

Dichromate fixatives

There is a variation among the names attributed to the formulas of dichromate fixatives but not in the formulas themselves. Time of fixation (24 hours) is critical for dichromate fixatives. Tissue should be washed after fixation and transferred to 70% ethanol. Failure to wash the tissue after fixation may cause pigments to be precipitated. Extensive shrinkage occurs when tissues are processed to paraffin blocks.

Miller's solution or Möller's solution

Potassium dichromate	2.5 g
Sodium sulfate	1 g
Distilled water	100 ml

Möller's or Regaud's solution

Potassium dichromate	3 g
Distilled water	80 ml

At time of use add 20 ml of formaldehyde (37%).

Orth's solution

Potassium dichromate	2.5 g
Sodium sulfate	1 g
Distilled water	100 ml

At time of use add 10 ml of formaldehyde (37%).

Lead fixatives

See special fixatives.

Picric acid fixatives

Many picric acid fixatives require a saturated aqueous solution of picric acid. Aqueous picric acid 2.1% will produce a saturated solution and 5% picric acid a saturated solution in absolute ethanol.

Bouin's solution

Saturated aqueous solution of picric acid	1500 ml
Formaldehyde (37%)	500 ml
Glacial acetic acid	100 ml

Bouin's solution is an excellent general fixative for connective tissue stains. The yellow color can be removed with 70% ethanol, lithium carbonate, or another acid dye, separately or during the staining sequence. Bouin's solution destroys membranes, therefore intact nuclei cannot be recovered from Bouin's fixed tissue and there may be extensive shrinkage of larger specimens.

Hollande's solution

Distilled water	1000 ml
Formaldehyde 37%	100 ml
Acetic acid	15 ml
Picric acid	40 g
Copper acetate	25 g

A useful fixative for gastrointestinal biopsies and endocrine tissue; specimens are washed before exposure to NBF.

Dehydrant fixatives

Dehydrant fixatives act to remove free and bound water and change the tertiary structure of proteins so that proteins precipitate but leave nucleic acids relatively unchanged. Histopathology of tissues is almost as good as NBF. Ultrastructure is destroyed by any of these four

dehydrants due to the extraction of lipids, and each may cause excessive shrinking of tissue components after more than 3–4 hours of fixation. Each of these fixatives can be modified by adding other chemicals to produce specific effects.

1 ethanol, absolute
2 ethanol, 95%
3 ethanol, 70%–95%
4 methanol, 100%
5 acetone, 100%

Methanol is useful for touch preparations and smears, especially blood smears. Many alcohol mixtures may undergo slow reactions among ingredients upon long-term storage; in general most alcohol-based fixatives should be prepared no more than 1–2 days before use. Acetone fixation should be short (1 hour) at 4°C only on small specimens. Acetone produces extensive shrinkage and hardening, and results in microscopic distortion. It is used for immunohistochemistry, enzyme studies, and in the detection of rabies. Cold acetone is especially useful to 'open' membranes of intact cells (e.g. grown on coverslips or microscope slides) to facilitate entrance of large molecules (e.g. antibodies for immunohistochemical studies). 'Trade secret' ingredients stabilize commercial formulations.

Clarke's solution

Absolute ethanol	60 ml
Glacial acetic acid	20 ml

This solution produces good general histological results for H&E stains. It has the advantage of preserving nucleic acids while lipids are extracted. A short fixation is recommended and tissues are transferred to 95% ethanol following fixation.

Carnoy's fixative

Acetic acid	10 ml
Absolute ethanol	60 ml
Chloroform	30 ml

Useful in cytology to clear bloody specimens.

Carnoy's fixative is useful for RNA stains, e.g. methyl green pyronine, and for glycogen preservation. It shrinks and hardens tissues and hemolyzes red blood cells. It may destroy the staining of acid-fast bacilli.

Methacarn

Acetic acid	10 ml
100% methanol	60 ml
Chloroform	30 ml

Causes less hardening and less shrinkage than Carnoy's but with the same pattern of staining.

Dehydrant—cross-linking fixatives

Compound fixatives with both dehydrant and cross-linking actions include alcohol–formalin mixture. These produce excellent results in the immunohistochemical identification of specific antigens (Arnold et al 1996). In some situations the results may be too good, e.g. the Herceptin test by DAKO to identify the membrane expression of p185^{erbB-2} depends upon the paraffin-embedded tissue being fixed in NBF. This test is used to identify patients whose tumors (e.g. breast) are likely to respond to therapy with the monoclonal antibody therapy Herceptin. Fixation in alcoholic formalin will produce a stronger membrane pattern of staining than in tissues fixed in NBF. The mechanism of this is unknown, but may involve less immunorecognition of cytoplasmic p185^{erbB-2} antigens in tissues fixed in ethanol, together with increased immunorecognition of p185^{erbB-2} on membranes (Arnold et al 1996). Some breast tissue should be fixed in NBF without a post-fixation step in alcoholic formation in order to reduce false-positive Herceptin tests.

Alcohol–formalin fixation or post-fixation is advantageous in large specimens with extensive fat (e.g. breast specimens). Lymph nodes can be detected much more easily in specimens with alcohol–formalin fixation due to the extraction of lipids and to texture differences compared with tissues fixed in NBF. The preparation of alcohol–formaldehyde solutions is complex, especially buffered forms of this compound fixative. It is probably best to purchase commercial preparations of buffered alcohol–formaldehyde. For use in post-fixation (e.g. after 10% NBF), Carson (1990) recommends the following formula:

Absolute ethanol	650 ml
Distilled water	250 ml
Formaldehyde (37%)	100 ml

Carson recommends this formula because she noted that the concentration of ethanol should be less than 70% to prevent the precipitation of phosphates in 10% NBF sat-urated tissues. For initial fixation the following formulas can be used:

Alcoholic formalin

Ethanol (95%)	895 ml
Formaldehyde (37%)	105 ml

Alcohol–formalin–acetic acid fixative

Ethanol (95%)	85 ml
Formaldehyde (37%)	10 ml
Glacial acetic acid	5 ml

Methanol may be substituted with care for ethanol; similarly various mixtures of ethanol, acetic acid, and formalin may be used.

Alcoholic Bouin's (Gendre's solution)

This fixative is similar to Bouin's except it is less aqueous and there is better retention in tissues of some carbohydrates (e.g. glycogen). Fixation should be between 4 hours and overnight followed by washing in 70% ethanol, followed by 95% ethanol (several changes). This is the one alcoholic fixative that improves upon aging (Lillie & Fullmer 1976).

Gendre's solution

95% ethanol saturated with picric acid	
(5 g per 100 ml)	800 ml
Formaldehyde (37%)	150 ml
Glacial acetic acid	50 ml

To increase the effectiveness of alcoholic Bouin's, if there is no time for aging, the following formula has been recommended (Gregory 1980):

Equivalent to aged alcoholic Bouin's

Picric acid	0.5 g
Formaldehyde	15 ml
95% ethanol	25 ml
Glacial acetic acid	5 ml
Ethyl acetate	25 ml
Tap water	30 ml

Another alcoholic form of Bouin's solution is as follows:

Stock Bouin's solution	75 ml
95% ethanol	25 ml

This solution is excellent for lymph nodes (24 hours) and for fatty tissue (48 hours).

A closely related fixative is:

Rossman's solution

Tap water	10 ml
Formaldehyde (37%)	10 ml
Absolute ethanol	80 ml
Lead nitrate	8 g

Fix for 24 hours at room temperature. This is a good fixative for connective tissue mucins and umbilical cord.

FOR METABOLIC BONE DISEASE

Phosphate buffer

Tap water	1000 ml
$NaH_2PO_4 \cdot H_2O$	1.104 g
$NaHPO_4$ (anhydrous)	4.675 g

Fixative

Phosphate buffer	900 ml
Formaldehyde (37%)	100 ml

Adjust pH to 7.35.

FIXATION AND DECALCIFICATION

Bouin's decalcifying solution

Saturated aqueous solution of picric acid (10.5 g per 500 ml)	500 ml
Formaldehyde (37%)	167 ml
Formic acid	33 ml

FIXATION FOR FATTY TISSUE

Bouin's solution	75 ml
95% ethanol	25 ml

May require up to 48 hours for good sections of lipomas or well differentiated liposarcomas.

Note

This chapter is an introduction to fixation. More detailed and advanced issues related to fixation are included in several other texts/references (Sheehan & Hrapchak 1980; Eltoum et al 2001a, 2001b; Grizzle et al 2001). As discussed, various formulas may vary within a few percentages, but most of these formulas produce equivalent results.

Acknowledgment

David Hopwood contributed this chapter for the first five editions. Our acknowledgments are due to him for his contribution.

REFERENCES

Adickes E.D., Folkerth, R.D., Sims, K.L. (1997) Use of profusion fixation for improved neuropathologic fixation. Archives of Pathology and Laboratory Medicine 121:1199–1206.

Anonymous (2001) Preserve for microwave fixation, vol. 2001. Energy Beam Sciences. Online. Available: http://www.ebsciences.com/microwave/preserve.htm.

Arnold M.M., Srivastava S., Fredenburgh J. et al. (1996) Effects of fixation and tissue processing on immunohistochemical demonstration of specific antigens. Biotechnic and Histochemistry 71:224–230.

Bayliss High O.B., Lake B. (1996) Lipids. In: Bancroft J.D., Stevens A., eds. Theory and practice of histological techniques. Edinburgh: Churchill-Livingstone, pp. 213–242.

Bhakuni V. (1998) Alcohol-induced molten globule intermediates of proteins: are they real folding intermediates or off pathway products? Archives of Biochemistry and Biophysics 357:274–284.

Carson F.L. (1990) Histotechnology: a self-instructional text. Chicago, IL: American Society of Clinical Pathologists.

Dapson R.W. (1993) Fixation for the 1990s: a review of needs and accomplishments. Biotechnic and Histochemistry 68:75–82.

Eltoum I.-E., Fredenburgh J., Grizzle W.E. (2001a) Advanced concepts in fixation: effects of fixation on immunohistochemistry and histochemistry, reversibility of fixation and recovery of proteins, nucleic acids, and other molecules from fixed and processed tissues, special methods of fixation. Journal of Histotechnology 24:201–210.

Eltoum I., Fredenburgh J., Myers R.B., Grizzle W. (2001b) Introduction to the theory and practice of fixation of tissues. Journal of Histotechnology 24:173–190.

Fox C.H., Johnson F.B., Whiting J., Roller P.P. (1985) Formaldehyde fixation. Journal of Histochemistry and Cytochemistry 33:845–853.

Fraenkel-Conrat H., Mecham D.K. (1949) The reaction of formaldehyde with proteins. VII. Demonstration of intermolecular cross-linking by means of osmotic pressure measurements. Journal of Biological Chemistry 177:477–486.

Fraenkel-Conrat H., Olcott H.S. (1948a) The reaction of formaldehyde with proteins. V. Cross linking between amino and primary amide or guanidyl groups. Journal of the American Chemical Society 70:2673–2684.

Fraenkel-Conrat H., Olcott H.S. (1948b) Reactions of form-aldehyde with proteins. VI. Cross-linking of amino groups with phenol, imidazole, or indole groups. Journal of Biological Chemistry 174:827–843.

Fraenkel-Conrat H., Cooper M., Olcott H.S. (1945) The reaction of formaldehyde with proteins. Journal of the American Chemical Society 67:950–954.

Fraenkel-Conrat H., Brandon B.A., Olcott H.S. (1947) The reaction of formaldehyde with proteins. IV. Participation of indole groups. Gramacidin. Journal of Biological Chemistry 168:99–118.

French D., Edsall J.T. (1945) The reactions of formaldehyde with amino acids and proteins. Advances in Protein Chemistry 2:277–333.

Gray P. (1954) The microanatomist's formulary and guide. New York, NY: The Blakiston Co., McGraw-Hill.

Gregory R.E. (1980) Alcoholic Bouin fixation of insect nervous systems for Bodian silver staining. I. Composition of 'aged' fixative. Stain Technology 55:143–149.

Grizzle W.E. (1996a) Theory and practice of silver staining in histopathology. Journal of Histotechnology 19: 183–195.

Grizzle W.E. (1996b) Silver staining methods to identify cells of the dispersed neuroendocrine system. Journal of Histotechnology 19:225–234.

Grizzle W.E., Fredenburgh J. (2001) Avoiding biohazards in medical, veterinary and research laboratories. Biotechnic and Histochemistry 76:183–206.

Grizzle, W.E., Fredenburgh, J. (2005) Safety in biomedical and other laboratories. In: Patrinos G., Ansorg W., eds. Molecular diagnostics, Ch. 33, pp. 421–428.

Grizzle W.E., Myers R.B., Oelschlager D.K. (1995) Prognostic biomarkers in breast cancer: factors affecting immunohistochemical evaluation. Breast 1:243–250.

Grizzle W.E., Myers R.B., Manne U. (1997) The use of bio-marker expression to characterize neoplastic processes. Biotechnic and Histochemistry 72:96–104.

Grizzle W.E., Myers R.B., Manne U. et al. (1998a) Factors affecting immunohistochemical evaluation of biomarker expression in neoplasia. In: Hanausek M., Walaszek Z., eds. John Walker's methods in molecular medicine—tumor marker protocols. Totowa, NJ: Humana Press, Vol. 14, pp. 161–179.

Grizzle, W.E., Myers, R.B., Manne, U., Srivastava, S. (1998b) Immunohistochemical evaluation of biomarkers in prostatic and colorectal neoplasia. In: Hanausek M., Walaszek Z., eds. John Walker's methods in molecular medicine—tumor marker protocols. Totowa, NJ: Humana Press, Vol. 14, pp. 143–160.

Grizzle W.E., Stockard C., Billings P. (2001) The effects of tissue processing variables other than fixation on histochemical staining and immunohistochemical detection of antigens. Journal of Histotechnology 24:213–219.

Gustavson K.H. (1956) The chemistry of tanning processes. New York, NY: Academic Press.

Habeeb A.F. (1966) Determination of free amino groups in proteins by trinitrobenzenesulfonic acid. Analytical Biochemistry 14:328–336.

Hayat M.A. (1981) Principles and techniques of electron microscopy. Biological applications, 2nd edn. Baltimore, MD: University Park Press, Vol. 1.

Helander K.G. (1994) Kinetic studies of formaldehyde binding in tissue. Biotechnic and Histochemistry 69: 177–179.

Herskovits T.T., Gadegbeku B., Jaillet H. (1970) On the structural stability and solvent denaturation of proteins. I. Denaturation by the alcohols and glycols. Journal of Biological Chemistry 245:2588–2598.

Hopwood D. (1969) Fixatives and fixation: a review. Histochemical Journal 1:323–360.

Hopwood D. (1973) Fixation with mercury salts. Acta Histochemica (Suppl) 13:107–118.

Hopwood D. (1985) Cell and tissue fixation, 1972–1982. Histochemical Journal 17:389–442.

Hopwood D. (2002) Fixation and fixatives. In: Bancroft J.D., Gamble M., eds. Theory and practice of histological techniques. London: Churchill Livingstone, pp. 63–84.

Hopwood D., Milne G., Penston J. (1990) A comparison of microwaves and heat alone in the preparation of tissue for electron microscopy. Journal of Histochemistry 22:358–364.

Horobin R.W. (1982) Histochemistry: an explanatory outline of histochemistry and biophysical staining. Stuttgart: Gustav Fischer.

Jewell S.D., Srinivasan M., McCart L.M. et al. (2002) Analysis of the molecular quality of human tissues: an experience from the Cooperative Human Tissue Network. American Journal of Clinical Pathology 118:733–741.

Jones W.T., Stockard C.R., Grizzle, W.E. (2001) Effects of time and temperature during attachment of sections to microscope slides on immunohistochemical detection of antigens. Biotechnic and Histochemistry 76:55–58.

Kiernan J.A. (1999) Histological and histochemical methods: theory and practice, 3rd edn. Oxford UK: Butterworth-Heinemann.

Kok L.P., Boon M.E. (2003) Microwaves for the art of microscopy. Leyden: Coulomb Press.

Leong A.S.-Y. (2005) Microwave technology for light microscopy and ultrastructural studies. Bangkok: Milestone.

Lhotka J.F., Ferreira A.V. (1949) A comparison of deforma-linizing technics. Stain Technology 25:27–32.

Lillie R.D., Fullmer H.M. (1976) Histopathologic technic and practical histochemistry, 4th edn. New York: McGraw-Hill.

McGhee J.D., von Hippel P.H. (1975a) Formaldehyde as a probe of DNA structure. I. Reaction with exocyclic amino groups of DNA bases. Biochemistry 14:1281–1296.

McGhee J.D., von Hippel P.H. (1975b) Formaldehyde as a probe of DNA structure. II. Reaction with endocyclic imino groups of DNA bases. Biochemistry 14:1297–1303.

McGhee J.D., von Hippel P.H. (1977a) Formaldehyde as a probe of DNA structure. 3. Equilibrium denaturation of DNA and synthetic polynucleotides. Biochemistry 16:3267–3276.

McGhee J.D., von Hippel P.H. (1977b) Formaldehyde as a probe of DNA structure. 4. Mechanism of the initial reaction of formaldehyde with DNA. Biochemistry 16:3276–3293.

Means G.E., Feeney R.E. (1995) Reductive alkylation of proteins. Analytical Biochemistry 224:1–16.

Medawar P.B. (1941) The rate of penetration of fixatives. Journal of the Royal Microscopical Society 61:46–57.

O'Leary T.J., Mason J.T. (2004) A molecular mechanism of formalin fixation and antigen retrieval. American Journal of Clinical Pathology 122:154; author reply 154–155.

Papanikolau Y., Kokkinidis M. (1997) Solubility, crystallization and chromatographic properties of macromolecules strongly depend on substances that reduce the ionic strength of the solution. Protein Engineering 10:847–850.

Pearse A.G. (1980) Histochemistry, theoretical and applied, Volume I. Edinburgh: Churchill Livingstone.

Pearse A.G.E., Stoward P.J. (1980) Histochemistry, theoretical and applied. Vol. 1. Preparative and optical technology. Vol. 2. Analytical technique. Vol. 3. Enzyme histochemistry. Edinburgh: Churchill-Livingstone.

Rait V.K., O'Leary T.J., Mason J.T. (2004) Modeling formalin fixation and antigen retrieval with bovine pancreatic ribonuclease A: I—structural and functional alterations. Laboratory Investigations 84:292–299.

Rait V.K., Zhang Q., Fabris D. et al. (2005) Conversions of formaldehyde-modified 2-deoxyadenosine 5′-monophosphate in conditions modeling formalin-fixed tissue dehydration. Journal of Histochemistry and Cytochemistry 54:301–310.

Sheehan D.C., Hrapchak B.B. (1980) Theory and practice of histotechnology, 2nd edn. St. Louis, MO: C.V. Mosby.

Singer S.J. (1962) The properties of proteins in nonaqueous solvents. Advances in Protein Chemistry 17:1–68.

Steg A., Wang W., Blanquicett C. et al. (2006) Multiple gene expression analyses in paraffin-embedded tissues by taqman low-density array: application to hedgehog and wnt pathway analysis in ovarian endometrioid adenocarcinoma. Journal of Molecular Diagnostics 8:76–83.

Tome Y., Hirohashi S., Noguchi M., Shimosato, Y. (1990) Preservation of cluster 1 small cell lung cancer antigen in zinc–formalin fixative and its application to immunohistological diagnosis. Histopathology 16:469–474.

5

The Gross Room/Surgical Cutup

Paul E. Billings and William E. Grizzle

INTRODUCTION

The Gross Room or Specimen Reception Laboratory is where tissue specimens from the operating theaters and clinics are received. An accurate diagnosis from this tissue is dependent upon the correct identification, handling, and processing in this busy area. Numerous different specimens and types of tissue arrive, each of which must be reviewed carefully (Grizzle et al 1998; Grizzle & Sexton 1999; Debski et al 2004). Histotechnologists, biomedical scientists, and medical assistants work in this area with the pathologist ensuring that the specimen is handled correctly, as the diagnosis is essential to the patient's clinical outcome. Dermatological specimens are discussed in more depth in this chapter as they require more specific handling than most other tissues. The processing of dermatological as well as pediatric specimens can serve as a model for processing other types of tissue.

SPECIMEN HANDLING AND IDENTIFICATION

Each laboratory has its own way of specimen identification, giving the tissue a unique accession number. This may include the year and month the specimen was received (Grizzle et al 1998; Grizzle & Sexton 1999), e.g. 04-05-06 could represent a specimen that was the fourth case received in May 2006; the laboratory computer usually generates this number. If multiple specimens are received on the same patient from the same operation/procedure, then specimens may be given the same number followed by a numerical or alphabetical designation. Bar codes are frequently used by clinical labora-

tories; the bar code on the request card is read into the departmental computer and the complete information on the patient is then generated from the hospital information system. The gross description of the specimen is entered at a later stage.

The correct identification of the specimen(s) with its unique number is the link between the specimen and the patient. The specimen container label and the accompanying request form should arrive in the laboratory already completed and typically include the patient's name, age or birth date, and a medical record number. For hospitals with diverse populations, race and ethnicity are important parameters to record, because diseases may vary with race/ethnicity (Manne et al 1998). The label should be firmly attached to the body of the container so that it cannot be separated; labels should not be attached just to the lid of the container. The request form should have a provisional diagnosis and brief clinical details. Any discrepancies in specimen identification or labeling are resolved prior to processing and the discrepancy noted on the request form and in the computer details. Incorrect identification of any specimen results in the wrong diagnoses and incorrect treatment to potentially two patients.

GROSSING

A pathologist, resident, physician assistant, histotechnologist, or biomedical scientist can gross specimens. This is dependent upon the nature of the specimen and the local and national regulations in place in the laboratory. The routine surgical laboratory receives many different tissue specimens ranging from small biopsies (e.g. of breast, bladder, bone marrow) to complete resections (e.g. larynx, uterus, large bowel). Small amounts of tissue can be unidentifiable as to their anatomical source and, thus, gross descriptions are important. The type of biopsy and the number of fragments received should be documented. The exact dimensions of each fragment can be specified if there are only a few. The features of the biopsy should be described including the color and consistency of the tissue and the presence of blood clot or foreign material. Most laboratories have developed standardized formats that describe the gross examination and processing of specimens. By following these, it is clear how specimens should be grossed. Unless the tissue specimens are oriented correctly, the margins of the specimens may be confused and an inaccurate diagnosis made. The use of drawings and photographs to indicate the source of sections is useful, and, on occasion, it may be useful to contact the surgeon/clinician to ensure the correct orientation of complex specimens.

There are seven major components in grossing a specimen:

- Reliable and rapid transfer of the specimen from surgery to pathology
- Accurate identification of the specimen
- Description of additional specimens received from the same patient
- Gross description of the specimen's normal and abnormal features
- Recording the sites from which blocks of tissue are taken
- Recording markers (e.g. sutures) that help with the correct orientation
- Identifying special studies requested and/or needed.

SPECIMENS FROM DERMATOLOGY

Dermatological specimens are often small and can be excisional, shave, core, or re-excisional biopsies. Each type of biopsy is handled differently and is often processed separately from other tissues. It is good practice to have a separate gross sheet where the type of specimen and how it should be oriented is noted (Fig. 5.1). It may be difficult to visualize some lesions on core biopsies, so attention to cutting and orientation is important. Tissue should be oriented to determine the depth of invasion of the lesion and the margins of resection. Pigmented lesions may represent melanomas and need to be

processed to demonstrate the maximum thickness of the lesion. This is discussed below.

Small specimens

Small specimens should not be cut, bisected, or inked while fresh and unfixed. The accurate cutting of unfixed tissue can be difficult, and an irregular cut can cause problems at the embedding stage. Small specimens are processed in cassettes either with a fine mesh (Fig. 5.2b), in lens paper, or in a 'tea bag' (Fig. 5.2d) so they are not lost during processing. The use of sponges is an alternative but specimens may dry out when sponges are used and tiny fragments of tissue may dry, harden, and stick to the sponge (Fig. 5.2c). However, if the biopsy is large enough, processing using sponges can help with orientation. Similarly tiny specimens of skin should not be bisected; instead, the whole biopsy is embedded on its edge and this noted appropriately on the gross sheet.

Core biopsies

Core biopsies are usually taken of a larger lesion or of a generalized inflammatory or other disease process. The core biopsy should be taken with the lesion at its center. Larger core biopsies (= 4 mm) should be bisected eccentrically, perhaps $2/3$ or $1/3$, and the specimen embedded with cut surfaces down. This permits the initial paraffin sections to sample the center of the core and ensures these lesions are not missed. Bisecting the core of small biopsies (= 2 mm) may cause damage, e.g. the surface epithelium may be lost, so the core is embedded totally without cutting it (Fig. 5.3).

Shave biopsies of skin

The dermatologist uses shave biopsies to remove or sample skin lesions. Even if the lesion extends throughout the biopsy it may have been totally removed because the base of the area may have been treated further, e.g. by cautery. Depending upon the size of the biopsy, it may be bisected, trisected, or cut into sections. Generally, most specimens of skin or other epithelial surfaces should be cut so that all aliquots are embedded on edge (Fig. 5.4). Care should be taken with any pigmented lesions of the skin. Excision biopsy is the method of choice for surgical removal of melanomas but they are sometimes inadvertently removed by shaving. The width of a tumor and depth of invasion are of prognostic importance so

Type of Specimen and Description

☐   Pigmented lesion—take great care

☐   Core biopsy   size ____mm

☐   Shave biopsy ___ x ___ x ___ mm   Oriented _____
Yes ___No

☐   Excision size ___ x ___ x ___   Oriented _____
Yes ___No

Description

—   _____

—   _____

Gross action

☐   Submitted totally—embed as core

☐   Submitted in total, uncut—embed on edge

☐   Bisected eccentrically and submitted in
total—embed each aliquot on edge

☐   Bisected eccentrically and submitted in
total—embed cut surface down

☐   Bisected, trisected, or otherwise cut—embed all aliquots on edge

☐   Specimen is oriented; the labeling of margins
follows the orientation of the specimen

☐   Other _____
(specify)

_____

Fig. 5.1   A suggested form for collecting specimen data to aid in diagnosis of dermatology specimens.

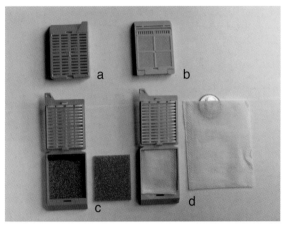

Fig. 5.2 Supplies that can be used for processing small specimens. (a) A standard cassette used in tissue processing. (b) A cassette with very small holes permitting fluid exchange but minimizing the likelihood of loss of small specimens. Note that air bubbles may form in this type of cassette and may cause inhomogeneous processing of tissue. (c) The use of sponges in a standard cassette. (d) The use of a tea bag to minimize the likelihood of specimen loss during tissue processing.

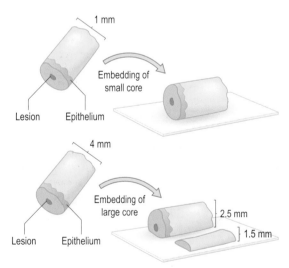

Fig. 5.3 An approach to processing punch biopsies, which are typical, cores ranging in diameter from 1 mm to 5 mm. The center of the core usually represents the lesion. Small cores (top) should not be cut, but should be embedded on their side because cutting the core prior to processing is likely to result in missing the lesion. Larger cores (bottom) should be cut excentrically and both parts embedded, cut side down, to best ensure that the central lesion is captured in initial levels.

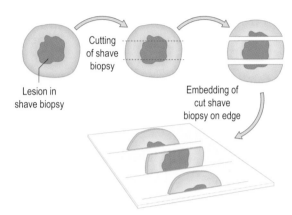

Fig. 5.4 One approach to a shave biopsy. Un-oriented shave biopsies usually are not taken to demonstrate margins. A large shave biopsy can be trisected and embedded on edge to best demonstrate the whole lesion.

the biopsy should be processed to demonstrate the thickness of the lesion, and the tissue cut eccentrically so that the thickest part of the lesion can be evaluated.

Excisional biopsies

These biopsies of skin or other epithelial surfaces (e.g. oral mucosa) are examined to ensure that the lesion has been completely removed and that the original clinician's diagnosis was correct. The biopsies can be oriented using sutures or dyes. When the specimen is oriented, the margins should be marked prior to grossing with inks, or other pathology stains. This is useful if a tumor comes close to, but does not involve, a margin. It is helpful to photograph the specimen to record its orientation. If shave margins are to be taken on an oriented specimen (Fig. 5.5), half the specimen from 12 to 3 to 6 on the clock face could be stained with red dye and the other half from 6 to 9 to 12 with green dye. Shave margins should cover areas such as 12 to 3, 3 to 6, 6 to 9, and 9 to 12. Multiple shave margins of specimens that do not need orienting may be taken and combined in a single cassette but evaluation of the involvement of lateral and deep margins is still important. Alternatively, with a well localized lesion, radial sections may be cut to demonstrate margins.

Re-excision specimens

The original site of a lesion may need to be re-excised if the histopathology has shown that the margins are

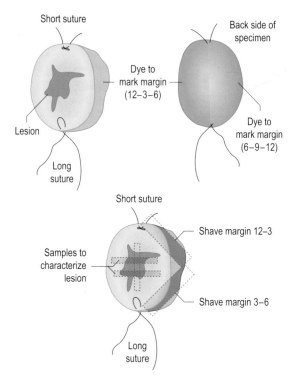

Fig. 5.5 Oriented specimens are submitted to diagnose the lesion and to ensure the lesion has been removed completely. The specimen should be inked on its deep margins to the edge of the surface of the skin. Specimens approximating an ellipse can be oriented like a clock with a specific orientation at 12 (e.g. short suture). Four shave margins can then conveniently be taken from 12 to 3, 3 to 6, 6 to 9, and 9 to 12, according to the time on a clock face. Next, sections to represent the lesion can be obtained so that a transition between uninvolved skin and the lesion is taken. Also, one cut of the lesion should demonstrate its deepest point of invasion.

invaded by tumor, or are too close to the tumor in the case of a melanoma or basal cell carcinoma. The evaluation of the area of the scar determines whether the original excision was adequate. A wide re-excision is often performed for melanomas even if the margins of the original excision are histopathologically free of tumor. This re-excision is performed because there is rapid and extensive radial spread of melanomas from the original primary and this may produce satellite lesions. In all re-excisions the scar is evaluated carefully to determine if residual disease is present, and the new

margins are evaluated for surface, satellite, and metastatic tumors.

NON-SKIN SPECIMENS

Excisional biopsies

Operative specimens may be tumors, unidentifiable inflammatory masses, tissues removed prior to transplantation, traumatic, congenital malformations, or cosmetic surgical specimens. Evaluation of tumors or masses requires the greatest attention to detail; nevertheless, all specimens must be examined carefully because even cosmetic specimens and tissues removed as part of transplantation may harbor unsuspected malignant tumors. Excision specimens from areas other than skin can be complex. Tumor specimens may be oriented just like excisional specimens of skin. In such cases, all surgical cuts are potential surgical margins and each surgical margin must be evaluated. This can follow the general approaches discussed under the section on skin excisions. It is necessary to orient the specimen correctly in order that the true margins are identified. The overall size of the tumor, depth of invasion into or through tissue walls, and the involvement of margins and lymph nodes are important determinants in neoplastic specimens.

The majority of specimens that are received unoriented can be easily identified, e.g. removal of a kidney. Others can be identified by their anatomical features, e.g. a colorectal adenocarcinoma of the cecum can be oriented by the ileocecal valve, section of ileum, the appendix, and the surgical cut across the ascending right side of the colon. Margins are the ileum, peritoneal area beneath the tumor, and the transection site of the ascending right colon. Other features to evaluate are involvement of lymph nodes, spread to peritoneal or pleural surfaces, and liver metastases.

PEDIATRIC SPECIMENS

The gross examination and processing of pediatric biopsies requires special care due to diagnostic difficulties of pediatric lesions/diseases (Debski et al 2004). Pediatric tumors are rare and some types appear histologically similar as 'small, round blue-cell tumors'; it is therefore often necessary to use immunohistochemistry, electron microscopy, flow cytometry, cytogenetics, and molecular genetics to confirm the diagnosis. These studies may require fresh, frozen or other specially processed tissues (see later chapters). Photographs of the gross specimen are taken marking clearly where tissues were selected for specialized techniques.

The specialized techniques required should be identified prior to the final resection in order that optimal tissue handling is performed. An initial working diagnosis is based on the demographics of the patient, clinical presentation, laboratory results, radiographic features, and the histology of any biopsies. There may also be additional requirements for special studies needed for clinical trials under which the patient may be treated.

The College of American Pathologists and the UK Royal College of Pathologists have developed specific protocols for pediatric tumors including hepatoblastoma, neuroblastoma, Ewing's sarcoma, Wilms' tumor, retinoblastoma, and rhabdomyosarcoma (Devoe & Weidner 2000; Albert & Syed 2001; Peydro-Olaya et al 2003; Qualman et al 2003a, 2003b, 2005; Carpentieri et al 2005; Finegold et al 2006).

FIXATION FOR GROSSED SPECIMENS

Prior to processing to paraffin blocks, tissue specimens are placed in fixative, usually neutral buffered 10% formaldehyde or neutral buffered formalin (NBF) (see Chapter 6). Fixation preserves the morphology, minimizes the loss of molecular components, and prevents decomposition, autolysis, and microbial growth. It is important to ensure adequate fixation by covering the specimen with at least 10 times its volume of the fixative (Eltoum et al 2001a, 2001b). It may be necessary to replace the fixative with fresh solution when the specimen contains a high percentage of blood. Fixatives penetrate slowly, approximately 1 mm per hour; covering large specimens with fixative-soaked gauze or cloth may help penetration and reduce surface drying (Eltoum et al 2001a, 2001b; Grizzle et al 2001; Jones et al 2001). Large specimens may require fixation overnight. Inadequate fixation produces poor results with subsequent processing, embedding, cutting, and staining (Grizzle et al 2001; Jones et al 2001).

GROSS ONLY EXAMINATION

Some specimens are only examined grossly. Non-tissue examples include bullets, implants, and foreign bodies. It may be necessary medico-legally to maintain a chain of evidence for some of these and there should be a written procedure to ensure this. Tissues that are unlikely to require a detailed diagnosis and may be examined grossly to reduce costs include tonsils, traumatic injuries, teeth, and incidental resections such as ribs, fat, and vessels. Organizations have guidelines to deal with non-diagnostic specimens and these are followed as well as national and other regulatory guidelines. Tissues removed secondary to traumatic injuries require photographic documentation using standard operating procedures (SOPs).

VERBAL REPORTS

The final diagnostic report signed by the pathologist is ideal but such reports are not always provided fast enough to meet the surgeon's needs, so verbal reports are occasionally necessary. These can be from an operating room consultation on frozen sections or the report of an urgent biopsy specimen. Problems can arise with accuracy such as patient misidentification and interpretive errors, so the SOPs for the laboratory should be followed and all verbal contacts clearly documented. It is important in practice to make sure one reaches the appropriate person to report to by phone and, if they are not available, document with whom you spoke. Verbal reports should be immediately followed by written confirmation (e-mail or fax).

SAFETY

The histopathology area is potentially one of the higher injury-risk areas of the hospital, even after safety risks have been minimized (Grizzle & Fredenburgh 2001; Grizzle et al 2005) (see Chapter 2). Staff working in the gross room encounter many possible risks including infection, chemicals that may be flammable, toxic, allergenic, or carcinogenic, electrical and physical hazards as well as cuts and needlestick injuries. Formaldehyde is one of the most common hazards in this area (see p. 27). Safety within a laboratory is the responsibility of the safety committee, which develops a safety plan administered by a safety officer (Grizzle & Fredenburgh 2001; Grizzle et al 2005). Each institution has different safety rules, but the most commonly used in all areas are as follows (Grizzle & Fredenburgh 2001; Grizzle et al 2005):

- Treat all tissues/specimens with universal precautions
- Wear aprons or disposable gowns in the grossing laboratory
- Wear gloves when handling or processing specimens
- Wear facemask and goggles when handling or processing specimens
- Clean all instruments with a disinfectant
- Do not touch 'clean' areas (e.g. telephone receiver) when wearing gloves
- Dispose of gowns, facemasks, eye protection, and gloves in a designated area before you leave contaminated areas
- Wash hands frequently
- Minimize contact (skin and vapors) with chemicals; be aware of toxicities of chemicals in the workplace.

By following these steps, obtaining training in safety, and following the requirements of the safety manual, employees of a pathology department can minimize their exposure to safety hazards. Safety for all employees should be the most important concern for any institution.

Note

This chapter discusses the most important issues related to the operation of a gross room. Each laboratory will have written standards and procedures of their own. Following standard operating procedures minimizes risks and produces the best results.

REFERENCES

Albert D., Syed N. (2001) Protocol for the examination of specimens from patients with retinoblastoma: a basis for checklists. Archives of Pathology and Laboratory Medicine 125:1183–1188.

Carpentieri D.F., Qualman S.J., Bowen J. et al. (2005) Protocol for the examination of specimens from pediatric and adult patients with osseous and extra-osseous Ewing sarcoma family of tumors, including peripheral primitive neuroectodermal tumor and Ewing sarcoma. Archives of Pathology and Laboratory Medicine 129:866–873.

Debski R.F., Rutledge J.C., Kapur F.P. (2004) A plea for the masses: a gross room approach to pediatric tumors. Journal of Histotechnology 27(4):221–228.

Devoe K., Weidner N. (2000) Immunohistochemistry of small round-cell tumors. Seminars in Diagnostic Pathology 17:216–224.

Eltoum I., Fredenburgh J., Myers R.B., Grizzle W.E. (2001a) Introduction to the theory and practice of fixation of tissues. Journal of Histotechnology 24(3):173–190.

Eltoum I., Fredenburgh J., Grizzle W.E. (2001b) Advanced concepts in fixation: effects of fixation on imunohistochemistry, reversibility of fixation and recovery of proteins, nucleic acid, and other molecules from fixed and processed tissues, developmental methods of fixation. Journal of Histotechnology 24(3): 201–210.

Finegold M.J., Lopez-Terrada D, Bowen J. et al. (2007) Protocol for the examination of specimens from pediatric patients with hepatoblastoma. Archives of Pathology and Laboratory Medicine 131(4):520–529.

Grizzle W.E., Fredenburgh, J. (2001) Avoiding biohazards in medical, veterinary and research laboratories. Biotechnic and Histochemistry 76(4):183–206.

Grizzle W.E., Sexton K.C. (1999) Development of a facility to supply human tissues to aid in medical research. In: Srivastava S., Henson D.E., Gazdar A., eds. Molecular pathology of early cancer. Van Diemenstratt, Amsterdam, the Netherlands: IOS Press, Ch. 24, pp. 371–383.

Grizzle W.E., Aamodt R., Clausen K. et al. (1998) Providing human tissues for research: how to establish a program. Archives of Pathology and Laboratory Medicine 122(12): 1065–1076.

Grizzle W.E., Stockard C.R., Billings, P.E. (2001) The effects of tissue processing variables other than fixation on histochemical staining and immunohistochemical detection of antigens. Journal of Histotechnology 24(3):213–219.

Grizzle W.E., Bell W., Fredenburgh J. (2005) Safety in biomedical and other laboratories. In: Patrinos G., Ansorg W., eds. Molecular diagnostics, Ch. 33, pp. 421–428.

Jones W.T., Stockard C.R., Grizzle W.E. (2001) Effects of time and temperature during attachment of sections to microscope slides on immunohistochemical detection of antigens. Biotechnic and Histochemistry 76(2): 55–58.

Manne U., Weiss H.L., Myers R.B. et al. (1998) Nuclear accumulation of p53 in colorectal adenocarcinoma: prognostic importance differs with race and location of the tumor. Cancer 83(12):2456–2467.

Peydro-Olaya A., Llombart-Bosch A, Carda-Batalla C., Lopez-Guerrero J.A. (2003) Electron microscopy and other ancillary techniques in the diagnosis of small round cell tumors. Seminars in Diagnostic Pathology 20: 25–45.

Qualman S.J., Bowen J., Amin M.B. et al. (2003a) Protocols for the examination of specimens from patients with Wilms tumor (nephroblastoma) or other renal tumors of childhood. Archives of Pathology and Laboratory Medicine 127:1280–1289.

Qualman S.J., Bowen J., Parham D.M. et al. (2003b) Protocol for the examination of specimens from patients (children and young adults) with rhabdomyosarcoma. Archives of Pathology and Laboratory Medicine 127: 1290–1297.

Qualman S.J., Bowen J., Fitzgibbons P.L. et al. (2005) Protocol for the examination of specimens from patients with neuroblastoma and related neuroblastic tumors. Archives of Pathology and Laboratory Medicine 129:874–883.

6

Tissue Processing

Lena T. Spencer and John D. Bancroft

INTRODUCTION

After the removal of a tissue sample from the patient, a series of processes must take place to ensure the final microscope slides are of a diagnostic quality. Tissues are exposed to a series of reagents that fix, dehydrate, clear, and infiltrate, with final embedding in a medium that provides support for the tissue. The quality of the structural preservation of tissue components is determined by the choice of reagent and exposure times to the reagents during processing. Each step in the tissue processing is important from procurement of the specimen and the selection of the sample, determining the appropriate protocols and reagents to use, to staining and final diagnosis. Producing quality slides for diagnosis is not an accident; it requires skills that are developed through continued practice and experience. As new technology and instrumentation develops, the role of the histology laboratory in patient care will continue to evolve.

Labeling of tissues

A unique identification number or code is assigned to the tissue sample accessioned in the laboratory. This number may be electronically or manually generated and should accompany the specimens throughout the entire laboratory process, including documentation in the pathology report. Recent technology has made bar code and character recognition systems readily available to most laboratories. Automated pre-labeling systems that permanently etch or emboss tissue cassettes and slides, as well as chemically resistant pens, pencils, slides, and labels, are routinely used in pathology laboratories. Regardless of whether an automated or manual labeling

system is used, adequate policies and procedures have to be in place to ensure positive identification of the tissue blocks and slides during processing, diagnosis, and filing.

Completion of fixation before processing

Fixation is the most important step in the processing of the tissue sample. If fixation is not complete prior to processing, stations should be designated on the processor for this purpose. If tissue is inadequately fixed, the subsequent dehydration solutions may complete the process, possibly altering the staining characteristics of the tissue. The size and type of specimen in the tissue cassette determines the time needed for complete fixation and processing. The tissue should be dissected to 3–4 mm in thickness; a rule of thumb for most specimens is the size of a small 'coin'. Care must be taken not to overfill the cassette during gross dissection, impeding the flow of reagents around the tissue. If possible, larger or smaller pieces of tissue should be separated and processed using different schedules.

Post-fixation treatment

Special fixation techniques may require additional steps before processing is initiated. Picric acid fixatives form water-soluble picrates making it necessary to place the tissue cassettes directly into 70% alcohol for processing. Alcoholic fixatives, such as Carnoy's fluid, should be placed directly into 100% alcohol. To help in the visualization of small fragments of tissue during embedding, a few drops of 1% eosin can be added to the specimen container 30 minutes prior to processing. The pink coloration of the tissue remains during processing, but washes out during subsequent staining.

PRINCIPLES OF TISSUE PROCESSING

Tissue processing is designed to remove all extractable water from the tissue, replacing it with a support medium that provides sufficient rigidity to enable sectioning of the tissue without damage or distortion.

Stages of tissue processing are:

- dehydration: removal of water and fixative from the tissue
- clearing: removal of dehydrating solutions, making the tissue components receptive to the infiltrating medium
- infiltrating: permeating the tissue with a support medium
- embedding: orienting the tissue sample in a support medium and allowing it to solidify.

Factors influencing the rate of processing

When tissue is immersed in fluid, interchange occurs between the fluid within the tissue and the surrounding fluid. Several factors, discussed below, influence the rate at which interchange occurs.

Agitation

The rate of fluid exchange is dependent upon the exposed surface of the tissue that is in contact with the processing reagent. Agitation increases the flow of fresh solutions around the tissue. Automated processors incorporate vertical or rotary oscillation or pressurized removal and replacement of fluids at timed intervals as the mechanism for agitation. Efficient agitation can reduce the overall processing time by 30%.

Heat

Heat increases the rate of penetration and fluid exchange. It must be used sparingly to reduce the possibility of shrinkage, hardening, and brittleness of the tissue. Temperatures limited to 45°C can be used effectively; higher temperatures may be deleterious to subsequent immunohistochemical staining.

Viscosity

Viscosity is the property of resistance to the flow of a fluid. The smaller the size of the molecules in the solution, the faster the rate of fluid penetration (low viscosity). Conversely, if the molecular size is larger, the rate of exchange is slower (high viscosity). Most of the solutions used in processing, dehydrates and clearants, have similar viscosities, with the exception of cedar wood oil. Embedding mediums have varying viscosities. Paraffin has a lower viscosity in the fluid (melted) state, enhancing the rapidity of the impregnation.

Vacuum

Using reduced pressure to increase the rate of infiltration decreases the time necessary to complete each step in the processing of tissue samples. Vacuum will remove reagents from the tissue only if they are more volatile than the reagent it is replacing. Vacuum used on the automated processor should not exceed 15 inches of Hg (mercury) to prevent damage and deterioration to the tissue. Vacuum can aid in the removal of trapped air in porous tissue. Impregnation time of dense, fatty tissue can be greatly reduced with the addition of vacuum during processing.

Fixation

Preserving cells and tissue components with minimal distortion is the most important step in the processing of tissue samples and is discussed in detail in Chapter 4. Fixation stabilizes proteins, rendering the cell and its components resistant to further autolysis by inactivating lysosomal enzymes, and changes the tissues receptiveness to further processing. Fixation must be complete before subsequent steps in the processing schedule are initiated.

DEHYDRATION

The first stage of processing is the removal of unbound water and aqueous fixatives from the tissue components. Many dehydrating reagents are hydrophilic ('water loving'), possessing strong polar groups that interact with the water molecules in the tissue. Other reagents affect dehydration by repeated dilution of the aqueous tissue fluids. Dehydration should be accomplished slowly. If the concentration gradient between the fluid inside and outside the tissue is excessive, diffusion currents cross the cell membranes during fluid exchange, increasing the possibility of cell distortion. For this reason specimens are always processed through a graded series of reagents of increasing concentration. Excessive dehydration may cause the tissue to become hard, brittle, and shrunken. Incomplete dehydration will prohibit the penetration of the clearing reagents into the tissue, leaving the specimen soft and non-receptive to infiltration. There are numerous dehydrating agents: ethanol, ethanol acetone, methanol, isopropyl, glycol, and denatured alcohols. If the dehydrant of choice is ethanol, the tissue is first immersed in 70% ethanol in water, followed by 95% and 100% solutions. For delicate tissue it is recommended that the processing start in 30% ethanol.

Dehydrating fluids

Ethanol C_2H_5OH

This is a clear, colorless, flammable liquid. It is hydrophilic, miscible with water and other organic solvents, fast acting, and reliable. Ethanol is taxable, controlled by the federal government, and requires careful record keeping. Graded concentrations of ethanol are used for dehydration. Ethanol ensures total dehydration, making it the reagent of choice for the processing of electron microscopy specimens.

Industrial methylated spirit (denatured alcohol)

This has the same physical properties as ethanol. Denatured alcohol consists of ethanol, with the addition of methanol (about 1%), isopropyl alcohol, or a combination of alcohols. For purposes of tissue processing it is used in the same manner as ethanol.

Methanol

This is a clear, colorless and flammable fluid which is highly toxic; it is miscible with water, ethanol, and most organic solvents. It can be substituted for ethanol.

Propan-2-ol, isopropyl alcohol $CH_3CHOHCH_3$

Isopropyl alcohol is miscible with water, ethanol, and most organic solvents. It is often used in microwave processing schedules. Isopropyl alcohol does not cause over-hardening or shrinkage of the tissue.

Butyl alcohol (butanol)

This is used primarily for plant and animal histology; it is a slow dehydrant with less shrinkage and hardening of the tissue.

Acetone CH_3COCH_3

Acetone is a clear, colorless, flammable fluid, miscible with water, ethanol, and most organic solvents. It is rapid in action, with poor penetration, and causes brittleness in tissues if use is prolonged. Acetone removes lipids from tissue during processing.

Additives to dehydrating agents

When added to dehydrating agents, phenol acts as a softening agent for hard tissues such as tendon, nail, dense fibrous tissue, and keratin masses. A 4% solution is added to each of the 95% ethanol stations. Alternatively, hard tissue can be immersed in a glycerol–alcohol mixture.

Universal solvents

Universal solvents dehydrate and clear during tissue processing. Dioxane, tertiary butanol, and tetrahydrofuran are considered to be universal solvents; they are not recommended for processing delicate tissues due to their hardening properties (Carson 1977; Sheehan & Hrapchak 1980). For safety issues see Chapter 2.

CLEARING

A clearing reagent acts as an intermediary between the dehydration and infiltration solutions. It should be miscible with both solutions. Most clearants are hydrocarbons with refractive indices similar to protein. When the dehydrating agent has been entirely replaced by most of these solvents the tissue has a translucent appearance, hence the term 'clearing agent'.

The criteria for choosing a suitable clearing agent are:

- rapid removal of dehydrating agent
- ease of removal by melted paraffin
- minimal tissue damage
- flammability
- toxicity
- cost.

Most clearing agents are flammable liquids, which warrants caution in their use. The boiling point of the clearing agent gives an indication of its speed of replacement by melted paraffin. Fluids with a low boiling point are generally more readily replaced. Viscosity influences the speed of penetration of the clearing agent. Prolonged exposure to most clearing agents causes the tissue to become brittle. The time in the clearing agent should be closely monitored to ensure that dense tissue blocks are sufficiently cleared and smaller, more fragile, tissue blocks are not damaged (Carson 1977; Sheehan & Hrapchak 1980; Luna 1992). Cost should be considered, especially as it relates to disposal of the reagent. Since most clearing agents are aromatic hydrocarbons or short-chain aliphatic hydrocarbons, environmental issues have to be addressed. Most institutions have a policy for the storage, disposal, and safety requirements for all flammables used in the laboratory.

Clearing agents suitable for routine use

Xylene

A flammable, colorless, liquid with a characteristic petroleum or aromatic odor, miscible with most organic solvents and paraffin. Suitable for blocks that are less than 5 mm in thickness. Over-exposure during processing will cause over-hardening. Xylene is commonly used in routine histology laboratories and is recyclable.

Toluene

Similar properties to xylene, although it is less damaging with prolonged immersion of tissue. It is flammable and more volatile than xylene.

Chloroform

Chloroform is slower in action than xylene but causes less brittleness. Thicker tissue blocks can be processed, greater than 1 mm in thickness. Tissues placed in chloroform do not become translucent. It is non-flammable but highly toxic, and phosgene gas is given off when chloroform is heated. Often used when processing specimens of the central nervous system.

Methyl benzoate and methyl salicylate

These are slow-acting clearing agents and can be used when double embedding techniques are required.

Citrus fruit oils—limonene reagents

Limonene reagents are extracts from orange and lemon rinds; they are non-toxic and miscible with water. Disposal is dependent upon the water treatment center's standards at the site of the laboratory. Their main disadvantages are a strong pungent odor and small tissue deposits of minerals such as copper or calcium, which may dissolve.

Safety

Safe handling of common histological chemicals is discussed in Chapter 2. Every histology laboratory should have a chemical hygiene plan that incorporates specific work practices to protect workers from potentially hazardous chemicals. Information sheets should be available for all the chemicals used in the laboratory. The basic information includes exposure limits, target organs, storage, disposal, and how to handle spills. These sheets are placed in an easily accessible place for quick reference.

RECYCLING REAGENTS

Distillation equipment is used in many laboratories to recycle alcohol and xylene using fractional distillation heat to separate different waste products in the solvents by boiling points; the component with the highest boiling point is purified.

Advantages include:

- reduced cost
- rapid
- efficient
- eliminates the need to have chemicals removed by a waste disposal company, and
- environmentally unsafe chemicals are not being sent to land-fills for disposal.

The recycled reagents must be tested for quality (Dapson & Dapson 2005).

PARAFFIN WAX

Paraffin continues to be the most popular infiltration and embedding medium in the histology laboratory. The tissue is impregnated with wax, which forms a matrix preventing tissue structure distortion during microtomy. Paraffin wax has a wide range of melting points, which is important for use in the different climatic regions of the world. It is inexpensive, provides quality sections, and is easily adaptable to a variety of uses. It can be used for most routine and special stains.

Paraffin wax properties

Paraffin wax is a mixture of long-chain hydrocarbons produced in the cracking of mineral oil. Its properties are varied depending on the melting point; low melting point paraffin is usually softer, higher melting point paraffin is usually harder, which can effect microtomy. Melting points range from 40 to 70°C. Heating the paraffin to a high temperature alters the properties of the wax. To promote good ribboning during microtomy, paraffin wax of suitable hardness at room temperature should be chosen.

Paraffin wax additives

Paraffin waxes that contain plasticizers or other resin additives are commercially available, providing a selection that is appropriate for most laboratories. These mixtures create paraffin with the desired hardness for the tissue to be embedded. Substances that were added to paraffin in the past included beeswax, rubber, ceresin, plastic polymers, and diethylene glycol distearate. Many of these additives have a higher melting point than paraffin wax, consequently making the tissue more brittle.

Embedding tissue in paraffin wax

Embedding involves the enclosing of properly processed, correctly oriented specimens in a support medium that provides external support during microscopy. The embedding medium must fill all the spaces within the tissue, supporting cellular components. It should provide elasticity, resisting section distortion while facilitating sectioning.

Most laboratories use embedding centers, consisting of three modules: a paraffin dispenser, a cold plate, and a heated storage area for molds and tissue cassettes. Paraffin is dispensed automatically from a nozzle into a suitably sized mold. The tissue is oriented in the mold; a cassette is attached, producing a flat block face with parallel sides. The mold is placed on a small cooling area to allow the paraffin to solidify. The quick cooling of the wax ensures a small crystalline structure, producing fewer artifacts when sectioning the tissue.

The advantages of using an embedding system are:

- ease of use
- speed
- tissue and holder are firmly attached, creating a single unit
- blocks filed immediately after sectioning
- permanent identification.

Cassettes and molds that accommodate larger or smaller specimens may be purchased from scientific supply companies.

Quality control

Temperature of all paraffin dispensers, flotation water baths, and automated processors are carefully monitored and documented. The histology laboratory should have a policy and procedure manual that addresses quality issues and corrective actions.

Orientation of tissues

Specimen orientation during embedding is important for the demonstration of proper morphology. Improper orientation may result in diagnostic tissue elements being damaged during microscopy (see Chapter 5). Products are available that help ensure proper orientation: marking systems, tattoo dyes, biopsy bags, sponges, and papers.

Orientation of the tissue should offer the least resistance of the tissue against the knife during sectioning. Most tissue are embedded flat; the margin of embedding medium around the tissue will assure support of the tissue.

Tissues requiring special orientation include:

- Tubular structures: arteries, veins, fallopian tubes, and vas deferens—cut in cross-section of the lumen.
- Skin, intestine, gallbladder, and other epithelial biopsies—cut in a plane at right angles to the surface, and oriented so the epithelial surface is cut last, minimizing compression and distortion of the epithelial layer.
- Muscle biopsies—sections containing both transverse and longitudinal planes.
- Multiple pieces of a tissue—oriented side by side with the epithelial surface facing in the same direction.

AUTOMATED TISSUE PROCESSING

The basic principle for tissue processing requires the exchange of fluids using a series of solutions for a predetermined length of time in a controlled environment. For decades instrumentation used in tissue processing was relatively unchanged. Recent advances now include specialty microwave ovens and the emergence of constant through-put processors.

Tissue processors

The carousel-type processor (tissue transfer) and the self-contained fluid exchange systems were the first automated tissue processors used in the histology laboratory. This type of processor transported tissue blocks contained in baskets through a series of reagents housed in stationary containers. The length of time the specimens were submerged in each reagent container was electronically programmed. Earlier models accomplished this step by notching the face of a clock disc. Vertical oscillation or the mechanical raising and lowering of the tissue into the reagent containers provided the agitation needed for the processing of the tissue.

The enclosed, self-contained vacuum tissue processor later became the mainstay in most laboratories. A microprocessor is used to program the instrument. Tissues are loaded into a retort chamber where they remain throughout the process. Reagents and melted paraffin are moved sequentially into and out of the retort chamber using vacuum and pressure. Each step is customized by adding time, temperature, or vacuum/pressure. The advantages of this system are that vacuum and heat can be applied at any stage, customized schedules for tissue processing produced, fluid spillage contained, and fumes eliminated. These processors employ alarm systems and diagnostic programs for trouble-shooting instrumentation malfunction.

Specially designed microwave ovens for tissue processing are now common. The microwave oven shortens the processing time from hours to minutes. Microwave exposure stimulates the diffusion of the solutions into the tissue by increasing the internal heat of the specimen, accelerating the reaction time. Tissues are manually transferred from container to container of reagent. Most laboratory microwave ovens contain precise temperature controls, timers, and fume extraction systems. The time for processing is dependent on the thickness and density of the specimen. Reagents used for microwave processing include ethanol, isopropanol or proprietary mixtures of alcohol, and paraffin. Graded concentration of solutions is not required. Clearing agents are not necessary because the temperature of the final paraffin step facilitates evaporation of the alcohols from the tissue. Xylene and formalin are not used in this process, which eliminates toxic fumes and carcinogens. Properly controlled processing provides uncompromised morphology and antigenicity of the specimens. Increased efficiency through improved turnaround times, environmentally friendly reagents, and greater profitability due to reduction in number and volume of reagents, are advantages of this system. Disadvantages of the system are: the process is labor intensive because the solutions are manually manipulated, the cost of laboratory-grade microwaves may be prohibitive, and proper use of the microwave oven requires calibration and monitoring (Kok & Boon 1992; Willis & Minshew 2005).

Recent advances in technology have led to the development of an enclosed processor, called a continuous input, rapid tissue processor, that uses microwave technology, vacuum infiltration, and proprietary reagents described as being 'molecular-friendly'. The tissue cassettes are moved through four stations that contain acetone, isopropanol, polyethylene glycol, mineral oil, and paraffin. Microwaves and agitation are used to accelerate the diffusion of solvents in the tissue. A patented microwave technology is utilized operating at a continuous low power instead of pulsing high levels of microwave energy. The advantage of this system is the acceptance of tissues into the system at timed intervals, improving turnaround time. The reagents used are environmentally safe, eliminating toxic vapors in the laboratory. The morphology and quality of the specimens is consistent with that of traditional tissue processing. Disadvantages include the cost of the processor and that grossing of the tissue sample requires standardized specimen dissection (Morales et al 2004).

Processor maintenance

Every institution should have a policy outlining the rotation and changing of solutions for each tissue processor. The numbers, sizes, types of tissue processed and the reagents used will play a role in the determination of this policy. Solutions should be carefully monitored to ensure quality. Every manufacturer has a handbook outlining a preventive maintenance schedule.

Important maintenance tips

- Any spillage or overflow should be wiped away immediately
- Accumulation of wax on any surface should be removed
- Temperature of the paraffin bath should be set to 3°C above the melting point of the paraffin
- Timing should be checked when placing tissue cassettes in the processor, especially when delayed schedules are selected.

Advantages of the newer technology in processing:

- Custom programs specific to tissues being processed; addition of vacuum, agitation, or heat at any stage
- Rapid schedules
- Fluid and fume containment
- Environmentally friendly reagents
- Delay schedules.

Automated processing schedules

Overnight schedules for tissue processing are still popular in laboratories, but schedules have changed to reflect the emphasis on reducing turnaround time for the specimen. Rapid processing for small biopsies or stat specimens is easily accommodated.

Overnight processing

For many laboratories, this is considered the routine processing schedule. Tissues continue fixation by being submerged in 10% formalin, buffered or unbuffered. The process may include alcoholic formalin, varying concentrations of alcohol, xylene, or a xylene substitute, followed by infiltration in paraffin.

Schedules are customized for the tissues being processed; factors influencing the processing schedule include the end-time required, reagents used, the inclusion of heat and vacuum, the size and number of tissues. The schedule in Table 6.1 can be modified, adjusting times from the various stations, keeping in mind the end-time needed for completion and prior fixation.

Specialized tissues

Tissues such as brain, eyes, and bone require specialized processing (see Chapter 19 for brain, Chapters 18 and 29 for bone). A schedule for eyes is shown in Table 6.2.

Table 6.1	Overnight processing			
Station	Reagents	Time	Pressure/Vacuum	Temp
1	10% Formalin	1 h	On	38° C
2	10% Formalin	1 h	On	38°C
3	50% Alcohol/formalin	1 h	On	38°C
4	70% Alcohol	30 min	On	38°C
5	95% Alcohol	30 min	On	38°C
6	95% Alcohol	40 min	On	38°C
7	100% Alcohol	40 min	On	38°C
8	100% Alcohol	40 min	On	38°C
9	Xylene	40 min	On	38°C
10	Xylene	40 min	On	38°C
11	Paraffin	30 min	On	60°C
12	Paraffin	20 min	On	60°C
13	Paraffin	20 min	On	60°C
14	Paraffin	40 min	On	60°C

Schedule for processing eyes

Eyes require special processing; this is dictated by the delicate nature of some parts of the structures and toughness of others. Ideally, a separate processor should be dedicated for tissues that require special handling because of the reagents used. The eye must be thoroughly fixed, prior to dissection and subsequent processing. Phenol is added to the lower percentage alcohols to soften the sclera and lens. Reagents are selected that provide the best dehydration and clearing of the tissue (chloroform has been used as the clearing agent because it is less harsh than xylene and causes minimal shrinkage), keeping the retina attached. Large tissue cassettes and molds are specifically made for use in processing eyes.

Rapid processing schedules for small biopsies

Recently excised endoscopic biopsies and needle biopsies can be adequately processed in 2–5 hours using heat (37–45°C) and vacuum. Tissues requiring dissection should be trimmed to 2 mm in thickness. Most small specimens will fix prior to processing. If fixation is not complete, processing should begin in a station containing 10% formalin. Table 6.3 shows an example of a shortened process for an enclosed processor. The enclosed processor drain time is approximately 3–5 minutes at each station. The program can be amended, changing times at various stations; drain times should be taken into consideration when determining the end time. After each run the instrument must be cleaned to purge the lines of any residual paraffin. The clean cycle will flush the lines using xylene, 100% alcohol, and water.

MANUAL TISSUE PROCESSING

Manual tissue processing is rarely used today. There can be circumstances requiring the tissue sample to be manually processed, including:

- Power failure or equipment malfunction
- Large tissue samples requiring more time than can be allocated on an automated processor
- Small biopsies, such as transplant specimens, needing a rapid diagnosis.

Manual processing schedules

The schedule in Table 6.4 is adaptable for large, dense tissue blocks. Times should be extended in each container, or more containers may be added to the schedule.

Table 6.3 Short processing schedule for biopsies

Station	Reagents	Time	Pressure/ Vacuum	Temp
1	10% Formalin	10 min	On	38°C
2	10% Formalin	10 min	On	38°C
3	70% Alcohol	10 min	On	38°C
4	95% Alcohol	10 min	On	38°C
5	95% Alcohol	10 min	On	38°C
6	100% Alcohol	10 min	On	38°C
7	100% Alcohol	10 min	On	38°C
8	Xylene	10 min	On	38°C
9	Xylene	10 min	On	38°C
10	Paraffin	10 min	On	38°C
11	Paraffin	10 min	On	58°C

Table 6.2 Processing eyes

Station	Reagents	Time
1	10% Formalin	0 h
2	4% Phenol/70% Alcohol	1 h
3	4% Phenol/70% Alcohol	1 h
4	95% Alcohol	1 h
5	95% Alcohol	1 h
6	100% Alcohol	1.5 h
7	100% Alcohol	1.5 h
8	100% Alcohol/Chloroform	2 h
9	Chloroform	2 h
10	Chloroform	2 h
11	Paraffin	2 h
12	Paraffin	3 h

Table 6.4 Manual tissue processing for small biopsies

Step	Time
10% Formalin	10 min
95% Alcohol	10 min
100% Alcohol	10 min
Xylene	10 min
Paraffin	10 min

1. Place tissue in cassette. Drop cassette in 10% formalin. Formalin container placed under warm tap water.
2. Remove tissue cassette from formalin and place in container with 95% alcohol, on a stir plate with a stir bar.
3. Continue through 100% alcohol and xylene using stir plate and stir bar.
4. Place tissue cassette in melted paraffin.
5. Embed as usual.

ALTERNATIVE EMBEDDING MEDIA

There are occasions when paraffin is an unsuitable medium for the type of section required, including:

- Processing reagents remove or destroy tissue components, the object of investigation
- Sections are required to be thinner
- The use of heat may adversely affect tissue
- The infiltrating medium is not sufficiently hard to support the tissue.

Resin

Resin is used exclusively as the embedding medium for electron microscopy (see Chapter 30), ultra-thin sectioning for high resolution and for undecalcified bone (see Chapters 18 and 29).

Agar

Agar gel alone does not provide sufficient support for sectioning of tissues. Its main use is as a cohesive agent for small friable pieces of tissue after fixation. Fragments of tissue are embedded in melted agar, allowed to solidify, and trimmed for routine processing. One method providing superior results is as follows: filter the fixative with the tissue fragments through a Millipore filter using suction, carefully pour melted agar into the tube, allow solidification of the agar, and follow with routine processing and embedding in paraffin.

Gelatin

Gelatin is used primarily in the production of sections of whole organs in the Gough-Wentworth technique and in frozen sectioning.

Celloidin

The use of celloidin or LVN (low viscosity nitrocellulose) is discouraged because of the special requirements

needed to house the processing reagents and the limited use these types of section have in neuropathology. It is included here for historical purposes only.

Restoration of tissue dried in processing

Despite precautions taken during processing, technical or mechanical malfunctions may occur, resulting in tissue drying out prior to paraffin impregnation. The tissue will never be regarded as normal, but the following treatment may help provide slides of diagnostic quality.

Tissue restoration

70% ethanol	70 ml
Glycerol	30 ml
Dithionite	1 g

Tissues remain in the solution for several hours or overnight. Processing begins with the dehydrating solutions and continues to completion. Tissue may be difficult to section; coated or plus slides should be used.

Summary

Technological advances have been made in the instrumentation of tissue processors, in part due to increased workload, the demand for faster turnaround time for diagnostic samples, and shortages in the workforce. The addition of microprocessors, microwaves, and environmentally friendly chemicals are only a few of the improvements that will eventually revolutionize tissue processing.

Acknowledgments

This chapter is a development of the chapter that appeared in the first five editions. In those editions, Tissue processing was written by Keith Gordon and Paul Bradbury, with successful merging for later editions by Graeme Anderson and John Bancroft. Our acknowledgments go to the previous contributors.

REFERENCES

Carson F.L. (1977) Histotechnology, a self-instructional text, 2nd edn. Chicago: ASCP Press, pp. 26–42.

Dapson J.C., Dapson R.W. (2005) Hazardous materials in the histopathology laboratory, regulations, risks, handling and disposal, 4th edn. Battle Creek, MI: Anatech, pp. 157–164.

Kok L.P., Boon M.E. (1992) Microwave cookbook of microscopists, 3rd edn. Leiden: Coulomb Press.

Luna L.G. (1992) Histopathologic methods and color atlas of special stains and tissue artifacts. Downers Grove: Johnson Printers, pp. 1–66.

Morales A.R., Nassiri M., Kanhoush R. et al. (2004) Experience with an automated microwave-assisted rapid tissue processing method: validation of histologic quality and impact on the timeliness of diagnostic surgical pathology. American Journal of Clinical Pathology 121:528–536.

Sheehan D.C., Hrapchak B. (1980) Theory and practice of histotechnology, 2nd edn. St Louis: C.V. Mosby, pp. 59–85.

Vernon S.E. (2005) Continuous throughput rapid tissue processing revolutionizes histopathology workflow. Laboratory Medicine 36:300–302.

Willis D., Minshew J. (2005) The whole enchilada with the rice and beans. Ft. Lauderdale: National Society for Histotechnology.

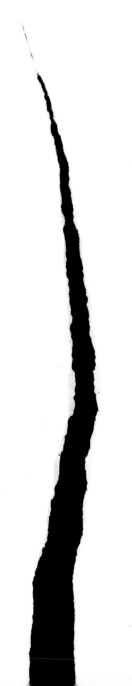

7

Microtomy: Paraffin and Frozen

Lena T. Spencer and John D. Bancroft

MICROTOMY

Microtomy is the means by which tissue can be sectioned and attached to a surface for further microscopic examination. Most microtomy is performed on paraffin-embedded tissue blocks. The basic instrument used in microtomy is the microtome; an advancing mechanism moves the object (paraffin block) for a predetermined distance until it is in contact with the cutting tool (knife or blade). The specimen moves vertically past the cutting surface producing a tissue section. Good technique is mastered through continuous practice.

Types of microtome

There are several types of microtome, each designed for a specific purpose, although many have multifunctional roles.

Rotary microtome

The rotary microtome is often referred to as the 'Minot' after its inventor. The basic mechanism requires the rotation of a fine advance hand-wheel through 360°, moving the specimen vertically past the cutting surface and returning it to the starting position. The rotary microtome may be: manual (completely manipulated by the operator), semi-automated (one motor to advance either the fine or coarse hand-wheel), or fully automated (two motors that drive both the fine and the coarse advance hand-wheel). The mechanism for block advancement may be retracting or non-retracting. Advantages include: the ability to cut thin 2–3-mm sections, and easy adaptation to all types of tissue (hard, fragile, or fatty) sectioning (Mailhiot 2005).

Technological advances in the automation of microtomy have improved section quality, increased productivity, and improved occupational safety for the technologist. Eliminating manual hand-wheel operation of the microtome reduces the incidence of repetitive motion disorders, a common occupational health problem in the histology laboratory.

Base sledge microtome

With the sledge microtome, the specimen is held stationary and the knife slides across the top of the specimen during processing. Used primarily for large blocks, hard tissues, or whole mounts, it is especially useful in neuropathology and ophthalmic pathology. Three-micron sections are difficult to produce. Further information regarding sectioning of undecalcified bone is available in Chapters 18 and 29.

Rotary rocking microtome

Common in early cryostats, the retracting action moves the tissue block away from the knife on the upstroke, producing a flat face to the tissue block.

Sliding microtome

The knife or blade is stationary and the specimen slides under it during sectioning. This microtome was developed for use with celloidin-embedded tissue blocks.

Ultramicrotomes

Used almost exclusively for electron microscopy (Chapter 30).

Microtome knives

There are many shapes, sizes, and materials for microtome knives. Knives were developed to fit specific types of microtome and to cope with different degrees of hardness of tissues and embedding media. Most steel knives have been replaced with disposable blades; exceptions include the tool-edge knives for resin, and steel knives for some cryostats.

Disposable blades

The introduction of disposable blades has revolutionized microtomy in the laboratory. Disposal blades are used for routine microtomy and cryotomy, providing a sharp cutting edge that can produce flawless 2–4-mm sections. Disposable blade holders are incorporated into the microtome or an adaptor may be purchased. The blade is coated with a special PTFE (polytetrafluoroethylene), allowing ribbons to be sectioned with ease. Disposable blades are purchased in dispensers, a convenience feature. Over-tightening the disposable blade in the clamping device may cause cutting artifact, such as thick and thin sections. The clamping device must be clean and free of defects. During sectioning the handwheel must be turned slowly. Reliability of a constant sharp edge, ease of use, low or high profiles adaptable to a variety of tissue and paraffin types, and low cost relative to steel knife sharpening make these blades a mainstay in most laboratories.

Glass and diamond knives

Glass and diamond knives are used in electron microscopy and with plastic resin-embedded blocks.

PARAFFIN SECTION CUTTING

Equipment required

- Floatation (water) bath.
- Slide drying oven or hot plate.
- Fine pointed or curved forceps.
- Sable or camel haired brush.
- Scalpel.
- Slide rack.
- Clean slides.
- Teasing needle.
- Ice tray.
- Chemical resistant pencil or pen.

Floatation (water) bath

A thermostatically controlled water bath is used for floating out tissue ribbons after sectioning. The temperature of the water in the bath should be 10°C below the melting point of the paraffin to be sectioned. Care should be taken to prevent water bubbles from being trapped under the section; this can be accomplished by using distilled water in the bath. Alcohol or a small drop of detergent may be added to the water to reduce the surface tension, allowing the section to flatten out with greater ease.

Drying oven or hot plate

Drying ovens incorporate fans that keep the warm air circulating around the slides. The temperature setting should be approximately that of the melting point of the paraffin. If the oven is too hot there may be distortion to the cells, causing dark pyknotic nuclei or nuclear bubbling, and cells that are completely devoid of nuclear detail (Carson 1997). Drying time varies depending on the type of tissue, number of slides to be dried, and size of the drying device. Many automated stainers incorporate drying ovens as part of the instrument; the time and temperature are easily regulated.

Special care should be taken when drying delicate tissues or tissues from the central nervous system; a lower temperature is required to prevent splitting and cracking of the section (a recommendation is 37°C for 24 hours).

Brush and forceps

Forceps, brushes, or teasing needles are helpful in the removal of folds, creases, and bubbles that may form during the floating out of the section on the water bath. They are also helpful for manipulating the section as it passes across the edge of the blade.

Slides

For normal routine work, 76 × 25-mm slides are universally used. Although slides are available in a variety of thicknesses, those specified as 1.0–1.2 mm in thickness are preferred because they do not break as easily. Most slide racks are made to accommodate this slide size. Larger slides are available for use with specialty tissues such as eyes or brains.

Unique identification numbers or codes, patient name or other accessioning information should be etched, embossed, or written on each slide. Automated instruments that imprint the patient's information on the glass slide are readily available. Chemical resistant pens and pencils are routinely used to label the slide.

Slides that are positively charged or pre-treated with an adhesive resist detachment of the tissue from the slide during staining. Colored, frost-end slides may be used to identify special handling (decalcified, special stains, immunohistochemistry, etc.).

Section adhesives

Provided clean slides are used and sections are adequately dried, the problem of sections detaching from the slide during staining should not occur. There are occasions when sections may detach from the slide:

- Exposure to strong alkali solutions during staining
- Cryostat sections for immunofluorescence, immuno-histochemistry, or intraoperative diagnosis
- Central nervous system (CNS) tissues
- Sections are submitted to extreme temperatures
- Tissues containing blood and mucus
- Decalcified tissues.

Adhesives may alleviate the problem of tissue loss. Protein adhesives such as albumen, gelatin, and starch may be prone to bacterial overgrowth or heavy staining; close monitoring will prevent these problems. Adhesives that may be used include the following:

Poly-L-lysine

Poly-L-lysine is bought as a 0.1% solution which is further diluted for use, 1 in 10 with distilled water. Slides are coated with the diluted solution and allowed to dry. The effectiveness of the coating in adhering the tissue to the slide will diminish within a few days.

3-Aminopropyltriethoxysilane (APES)

Slides are dipped in a 2% solution of APES in acetone, drained, dipped in acetone, drained again. The process is complete when the slides are dipped in distilled water. Slides are placed upright in a rack to dry. These slides are useful for cytology, especially specimens that may be bloody or contain proteinaceous material.

Charged or plus slides

Laboratories use slides that have been manufactured with a permanent positive charge. Placing a positive charge on the slides is accomplished by coating the slide with a basic polymer in which a chemical reaction occurs leaving the amino groups linked by covalent bonds to the silicon atoms of the glass. These slides have proven to be superior in their resistance to cell and tissue loss during staining or pre-treatments such as enzyme and antigen retrieval.

Practical microtomy

The expertise that must be gained to become a competent microtomist cannot be achieved from textbooks. Practical experience under the guidance of a skilled tutor is the best way to gain the confidence and coordination necessary to manipulate the microtome and the sections produced. Techniques will be described, providing information and helpful hints for use during microscopy.

Setup of the microtome

Maintenance of the microtome is important to the production of quality slides for diagnosis. The manufacturer's recommendation regarding the proper care of the instrument should be closely followed. A departmental policy should be implemented outlining daily, weekly, quarterly, and yearly preventive maintenance procedures.

The water bath and the microtome should be ergonomically positioned to reduce stress and tension on the neck and shoulders.

The water bath may be filled with distilled or tap water, and adjusted to the proper temperature of the paraffin. Care should be taken to reduce air bubbles that may distort the tissue section.

The blade should be sharp and defect free. The blade or knife holder should be adjusted to optimize the clearance angle, the distance between the lower facet angle, and the surface of the block face. Clamps and screws must be firmly tightened. If a disposable blade is to be used, care should be taken to ensure enough pressure is being exerted on the blade to provide support, but not over-tightened causing thick and thin sectioning.

Sectioning

Trimming the tissue blocks

The paraffin block may be faced or 'rough cut' by setting the micrometer at 15–30 mm or by advancing the block using the coarse feed mechanism. Aggressive trimming will cause 'moth-holes' artifact. Care must be taken to ensure that the block clamped in the chuck has been retracted so there is no contact with the blade on the initial downstroke. It is possible to damage the tissue by gouging or scoring when trimming the block.

Cutting sections

Blocks should be arranged in numerical order on a cooling device, cooling both the tissue and the paraffin, giving them a similar consistency. A small amount of water is absorbed into the tissue, causing slight swelling, making sectioning easier. Over-soaking may cause expansion and distortion of the tissue section. Proper processing eliminates the need to pre-soak blocks. Routine surgical material should be cut at 3–4 microns. Experience will determine the speed of the stroke, but in general one should use a smooth, slow stroke. If there is difficulty cutting a smooth flat section, warming the block face with warm water or gently exhaling breath onto the block surface during sectioning may help. This has the effect of expanding the block, giving a slightly thicker section. Ideally, successive sections will stick edge-to-edge due to local pressure with each stroke, forming a ribbon. If the entire block is to be sectioned and retained, the ribbons are stored in a box for future use. Ribbons of sections are the most convenient way of handling sections. When a ribbon of several sections has been cut, the first section is held by forceps, or teasing needle, and the last section eased from the knife edge with a small brush.

Floating out sections

The floating out of the ribbon must be smooth, with the trailing end of the ribbon making contact with the water first. The slight drag produced when the rest of the ribbon is laid on the water is sufficient to remove most, if not all, of the folds that occur. Sections are floated on the water bath, shiny side down. Folds in the section may be removed by simply teasing with the forceps. Approximately 30 seconds should be long enough for a ribbon to flatten; prolonged time on the water causes excessive expansion, distorting the tissue. Individual sections or ribbons may be floated onto the slide.

Circular structures such as eyes are difficult to flatten. Various techniques are useful in these situations, such as placing the section on the slide that has been pre-flooded with 50% alcohol. The slide is gently immersed in the water bath and the section of eye will float on the surface. The presence of the alcohol will set up diffusion currents that help to flatten the tissue section. The water bath should be cleaned after each block is cut, removing debris and tissue fragments, by dragging tissue paper across the surface. Cleanliness cannot be over-emphasized: 'pick-up' material from different blocks presents a serious problem.

Drying sections

The small amount of water held under the section will allow further flattening to occur when heat is applied to dry the section. The temperature should be at the melting point of the paraffin. Many automated stainers include drying ovens as part of the instrumentation. Slides may be attached to the stainer with individual slide holders or in racks that are designed for the instrument. It is important to eliminate over-heating during the slide drying stage, cellular details may be compromised. Hot plates may cause localized overheating of the slide. When delicate tissues are to be dried, less distortion will occur if the temperature is reduced and the time prolonged. Overnight at 37°C is recommended for many tissues.

Cutting hard tissues

Since the introduction of disposable blades, cutting hard tissues is less problematic. The reason for cutting difficulties is more likely poor fixation or over-processing. Prolonged soaking of the block, or exposing the block surface to running tap water for 30 minutes, will often overcome many of the problems associated with cutting hard tissues. A slight reduction in the knife slant may also yield results. If these remedies fail, softening agents may be used on the surface of the block.

Surface decalcification

When small foci of calcium are present in the tissue section, cutting a quality section may be difficult. The block may be removed from the chuck after rough cutting of the tissue and placed face down in a dish that contains a small amount of decalcification solution.

The time for exposure to the decal will vary depending on the tissue; closely monitor the progress of the decal to determine endpoint. The block is rinsed well, blotted dry, and returned to the microtome. An immediate section should be taken since the decalcification achieved will be limited. Diagnostic materials may be compromised if over-decalcification occurs. It must be noted that the staining properties of the tissue will be affected after this treatment and allowances must be made to achieve optimal results.

Problems and solutions

Table 7.1 addresses the most common problems encountered during microtomy and possible solutions (Sheehan & Hrapchak 1980; Carson 1997; Anderson & Bancroft 2002).

Table 7.1   Problems and solutions for paraffin section

Causes	Solutions
Problem: Ribbon/consecutive sections curved	
1. Block edges not parallel	1. Trim block until parallel
2. Dull blade edge	2. Replace blade or move to a different area
3. Excessive paraffin	3. Trim away excess paraffin
4. Tissue varying in consistency	4. Re-orient block
Problem: Thick and thin sections	
1. Paraffin too soft for tissue or conditions	1. Remove excess paraffin from the edge of blade
2. Insufficient clearance angle	2. Maintain microtome—lubricate and calibrate. Check for obvious faults with microtome; parts may be worn
3. Faulty microtome mechanisms	3. Tighten block and blade
4. Blade or block loose in holder	4. Increase clearance angle
Problem: Chatter—thick and thin zones parallel to blade edge	
1. Knife or block loose in holder	1. Clean blade edge to remove excess paraffin
2. Excessively steep clearance angle or knife tilt	2. Replace or use new area of blade
3. Tissue or paraffin too hard for sectioning	3. Tighten the blade levers
4. Calcified areas in tissue	4. Reduce angle
5. Over-dehydration of tissue	5. Rehydrate and surface decalcify
6. Dull blade	6. Re-embed in fresh paraffin
Problem: Splitting of sections at right angles to knife edge	
1. Nicks in blade	1. Use different part of blade or replace
2. Hard particles in tissue	2. If calcium deposit—surface decal
3. Hard particles in paraffin	3. If mineral or other particle, remove with fine sharp-pointed scalpel
Problem: Sections will not form ribbons	
1. Paraffin too hard for sectioning conditions	1. Re-embed in lower melting point paraffin
2. Debris on knife edge	2. Warm surface of block
3. Clearance angle incorrect	3. Clean blade and back of blade holder
	4. Adjust to optimal angle
Problem: Sections attach to block on return stroke	
1. Insufficient clearance angle	1. Increase clearance angle
2. Debris on blade edge	2. Clean blade edge
3. Debris on block edge	3. Trim edges of block
4. Static electricity on ribbon	4. Humidify the air around the microtome
	5. Place static guard or dryer sheets near microtome
Problem: Incomplete section	
1. Incomplete impregnation of tissue with paraffin	1. Re-process tissue block
2. Tissue incorrectly embedded	2. Re-embed tissue; make sure orientation is correct and tissue is flat in mold
3. Sections superficially cut	3. Re-face block, cut deeper into the tissue

Table 7.1 (continued)	
Causes	Solutions
Problem: Excessive compression 1. Dull blade 2. Paraffin too soft for the tissue	 1. Replace blade 2. Cool block face and re-cut
Problem: Sections expand or disintegrate on water bath 1. Incomplete tissue processing 2. Water temperature too high in floatation bath	 1. Re-process tissue 2. Turn down the temperature in the floatation bath
Problem: Sections roll into a tight coil instead of remaining flat on knife edge 1. Blade dull 2. Rake angle too small 3. Section too thick	 1. Use a new blade 2. Reduce blade tilt if clearance angle is excessive 3. Reduce section thickness

FROZEN AND RELATED SECTIONS

This section is a discussion of the methods that produce sections without the use of dehydrating and clearing solutions, and, in the case of frozen section, without embedding media. Frozen sections have many uses, including the demonstration of soluble substances, histochemical analysis, and intraoperative diagnosis. The standard processing methods have many deleterious effects on tissue constituents (Bancroft & Cook 1994).

USES FOR FROZEN SECTIONS

The production of frozen sections has many applications in routine histology laboratories:

- Rapid production of sections for intraoperative diagnosis
- Diagnostic and research enzyme histochemistry; enzymes are labile
- Immunofluorescent methods (see Chapter 24)
- Immunohistochemistry methods; heat and fixation may inactivate or destroy many of the antigens (see Chapter 21)
- Diagnostic and research non-enzyme histochemistry, e.g. lipids and some carbohydrates (see Chapters 11 and 12)
- Silver methods, particularly in neuropathology (see Chapter 19).

Theoretical considerations

The principle of cutting frozen section is simple: when the tissue is frozen, the water in the tissue turns to ice, and in this state the tissue is firm, the ice acting as the embedding medium. The consistency of the frozen block can be altered by varying the temperature of the tissue. Reducing the temperature will produce a harder block, raising the temperature makes the tissue softer. The majority of non-fatty unfixed tissues section well at -20 to $-25°C$. The sectioning of fixed tissue requires a block temperature of approximately $-10°C$ or warmer. There is more water in fixed tissue; consequently the tissue will have a harder consistency, requiring a higher temperature to obtain the ideal consistency for sectioning.

The cryostat

The use of the cryostat in the histology laboratory has been instrumental to the expansion of the field of histochemistry, while improving sections for intraoperative consultation. The cryostat is a refrigerated cabinet in which a specialty microtome is housed. All the controls to the microtome are operated outside the cabinet. The first cryostats were introduced in 1954; improvements in design have facilitated sectioning and safety:

- Electronic temperature control
- Electronically controlled advance and retraction of the block
- Specimen orientation facility
- Digital visualization of chuck and cabinet temperature
- Mechanical cutting speed control and section thickness
- Automatic defrost mechanism
- Automated de-contamination and sterilization.

Cryostat technique

To produce thin, high-quality frozen sections, the tissue must be well prepared, the conditions of the cryostat must be optimal, and the block temperature must be correct for the tissue being cut. The best quality frozen sections are produced from fresh unfixed tissue that has been rapidly frozen. Freezing tissue in the cryostat may produce freeze artifact because the process is slower than other methods.

Freezing of fresh unfixed tissue

Tissue for freezing should be fresh. The specimen should be frozen as rapidly as possible without creating freeze artifact. Techniques for suitable freezing include:

- Liquefied nitrogen ($-190°C$)
- Isopentane (2-methylbutane) cooled by liquid nitrogen ($-150°C$)
- Dry ice ($-70°C$)
- Carbon dioxide gas ($-70°C$)
- Aerosol sprays ($-50°C$).

When freezing tissue for frozen sections, freeze artifact may occur. The water in the tissue freezes and forms ice crystals; the crystal size and the quantity of crystals is proportional to the speed at which the tissue is frozen. The tissue is cut and placed on a room temperature slide; at this point the tissue is thawed. The thawing of the ice crystals produces freeze artifact that appears as holes when viewed microscopically.

The best frozen sections are obtained when the tissue is frozen quickly. The method of choice is isopentane and liquid nitrogen. The problem with using liquid nitrogen alone is the formation of a vapor bubbles around the tissue, acting as an insulator, inhibiting rapid even cooling of the tissue. This can produce freeze artifact in the tissue, which may make diagnostic interpretation difficult; this is especially true for muscle biopsies. The problem can be overcome by freezing the tissue in an agent with a high thermal conductivity which has been cooled to approximately $-160°C$ by immersion in liquid nitrogen; an example is isopentane. A beaker of isopentane is suspended in a flask of liquid nitrogen. When the temperature of the isopentane reaches $-160°C$ the tissue is submerged in the isopentane (affixed to a cork disc, aluminum foil, or a cryostat chuck). The tissue may be rolled in talc prior to snap freezing to reduce freezing artifact.

Solid carbon dioxide (dry ice) may be used for freezing tissue blocks. Two pieces of dry ice are held in gloved hands against the cryostat block holder containing the tissue which has been oriented in a support medium, such as OCT. As the tissue is frozen a white line will be seen to pass through the tissue, the dry ice should be removed, to avoid over-freezing of the tissue. This method is not economical as the dry ice will return to the gaseous state upon storage. Regular deliveries and wasting of large amount of dry ice are disadvantages of this method.

Carbon dioxide gas from a CO_2 cylinder has been successful in the past. Tissue block are frozen by adapting a conventional freezing microtome with a gas supply or by using a special adaptor for the CO_2 tank that holds the tissue chuck.

Aerosol sprays have gained popularity as a means of freezing small tissue blocks. These sprays are available from a number of vendors, having the advantage of being readily available and easily stored. A major problem is the environmental issue of aerosol emissions and the safety issue involved with inhaling the aerosol emissions while cutting the tissue.

Fixed tissue and the cryostat

For most diagnostic purposes in a routine laboratory, cryostat sections of unfixed tissue are suitable. The effect of freezing unfixed tissue causes the diffusion of labile substances. This is enhanced during sectioning, which produces heat causing a temporary slight thawing of the cut section. This may not cause a problem for diagnosis, but affects the accurate localization of enzymes, e.g. acid and alkaline phosphatases. To localize hydrolytic enzymes and other antigens the tissue is fixed prior to sectioning. The tissue must be fresh and placed in formal calcium at $4°C$ for 18 hours. The technique is outlined below.

Gum sucrose

Gum acacia	2 g
Sucrose	60 g
Distilled water	200 ml
Store at 4°C	

Method

1. Fix fresh tissue block in formal calcium, at 4°C for 18 hours.
2. Rinse in running water, or for a short time in distilled water if the tissue fragment is small or fragile, e.g. jejunal biopsy.
3. Blot dry.
4. Place tissue in the gum sucrose solution at 4°C for 18 hours, or less with small fragments.
5. Blot dry.
6. Freeze tissue onto the block holder.

Following fixation, the block is frozen slowly to avoid damage caused by the rapid expansion of ice within the tissue. Freezing the block by standing it in the cryostat cabinet gives acceptable results for the majority of fixed tissue. The length of time required for this procedure limits its value as a diagnostic tool.

Cryostat sectioning

Cabinet temperature

The temperature of the microtome and the cryostat chamber should be monitored. Many cryostats have digital read-outs of the block temperature and the cabinet temperature. The temperature should be suitable for the tissue type and the type of preparation to be cut. Most unfixed material will section well between −15°C and −23°C. Tissues containing large amounts of water will section best at the warmer temperature, and harder tissues and those that contain fat require a colder temperature. Table 7.2 gives an indication of the optimal cutting temperatures for a variety of tissue types. If sections are shattered, with chatter lines, this is an indication that the block is too cold.

Most fixed tissues will section best within the range of −7°C to −12°C, depending on the hardness of the tissue. Small blocks of undecalcified cancellous bone can be sectioned, but care must be taken to remove any cortical bone fragments prior to freezing.

Microtome

If cutting problems are encountered the microtome should be defrosted and oiled according to manufacturer's recommendation. A policy should be in place that outlines a routine maintenance schedule for each cryostat.

Blade or knife

Stainless steel knives have been replaced by disposable blades in many clinical settings, although they still have a place in research and animal pathology laboratories. The type of tissue and the procedures to be performed may dictate the use of a steel knife. If a knife is used, sharpening techniques should be addressed in the procedure manual. A sharp edge is paramount in obtaining a quality frozen section.

Disposable blades have become routine in most laboratories; they produce a perfect edge and are instantly available. In addition to the advantage of sharpness, the blades are rapidly cooled as a result of their size. Tissues that are extremely hard or dense may be troublesome for a disposable blade.

Anti-roll plate

This piece of equipment, which is attached to the front of the microtome, is intended to stop the natural tendency of frozen sections to curl upwards on sectioning. The device is usually made of plexiglass or a hard plastic material. The anti-roll plate is aligned parallel to the blade edge and fractionally above it. The plate can be raised or lowered against the knife, to increase the angle between the knife and the blade. It is the microadjusting of the anti-roll plate that determines the success of sectioning the tissue block. Anti-roll adjustments include:

- Correct height of blade edge
- Correct angle of blade
- Edge of plate should not be nicked or damaged
- Cabinet temperature.

If the anti-roll plate is not working correctly, a sable hair brush can be used to manipulate the section.

Sectioning technique

Frozen sectioning may require practice to master the technique. Speed, tissue type, and temperature of the block and the cabinet play important roles in frozen sectioning. The cut section will rest on the surface of the blade holder after cutting. A room temperature slide is held above the section, and electrostatic attraction

Table 7.2 Optimal tissue freezing temperatures

Tissue	−7° to −10°C	−10° to −13°C	−13° to −16°C	−16° to −20°C	−20° to −25°C	−25° to −30°C
Heart				X		
Lung				X		
Brain	X					
Skin			X			
Muscle			X			
Bone marrow					X	
Kidney			X			
Lymphoid						
Testicular		X	X			
Intestinal				X		
Rectal			X			
Fat					X	X
Breast					X	
Breast with fat						X
Liver	X	X				
Uterine scrapings	X					
Spleen	X					
Adrenal			X			
Thyroid		X				
Bladder		X				
Cervix				X		
Pancreas				X		
Ovary				X		
Prostate				X		
Uterus			X			

causes the tissue to adhere to the slide. If tissues are being cut that will require harsh or lengthy staining procedures; positively charged or coated slides should be used. Several coatings can be used if coated slides are required, e.g. gelatin–formaldehyde or poly-L-lysine (0.01% aqueous solution). Difficult sections may also be cut and placed on the slide by use of a tape transfer system. This system is valuable for tissue sections that will not adhere to the slide.

Gelatin–formaldehyde mixture

1% gelatin	5 ml
2% formaldehyde	5 ml

Coat slides with the above mixture. Allow to dry at 37°C for 1 hour or overnight before picking up sections. Another suitable adhesive is poly-L-lysine.

Poly-L-lysine coating

0.01% poly-L-lysine (PLL) aqueous

1. Wash slides in detergent for 30 min.
2. Wash slides in running tap water 30 min.
3. Rinse slides in distilled water two times, 5 min each.
4. Wash slides in 95% alcohol two times, 5 min each.
5. Air dry slides 10 min.
6. Smear 20 µl of PLL over each slide.
7. Air dry and store dust free.

This is used as a section adhesive in immunohistochemistry.

Rapid biopsy for intraoperative diagnosis

Frozen sections provide a valuable tool in the rapid diagnosis of tissues during surgery. The pathologist selects a piece of tissue and the tissue is frozen using one of several techniques that have previously been discussed. The slide is immediately submerged in cold acetone or 95% alcohol. The sections are stained immediately by a rapid hematoxylin and eosin, methylene blue, or polychrome stain. With properly cut and stained slides an immediate diagnosis can be made in the operating suite.

Ultracryotomy

Ultracryotomy is used primarily in research laboratories. It involves rapid freezing of fixed or unfixed tissue by using isopentane and liquid nitrogen and cutting sections at 50–150 nm. Much success has been gained by pre-fixing the tissue in glutaraldehyde prior to sectioning.

Equipment

There are two basic types of equipment for frozen ultrathin sectioning. The first uses a standard or slightly modified ultra-microtome in a deep freeze, and the second utilizes a microtome specially designed for ultrathin sectioning at low temperatures. The temperature control on these ultra-cryotomes is between −20°C and −212°C. The sections are cut with a glass knife and picked up on grids. A cutting temperature of approximately −180°C is suitable for most tissues. These sections are useful in the localization of enzyme activity at the ultrastructural level.

Freeze drying and freeze substitution

Freeze drying is the technique of rapid freezing (quenching) of fresh tissue at −160°C, and the subsequent removal of water molecules (in the form of ice) by sublimation in a vacuum at a higher temperature (−40°C). The blocks are raised to room temperature and fixed by vapor or embedded in a suitable medium. This technique is usually restricted to research laboratories, and is not widely used in clinical laboratories. The technique minimizes:

- Loss of soluble substances
- Displacement of cell constituents
- Chemical alteration of reactive groups
- Denaturation of proteins
- Destruction or inactivation of enzymes.

Four stages to freeze drying

Quenching

Quenching instantly stops chemical reactions and diffusion in the tissue, bringing the tissue into a solid state in which unbound water in the tissue is changed into small ice crystals, which are subsequently removed in the drying phase.

Drying

This stage in the technique is the most time consuming because the tissues contain 70–80% water by weight that has to be removed without damage to the tissue. Drying is divided into three distinct steps.

- Introduction of heat to the tissue to cause sublimation of ice
- Transfer of water vapor from the ice crystals through the dry portion of the tissue
- Removal of water vapor from the surface of the specimen.

Drying of tissue takes place when heat is supplied to the frozen tissue in a vacuum of 133 mPa or greater. The heat vaporizes the water molecules that pass through the tissue to the surface. For drying to continue there must be efficient removal of the water molecules from the surface of the specimen. The water molecules leaving the tissue are removed by a vapor trap, either a 'cold finger' trap filled with liquid nitrogen or a chemical trap containing a dehydrant chemical such as phosphorus pentoxide.

Fixation and embedding

When the tissue is completely dry, it is allowed to come to room temperature. At atmospheric pressure it will not absorb moisture unless drying is incomplete, when the tissue will rapidly reabsorb water. The dried piece of tissue is extremely friable, and any undue pressure will cause the tissue to disintegrate into a fine powder. The delicate tissue is ready for embedding and sectioning or for fixing in a suitable vapor.

Vapor fixation

A number of fixatives can be used in their vapor form including formaldehyde, glutaraldehyde, and osmium tetroxide. The most important is formaldehyde; this gives excellent preservation of the tissue components, and the tissue can be used for histochemical techniques, with the exception of enzymes. Following fixation the tissue is embedded in paraffin.

Applications and uses of freeze-dried material

Initially, the technique of freeze drying was used as a method of demonstrating fine structural details. Other applications include:

- Immunohistochemical methods
- Demonstration of hydrolytic enzymes
- Fluorescent antibody studies
- Autoradiography
- Microspectrofluorimetry of autofluorescent substances
- Formaldehyde-induced fluorescence
- Mucosubstances
- Proteins
- Scanning electron microscopy.

Fluorescent antibody studies

These studies are usually carried out on cryostat sections. Many polypeptides and polypeptide hormones are better demonstrated on freeze-dried sections (see Chapter 24).

Autoradiography

This technique provides excellent results with freeze-dried sections, and accurate localization of soluble substances. Water-soluble isotopes can be used if the sections are dry mounted onto the slides.

Microspectrofluorimetry of autofluorescent substances

This technique requires sections that are unaltered by processing methods. Frozen sections give adequate results, but are affected by thawing of the water in the section. The effect of the embedding medium on freeze-dried sections appears to cause less damage.

Formaldehyde-induced fluorescence (FIF)

Used in the demonstration of biogenic amines. This technique, known as the Falck method (1962), involves the use of blocks of tissue freeze-dried and subjected to formal vapor at room temperature between 60°C and 80°C with controlled humidity. Formaldehyde-induced fluorescence (FIF) is used to demonstrate 5-hydroxytryptamine,

epinephrine (adrenaline), norepinephrine (noradrenaline), and other catecholamines. When these amines react with formalin they are converted to fluorescent compounds (see Chapter 14).

Mucosubstances

Formal vapor fixation, after freeze drying, produces good staining of mucosubstances. The reactivity of mucins appears unaltered while the localization is improved, compared to frozen or paraffin sections. The uses of freeze-dried sections are recommended for the accurate demonstration and localization of glycogen (see Chapter 11).

Proteins

Many proteins can be satisfactorily demonstrated on suitably fixed freeze-dried sections. Formal vapor fixation may remove some protein sections (see Chapter 13).

Scanning electron microscopy (SEM)

Standard processing procedures do not work well for electron microscopy. Processing causes alteration as water present in tissue will evaporate when placed under a vacuum condition, leading to distortion of the tissue. Frozen tissue, under vacuum, will slowly freeze dry, and the sublimation of the ice from the tissue surface will distort the picture (see Chapter 30).

FROZEN SECTION SUBSTITUTION

The technique of frozen section substitution involves the rapid freezing of the tissue to −160°C in isopentane supercooled by liquid nitrogen. Cryostat sections are cut at 8–10 μm and placed in a cold container maintained at cryostat temperature. The sections are transferred to water-free acetone and cooled to −70°C for 12 hours. The sections are floated onto slides and allowed to dry. The histochemical method is applied. For most diagnostic purposes, cryostat sections preserve most tissue components. This method is easy, convenient, and labor-saving, and is easy to implement in the laboratory. Freeze drying and freeze substitution are too labor-intensive, time-consuming, and capricious for clinical diagnostic use. These techniques are more widely used in research.

Acknowledgments

This chapter is an amalgamation of the three chapters that appeared in the first three editions. In those editions Paraffin microtomy was written by Keith Gordon and Paul Bradbury, and Frozen sections was written by John Bancroft. In the fourth edition, Graeme Anderson successfully merged the Processing and Microtomy chapters, and John Bancroft and Janet Palmer updated the Frozen section chapter. Our acknowledgments go the previous contributors.

REFERENCES

Anderson G., Bancroft J.D. (2002) Tissue processing and microtomy including frozen. In: Bancroft J.D., Gamble M., eds. Theory and practice of histological techniques, 5th edn. Edinburgh: Churchill Livingstone, pp. 85–107.

Bancroft J.D., Cook H.C. (1994) Manual of histological techniques and their diagnostic application. Edinburgh: Churchill Livingstone.

Carson F.L. (1997) Histotechnology, a self-instructional text, 2nd edn. Chicago: ASCP Press, pp. 35–42.

Falck B. (1962) Observations on the possibilities of the cellular localization of monoamines by a fluorescence method. Acta Physiologica Scandinavica 56(Suppl): 197.

Mailhiot M.A. (2005) Microtomy, it's all about technique! (workshop handout) Bowie, MD: National Society for Histotechnology.

Sheehan D.C., Hrapchak B. (1980) Theory and practice of histotechnology, 2nd edn. St. Louis: C.V. Mosby, pp. 79–82.

8

How do Histological Stains Work?

Richard W. Horobin

INTRODUCTION

The physicochemical principles underlying all histological staining methods, from acid dyeing to silver impregnation, will be described in this chapter. Examples are provided from many of the application areas discussed in this book, although methods using dyestuffs are emphasized. Further information concerning dyes, and a troubleshooting guide, are found at the end of the chapter. The key questions to bear in mind throughout this chapter are:

a. Why do *any* tissue components stain?
b. Why do stained components *remain* stained?
c. Why are *all* components not stained?

Answers reflect the multiphase nature of the staining process—of solid cells and tissues interacting with solutions of staining reagents. Thus the periodic acid–Schiff (PAS) procedure is not merely organic chemistry, immunostaining is not just immunochemistry, nor is enzyme histochemistry merely biochemistry. Staining methods are also influenced by selective uptake of reagents into tissues, and selective losses of products and/or reagents from the tissue. These uptakes and losses depend on both affinity and rate factors. Note: *staining* always involves the visual labeling of some entity by attaching, or depositing in its vicinity, a marker of characteristic color or shape. The *stain* is the marker, or the reagent used to generate the marker.

A GENERAL THEORY OF STAINING

Why are stains taken into the tissues?

Often, stain uptake is due to dye–tissue or reagent–tissue affinities. In biological staining and histochemical usage the word affinity has two distinct emphases. To say a tissue component has a high affinity for a dye may merely mean that, under the conditions of use, the component becomes intensely stained. Affinity is also used to describe attractive forces binding dye to tissue. Physical chemists use the term in the former sense, and their usage is adopted here.

So in this chapter affinity describes the tendency of a stain to transfer from solution onto a section. The affinity's magnitude depends on every factor aiding or hindering this process. Consequently stain–tissue, solvent–solvent, stain–solvent, and stain–stain interactions will all be considered. This approach assumes staining continues until equilibrium is reached, and in practice this is often not so. Moreover uptake of dyes and reagents may well be multistep, in both time and space. A reagent may initially enter tissues due to, say, coulombic attractions. Once inside it may form covalent bonds with some tissue grouping.

Various contributions to stain–tissue affinity are outlined in Table 8.1, and discussed below. Practical staining processes commonly involve several such factors.

Reagent–tissue interactions

Coulombic attractions, also termed salt links or electrostatic bonds, are widely discussed reagent–tissue interactions. These arise from electrostatic attractions of unlike ions, e.g. the colored cations of basic dyes and tissue structures rich in anions such as phosphated DNA, or sulfated mucosubstances (Lyon 1991; Prentø 2001). In practice, the amount of dye ion binding to a tissue substrate depends not only on the charge signs of dye and tissue but also on their magnitude, on the amount of non-dye electrolyte present in the dyebath, and on the

Table 8.1 Factors contributing to dye–tissue affinities	
Interactions	**Practical examples where the factor is important**
Solvent–solvent interactions	
The hydrophobic effect	Staining systems using aqueous solutions of dyes or other organic reagents; enzyme substrates for example
Reagent–reagent interactions	Metachromatic staining with basic dyes, Gomori-type enzyme histochemistry, silver impregnation
Reagent–tissue interactions	
Coulombic attractions	Acid and basic dyes, and other ionic reagents, including inorganic salts
Van der Waals' forces	Most important with large molecules such as the elastic fiber stains, and final reaction products such as bisformazans in enzyme histochemistry
Hydrogen bonding	Staining of glycogen by carminic acid, and collagen by Sirius red
Covalent bonding	Methods such as the Feulgen nucleal, PAS, and mercury orange

ability of the tissue substrate to swell or shrink (Scott 1973; Bennion & Horobin 1974; Goldstein & Horobin 1974b; Horobin & Goldstein 1974).

Such phenomena are important for all ionic reagents not just dyestuffs, e.g. the periodate anions used in the periodic acid–Schiff procedure (Scott & Harbinson 1968). Even initially uncharged tissue substrates can acquire ionic character after binding ionic reagents, e.g. glycogen staining by the PAS procedure and with Best's carmine.

Van der Waals' forces include such intermolecular attractions as dipole–dipole, dipole-induced dipole and dispersion forces. These occur between all reagents and tissue substrates, but since molecules with extensively delocalized electronic systems tend to have larger dipoles and be more polarizable, van der Waals' forces are usually most important when tissues or stains contain such moieties.

Consequently substrate groupings such as tyrosine and tryptophan residues of proteins, and heterocyclic bases of nucleic acids, favor van der Waals' attractions, as do the large aromatic systems of stains such as bisazo dyes and bistetrazolium salts, halogenated dyes such as rose Bengal and phloxine, and enzyme substrates based on naphthyl and indoxyl systems (Horobin & Bennion 1973). For instance, van der Waals' attractions contribute substantially to stain–tissue affinity when staining elastic fibers—rich in aromatic desmosine and isodesmo-

sine residues—with polyaromatic acid and basic dyes such as Congo red and orcein.

Hydrogen bonding is a dye–tissue attraction arising when a hydrogen atom lies between two electronegative atoms (e.g. oxygen or nitrogen), though is covalently bonded only to one. Water is hydrogen bonded extensively to itself, forming the clusters important for the hydrophobic effect discussed below, and also to other molecules with hydrogen bonding groups, such as many dyes and tissue components. Consequently hydrogen bonding is not usually important for stain–tissue affinity when aqueous solvents are used, except when particularly favored by the substrate, as is so with connective tissue fibers (Prentø 2007). In wholly or partially non-aqueous solutions, hydrogen bonding can also be significant, as with Best's carmine stain for glycogen, and the staining of amyloid by Congo red and similar dyes; these procedures use largely non-aqueous solvents.

Covalent bonding between tissue and stain also occurs. Covalent bonds may be viewed merely as another source of stain–tissue affinity. Practical reactive methods, e.g. the Feulgen nucleal and the periodic acid–Schiff procedures, are discussed elsewhere in this volume. The polar covalent bonds between metal ions and 'mordant' dyes are a special case. Such bonds were thought to facilitate dye–tissue binding; however, such *mordanting* is largely speculative, and the characteristic staining properties of mordant dyes may have other, or additional, causes. For instance, metal-complex dyes are usually hydrophilic (Bettinger & Zimmermann 1991) and so resist extraction into alcoholic dehydration fluids (Marshall & Horobin 1973).

Solvent–solvent interactions

A major contribution to stain–tissue affinity, when using organic reagents or dyes in aqueous solution, is the *hydrophobic effect*. This is the tendency of hydrophobic groupings (such as leucine and valine side chains of proteins, or biphenyl and naphthyl groupings of enzyme substrates and dyes) to come together, even though initially dispersed in an aqueous environment. The process occurs because water is a highly structured liquid. Many water molecules are held together by hydrogen bonding (see above) in transient clusters, whose formation is favored by the presence of hydrophobic groups. Processes breaking clusters into individual water molecules occur spontaneously, because these events increase the entropy of the system. Consequently, removing cluster-stabilizing hydrophobic groups from contact with water, by placing them in contact with each other, is thermodynamically favored. For background on the hydrophobic effect see textbooks of biochemistry or chemical thermodynamics, or, more enjoyably if less scholarly, a book by Tanford (2004). The effect becomes more important as the substrate and reagent become more hydrophobic, as with staining of fats by Sudan dyes. When these hydrophobic dyes are applied from substantially aqueous solutions, the hydrophobic effect will be a major contribution to affinity. Nomenclature note: the hydrophobic effect is sometimes termed 'hydrophobic bonding', even though no special bonds are involved, only water–water hydrogen bonds and, sometimes, stain–tissue van der Waals' attractions.

Some Sudan staining procedures, however, use solvents in which water is only a minor constituent. Here the second law of thermodynamics—the tendency of a system to change spontaneously to maximize its disorder, i.e. for *entropy* to increase as described in texts of chemical thermodynamics—may again be invoked. Dye dispersed through fat *and* solvent constitutes a more disordered system than dye restricted to a single phase. Consequently dye becomes dispersed, and staining occurs. Of course such increases in entropy involving substrate and dye occur in all types of staining system.

Stain–stain interactions

Dye–dye interactions can also contribute to affinity. Dye molecules tend to attract each other, forming aggregates. Even in dilute solutions, and especially in aqueous solutions where the hydrophobic effect is important, dimers of dye ions are often present. Van der Waals' attractions (see above) between dye molecules will be important in both aqueous and non-aqueous solutions. Dye aggregation increases with concentration, e.g. when high dye concentrations build up on tissue sections. With basic (cationic) dyes this occurs on substrates of high negative charge density, e.g. sulfated polysaccharides in mast cell granules, a classic site for *metachromatic staining* by dyes such as toluidine blue. This phenomenon occurs because dye aggregates have spectral properties different from the monomeric dye. That dye–dye interactions contribute to affinity was demonstrated quantitatively by Goldstein (1962).

Other examples of stain–stain interactions contributing to affinity include microcrystals of metallic silver generated following silver impregnation, metal sulfide precipitates formed in Gomori-type enzyme histochemistry, and the purple azure–eosin charge transfer complex produced during Romanowsky–Giemsa staining of cell nuclei.

Some oddball possibilities

Some effective stains are not taken up into the tissues. In *negative staining* the shapes of structures are disclosed by outlining or filling them with a stain. Examples range from visualizing individual microorganisms using nigrosine, to demonstrating canaliculi of bone matrix using picro-thionine.

Sometimes the stains are taken into live creatures, in ways that reflect the biochemical composition and physiological activities of the living cell or organism. Traditionally termed *vital staining* or supravital staining, this is now called the *use of fluorescent probes*. This methodology has undergone a renaissance; for a recent overview see Mason (1999).

Why do stains remain in tissue after its removal from the staining bath?

This is because the stains either have no affinity for processing fluids and mounting media, or dissolve in these materials very slowly. To illustrate these points, consider some common stains.

Inorganic pigments—such as Prussian blue in the Perls' method for iron, and lead sulfide in enzyme histochemistry—are virtually insoluble in routine solvents. This is also true for microcrystals of silver and gold produced by metal impregnation. Other pigments are less satisfactory. Azodyes, formazans, and substituted indigos produced as final reaction products in enzyme histochemistry are of low solubility in water, but may dissolve in hydrophobic media such as alcohols, xylene, and polystyrene. If so, hydrophilic mounting media are used, and moreover staining of lipid-rich tissue elements should be regarded with suspicion. Solubilities of formazans and azodyes are sometimes reduced by in situ conversion to metal complexes.

Other routine metal complex stains are the Al, Cr, and Fe complexes of hematein, and the Cr complex of gallocyanine. These metal complex dyes are not readily removed from tissues by routine processing fluids or mounting media (see above).

This contrasts with routine cationic (basic) dyes such as crystal violet or methylene blue, which freely and rapidly dissolve in the lower alcohols (see Fig. 8.3, p. 115). Anionic (acid) dyes, such as eosin Y or orange G, are often less soluble in alcohols, as indeed are hydrophilic basic dyes with large aromatic systems, such as alcian blue (see Fig. 8.3). Non-ionic dyes such as Sudan fat stains are soluble in common dehydrating agents and clearing solvents, and in resin mountants.

Sections stained with routine basic dyes must therefore be dehydrated rapidly through the alcohols, or by using non-alcoholic solvents, or by air-drying, whereas dehydration is less critical with acid dyes. Sections stained with either acid or basic dyes are usually mounted in non-aqueous media to prevent loss of dye. Alternatively dyes may be immobilized, e.g. by formation of metal coordination compounds, phosphotungstates, or iodine complexes. Non-ionic dyes must be mounted in aqueous media.

Why are the stains not taken up into every part of the tissue?

This question of selectivity is fundamental to histochemistry, and even routine histological oversight stains such as hematoxylin and eosin (H&E) distinguish nuclei from cytoplasm. What factors control such selectivities?

Numbers and affinities of binding sites

Stain–tissue affinities and numbers of binding sites present in tissues can both vary. For instance, Sudan dyes have high affinities for fat but low affinities for the surrounding hydrated proteins. In staining systems forming covalent bonds, reagents give colored products only with a limited range of tissue chemical groupings. For example, the acid hydrolysis–Schiff reagent sequence of the Feulgen nucleal technique gives red derivatives only with DNA.

An understanding of staining systems often requires consideration of patterns of affinities. Consider the traditional acid dye–basic dye pairs: H&E, Papanicolaou, and Romanowsky. The negatively charged acid dyes have high affinities for tissue structures carrying cationic charges (proteins, under acidic conditions), but low affinities for structures carrying negative charges (those rich in sulfated glycosaminoglycans, or in phosphated nucleic acids), with the opposite being the case for basic dyes. This produces two-tone staining patterns in which cytoplasms contrast with nuclei.

Practical staining conditions maximize selective affinities. In the above examples pH is important, and basic dyes are applied from neutral or acidic solutions, since under alkaline conditions proteins carry an overall negative charge and so also bind basic dyes. Affinities are also influenced by varying the concentration of inorganic salt present. The various aluminum-hematoxylins, for instance, differ substantially in their inorganic salt content. The critical electrolyte concentration methodology (Scott 1973) and several other empirical procedures are based on control of electrolyte content. However, staining that distinguishes two structures is still possible even when stain–tissue affinities and the number of stain-binding sites are the same. This is because rate of reagent uptake, or rate of subsequent reaction, or rate of loss of reagent or product may not be the same in the two structures.

Rates of reagent uptake

Progressive dyeing methods may be *rate controlled*, for instance mucin staining using alcian blue or colloidal iron. Selectivity requires short periods of dyeing during which only fast-staining mucins acquire color (Goldstein 1962, Goldstein & Horobin 1974a). If staining is prolonged, additional basophilic materials such as nuclei and RNA-rich cytoplasms can also stain.

Rate of reaction

Selective staining by reactive reagents, yielding colored derivatives, may depend on differential *rates of reaction*. For instance, periodic acid can oxidize a variety of substrates present in tissues. In histochemical applications of the periodic acid–Schiff procedure, however, a short oxidation time limits subsequent coloration to fast reacting 1,2-diol groupings of polysaccharides. Enzyme histochemistry also provides examples of reaction rate controlling selectivity. When incubating at low pH, hydrolysis of an organic phosphate is rapid in tissues containing acid phosphatases, whereas in structures containing alkaline phosphatases, with higher pH optima, hydrolysis rates are slow.

Rate of reagent loss

Differentiation or *regressive staining* involves selective losses of stain from tissues. Many dyeing methods exploit this, e.g. staining of muscle striations with iron–hematoxylin, and of myelin sheaths with luxol fast blue. In such procedures an initial non-selective staining is followed by extraction in a solvent. Dye is first lost from permeable structures such as collagen fibers. Relatively impermeable structures such as the A and Z bands of muscle, and myelin sheaths, retain stain longest.

Rate control of reagent loss is critical in a very different methodology, namely silver staining of nerve fibers. During an impregnation step, silver ions bind non-selectively to many tissue groupings. Then the tissue is treated with a developer capable of reducing silver cations to silver metal. The rate of action of this reducing agent is critical. If the rate is too fast, because of high concentration or high reactivity of the reagent, silver grains are deposited non-selectively throughout the tissue. If reduction is too slow, no staining occurs because most silver ions diffuse away into the solvent before they are reduced. Selective staining occurs when silver ions diffuse from the background quickly, being retained in less permeable entities (e.g. nerve fibers, nucleoli, red blood cells) where they are then reduced (Peters 1955a, 1955b).

Such rate-controlled methods are bedeviled by a wide range of technical artifacts. Any factor affecting rate of reagent loss (e.g. variation in section thickness, temperature, stirring of the reagent solution, presence of cavities in the tissue) can alter the staining pattern.

Metachromasia and related phenomena

Even if a stain is not selectively bound, it may nevertheless give selective coloration. Such effects arise with dyes and with reactive stains. For instance basic dyes such as methylene blue and toluidine blue are absorbed by a variety of basophilic substrates in the tissues. Whilst chromatin stains orthochromatically blue, cartilage matrix, mast cell granules, and mucins stain metachromatically reddish purple (reviewed by Pearse 1968).

What are the effects of tissue modification prior to staining?

Modifications include fixation, whose effects on staining are adventitious, as well as blocking and extraction techniques intended to alter staining patterns. The case of resin embedding is discussed later.

Effects of fixation

Fixation is carried out to prevent losses of tissue constituents into processing and staining solutions, and to reduce postmortem morphological changes of the tissue. Fixation converts soluble tissue components into insoluble derivatives, resistant to autolysis or attack by bacteria and fungi. (For a general account of fixation see Chapter 4; here only the influences on staining are discussed.)

A given substance is often retained to different extents by different fixative agents, and nothing can be stained that is not retained. For instance, many lipids are well preserved after fixation in osmium tetroxide or dichromates, poorly preserved after formalin, and actively extracted during alcoholic or acetone fixation. Staining lipids after alcoholic fixation is therefore ineffective.

Moreover, whilst retention of a substance is necessary, mere retention may be insufficient for subsequent histochemical demonstration. Thus glutaraldehyde often retains more protein than do other fixative agents, although its use in immunostaining and enzyme histochemistry (and most antigens and all enzymes are proteins) is limited. The same chemical reactions that insolubilize proteins also modify haptenic and enzymic activity. Alcohol and acetone on the other hand, although poor at retaining proteins in the tissues, are also poor at destroying the activity of what antigen or enzyme is retained. So both retention and reactivity of substances affect staining, and both may be fixative dependent.

Fixation has additional, more subtle, influences on staining patterns. As an example, consider the basophilia–acidophilia balance of a tissue. Formalin and osmium tetroxide generally induce tissue basophilia, whilst acidic dichromate solutions and alcoholic cyanuric chloride raise tissue acidophilia (Baker 1958). Such global differences, however, mask complex detail. Formalin, for example, lowers the number of potentially cationic (acidophilia inducing) amino groups, by converting them to non-ionizing N-methylols and other compounds. Chromation reduces the number of anionic (basophilia inducing) tissue carboxylate groups by converting them to cationic (acidophilia inducing) chromium complexes. Osmium tetroxide oxidizes both amines, reducing the number of potential tissue cations, and thiol and disulfide groups, which latter yield anionic (basophilia inducing) sulfonic acids. Alcoholic cyanuric chloride gives a predominantly basophilic staining only with short staining times; longer times produce an acidophilia very like that of formalin—indeed cyanuric chloride and formalin react with much the same tissue moieties.

Effects of histochemical blocking and extraction procedures

Such procedures intentionally modify tissue components to eliminate staining, with any subsequent staining indicating lack of staining specificity. Tissue modifications, however, may be incomplete, or may result in changes other than those expected, so invalidating the test, as illustrated below.

Incomplete blockade occurs with van Slyke's nitrous acid reagent (used to convert tissue amino groups to hydroxyls). The efficacy of this reagent is tissue and fixative dependent. However, suppose that, in a given structure, 75% of the amino groups are converted to hydroxyls. Will the staining intensity be correspondingly reduced? Uptake of acid dyes will be much reduced, since the overall charge carried by the tissue (dependent on the numbers of $-NH_3^+$ and of $-CO_2^-$ groupings) will have altered radically. However, staining by reagents forming covalent bonds with amino groups, such as procion dyes, is little affected, since such reagents may give an intense staining after reacting with only a small proportion of available amino groups. Incomplete blocking also arises when a stain reverses the blockade. An example is blocking thiol groups by treatment with mercuric chloride, giving rise to -S-Hg-Cl derivatives. These are unreactive with the disulfide groups of disulfide–dinaphthyl type reagents, but mercury orange is able to react with them and so its staining is not blocked.

Analogous effects occur with histochemical extraction procedures. The lipid components of lipoproteins, unlike those of fat droplets, are not readily removed from tissues by treatment with organic solvents. Removal of RNA from ribosomes by RNase is fixative dependent and does not occur readily after formalin fixation; perhaps there is cross-linkage to protein.

Unexpected tissue modifications due to blockade and extractive procedures also occur, removing substances additional to those intended. When using trichloracetic or perchloric acids to extract nucleic acids, losses of polysaccharides and some proteins can also occur. Analogous problems arise during enzymic extractions when trace enzyme impurities are present. Polysaccharides may also be lost by chemical solvolysis during 'methylation' of tissue acids by methanolic-HCl, and DNA and RNA are extracted by the acetic anhydride–pyridine used to blockade nuclear histones. In fact material can be extracted by staining solutions, especially if acidic or alkaline or when tissues are poorly fixed.

In addition to these narrowly chemical effects, all such procedures modify the physical properties of a tissue section, e.g. its permeability. So after exposure to swelling agents or proteases, tissues may stain more rapidly, e.g. nuclei may be stained by alcian blue, and cytoplasms by the 'collagen' dye of a trichrome stain.

What are the effects of specimen geometry on staining?

The varied three-dimensional features of specimens

In this section 'specimen' means the material that is stained, e.g. a deparaffined section, a cervical smear, or a lymph node dab. When observing on a screen or down the microscope it is easy to forget that a specimen has thickness, not just breadth and width. Many people find it hard to believe that differences in thickness of a few µm or less influence staining patterns. However, dispersed cells prepared by smearing often stain differently to cells of the same type cut from a tissue block, and thin sections stain differently from thick. Indeed sections with irregular surface profiles can stain differently to the same biological material cut in sections with smooth surfaces.

Simple geometrical influences on staining

Other things being equal, thin specimens stain faster than thick; specimens with irregular surfaces stain faster than smooth; and dispersed specimens stain faster than uniform slabs. In a given staining procedure, therefore, dispersed specimens such as smears or dabs require shorter staining times than sections of similar cells cut from a solid tissue. Moreover cryosections, which usually have irregular surfaces, will typically stain faster than paraffin sections, which usually have smoother profiles. Resin sections typically have even smoother profiles (see below).

In systems with rate-controlled staining mechanisms such effects can result in loss of selectivity. Thus trichrome stains require shorter staining times with cryo- than with paraffin sections, otherwise cryosections become overstained by the higher ionic weight dye.

More complex effects of specimen geometry

The more complex geometries considered here may originate in the biological structures, or may arise during specimen preparation. These latter artifactual geometries are considered first. A well known modification of section geometry induced by microtomy is chatter. This results in sections containing alternating thick and thin strips. Possible staining outcomes include the occurrence of alternate strips of strong and weak staining or, with trichromes, alternate strips of varying color.

Complex geometries also arise when thin specimens are formed in ways other than sectioning. For instance, smears from epithelia often contain multicellular clumps of cells, as well as monocellular dispersions. Cells at the centers of such clumps are less accessible to stains than are peripheral cells. Consequently, in rate-controlled methods such as the Papanicolaou stain, centrally situated cells can stain artifactually with the smallest dye present, as if they were hyperkeratinized.

A section's profile is also influenced by fixation. Coagulant fixatives such as Carnoy's fluid tend to shatter cells and tissues, giving rise to more dispersed specimens, whilst fixatives such as formalin give more integral forms. Consequently if a rate-controlled method such as a trichrome stain gives rise to the correct color balance when applied to formalin-fixed tissue, it will tend to show overstaining by the collagen fiber stain (usually the larger dye) if applied without modification to material fixed in Carnoy's fluid.

The size of a biological structure relative to the thickness of a section is also significant. Compare secretion granules much larger than the section thickness to granules that are much smaller. All large granules will be sliced through, their contents exposed on a surface of the section, whereas many small granules will be

intact, enclosed within the section. This has marked consequences for methods strongly influenced by stain accessibility, e.g. immunostaining, in which stains are macromolecular. Thus the 'two types of secretion granule' reported in a number of studies may represent intact versus sliced granules. The same may hold for dyeing systems demonstrating 'two types' of erythrocyte, mast cell, mitochondrion, and so on. Such effects can be even more pronounced in resin sections (see below).

Geometrical complexity also results from swelling of cell and tissue components in staining solvents. Structures rich in glycosaminoglycans, e.g. mucus and cartilage matrix, swell markedly in aqueous solutions, whilst collagen fibers swell grossly at extremes of pH. Such swelling can increase rates of staining of these structures, compared to unswollen material. This probably contributes to the high selectivity of aqueous alcian blue for mucins, nuclear staining usually being absent after short staining times, and to the high selectivity of strongly acidic picro-trichrome stains for collagen fibers. Such effects may partially account for changes in staining patterns seen when a dye is used from alcoholic rather than aqueous solution. Luxol fast blue, for instance, stains myelin selectively from aqueous solution, but from alcoholic solutions gives selective staining of collagen fibers. Such effects are often more marked in resin sections, as noted later.

What are the effects of resin embedding on staining?

What is meant by resin embedding?

Typically this involves infiltration of biological material with a reactive monomer, most commonly an acrylate or epoxide. Subsequent polymerization yields a block of resin enclosing the specimen. Sections cut from such blocks are termed resin, or plastic, sections. The peculiarities of staining such sections result from the presence of resin, as well as biological material, during the staining process. If resin is removed prior to staining, as is usually done with methylmethacrylate sections, staining patterns closely resemble those of paraffin sections, so are not discussed here. Specimens may also be embedded in a preformed polymer, usually nitrocellulose, i.e. celloidin. These sections are routinely stained with the polymer present, and behave much like resin sections.

Resins as stain excluders

As resin sections contain both biological material and resin, penetration of staining reagents is usually slower than into paraffin or cryosections. The biological material is said to be occluded. If resin cross-linking is increased, rates of stain penetration fall further.

Resin embedding often has more complicated effects than a mere reduction in staining rate. For example, resin usually infiltrates biological specimens unevenly, with dense and/or hydrophilic structures being poorly infiltrated. This is because even water-miscible or low-viscosity resin systems use monomers which are slightly lipophilic and quite viscous, although less so than the highly lipophilic and viscous media originally developed for transmission electron microscopy. The consequences of uneven resin infiltration are complex. In glycolmethacrylate-embedded specimens structures such as dense secretion granules are often poorly infiltrated, so they may be resin free and stain readily. Moreover, if the surrounding cytoplasm is better infiltrated, granules may stand out more clearly and crisply than in paraffin sections.

Resins as stain binders

Resins can themselves bind stains. For instance, methacrylic acid is sometimes present as a contaminant of glycolmethacrylate monomer, resulting in formation of carboxylated glycolmethacrylate resins. Such anionic resin samples can give rise to strong background basophilia, avoided by using pure monomer. However, background staining due to binding of lipophilic dyes, such as aldehyde fuchsine or Janus green, to glycolmethacrylate is unavoidable because the resin itself is somewhat lipophilic, despite the resin monomer being water miscible (Horobin et al 1992). In addition to background artifacts, stain–resin binding can give negative staining artifacts since the amount of reagent reaching the biological staining target may be reduced by binding to resin. An example is the weak enzyme histochemical staining seen with certain lipophilic enzyme substrates.

Glycolmethacrylate, the major constituent of many light microscopic resin embedding kits, illustrates another dye binding artifact, namely the 'irreversible' binding of certain dyes. This arises with dyes of moderate size, e.g. aluminum hematoxylin or eosin. These can enter the resin and modify the polymer structure, making it less permeable. This antiplasticizing effect traps excess dye, which, however, can sometimes be removed by differentiating in a solvent (such as ethanol) with a plasticizing action.

How stain chemistry influences staining patterns

For small reagents, which diffuse through resins rapidly, staining methods developed for paraffin or cryostat sections can be used without modification. When working with glycolmethacrylate embedding media 'small' means <550 daltons, and includes such common reagents as methylene blue, naphthyl phosphate, and Schiff reagent. However, large reagents may be totally excluded from the resin, restricting staining to resin-free structures. When using glycolmethacrylate resins 'large' reagents are those with sizes >1000 daltons, and include alcian blue, Sirius red, and labeled antibodies.

The possibility of stains binding to lipophilic embedding media, resulting in both positive and negative staining artifacts, was noted above. Such problems occur only with lipophilic reagents. When glycolmethacrylate resin is being used, 'lipophilic' implies reagents whose log P > 1 (see below for explanation of this parameter). Examples include eosin, which has to be differentiated with alcohol, and Gomori's aldehyde fuchsine, which cannot be satisfactorily differentiated.

By considering both size and hydrophilicity–lipophilicity, guidelines may be specified for staining specimens in water-miscible resins such as glycolmethacrylate:

- Small hydrophilic stains, e.g. methylene blue and Schiff reagent, behave much as they do in paraffin or cryosections, though staining a little more slowly.
- Stains of moderate size and/or lipophilicity, e.g. eosin Y and aluminum hematoxylin, often stain more slowly in resin. They also color the resin, and removing this background requires differentiation with plasticizing solvents such as ethanol.
- Lipophilic stains, e.g. Gomori's aldehyde fuchsine, give intense resin coloration, which may prove difficult to remove without de-staining the tissue.
- Coloration of tissues by large hydrophilic stains, e.g. alcian blue, Sirius red, or a labeled antibody, is limited to structures poorly infiltrated with resin.

How resin chemistry influences staining patterns

Two aspects will be considered. The first involves the processes of resin formation, around and within the tissues; the second concerns the nature of the resin itself.

Occurrence of high temperatures within tissue blocks during embedding is considered to cause loss of antigenicity and enzymic activity. Consequently low temperature embedding is used to increase the sensitivity of immunohistochemical and enzyme histochemical methods with resin-embedded tissues. It is also probable that organic solvents and reagents used for dehydration, infiltration, and polymerization cause increased protein denaturation. Hence, partial dehydration and short infiltration times have been adopted to enhance staining sensitivity. These maneuvers may also lower the amount of resin in a section, and hence reduce stain exclusion.

The properties of the resin itself also influence staining processes: ionic character, cross-linking, and lipophilicity were mentioned above. Carry over of plasticizers and polymerization catalysts into the resin block is another factor. Variations in amount and type of plasticizer influence the permeability of resin to stains. Presence of a basic polymerization catalyst results in binding of anionic staining reagents (e.g. acid dyes) to the resin at low pHs, when the base is protonated and so cationic.

SOME DYESTUFF PROPERTIES

Why are dyes colored?

Dyes appear colored because they absorb radiation in the visible region of the electromagnetic spectrum ('light'), between wavelengths of about 400 and 650 nm. Since we perceive the totality of the visible spectrum as white, a dye absorbing right across this range is seen as gray or black. Dyes absorbing light over more limited wavelength ranges have more precise colors. For example, picric acid absorbs predominantly blue–violet light from the short wavelength end of the visible spectrum, and transmits yellow light. Acid fuchsine absorbs blue–green light strongly, from the middle of the visible spectrum, and transmits predominantly red light.

Light absorption is complex; for detailed and up-to-date accounts see color chemistry texts such as Zollinger's (2003). Here highly simplified answers to the question in the heading are sketched around an energy level model. Electrons most weakly attached to a dye molecule —bonding electrons, and non-bonding lone pairs on atoms such as nitrogen, oxygen, or sulfur—have certain specific energies. It is as if electrons stand upon the rungs of an energy ladder, with no footholds in between. Light, and indeed other radiation, comes in packets or quanta of specific energies, with the energies of a quantum increasing as the wavelength decreases. The energies of electrons and the absorption of light quanta are related, as follows. An electron may jump up from a given energy level to a higher one, but for such a jump to take place a quantum must be absorbed whose energy is equal to the energy difference between the two levels. Light absorption corresponds to pushing electrons into higher energy levels.

Now consider why dyes come in different colors and, since all molecules contain bonding electrons if not lone pairs, why all compounds are not colored. The reason is the spacing of energy levels, which is different in different molecules. Consequently the energy of the quanta required to cause electron jumps (i.e. the wavelengths of light absorbed) also varies. When energy of quanta corresponds to wavelengths in the visible spectrum, then absorption is of light, and the compound appears colored. When quanta are of higher energies, the corresponding wavelengths are in the ultraviolet spectrum and the compound appears colorless. The physics is the same, the difference is in our retinal apparatus.

So dyestuffs absorb in the visible spectrum, whilst other compounds do not, because of the spacing of their energy levels. On what do the spacings depend? A critical factor is the degree of delocalization of the bonding electrons. Consider the set of compounds illustrated in Figure 8.1, all containing carbon–carbon double bonds: ethylene, butadiene, benzene, naphthalene, anthracene, and naphthacene. In ethylene the electrons of the π-bond are located between two specific carbon atoms. In butadiene the electrons of the two π-bonds are distributed in orbitals covering all four carbon atoms. In benzene the electrons of three π-bonds are delocalized over six carbon atoms . . . and so on. Parallel changes occur in the spacings of the electronic energy levels of the π-bond component of the carbon–carbon double bonds in this series. Ethylene has the largest spacings and absorbs in the ultraviolet, as do butadiene, benzene, naphthalene, and anthracene. However, the energy level spacings become smaller as the number of conjugated double bonds in each molecule increases. Paralleling this, absorption occurs at longer wavelengths. Finally, with naphthacene, the electron delocalization is so extensive that energy level spacings are small enough for absorption to occur in the visible spectrum, and naphthacene is orange in color. Dyestuffs all possess extensively delocalized electronic systems. Much detailed work has been done to correlate the molecular structures of dyes with electronic absorption spectra (Zollinger 2003).

$$CH_2 = CH_2$$

Ethylene

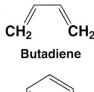

Butadiene

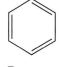

Benzene

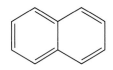

Naphthalene

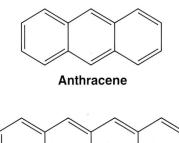

Anthracene

Naphthacene

Fig. 8.1 The molecular structures of a series of compounds containing carbon–carbon double bonds, drawn using the Kekulé structures. Although these formulas cannot show this, the electrons of the double bonds become progressively more delocalized as the series is descended. Paralleling this, the wavelengths of natural absorption increase until, with naphthacene, absorption occurs in the visible spectrum and this compound appears orange.

The energy level model can also be used to understand *fluorescence*, the emission of light by a molecule following prior absorption of ultraviolet radiation or light of a shorter wavelength. In the energy level model (see Figure 8.2 for a simplified version) fluorescence entails falling back of an electron from a higher electronic level to a lower one. But why is visible light emitted when ultraviolet radiation is absorbed? Why are the emitted quanta of lower energy than those absorbed? In fact electronic energy levels, contrary to the impression given so far, contain sublevels. Electrons usually jump from a lower sublevel of a given electronic energy level, to an upper sublevel of a higher electronic energy level. However electrons typically fall back from a lower sublevel of the higher energy level to a higher sublevel of the lower. This smaller jump corresponds to a quantum of lower energy, and so light of longer wavelength is emitted.

Finally consider *metachromasia*, involving dye molecules absorbing light at different wavelengths depending on dye concentration and surroundings. Toluidine blue, for example, transmits in the blue (i.e. is orthochromatic) at low concentrations and when absorbed onto nuclear chromatin. At higher concentrations, or when absorbed into such substrates as cartilage matrix, it transmits in the purple, i.e. is metachromatic. Such spectral variations arise from dye–dye interactions. When two or more dye molecules come into close proximity, their interaction

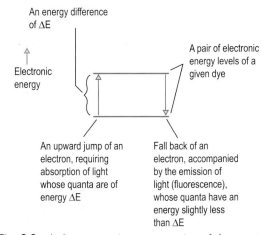

Fig. 8.2 A diagrammatic representation of the movement of an electron between two energy levels: to move upwards quanta are absorbed, on moving downwards quanta are emitted (i.e. fluorescence).

gives rise to a new set of energy level spacings, and thus a new wavelength of light absorption. Often the orthochromatic color derives from the unperturbed levels and the metachromatic color from the new energy levels produced by dye–dye interaction. Any factor favoring dye–dye interactions, such as high charge density substrates or salty dyebaths, will therefore favor metachromatic staining.

Influence of dye chemistry on staining

When those physicochemical features of dyes that influence dye–tissue affinity and staining rates are described using numerical parameters, systematic correlations can be demonstrated between dye chemistry and staining outcomes. Physicochemical parameters include electric charge; overall size, as represented by ionic or molecular weight; and hydrophilic/lipophilic character, modeled by the log P value, i.e. the logarithm of the octanol–water partition coefficient. To appreciate the advantages of numerical parameters inspect Figure 8.3, where chemical information concerning two widely used basic dyes is presented in two modes, graphical and numerical.

When considering relative sizes of the dyes, information provided graphically by structural formulas is satisfactory: alcian blue is obviously a much larger dye than crystal violet. The fact that the staining pattern of alcian blue is highly dependent on staining time (Goldstein & Horobin 1974a) is thus not surprising. The relative hydrophilic/lipophilic character of the two dyes cannot however be readily assessed by visual inspection of formulas, whilst the log P values of the two dyes are clearly different. Negative values imply hydrophilicity, and positive values imply lipophilicity. In keeping with this, sections stained with alcian blue are dehydrated through the alcohols with no removal of dye, but crystal violet is easily lost into the alcohols.

Several dye properties are usually required to predict the performance of a stain. Detailed discussion being inappropriate, note that structure–staining correlations can illuminate diverse issues in histotechnology, from fixation effects in the staining of phospholipids (Horobin 1989), through staining mechanisms of trichromes (Horobin & Flemming 1988), to assessing effects of resin embedding on histochemical staining procedures (Horobin et al 1992). Indeed such correlations have also proved applicable to vital staining by fluorescent probes, e.g. to develop a stain to demonstrate fluid phase pino-

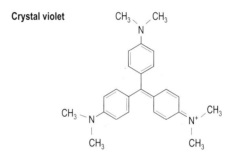

Dye	Ionic weight	Log P
Alcian blue 8G	1380	−9.7
Crystal violet	372	+1.9

Fig. 8.3 Structural formulas of two widely used basic dyes, plus numerical descriptions of certain of their physicochemical properties.

cytosis (Espada et al 1997), and to predict localization of fluorescent probes in bacterial cell walls (Christensen et al 1999). (For more general accounts of such structure–staining correlations see Horobin 1982, 1988, 2001, 2004.)

Effects of dye impurities on staining

Almost all dyes used as stains are impure, which has provoked experimental investigations and polemical editorials. But what is an 'impure' dye?

A batch of dye is considered impure if it does not contain the compound named on the label, or if it contains substantial amounts of other colored substances additional to the named dye. Or the batch may contain very little dye, most of the contents being inorganic salt. Dyes that are pure when purchased may decompose on storage, or after being made up as a staining solution, or during staining itself. Impurities influence staining in two ways. First they may alter staining intensity. Typically staining is reduced, but occasionally impurities result in a more intense coloration. Second, impurities may change staining patterns, the nature and mechanisms of such effects depending on the type of impurity, the particular staining procedure, and the tissue substrate.

Unfortunately there is no simple way to identify, and so avoid, such impure products. A practical tip is to purchase dye batches certified by the *Biological Stain Commission*. These have been tested in the *Commission's* laboratory, and met purity and staining efficacy criteria. Surprisingly, *Commission* certified dyes are on average no more expensive than non-certified dyes. (For a recent example of the benefits of certified dyes see Henwood 2003.) Another practical tip is to check if staining problems are due to impure stains, e.g. by retaining samples of effective dye batches. Faced with an unexpected staining pattern, a specimen can then be stained with the effective dye. If this gives satisfactory coloration, there may be problems due to dye impurity.

What can you do about impure dye batches? Few have the resources, or the inclination, to engage in analysis or purification. The most useful advice is to buy another batch of dye, preferably *Biological Stain Commission* certified. If analysis or purification does prove necessary, there is an extensive literature, some cited in the present book. For further information Chayen and Bitensky's book (1991) is a useful source, as is a review article by the present author (Horobin 1969).

Dye nomenclature

Names of individual dyes, and terms used to describe dye properties, are sometimes inconsistent and are often confusing. As dyes are complex molecules nearly all have trivial names, which do not describe their structures. Moreover most biological stains were first manufactured as textile dyes, when each manufacturer gave the dye their own trade name. A biologist may therefore say 'Use Congo blue', to which his colleagues reply 'But we haven't got any of *that*'. And yet they have, but on their shelves it is labeled trypan blue. Even worse is the surfeit of suffixes. Sometimes these are merely flourishes of a copywriter's pen, so pyronines G and Y are synonyms. Sometimes suffixes indicate dye content, and a standard product may be labeled 'A 100' whilst a grade containing a higher content of dye is termed 'A 150' or merely 'A extra'. Sometimes, however, suffixes indicate substantial chemical differences, e.g. rhodamines B and 6G respectively describe zwitterionic and cationic dyes.

To reduce confusion, industrial dye users established the *Colour Index* (Society of Dyers and Colourists 1999). Dyes were given unique code numbers—the *Colour Index*, or C.I., number—and code names. Thus eosins G, WG, and Y are identified as a single dye, C.I. 45380, Acid Red 87, whilst eosin B is a chemically different dye, C.I. 45400, Acid Red 91.

When biologists synthesize dyes they name them equally idiosyncratically. A traditional example is Gomori's aldehyde fuchsine, and a recent one YOYO-1. Since these products are not of industrial significance, most do not have a *Colour Index* entry. In such cases the puzzled should peruse *Conn's Biological Stains* (see Lillie 1977 and Horobin & Kiernan 2002 for the 9th and 10th editions respectively).

Various terms used to classify dyestuffs are given in Table 8.2, and comments on points sometimes confused in the histochemical literature follow. *Acid* and *basic* dyes are not acids and bases but salts, whose colored species are anionic and cationic respectively. *Neutral* dyes are not non-ionic, but salts in which both the anion and cation are dyes. *Vital stains*, used to stain living cells, are nowadays often called *fluorescent probes*. Any dye can be described by many terms. Thus alcian blue 8G is a *synthetic basic* dye, structurally a *metal complex*, though not a *mordant dye*, of copper with *phthalocyanine*, substituted by *thioguanidinium groups*, and is typically used as a *mucin stain*.

PROBLEM AVOIDANCE AND TROUBLESHOOTING

Avoiding problems and recognizing and correcting errors are perennial laboratory concerns. Typical strategies are sketched below, and detailed information for several dozen routine and special histopathology stains may be found in Horobin and Bancroft (1998).

Table 8.2 Some descriptive terms used in classifying dyestuffs used in biology

Categories of terms	Examples of terms (and of dyes)
Describing the origins of a dye	Natural (hematoxylin and carmine), synthetic or aniline (almost any other)
Describing physicochemical properties of a dye	Fluorescent (acridine orange), metachromatic (toluidine blue), leuco (leuco methylene blue), neutral (azure-eosinate)
Giving some kind of description of the dye's structure	Metal complex (aluminum or iron complexes of hematein), azo (orange G), xanthene (pyronine Y)
Describing the dye's usage in biological staining	Fluorescent probe (YOYO-1), fat (oil red), mucin (alcian blue)
Describing the dye's usage in textile dyeing	Acid (eosin), basic (safranine), direct (Congo red)
Describing the supposed mode of action of the dye	Mordant (gallocyanine chrome alum), reactive (mercury orange)

Strategies for avoiding problems—to minimize the need for troubleshooting

Issues concerning staining procedures

- Choose fixative and embedding media suitable for the proposed stains. *Case example*: water-miscible resin sections do not allow selective staining of elastic fibers with aldehyde fuchsine.
- Use a routine, preferably a standardized, staining protocol. *Tip*: see listing of such at the back of Horobin and Bancroft (1998).
- Use controls to detect problems proactively, not merely to investigate mistakes retrospectively. *Tip*: keep samples of effective batches of stain to use when you suspect inadequate stain purity.
- Consider whether you have necessary skills and knowledge, or if not is a mentor available? *Tip*: many silver stains are tricky; expect problems with their use.

Issues concerning staining reagents

- Obtain reliable stains and reagent. *Tip*: use *Biological Stain Commission* certified dyes, as they are on average no more expensive.
- Ensure stains remain reliable. *Tips*: store Schiff reagent in a gas-tight container; store dye solutions in light-proof containers.

Cues for recognizing errors—before mistakes can be rectified, they must be noticed

1. Stain or staining solution is not as expected in terms of color, solubility, or stability. *Case example*: some alcian blue samples dissolve, but then precipitate from solution within an hour or less.
2. The expected structures stain, but only weakly. *Case example*: unexpectedly weak staining of calcium by alizarin red S results from loss of calcium ions into aqueous fixatives.
3. Color of staining is unexpected. *Case example*: excessively red staining seen with Gomori's trichrome may arise from insufficiently acidic staining solutions.
4. Unexpected structures stain. *Case example*: granular material stained by the Feulgen nucleal procedure may be carbonate deposits.
5. Nature of the staining is unusual. *Case example*: if differential staining of Gram positive and negative organisms is poor, the preparation may be too thick.
6. And there are always *other* problems! *Case examples*: loss of sections from slides in the Grocott hexamine silver method for fungi, due to overheating; and black deposits on slides and sections in the Von Kossa procedure, due to contaminated glassware.

Once an error has been noticed, and a plausible cause identified, a solution can be sought. This is sometimes simple. Perhaps the trickiest situations arise when staining specimens prepared in another laboratory. Again a variety of practical problem-solving suggestions, for a range of routine and special histopathology stains, is given in Horobin and Bancroft (1998).

REFERENCES

Baker J.R. (1958) Principles of biological microtechnique. London: Methuen.

Bennion P.J., Horobin R.W. (1974) Some effects of salts on staining: the use of the Donnan equilibrium to describe staining of tissue sections with acid and basic dyes. Histochemistry 39:71–82.

Bettinger C.H., Zimmermann H.W. (1991) New investigations on hematoxylin, hematein, and hematein–aluminium complexes. 2. Hematein–aluminium complexes and hemalum staining. Histochemistry 96:215–228.

Chayen J., Bitensky L. (1991) Practical histochemistry, 2nd edn. Chichester: Wiley.

Christensen H., Garton N.J., Horobin R.W. et al. (1999) Lipid domains of mycobacteria studied with fluorescent molecular probes. Molecular Microbiology 31:1561–1572.

Espada J., Horobin R.W., Stockert J.C. (1997) Fluorescent cytochemistry of acid phosphatases and demonstration of fluid-phase endocytosis using an azo dye method. Histochemistry and Cell Biology 108:481–487.

Goldstein D.J. (1962) Correlation of size of dye particle and density of substrate, with special reference to mucin staining. Stain Technology 37:79–93.

Goldstein D.J., Horobin R.W. (1974a) Rate factors in staining with alcian blue. Histochemical Journal 6:157–174.

Goldstein D.J., Horobin R.W. (1974b) Surface staining of cartilage by alcian blue, with reference to the role of microscopic aggregates in histological staining. Histochemical Journal 6:175–184.

Henwood A. (2003) Current applications of orcein in histochemistry. A brief review with some new observations concerning influence of dye batch variation and aging of dye solutions on staining. Biotechnic and Histochemistry 78:303–308.

Horobin R.W. (1969) The impurities of biological dyes: their detection, removal, occurrence and histological significance—a review. Histochemical Journal 1:231–265.

Horobin R.W. (1982) Histochemistry: an explanatory outline of histochemistry and biophysical staining. Stuttgart: Fischer, and London: Butterworths.

Horobin R.W. (1988) Understanding histochemistry: selection, evaluation and design of biological stains. Chichester: Horwood.

Horobin R.W. (1989) A numerical approach to understanding fixative action: being a reanalysis of the fixation of lipids by the dye-glutaraldehyde system. Journal of Microscopy 154:93–96.

Horobin R.W. (2001) Uptake, distribution, and accumulation of dyes and fluorescent probes within living cells. A structure–activity modelling approach. Advances in Colour Science and Technology 4:101–107.

Horobin R.W. (2004) Staining by numbers: a tool for understanding and assisting use of routine and special histopathology stains. Journal of Histotechnology 27:23–28.

Horobin R.W., Bancroft J.D. (1998) Troubleshooting histology stains. New York: Churchill Livingstone.

Horobin R.W., Bennion P.J. (1973) The interrelation of the size and substantivity of dyes: the role of van der Waals' attractions and hydrophobic bonding in biological staining. Histochemie 33:191–204.

Horobin R.W., Flemming L. (1988) One-bath trichrome staining: investigation of a general mechanism based on a structure-staining correlation analysis. Histochemical Journal 20:29–34.

Horobin R.W., Goldstein D.J. (1974) The influence of salt on the staining of sections with basic dyes; an investigation into the general applicability of the critical electrolyte concentration theory. Histochemical Journal 6:599–609.

Horobin R.W., Kiernan J.A. (2002) Conn's biological stains. A handbook of dyes and fluorochromes for use in biology and medicine, 10th edn. Oxford: BIOS Scientific Publishers.

Horobin R.W., Gerrits P.O., Wright D.J. (1992) Staining sections of water-miscible resins. 2. Effects of staining-reagent lipophilicity on the staining of glycolmethacrylate-embedded tissues. Journal of Microscopy 166:199–205.

Kiernan J.A. (2007) Histological and histochemical methods: theory and practice, 4th edn. Bloxham: Scion.

Lillie R.D. (1965) Histopathologic technic and practical histochemistry, 3rd edn. New York: McGraw-Hill.

Lillie R.D. (1977) H.J. Conn's biological stains, 9th edn. Baltimore: Williams & Wilkins.

Lyon H. (1991) Theory and strategy of histochemistry: a guide to the selection and understanding of techniques. Berlin: Springer-Verlag.

Mann G. (1902) Physiological histology. Methods and theory. Oxford: Clarendon.

Marshall P.N., Horobin R.W. (1973) The mechanism of action of 'mordant' dyes—a study using preformed metal complexes. Histochemie 35:361–371.

Mason W.T. (1999) Fluorescent and luminescent probes for biological activity, 2nd edn. San Diego: Academic Press.

Pearse A.G.E. (1968) Histochemistry, theoretical and applied, Vol. 1, 3rd edn. Edinburgh: Churchill Livingstone.

Peters A. (1955a) Experiments on the mechanism of silver staining. 1. Impregnation. Quarterly Journal of Microscopical Science 96:84–102.

Peters A. (1955b) Experiments on the mechanism of silver staining. 2. Development. Quarterly Journal of Microscopical Science 96:103–115.

Prentø P. (2001) A contribution to the theory of biological staining based on the principles for structural organization of biological macromolecules. Biotechnic and Histochemistry 76:137–161.

Prentø P. (2007) The structural role of glycine and proline in connective tissue fiber staining with hydrogen bonding dyes. Biotechnic and Histochemistry 82:170–173.

Scott J.E. (1973) Affinity, competition and specific interactions in the biochemistry and histochemistry of polyelectrolytes. Biochemical Society Transactions 1:787–806.

Scott J.E., Harbinson J. (1968) Periodic oxidation of acid polysaccharides. Inhibition by the electrostatic field of the substrate. Histochemie 14:215–220.

Sheehan D.C., Hrapchak B.B. (1987) Theory and practice of histotechnology, 2nd edn. Columbus, OH: Battelle Press.

Society of Dyers and Colourists (1999) Colour Index International, 3rd edn. Issue 3 on CD ROM. Bradford, UK: The Society of Dyers and Colourists.

Tanford C. (2004) Ben Franklin stilled the waves: an informal history of pouring oil on water with reflections on the ups and downs of scientific life in general. Oxford: Oxford University Press.

Zollinger H. (2003) Colour chemistry, 3rd edn. Weinhein: Wiley-VCH, and Zurich: VHCA.

FURTHER READING

Few accounts of histochemistry emphasize the physicochemical unity underlying the technical diversity of the various staining technologies. There are many published protocols but a paucity of critical accounts and summations. Thus encyclopedic texts like the present one—and earlier examples such as those of Lillie (1965), Pearse (1968), and Sheehan and Hrapchak (1987)— summarize a remarkable amount of information and provide extensive bibliographies. Some staining manuals also set out to integrate theoretical background with procedural information, e.g. Chayen and Bitensky (1991) and Kiernan (2007). A few authors have attempted to provide modern physicochemical accounts of staining methods as a whole; for instance Horobin (1982, 1988), Horobin and Bancroft (1998), Lyon (1991), and Prentø (2001). Some classic works can also be recommended: read Baker (1958) for his early integrative account, and his elegant English; read Lillie (1965) for his hard-won personal experience, and historical longview; and then read Mann (1902) to be astonished at why it took us so long to follow up his experimental investigations.

9

The Hematoxylins and Eosin

Marilyn Gamble

INTRODUCTION

The hematoxylin and eosin stain (H&E) is the most widely used histological stain. Its popularity is based on its comparative simplicity and ability to demonstrate clearly an enormous number of different tissue structures. Hematoxylin can be prepared in numerous ways and has a widespread applicability to tissues from different sites. Essentially, the hematoxylin component stains the cell nuclei blue–black, with good intranuclear detail, while the eosin stains cell cytoplasm and most connective tissue fibers in varying shades and intensities of pink, orange, and red. While automated staining instruments and commercially prepared hematoxylin and eosin solutions are more commonly used in today's laboratories for routine staining, students of histological techniques must have a basic knowledge of the dyes and preparation techniques in order to troubleshoot and/or modify procedures for specialized use. Hematoxylin has many more uses than in the hematoxylin and eosin combination.

Hematoxylin

Hematoxylin is extracted from the heartwood ('logwood') of the tree *Haematoxylon campechianum* that originated in the Mexican State of Campeche, but is now mainly cultivated in the West Indies. The hematoxylin is extracted from logwood with hot water, and then precipitated out from the aqueous solution using urea (Lamb, personal communication 1974). Hematoxylin itself is not a stain. The major oxidization product is hematein, a natural dye that is responsible for the color properties. Hematein can be produced from hematoxylin in two ways:

Natural oxidation ('ripening') by exposure to light and air. This is a slow process, sometimes taking as long as 3–4 months, but the resultant solution seems to retain its staining ability for a long time. Ehrlich's and Delafield's hematoxylin solutions are examples of naturally ripened hematoxylins.

Chemical oxidation using sodium iodate (e.g. Mayer's hematoxylin) or mercuric oxide (e.g. Harris's hematoxylin). The use of chemical oxidizing agents converts the hematoxylin to hematein almost instantaneously, so these hematoxylin solutions are ready for use immediately after preparation. In general, they have a shorter useful life than the naturally oxidized hematoxylins, probably because the continuing oxidation process in air and light eventually destroys much of the hematein, converting it to a colorless compound. Hematein is anionic, having a poor affinity for tissue, and is inadequate as a nuclear stain without the presence of a mordant. The most useful mordants for hematoxylin are salts of aluminum, iron, and tungsten, although hematoxylin solutions using lead as a mordant are occasionally used (for example in the demonstration of argyrophil cells). The mordant/metal cation confers a net positive charge to the dye–mordant complex and enables it to bind to anionic tissue sites such as nuclear chromatin. The type of mordant used influences strongly the type of tissue components stained and their final color. Most mordants are incorporated into the hematoxylin staining solutions, although certain hematoxylin stains required the tissue section to be pre-treated with the mordant before staining; an example is Heidenhain's iron hematoxylin. Hematoxylin solutions can therefore be arbitrarily classified according to which mordant is used:

- alum hematoxylins
- iron hematoxylins
- tungsten hematoxylins
- molybdenum hematoxylins
- lead hematoxylins
- hematoxylin without mordant.

ALUM HEMATOXYLINS

This group comprises most of those that are used routinely in the hematoxylin and eosin stain, and produce good nuclear staining. The mordant is aluminum, usually in the form of 'potash alum' (aluminum potassium sulfate) or 'ammonium alum' (aluminum ammonium sulfate). All stain the nuclei a red color, which is converted to the familiar blue–black when the section is washed in a weak alkali solution. Tap water is usually alkaline enough to produce this color change, but occasionally alkaline solutions such as saturated lithium carbonate, 0.05% ammonia in distilled water, or Scott's tap water substitute (see Appendix II) are necessary. This procedure is known as 'bluing'.

The alum hematoxylins can be used *regressively*, meaning that the section is over-stained and then differentiated in acid alcohol, followed by 'bluing', or *progressively*, i.e. stained for a predetermined time to stain the nuclei adequately but leave the background tissue relatively unstained. The times for hematoxylin staining and for satisfactory differentiation will vary according to the type and age of alum hematoxylin used, the type of tissue, and the personal preference of the pathologist. For routine hematoxylin and eosin staining of tissues, the most commonly used hematoxylins are Ehrlich's, Mayer's, Harris's, Gill's, Cole's, and Delafield's. Carazzi's hematoxylin is occasionally used, particularly for urgent frozen sections.

Ehrlich's hematoxylin (Ehrlich 1886)

This is a naturally ripening alum hematoxylin which takes about two months to ripen; the ripening time can be shortened somewhat by placing the unstoppered bottle in a warm sunny place such as a windowledge, and is shorter in the summer than in winter. Once satisfactorily ripened this hematoxylin solution will last in bulk for years, and retains its staining ability in a Coplin jar for some months. Ehrlich's hematoxylin, as well as being an excellent nuclear stain, also stains mucins including the mucopolysaccharides of cartilage; it is recommended for the staining of bone and cartilage (see Chapter 18).

Preparation of solution

Hematoxylin	2 g
Absolute alcohol	100 ml
Glycerin	100 ml
Distilled water	100 ml
Glacial acetic acid	10 ml
Potassium alum	15 g approx.

The hematoxylin is dissolved in the alcohol, and the other chemicals are added. Glycerin is added to slow the oxidation process and prolong the hematoxylin shelf life. Natural ripening in sunlight takes about two months, but in an emergency the stain can be chemically ripened by the addition of sodium iodate, using 50 mg for every gram of hematoxylin; this will inevitably shorten the bench life of the stain. By definition this chemically oxidized variant is not a true Ehrlich's hematoxylin and will not have the same longevity as naturally oxidized Ehrlich's hematoxylin. Always filter before use.

Ehrlich's hematoxylin, being a strong hematoxylin solution, stains nuclei intensely and crisply, and stained sections fade much more slowly than those stained with other alum hematoxylins. It is particularly useful for staining sections from tissues that have been exposed to acid. It is suitable for tissues that have been subjected to acid decalcification or, more valuably, tissues that have been stored for a long period in formalin fixatives which have gradually become acidic over the storage period, or in acid fixatives such as Bouin's fixative. Ehrlich's hematoxylin is not ideal for frozen sections.

Delafield's hematoxylin (Delafield 1885)

A naturally ripened alum hematoxylin, Delafield's has similar longevity to Ehrlich's hematoxylin.

Preparation of solution

Hematoxylin	4 g
95% alcohol	125 ml
Saturated aqueous ammonium alum (15 g/100 ml)	400 ml
Glycerin	100 ml

The hematoxylin is dissolved in 25 ml of alcohol, and then added to the alum solution. This mixture is allowed to stand in light and air for 5 days, then filtered, and to it are added the glycerin and a further 100 ml of 95% alcohol. The stain is allowed to stand exposed to light and air for about 3–4 months or until the stain is sufficiently dark in color, then filtered and stored. Filter before use.

Mayer's hematoxylin (Mayer 1903)

This alum hematoxylin is chemically ripened with sodium iodate. It can be used as a regressive stain like any alum hematoxylin. However, it is also useful as a progressive stain, particularly in situations where a nuclear counterstain is needed to emphasize a cytoplasmic component which has been demonstrated, by a special stain, and where the acid–alcohol differentiation might destroy or de-color the stained cytoplasmic component. It is used as a nuclear counterstain in the demonstration of glycogen, in various enzyme histochemical techniques, and in many others. The stain is applied for a short time (usually 5–10 minutes), until the nuclei are stained, and is then 'blued' without any differentiation.

Preparation of solution

Hematoxylin	1 g
Distilled water	1000 ml
Potassium or ammonium alum	50 g
Sodium iodate	0.2 g
Citric acid	1 g
Chloral hydrate SLR	50 g *or*
Chloral hydrate AR	30 g

The hematoxylin, potassium alum, and sodium iodate are dissolved in the distilled water by warming and stirring, or by allowing to stand at room temperature overnight. The chloral hydrate and citric acid are added, and the mixture is boiled for 5 minutes, then cooled and filtered. If higher purity chloral hydrate AR grade is used then the amount used may be reduced, as shown above. The stain is ready for use immediately. Filter before use.

Harris's hematoxylin (Harris 1900)

An alum hematoxylin, Harris's was traditionally chemically ripened with mercuric oxide. As mercuric oxide is highly toxic, environmentally unfriendly, and can have detrimental, corrosive long-term effects on some automated staining machines, sodium or potassium iodate is frequently used as a substitute for oxidation. Harris's is a useful general-purpose hematoxylin and gives particularly clear nuclear staining, and for this reason has been used, as a progressive stain, in diagnostic exfoliative cytology. In routine histological practice, it is generally used regressively, but can be useful when used progressively. When using Harris's hematoxylin as a progressive stain, an acetic acid–alcohol rinse provides a more controllable method in removing excess stain from tissue components and the glass slide. The traditional hydrochloric acid–alcohol acts quickly and indiscriminately, is more difficult to control, and can result in a light nuclear stain. A 5–10% solution of acetic acid, in 70–95% alcohol, detaches dye molecules from the cytoplasm/nucleoplasm while keeping nucleic acid complexes intact (Feldman & Dapson 1985).

Preparation of solution

Hematoxylin	2.5 g
Absolute alcohol	25 ml
Potassium alum	50 g
Distilled water	500 ml
Mercuric oxide	1.25 g *or*
Sodium iodate	0.5 g
Glacial acetic acid	20 ml

The hematoxylin is dissolved in the absolute alcohol, and is then added to the alum, which has previously been dissolved in the warm distilled water in a 2-liter flask. The mixture is rapidly brought to the boil and the mercuric oxide or sodium iodate is then slowly and carefully added. Plunging the flask into cold water or into a sink containing chipped ice rapidly cools the stain. When the solution is cold, the acetic acid is added, and the stain is ready for immediate use. The glacial acetic acid is optional but its inclusion gives more precise and selective staining of nuclei.

As with most of the chemically ripened alum hematoxylins, the quality of the nuclear staining begins to deteriorate after a few months. This deterioration is marked by the formation of a precipitate in the stored stain. At this stage, the stain should be filtered before use, and the staining time may need to be increased. For the best results, it is wise to prepare a fresh batch of stain every month, although this may be uneconomical unless only small quantities are prepared each time.

Cole's hematoxylin (Cole 1943)

This is an alum hematoxylin, artificially ripened with an alcoholic iodine solution.

Preparation of solution

Hematoxylin	1.5 g
Saturated aqueous potassium alum	700 ml
1% iodine in 95% alcohol	50 ml
Distilled water	250 ml

The hematoxylin is dissolved in warm distilled water and mixed with the iodine solution. The alum solution is added, and the mixture brought to the boil, then cooled quickly and filtered. The solution is ready for immediate use, but may need filtering after storage, for the same reason as described above for Harris's hematoxylin. Filter before use.

Carazzi's hematoxylin (Carazzi 1911)

Carazzi's is an alum hematoxylin which is chemically ripened using potassium iodate.

Preparation of solution

Hematoxylin	5 g
Glycerol	100 ml
Potassium alum	25 g
Distilled water	400 ml
Potassium iodate	0.1 g

The hematoxylin is dissolved in the glycerol, and the alum is dissolved in most of the water overnight. The alum solution is added slowly to the hematoxylin solution, mixing well after each addition. The potassium iodate is dissolved in the rest of the water with gentle warming and is then added to the hematoxylin–alum–glycerol mixture. The final staining solution is mixed well and is then ready for immediate use; it remains usable for about 6 months. Care must be taken in preparing the hematoxylin to avoid over-oxidation; it is safer if heat is not used to dissolve the reagents. Filter before use.

Like Mayer's hematoxylin, Carazzi's hematoxylin may be used as a progressive nuclear counterstain using a short staining time, followed by bluing in tap water. It is particularly suitable since it is a pale and precise nuclear stain and does not stain any of the cytoplasmic components.

Our experience with Carazzi's hematoxylin is largely confined to its use with frozen sections from an urgent surgical biopsy. Its advantage in this situation is the excellent and clear nuclear staining when used as a double or triple strength solution (i.e. using 10 g or 15 g of hematoxylin in the above) with a short staining time; only the nuclei stain. This short staining time is important where speed and accuracy are essential. The method for urgent frozen sections using Carazzi's hematoxylin is given on p. 127.

Gill's hematoxylin (Gill et al 1974 modified)

Preparation of solution

Hematoxylin	2 g
Sodium iodate	0.2 g
Aluminum sulfate	17.6 g
Distilled water	750 ml
Ethylene glycol (ethandiol)	250 ml
Glacial acetic acid	20 ml

The distilled water and ethylene glycol are mixed, and then the hematoxylin is added and dissolved. The ethylene glycol is an excellent solvent for hematoxylin and it prevents the formation of surface precipitates (Carson 1997). Sodium iodate is added for oxidation, and the aluminum sulfate mordant is then added and dissolved. Finally, the glacial acetic acid is added and stirred for 1 hour. The solution is filtered before use. Carson reported that, although the stain can be used immediately, it provides a better intensity if allowed to ripen for 1 week in a 37°C incubator. It should be noted that the popularity of Gill's solution has made it one of the more commercially successful formulas.

Double or triple hematoxylin concentrations may be used as preferred. These are usually referred to as Gill's I (normal), Gill's II (double), and Gill's III (triple), with the Gill III being the most concentrated. Gill's hematoxylin is more frequently used for routine H&E staining than Mayer's hematoxylin, and is more stable than Harris's hematoxylin, as auto-oxidation is inhibited to the extent that no measurable changes occur over many months. Disadvantages associated with Gill's hematoxylin include staining of gelatin adhesive and even the glass itself. Some mucus may also stain darkly, as compared to Harris's, where mucus generally remains unstained, and the glass usually fails to attract the stain. Feldman and Dapson (1987) theorized that the aluminum sulfate mordant is responsible. Certain charged sites in the tissue, in the adhesive, and on the glass are masked by the Harris mordant, leaving them unavailable for staining. Gill's mordant system fails to do that, and the sites attract the dye–mordant complex.

Staining times with alum hematoxylins

It is not possible to give other than a rough guide to suitable staining times with alum hematoxylins because the time will vary according to the following factors:

1. Type of hematoxylin used, e.g. Ehrlich's 20–45 min, Mayer's 10–20 min.
2. Age of stain. As the stain ages, the staining time will need to be increased.
3. Intensity of use of stain. A heavily used hematoxylin will lose its staining powers more rapidly and longer staining times will be necessary.
4. Whether the stain is used progressively or regressively, e.g. Mayer's hematoxylin used progressively 5–10 min, used regressively 10–20 min.
5. Pre-treatment of tissues or sections, e.g. length of time in fixative or acid decalcifying solution, or whether paraffin or frozen sections.
6. Post-treatment of sections, e.g. subsequent acid stains such as van Gieson.
7. Personal preference.

The times given in Table 9.1 are, therefore, only a general indication of a suitable range for each type of stain; the optimal time must be determined by trial and error. Except where stated, these figures refer to normally fixed paraffin sections. As a rule, the times need to be considerably shortened for frozen sections, and increased for decalcified tissues and those that have been stored for a long time in non-buffered formalin.

Disadvantages of alum hematoxylins

The major disadvantage of alum hematoxylin nuclear stains is their sensitivity to any subsequently applied

Table 9.1 Staining times with alum hematoxylins

Cole's	20–45 min
Delafield's	15–20 min
Ehrlich's (progressive)	20–45 min
Mayer's (progressive)	10–20 min
Mayer's (regressive)	5–10 min
Harris's (progressive in cytology)	4–30 s
Harris's (regressive)	5–15 min
Carazzi's (progressive)	1–2 min
Carazzi's (regressive)	45 s
Carazzi's (frozen sections, see text)	1 min
Gill's I (regressive)	5–15 min

acidic staining solutions. The most common examples are in the van Gieson and other trichrome stains. The application of the picric acid–acid fuchsin mixture in van Gieson's stain removes most of the hematoxylin so that the nuclei are barely discernible. In this case satisfactory nuclear staining can be achieved by using an iron-mordanted hematoxylin such as Weigert's hematoxylin (see below), which is resistant to the effect of picric acid. A suitable, and now more popular, alternative is the combination of a celestine blue staining solution with an alum hematoxylin. Celestine blue is resistant to the effects of acid, and the ferric salt in the prepared celestine blue solution strengthens the bond between the nucleus and the alum hematoxylin to provide a strong nuclear stain which is reasonably resistant to acid.

Celestine blue–alum hematoxylin procedure

Celestine blue solution

Celestine blue B	2.5 g
Ferric ammonium sulfate	25 g
Glycerin	70 ml
Distilled water	500 ml

The ferric ammonium sulfate is dissolved in the cold distilled water with stirring, the celestine blue is added to this solution, and the mixture is boiled for a few minutes. After cooling, the stain is filtered and glycerin is added. The final stain should be usable for over 5 months. Filter before use.

Method
1. Deparaffinize sections, hydrate through graded alcohols to water.
2. Stain in celestine blue solution for 5 min.
3. Rinse in distilled water.
4. Stain in an alum hematoxylin (e.g. Mayer's or Cole's) for 5 min.
5. Wash in water until blue.
6. Proceed with required staining technique.

EOSIN

Eosin is the most suitable stain to combine with an alum hematoxylin to demonstrate the general histological architecture of a tissue. Its particular value is its ability, with proper differentiation, to distinguish between the cytoplasm of different types of cell, and between the different types of connective tissue fibers and matrices, by staining them differing shades of red and pink.

The eosins are xanthene dyes and the following types are easily obtainable commercially: eosin Y (eosin yellowish, eosin water-soluble) C.I. No. 45380 (C.I. Acid Red 87); ethyl eosin (eosin S, eosin alcohol-soluble) C.I. No. 45386 (C.I. Solvent Red 45); eosin B (eosin bluish, erythrosin B) C.I. No. 45400 (C.I. Acid Red 91).

Of these, eosin Y is much the most widely used, and despite its synonym it is also satisfactorily soluble in alcohol; it is sometimes sold as 'water and alcohol soluble'. As a cytoplasmic stain, it is usually used as a 0.5 or 1.0% solution in distilled water, with a crystal of thymol added to inhibit the growth of fungi. The addition of a little acetic acid (0.5 ml to 1000 ml stain) is said to sharpen the staining. Differentiation of the eosin staining occurs in the subsequent tap water wash, and a little further differentiation occurs during the dehydration through the alcohols. The intensity of eosin staining, and the degree of differentiation required, is largely a matter of individual taste. Suitable photomicrographs of H&E-stained tissues are easier to obtain when the eosin staining is intense and the differentiation slight (at least double the routine staining time is advisable). Ethyl eosin and eosin B are now rarely used, although occasional old methods specify their use, for example the Harris stain for Negri bodies. Alternative red dyes have been suggested as substitutes for eosin, such as phloxine,

Biebrich scarlet, etc., but, although these substitutes often give a more intense red color to the tissues, they are rarely as amenable to subtle differentiation as eosin and are generally less valuable.

Under certain circumstances eosin staining is intense and difficulty may be experienced in obtaining adequate differentiation; this may occur after mercuric fixation. Over-differentiation of the eosin may be continued until only the red blood cells and granules of eosinophil polymorph are stained red. This is, occasionally, used to facilitate the location and identification of eosinophils. Combining eosin Y and phloxine B (10 ml 1% phloxine B, 100 ml 1% eosin Y, 780 ml 95% alcohol, 4 ml glacial acetic acid) produces a cytoplasmic stain, which more dramatically demonstrates various tissue components. Muscle is clearly differentiated from collagen, and red cells stain bright red. According to Luna (1992), eosin dye content should be 88% and not contain sodium sulfate (sometimes used as a filler). When using this dye in solution, a fine granular precipitate forms, and the staining of the cytoplasm will be poor.

Routine staining procedures using alum hematoxylins

Hematoxylin and eosin stain for paraffin sections

Method
1. Deparaffinize sections, hydrate through graded alcohols to water.
2. Remove fixation pigments (see p. 253) if necessary.
3. Stain in an alum hematoxylin of choice for a suitable time (see p. 125).
4. Wash well in running tap water until sections 'blue' for 5 minutes or less.
5. Differentiate in 1% acid alcohol (1% HCl in 70% alcohol) for 5–10 seconds.
6. Wash well in tap water until sections are again 'blue' (10–15 min), or
7. Blue by dipping in an alkaline solution (e.g. ammonia water), followed by a 5-min tap water wash.
8. Stain in 1% eosin Y for 10 min.
9. Wash in running tap water for 1–5 min.
10. Dehydrate through alcohols, clear, and mount.

Results

Nuclei	blue/black
Cytoplasm	varying shades of pink
Muscle fibers	deep pink/red
Red blood cells	orange/red
Fibrin	deep pink

Notes

Note that structures and substances other than nuclei may be hematoxyphilic to varying degrees. Examples include fungal hyphae, which are faintly hematoxyphilic, and calcium deposits, which are often deep blue–black.

Rapid hematoxylin and eosin stain for urgent frozen sections

1. Freeze suitable tissue block onto a chuck.
2. Cut cryostat sections at 3–6 mm thickness.
3. Fix section in 10% neutral buffered formalin at room temperature for 20 seconds.
4. Rinse in tap water.
5. Stain in double strength Carazzi's hematoxylin (see p. 124) for 1 minute.
6. Wash well in tap water for 10–20 seconds.
7. Stain in 1% aqueous eosin for 10 seconds.
8. Rinse in tap water.
9. Dehydrate, clear, and mount.

Suitably modified techniques for routine H&E sections of resin-embedded tissues are given in Chapter 29, and for other types of tissue preparation in various chapters in this book.

Papanicolaou stain for cytological preparations

The universal stain for cytological preparations is the Papanicolaou stain. Harris's hematoxylin is the optimal nuclear stain and the combination of OG 6 and EA 50 gives the subtle range of green, blue, and pink hues to the cell cytoplasm.

Most laboratories use commercial stains and each will consider their modification of the original technique to be the optimum. The result, however, should retain the transparent quality of the cytoplasmic stain, and the nuclear chromatin should be easily distinguished.

Papanicolaou formula

Harris's hematoxylin (see p. 123)

Orange G 6

10% aqueous Orange G	50 ml
Alcohol	950 ml
Phosphotungstic acid	0–15 g

EA 50

0.04 M light green SF	10 ml
0.3 M eosin Y	20 ml
Phosphotungstic acid	2 g
Alcohol	750 ml
Methanol	250 ml
Glacial acetic acid	20 ml

Filter all stains before use.

Papanicolaou staining method

1. a. Remove polyethylene glycol fixative in 50% alcohol, 2 min.
   b. Hydrate in 95% alcohol, 2 min, and 70% alcohol, 2 min.
2. Rinse in water, 1 min.
3. Stain in Harris's hematoxylin, 5 min.
4. Rinse in water, 2 min.
5. Differentiate in 0.5% aqueous hydrochloric acid, 10 seconds approx.
6. Rinse in water, 2 min.
7. 'Blue' in Scott's tap water substitute, 2 min.
8. Rinse in water, 2 min.
9. Dehydrate, 70% alcohol for 2 min.
10. Dehydrate, 95% alcohol, 2 min.
11. Dehydrate, 95% alcohol, 2 min.
12. Stain in OG 6, 2 min.
13. Rinse in 95% alcohol, 2 min.
14. Rinse in 95% alcohol, 2 min.
15. Stain in EA 50, 3 min.
16. Rinse in 95% alcohol, 1 min.

The staining times can be adjusted to suit personal preference for a darker or paler stain. Alternatives to Scott's tap water substitute include 0.1% ammoniated water or a weak aqueous solution of lithium carbonate.

Results

The nuclei should appear	blue/black
Cytoplasm (non-keratinizing squamous cells)	blue/green
Keratinizing cells	pink/orange

Note

Change stains frequently.

IRON HEMATOXYLINS

In these hematoxylin solutions, iron salts are used both as the oxidizing agent and as mordant. The most commonly used iron salts are ferric chloride and ferric ammonium sulfate, and the most common iron hematoxylins are:

- Weigert's hematoxylin
- Heidenhain's hematoxylin
- Loyez hematoxylin for myelin
- Verhöeff's hematoxylin for elastin fibers.

Over-oxidation of the hematoxylin is a problem with these stains, so it is usual to prepare separate mordant/oxidant and hematoxylin solutions and mix them immediately before use (e.g. in Weigert's hematoxylin) or to use them consecutively (e.g. Heidenhain's and Loyez hematoxylins). Because of the strong oxidizing ability of the solution containing iron salts, it is often used as a subsequent differentiating fluid after hematoxylin staining, as well as for a mordanting fluid before it.

The iron hematoxylins are capable of demonstrating a much wider range of tissue structures than the alum hematoxylins, but the techniques are more time-consuming and usually incorporate a differentiation stage which needs microscopic control for accuracy. The use of iron hematoxylin-based methods for the specific identification of phospholipids is discussed in Chapter 12.

Weigert's hematoxylin (Weigert 1904)

This is an iron hematoxylin in which ferric chloride is used as the mordant/oxidant. The iron and the hematoxylin solutions are prepared separately and are mixed immediately before use. They are prepared as follows.

Weigert's iron hematoxylin

Preparation of solutions

a. *Hematoxylin solution*

Hematoxylin	1 g
Absolute alcohol	100 ml

This is allowed to ripen naturally for 4 weeks before use.

b. *Iron solution*

30% aqueous ferric chloride (anhydrous)	4 ml
Hydrochloric acid (concentrated)	1 ml
Distilled water	95 ml

This solution is filtered and added to an equal volume of the hematoxylin solution immediately before the stain is used. The mixture should be a violet–black color and must be discarded if it is brown. The main use of Weigert's hematoxylin is as a nuclear stain in techniques where acidic staining solutions are to be applied to the sections subsequently (e.g. van Gieson stain). A staining time of 15–30 minutes is usual. In this role, Weigert's hematoxylin has been largely replaced by the more convenient celestine blue–alum hematoxylin procedure (see p. 125). It remains a useful stain, with eosin, for CNS tissues. For the purist who prefers a black nuclear counterstain with a van Gieson technique, the ferrous hematein technique of Slidders (1969) is satisfactory.

Heidenhain's hematoxylin (Heidenhain 1896)

This iron hematoxylin uses ferric ammonium sulfate as oxidant/mordant, and the same solution is used as the differentiating fluid. The iron solution is used first and the section is then treated with the hematoxylin solution until it is over-stained, and is then differentiated with iron solution under microscopic control.

Heidenhain's hematoxylin can be used to demonstrate many structures according to the degree of differentiation. After staining, all components are black or dark gray–black. The hematoxylin staining is removed progressively from different tissue structures at different rates using the iron alum solution. Mitochondria, muscle striations, nuclear chromatin, and myelin can all be demonstrated; the black color disappears first from mitochondria, then from muscle striations, then from nuclear chromatin. Differentiation that is more prolonged will remove the stain from almost all structures, although red blood cells and keratin retain the stain the longest. More easily controllable differentiation can be achieved if the differentiating iron alum solution is diluted with an equal volume of distilled water or an alcoholic picric acid solution.

Heidenhain's iron hematoxylin

Preparation of solutions

a. *Hematoxylin solution*

Hematoxylin	0.5 g
Absolute alcohol	10 ml
Distilled water	90 ml

The hematoxylin is dissolved in the alcohol, and the water is then added. The solution is allowed to ripen naturally for 4 weeks before use.

b. *Iron solution (5% iron alum)*

Ferric ammonium sulfate	5 g
Distilled water	100 ml

It is important that only the clear violet crystals of ferric ammonium sulfate be used.

Method

1. Deparaffinize sections, hydrate through graded alcohols to water.
2. Mordant in iron solution (5% iron alum) for 1 hour (see Note a).
3. Rinse in distilled water.
4. Stain in Heidenhain's hematoxylin solution for 1 hour (see Note a).
5. Wash in running tap water.
6. Differentiate in the iron solution (5% iron alum), or the iron solution diluted with an equal volume of distilled water. Alternate a rinse in differentiator with a rinse in tap water. The degree of differentiation is controlled microscopically until the desired structure is clearly demonstrated (see Note b).
7. Wash in running tap water for 10 min.
8. Dehydrate, clear, and mount.

Results

Mitochondria, muscle striations, myelin, chromatin etc. gray–black.

Notes

a. The time needed in the mordant and stain will vary according to the fixative used; for most purposes, 1 hour in each solution is satisfactory, but tissues fixed in dichromate solutions need longer. The following times are a rough guide. Tissues fixed in formalin solutions, formal sublimate, Susa, Bouin's, and Carnoy's, 1 hour. Tissues fixed in Helly's or Zenker's, 3 hours. Tissues fixed in osmium tetroxide and Flemming's fluid, up to 24 hours.
b. If the differentiation proceeds beyond the desired end, the section can be restained in the hematoxylin solution for the same length of time and differentiation attempted again.
c. Cytoplasmic counterstains are rarely necessary, although they may be used to accentuate nuclear chromatin, particularly in the demonstration of chromosomes or mitoses. Aqueous eosin or Orange G is satisfactory.
d. Sections stained with Heidenhain's iron hematoxylin are resistant to fading only if the section is washed well after the differentiation stage to remove all traces of iron alum.

Loyez hematoxylin (Loyez 1910)

This iron hematoxylin uses ferric ammonium sulfate as the mordant. The mordant and hematoxylin solutions are used consecutively, and differentiation is by Weigert's differentiator (borax and potassium ferricyanide). It is used to demonstrate myelin and can be applied to paraffin, frozen, or nitrocellulose sections. Two methods similar to that of Loyez are given in Chapter 19; one, the so-called Heidenhain myelin stain (not to be confused with Heidenhain's iron hematoxylin), is essentially the Loyez technique but judicious selection of staining time removes the need for separate differentiation. The second variant is the short Weil technique in which the mordant and dye are mixed before use, rather than used consecutively. Both these techniques are shorter than the Loyez.

Verhöeff's hematoxylin (Verhöeff 1908)

This iron hematoxylin is used to demonstrate elastic fibers. Ferric chloride is included in the hematoxylin staining solution, together with Lugol's iodine, and 2% aqueous ferric chloride is used as the differentiator. Coarse elastic fibers stain black.

Other elastin methods may stain finer fibers, but for the high contrast required for photomicrography the intense black staining produced by Verhöeff's is ideal. Verhöeff's is also used to stain elastin fibers as part of the Movat's pentachrome. The composition of the staining solution, and the staining procedure, are given on page 152, Chapter 10.

TUNGSTEN HEMATOXYLINS

There is only one widely used tungsten hematoxylin, although there are many variants on the original Mallory PTAH technique. Mallory (1897, 1900) combined hematoxylin with 1% aqueous phosphotungstic acid, the latter acting as the mordant. It is possible to prepare a staining solution using hematein instead of hematoxylin; the oxidation process is unnecessary and the staining solution can be used immediately, but its activity is comparatively short-lived. The hematoxylin can be oxidized chemically by using a potassium permanganate solution; again, the solution is usable within 24 hours. The most satisfactory method of preparation, albeit time-consuming, is to allow natural ripening of the tungsten hematoxylin solution in light and air; PTAH solution so produced may take some months to ripen, but will remain usable for many years. Its use is applicable to both CNS material and general tissue structure, and to

tissues fixed in any of the standard fixatives. Staining times will vary according to the method of preparation, the fixative used, and the tissue structure to be demonstrated. Staining is more precise after the section has been treated with an acid dichromate solution, and after a Mallory bleach procedure (which also aids differential staining).

PTAH staining technique solution using hematein (Shum & Hon 1969)

Solution A

Hematein	0.8 g
Distilled water	1 ml

Grind the 0.8 g hematein to a paste with 1 ml distilled water. (The paste should be chocolate brown. Lighter colors are usually indicative of an unsuitable batch of hematein and should be discarded.)

Solution B

Phosphotungstic acid	0.9 g
Distilled water	9 ml

Mix solution A and solution B, bring to the boil, then cool and filter.

Method

1. Deparaffinize, hydrate through graded alcohols to water.
2. Treat with acid permanganate (see Note b) for 5 min.
3. Rinse in tap water.
4. Bleach with 5% aqueous oxalic acid.
5. Wash well in tap water.
6. Stain in PTAH solution for 12–24 hours at room temperature.
7. Wash in distilled water.
8. Dehydrate rapidly, clear, and mount.

The solution may be used at 56°C for several hours, but staining for the longer time at room temperature gives results that are more precise and is preferable.

PTAH solution, chemically oxidized with potassium permanganate

Solution

Hematoxylin	0.5 g
Phosphotungstic acid	10 g
Distilled water	500 ml
0.25% aqueous potassium permanganate	25 ml

The hematoxylin is dissolved in 100 ml of the distilled water, and the phosphotungstic acid in the remaining 400 ml; the two solutions are mixed and the potassium permanganate solution is added. The stain can be used next day, but peak staining activity is not reached until after 7 days. Continuing oxidation of the hematoxylin means that this stain has a comparatively short life.

PTAH solution, naturally oxidized

a. *Acid dichromate solution*

10% HCl in absolute alcohol	12 ml
3% aqueous potassium dichromate	36 ml

b. *Acid permanganate solution*

0.5% aqueous potassium permanganate	50 ml
3% sulfuric acid	2.5 ml

c. *Staining solution*

Hematoxylin	0.5 g
Phosphotungstic acid	5 g
Distilled water	500 ml

The solids are dissolved in separate portions of the distilled water, and then mixed as in the recipes above. The stain is allowed to ripen naturally in a loosely stoppered bottle in a warm, light place for several months.

Method

1. Deparaffinize, hydrate through graded alcohols to water.
2. Place in acid dichromate solution for 30 min.
3. Wash in tap water.
4. Treat with acid permanganate solution for 1 min.
5. Wash in tap water.
6. Bleach in 1% oxalic acid.
7. Rinse in tap water.
8. Stain in Mallory's PTAH stain overnight.
9. Dehydrate through graded alcohols, clear, and mount.

Results

Muscle striations, neuroglia fibers, fibrin and amoebae	dark blue
Nuclei, cilia, red blood cells	blue
Myelin	lighter blue
Collagen, osteoid, cartilage, elastic fibers	deep brownish-red
Cytoplasm	pale pinkish-brown

Notes

The acid dichromate treatment (post chroming) can be omitted if fixation has been by a chromate-containing fixative.

Dehydration should be rapid since water and alcohol may remove some of the stain. If the sections are too blue, some degree of differentiation can be achieved during dehydration. Dehydration may be commenced in 95% alcohol, and CNS sections may need thorough washing in 95% alcohol for several minutes to remove excess red stain. The times in dichromate, permanganate, and stain may need to be modified depending on the nature of the tissue and the feature to be demonstrated. A suitable variant for CNS material is given in Chapter 19.

MOLYBDENUM HEMATOXYLINS

Hematoxylin solutions that use molybdic acid as the mordant are rare, and the only technique that gained any acceptance was the Thomas (1941) technique which was mentioned by McManus and Mowry (1964). They recommend the method for the demonstration of collagen and coarse reticulin, although more valuable and widely accepted techniques for these connective tissue fibers exist (see Chapter 10); the Thomas method also stains argentaffin cell granules and may have a potential use for this purpose.

Phosphomolybdic acid hematoxylin stain (Thomas 1941)

Preparation of solutions

a. *Hematoxylin solution*

Hematoxylin	2.5 g
Dioxane	49 ml
Hydrogen peroxide	1 ml

b. *Phosphomolybdic acid solution*

Phosphomolybdic acid	16.5 g
Distilled water	44 ml
Diethylene glycol	11 ml

The phosphomolybdic acid solution is filtered and 50 ml of the filtrate is added to the hematoxylin solution. The resultant solution, which should be dark violet in color, is allowed to stand for 24 hours before use.

Method

1. Deparaffinize, hydrate through graded alcohols to water.
2. Stain with phosphomolybdic acid hematoxylin for 2 min.
3. Wash with distilled water.
4. Drop picro-acetic alcohol (see Note a) onto section, then wash away immediately with distilled water.
5. Rinse in tap water, dehydrate in 95% and absolute alcohol, clear, and mount.

Results

Collagen and coarse reticulin	violet to black
Argentaffin cells	black
Nuclei	pale blue
Paneth cells	orange

Notes

a. Picro-acetic alcohol (picric acid 0.5 g, glacial acetic acid 0.5 ml, 70% alcohol 100 ml) acts as a differentiator; this can be omitted.
b. Tissues fixed in dichromate do not give good results.

LEAD HEMATOXYLINS

Hematoxylin solutions that incorporate lead salts have recently been used in the demonstration of the granules in the endocrine cells of the alimentary tract and other regions. The most practical diagnostic application is in the identification of endocrine cells in tumors of doubtful origin, but it is also used in research procedures such as in the localization of gastrin secreting cells in stomach (Beltrami et al 1975).

Its value in the investigation of the diffuse endocrine system is discussed in Chapter 16, where the most reliable technique, that of Solcia et al (1969), is given. This empirical method has largely been superseded by the use of more reliable and specific immunohistochemical methods for neurocrine cells.

HEMATOXYLIN WITHOUT A MORDANT

Freshly prepared hematoxylin solutions, used without a mordant, have been used to demonstrate various minerals in tissue sections. Mallory (1938) described a method for lead, and later published a similar method capable of demonstrating iron and copper (Mallory & Parker 1939); these methods have now been superseded by techniques that are more specific. The basis of the Mallory methods is the ability of unripened hematoxylin to form blue–black lakes with these metals. The methods are given by Lillie and Fulmer (1976).

One final hematoxylin method is worthy of note. The Weigert–Pal technique discussed in elsewhere in the book, for the demonstration of myelin, is a hematoxylin method in which the tissue block is mordanted in a chromate solution before embedding and sectioning. Further mordanting of the section in a copper acetate solution is often performed before the hematoxylin is applied. It is likely that the major mordant is a chromium compound.

The uses of hematoxylin stains are briefly summarized in Table 9.2.

QUALITY CONTROL IN ROUTINE H&E STAINING

Accurate diagnosis depends on a pathologist or cytologist examining stained microscope slides—usually H&E paraffin sections, the H&E staining having been carried out in bulk by an automated staining machine. The need for consistency of staining is vital to avoid difficult histological interpretation. In general, automated staining machines allow accurate and consistent staining, differentiation, and dehydration by adjusting the times of each step. However, variability in the stains may necessitate adjustment of the staining times. In staining machines, the problems are usually associated with the hematoxylin staining rather than eosin. Variation in batch number of the hematoxylin, a change of supplier, and pH differences are the most common variables. A different person following the same preparation instructions can also result in a stain such as hematoxylin

Table 9.2 The uses of hematoxylin stains

Mordant	Oxidant	Examples	Applications
Alum	Natural	Ehrlich	Nuclear stain used with eosin. Stains some mucins
Alum	Natural	Delafield	Nuclear stain used with eosin
Alum	Sodium iodide	Mayer	Nuclear stain used with eosin. Nuclear counterstain
Alum	Mercuric oxide	Harris	Nuclear stain used with eosin
Alum	Iodine	Cole	Nuclear stain used with eosin
Alum	Potassium iodate	Carazzi	Nuclear stain used with eosin (used with frozen sections)
Alum	Sodium iodate	Gill	Nuclear stain used with eosin
Iron	Natural	Weigert	Nuclear stain used with acid dyes
Iron	Natural	Heidenhain	Intranuclear detail, muscle striations
Iron	Natural	Verhöeff	Elastic fibers
Iron	Natural	Loyez	Myelin
Tungsten	Natural	Mallory PTAH	Fibrin, muscle striations, glial fibers
Molybdenum	Hydrogen peroxide	Thomas	Collagen, endocrine cell granules
Lead		Solcia	Endocrine cell granules
Without mordant		Mallory	Iron, copper, lead
Chromium–copper		Weigert–Pal	Myelin (in block preparation)

having slightly different staining properties each time it is made up. The age of the stain, and the degree of usage, will also affect the staining properties. New batches of stain must be checked for efficacy against current or earlier batches, and staining times must be adjusted to give uniformity. It is also important to realize that other factors, such as fixation, variations in processing schedules, section thickness, and excessive hot plate temperatures, may all lead to variation in staining.

DIFFICULT SECTIONS

The problem of using hematoxylin as a nuclear counterstain when other acidic dyes are to be used (for example van Gieson) has already been mentioned. A similar problem occurs when attempting to stain paraffin sections when the tissue has been fixed for a long time in a formalin fixative that has gradually become more acid. Tissues and/or paraffin blocks sent from countries with hot climates compound the problem. This may occur, particularly in third world countries, because tissues may be fixed in poor quality, unbuffered, non-neutral formalin fixative that deteriorates in the heat, and progressively becomes more acidic. The major problem is getting adequate nuclear staining with hematoxylin without also staining the cytoplasm; this phenomenon

gives a uniformly muddy purple to the finished section after eosin has been applied.

There are two main ways in which diagnostically acceptable H&E sections can be obtained in these circumstances: one is the use of the celestine blue–alum hematoxylin sequence (see p. 125); the other is the use of an iron hematoxylin such as Weigert's.

Acknowledgments

Alan Stevens wrote this chapter for the first three editions. Ian Wilson was his co-author in the fourth edition. Our acknowledgments are due to Alan Stevens for his considerable contribution.

REFERENCES

Beltrami C.A., Fabris, G., Marzola, A. et al. (1975) Staining of gastrin cells with lead hematoxylin. Histochemical Journal 7:95.

Carazzi D. (1911) Eine neue Hämatoxylinlösung. Zeitschrift für wissenschaftliche Mikroskopie und für mikroskopische Technik 28:273.

Carson F.L. (1997) Histotechnology: a self-instructional text. Chicago: American Society for Clinical Pathology 6:93.

Cole E.C. (1943) Studies in hematoxylin stains. Stain Technology 18:125.

Cox G. (1973) Neuroglia and microglia. In: Cook H.C., ed. Histopathology: selected topics. London: Baillière Tindall.

Delafield J., cited by Prudden J.M. (1885) Zeitschrift für wissenschaftliche. Mikroskopie und für mikroskopische Technik 2:228.

Ehrlich P. (1886) Fragekasten. Zeitschrift für wissenschaftliche. Mikroskopie und für mikroskopische Technik 3:150.

Feldman A., Dapson R. (1985) Newsletter, Winter. ANATECH.

Feldman A., Dapson R. (1987) Newsletter, Winter. ANATECH.

Gill G.W., Frost J.K., Miller K.A. (1974) A new formula for half-oxidised hematoxylin solution that neither overstains or requires differentiation. Acta Cytologica 18: 300.

Harris H.F. (1900) On the rapid conversion of hematoxylin into haematein in staining reactions. Journal of Applied Microscopic Laboratory Methods 3:777.

Heidenhain M. (1896) Noch einmal über die Darstellung der Centralkörper durch Eisenhämatoxylin nebst einigen allgemeinen Bemerkungen über die Hämatoxylinfarben. Zeitschrift für wissenschaftliche. Mikroskopie und für mikroskopische Technik 13:186.

Lillie R.D., Fulmer H.M. (1976) Histopathologic technic and practical histochemistry, 4th edn. New York: McGraw-Hill.

Loyez M. (1910) Coloration des fibres nerveuses par la méthode à l'hématoxyline au fer après inclusion à la celloidine. Compte Rendu des Séances de la Société de Biologie 69:511.

Luna L. (1992) Histopathologic methods and color atlas of special stains and tissue artefacts. Downers Grove, IL: Johnson Printers 67, 73, 77, 78.

Mallory F.B. (1897) On certain improvements in histological technique. Journal of Experimental Medicine 2: 529.

Mallory F.B. (1900) A contribution to staining methods. Journal of Experimental Medicine 5:15.

Mallory F.B. (1938) Pathological technique. Philadelphia: Saunders.

Mallory F.B., Parker F. (1939) Fixing and staining methods for lead and copper in tissues. American Journal of Pathology 15:517.

Mayer P. (1903) Notiz über Hämatein und Hämalaun. Zeitschrift für wissenschaftliche Mikroskopie und für mikroskopische Technik 20:409.

McManus J.F.A., Mowry R.W. (1964) Staining methods, histologic and histochemical. London: Harper & Row, p. 268.

Shum M.W., Hon J.K.Y. (1969) A modified phosphotungstic acid hematoxylin stain for formalin fixed tissue. Journal of Medical Laboratory Technology 26:38.

Slidders W. (1969) A stable iron–hematoxylin solution for staining the chromatin of cell nuclei. Journal of Microscopy 90:61.

Solcia E., Capella C.C., Vassallo G. (1969) Lead–hematoxylin as a stain for endocrine cells. Significance of staining and comparison with other selective methods. Histochemie 20:116–126.

Thomas J.A. (1941) Un nouveau colorant élécrif des structures collagènes et réticulaires: l'hématoxyline phosphomolybdique au dioxane. Technique de coloration. Comptes Rendus des Séances de la Société de Biologie et de ses Filiales 135:935.

Verhöeff F.H. (1908) Some new staining methods of wide applicability. Including a rapid differential stain for elastic tissue. Journal of the American Medical Association 50: 876.

Weigert K. (1904) Eine kleine Verbesserung der Hämatoxylin van-Gieson-methode. Zeitschrift für wissenschaftliche Mikroskopie und für mikroskopische Technik 21:1.

10

Connective Tissues and Stains

M. Lamar Jones, John D. Bancroft and Marilyn Gamble

INTRODUCTION

Connective tissue is one of the four tissue types found throughout the body. The term connect comes from the Latin word connectere meaning 'to bind'. Its main function is to connect together and provide support to other tissues of the body. During embryonic development, the ectoderm and endoderm are divided by a germ layer called the mesoderm, known as mesenchyme; this comes from the Greek words *mesos* meaning middle and *enchyma* meaning infusion. It is from the mesenchyme that the connective tissues develop.

Connective tissue usually consists of a cellular portion in a surrounding framework of a non-cellular substance. The ratio of cells to intercellular substance varies from one type of connective tissue to another, as does the primary function of the connective tissue. For example, bone has only a few cells in a usually dense, rigid intercellular substance with its main function being that of providing strength and support. The cell types of connective tissue can include entities such as fibroblasts, mast cells, histiocytes, adipose cells, reticular cells, osteoblasts and osteocytes, chondroblasts and chondrocytes, blood cells and blood-forming cells. Some connective tissue has little substance and consists primarily of cells whose functions are not those of production of intercellular substance such as adipose tissue. Since they do not connect or support the other body tissues they are included under connective tissues as they probably derive from the same parent cell. The parent cell of the entire series is the embryonic mesenchyme cell, which is rarely found in adults.

The intercellular substance is usually composed of both amorphous (non-sulfated and sulfated mucopolysaccharides) and formed elements (collagen reticular fibers and elastic fibers). These are the non-living parts of the connective tissues and represent the functional part of many of them. The nature of the intercellular substance varies according to its function: it may be extremely hard and dense, in cortical bone, or soft as in umbilical cord. The microscopical appearances are also variable, some being fibrillar whereas others are completely homogeneous. Intercellular substances may be readily classified into two main groups by their microscopical appearance:

- formed or fibrous types
- amorphous or gel types.

FORMED OR FIBROUS INTERCELLULAR SUBSTANCES

A frequent fault among histologists is to speak of collagen, reticulin, and elastin, when in reality they mean collagenic fibers, reticular fibers, and elastic fibers. The former terms relate to the protein compound that is predominant in the particular fiber and should not be used to describe the connective tissue fiber itself.

Collagenic fibers

These are the most frequently encountered of all the fibrous types of intercellular substance, and are found in large quantities in most sites in the body. They may occur as individual fibers, as in loose areolar tissues, arranged in a open weave system, or as large bundles of fibers clumped together to form structures of great tensile strength, such as tendon. Individual collagenic fibers are never seen to branch, although bundles of fibers do

135

branch frequently. When viewed by polarized light, they are strongly birefringent. In almost any type of connective tissue there are three elements, the cells, the fibers, and the amorphous ground substance. The identification of the cells may be based upon their appearance in areolar and loose tissues that can be considered the main 'packing' material in the adult. This can also be considered as a prototype of the connective tissue. The connective tissues are divided into the following groups:

- Connective tissue proper—includes loose or areolar, dense, regular and adipose irregular, reticular
- Cartilage—hyaline elastic and fibrocartilage
- Bone—spongy or cancellous and dense or cortical
- Blood
- Blood-forming—hemopoietic.

Types of collagen

Four major types of collagen and several minor types have been characterized and described by a number of authors. It is apparent that the production of the different types is under genetic control, each reflecting slight variations in the α-chain composition. They all display the characteristic amino acid content.

Type I

This collagen forms the thick collagenous fibers that have been demonstrated histologically and form the bulk of the body's collagen. This type accounts for most of the organic matrix of bases, but is also a major structural protein in the lung. The electron microscopic appearances of Type I collagen are of bundles of tightly packed, thick fibrils (75 nm diameter) with little interfibrillar substance. The fibrils show the characteristic 64 nm axial periodicity (Fig. 10.1). The prominence of the 'cross banding' in Type I collagen is thought to be due to the lack of interference from interfibrillar ground substance. However, the presence of a partially processed form of Type III precollagen, pN collagen III, helps to regulate the diameter of fibrils formed by collagen Type I, by

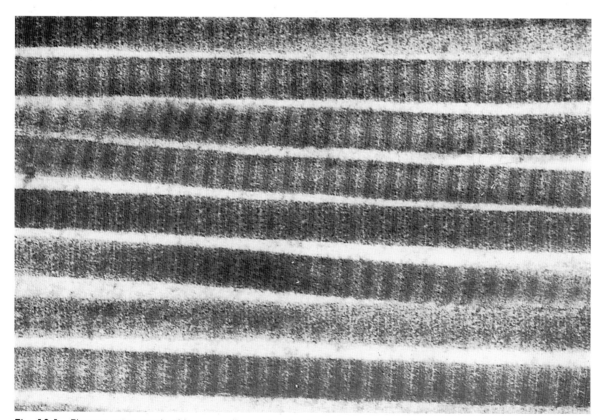

Fig. 10.1 Electron micrograph of human collagen showing transverse cross-banding.

forming co-polymers with the fibrils. pN collagen III inhibits the rate at which collagen Type I is assembled into fibrils and also decreases the amount of collagen Type I that is incorporated into the fibrils.

Type II

This collagen is found in hyaline and elastic cartilage and is produced by chondroblast activity. The fibers are thin and composed of fibrils arranged in a meshwork with copious amounts of proteoglycans. Type II collagen is usually not readily visible by light microscopic methods. The Type II fibers found in articular cartilage are thicker and resemble, ultrastructurally, Type I fibers. The cross-banding of Type II collagen is less evident due to the masking effect of the abundant interfibrillar material. Treatment with hyaluronidase may unmask Type II fibers to render them accessible for immunohistochemical evaluation.

Type III

This collagen is found only in those tissues that also contain Type I collagen (e.g. lung, liver, spleen, kidney, etc.). The fibers that have been classically known as 'reticular fibers' contain Type III collagen. EM studies of reticular fibers reveal loosely packed fibrils surrounded by abundant carbohydrate-rich interfibrillar material. The argyrophilia of reticulin fibers is due to the proteoglycan content of the fibers and is not dependent upon the proteins of the fibrils themselves. Type III collagen appears to provide a limited amount of support, but also to allow some motility and the easy diffusion and exchange of metabolites. In some references, Type III collagen is referred to as 'fetal collagen'; this term is, however, misleading as Type III collagen constitutes a significant proportion of the collagen present in adults. Fetal tissues do contain quite large amounts of Type III collagen in comparison to adult tissues from the same site (e.g. 60% of the collagen in fetal skin is Type III, compared to only 20% in adult skin).

Type IV

This collagen has been characterized in structures identified morphologically as basement membranes. It is generally accepted that Type IV collagen does not form fibers or fibrils visible on light microscopic examination. Electron microscopy reveals a random organization of fine fibrils forming a feltwork-like structure in all basement membranes. Type IV collagen is closely associated with significant amounts of carbohydrate complexes, which explains the strong reaction of basement membranes to the periodic acid–Schiff method.

Types V and VI

Type V collagen is produced in small quantities by a wide range of cells, including connective tissue cells, endothelial cells, and some epithelial cells. It remains in close contact with the cell surface and is presumed to be involved in the attachment of cells to adjacent structures and in the maintenance of tissue integrity. Type VI collagen is a disulfide-rich variant which has been identified in boundary zones where interstitial collagenous fibers (Types I and II) are linked to non-collagenous elements.

Staining reactions of collagen

Type I collagen stains strongly with acid dyes, due to the affinity of the cationic groups of the proteins for the anionic reactive groups of the acid dyes. They may be demonstrated more selectively by compound solutions of acid dyes (e.g. van Gieson) or by sequential combinations of acid dyes (e.g. Masson's trichrome, Lendrum's MSB, etc.) The different types of collagen may be differentiated immunohistochemically.

Reticular fibers

These are the fine and delicate fibers that are found connected to coarser and stronger collagenous fibers (Type I fibers). They provide the bulk of the supporting framework of the more cellular organs, e.g. spleen, liver, lymph nodes, etc., where they are arranged in a three-dimensional network to provide a system of individual cell support (Fig. 10.2). On light microscopic examination, reticular fibers are weakly birefringent, the weak reaction being attributed to their lack of physical size and the masking effect of the interfibrillar substance. They are seen to branch frequently and appear indistinct in H&E-stained preparations. The characteristics of reticulin fibers in human kidney cortex have been studied using immunohistochemical means. Antibodies directed against Type I and Type III collagens, their corresponding amino peptides and decorin (PG-II), revealed that in this organ the reticulin fibrils consist of hybrids of Type I and Type III collagens. Double immuno-electron microscopy shows that 20–25-nm fibrils consist mainly of Type I collagen, whereas the larger fibrils, 30–35 nm, label simultaneously for Type I and Type III collagens. Most fibrils larger than 40 nm in diameter label for Type

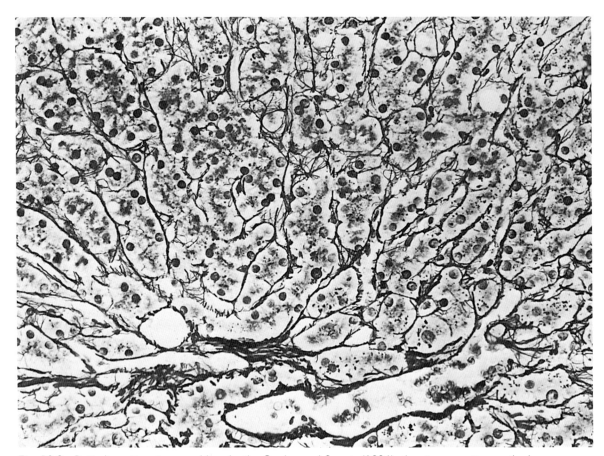

Fig. 10.2 Reticulin pattern in normal liver by the Gordon and Sweets (1936) silver impregnation method.

III collagen. Reticular fibers may be demonstrated distinctly, in paraffin sections, using one of the many argyrophil-type silver impregnation techniques available or, in frozen section, by the periodic acid–Schiff technique. Both methods of demonstration are dependent upon the reactive groups present in the carbohydrate matrix, and not upon the fibrillar elements of the fiber.

Elastic fibers

The elastic system fibers, i.e. oxytalan, elaunin, and elastic fibers, have respectively a fibrillar, amorphous, or mixed structure. The elastic fibers may be found throughout the body but are especially associated with the respiratory, circulatory, and integumentary systems. Their light microscope appearances may vary considerably according to location, from fine, single fibers, as in the upper dermis, to membrane-like structures ('internal and external elastic laminae') in the large arteries. In the latter situation, the elastic membranes are interrupted by minute holes called fenestrae (Latin *fenestra*—window) which permit diffusion of materials through the otherwise impermeable membrane. Recent high-resolution electron microscopic examination has demonstrated that elastic fibers consist of two quite distinct components. There is an amorphous substance which, biochemically, is consistent with the protein, elastin, and a second component, which shows a periodicity of 4–13 nm, is microfibrillar in nature, and has been termed elastic fiber microfibrillar protein (EFMP). These microfibrils, sometimes also called elastin-associated microfibrils (EAMF), are ubiquitous connective tissue structures that are believed to provide tensile strength and flexibility to numerous tissues. They may also act as a scaffold for elastin deposition.

When viewed in transverse section, the central core of the elastic fiber is seen to be composed of the amorphous protein, elastin, surrounded by a ring or band of EFMP. The proportions of the two components seem to alter with the age of the fiber (and probably also with the age of the subject). In young fibers, the dominant fraction is the microfibrillar protein. In older fibers, the amorphous protein accounts for over 90% of the fiber content. The basic molecular unit of elastin is a linear polypeptide with a molecular weight of approximately 72 kilodaltons (kDa). This subunit has been referred to as 'soluble elastin' or 'tropoelastin'. One of the characteristic features of elastic fibers is the presence of cross-linking which binds the polypeptide chains into a fiber network. Desmosine and its isomer, isodesmosine, are the cross-linking compounds involved. The polypeptides are transported out of the fibroblasts or smooth muscle cells and the cross-linking occurs in the extracellular spaces.

Elastic fiber microfibrillar protein (EFMP) has an amino acid content that is quite distinct, biochemically, from that of elastin protein. It is particularly rich in amino acids, which are lacking or present in only small quantities in elastin. The content of cysteine in EFMP is high, reflecting the presence of numerous disulfide linkages that will be of significance when the staining properties of elastic fibers are considered later. Associated with EFMP are a number of carbohydrate complexes, termed 'structural glycoproteins' (Cleary & Gibson 1983); the significance of these in the staining of elastic fibers will also be considered later. For a more detailed account of elastic fiber composition and biochemistry, reference should be made to the work of Cleary and Gibson (1983), Uitto (1979), or Bailey (1978). Elastic fibers are acidophilic, congophilic, and refractile. Following oxidation, they are quite strongly basophilic due to the formation of sulfonic acid groups from the disulfide linkages of the EFMP. Young fibers with a high content of EFMP show a positive periodic acid–Schiff reaction. They may be seen in routine H&E-stained sections, but, for exacting studies, numerous more selective techniques are available. These may be relatively simple, e.g. the Taenzer–Unna orcein method, or more lengthy and complex, e.g. Weigert resorcin–fuchsin methods. With increasing age of the elastic fibers, physical and biochemical changes are seen to occur. These may include splitting and fragmentation, alteration of the ratio of EFMP to elastin, and increases in the levels of glutamic and aspartic acids and calcium.

These changes are readily visible in the skin of the subject, which becomes wrinkled and 'loose-fitting'. A more serious problem occurs with the loss of elasticity of the elastic arteries.

Oxytalan fibers

Oxytalan fibers were first described by Fullmer and Lillie (1958) in periodontal membranes. More recently they have been demonstrated in a wide variety of tissues, both normal and abnormal (Alexander & Garner 1977; Cleary & Gibson 1983; Goldfischer et al 1983). On light microscopic examination, oxytalan fibers may be distinguished from mature elastic fibers by their failure to stain with aldehyde fuchsin solutions, unless they have been previously oxidized by potassium permanganate, performic acid, or peracetic acid. They have also been reported to remain unstained following Verhöeff's hematoxylin, with or without prior oxidation. Following electron microscopic examination by a number of workers, it has been suggested that oxytalan fibers are similar to, if not identical to, elastic fiber microfibrillar protein fibers. They appear to be composed of microfibrillar units, 7–20 nm in diameter, with a periodicity of 12–17 nm. Their periodicity is made more conspicuous by pretreatment with ruthenium red. From their morphology, localization, and staining properties, it seems possible that oxytalan fibers may represent an immature form of elastic tissue. It has also been suggested by Goldfischer et al (1983) that microfibrils and oxytalan fibers may have a role beyond that of elastogenesis and may involve 'anchoring' mechanisms between collagen fibers, stromal cells, lymphatic capillary walls, mature elastic fibers, muscle cells, etc.

Elaunin fibers

Gawlik (1965) first described elaunin fibers; the term 'elaunin' is derived from the Greek 'I stretch'. Unlike oxytalan fibers, elaunin fibers stain with orcein, aldehyde fuchsin, and resorcin–fuchsin without prior oxidation, but do not stain with Verhöeff's hematoxylin.

Classification of fiber types

It is often suggested that the mechanisms of the stains used to classify elaunin and oxytalan fibers are too empirical, that the terms 'elaunin' and 'oxytalan' lack structural or functional significance, and that the three fiber types, oxytalan, elaunin, and elastic, correspond to consecutive stages of normal elastogenesis. It has been shown that there is continuity between the coarse, mature elastic fibers deep in the dermis, through the intermediate elaunin fibers, to the fine oxytalan fibers in the most superficial aspects of the papillary dermis.

Basement membranes

Basement membranes are found throughout the body as a resilient matrix, separating connective tissues from epithelial, endothelial or mesothelial cells, muscle cells, fat cells, and nervous tissues. They support the epithelial cells of mucosal surfaces, glands, and several other structures, for example renal tubules. They also support the endothelial cells lining blood vessels, capillaries, etc. The basement membrane is not homogeneous, but is divided into three zones or layers:

- lamina rara (or lamina lucida);
- lamina densa (basal lamina);
- lamina reticularis.

The lamina rara (lucida) is adjacent to the surface cells and is composed mainly of carbohydrate complexes. This layer is apparently continuous with the glycocalyx of the surface cells and it has been suggested that the lamina rara is produced by the surface cells and not by the underlying connective tissue cells. The lamina densa is composed of a feltwork of microfibrils which have been immunohistochemically identified as predominantly Type IV collagen with a lesser amount of Type V collagen. Type IV collagen is associated with relatively large amounts of structural glycoproteins, mainly laminin and fibronectin, and small amounts of proteoglycans, principally heparan sulfate (Junqueira & Montes 1983; Laurie & Leblond 1983). The lamina reticularis is seen as a layer containing fibrous elements, which are continuous with the underlying connective tissue fibers.

The thickness of the basement membrane varies from site to site; most are in the range 15–50 nm. The glomerular basement membrane (GBM) is particularly thick, up to 350 nm in a healthy adult. The ultrastructural appearance of the GBM also differs from that of other basement membranes, in that the central lamina densa is bordered on both sides by a lamina rara. The sequence of the ultrastructural elements in the GBM is thus, from the capillary lumen outwards: endothelial cell, endothelial-associated lamina rara, lamina densa, epithelial-associated lamina rara, epithelial cell (podocyte). In H&E-stained sections of most tissues, basement membranes are difficult to distinguish; in the glomerulus, they are more conspicuous, particularly in disorders such as membranous nephropathy or diabetes where they can be markedly thickened. For more critical examination, a number of techniques are available. As a result of their carbohydrate content, the membranes are strongly positive by the periodic acid–Schiff reaction and by any other oxidation–aldehyde demonstration techniques, e.g. methenamine silver, Gridley, Bauer–Feulgen, etc. In sections by the MSB or Azan trichrome methods, the basement membrane stains intensely by the larger molecule, acid dye.

METHENAMINE SILVER MICROWAVE METHOD

This method delineates the glomerular basement membranes. Methenamine silver demonstrates the carbohydrate component of basement membranes by oxidizing the carbohydrates to aldehydes. Silver ions from the methenamine–silver complex are first bound to carbohydrate components of the basement membrane and then reduced to visible metallic silver by the aldehyde groups. Toning is with gold chloride, and any unreduced silver is removed by sodium thiosulfate. The use of a microwave oven is recommended for the method and the technique followed exactly for optimal results. The method below is for five slides; if you do not have five slides, then include blank slides but do not use more than five.

Periodic acid–methenamine silver microwave method for basement membranes (Brinn 1983; Carson 1997)

Fixative
10% neutral buffered formalin is preferred. Mecury-containing fixatives are not recommended.

Sections
Paraffin-processed tissue cut at 2 microns.

Solutions

Stock methenamine silver
3% aqueous methenamine	400 ml
Silver nitrate, 5% aqueous	20 ml

Keep refrigerated at 4°C.

5% borax (sodium borate) solution

Working methenamine silver solution
Stock methenamine silver	25 ml
Distilled water	25 ml

5% borax (sodium borate)	2 ml

1% periodic acid solution

0.02% gold chloride solution

1% gold chloride	1 ml
Distilled water	49 ml

Stock light green solution

Light green SF (yellowish)	1 g
Distilled water	500 ml
Glacial acetic acid	1 ml

Working light green solution

Light green stock solution	10 ml
Distilled water	50 ml

Method

1. Deparaffinize sections and hydrate to distilled water.
2. Place sections in 1% periodic acid solution for 15 minutes at room temperature.
3. Rinse in distilled water.
4. Place slides (five) in a plastic Coplin jar containing 50 ml of methenamine working solution. Loosely apply the screw cap and place in the microwave oven, and place a loosely capped plastic Coplin jar containing exactly 50 ml (measured) of distilled water in the oven. Microwave on full power for exactly 70 seconds (see Note 2). Remove both jars from the oven, mix the solution with a plastic Pasteur pipette, and let stand. Check the slides frequently until the desired staining intensity is achieved. This will take approximately 15–20 minutes.
5. Rinse slides in the heated distilled water.
6. Tone sections in 0.02% gold chloride for 30 seconds.
7. Rinse slides in distilled water.
8. Treat sections with 2% sodium thiosulfate for 1 min.
9. Wash in tap water.
10. Counterstain in the working light green solution for 1½ min.
11. Dehydrate with two changes each of 95% and absolute alcohols.
12. Clear with xylene and mount with synthetic resin.

Results

Basement membrane	black
Background	green

If a microwave oven is not used, substitute the following solutions and staining times:

Methenamine silver solution

Stock methenamine silver solution	50 ml
Borax, 5%	5 ml

Preheat the solution and stain slides at 56–60°C for 40–90 minutes.

0.2% gold chloride solution

Gold chloride, 1% solution	10 ml
Distilled water	40 ml

Notes

a. Sharper staining of the basement membrane and less background staining can be obtained with the use of the microwave oven for silver techniques.
b. The temperature is critical and should be just below boiling, or approximately 95°C, immediately after removal from the oven. Each oven should be calibrated for the time required to reach the correct temperature.
c. This is a difficult stain to perform correctly. The glomerular basement membrane should appear as a continuous black line. Stopping the silver impregnation too soon will result in uneven or interrupted staining. The application of too much counterstain will mask the silver stain and decrease contrast.

CONNECTIVE TISSUE CELLS

Connective tissues consist of a non-living framework in which cells function and live; the cellular component is an important aspect of this group of tissues. The parent cell of the entire series of connective tissues is the undifferentiated mesenchymal cell. From this develop many varied cells, each with its different function.

Fibroblasts

The fibroblast is the cell responsible for the production of the collagenic fibers, and also probably the amorphous intercellular substance, which binds the fibers together. Many authors refer to the young active secretory cell as the fibroblast, and reserve the term fibrocyte for the older non-secretory stage of development. The two stages may be distinguished easily by examining the cells. In the active spindle-shaped fibroblast the nucleus contains a prominent nucleolus and is surrounded by abundant, slightly basophilic cytoplasm; the even thinner spindle-shaped fibrocyte has an ovoid flattened nucleus with scanty chromatin and no nucleolus, and the cytoplasm is difficult to distinguish. The fibroblasts are responsible for repair processes in the body and will accumulate at the edges of sites of injury and secrete fibrous intercellular substances which ultimately form scar tissue.

Fat cells

Among the cells that differentiate from the mesenchymal cell, fat cells are exceptional in that their main function is not one of production of intercellular substances or of defense mechanisms, but is one of storage. The first sign of development of a fat cell is the accumulation within its cytoplasm of tiny droplets of lipid material; these gradually increase in size until the cell loses its previous shape and appears as a swollen object with the nucleus forced to one side.

CONNECTIVE TISSUES

The physical characteristics of the cells and the intercellular substances vary considerably and they may be divided into groups, according to the ratio of cells to intercellular substance, and the types of cells and intercellular substance:

- areolar tissue
- adipose tissue
- myxoid connective tissue
- dense connective tissue
- cartilage
- bone
- blood.

Areolar tissue

This is probably the most widespread of all the connective tissue types. It connects the epithelial surfaces to the underlying structures; it fills any spaces between organs, and forms the fascia of intermuscular planes. Its construction is such that, although it has considerable strength, it allows movement of adjacent structures relative to each other. The loose pattern of areolar tissue permits free passage of nutrients and waste products. In a stained section, areolar tissue appears as an open-weave network of numerous single or small bundles of collagenic fibers running in all directions, with some

elastic fibers and reticular fibers; the most frequent cells are the fibroblasts which lie adjacent to a fiber or bundle. Also present are small numbers of mast cells and macrophages. In some sites, plasma cells may also be present. There is a liberal supply of arterioles, blood vessels, and lymphatic vessels.

Adipose tissue

Adipose tissue is found among the tissues forming the connective tissues, as it is not directly concerned with support or defense functions. It derives from areolar tissue, and evolves as fat cells to replace almost all other cells and many of the fibers. There is a well developed network of reticular fibers surrounding the fat cells that are collagenic and the elastic fibers are almost absent. Adipose tissue is well supplied with capillaries and lymphatic capillaries, as it is so closely associated with storage of excess nutriments. Microscopically, it resembles no other body tissue and appears as a collection of cells with flattened eccentric nuclei and, in paraffin wax preparations, clear spaces from where the lipid has been removed during processing. The overall appearance is rather similar to that of nucleated chicken-wire.

'Myxoid' connective tissue

One of the less commonly encountered connective tissues, this is not normally found in adult humans. It is found in embryonic specimens and in umbilical cord as 'Wharton's jelly'. It is a cellular tissue with stellate fibroblasts which anastomose and are embedded in a mucinous intercellular matrix containing hyaluronic acid. There are few collagenic fibers apart from those in blood vessels.

Dense connective tissue

Dense connective tissue is often seen as the capsules enclosing organs and, in particular, tubular structures, but is most strikingly characterized in its appearance as tendons and ligaments. These are basically dense masses of collagenic fibers and fibroblasts arranged in an orderly manner, the cells and fibers being oriented in the same direction, i.e. parallel to the long axis of the tendon. Primarily there is a predominance of fibroblasts, but these secrete increasing amounts of collagen and the bulk of the tendon becomes collagenic and fibrous. Structures of this composition possess enormous tensile strength and are perfectly suited for connecting the skeletal muscles to the skeleton and so transmitting power. Immature dense connective tissue contains capillaries, but as the fibroblasts mature to become fibrocytes and stop producing intercellular substances, the need for nutriments in quantity is much reduced and the capillary blood supply disappears.

Cartilage

The connective tissues discussed previously possess great tensile strength (that is, will resist diverging forces) but, when placed under pressure, they will bend. The structural characteristics of cartilage partly overcomes this problem; it consists of a fairly dense network of collagenic fibers encased in, or bonded with, an amorphous intercellular substance of the chondroitin sulfate type which is in the form of a thin gel. Cartilage is distributed throughout the body in sites where the functions it is required to perform are slightly different. Hence, although it has an almost 'standard' form known as hyaline cartilage, it does have two other modified forms, elastocartilage and fibrocartilage. These will be considered later.

Microscopically, cartilage is composed of a matrix of apparently homogeneous intercellular substance, and, under high power microscopy, it can be seen to be fibrillar in structure, containing large numbers of collagenic fibers. In the matrix are the cellular components of cartilage, the chondrocytes, which reside in spaces in the matrix known as 'lacunae'. There may be one cell or as many as six cells in each lacuna. In a fresh state the chondrocytes will fill the lacunae, whereas in stained sections they will often appear rather shrunken. The cytoplasm contains glycogen and lipid, and the nuclei are spherical with one or more nucleoli. Young immature chondrocytes tend to be rather small and flattened; as they mature they become larger and more rounded. Immediately surrounding the cell lining the lacuna is what appears to be an intercellular substance of a different type from that which comprises the bulk of the matrix.

Hyaline cartilage is the most common cartilage and is found in the larynx, the bronchus, the nose and as the articulatory surface of joints. When thoroughly lubricated with synovial fluid, the surface of cartilage will take on a high polish, with little friction, and is ideally suited for the bearing surfaces of joints. Although hyaline cartilage is slightly elastic, in some instances this is not adequate. Elastocartilage is found where more elasticity is required; it contains as many collagenic fibers but has the addition of elastic fibers. It is found in the external ear and the epiglottis.

Fibrocartilage is found in sites such as tendon inserts where the tensile strength of hyaline cartilage is insufficient. The collagenic fibers of hyaline cartilage are arranged with no regular pattern; in fibrocartilage they are packed in rows parallel to the direction of the force. Between the collagenic fiber bundles lie fibroblasts and rows of chondrocytes and intercellular substance. Cartilage develops from the mesenchymal cells that differentiate into chondroblasts and lay down intercellular substance; they mature into chondrocytes and the cartilage in this form can live for long periods, as it does in joints. Mature, hypertrophied chondrocytes will produce alkaline phosphatase, which brings about a reaction whereby insoluble calcium salts are precipitated in the matrix of the cartilage. As the calcification proceeds, the nutriments needed by the chondrocytes are cut off and the cells use up their stored glycogen and die. The calcified cartilage is not a permanent formation as it has no living cellular component, and it soon breaks down and the tissue loses all its supporting structures.

Bone

Cartilage in its several forms is capable of providing support and resisting converging forces; calcified cartilage is much stronger, but as the process of calcification occurs the chondrocytes are cut off from their nutriments, which come through the permeable intercellular structure, and so they die. A permanent rigid type of connective tissue is required to support the body's weight, to maintain its optimal shape and to shield its delicate structures from external damage; this tissue is bone. The structure of bone is discussed in detail in Chapter 18.

Muscular tissue

The purpose of muscular tissue is to provide the power to enable the body to move and to function. Although muscular tissues are readily divided into three distinct categories, all types are composed of similar constituents and their mode of providing power and movement is also similar. Muscles provide power and movement by contracting their cells, so shortening their overall length, thus pulling closer together the points to which the muscle is attached. Many cells in the body share this ability to contract and change shape. This phenomenon is due to the presence of three proteins and the interactions between them:

- α-actin
- actin
- myosin.

α-Actin forms a base, which allows a strand of actin to become attached. Myosin in turn attaches to this actin strand and is able to move up the strands towards the base by means of a ratchet-like mechanism. Because myosin is double-headed, it interacts simultaneously with two separate actin strands. The movement up the strands from these different base plates pulls the strands together, causing the fiber to contract. A single muscle fiber of skeletal muscle is long and thin and comprises many myofibrils. These subcellular components run parallel to the fiber's long axis. Each myofibril is built up of a large number of identical contractile units called sarcomeres. Neither the fiber nor the sarcomere contracts simultaneously, and on full contraction can shorten by about 30% of its resting length. The three types into which muscular tissues may be classified are:

- involuntary smooth muscle
- voluntary striated muscle
- striated cardiac muscle.

Involuntary smooth muscle

Smooth muscle is developed from mesenchymal cells, which elongate themselves to form tapered cells of 20–50 μm in length. The size of the muscle cell, or fiber as it is often called, varies enormously and depends upon the site in which the cells are found. Microscopically, the cells appear eosinophilic with areas of paler staining denoting the presence of glycogen. The cytoplasm contains bundles of myofilaments called myofibrils, which may be up to 1 mm in diameter; these are surrounded by the sarcoplasm, which constitutes the remainder of the cell. The centrally situated nuclei with their fine chromatin pattern are palely stained with hematoxylin and have an elongated appearance; they may contain one or two nucleoli. In cells that contract extensively and regularly, the nuclei may take on a 'concertina' shape which enables them to fit comfortably into the cell when it is in a state of full contraction.

Voluntary striated muscle

Striated or voluntary muscle makes up the bulk of the body's shape and is widely distributed over all parts of the skeleton—hence its alternative name of skeletal muscle. It is the type of muscle over which a person has voluntary control. It is capable of briefly producing tremendous forces when called upon to do so, and also of maintaining a state of 'semi-contraction' for long periods of time, i.e. holding the body upright while standing. Some functions become almost automatic although the person still maintains voluntary control, such as respiration, swallowing, blinking, etc. Like smooth muscle, it is composed of elongated eosinophilic cells, but in striated muscle these are much larger and longer, up to 40 mm in length and up to 40 μm in diameter. The cells themselves do not taper towards the ends but are more cylindrical. The nuclei are elongated and stain palely with hematoxylin. There is often more than one nucleus present in each cell and these are situated peripherally and often in contact with the sarcolemma or cell membrane.

The most obvious and striking characteristic of striated muscle is the striations or stripes that cross the cells at right angles to their long axes. On closer examination, and by polarized light, the striations can be seen to be alternating light and dark bands or discs. The darker bands are birefringent and are referred to as A-bands or Q-bands; the paler bands are isotropic and are known as I-bands. On occasions, running through the center of the paler I-bands may be seen a narrow, dark band, known as the Z-line. Studies of relaxed voluntary muscle with the electron microscope have shown the presence of a fourth band, an extremely thin band running through the A-band; this is called the H-line or H-disc (Fig. 10.3). Again with the aid of the electron microscope it may be seen that these numerous discs or bands are not, in fact, complete structures crossing the muscle cells, but are composed of myofibrils which are striated, and it is the organized arrangement of these striae that gives the appearance of discs. Between these myofibrils is a well developed system of mitochondria and sarcoplasmic reticulum. Stored in the sarcoplasm, adjacent to the sarcoplasmic reticulum, is an abundant store of glycogen to provide an immediate source of energy.

Striated cardiac muscle

Cardiac muscle constitutes the myocardium and this is the only situation in which it is found. It differs from

Z-line   H-disc containing
         dark M-line

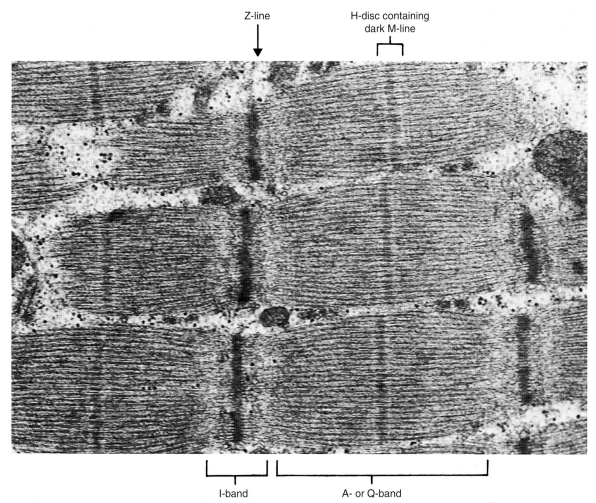

I-band   A- or Q-band

Fig. 10.3 Electron micrograph of human striated muscle showing characteristic pattern of striations.

smooth muscle and striated muscle in a number of ways. It is not composed of distinctly separate cells which branch and anastomose with great frequency. The cytoplasm contains myofibrils and sarcoplasm and exhibits a 'striated' appearance similar to that of voluntary muscle. The striations are less distinct as the myofibrils are not arranged to coincide as regularly as in voluntary striated muscle.

One feature unique to cardiac muscle is the presence of intercalated discs. These were originally believed to be another type of striation or stripe. From studies of these bands with the electron microscope it can be seen that these discs represent the end-to-end junction of adjacent cardiac muscle cells. The nuclei are placed centrally in the cells and stain palely with hematoxylin. Situated in

the intercellular spaces created by the branching and anastomosing of the cells are the blood vessels, lymphatics, and nerves to maintain and nourish the cardiac muscle.

General structure of muscle

The muscles of the body, whether they are of voluntary, involuntary, or cardiac type, contain considerable amounts of connective tissue. Each complete muscle is surrounded by an envelope of collagenic and elastic fibers known as the 'epimysium'. Arising from the epimysium are numerous bands or sheets of connective tissue which divide the whole muscle into bundles of muscle cells; this is the 'perimysium'. A connective tissue sheath called the 'endomysium' covers each individual muscle cell. This complex system of interconnecting collagenic fibers is continuous with the attachment points of the muscle; the fine sheets of collagenic fibers give way to broader, stronger bands of dense connective tissue which continue to form the tendon.

Fibrin and fibrinoid

Fibrin is an insoluble fibrillar protein formed by polymerization of the smaller soluble fibrillar protein, fibrinogen, which is one of the plasma proteins. Fibrin is most commonly seen in tissues where there has been tissue damage, in an acute inflammatory reaction, resulting in transudation of fluid and plasma proteins out of damaged vessels. The plasma fibrinogen polymerizes to form insoluble fibrin outside the vessels. Fibrin is an important constituent of the acute inflammatory exudate and may be found wherever there is recent tissue damage.

In paraffin sections fibrin is strongly eosinophilic and stains blue–black with Mallory's PTAH. Lendrum et al (1962) devised a trichrome method, the MSB, to demonstrate fibrin and to attempt to distinguish between fibrin of varying ages. 'Fibrinoid' is an eosinophilic material which has identical staining reactions to fibrin, but occurs in tissues in different situations and disorders. It is frequently found within vessel walls where the vessel has undergone acute damage ('necrotizing vasculitis'), and sometimes as plugs in capillaries. There is much controversy about the nature of fibrinoid, but many regard it as a mixture of forming fibrin with other protein components of the plasma. A more detailed discussion of the nature of fibrin, collagen, and basement membranes may be found in the 'Further reading' section.

CONNECTIVE TISSUE STAINS

See Table 10.1.

Trichrome stains

Many techniques available for the differential demonstration of the connective tissues fall into the category of 'trichrome stains'. The term 'trichrome stain' is a general name for a number of techniques for the selective demonstration of muscle, collagen fibers, fibrin, and erythrocytes (Fig. 10.4). By implication three dyes are employed, one of which may be a nuclear stain. The original methods were used to differentiate between collagen and muscle fibers, and some are satisfactory for this application. One of the earlier techniques still in constant use is the van Gieson method.

Table 10.1	Connective tissue stains and their reactions										
Tissue	van Gieson	Masson trichrome	MSB	PTAH	PAS	Retic	Meth. silver	Auto fluor.	Refrac.	Biref.	H&E
Muscle	Yellow	Red	Red	Blue	+	Gray	Gray	−	−	−	Deep pink
Collagen	Red	Blue green	Blue	Orange red	+	Gray	−	−	−	+	Deep pink
Elastin	Yellow		Blue	Orange brown	−	−	−	+	+	−	Pink
Reticulin	Yellow	Blue green	Blue	Orange brown	++	Black	−	−	−	−	
Basement membranes	Yellow	Blue green	Blue	Orange	+++	Gray	Black	−	−	−	Pink
Osteoid	Red	Blue green	Blue	Orange red	+	Gray	−	−	−	+	Deep pink
Cartilage	Varies	Varies	Varies	Varies	++	Varies	Varies	−	−	−	Purple
Fibrin	Yellow	Red	Red	Blue	+/−	Gray	−	−	−	−	Pink

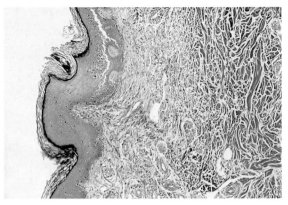

Fig. 10.4 Masson trichrome on a section of skin demonstrating collagen.

Factors affecting trichrome staining

Tissue permeability and dye molecular size

Although little work has been published on the permeability of tissues and the 'pore' size of fixed tissues, some deductions may be made from the reactions of various tissue elements with a range of anionic dyes of differing molecular size (Table 10.2). When the protein component of a tissue is exposed to a fixative agent, an interaction between the protein chains and the fixative occurs. The nature of the reaction and the end result will vary according to the exact composition of the protein and the fixative in use. As a general rule, a three-dimensional, insoluble protein 'network' is formed; different proteins

Table 10.2 Dyes in connective tissue stains

Dye	Alternate name	Color index number	Dye formula weight
Picric acid	Trinitrophenol	—	229
Martius yellow	Acid yellow 24	13015	251
Lissamine fast yellow	Xylene yellow G	18965	551
Sun yellow	Direct yellow 11	4000	837
Orange G	Acid orange 10, Lissamine orange 2G	16230	452
Fast green FCF	Food green 3	42053	809
Fast light green	Cyanol green B, Acid green 50	44090	577
Light green SF	Acid green 5	42095	793
Acid fuchsin	Acid violet 19, Acid magneta	42685	586
Ponceau 2R	Acid red 26	16150	480
Ponceau 3R	Ponceau de xylidine, Acid red 18	16155	494
Azocarmine B	Acid red 103	50085	682
Azofuchsin	Acid red 33	16550	467
Azophloxine	Acid red 1, Amidonaphthol red	18050	509
Biebrich scarlet	Acid red 66, Ponceau B	26905	556
Congo red	Direct red 28, Direct red Y	22120	697
Crystal ponceau 6R	Acid red 44	16250	502
		22145	698
Direct garnet	Direct red 10, Congo Corinth		
Azo eosin	Acid red 4	14710	380
Lissamine red 3GX	Acid red 57, Propalan red 3 GX		
Sirius	Direct red 80, Chlorantine fast red	35780	1373
Methyl blue	Aniline blue, Acid blue 93, Cotton blue	42780	800
Alkali blue		42750	574
		42765	
Durazol brilliant blue	Direct blue, Direct blue 109	51310	
Naphthol blue black	Amido black 10B, Acid black 1	20470	617
Pontamine sky blue	6BX Chicago blue 6B, Direct blue 1	24410	993
Isamine blue	Direct blue 41, Pyrrol blue	42700	786
Azocarmine G	Acid red 101	50085	580

will form networks with different physical features. For example, erythrocyte protein will produce a dense network, with only small pores between the protein elements. Muscle cells will form a more open structure with larger pores. Collagen will show the least dense network and is seemingly quite porous.

The structure and density of the protein network may relate directly to the staining reactions of the tissue components. The smaller molecule dyes will penetrate (and stain) any of the three tissue types. Medium size dye molecules will penetrate muscle and collagen, but will not react with erythrocytes. The larger dye molecules will penetrate only collagen, leaving muscle and erythrocytes unstained. In practice, the rules seem less rigid and the size of the dye molecule seems to be significant. For example, acid will stain collagen when used in combination with picric acid in van Gieson's stain, but, when used with light green SF in Masson's trichrome, it stains erythrocytes and muscle. Some of the large molecular size dyes, such as sun yellow, pontamine sky blue 6BX, will fail to stain erythrocytes even when the tissues are exposed to the dye solution for long periods due to the incompatibility between the dye molecule size and the permeability of the red cell protein.

The general rule in trichrome staining is that a smaller dye molecule will penetrate and stain a tissue element, but whenever a larger dye molecule can penetrate the same element, the smaller molecule will be replaced by it. Detailed information regarding molecular size of dyes is not readily available. However, the molecular weight may be used as an indication of the relative sizes. It is also possible to calculate the ionic weight of a dye from the molecular weight; this is also of value in estimating relative sizes. Horobin (1980) presents a number of interesting hypotheses relating to tissue structure and its influence on staining mechanisms. For an in-depth review, reference should be made to this work. (See also Chapter 8.)

Heat

Heat has been shown to increase the rate at which staining occurs and also to influence penetration by the larger dye molecules.

pH

In order to achieve adequate and even staining of connective tissue fibers, dyes utilized in trichrome methods are prepared as low pH solutions (often in the range pH 1.5–3.0).

Nuclear stains for trichrome

Due to the acidity of dye solutions used in the differential staining of connective tissue fibers, standard alum hematoxylins are decolorized in the subsequent treatment. Iron hematoxylins are more resistant to acid solutions and are prescribed in most of the techniques. An improved and resistant stain can be achieved by sequential staining with celestine blue or solochrome prune in iron alum solution, followed by a conventional alum hematoxylin (for details see Chapter 9).

Effects of fixation

The use of routine, formaldehyde-fixed tissues for trichrome techniques will not produce optimal results. If fixation in formaldehyde has been prolonged the results will be even less satisfactory, due to the saturation of tissue groups with formaldehyde, thus leaving few groups available to react with the trichrome dyes. Treatment of formaldehyde-fixed tissues with picric acid, mercuric chloride solutions, or both, will enhance trichrome intensity and brilliance. Lendrum et al (1962) recommended 'degreasing' sections for 24–48 hours in trichlorethylene prior to staining; this was claimed to improve further the intensity of the staining reactions. Zenker's solution, formal mercury, Bouin's fixative, or picro-mercuric alcohol are the most satisfactory fixatives for trichrome techniques. The staining reactions following these fixatives will be much brighter and more saturated than those following formaldehyde fixation.

---

van Gieson technique (van Gieson 1889)

Sections
Paraffin. For celloidin or low-viscosity nitrocellucose (LVN) sections see Notes d and e below.

Solution
Saturated aqueous picric acid solution	50 ml
1% aqueous acid fuchsin solution	9.0 ml
Distilled water	50 ml

Method
1. Deparaffinize sections and bring to water.
2. Stain nuclei by the celestine blue–hematoxylin sequence (see p. 125).
3. Wash in tap water.
4. Differentiate in acid alcohol.
5. Wash well in tap water.

6. Stain in van Gieson solution for 3 minutes.

7. Blot and dehydrate through alcohols.

8. Clear in xylene and mount in permanent mounting medium.

Results

Nuclei	blue/black
Collagen	red
Other tissues	yellow

Notes

a. Fixation is not critical, buffered formalin being satisfactory.

b. Washing in water after van Gieson solution should be avoided, the color balance being impaired by this.

c. Nuclear staining should be intense before application of van Gieson solution; the picric acid will act as a differentiator.

d. Celloidin sections are washed in distilled water after van Gieson solution.

e. Celestine blue may stain the celloidin intensely. In such circumstances, Weigert's iron hematoxylin should be used.

Role of phosphotungstic and phosphomolybdic acids (PTA and PMA)

Although phosphomolybdic and phosphotungstic acids do not give identical reactions in trichrome staining techniques, their properties are similar. Experimental work indicates that the principles involved are identical, but it is not suggested that the two substances are interchangeable in any given technique. Throughout the literature on trichrome staining, reference is frequently made to mordanting in phosphotungstic or phosphomolybdic acid. There remains some controversy about the precise roles of these two substances, but it is unlikely that they act as mordants towards the anionic dyes used in these techniques. Everett and Miller (1974) have shown that treatment of formalin-fixed sections with PMA or PTA greatly reduces staining of all tissue components, other than collagen fibers, with aniline blue and other similar anionic dyes. Blocking towards smaller dye molecules such as Biebrich scarlet

was shown to be less complete. Binding of PTA to epithelium and connective tissue fibers was demonstrated by the quenching of autofluorescence and by the reduction of the bound PTA to a blue color by means of titanium trichloride solution. These workers postulated that the differential staining by the trichrome methods occurs by binding of aniline blue to basic residues in the connective tissues not already blocked by PTA. Baker (1958) stated that PMA acts as a 'colorless acid dye', of large molecular size and hence slowly diffusing.

Practical uses of PMA and PTA

In trichrome staining, there are three stages at which PMA or PTA may be used: firstly before treatment with the small molecule dye, secondly combined in solution with the small molecule dye, and thirdly before treatment with the large molecule dye. Any combination of these techniques is possible. If a section is first treated with PMA or PTA solution and then with a low concentration of a 'leveling' dye in the same solution, the leveling dye will color nothing but the erythrocytes. In practice, the first treatment with the PMA or PTA is frequently omitted without detriment to the final results. When a section is first treated with a leveling dye or other suitable small molecule anionic dye and then with PMA or PTA solution, the PMA or PTA competes with the dye and gains access to the collagen easily, expelling the dye in the process. If treatment is stopped at the right moment, only collagen will be free to stain when treated with a 'milling' or other large molecule dye. If treatment with the large molecule dye is greatly prolonged, some staining of muscle and cytoplasm may take place. In addition to the rather complex role played by PMA and PTA in connective tissue staining, it must not be forgotten that both are quite capable of acting simply as conventional acidifying agents, a 10% solution of PTA having a pH of less than 1; indeed, PTA is unstable at a pH greater than about 2.

Identification of dyes

There is little standardization between manufacturers in the naming of dyes, and consequently the chemically identical dye may be obtained from different suppliers under a wide range of names (see Dye nomenclature in Chapter 8, and Table 8.2).

Masson trichrome technique
(Masson 1929)

Fixation
Formal sublimate or formal saline.

Sections
All types.

Solution a
Acid fuchsin	0.5 g
Glacial acetic acid	0.5 ml
Distilled water	100 ml

Solution b
Phosphomolybdic acid	1 g
Distilled water	100 ml

Solution c
Methyl blue	2 g
Glacial acetic acid	2.5 ml
Distilled water	100 ml

Method
1. Deparaffinize sections and bring to water.
2. Remove mercury pigment by iodine, sodium thiosulfate sequence.
3. Wash in tap water.
4. Stain nuclei by the celestine blue–hematoxylin method.
5. Differentiate with 1% acid alcohol.
6. Wash well in tap water.
7. Stain in acid fuchsin solution a, 5 minutes.
8. Rinse in distilled water.
9. Treat with phosphomolybdic acid solution b, 5 minutes.
10. Drain.
11. Stain with methyl blue solution c, 2–5 minutes.
12. Rinse in distilled water.
13. Treat with 1% acetic acid, 2 minutes.
14. Dehydrate through alcohols.
15. Clear in xylene, mount in permanent mounting medium.

Results
Nuclei	blue/black
Cytoplasm, muscle, and erythrocytes	red
Collagen	blue

Notes
a. The celestin blue–hematoxylin sequence provides a satisfactory alternative to the iron alum hematoxylin used in the original method.
b. Light green may be substituted for methyl blue.

Heidenhain's 'Azan'

Due to prolonged staining times the 'Azan' technique is not recommended as a general connective tissue method. In the demonstration of 'wire loop lesions', in the diagnosis of lupus nephritis in renal biopsies, the method may be found useful.

The demonstration of fibrin

Techniques for the selective demonstration of fibrin are of three types:

- Gram–Weigert
- phosphotungstic acid–hematoxylin
- trichrome methods.

Although there would appear to be little similarity between these methods, they all depend for their selectivity upon the use of dyes or dye complexes of suitable molecular size. Trichrome techniques of the Masson type may prove satisfactory for the demonstration of fibrin, although older deposits tend to stain as collagen. Lendrum et al (1962) showed that modifications to the Masson technique enable older deposits of fibrin to be demonstrated. The main features of the Martius, scarlet, blue (MSB) technique are the use of a small-molecule yellow dye, together with phosphotungstic acid in alcoholic solution, selectively to stain red cells. Early fibrin deposits may be stained by this dye, although the phosphotungstic acid blocks the staining of muscle, collagen, and most connective tissue fibers. On treatment with the medium-sized molecule red dye, muscle and mature fibrin are stained, gross staining of collagen being prevented by phosphotungstic acid remaining from the first stage. Further treatment with aqueous phosphotungstic acid removes any trace of red from the collagen fibers. Final treatment with a large-molecule blue dye demonstrates collagen and old fibrin deposits.

MSB technique for fibrin (Lendrum et al 1962)

The standard MSB technique employs Martius yellow (acid yellow 24) CI 10315, brilliant crystal scarlet (acid red 44) CI 16250, and soluble blue (methyl blue) (acid blue 93) CI 42780.

Preparation of solutions

Solution a
Martius yellow	0.5 g
Phosphotungstic acid	2 g
95% alcohol	100 ml

Solution b
Brilliant crystal scarlet	1 g
Glacial acetic acid	2 ml
Distilled water	100 ml

Solution c
Phosphotungstic acid	1 g
Distilled water	100 ml

Solution d
Methyl blue	0.5 g
Glacial acetic acid	1 ml
Distilled water	100 ml

Solution e
Glacial acetic acid	1 ml
Distilled water	100 ml

Notes on solutions

Martius yellow is dissolved in alcohol before adding the phosphotungstic acid. A satisfactory substitute for Martius yellow is the larger-molecule dye, lissamine fast yellow, which has the advantage of being less easily removed by the subsequent red dye. A number of medium-sized molecule anionic red dyes may be substituted for the brilliant crystal scarlet, and Ponceau de xylidine and azofuchsin have been found satisfactory. Many large-molecule blue or green dyes may be substituted for the methyl blue, including the following: durazol blue, pontamine sky blue, fast green FCF, and naphthalene black 10B. The replacement of methyl blue by pontamine sky blue reduces the tendency of fibrin coloring by the blue dye, due to the larger molecular size.

Method

1. Deparaffinize sections and bring to water.
2. Remove mercury pigment with iodine, sodium thiosulfate treatment.
3. Stain nuclei by the celestine blue–hematoxylin sequence.
4. Differentiate in 1% acid alcohol.
5. Wash well in tap water.
6. Rinse in 95% alcohol.
7. Stain in Martius yellow solution, 2 minutes.
8. Rinse in distilled water.
9. Stain in brilliant crystal scarlet solution, 10 minutes.
10. Rinse in distilled water.
11. Treat with phosphotungstic acid solution until no red remains in the collagen.
12. Rinse in distilled water.
13. Stain in methyl blue solution until collagen is sufficiently stained.
14. Rinse in 1% acetic acid.
15. Dehydrate through alcohols.
16. Clear in xylene and mount in permanent mounting medium.

Results

Nuclei	blue
Erythrocytes	yellow
Muscle	red
Collagen	blue
Fibrin	red (early fibrin may stain yellow and old fibrin, blue)

Notes

a. At stage 11 the time required may be up to 10 minutes, although sufficient selectivity may be achieved by using a standard time of 5 minutes.
b. At stage 13, examine after 2 minutes and at successive 2-minute intervals; excessive stain cannot readily be removed.

Demonstration of muscle striations

Muscle striations can be demonstrated by hematoxylin and eosin, and trichrome methods. They may also be stained by using Heidenhain's iron hematoxylin (see p. 128) and Mallory's phosphotungstic acid hematoxylin (see p. 130). Both these methods will give better definition of muscle striations than the trichromes.

Staining of elastic tissue fibers

Numerous techniques have been evolved for the demonstration of elastic tissue fibers, although few are in current use. Of these, the most popular are Verhöeff's method, the orcein technique, Weigert's resorcin–fuchsin, and the aldehyde fuchsin method. In addition to these methods, use has been made of the dyes chlorazol black E and luxol fast blue, mainly as techniques to determine the mechanism of elastic tissue staining.

General notes on the mechanism of elastic staining

Elastic fibers will stain quite intensely, but not always selectively, by a number of sometimes unrelated techniques, e.g. H&E, hematoxylin–phloxine–saffron, Congo red, periodic acid–Schiff (PAS), Verhöeff's hematoxylin, resorcin–fuchsin, aldehyde fuchsin, Taenzer–Unna orcein, etc. The reaction of elastic fibers with eosin, phloxine, or Congo red may be attributed to coulombic reactions between elastin protein and the acid dyes. The positive PAS reaction, seen particularly in immature, fine fibers, may be accounted for by the presence of carbohydrate-containing glycoproteins, associated with the elastic fiber microfibrillar protein which is a major component of young elastic fibers (and possibly oxytalan and elaunin fibers also).

As stated previously, elastin and the 'pre-elastin' fibers are highly cross-linked by disulfide bridges. Following oxidative treatment, for instance by permanganate in Weigert-type methods and aldehyde fuchsin, or by iodine as in Verhöeff's hematoxylin, these disulfide bridges may be, in part, converted to anionic sulfonic acid derivatives (Horobin & Flemming 1980). These derivatives will be strongly basophilic and capable of relatively selective reactions with the basic dye compounds of the above solutions. These reactions are further enhanced by the high electrolyte concentrations of the staining solutions, which will inhibit dye uptake by chromatin, ribosomal RNA, etc. Goldstein (1962) showed that elastic tissue staining by orcein, resorcin–fuchsin and aldehyde fuchsin was reduced or inhibited by the presence of urea, a strong hydrogen bonding agent, in the stain solution. He further considered that, if hydrogen bonding was responsible for elastic staining, the stain molecule must be the hydrogen donor and the tissue the hydrogen acceptor. For an informative discussion on the mechanisms of elastic fiber staining, the work of Horobin and Flemming (1980) should be consulted.

Verhöeff's method is the classical method for elastic fibers and works well after all routine fixatives. Coarse fibers are intensely stained, but the staining of the fine fibers may be less than satisfactory. The differentiation step is critical to the success of this method, and some expertise is necessary to achieve reproducible results; it is easy to over-differentiate (and lose) the finer fibers. Although some older texts state that the prepared working solution has a usable life of only 2–3 hours, satisfactory results have been obtained using solutions up to 48 hours old.

Verhöeff's method for elastic fibers (Verhöeff 1908)

Preparation of stain

Solution a

Hematoxylin	5 g
Absolute alcohol	100 ml

Solution b

Ferric chloride	10 g
Distilled water	100 ml

Solution c, Lugol's iodine solution

Iodine	1 g
Potassium iodide	2 g
Distilled water	100 ml

Solution d, working solution

Solution a	20 ml
Solution b	8 ml
Solution c	8 ml

Add in the above order, mixing between additions.

Method

1. Deparaffinize sections and bring to water.
2. Verhöeff's solution, 15–30 minutes.
3. Rinse in water.
4. Differentiate in 2% aqueous ferric chloride until elastic tissue fibers appear black on a gray background.
5. Rinse in water.
6. Rinse in 95% alcohol to remove any staining due to iodine alone.
7. Counterstain as desired (van Gieson is conventional, although eosin may be used).
8. Blot to remove excess stain.
9. Dehydrate rapidly through alcohols.
10. Clear in xylene and mount in permanent mounting medium.

Results

Elastic tissue fibers   black

Other tissues according to counterstain.

Notes

a. Pre-treatment with 1% potassium permanganate for 5 minutes, followed by oxalic acid, improves sharpness and intensity of staining.
b. Removal of mercury pigment is unnecessary, this being carried out by the iodine in the staining solution.
c. Rinsing in warm tap water improves intense staining of fibers.

Orcein methods

Orcein is a naturally occurring vegetable dye, which has now been synthesized. Variations between batches of dye may produce erratic results with insufficient depth of stain on occasions. The main advantage of this stain is the simplicity of preparation. The choice of fixative appears unimportant.

Weigert's resorcin–fuchsin method

Although the standard Weigert technique employs basic fuchsin, a number of related cationic dyes of the triphenyl-methane group may be substituted; indeed, the composition of basic fuchsin is variable, at least three dyes being present in many batches of this dye. These variations considerably affect the staining and storage properties of the prepared solution as well as the stain imparted to elastic fibers. Another variable is the impurities in the ferric chloride. Even fresh ferric chloride contains the ferrous salt, which does not produce a satisfactory staining solution. Ferric nitrate has been found to be consistently free from the ferrous salt, and should be substituted for the chloride in the Weigert technique and its variations.

Resorcin–fuchsin method (Weigert 1898)

Preparation of Weigert resorcin–fuchsin

To 100 ml of distilled water, add 1 g of basic fuchsin and 2 g of resorcin. Boil. Add 12.5 ml of freshly prepared 30% ferric chloride solution (see previous note on the use of ferric nitrate). Continue boiling for 5 minutes. Cool and filter, discarding the filtrate. Dissolve the whole of the precipitate in 100 ml of 95% ethanol, using a hotplate or water bath for controlled heating, and add 2 ml of concentrated hydrochloric acid.

As an improved solvent, the precipitate may be dissolved in:

2-methoxyethanol	50 ml
Distilled water	50 ml
Concentrated hydrochloric acid	2 ml

Staining time is reduced with this solvent.

Method

1. Deparaffinize sections and bring to alcohol.
2. Place in staining solution in a Coplin jar, 1–3 hours at room temperature or 1 hour at 56°C.
3. Rinse in tap water.
4. Remove background staining by treating with 1% acid alcohol.
5. Rinse in tap water.
6. Counterstain as desired (van Gieson, eosin or tri-chrome methods are applicable).
7. Dehydrate through alcohols.
8. Clear in xylene and mount in permanent mounting medium.

Notes

a. Staining may be carried out after most fixatives. Those containing chromium salts produce less intense and more diffuse staining.
b. Acid alcohol treatment for removal of background staining can be brief, a few seconds, but may be prolonged without harm.
c. Treatment before stage 2, for 5 minutes with 1% potassium permanganate followed by oxalic acid, improves the staining.

Results

Elastic tissue fibers   brown to purple

Modification of the Weigert technique

Hart's modification has been recommended for use after fixatives containing potassium dichromate and is simply prepared by making a dilution of between 5 and 20% of the Weigert solution in 70% alcohol containing 1% hydrochloric acid. Staining time must be increased to overnight. Sheridan's resorcin–crystal violet method uses a solution as for the Weigert, but substituting the basic fuchsin by 1 g of crystal violet and 1 g dextrin. The methyl violet/ethyl violet–resorcin method for elastic fibers (given below) has replaced the dahlia elastic tissue stain given in earlier editions, this substitution being necessary due to the withdrawal of dahlia from the commercial market.

Methyl violet/ethyl violet–resorcin method for elastic fibers

Preparation of staining solution
Dissolve 0.5 g of methyl violet (CI 42535) and 0.5 g of ethyl violet (CI 42600) in 100 ml of boiling distilled water. Add 2 g of resorcin and 25 ml of 30% ferric nitrate solution; continue boiling for an additional 3 minutes. Cool and filter. Discard the filtrate and dissolve the whole of the precipitate by gentle heating on hotplate or water bath in:

2 methoxyethanol	50 ml
Distilled water	50 ml
Concentrated hydrochloric acid	2 ml

Preparation of staining solution may be speeded by the use of a microwave oven at both heating stages.

Method
The same technique as for the Weigert method (p. 154) is employed, using the potassium permanganate and oxalic acid pre-treatment. Staining may be adequate, with formalin-fixed tissues, in 15 minutes at room temperature.

Results
Elastic tissue fibers	blue–black

Mechanism of Weigert elastin staining

It has been shown that acetylation, sulfation, and phosphorylation of tissues induce binding of resorcin–fuchsin to glycogen, basement membranes, reticular fibers, collagen, and other tissue structures containing polysaccharides. These structures are unstained by resorcin–fuchsin without prior treatment, indicating that this binding is due to the introduction of ester groups. Extraction procedures designed to remove dyes bonded by salt or ionic linkages indicate that non-ionic bonds are involved.

Aldehyde fuchsin

Aldehyde fuchsin was first introduced into histology as an elastic tissue stain by Gomori (1950). Coarse and fine fibers are stained adequately with a suitably ripened solution although a number of other tissue components are equally well stained, including beta cell granules of pancreas, and sulfated mucosubstances. With prior oxidation in periodic acid, peracetic acid, or potassium permanganate, other components are demonstrated, such as glycogen and neutral mucosubstances, but with increased intensity of elastic tissue staining.

Aldehyde fuchsin method for elastic fibers

Preparation of staining solution
Dissolve 1 g of basic fuchsin in 100 ml of 70% ethanol; heat may be used to speed the process. After cooling and filtering add 1 ml of concentrated hydrochloric acid and 2 ml of paraldehyde. Stand at room temperature for 2 days to complete the ripening process, which is indicated by a conversion from red to purple. Ripening time may be reduced by increased temperature at 50–60°C. The ripened solution should be refrigerated for storage. Batches of basic fuchsin suitable for the production of Schiff's reagent are usually satisfactory for the preparation of aldehyde fuchsin. Paraldehyde may lose some potency upon storage but this may be partially compensated by the addition of an extra 0.5 ml of this solution. The staining potential of aldehyde fuchsin is greatest at between 2 and 4 days after preparation, but may be adequate for the demonstration of elastic tissue fibers for several weeks if stored at 4°C.

Method
1. Deparaffinize sections and bring to water.
2. Oxidize in 1% potassium permanganate, 5 minutes.
3. Rinse in tap water.
4. Remove permanganate staining by treatment with 1% oxalic acid.
5. Rinse in tap water.
6. Rinse in 70% ethanol.
7. Place in sealed container of aldehyde fuchsin for 15 minutes.
8. Rinse well in 70% ethanol.
9. Rinse in tap water.

10. Counterstain as desired (eosin, van Gieson or neutral red are suitable).
11. Dehydrate through alcohols.
12. Clear in xylene and mount in permanent mounting solution.

Results

Elastic tissue fibers	blue–purple

Also stained are beta cell granules of pancreas, some mucosubstances, some fungi, cartilage matrix, and mast cell granules. Other tissues, according to counterstain.

Note

Contrast between the collagen and fine elastic tissue fibers may be inadequate following van Gieson counterstain, and a purely nuclear counterstain may be considered more suitable.

The demonstration of reticular fibers

Techniques for the demonstration of reticular fibers may be divided into those using dyes as a means of staining, and the metal impregnation methods. Dye techniques for reticular demonstration cannot be considered completely reliable, the density of stain being insufficient to resolve the fine fibers. Staining techniques do not readily differentiate between collagen and reticular fibers. Metal impregnation techniques provide contrast, enabling even the finest fibers to be resolved (see Fig. 10.2, p. 138).

Metal impregnation techniques

Many techniques for the demonstration of reticular fibers, mainly employing silver salts, have been published. Whilst the composition of these solutions varies widely, all have in common the silver in alkaline solution in a state readily able to precipitate as metallic silver. Reticular fibers have only a low natural affinity for silver salts and require suitable pretreatment in order to enhance the selectivity of the impregnation. Pretreatment baths are frequently heavy metal salt solutions, commonly ferric ammonium sulfate. Treatment with silver solution has a twofold effect: submicroscopic sensitized sites of silver in reduced form are created on the reticular fibers, and a considerable quantity of silver is taken up by tissues in unreduced form. These reactions are both optimized at around pH 9.0 and are quite rapid.

Upon treatment with a reducing agent, silver taken up by the tissue in unreduced form is converted to metallic silver which is deposited at the sensitized sites. Any remaining unreacted silver may be removed by treatment with sodium thiosulfate solution. For a completely permanent preparation, the silver may be partially converted to a gold impregnation by treatment with gold chloride solution, at the same time slightly increasing the contrast. Ammoniacal silver salts, when in the dry state, are potentially dangerous due to their explosive properties; they should be stored, only in solution, in plastic rather than glass bottles.

Preparation of silver solutions

All aqueous silver solutions require the solvent to be glass-distilled or deionized water to prevent precipitation of insoluble silver salts. The literature abounds with formulas for suitable silver solutions; the majority follow the same pattern. To a solution of silver nitrate is added a carbonate or hydroxide solution to produce a precipitate. The precipitate is re-dissolved, usually by the addition of ammonia solution. All of these formulas require great attention to detail: glassware must be perfectly clean and solutions prepared from the purest of reagents with weights and volumes accurately measured. Any excess of ammonia in the solution results in a great loss of sensitivity, giving only weak or complete lack of reticular fiber impregnation. The most reliable procedure is to add rather less ammonia than is needed to dissolve the precipitate, and filter to remove remaining turbidity. Alternatively, back titration with silver nitrate may be employed to react with any excess ammonia.

Sections for reticular fiber silver impregnation

Frozen, cryostat, and celloidin sections may be employed for the demonstration of reticular fibers; most of the published techniques are intended for use with paraffin sections. Impregnation is carried out on tissues after a wide range of fixatives. Fixatives containing the heavy metal salts of mercury or osmium occasionally cause a little non-specific background precipitation of silver. Silver impregnation fluids having sufficient sensitivity for these techniques are mainly alkaline, frequently causing sections to become detached from the slide. Adhesives, previously mentioned in Chapter 7, may be used, although any excess adhesive may cause unwanted precipitate around and beneath the tissue.

Gordon & Sweets' method for reticular fibers (Gordon & Sweets 1936)

Preparation of silver solution

To 5 ml of 10% aqueous silver nitrate solution add concentrated ammonia, drop by drop, until the precipitate first formed dissolves, taking care to avoid any excess of ammonia. Add 5 ml of 3% sodium hydroxide solution. Re-dissolve the precipitate by the addition of concentrated ammonia, drop by drop, until the solution retains a trace of opalescence. If at this stage any excess of ammonia is present, indicated by the absence of opalescence, add a few drops of 10% silver nitrate solution, to produce a light precipitate. Make up the volume to 50 ml with distilled water. Filter before use. Store in a dark bottle.

Method

1. Deparaffinize sections and bring to water.
2. Treat with 1% potassium permanganate solution, 5 minutes.
3. Rinse in tap water.
4. Bleach in 1% oxalic acid solution.
5. Rinse in tap water.
6. Treat with 2.5% iron alum solution for at least 15 minutes.
7. Wash well in several changes of distilled water.
8. Place in a Coplin jar of silver solution, 2 minutes.
9. Rinse in several changes of distilled water.
10. Reduce in 10% aqueous formalin solution, 2 minutes.
11. Rinse in tap water.
12. Tone in 0.2% gold chloride solution, 3 minutes.
13. Rinse in tap water.
14. Treat with 5% sodium thiosulfate solution, 3 minutes.
15. Rinse in tap water.
16. Counterstain as desired.
17. Dehydrate through alcohols.
18. Clear in xylene and mount in permanent mounting medium.

Results

Reticular fibers	black
Nuclei	black or unstained (see Note a below)
Other elements	according to counterstain

Notes

a. A short treatment with iron alum solution, of less than 5 minutes, gives less staining of nuclei.
b. The use of a Coplin jar for the silver solution greatly reduces the possibility of precipitation on the slide. Sections can be counterstained with eosin, nuclear fast red, tartrazine, or van Gieson.

Gomori's method for reticular fibers (Gomori 1937)

Preparation of silver solution

To 10 ml of 10% potassium hydroxide solution add 40 ml of 10% silver nitrate solution. Allow the precipitate to settle and decant the supernatant. Wash the precipitate several times with distilled water. Add ammonia drop by drop until the precipitate has just dissolved. Add further 10% silver nitrate solution until a little precipitate remains. Dilute to 100 ml and filter. Store in a dark bottle.

Method

1. Deparaffinize sections and bring to water.
2. Treat with 1% potassium permanganate solution, 2 minutes.
3. Rinse in tap water.
4. Bleach in 2% potassium metabisulfate solution.
5. Rinse in tap water.
6. Treat with 2% iron alum, 2 minutes.
7. Wash in several changes of distilled water.
8. Place in Coplin jar of silver solution, 1 minute.
9. Wash in several changes of distilled water.
10. Reduce in 4% aqueous formalin solution, 3 minutes.
11. Rinse in tap water.
12. Tone in 0.2% gold chloride solution, 10 minutes.
13. Rinse in tap water.
14. Treat with 2% potassium metabisulfite solution, 1 minute.
15. Rinse in tap water.
16. Treat with 2% sodium thiosulfate solution, 1 minute.
17. Rinse in tap water.
18. Counterstain as desired (van Gieson or eosin is suitable).

19. Dehydrate through alcohols.
20. Clear in xylene and mount in permanent mounting medium.

Results

Reticular fibers	black
Nuclei	gray
Other tissues	according to counterstain

Russell modification of the Movat pentachrome stain (Carson 1997) See Figure 10.5

Fixation

10% neutral buffered formalin or acetic formalin sublimate (mercuric chloride, 4 g; 37–40% formaldehyde, 20 ml; distilled water, 80 ml; glacial acetic acid, 5 ml).

Sections

5 microns

Solutions

1% alcian blue solution

Alcian blue, 8 GS	1 g
Distilled water	100 ml
Glacial acetic acid	2 ml

Mix well and store at room temperature.

Alkaline alcohol

Ammonium hydroxide	10 ml
95% alcohol	90 ml

Iodine solution

Iodine	2 g
Potassium iodide	2 g
Distilled water	100 ml

Add the iodine and potassium iodide to about 25 ml of distilled water and mix until dissolved, and add the remaining water.

10% absolute alcoholic hematoxylin

Hematoxylin	10 g
Absolute alcohol	100 ml

Mix until dissolved. Cap tightly and store at room temperature.

10% ferric chloride

Ferric chloride	10 g
Distilled water	100 ml

Mix until dissolved and store at room temperature.

Hematoxylin solution

10% absolute alcoholic hematoxylin	25 ml
Absolute alcohol	25 ml
10% aqueous ferric chloride	25 ml
Iodine solution	25 ml

Prepare just before use.

2% ferric chloride (for differentiation)

10% ferric chloride	10 ml
Distilled water	40 ml

Prepare just before use.

5% sodium thiosulfate

Sodium thiosulfate	5 g
Distilled water	100 ml

Mix until dissolved and store at room temperature.

Crocein scarlet–acid fuchsin

Solution A (stock)

Crocein scarlet	1 g
Distilled water	99.5 ml
Glacial acetic acid	0.5 ml

Mix until dissolved and store at room temperature.

Working solution

Solution A	8 parts
Solution B	2 parts

Prepare just before use.

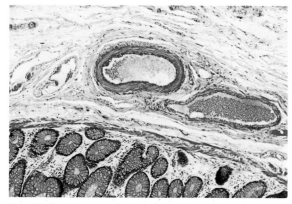

Fig. 10.5 Movat method demonstrating fibrin, muscle, collagen and muscle in a small intestine section.

5% phosphotungstic acid solution

Phosphotungstic acid	5 g
Distilled water	100 ml

Mix until dissolved and store at room temperature.

Alcoholic safran

Safran du Gatinais	6 g
Absolute alcohol	100 ml

Keep tightly closed to prevent hydration.

Method

1. Deparaffinize and hydrate to distilled water.
2. Stain in alcian blue for 20 minutes.
3. Wash in running tap water for 5 minutes.
4. Place sides in alkaline alcohol for 1 hour.
5. Wash in running tap water for 10 minutes.
6. Rinse in distilled water.
7. Stain in hematoxylin solution for 15 minutes.
8. Rinse in several changes of distilled water.
9. Differentiate in 2% aqueous ferric chloride until the elastic fibers contrast sharply with the background.
10. Rinse in distilled water.
11. Place slides in sodium thiosulfate for 1 minute.
12. Wash in running tap water for 5 minutes, and rinse in distilled water.
13. Stain in crocein scarlet–acid fuchsin for 1–5 minutes.
14. Rinse in several changes of distilled water.
15. Rinse in 0.5% acetic acid water.
16. Place slides in 5% aqueous phosphotungstic acid, two changes of 5 minutes each.
17. Rinse in 0.5% acetic acid water.
18. Rinse in three changes of absolute alcohol.
19. Stain in alcoholic safran solution for 15 minutes.
20. Rinse in three changes of absolute alcohol.
21. Clear in two or three changes of xylene and mount with a synthetic resin.

Results

Nuclei and elastic fibers	black
Collagen and reticular fibers	yellow
Ground substance, mucin	blue
Fibrinoid, fibrin	intense red
Muscle	red

Notes

The differentiation of the elastic fibers is usually complete in 2–3 minutes. The complete removal of alkaline alcohol with running water is important. Failure to remove all of the alkaline alcohol will inhibit the subsequent staining steps. This stain may be used to demonstrate *Cryptococcus neoformans*, staining the organism a brilliant blue.

Acknowledgments

Paul Bradbury and Keith Gordon wrote this chapter for the first three editions, and Kenny Rae updated the text for the fourth edition. Our acknowledgments are due to them for their contributions.

REFERENCES

Alexander R.A., Garner D. (1977) Oxytalan fiber formation in the cornea: a light and electron microscopical study. Histopathology 1:189.

Bailey A.J. (1978) Collagen and elastin fibers. Journal of Clinical Pathology 31(Suppl 12):49–58.

Baker J.R. (1958) Principles of biological microtechnique. London: Methuen.

Brinn N.T. (1983) Rapid metallic histological staining using the microwave oven. Journal of Histotechnology 6:125.

Carson F.L. (1997) Histotechnology: a self instruction text, 2nd edn. Chicago: ASCP Press, pp. 151–154.

Cleary E.G., Gibson M.A. (1983) Elastin-associated microfibrils and microfibrillar proteins. International review of connective tissue research 10. New York: Academic Press.

Everett M.M., Miller W.A. (1974) The role of phosphotungstic and phosphomolybdic acids in connective tissue staining 1. Histochemical studies. Journal of Histochemistry 6:25.

Fullmer H.M., Lillie R.D. (1958) The oxytalan fiber: a previously undescribed connective tissue fiber. Journal of Histochemistry and Cytochemistry 6:425.

Gawlik Z. (1965) Morphological and morphochemical properties of the elastic system in the motor organ of man. Folia Histochemistry and Cytochemistry 3:233.

Goldfischer S., Coltoff-Schiller B., Schwartz E., Blumenfeld O.O. (1983) Ultrastructure and staining properties of aortic microfibrils (oxytalan). Journal of Histochemistry and Cytochemistry 31:382–390.

Goldstein D.G. (1962) Ionic and non ionic bonds in staining with special reference to the action of urea and sodium chloride on the staining of elastic fibers and glycogen. Quarterly Journal of Microscopical Science 103:477.

Gomori G. (1937) Silver impregnation of reticulum in paraffin sections. American Journal of Physiology 13: 993.

Gomori G. (1950) Aldehyde–fuchsin, a new stain for elastic tissue. American Journal of Clinical Pathology 20:665.

Gordon H., Sweets H.H. (1936) A simple method for the silver impregnation of reticulum. American Journal of Pathology 12:545.

Horobin R.W. (1980) Structure–staining relationships in histochemistry and biological staining. I. Journal of Microscopy 119:345–355.

Horobin R.W., Flemming L. (1980) Structure–staining relationships in histochemistry and biological staining. II. Journal of Microscopy 119:357–372.

Junqueira L.C.U., Montes G.S. (1983) Biology of collagen–proteoglycan interaction. Archivum Histologicum Japonicum 46:589–629.

Laurie G.W., Leblond C.P. (1983) What is known of the production of basement membrane components. Journal of Histochemistry and Cytochemistry 31(Suppl):159–163.

Lendrum A.C., Fraser D.S., Slidders W., Henderson R. (1962) Studies on the character and staining of fibrin. Journal of Clinical Pathology 15:401.

Masson P. (1929) Some histological methods. Trichrome stainings and their preliminary technique. Bulletin of the International Association of Medicine 12:75.

Uitto J. (1979) Biochemistry of the elastic fibers in normal connective tissue and its alterations in diseases. Journal of Investigative Dermatology 72:1–10.

van Gieson I. (1889) Laboratory notes of technical methods for the nervous system. New York Medical Journal 50:57.

Verhöeff F.H. (1908) Some new staining methods of wide applicability, including a rapid differential stain for elastic tissue. Journal of American Medical Association 50:876.

Weigert C. (1898) Über eine Methode zue Färbung elastischer Fasern. Zentralblatt für Allgemeine Pathologie und Pathologische Anatomie 9:289.

FURTHER READING

Chavrier C. (1990) Elastic system fibers of healthy human gingiva. Journal de Paradontologie 9:29–34.

Clemmensen I. (1984) Significance of plasma fibronectin. Haematologia 17:101–106.

Courtoy P.J., Timpl, R., Farquhar, M.G. (1982) Comparative distribution of laminin, type IV collagen and fibronectin in the rate glomerulus. Journal of Histochemistry and Cytochemistry 30:874–886.

Fleischmajer R., Jacobs L., Perlish J.S., Katchen B. (1992) Immunochemical analysis of human kidney reticulin. American Journal of Pathology 140:1225–1235.

Gay S., Miller, E.J. (1983) What is collagen, what is not: an overview. Ultrastructural Pathology 4:365–377.

Godfrey M., Nejezchleb P.A., Schaefer G.B. et al. (1993) Elastin and fibrillin mRNA and protein levels in the ontogeny of normal human aorta. Connective Tissue Research 29:61–69.

Goldstein R.H. (1991) Control of type I collagen formation in the lung. American Journal of Physiology 261:29–40.

Horton W.A. (1984) Histochemistry, a valuable tool in connective tissue research. Collagen Related Research 4: 231–237.

Horton W.A., Dwyer C., Goering R., Dean D.C. (1983) Immunohistochemistry of types I and II collagen in undecalcified skeletal tissues. Journal of Histochemistry and Cytochemistry 31:417–425.

Jackson D.S. (1978) Collagens. Journal of Clinical Pathology 31(Suppl 12):44–48.

Laurie G.W., Leblond C.P. (1982a) Intracellular localization of basement membrane precursors in the endodermal cells of the rat parietal yolk sac: I, Ultrastructure and phosphatase activity of endodermal cells. Journal of Histochemistry and Cytochemistry 30:973–982.

Laurie G.W., Leblond C.P. (1982b) Intracellular localization of basement membrane precursors in the endodermal cells of the rat parietal yolk sac: II, Immunostaining for type IV collagen and its precursors. Journal of Histochemistry and Cytochemistry 30:983–990.

Laurie G.W., Leblond C.P., Martin G.R., Silver M.H. (1982) Intracellular localization of basement membrane precursors in the endodermal cells of the rat parietal yolk sac: III, Immunostaining for laminin and its precursors. Journal of Histochemistry and Cytochemistry 30: 991–998.

Martinez-Hernandez A., Chung A.E. (1984) The ultrastructural localization of two basement membrane components: entactin and laminin in rat tissues. Journal of Histochemistry and Cytochemistry 32:289–298.

Minor R.R. (1980) Collagen metabolism: a comparison of diseases of collagen and diseases affecting collagen. American Journal of Pathology 98:227–271.

Reale E., Luciano L., Kühn K.W. (1983) Ultrastructural architecture of proteoglycans in the glomerular basement membrane: a cytochemical approach. Journal of Histochemistry and Cytochemistry 31:662–668.

Risteli J., Melkko J., Niemi S., Ristell L. (1991) Use of a marker of collagen formation in osteoporosis studies. Calcified Tissue International 49(Suppl):S24–S25.

Robert L., Jacob M.P., Frances C. et al. (1984) Interaction between elastin and elastases and its role in the aging of the arterial wall, skin and other connective tissues: a review. Mechanisms of Aging and Development 28:155–166.

Rojkind M., Cordero-Hernandez J., Ponce, P. (1984) Non-collagenous glycoproteins of the connective tissues and biomatrix. Myelofibrosis and the biology of connective tissue. New York: A.R. Liss, pp. 103–122.

Sternberg M., Cohen-Forterre L., Peyroux J. (1985) Connective tissue in diabetes mellitus: biochemical alterations of the intercellular matrix with special reference to proteoglycans, collagens and basement membranes. Diabète et Métabolisme (Paris) 11:27–50.

Timpl R. (1993) Proteoglycans of basement membranes. Experientia 49:417–428.

Warburton M.J., Mitchell D., Ormerod E.J., Rudland P. (1982) Distribution of myoepithelial cells in the resting, pregnant, lactating, and involuting rat mammary gland. Journal of Histochemistry and Cytochemistry 30: 667–676.

11

Carbohydrates

Russell B. Myers, Jerry L. Fredenburgh and William E. Grizzle

INTRODUCTION

The word 'carbohydrate' was coined more than 100 years ago to describe a large group of compounds of the general formula $C_n(H_2O)_n$. While the role of carbohydrates in cellular metabolism has been known for many years, more recently carbohydrates have been implicated in a wide range of cellular functions including protein folding, cell adhesion, enzyme activity, and immune recognition (Varki et al 1999). Today the study of carbohydrates or glycobiology is a complex discipline that permeates such diverse fields as cell biology, microbiology, enzymology, and molecular biology. Histochemical techniques for the detection and characterization of carbohydrates and carbohydrate-containing macromolecules (glycoconjugates) are common practices in the histology laboratory. These techniques often provide invaluable information which may aid the pathologist in diagnosing and characterizing various pathological conditions including neoplasia, inflammation, autoimmune disorders, and infectious diseases.

This chapter includes instructions and references for the more commonly used techniques for the evaluation of carbohydrates. Furthermore, this chapter was written to provide the reader with a deeper and more thorough understanding of the mechanisms upon which the techniques are based. It is important to begin such an endeavor, however, with a basic review of the chemistry of carbohydrates as well as the classification of carbohydrates or glycoconjugates.

CLASSIFICATION OF CARBOHYDRATES

The classification of carbohydrates is a complicated subject due in part to the numerous classification schemes or systems used in the past. Descriptions or classifications presented in many texts of histological or histochemical techniques are based upon the reaction of various dyes or dyes under different conditions of ionic strength or pH with tissue components. Classifications based solely upon reactivity with histochemical stains may be of value to the histologist but they lead to identifications that are difficult to correlate with known chemical structures. For a review of these classification systems, the reader is referred to the publications of Spicer (1961), Culling et al (1985), and Cook (1974).

In the present text, a more broad or generalized scheme of categorization is applied (Table 11.1). In this scheme, classification is based upon structure of the monosaccharide moieties within the molecule, the structure of the polysaccharide components, as well as the structure or nature of molecules attached to the polysaccharide. In addition some carbohydrate-containing molecules (i.e. mucins) are characterized or classified in part based upon genetic or molecular criteria. Carbohydrates are broken down into two broad categories: simple carbohydrates or those molecules composed purely of carbohydrates, and glycoconjugates, those molecules composed of carbohydrates and other molecules such as protein or lipid (Table 11.1). The simple carbohydrates are further categorized as monosaccharides, oligosaccharides, or polysaccharides. Glycoconjugates may further be broken down into proteoglycans, mucins, and 'other' glycoproteins. Although lipid–carbohydrate complexes are widely distributed in cells and tissues, these types of molecule are not discussed here as they are not detectable by routine histochemical techniques described in this chapter.

Table 11.1 Basic classification of carbohydrates and glycoconjugates

Simple carbohydrates
Monosaccharides
glucose, mannose, galactose
Oligosaccharides
sucrose, maltose
Polysaccharides
glycogen, starch

Glycoconjugates
Connective tissue glycoconjugates
proteoglycans
hyaluronic acid

Mucins
neutral mucins
sialomucins
sulfomucins

Other glycoproteins
membrane proteins (receptors, cell adhesion molecules)
blood group antigens

Glycolipids
cerebrosides
gangliosides

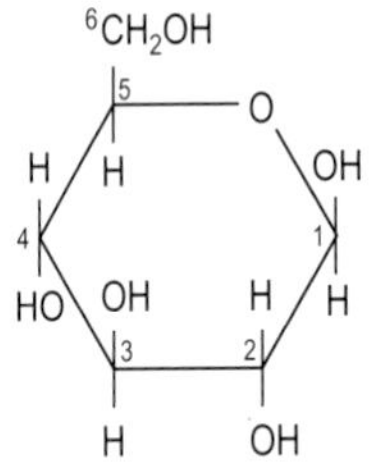

Fig. 11.1 Structure of β-D-glucose.

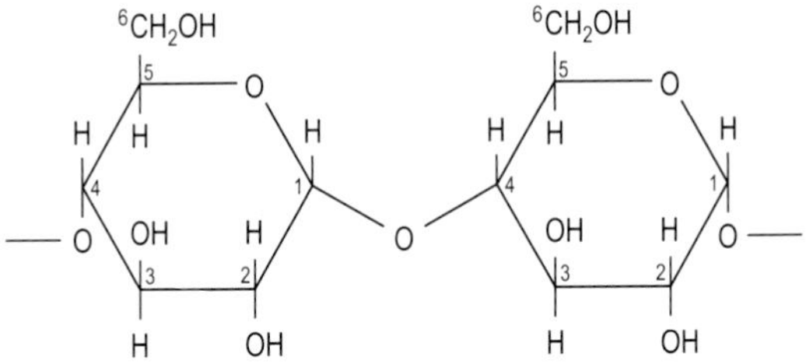

Fig. 11.2 Stucture of two glucose units joined by an α1–4 glycosidic linkage.

Monosaccharide, the basic carbohydrate structure

The most basic or simple form of a carbohydrate is the monosaccharide. Typical monosaccharides are of the empirical formula $(CH_2O)_n$, where n is a value between 3 and 9. The basic or archetypal monosaccharide is the six-carbon simple carbohydrate glucose (Fig. 11.1). Glucose is not charged or ionized and for this reason is referred to as a neutral sugar. Other neutral sugars include mannose, galactose, and fructose. Monosaccharides contain asymmetric carbons referred to as chiral centers. The letters D or L at the beginning of a name refer to the conformation of one of the chiral carbons within the molecule. This is of little interest to the reader with the exception that monosaccharides of the D conformation predominate in nature.

The high number of hydroxyl (OH) groups present on the monosaccharide renders most monosaccharides extremely water soluble. Monosaccharides within a tissue specimen are lost during fixation and tissue pro-

cessing due to the small size and the water solubility of these molecules. As a result, the monosaccharides are not easily demonstrated with most histochemical techniques. Regardless, the reader should familiarize themself with the basic monosaccharide structure as the monosaccharides represent the building blocks of larger more complex carbohydrates. The chemical and physical properties or characteristics of the polysaccharides and glycoconjugates are determined largely by the types of monosaccharide that make up these molecules as well as various reactive groups within the monosaccharides.

Polysaccharides

A polysaccharide is a large macromolecule composed of multiple monosaccharides joined by covalent bonds referred to as glycosidic linkages. Figure 11.2 demonstrates an α1–4 glycosidic linkage connecting molecules of glucose in a large polysaccharide. The α1–4 glycosidic linkage of glucose units is the predominant linkage in the polysaccharides starch and glycogen. In addition, some of the glucose units of these polysaccharides may be involved in more than one glycosidic linkage, thus forming a branching type of structure which may resemble a tree. Both glycogen and starch consist of glucose units with $\alpha 1$–4 as well as $\alpha 1$–6 glycosidic linkages. Starch and glycogen differ only in size and branching structure. Starch and glycogen are extremely large macromolecules with molecular weights that surpass 1×10^6 Da.

Glycogen is the only polysaccharide found in animals that frequently is evaluated by histochemical techniques. Glycogen serves as a major form of stored energy reserves in humans. Carbohydrates absorbed following a meal are converted to glycogen by the hepatocytes of the liver. Between meals or in times of fasting, glycogen is broken down into glucose units that can be used as an immediate source of energy. Glycogen occupies a significant volume of the cytoplasm of hepatocytes and may even form intranuclear inclusions. Skeletal and cardiac muscle cells also store significant quantities of glycogen.

There are a number of disease processes or pathological conditions in which histochemical assessment of glycogen content or accumulation may be of value diagnostically (Table 11.2). There are several well-characterized glycogen storage diseases which are the result of inherited defects of one or more of the enzymes involved in the synthesis or breakdown of glycogen (Cori & Cori 1952; Hers 1963). In most of these disorders, the liver shows massive accumulation of glycogen. In some diseases, glycogen accumulation also is observed in skeletal and cardiac muscle.

Histochemical detection of glycogen also may prove helpful in the differential diagnosis of several malignancies. Seminomas, rhabdomyosarcomas, and tumors of the Ewing's or primitive neuroectodermal tumor (PNET) family frequently contain detectable glycogen (Angervall & Enzinger 1975; Ro et al 2000). Histochemical detection of glycogen may be particularly valuable in differentiating rhabdomyosarcomas and the Ewing/PNET neoplasms from lymphomas and neuroblastomas. As would be expected, the malignant hepatocytes of hepatocellular carcinomas also frequently demonstrate glycogen on histochemical evaluation.

CONNECTIVE TISSUE GLYCOCONJUGATES—THE PROTEOGLYCANS

Proteoglycans also are commonly referred to in the older literature as connective tissue mucins or mucopolysac-charides. These molecules are large glycoconjugate complexes that are found in high concentrations within the extracellular matrix of connective tissues. Proteoglycans are highly glycosylated and, in many cases, 90–95% of the molecular weight of the typical proteoglycan is due to the carbohydrate components.

The carbohydrate components of proteoglycans are known as glycosaminoglycans. Glycosaminoglycans are large polysaccharide polymers that are covalently bound to the protein core of proteoglycans. The glycosaminoglycans contain high concentrations of acidic monosaccharides which contain a sulfate ester linkage or a carboxyl group. At a neutral pH both of these groups are ionized and carry a negative charge. The typical glycosaminoglycan is a long unbranched polysaccharide composed of repeating disaccharide units each made up of two different monosaccharides. Each disaccharide typically is composed of a carboxylated uronic acid (glucuronic or iduronic acid) and a hexosamine such as N-acetyglucosamine or N-acetylgalactosamine. The hexosamines frequently contain highly acidic sulfate groups. There are six distinct classes of glycosaminoglycans (Table 11.3). The chondroitin sulfates are the most abundant of the glycosaminoglycans in the human. Figure 11.3a illustrates the structure of the repetitive disaccharide unit of chondroitin 4-sulfate.

The glycosaminoglycan chains are covalently bound to a protein core of the proteoglycan via the side chain of the amino acids serine or threonine (O-glycosidic linkage) and to a lesser extent to asparagine (N-glycosidic linkage). The number of glycosaminoglycan chains varies greatly among different proteoglycans. While some proteoglycans may contain only one or two glycosaminoglycans per protein core, other proteoglycans may contain as many as 100 glycosaminoglycans (Varki et al 1999). An exception to this structural motif is hyaluronic acid which does not contain a covalently bound protein core (Mason et al 1982).

Hyaluronic acid (Fig. 11.3b) is a polymer of repeating N-acetylglucosamine and glucuronic acid disaccharide units (Roden 1980). Hyaluronic acid also differs from the other glycosaminoglycans in the absence of sulfate groups. In spite of these differences, hyaluronic acid is classified as a glycosaminoglycan because of its overall structural similarity to the other glycosaminoglycans.

The negatively charged sulfate and/or carboxyl groups together with numerous hydroxyl groupings render most proteoglycans extremely hydrophilic. This property accounts for the gel-like consistency of the

Table 11.2 Summary of the different types of carbohydrates and glycoconjugates

Type	Location	Function	Associated pathological condition
Glycogen	Liver, skeletal muscle, cardiac muscle, hair follicles, cervical epithelium, etc.	Storage form of carbohydrate	Found in a wide range of malignancies—Ewing's sarcoma/PNET, rhabdomyosarcoma, seminoma etc. Abnormal accumulation in tissues of patients with glycogen storage diseases
Proteoglycans and hyaluronic acid	Cartilage, heart valves, blood vessels, tendons, ligaments, extracellular matrices, and ubiquitously expressed on the membranes of many cell types	Support, lubrication, cell adhesion, etc.	Found in certain sarcomas—myxoid chondrosarcomas, myxoid liposarcomas, myxoid fibrous histiocytomas, etc. Abnormal accumulation in tissues of patients with mucopolysaccharidoses
Mucins	Epithelia of the gastrointestinal tract, respiratory tract, reproductive tract	Secreted mucins—lubrication and protection Membrane-bound mucins—cell adhesion and regulation of proliferation	Frequently found in adenocarcinomas of the gastrointestinal tract Aberrant or inappropriate expression of specific mucin types occurs frequently in the neoplastic process
Glycoproteins	Ubiquitously expressed on cell membranes Blood group antigens Secreted products such as peptide hormones and immunoglobulins	Multiple and diverse functions such as cell adhesion, immune recognition, regulation of receptor ligand binding, etc.	Aberrant expression of blood group antigens in various malignancies

Table 11.3 Characterization of glycosaminoglycans

Glycosaminoglycan	Disaccharide repeat	Location
Chondroitin sulfate[a]	Glucuronic acid and N-acetylgalactosamine	Cartilage, tendons, ligaments, aorta, cell membranes
Dermatan sulfate	Iduronic acid and N-acetylgalactosamine	Skin, blood vessels, heart valves
Keratan sulfate	Galactose and N-acetylglucosamine	Cartilage, cornea
Heparin sulfate[b]	Glucuronic acid and N-acetylglucosamine or N-sulfate glucosamine	Blood vessels, aorta, cell membranes
Heparin	Glucuronic acid and N-acetylglucosamine or N-sulfate glucosamine	Mast cell granules
Hyaluronic acid	Glucuronic acid and N-acetylglucosamine	Synovial fluid, vitreous humor, loose connective tissues. Small amounts are found in cartilage where it serves as a scaffold for the proteoglycans

[a] Chondroitin sulfates may be subcategorized as chondroitin 4-sulfate or chondroitin 6-sulfate depending upon the position of the sulfate group in the N-acetylgalactosamine.
[b] Heparin and heparin sulfate differ structurally in the degree of sulfation of the glucosamine units. Heparin contains more sulfate and fewer N-acetyl groups in this unit.

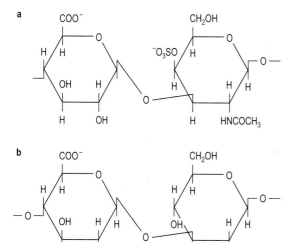

Fig. 11.3 The repeating disaccharide units of the glycosaminoglycans, chondroitin 4-sulfate (a) and hyaluronic acid (b).

extracellular matrix and connective tissues such as cartilage. The proteoglycans of cartilage in particular contain many glycosaminoglycan chains and thus are capable of binding a large volume of water. Proteoglycans act in stabilizing and supporting fibrous elements of connective tissue. Tissues that contain high concentrations of proteoglycans include cartilage, tendons, ligaments, blood vessels, heart valves, and skin (Table 11.3). Hyaluronic acid is found in high concentrations in synovial fluid and in the ground substance and connective tissue matrices where other proteoglycans are found.

While it is convenient to classify or categorize proteoglycans as connective tissue glycoconjugates, proteoglycan expression is not limited to the extracellular matrix or connective tissues. Heparin is found within the secretory granules of mast cells, and upon release acts as an anticoagulant. Proteoglycans also are ubiquitously expressed on the surface of cell membranes of many different cell types (Mali et al 1990; David 1993). Membrane-bound proteoglycans typically are composed exclusively of heparin sulfate although in some cases chondroitin sulfate may predominate. These proteoglycans are known to modulate the response of the cells to growth factors and are involved in the modulation of cell adhesion (Gallo et al 1994). The CD44 cell adhesion molecule is an example of a membrane-bound proteoglycan that is expressed on lymphocytes and a wide range of epithelial cell types (Hollenbaugh et al 1999). Aberrant expression of CD44 has been observed in a wide range of neoplasms (Woodman et al 1996).

Several pathological conditions involve accumulation of glycosaminoglycans or proteoglycans (see Table 11.2). The mucopolysaccharidoses are a group of genetic disorders that result from a deficiency of one or more of the enzymes that are involved in the degradation of heparin sulfate and dermatan sulfate (McKusick & Neufeld 1983). This results in the abnormal accumulation of glycosaminoglycans in connective tissues as well as cell types such as neurons, histiocytes, and macrophages.

Glycosaminoglycans and proteoglycans are expressed by a number of different sarcomas. Hyaluronic acid and chondroitin sulfates in particular may be found in high concentrations in myxoid chondrosarcomas as well as the myxoid variants of liposarcoma and malignant fibrous histiocytoma (Tighe 1963; Kindblom & Angervall 1975; Weiss & Goldblum 2001). In addition, proteoglycans may be observed in the stromal components of sarcomas as well as some carcinomas.

MUCINS

Mucins, like the proteoglycans, consist of polysaccharide chains covalently linked to a protein core (Gendler & Spicer 1995). Typically, the carbohydrate component is attached via an O-glycosidic linkage to serine or threonine. The serine and threonine-rich protein core may contain anywhere from several hundred to several thousand amino acids. A defining structure of the epithelial mucins is the presence of tandemly repeated amino acid sequences within the protein core. Mucins are categorized into functionally distinct families (muc1, muc2, muc3, etc.) based in part upon differences in the amino acid sequences within the tandem repeats and the structure of the protein core of mucins (Perez-Vilar & Hill 1999). Two of the families are composed of membrane-

bound mucins (muc1 and muc4) while others (muc2, muc5A, muc5B, and muc7) are produced within the cell and secreted (Moniaux et al 1999; Perez-Vilar & Hill 1999). Although the classic mucin genes (*Muc* series) are primarily expressed by epithelial cells, various glycoproteins (e.g. CD34, CD43 and an alternate exon of CD45) expressed in other cellular systems can demonstrate mucin-like characteristics such as clustered O-linked glycans with or without the tandem repeat sequences (Baeckstrom 1997).

The carbohydrate content of a mucin may account for up to 90% of its molecular weight. In contrast to the glycosaminoglycans, which are strongly acidic polyanions, the polysaccharide chains of the mucins vary from neutral or weakly acidic to strongly acidic sulfomucins. In addition, mucins demonstrate a more varied composition of monosaccharide units than the glycosaminoglycans.

The neutral mucins contain a high content of uncharged monosaccharides such as mannose, galactose, and galactosamine. Neutral mucins are found in high concentrations in the surface epithelia of the gastric mucosa, Brunner's glands of the duodenum, and in the prostatic epithelia.

The sialic acids are a diverse group of nine-carbon monosaccharides that contain a carboxylate group at the carbon in position 1 (Schauer 1982; Varki et al 1999). The carboxylate group is ionized at a physiological pH and imparts an overall negative charge on the molecule. The sialic acids are unique among the monosaccharides in that they contain a polyhydroxy chain at carbons 7–9 (Varki et al 1999). The sialic acids found in vertebrates also contain an N-acetyl group at the 5-carbon position. Figure 11.4 illustrates the structure of

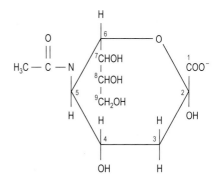

Fig. 11.4 Structure of N-acetylneuraminic acid, a common sialic acid in humans.

N-acetylneuraminic acid, a common sialic acid in the human. The sialic acids typically are found at the outermost ends of the carbohydrate chains of the mucins and other glycoproteins.

The diversity observed in sialic acids is due to modifications or additions to the core of the basic nine-carbon structure as well as the polyhydroxy side chain. One such modification that is of interest histochemically is the incorporation of O-acetyl groups in the polyhydroxy side chain (Varki et al 1999). Sialic acids of this type are frequently found in the mucins of the large intestine and are resistant to cleavage with the enzyme sialidase (Drzeniek 1973; Culling et al 1974). Sialic acids are categorized histochemically as sialidase labile or resistant based upon the presence or absence of the O-acetyl groups. Sialidase-resistant sialic acids are not detectable by the standard periodic acid–Schiff technique (PAS), while the sialidase labile sialic acids are clearly visible with this technique (Culling et al 1974; Jass 1996).

Epithelial mucins that contain sialic acids (sialomucins) demonstrate a weak or intermediate level of acidity. The sialomucins are found in a wide range of cell types or mucous glands but are particularly prevalent in the bronchial submucous glands, goblet cells of the intestines, and in the salivary glands. Within the gastrointestinal tract, transformation of the epithelium to the malignant phenotype often is accompanied by striking changes in the quantity or type of sialic acid expressed by the neoplastic cells (Habib et al 1985; Turani et al 1986).

Mucins containing carbohydrate-bound sulfate groups are significantly more acidic than the sialomucins. The sulfomucins are found in the goblet cells of the large intestine and in bronchial mucous glands.

The function of the mucins varies in part upon the tissue location of the mucin-producing cell as well as the mucin type. In most cases, the secreted mucins provide lubrication and protection for the secreting cells or tissues in the immediate area. The function or role of the membrane-bound mucins is not well understood. These mucins are likely involved in the regulation of cellular functions such as cell proliferation and cell adhesion (Wesseling et al 1995; Moniaux et al 1999; Schroeder et al 2001).

While immunohistochemistry has largely replaced special stains in the differential diagnosis of anaplastic tumors or tumors of unknown origin, detection of mucin in a tumor may be a valuable clue in the identification of a malignancy. Malignancies derived from simple epithelial tissues (carcinomas) frequently contain detectable mucin. In contrast, melanomas, lymphomas, and sarcomas rarely exhibit significant levels of mucins. In addition, determining the type of mucin (i.e. neutral or acidic) may be helpful in evaluating neoplastic changes within a tissue. The detection of acid or sulfomucins within the gastric mucosa may aid in the detection and characterization of intestinal metaplasia, a lesion associated with gastric carcinoma (Turani et al 1986).

OTHER GLYCOPROTEINS

There is a wide range of protein carbohydrate conjugates that are not easily categorized and fall under the general heading of glycoprotein. This is an extremely varied group of molecules with respect to carbohydrate composition, protein structure, and function. These molecules frequently contain relatively short oligosaccharide or polysaccharide chains attached to a protein core. Common carbohydrate moieties include neutral sugars such as mannose and N-acetylglucosamine, and the carboxylated sialic acids also may be present.

Glycoproteins are ubiquitously expressed throughout the cells and tissues of the body. Many of the proteins on the external surface of the cell membrane contain carbohydrates. The cluster of differentiation or CD markers found on the surface of lymphocytes frequently contain numerous glycosylation sites. These glycoproteins are involved in a varied array of cellular functions including cell adhesion and lymphocyte activation. In addition, many of proteins and peptides secreted from cells contain sites of glycosylation. These include cytokines, growth factors, and hormones.

FIXATION

The selection of an appropriate fixative for the histochemical detection of carbohydrates depends largely on the type of carbohydrate to be demonstrated. The fixation of glycogen is somewhat more demanding than the glycoconjugates such as the mucins and proteoglycans. Due to the aqueous solubility of glycogen, many of the older studies recommended the avoidance of aqueous based fixatives such as formalin (Lillie 1954). It is now accepted that glycogen loss during formalin fixation usually does not compromise the ability to detect glycogen with techniques such as the periodic acid–Schiff

(PAS) method. This is likely due to the retention of a portion of the cellular glycogen by non-covalent association with adjacent proteins (Manns 1958).

While neutral buffered formalin (NBF) is an acceptable fixative for glycogen, there is agreement that alcoholic formalins are superior fixatives for glycogen preservation (Lillie 1954). Rossman's fluid, alcoholic formalin with picric acid, also has been recommended for glycogen fixation (Bancroft & Cook 1994). Mercuric chloride containing fixatives such as Zenker's–acetic acid or Susa's are not recommended for fixation of glycogen-containing tissues (Manns 1958; Bancroft & Cook 1994).

Regardless of the fixative used, it is essential that tissues intended for glycogen analysis should be placed in a fixative promptly following removal. Glycogen present in many animal tissues is extremely labile to autolytic changes. If immediate fixation is not possible, the tissue should be refrigerated until adequate fixation in possible. When possible, fixation should be carried out at 4°C to minimize the streaming artifact which frequently occurs in fixed tissues (Lillie 1954).

The fixation requirements for the mucins and proteoglycans are less stringent than for glycogen. As these carbohydrates are covalently bound to proteins, the principal effect of fixation occurs on the protein portion of the molecule. In most cases, formalin or alcoholic formalin fixation is adequate for preservation. The carbohydrate deposits of the mucopolysaccharidoses have been reported to be less stable than typical mucins or proteoglycans (Bancroft & Cook 1994). In these cases, fresh or frozen sections are recommended although alcoholic formalin is also satisfactory.

TECHNIQUES FOR THE DEMONSTRATION OF CARBOHYDRATES

The histochemical techniques used for the demonstration of carbohydrates and glycoconjugates are outlined in Table 11.4. In the text that follows the potential mechanism(s) for each technique is discussed. Emphasis also is placed on the specificity of the techniques. For those techniques that are more frequently used in the histology laboratory a detailed method section that includes directions for the production of the solutions as well as directions for the staining procedure is included.

The periodic acid–Schiff (PAS) technique

The PAS technique is without question the most versatile and widely used technique for the demonstration of carbohydrates or glycoconjugates. The first histochemical use of this technique was by McManus (1946) for the demonstration of mucin. Subsequently other studies have demonstrated the utility of the PAS technique for demonstration of other carbohydrate-containing molecules such as glycogen and certain glycoproteins (Lillie 1947, 1951; McManus 1948). The list of PAS-reactive tissues and cell types is long and varied. Table 11.5 is a listing of the PAS-reactive tissues, cells, and cellular structures that are commonly evaluated in the histology laboratory. This listing is not intended to be all-inclusive and the reader is directed to several references (Lillie 1951; Thompson 1966; Bancroft & Cook 1994) for more extensive listings.

From a diagnostic perspective, PAS is one of the more useful and valuable special stains used in the pathology laboratory. The PAS technique may aid in the differential diagnosis of tumors through the detection of mucins or glycogen. The reactivity of Schiff reagent with glycoproteins within the basal lamina makes the PAS technique a valuable means of assessing basement membrane thickness (Hennigar 1987). Increased basement membrane thickness, particularly in the glomerular capillaries of the kidney, is indicative of a number of pathological conditions. The PAS technique also is a sensitive and relatively fast means of demonstrating viable fungi in tissue sections. This is due to the presence of periodic acid-reactive polysaccharides in the capsules or walls of many fungal species. Common fungal species that are PAS reactive include *Candida albicans*, *Histoplasma capsulatum*, *Cryptococcus*, and *Blastomyces* (Harley 1987).

Mechanism of the PAS technique

As typically employed in the histology laboratory, the PAS technique is based upon the reactivity of free aldehyde groups within carbohydrates with the Schiff reagent to form a bright red magenta end product. The initial step in the PAS technique is the oxidation of hydroxyl groups attached to adjacent carbon atoms (1,2 glycols) within the carbohydrate. The result is the formation of two free aldehyde groups and the cleavage of the adjoining carbon-to-carbon bond (Fig. 11.5). The oxidation of the 1,2 glycols to form adjacent aldehydes is produced by treatment of the sections with a dilute

Table 11.4 Summary of the specificity of the techniques for the detection of carbohydrates and glycoconjugates

	PAS	PAS-D	Ab 2.5	AB 1.0	Ab 2.5/PAS	Muc	Coll	HID	HID Ab 2.5	AF	AF Ab 2.5	Meta
Polysaccharides												
Glycogen	+	–	–	–	+(M)	–	–	–	–	–	–	–
Conn Tiss GC												
Proteoglycans	–	–	+	+	+(B)	V/–	+	+	+(BB)	+	+(P)	+
Hyaluronic acid	–	–	+	–	+(B)	V/–	+	–	+(B)	–	+(B)	+
Mucins												
Neutral	+	+	–	–	+(M)	–	–	–	–	–	–	–
Sialomucin (labile)	+	+	+	–	+(B)	+	+	–	+(B)	–	+(B)	+
Sialomucin (resist)	–	–	+	–	+(B)	+	+	–	+(B)	–	+(B)	+
Sulfomucin	V/–	V/–	+	+	+(B)	+	+	+	+(BB)	+	+(P)	+

PAS = conventional periodic acid–Schiff
D = diastase digestion
Ab 2.5 = alcian blue at pH 2.5
Ab 1.0 = alcian blue at pH 1.0
Muc = mucicarmine
Coll = colloidal iron
HID = high iron diamine
AF = aldehyde fuchsin
Meta = metachromatic techniques
V/– = variable to negative
Conn Tiss GC = connective tissue glycoconjugates
(labile) = digested with neuraminidase
(resist) = resistant to neuraminidase digestion
When two combined stains are used, the letter in parentheses represents the predominant color:
(B) = blue
(BB) = brown/black
(P) = purple
(M) = magenta

Table 11.5 PAS-reactive cells and tissue components

glycogen
starch
mucin (sialomucin, neutral mucin)
basement membranes
α-antitrypsin
reticulin
fungi (capsules)
pancreatic zymogen granules
thyroid colloid
corpora amylacea
Russell bodies

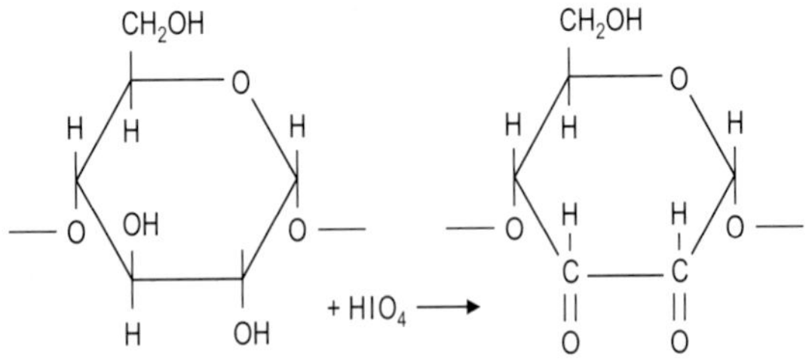

Fig. 11.5 Periodic acid (HIO_4) oxidation of a glucose unit within glycogen. Note the cleavage of the bond between carbons 2 and 3 and the formation of aldehyde groups at these carbons.

solution of periodic acid (HIO_4). In most protocols a 0.5–1.0% solution of periodic acid is used for 5–10 minutes. Other oxidants such as chromic acid and potassium permanganate have been used in variations of the technique (Bauer 1933; Thompson 1966). These oxidants, however, tend further to oxidize the aldehyde groups to carboxylic groups which are not reactive with Schiff reagent. As a result, the sensitivity of techniques using these oxidants is less than that of the PAS technique.

The intensity of the color that develops following reaction with Schiff reagent is dependent upon the tissue concentrations of reactive glycol structures (Leblond et al 1957). Monosaccharides that lack 1,2 glycols or contain hydroxyl groups that are involved in an ester or glycosidic linkage are not susceptible to periodic acid oxidation and hence cannot be detected with the PAS technique. Reactive monosaccharides include most of the neutral sugars such as mannose, fucose,

galactose, and glucose (Leblond et al 1957). The sialic acids with the three adjacent hydroxyl groups at C7, C8, and C9 also produce Schiff-reactive compounds following periodic acid oxidation. The neutral sugars and sialic acids are found in significant concentrations in glycogen (polymerized glucose), epithelial mucins, and various glycoproteins. This accounts for the reactivity of the Schiff reagent with these types of carbohydrates and glycoconjugates in tissue sections.

The connective tissue glycoconjugates and proteoglycans cannot be detected with the standard PAS technique. Several reports have suggested that hyaluronic acid and chondroitin sulfate, both of which contain 1,2 glycol groups within the glucuronic acid moieties (see Fig. 11.3), were PAS positive in tissue section. It subsequently has been demonstrated that periodic oxidation and/or aldehyde formation does not occur within these glycosaminoglycans when standard PAS techniques are used (Leblond et al 1957; Scott & Harbinson 1969). Periodic acid may not produce aldehydes in these molecules because of the electrostatic repulsion of the negatively charged periodate ions by the strong negative charge imparted by the ionized carboxylate groups of the glucuronic acids and the sulfate groups of adjacent hexosamine (Scott & Harbinson 1969).

Periodic acid also is known to oxidize substance other than carbohydrates to form reactive aldehydes. The α-amino alcohols of serine and threonine are oxidized by periodic acid but only when present at the end of the protein chain (Thompson 1966). It is also possible for periodic acid to oxidize hydroxylysine regardless of the position in the protein chain. It is doubtful, however, that the reactivity of these amino acids contributes significantly to the PAS reactivity in tissue sections.

Preparation of Schiff reagent

Schiff reagent is prepared from basic fuchsin. Basic fuchsin is not a specific dye but instead represents a mixture of triarylmethane dyes such as pararosaniline, rosaniline, and new fuchsin (Lillie 1977). The individual components of basic fuchsin also provide satisfactory starting points for the preparation of Schiff reagent.

A number of methods for the synthesis of Schiff reagent have been described since Schiff's original report in 1866. All of these methods, however, share a common theme in the production of an aqueous solution of sulfurous acid. The sulfurous acid may be generated from the reaction of sodium metabisulfite ($Na_2S_2O_5$) with a mineral acid such as hydrochloric acid (HCl), or by the reaction of thionyl chloride ($SOCl_2$) with water (Barger & DeLamater 1948; Longley 1952). Sulfur dioxide is the active agent in the production of Schiff reagent and the source of the sulfur dioxide is not critical as long as by-products of the reaction to produce sulfurous acid do not interfere with the reaction of sulfurous acid with basic fuchsin (Barger & DeLamater 1948).

The reaction of sulfur dioxide with basic fuchsin results in the addition of a sulfonic acid group to the central carbon of the triarylmethane molecule. The magenta or red coloration is lost due to the reduction of the quinoid configuration within the triarylmethane molecule. The free amino groups of the triarylmethane react with additional one or two equivalents of sulfur dioxide to form Schiff reagent (Lillie 1977).

As described above, Schiff reagent reacts with the free aldehydes generated from 1,2 glycol groups in periodic acid-treated carbohydrates. The initial monosaccharide–Schiff reagent conjugate is a colorless reaction intermediate. The loosely bound sulfonate of the central carbon is removed in a subsequent aqueous rinse. The re-establishment of the quinoid structure of the triarylmethane molecule results in the deposition of a deep red/magenta coloration in the site of the carbohydrate–Schiff reagent complex (Lillie 1977).

PAS technique (modified McManus 1946)

Periodic acid solution

Periodic acid	1 g
Deionized or distilled water	100 ml

Preparation of Schiff reagent

Dissolve 1 g of basic fuchsin and 1.9 g of sodium metabisulfite ($Na_2S_2O_5$) in 100 ml of 0.15 N hydrochloric acid (HCl). Shake the solution at intervals or on a mechanical shaker for 2 hours. The solution should be clear and yellow to light brown in color. Add 500 mg of activated charcoal and shake for 1 to 2 minutes. Filter the solution through a No. 1 Whatman filter into a bottle. The filtered solution should be clear and colorless. If the solution is yellow, repeat the charcoal decolorization using a fresh lot of activated charcoal. Store at 4°C. Solution is stable for several months.

Method

1. Deparaffinize in xylene and rehydrate through graded ethanols to deionized water.
2. Oxidize with periodic acid for 5 minutes.
3. Rinse in several changes of deionized water.
4. Cover the sections with Schiff reagent for 15 minutes.
5. Rinse in running tap water for 5–10 minutes.
6. Stain the nuclei with Harris's or Mayer's hematoxylin. Differentiate and blue the sections.
7. Dehydrate in graded ethanols and clear with xylene.
8. Coverslip.

Results

Glycogen, neutral/sialomucins	magenta
Various glycoproteins	magenta
Nuclei	blue

Notes

a. The intensity of stain is dependent to some extent on the length of treatment with the periodic acid and Schiff reagent. For basement membranes, a longer time in periodic acid (10 min) and Schiff reagent (20 min) may give better results.
b. Earlier descriptions of the PAS procedure frequently recommended post-Schiff bisulfite rinses for the reduction of background. This is not necessary provided the slides are adequately rinsed in tap water.
c. Fixatives containing glutaraldehyde should be avoided if tissues are to be stained with the PAS technique. This is because glutaraldehyde contains two aldehyde groups; tissues fixed in glutaraldehyde contain free aldehyde groups capable of undergoing the Schiff reaction. This results in nonspecific background staining.
d. Staining of glycolipids may be detected when frozen sections are used. In addition, staining of unsaturated lipids may occur in some cases due to the oxidation of carbon-to-carbon double bonds to produce Schiff-reactive aldehyde groups. Glycolipids and unsaturated lipids, however, rarely interfere with interpretation of results obtained from paraffin-embedded tissues as a significant loss of these molecules likely occurs during tissue processing.

Mild PAS technique

The mild PAS technique utilizes a weak periodic acid oxidation step to demonstrate N-acetyl sialic acid-containing mucins. The rationale for this technique is the high susceptibility of the hydroxyl groups on the 7–9 carbon side chain of sialic acids to periodic acid oxidation (Roberts 1977). It is possible selectively to oxidize the sialic acid residues of the sialomucins but not other hexoses that contain 1,2 glycols by using a dilute solution of periodic acid for a short period. For this protocol, specimens are oxidized with a 0.01% solution of aqueous periodic acid instead of the usual 1.0% solution (Bancroft & Cook 1994). As with the standard PAS technique, O-acetylated sialic acids are not demonstrated.

Alcian blue

Standard alcian blue technique

Alcian blue is a large conjugated dye molecule that initially was used for the dyeing of textile fibers. It is comprised of a central copper-containing pthalocyanine ring linked to four isothiouronium groups via thioether bonds (Scott et al 1964). The isothiouronium groups are moderately strong bases and account for the cationic nature of alcian blue (Scott et al 1964). A variety of different alcian blue dyes have been produced in the past that differ in the number of linked isothiouronium groups as well as the components of the diluent (Scott et al 1964: Horobin & Kiernan 2002). Alcian blue 8GX is the recommended dye for histological techniques (Scott & Mowry 1970).

While the exact mechanisms by which alcian blue stains carbohydrates are unknown, it is widely believed that the cationic isothiouronium groups bond via electrostatic linkages with polyanionic molecules within tissues (Pearse 1960; Quintarelli et al 1964). This is supported by the work of Scott et al (1964) in which alcian blue was demonstrated to bind and precipitate hyaluronic acid, chondroitin sulfate, and heparin from an aqueous solution. Alcian blue did not precipitate glycogen in this assay. The sulfate and carboxylate groups of chondroitin sulfate, dermatan sulfate, heparin sulfate, and hyaluronic acid are ionized at a pH of 2.5 and therefore carry a negative charge. This accounts for the staining of the proteoglycan/hyaluronic acid components of connective tissue and cartilage with alcian blue at a pH of 2.5. Similarly, the acidic epithelial mucins such as the sialomucins and sulfomucins of the large intestine are reactive

at pH 2.5. Neutral mucins such as those in the gastric mucosa and Brunner's glands are not reactive with alcian blue.

Alcian blue technique (modified Mowry 1956)

Alcian blue solution

Alcian blue 8GX	1 g
3% acetic acid solution	100 ml

Nuclear fast red

Aluminum sulfate $Al_2(SO_4)_3$ 18H_2O	5 g
Deionized water	100 ml
Nuclear fast red	0.1 g

Dissolve the aluminum sulfate in the water with heat. Add the nuclear fast red to water while still hot and filter.

Method

1. Deparaffinize in xylene and rehydrate through graded ethanols to deionized water.
2. Stain in the alcian blue solution for 30 minutes.
3. Rinse in running tap water for 5 minutes.
4. Counterstain in nuclear fast red for 10 minutes.
5. Wash in running tap water for 1 minute.
6. Dehydrate in graded ethanols.
7. Clear in xylene and mount in a miscible medium.

Results

Acid mucins (sulfomucins and sialomucins)	blue
Proteoglycans and hyaluronic acid	blue
Nuclei	red

Notes

To selectively identify sulfomucins and proteoglycans a low pH (pH 1) alcian blue solution should be used. Add 1.0 g alcian blue 8GX to 100 ml of 0.1 N hydrochloric acid. The staining procedure and incubation times are the same as those in the alcian blue pH 2.5 protocol.

Low pH alcian blue technique

Varying the pH of the alcian blue solution can be useful in the characterization of the subtypes of acidic mucins and proteoglycans present in a tissue (Spicer 1960; Lev & Spicer 1964; Sorvari & Sorvari 1969). The carboxylated sialomucins and hyaluronic acid do not demonstrate the same magnitude of acidity as the sulfomucins and sulfate-containing proteoglycans, and as a result these groups are not capable of ionization at a pH of 1 or less. The sialomucins and hyaluronic acid therefore are not charged at this pH. Conversely, the sulfomucins and sulfate-containing proteoglycans are ionized and negatively charged at a pH of 1. It follows that staining observed following incubation in an alcian blue solution at a pH of 1 is due predominately to sulfate groups among the mucins or proteoglycans. Examples of tissues or cell types that exhibit staining in an alcian blue solution at a pH of 1 include cartilage, goblet cell mucins of the large intestines, and the mucins of the bronchial serous glands.

Alcian blue with varying electrolyte concentrations

Alcian blue also may be used in a protocol in which the dye is mixed with varying concentrations of an inorganic salt such as magnesium chloride ($MgCl_2$). This modified technique is based upon phenomena known as the critical electrolyte concentration or CEC. The CEC may be defined as the point at which the amount of an electrolyte such as $MgCl_2$ is sufficient to prevent staining with alcian blue. This is believed to occur due to the competition of the cations of the salt with those of the dye for the polyanionic sites within the tissue (Scott & Dorling 1965). Although the mechanism of this effect has been questioned by some (Goldstein & Horobin 1974), nevertheless, independent of the mechanism, useful separations are possible as the various acidic carbohydrates have different CEC values.

Because of the numerous solutions of alcian blue and $MgCl_2$ that are necessary for this protocol as well as a lengthy overnight staining period, the alcian blue/CEC technique is time consuming and labor intensive. For these reasons, there is likely little use of the protocol in laboratories performing routine histology procedures. When performed correctly, however, the alcian blue/CEC procedure is an extremely useful means of differentiating mucins and proteoglycans based upon acidity of the carbohydrates in these molecules.

Combined alcian blue–PAS

The alcian blue and PAS techniques can be combined to differentiate neutral mucins from acidic mucins within a tissue section (Mowry 1963). This technique also is valuable in that it may be used as a broad means of detecting mucins. A lack of staining with the combined alcian blue–PAS technique strongly suggests that the substance in question is not a mucin.

In most protocols, sections are stained with a standard alcian blue (pH 2.5) method followed by PAS. The alcian blue stains sialomucins, sulfomucins, and proteoglycans blue. Neutral mucins are stained deep red/magenta with the PAS. Tissues and cells that contain both neutral and acidic mucins will stain varying shades of purple due to the binding of alcian blue and the reactivity with Schiff reagent. This is seen in the goblet cells of the small intestine that contain neutral and sialomucins (Spicer 1960).

Combined alcian blue–PAS technique
(Mowry 1956, 1963)

Alcian blue solution (in 3% acetic acid)
See page 172.

Periodic acid solution
See page 171.

Preparation of Schiff reagent
See page 171.

Method
1. Deparaffinize in xylene and rehydrate through graded ethanols to deionized water.
2. Stain in the alcian blue solution for 30 minutes.
3. Rinse in running tap water for 5 minutes and then briefly in deionized water.
4. Oxidize with periodic acid for 5 minutes.
5. Rinse in running tap water for 5 minutes.
6. Cover the sections with Schiff reagent for 15 minutes.
7. Rinse in running tap water for 10 minutes.
8. Stain lightly with Mayer's hematoxylin.
9. Rinse in running tap water for 5–10 minutes and blue in an appropriate bluing solution.
10. Rinse in tap water for 5 minutes.
11. Dehydrate in graded ethanols, clear with xylene, and mount with a miscible medium.

Results

Glycogen, neutral mucins, various glycoproteins	magenta
Acid mucins (sulfomucins and sialomucins)	blue
Proteoglycans and hyaluronic acid	blue

Cells or tissue that contains neutral mucins and acid mucins may stain various shades of blue–purple to purple.

Notes

a. It is important to stain lightly with hematoxylin in order to avoid cytoplasmic or mucin staining. Such staining could potentially mask the coloration of the alcian blue.

b. Several studies have shown that the staining sequence of the combined alcian blue/PAS technique can influence the end results (Johannes & Klessen 1984; Yamabayashi 1987). When the PAS technique is applied prior to the alcian blue, neutral mucins and glycogen may stain purple. In contrast, these substances are colored magenta, as would be expected, when stained with the alcian blue–PAS sequence. The reason that neutral carbohydrate moieties acquire an affinity for alcian blue following the PAS procedure is unknown. It has been suggested, however, that the aldehyde groups generated during periodic acid-mediated oxidation may react with sulfite present in the Schiff's solution to form an anionic group that subsequently may bind alcian blue (Johannes & Klessen 1984).

Mucicarmine

This technique is one of the oldest histochemical methods for the visualization of mucins in specimens (Mayer 1896; Southgate 1927). With the subsequent development of methods such as PAS, alcian blue, and colloidal iron the use of the mucicarmine technique has declined somewhat over the past 50 years. The mucicarmine technique, however, remains a valuable means for the demonstration of acidic mucins.

The active dye molecule used in the mucicarmine technique is an aluminum–carminic acid complex known as carmine (Lillie 1977). Carminic acid is a large multi-ring molecule that is produced from the dried bodies of female *Coccus cacti* insects (Lillie 1977). Although the exact mechanism by which this technique acts is unknown, it is believed that aluminum salts form a chelate complex with carminic acid thus conferring an overall positive charge on the carmine complex and an attraction for polyanionic molecules such as the sialomucins and sulfomucins. This theory is supported by a lack of staining of neutral mucin and the positive staining of neutral mucin following sulfation techniques (Lauren & Sorvari 1969).

Within tissue sections, carboxylated mucins and sulfomucins are colored a deep red with this technique. While it seems logical that proteoglycans with the densely packed negative charges of the carboxyl and sulfates would be detectable with this technique, this is not the case. In fact, in most situations, the proteoglycans and glycosaminoglycans demonstrate variable to weak reactivity with the mucicarmine technique (Tighe 1963). The reason for this is unknown.

Because the mucicarmine technique is specific for the mucins of epithelial origin, like PAS and alcian blue this technique may be useful for the identification of adenocarcinomas. This is particularly true of adenocarcinomas of the gastrointestinal tract. The capsule of the fungus *Cryptococcus neoformans* also may be detected with the mucicarmine technique.

Mucicarmine technique (modified Southgate 1927)

Southgate's mucicarmine stock solution

Carmine (alum lake)	1 g
Aluminum hydroxide	1 g
50% ethanol	100 ml

Add the above reagents and 50% ethanol to a 500 ml Pyrex flask. Shake well and add 0.5 g of anhydrous aluminum chloride. Place the flask in a boiling water bath; bring the solution to a boil. Agitate while boiling for 2.5 to 3 minutes. Cool the flask under running tap water. Filter and store at 4°C. Stable for several months.

Mucicarmine working solution

Southgate's mucicarmine stock solution	10 ml
Deionized water	90 ml

Alcoholic hematoxylin

Hematoxylin	1 g
Ethanol (95%)	100 ml

Acidified ferric chloride stock solution

Ferric chloride ($FeCl_3 \cdot 6H_2O$)	2.48 g
Deionized water	97 ml
Concentrated hydrochloric acid (HCl)	1 ml

Weigert's iron hematoxylin working solution

Alcoholic hematoxylin	50 ml
Acidified ferric chloride solution	50 ml

This solution should be mixed just before use.

Metanil yellow working solution

Metanil yellow	0.25 g
Deionized water	100 ml
Glacial acetic acid	0.25 ml

Mix and store in a brown bottle or a bottle completely wrapped with aluminum foil.

Method

1. Deparaffinize with xylene and rehydrate through graded ethanols to water.
2. Stain in Weigert's iron hematoxylin working solution for 10 minutes.
3. Rinse in running tap water for 10 minutes.
4. Stain in the mucicarmine working solution for 30 minutes.
5. Rinse slides in two changes of deionized water.
6. Stain in the metanil yellow working solution for 30–60 seconds.
7. Rinse quickly in distilled water.
8. Dehydrate in graded ethanols and clear in xylene.
9. Coverslip using a miscible mounting medium.

Results

Acidic epithelial mucins	deep rose to red
Nuclei	black
Other tissue elements	light yellow

Notes

The staining period with the mucicarmine working solution may be increased to 60 minutes if necessary.

Colloidal iron

The colloidal iron technique initially was described by Hale in 1946 as a technique for the detection of acid mucopolysaccharides. Since that time, numerous modifications of the original technique have been reported in the literature (Muller 1946; Rinehart & Abul-Haj 1951; Mowry 1958). All of the techniques, however, are based upon the attraction of ferric cations in a colloidal ferric oxide solution for the negatively charged carboxyl and sulfate groups of acid mucins and proteoglycans. The tissue-bound ferric ions subsequently are visualized by treatment with potassium ferrocyanide to form bright blue deposits of ferric ferrocyanide or Prussian blue.

Several investigators have demonstrated that the colloidal iron technique is as sensitive as alcian blue for the detection of acid mucosubstances (Mowry 1958; Korhonen & Makela 1968). There has been much debate, however, concerning the selectivity and specificity of the colloidal iron technique. When used as initially described by Hale the ferric ions of the solution likely react with a number of non-carbohydrate-based polyanionic polymers such as DNA and RNA (Pearse 1960). In addition, it has been suggested that the ferric ions may bind the anionic carboxyl groups of tissue-bound proteins (Pearse 1960). Several of the modifications made to Hale's original method were made in an attempt to improve the specificity or reduce background staining. Modifications that have proven beneficial to specificity include a reduction in the pH of the colloidal iron solution as well as the incorporation of acetic acid rinses following incubation with the colloidal iron (Mowry 1958; Pearse 1960). These modifications resulted in reduced nonspecific cytoplasmic staining. The colloidal iron technique also may be used with a PAS procedure. Sections are incubated with the colloidal iron solution and stained with potassium ferrocyanide prior to periodic acid oxidation. When used in this manner, acid mucins, proteoglycans, and hyaluronic acid stain bright blue with the colloidal iron/potassium ferrocyanide reaction while the neutral mucins and glycogen are colored red/magenta by the Schiff reaction.

Colloidal iron technique (modified Muller 1955; Mowry 1958)

Stock colloidal iron solution

Bring 250 ml of deionized water to a boil and add 4.4 ml of a 29% ferric chloride solution (USP XI). Continue to boil until the solution turns dark red, at which time the solution should be removed from the heat and allowed to cool. This solution is stable for one year.

Colloidal iron working solution

Stock colloidal iron solution	20 ml
Deionized water	15 ml
Glacial acetic acid	5 ml

Prepare just prior to use.

Acetic acid (12%) solution

Glacial acetic acid	24 ml
Deionized water to make	200 ml

Potassium ferrocyanide (5%) solution

Potassium ferrocyanide	5 g
Deionized water	100 ml

Hydrochloric acid (5%) solution

Concentrated hydrochloric acid (HCl)	5 ml
Deionized water	95 ml

Potassium ferrocyanide–hydrochloric acid

5% potassium ferrocyanide solution	50 ml
5% hydrochloric acid solution	50 ml

Mix just prior to use.

Acid fuchsin stock (1%)

Acid fuchsin	1 g
Deionized water	100 ml

van Gieson working solution

1% acid fuchsin stock	5 ml
Saturated picric acid	95 ml

Method

1. Deparaffinize in xylene and rehydrate through graded ethanols to water.
2. Rinse in 12% acetic acid solution for 1 minute.
3. Cover the sections with the colloidal iron working solution for 1 hour.
4. Rinse in four changes of the 12% acetic acid solution (3 minutes each).
5. Place in the potassium ferrocyanide–hydrochloric acid solution for 20 minutes.
6. Rinse in running tap water for 5 minutes.
7. Rinse briefly in deionized water.
8. Cover the specimens with the van Gieson working solution for 5 minutes.
9. Dehydrate the specimens in 95% ethanol and absolute ethanol, three changes each. Clear in xylene.
10. Coverslip using an appropriate mounting medium.

Results

Proteoglycans, hyaluronic acid, and acidic mucins	bright blue
Collagen	red
Muscle and cytoplasm	yellow

Notes

1. The pH of the colloidal iron working solution is critical. At a pH of 2.0 or higher nonspecific staining of structures other than acidic carbohydrate groups will occur.
2. Some protocols may recommend dialysis of the stock colloidal iron solution to remove free acid and unhydrolyzed (ionizable) iron salts. To dialyze the solution, transfer the stock colloidal ion solution in 25-ml portions to 41-mm dialysis tubes, suspended in deionized water. Dialyze for 24 hours, changing the water twice during this period. Filter the contents of the dialysis tubes through fine filter paper (Whatman No. 50 or equivalent) to remove any particulate matter (Lillie & Fulmer 1976).
3. Nuclear fast red may be used as an alternative counterstain for this technique. (See alcian blue technique page 172).
4. The colloidal iron technique may be performed in conjunction with the PAS protocol. The colloidal iron technique is performed first and after step 7 of the protocol the section may be subjected to periodic acid oxidation. The remainder of the PAS procedure is performed as described previously (see page 171).
5. A control slide for each test specimen should be included. This slide should be subjected to the potassium ferrocyanide–hydrochloric acid solution only. This is necessary to exclude the possibility that a positive result of the colloidal iron stain is due to the presence of hemosiderin.
6. If the official iron chloride solution is not available, a solution of 2.73 g of $FeCl_3 \cdot 6H_2O$ in 4.4 ml of deionized water may be used (Lillie & Fulmer 1976).

High iron diamine

The high iron diamine method of Spicer is a useful technique for the detection of the highly acidic sulfomucins. This technique is selective for carbohydrates carrying a high negative charge density due to ionized sulfate groups. Hyaluronic acid and sialomucins are not demonstrated by this technique (Spicer 1965; Gad & Sylven 1969). When combined with the alcian blue protocol the high iron diamine technique facilitates the differentiation of sulfomucins from sialomucins in tissue sections. Although the exact mechanism of action of this stain is unknown, Spicer (1965) suggested that oxidation of the diamine isomers results in the formation of a positively charged polymer. Ferric ions potentially catalyze the reaction and may form chelate complexes with the diamines. The ferric chloride also serves to lower the pH of the solution to 1.3–1.4. At this pH, the ionization of the carboxyl groups is inhibited or greatly reduced while the strongly acidic sulfate groups are fully ionized. This accounts to some extent for the specificity of this procedure for sulfomucins. The phosphate groups of the nucleic acids typically are not stained by this technique. Sorvari (1972) suggested that the phosphate ions preferentially attracted the ferric ions and excluded the diamine molecules.

When used together with the standard alcian blue procedure, sulfomucins and proteoglycans stain brown to black while sialomucins and hyaluronic acid stain blue. This combined technique is well suited to demonstrate the distribution of sialomucins and sulfomucins in the epithelia of the intestines (Spicer 1965).

Combined high iron diamine and alcian blue technique (modified Spicer 1965)

High iron diamine solution

N,N-dimethyl-m-phenylenediamine (HCl)$_2$	120 mg
N,N-dimethyl-p-phenylenediamine (HCl)	20 mg

Dissolve the above reagents in 50 ml of deionized water. Pour into a coplin jar containing 1.4 ml of N.F. 10% ferric chloride (FeCl$_3$).

Alcian blue solution (in 3% acetic acid)
See page 172.

Method
1. Deparaffinize in xylene and rehydrate through graded ethanols to deionized water.
2. Stain the sections in the high iron diamine solution for 18 hours.
3. Rinse in running tap water for 5 minutes.
4. Stain in the alcian blue solution (pH 2.5) for 30 minutes.
5. Rinse in running tap water for 10 minutes.
6. Dehydrate in graded ethanols and clear with xylene.
7. Coverslip with a miscible mounting medium.

Results
Sulfated mucins and proteoglycans	black–brown
Sialomucins and hyaluronic acid	blue

Notes
1. The diamine salts are potentially toxic and handling should be with great care and kept to a minimum.
2. Nuclear fast red may be used to enhance nuclear contrast (see Alcian blue technique, page 172).
3. The N.F. 10% ferric chloride solution is equivalent to a 62% w/v solution of FeCl$_3$·6H$_2$O (Lillie & Fulmer 1976).

Combined aldehyde fuchsin–alcian blue

Techniques utilizing aldehyde fuchsin have been used to demonstrate a wide array of tissue components including elastic fibers, β cells of the islets, and thyroid colloid to mention but a few (Gomori 1950; Thompson 1966). Several early studies also demonstrated that aldehyde fuchsin staining frequently was localized to tissue elements known either to contain highly sulfated mucosubstances or to demonstrate metachromasia (Halmi & Davies 1953; Scott & Clayton 1953). It is now generally accepted that aldehyde fuchsin reacts with sulfomucins and sulfated proteoglycans. This technique is largely empirical, as the attraction of the aldehyde fuchsin molecule for sulfate groups is poorly understood.

There is little value in using aldehyde fuchsin as a stand-alone technique as the low pH alcian blue technique is a more specific, reliable, and convenient means of detecting sulfated glycoconjugates. The aldehyde fuchsin technique together with the alcian blue procedure, however, may be used as an alternative to the high iron diamine–alcian blue procedure for the differentiation of sulfate and carboxylate-containing glycoconjugates (Spicer & Meyer 1960).

In the combined procedure, sections are first stained with the aldehyde fuchsin, which colors the strongly sulfated mucins and the sulfate-containing proteoglycans a deep purple. Weakly sulfated mucins, elastin, and pancreatic β cell cells stain a lighter purple. The subsequent application of alcian blue stains hyaluronic acid and sialomucins blue.

Combined aldehyde fuchsin–alcian blue technique (Spicer & Meyer 1960)

Aldehyde fuchsin solution

Basic fuchsin	1 g
70% ethanol	200 ml
Concentrated hydrochloric acid (HCl)	2 ml
Paraldehyde	2 ml

Dissolve the basic fuchsin in the alcohol and add the paraldehyde and HCl. Let stand at room temperature for 2–3 days, filter, and refrigerate. A fresh preparation should be made every 3–6 months. The pH of this solution should be 1.7.

Alcian blue solution (in 3% acetic acid)
See page 172.

Method
1. Deparaffinize in xylene and hydrate to 70% ethanol.
2. Stain in the aldehyde fuchsin solution for 20 minutes.
3. Rinse sections in 70% ethanol.
4. Rinse briefly is running tap water.
5. Stain in alcian blue (pH 2.5) for 30 minutes.
6. Rinse in running tap water for 2 minutes.
7. Dehydrate in graded ethanols and clear with xylene.
8. Coverslip using a miscible mounting medium.

Results

Proteoglycans and strongly acidic sulfomucins	deep purple
Weakly acidic sulfomucins	purple
Sialomucins and hyaluronic acid	blue

Note
a. As the aldehyde fuchsin solution ages, heavier background staining may occur while specific staining of sulfated carbohydrates may decrease in intensity.
b. For preparation of the aldehyde fuchsin solution, pararosanaline or a basic fuchsin sample that contains predominately this dye should be used (Mowry 1978).

Metachromatic methods

Metachromasia may be defined as the staining of tissue or tissue components such that the color of the tissue-bound dye complex differs significantly from the color of the original dye complex to give a marked contrast in color (Pearse 1960). Typically, there is a shift in the absorption of light by the tissue dye complex toward the shorter wavelengths with an inverse shift in color transmission or emission towards the longer wavelengths. Methylene blue, azure A, and toluidine blue are small planar cationic dyes that typically stain tissues blue. Under conditions of metachromasia, these dyes stain tissue components purple–red. The use of such dyes to identify charged mucins and proteoglycans is one of the oldest of the histochemical techniques for carbohydrates.

Metachromasia is believed to result from a specific form of dye aggregation that is characterized by the formation of new intermolecular bonds between adjacent dye molecules (Pearse 1960). The bonds between the dye molecules only occur in situations in which the molecules are brought into close proximity to one another (Sylven 1954; Bergeron & Singer 1958). In cases of acid mucins or proteoglycans, the anionic groups of the carbohydrates act to orient the cationic dye molecules. Simply put, the anionic carbohydrate structure serves as a template to induce the formation of a polymeric dye structure in which the dye molecules likely bind to one another through hydrogen bonds or van der Vaals' forces. Integration of water molecules between adjacent dye molecules is believed to be essential for the metachromatic phenomena (Sylven 1954; Bergeron & Singer 1958).

For metachromasia to occur a certain pattern of distribution and density of repeating anionic structures is necessary (Pearse 1960). The highly anionic proteoglycans with alternating sulfate and carboxylate groups meet these criteria and produce metachromatic stains with dyes such as toluidine blue, methylene blue, and azure. In general, the more strongly acidic or highly sulfated proteolglycans will produce the strongest and most stable metachromasia (Tonna & Cronkite 1959; Thompson 1966).

The post-treatment of sections following staining with metachromasia producing dyes can have a profound effect on the stability of the metachromasia. Metachromasia may be described as 'alcohol fast' if metachromasia is retained following dehydration, and as 'alcohol labile' if metachromasia is lost in the process (Pearse 1960). For this reason, it has been recommended by some that it is necessary to examine sections first in water prior to placement of the specimens in alcohol. The metachromasia generating techniques have largely been replaced by techniques such as alcian blue. The reader is directed to older texts such as those of Pearse, Lillie, and Fulmer as well as earlier publications in the literature (Kramer & Windrum 1955; Bergeron & Singer 1958) for more detailed information concerning these techniques.

Azure A technique (modified Kramer & Windrum 1955)

Alcoholic azure A solution

Azure A	0.01 g
Ethanol 30%	100 ml

Method

1. Deparaffinize sections in xylene and hydrate through graded ethanols to deionized water.
2. Cover sections with the azure A solution for 10 minutes.
3. Rinse in deionized water.
4. Dehydrate the sections in graded ethanols and clear in xylene.
5. Coverslip using a miscible mounting medium.

Results

Acid mucins and proteoglycans	purple to red
Tissue background	blue

Notes

0.1% azure A solution (0.1 g azure A in 100 ml of 30% ethanol) can be used to demonstrate the weakly metachromatic acid carbohydrate containing molecules.

LECTINS AND IMMUNOHISTOCHEMISTRY

Lectins

Lectins were initially characterized as proteins isolated from plants that were capable of agglutinating mammalian erythrocytes (Sharon & Lis 1972). Agglutination occurs because the lectin molecule binds multiple glycoprotein molecules on the cell surface and thus crosslinks the erythrocytes (Sharon & Lis 1972; Goldstein & Hayes 1978). From a histochemical perspective, lectins may be defined as plant or animal proteins which bind specific carbohydrate moieties in tissue specimens. Lectin

techniques, however, are not routinely performed in most histology laboratories. For this reason, the discussion of lectins provided is brief and the reader is directed to the following references for a more thorough discussion and review of lectins (Sharon & Lis 1972; Goldstein & Hayes 1978; Spicer & Schulte 1992).

Lectins have been isolated from a wide range of animal and plant sources. The more commonly used lectins include concanavalin A from the jack bean, peanut agglutinin, and *Ulex europaeus* (gorse). Lectins bind principally to the terminal carbohydrate molecules of the oligosaccharide or polysaccharide chains of glycoproteins (Goldstein & Poretz 1986). The affinity of a lectin, however, may be influenced by the monosaccharide unit adjacent to the terminal unit. Concanavalin A binds terminal mannose moieties while peanut agglutinin binds galactose or galactosamine (Hennigar et al 1987; Spicer & Schulte 1992). *Ulex europaeus* specifically binds L-fucose (Allen et al 1977).

Lectin molecules can be labeled with fluorochromes such as fluorescein or rhodamine as well as the histochemically detectable enzymes, horseradish peroxidase and alkaline phosphatase (Gonatas & Avrameas 1973). Lectins labeled in this manner have been used for a number of purposes in the histology or diagnostic pathology laboratory. *Ulex europaeus* in particular has been used as a valuable marker of normal and neoplastic endothelial cells (Walker 1985). The use of *Ulex* in this role, however, has diminished with the emergence of immunohistochemistry and specific antibodies to endothelial markers such as factor VIII, CD31, and CD34.

Immunohistochemistry

Immunohistochemical techniques are rarely used for the routine evaluation of tissue specimens for glycogen or the proteoglycans. In spite of the high sensitivity and specificity of immunohistochemistry, the special stains described in this chapter remain the standard means for the evaluation of these substances. Immunohistochemistry, however, has become an invaluable tool for the detection of a varied number of specific mucins as well as mucin-like molecules that are markers of the neoplastic process. Examples of these types of molecule include the epithelial membrane antigen (EMA) and the tumor-associated glycoprotein (TAG-72), to mention a few. As the list of mucins, mucin-like molecules, and glycoproteins that are evaluated by immunohistochemistry is long and varied and the discussion of immunohisto-chemical techniques is outside the scope of this chapter, the reader is referred to Chapter 23 in which the immuno-histochemistry of diagnostic pathology is discussed at length.

ENZYMATIC DIGESTION TECHNIQUES

Various enzymatic digestion techniques have been applied to increase or verify the specificity of carbohy-drate staining techniques. For example, the amylase or diastase techniques for glycogen digestion are commonly utilized in laboratories to enhance the specificity of the PAS technique. The other digestion techniques (neur-aminidase, hyaluronidase) described below, however, are not commonly performed in today's histology labo-ratories. They are more likely to be performed in research laboratories that possess an interest in a specific area of glycobiology.

Diastase digestion

The PAS technique is unique among the procedures described in this chapter in that PAS detects a varied number of mucosubstances such as glycogen, mucins, and glycoproteins. The distinction of mucins from glyco-gen can be problematic when using the PAS technique. The inclusion of a glycogen digestion step is necessary when the diagnosis requires the correct identification of mucosubstances such as mucin or glycogen. Typically α-amylase maybe used in such a situation. Alpha-amylase catalyzes the hydrolysis of the glycosidic bonds of glycogen and the breakdown of the large glycogen molecules to the water-soluble disaccharide known as maltose (Bernfeld 1951). The net result is the removal of glycogen from the tissue section prior to the PAS tech-nique. Malt diastase, which contains both α- and β-amylases, is frequently used for this purpose (Lillie et al 1947). Although human saliva is touted as an effective means of digesting glycogen, the use of saliva is discour-aged for reasons of safety and the lack of standardization of saliva preparations.

Duplicate slides are required when a glycogen digestion procedure is used. Following deparaffinization, one slide is treated with diastase in the appropriate buffer while the other slide is incubated with buffer only. Both slides are then subjected to the PAS procedure. Staining lost following digestion is indicative of glycogen.

Diastase digestion (Lillie & Fulmer 1976)

Phosphate buffer

Sodium phosphate (monobasic)	1.97 g
Sodium phosphate (dibasic)	0.28 g
Deionized water	1000 ml

This solution may be kept in the refrigerator for several months.

Diastase solution

Malt diastase	0.1 g
Phosphate buffer	100 ml

Method

1. Deparaffinize two serial sections in xylene and rehydrate through graded ethanols to water.
2. Place one slide in the diastase solution for 1 hour at 37°C. The other slide is an untreated control and may remain in water for 1 hour.
3. Wash both slides in running tap water for 5–10 minutes.
4. Proceed with the PAS technique.

Results (with PAS procedure)

Glycogen should demonstrate bright red/magenta staining in the untreated slide. Glycogen staining should be absent in the diastase-treated slide.

Notes

1. A known positive control should be included to verify the potency of the enzyme.
2. Commercial batches of diastase or amylase may vary widely in activity and purity. Contaminating enzymes may digest material other than glycogen.
3. Alpha-amylase may be used instead of malt diastase.

Sialidase

The enzyme sialidase or neuraminidase is isolated from the bacterium *Vibrio cholerae* (Kiernan 1999). This enzyme specifically cleaves the terminal sialic acid moi-eties from sialomucins and glycoproteins (Drzeniek 1973). The loss of PAS or alcian blue staining following sialidase treatment is clearly indicative of the presence of sialic acid in tissue specimens. If the combined alcian blue–PAS protocol is performed following sialidase treat-ment, sialomucins that normally would stain blue with alcian blue stain red with PAS. Removal of the alcian blue-reactive anionic carboxylate group containing sugars from these mucins renders the mucin reactive with PAS.

In contrast to the scenarios described above in which staining is lost following treatment, a lack of effect of sialidase is difficult to interpret. While it may indicate a lack of sialic acid in the specimen, such findings do not rule out the possibility of the sialidase resistant O-acetylated sialic acids. These resistant sialic acids can be converted to sialidase labile form by the deacetylation procedure (Ravetto 1968). This technique uses an alkaline (ammonia) alcohol solution to remove the O-acetyl groups from the sialic acid. Subsequent treatment with sialidase cleaves the previously enzyme-resistant sialic acids. A comparison of alcian blue (pH 2.5) staining in sections subjected to the deacetylation–sialidase combination to the staining of sections exposed only to sialidase will reveal the presence of O-acetyl group-containing sialic acids.

Sialidase digestion (Bancroft & Cook 1994)

Sialidase solution

One unit/ml sialidase (neuraminidase) ex. *V. cholerae* diluted 1 in 5 with 0.2 M acetate buffer pH 5.5. Add 1% calcium chloride w/v. The activity of the diluted enzyme will persist for a few weeks if stored at 4°C.

Method

1. Dewax two sections from a positive control and two sections from each test specimen. Bring sections to water.
2. Rinse the sections with buffer and treat one positive control section and one section from each test specimen with the sialidase solution for 16–24 hours at 37°C. The remaining slides (one positive control section and one section per test specimen) are incubated in buffer (37°C) alone for the same period of time.
3. Rinse in running tap water for 5 minutes.
4. Proceed to alcian blue (page 172) or the alcian blue–PAS (page 173) technique.

Results

Sialidase-labile sialic acids will stain bright blue in the untreated section. This staining is lost following sialidase treatment.

Alcian blue–PAS mucins containing sialidase-labile sialic acids will stain bright blue while neutral mucins stain red to magenta in the untreated sections. Following treatment, mucins containing sialidase-labile sialic acids will stain red to magenta secondary to the PAS stain (Spicer & Warren 1959).

Notes

1. Sialic acids containing an O-acetyl group usually are resistant to sialidase.
2. A known positive control should be included to verify the potency of the enzyme.

Hyaluronidase

The enzyme hyaluronidase cleaves the glycosidic linkages of hyaluronic acid and, depending upon the source of the enzyme, glycosidic linkages in other glycosaminoglycans. The most commonly used hyaluronidase is isolated from an extract of bull testis. This enzyme removes hyaluronic acid but also attacks the glycosidic linkages of the chondroitin sulfates (Meyer & Rapport 1952). The enzyme may be used as a pretreatment of specimens, prior to staining with alcian blue or colloidal iron. The loss of staining when compared to a non-treated duplicate section is indicative of the presence of hyaluronic acid or the chondroitin sulfates. If there is no effect of the pretreatment, this strongly suggests that the substance is not hyaluronic acid. Thus in spite of the lack of specificity a negative response to bull testis hyaluronidase can be used to rule out the possible presence of hyaluronic acid.

A form of hyaluronidase isolated from several bacterial species also has been used for the identification of hyaluronic acid (Meyer & Rapport 1952). These enzymes are more selective than bovine testicular hyaluronidase and have been shown to act specifically on hyaluronic acid.

Hyaluronidase digestion (Gaffney 1992)

Phosphate buffer solution	
Sodium chloride	8 g
Sodium phosphate, monobasic	2 g
Sodium phosphate, dibasic	0.3 g
Deionized water	1000 ml

Hyaluronidase solution

Bovine testicular hyaluronidase	50 mg
Phosphate buffer solution	100 ml

Method

1. Dewax two sections from a positive control and two sections from each test specimen. Bring sections to deionized water.
2. Incubate one positive control section and one section from each test specimen with the hyaluronidase solution for 3 hours at 37°C. The remaining slides (one positive control and one section per test specimen) should be treated with buffer alone for 3 hours at 37°C.
3. Wash all slides in running tap water for 5 minutes.
4. Perform staining technique such as alcian blue (see page 172).

Results

Alcian blue (pH 2.5)

Connective tissue proteoglycans containing chondroitin sulfate and/or hyaluronic acid stain bright blue in sections not treated with hyaluronidase. This staining is lost following hyaluronidase treatment.

Notes

A known positive control is necessary to verify the potency of the enzyme.

CHEMICAL MODIFICATION AND BLOCKING TECHNIQUES

There are a number of techniques that have been used to block the reactive groups of carbohydrates such as hydroxyls, carboxyls, and sulfate esters. Blocking these groups prevents the reaction with the reagents used in subsequent histochemical techniques. The blocking techniques, although infrequently used in today's histology laboratory, may be particularly useful for determining the specific types of carbohydrate present in a tissue specimen.

Methylation

There are a number of variations of this technique that have been used to identify the type (carboxyl or sulfate) of acid groups in mucins. All of these techniques, however, are based upon the treatment of the specimens with an acidified methanolic solution. In the so-called 'mild' technique, the sections are exposed to the solution for a relatively short period (4 hours) at 37°C (Spicer 1960). Under these conditions, the carboxylate groups of the mucins are converted to methyl esters. The loss of alcian blue (pH 2.5) reactivity within a specimen following this procedure is indicative of a preponderance of carboxylated carbohydrates in the tissue. Conversely, any staining following this procedure is likely due to sulfate containing carbohydrates.

Treatment of specimens with an acidified methanolic solution for 5 hours or more at 60°C converts carboxylate groups to methyl esters and also removes or hydrolyzes O-sulfate and N-sulfate groups in mucins and proteoglycans. Sections treated in this manner should demonstrate a total loss of alcian blue reactivity. This technique is of little value if performed alone and frequently is performed with the saponification technique.

Saponification

The alkaline alcoholic solution used in this technique cleaves the linkage of the O-acetyl groups within the enzyme-resistant sialic acids. As with the deacetylation procedure described above, this technique renders the O-acetylated sialic acids sensitive to neuraminidase. The removal of the O-acetyl group and the restoration of the hydroxyl groups on the C7–C9 side chain of sialic acid also restore the PAS reactivity of the sialic acids (Culling et al 1974).

This technique also is used for the reversal of the effects of methylation. Saponification cleaves the bonds of the methyl esters formed during methylation and restores the carboxylate groups (Spicer & Lillie 1959). Following the methylation protocol, saponification will restore the alcian blue staining of the carboxylated carbohydrates. Sulfate esters, however, that are lost due to the more aggressive methylation protocol are not restored by saponification. The restoration of alcian blue staining following saponification is due to the presence of sialomucins or hyaluronic acid.

Mild methylation technique (Spicer 1960)

Acid methanol solution

Concentrated hydrochloric acid (HCl)	0.8 ml
Methanol	99.2 ml

Method

1. Dewax two sections from a positive control and two sections from each test specimen. Bring sections to deionized water.
2. Place one positive control section and one section from each test specimen in preheated (37°C) acid methanol solution for 4 hours. The remaining slides (one positive control and one slide per test specimen) should be placed in deionized water at 37°C for 4 hours.
3. Wash in running tap water for 5 minutes.
4. Perform alcian blue (pH 2.5) stain.

Results

Alcian blue (pH 2.5)

Sulfated mucins and proteoglycans as well as sialomucins and hyaluronic acid will stain bright blue in the untreated specimen. A diminution of staining following treatment with the acid methanol reflects a loss of stainable sialomucins and/or hyaluronic acid. Any staining that remains following treatment is due to sulfomucins and/or sulfate proteoglycans.

Notes

Treatment beyond 4 hours may result in the hydrolysis of sulfate groups.

Positive control slides are necessary to verify the effectiveness of the methylation procedure.

Combined methylation–saponification technique (Spicer & Lillie 1959)

Acid methanol solution

Same as solution used for mild methylation (see section above).

Saponification solution

Potassium hydroxide	1 g
Ethanol	70 ml
Deionized water	30 ml

Method

1. Dewax three positive control sections and three sections from each test specimen. Bring sections to water.
2. Place two positive controls and two test sections in the acid methanol solution at 60°C for 5 hours. The additional positive control and test specimen should be placed in 60°C deionized water for 5 hours.
3. Wash all sections in running tap water for 5 minutes.
4. Place one each of the positive control sections and test sections that were treated with acid methanol (step 2) in the saponification solution for 30 minutes at room temperature. Place all other sections in 70% ethanol at room temperature for 30 minutes.
5. Wash for 5 minutes.
6. Stain with alcian blue (page 172).

Results

With alcian blue (pH 2.5) stain:

a. Sections without methylation or saponification: sulfated and carboxylated mucins as well as proteoglycans and hyaluronic acid will stain bright blue.
b. Sections treated with acid methanol but not subjected to saponification: there should be little or no alcian blue staining.
c. Sections treated with acid methanol and subjected to saponification: the carboxylated mucins and hyaluronic acid should demonstrate bright blue staining with alcian blue. Any loss of staining when compared to the sections that were not treated with acid methanol or subjected to saponification (group A) is due to the presence of sulfated mucins and/or sulfated proteoglycans.

Notes

1. Silanized slides should be used.
2. Celloidinization of slides has been recommended to reduce tissue loss during the saponification process.

REFERENCES

Allen H.J., Johnson E.A., Matta K.L. (1977) A comparison of the binding specificities of lectins from *Ulex europaeus* and *Lotus tetragonolobus*. Immunology Communications 6:585–602.

Angervall L., Enzinger F.M. (1975) Extraskeletal neoplasm resembling Ewing's sarcoma. Cancer 36:240–251.

Baeckstrom D. (1997) Post-translational fate of a mucin-like leukocyte sialoglycoprotein (CD 43) aberrantly expressed in a colon carcinoma cell line. Journal of Biological Chemistry 272:11503–11509.

Bancroft J.D., Cook H.C. (1994) Manual of histological techniques and their diagnostic applications. New York: Churchill Livingstone.

Barger J.D., DeLamater E.D. (1948) The use of thionyl chloride in the preparation of Schiff's reagent. Science 108:121–122.

Bauer H. (1933) Microskopisch-chemischer Natwer's von Glykogen und einigen anderen Polysaccharden. Zeitschrift für mikroskopische-anatomische Forschung 33:143.

Bergeron J.A., Singer M. (1958) Metachromasy: an experimental and theoretical re-evaluation. Journal of Biophysical and Biochemical Cytology 4:433–457.

Bernfeld P. (1951) Enzymes of starch degradation and synthesis. Advances in Enzymology 12:379–428.

Cook H.C. (1974) Manual of histological demonstration techniques. London: Butterworths.

Cori G.T., Cori C.F. (1952) Glucose-6-phosphatase of the liver in glycogen storage disease. Journal of Biological Chemistry 199:661–667.

Culling C.F.A., Reid P.E., Clay M.G., Dunn W.L. (1974) The histochemical demonstration of O-acylated sialic acid in gastrointerstinal mucin. Their association with the potassium hydroxide–periodic acid–Schiff effect. Journal of Histochemistry and Cytochemistry 22: 826–831.

Culling C.F.A., Allison R.T., Barr W.T. (1985) Cellular pathology technique, 4th edn. London: Butterworths.

David G. (1993) Integral membrane heparin sulfate proteoglycans. FASEB Journal 7:1023–1030.

Drzeniek R. (1973) Substrate specificity of neuraminidases. Histochemical Journal 5:271–290.

Gad A., Sylven B. (1969) On the nature of the high iron diamine method for sulfomucins. Journal of Histochemistry and Cytochemistry 17:156–160.

Gaffney E. (1992) Carbohydrates. In: Prophet E.B., Mills B., Arrington J.B., Sobin L.H., eds. Armed Forces Institute of Pathology: laboratory methods in histochemistry. Washington, D.C.: American Registry of Pathology.

Gallo R.L., Ono M., Povsic T. et al. (1994) Syndecans, cell surface heparin sulfate proteoglycans, are induced by a proline-rich antimicrobial peptide from wounds. Proceeding of the National Academy of Sciences (USA) 91:11035–11039.

Gendler S.J., Spicer A.P. (1995) Epithelial mucin genes. Annual Reviews of Physiology 57:607–634.

Goldstein I.J., Hayes C.E. (1978) The lectins: carbohydrate-binding proteins of plants and animals. Advances in Carbohydrate Chemistry and Biochemistry 35: 127–340.

Goldstein D.J., Horobin R.W. (1974) Rate factors in staining by alcian blue. Histochemical Journal 6:157–174.

Goldstein I.J., Poretz R.D. (1986) Isolation, physiochemical characterization, and carbohydrate-binding specificity of lectins. In: Liener I.E., Sharon N., Goldstein J.J., eds. The lectins: properties, functions and applications in biology and medicine. Orlando, FL: Academic Press, pp. 35–248.

Gomori G. (1950) Aldehyde–fuchsin: a new stain for elastic tissue. American Journal of Clinical Pathology 20:665–666.

Gonatas N.K., Avrameas S. (1973) Detection of plasma membrane carbohydrates with lectin peroxidase conjugates. Journal of Cell Biology 59:436–443.

Habib N.A., Smadja C., Dawson P., Wood C.B. (1985) Histochemical changes of the intestinal mucus in benign and malignant lesions of the colon and rectum. Gastroenterology and Clinical Biology 9:491–494.

Hale C.W. (1946) Histochemical demonstration of acid mucopolysaccharides in animal tissues. Nature (London) 157:802.

Halmi N.S., Davies J. (1953) Comparison of aldehyde fuchsin staining, metachromasia and periodic acid–Schiff reactivity of various tissues. Journal of Histochemistry and Cytochemistry 1:447–459.

Harley R.A. (1987) Histochemical and immunochemical methods of use in pulmonary pathology. In: Spicer S.S., ed. Histochemistry in pathologic diagnosis. New York: Marcel Dekker.

Hennigar G.R. (1987) Techniques in nephropathology. In: Spicer S.S., ed. Histochemistry in pathologic diagnosis. New York: Marcel Dekker.

Hennigar L.M., Hennigar R.A., Schulte B.A. (1987) Histochemical specificity of β galactose binding lectins from Arachis hypogaea (peanut) and Ricinus communis (castor bean). Stain Technology 62:317–325.

Hers H.G. (1963) Glucosidase deficiency in generalized glycogen storage disease (Pompe's disease). Biochemical Journal 86:11–16.

Hollenbaugh D., Bajorath J., Aruffo A. (1999) Cell adhesion molecules and their cellular targets. In: Hect S.M., ed. Bioorganic chemistry: carbohydrates. New York: Oxford University Press, pp. 313–334.

Hooghwinkel G.J., Smits G. (1957) The specificity of the periodic acid–Schiff technique studies by a quantitative test-tube method. Journal of Histochemistry and Cytochemistry 5:120–126.

Horobin R.W., Kiernan J.A. (2002) Conn's biological stains. A handbook of dyes, stains and flourochromes for use in biology and medicine, 10th edn. Oxford, UK: BIOS Scientific Publishers.

Jass J.R. (1996) Mucin staining. Journal of Clinical Pathology 49:787–790.

Johannes M.L., Klessen C. (1984) Alcian blue/PAS or PAS/alcian blue? Remarks on a classical technique used in carbohydrate histochemistry. Histochemistry 80:129–132.

Kiernan J.A. (1999) Histological and histochemical methods: theory and practice, 3rd edn. Oxford: Butterworth Heinemann.

Kindblom L.G., Angervall L. (1975) Histochemical characterization of mucosubstances in bone and soft tissue-tumors. Cancer 36:985–984.

Korhonen L., Makela V. (1968) Carbohydrate-rich components in lung cancer and normal bronchial tissue: a histochemical study. Histochemical Journal 1: 124–140.

Kramer H., Windrum G.M. (1955) The metachromatic staining reaction. Journal of Histochemistry and Cytochemistry 3:227–237.

Lauren P.A., Sorvari T.E. (1969) The histochemical specificity of mucicarmine staining in the identification of epithelial mucosubstances. Acta Histochemica 34:263–272.

Leblond C.P., Glegg R.E., Eidinger D. (1957) Presence of carbohydrates with free 1,2-glycol groups in sites stained by the periodic acid–Schiff technique. Journal of Histochemistry and Cytochemistry 5:445–458.

Lev R., Spicer S.S. (1964) Specific staining of sulfate groups with alcian blue at low pH. Journal of Histochemistry and Cytochemistry 12:309.

Lillie R.D. (1947) Reticulum staining with Schiff reagent after oxidation by acidified sodium periodate. Journal of Laboratory and Clinical Medicine 32:910–912.

Lillie R.D. (1951) Histochemical comparison of the Casella, Bauer and periodic acid oxidation leucofuchsin techniques. Stain Technology 26:123–136.

Lillie R.D. (1954) Histologic technique, 2nd edn. New York: McGraw-Hill.

Lillie R.D. (1977) H.J. Conn's biological stains. Baltimore, MD: Williams and Wilkins.

Lillie R.D., Fulmer H.M. (1976) Histopathologic technique and practical histochemistry, 4th edn. New York: McGraw-Hill.

Lillie R.D., Laskey A., Greco J., Jacquier H. (1947) Studies on the preservation and histologic demonstration of glycogen. Bulletin of the International Association of Medical Museums 27:23.

Longley J.B. (1952) Effectiveness of Schiff variants in the periodic Schiff and Feulgen nuclear technics. Stain Technology 27:161–169.

Mali M., Jaakkola P., Arilommi A.M., Jalkanen M. (1990) Sequence of human syndecan indicates a novel family of integral membrane proteoglycans. Journal of Biological Chemistry 265:6884–6889.

Manns E. (1958) The preservation and demonstration of glycogen in tissue sections. Journal of Medical Laboratory Technology 15:1–12.

Mason R.M., d'Arville C., Kimura J.H., Hascoll V.C. (1982) Absence of covalently linked core protein form newly synthesized hyaluronate. Biochemical Journal 207:445–457.

Mayer P. (1896) Uber schleimfarbung. Mitteilungeu aus der Zoologischen Station Zu Neapel 12:303.

McKusick V., Neufeld E.F. (1983) The mucodisaccharide storage diseases. In: Stanbury J.B., Wyngaarden J.B., Frederickson D.S. et al., eds. The metabolic basis of inherited disease, 5th edn. New York: McGraw-Hill.

McManus J.F.A. (1946) Histological demonstration of mucin after periodic acid. Nature (London) 158:202.

McManus J.F.A. (1948) The periodic acid routine applied to the kidney. American Journal of Pathology 24: 643–653.

Meyer K., Rapport M.M. (1952) Hyaluronidases. Advances in Enzymology 13:199–236.

Moniaux N., Nollet S., Porchet N. et al. (1999) Complete sequence of the human mucin MUC4: a putative cell membrane-associated mucin. Biochemical Journal 338:325–333.

Mowry R.W. (1956) Alcian blue techniques for the histochemical study of acid carbohydrates. Journal of Histochemistry and Cytochemistry 4:407.

Mowry R.W. (1958) Improved procedure for the staining of acidic polysaccharides by Muller's colloidal (hydrous) ferric oxide and its combination with the Feulgen and the periodic acid–Schiff reactions. Laboratory Investigation 7:566–576.

Mowry R.W. (1963) The special value of methods that color both acidic and vicinal hydroxyl groups in the histochemical study of mucins, with revised directions for the colloidal iron stain, and the use of alcian blue 8GX and their combinations with the periodic acid–Schiff reaction. Annals of the New York Academy of Sciences 106:402–423.

Mowry R.W. (1978) Aldehyde fuchsin staining, direct or after oxidation: problems and remedies with special reference to human pancreatic β cells, pituitaries and elastic fibers. Stain Technology 53:141–154.

Muller G. (1946) Über eine vereinfachung der reaction nach Hale. Acta Histochemie 2:68–70.

Muller G. (1955) [Simplification of the reaction after Hale (1946).] Acta Histochemica 2:68–70.

Pearse A.G.E. (1960) Histochemistry, theoretical and applied. Boston: Little, Brown.

Perez-Vilar J., Hill R.L. (1999) The structure and assembly of secreted mucins. Journal of Biological Chemistry 274:31751–31754.

Quintarelli G., Scott J.E., Dellovo M.C. (1964) The chemical and histochemical properties of alcian blue II. Dye binding of tissue polyanions. Histochemie 4:86–98.

Ravetto C. (1968) Histochemical identification of N-acetyl-O-diacetylneuraminic acid resistant to neuraminidase. Journal of Histochemistry and Cytochemistry 16:663.

Rinehart J.F., Abul-Haj S.K. (1951) Improved method for histochemical demonstration of acid mucopolysaccharides in tissues. Archives of Pathology 52:189–194.

Ro J.Y., Amin M.B., Sahin A.A., Ayala A.G. (2000) Tumors and tumorous conditions of the male genital urinary tract. In: Fletcher C.D.M., ed. Diagnostic histopathology of tumors. New York: Churchill Livingstone, pp. 733–838.

Roberts G.P. (1977) Histochemical detection of sialic acid residues using periodate oxidation. Histochemical Journal 9:97–102.

Roden L. (1980) Structure and metabolism of connective tissue proteoglycans. In: Lennarz W.J., ed. The biochemistry of glycoproteins and proteoglycans. New York: Plenum Press, pp. 267–371.

Schauer R. (1982) Sialic acids: chemistry, metabolism and function. Cell Biology Monographs, Vol. 10, New York: Springer-Verlag.

Schroeder J.A., Thompson M.C., Mockenstrum Gardner M., Gendler S.J. (2001) Transgenic MUC1 interacts with epidermal growth factor receptor and correlates with mitogen-activated protein kinase activation in the mouse mammary gland. Journal of Biological Chemistry 276:13057–13064.

Scott H.R., Clayton B.P. (1953) A comparison of the staining affinities of aldehyde–fuchsin and the Schiff reagent. Journal of Histochemistry and Cytochemistry 1:336–352.

Scott J.E., Dorling J. (1965) Differential staining of acid glycosaminoglycans (mucopolysaccharides) by alcian blue in salt solutions. Histochemie 5:221–233.

Scott J.E., Harbinson R.J. (1969) Periodate oxidation of acid polysaccharides. II Rates of oxidation of uronic acids in polyuronides and acid mucopolysaccharides. Histochemie 19:155–161.

Scott J.E., Mowry R.W. (1970) Alcian blue: a consumer's guide. Journal of Histochemistry and Cytochemistry 18:842.

Scott J.E., Quintarelli G., Dellovo M.C. (1964) The chemical and histochemical properties of alcian blue. I. The mechanism of alcian blue staining. Histochemie 4:73–85.

Sharon N., Lis H. (1972) Lectins: cell-agglutinating and sugar-specific proteins. Science 177:949–959.

Sorvari T.E. (1972) Histochemical observations on the role of ferric chloride in the high iron diamine technique for localizing sulfated mucosubstances. Histochemical Journal 4:193–204.

Sorvari T., Sorvari R.M. (1969) The specificity of alcian blue pH 1.0–alcian yellow pH 2.5 staining in the histochemical differentiation of acid groups in mucosubstances. Journal of Histochemistry and Cytochemistry 17:291–293.

Southgate H.W. (1927) Note on preparing mucicarmine. Journal of Pathology and Bacteriology 30:729.

Spicer S.S. (1960) A correlative study of the histochemical properties of rodent acid mucopolysaccharides. Journal of Histochemistry and Cytochemistry 8:18–35.

Spicer S.S. (1961) The use of cationic reagents in the histochemical differention of mucopolysaccharides. American Journal of Clinical Pathology 36:393–407.

Spicer S.S. (1965) Diamine methods for differentiating mucosubstances histochemically. Journal of Histochemistry and Cytochemistry 13:211–234.

Spicer S.S., Lillie R.D. (1959) Saponification as a means of selectively reversing the methylation blockade of tissue basophilia. Journal of Histochemistry and Cytochemistry 7:123–125.

Spicer S.S., Meyer D.B. (1960) Histochemical differentiation of acid mucopolysaccharides by means of combined aldehyde fuchsin–alcian blue staining. American Journal of Clinical Pathology 33:453–460.

Spicer S.S., Schulte B.A. (1992) Diversity of cell glycoconjugates shown histochemically: a perspective. Journal of Histochemistry and Cytochemistry 40:1–38.

Spicer S.S., Warren L. (1959) The histochemistry of sialic acid mucoproteins. Journal of Histochemistry and Cytochemistry 8:135–137.

Sylven B. (1954) Metachromatic dye–substrate interactions. Quarterly Journal of Microbiological Science 95:327–358.

Thompson S.W. (1966) Selected histochemical and histopathological methods. Springfield, IL: Charse C. Thomas.

Tighe J.R. (1963) The histological demonstration of mucopolysaccharides in connective-tissue tumors. Journal of Pathology and Bacteriology 86:141–149.

Tonna E.A., Cronkite E.P. (1959) Histochemical and autoradiographic studies on the effects of aging on the mucopolysaccharides of the periosteum. Journal of Biophyscial and Biochemical Cytology 6:171–178.

Turani H., Lurie B., Chaimoff C., Kessler E. (1986) The diagnostic significance of sulfated acid mucin content in gastric intestinal metaplasia with early gastric cancer. American Journal of Gastroenterology 81:343–345.

Varki A, Cummings R., Esko J. et al., eds. (1999) Essentials of glycobiology. Cold Spring Harbor, NY: Cold Spring Harbor Laboratory Press.

Walker R.A. (1985) *Ulex europeus* I-peroxidase as a marker of vascular endothelium: its application in routine histopathology. Journal of Pathology 146:123–127.

Weiss S.W., Goldblum J.R. (2001) Enzinger and Weiss's soft tissue tumors, 4th edn. St. Louis, MO: Mosby.

Wesseling J., van der Valk S.W., Vos H.L., Sonnenberg A. (1995) Episialin (MUC1) overexpression inhibits integrin-mediated cell adhesion to extracellular matrix components. Journal of Cell Biology 129:255–265.

Woodman A.C., Sugiyama M., Yoshida K. et al. (1996) Analysis of anomalous CD44 gene expression in human breast, bladder and colon cancer and correlation of observed mRNA and protein isoforms. American Journal of Pathology 149:1519–1530.

Yamabayashi S. (1987) Periodic acid–Schiff–alcian blue: a method for the differential staining of glycoproteins. Histochemical Journal 19:565–571.

FURTHER READING

Johnson W.C., Helwig E.B. (1963) Histochemistry of primary and metastatic mucus-secreting tumors. Annals of the New York Academy of Sciences 106:794–803.

12

Lipids

M. Lamar Jones

INTRODUCTION

Lipid comes from the Greek word *lipos* meaning fat. Lipids may be defined as any one of a group of fats or fat-like substances characterized by their insolubility in water. These fats would include:

- true fats—esters of fatty acids and glycerol
- lipids—phospholipids, cerebrosides, and waxes
- sterols—cholesterol and ergosterol
- hydrocarbons—squalene and carotene.

An ester is a fragrant compound formed by the reaction of an acid and an alcohol or phenol without water. Lipids have a vital role in the normal cell membrane, myelin, hormones, and secretions. The need to demonstrate lipids is important when they appear abnormal or fail to appear at all. Histochemical techniques are the most common method of choice for properly demonstrating lipids in tissue sections and cytological preparations. Ideally, histochemistry should be utilized with other techniques such as biochemistry and chromatography to demonstrate the exact nature of the lipid identified microscopically and then possibly quantified.

Not all lipids resemble fats. For example, free cholesterol with its melting point of 144°C is crystalline, and some of the phospholipids and gangliosides are even water soluble. Lovern's 1955 definition that lipids are 'actual or potential derivatives of free fatty acids and their metabolites' still holds true today.

Müller first demonstrated lipids in tissue sections in 1859 and a wide variety of fat stains, the Sudan dyes, have been utilized in histology since 1896. Today a panel of histochemical techniques is available to portray each group of lipids. This is an important step in the diagnosis of certain pathological conditions such as the disorders of lipid metabolism.

Classification

Lipids may be classified as a mixed group of substances with the common characteristics of solubility in organic solvents. Formaldehyde and formalin will fix most lipids and fats, but extended storage in these solutions may remove or alter some of the lipids. They can be classified as simple lipids, compound lipids, or derived lipids.

- *Simple lipids*: esters of fatty acids with alcohols, which include fats, oils, and waxes. Fats are neutral esters of glycerol with saturated or unsaturated fatty acids. Oils may be similar to fats but are liquid at room temperature. Waxes are esters of higher alcohols with long-chain fatty acids. Simple lipids are usually found in the body as energy stores in adipose tissue. Waxes are usually found in plant and animal species.
- *Compound lipids*: usually consist of a fatty acid, an alcohol, and one or more other groups such as phosphorus or nitrogen. These can be formed in the brain and central nervous system.
- *Derived lipids*: fatty acids that can originate from the simple and compound lipids by means of hydrolysis. Cholesterol, bile acids, and sex and adrenocortical hormones are examples.

Lipids can and do occur in cells in the form of droplets or bound to other tissue entities. Free lipid droplets can be demonstrated by standard procedures, but exposure to alcohols, acetone, chloroform, xylene, and paraffin will destroy them. Frozen sections best demonstrate simple fats. Some lipids such as phospholipids, lipofuscins, and granules of leukocytes can bind to other tissue elements

187

or entities and resist paraffin processing. These lipids must be fixed in neutral buffered formalin. For phospholipids, formal calcium is the fixative of choice. Chemical procedures utilizing oxidation or mordanting techniques or the Sudan dyes will demonstrate these types of lipid. Fixation of lipids will be discussed in greater detail later in this chapter. Table 12.1 outlines a simple classification of lipids with certain characteristics and properties for their identification.

Physicochemical properties

The physical state of a particular lipid is necessary in determining its behavior in the staining reactions to be described. Those lipids with a melting point below staining temperature can be demonstrated with the 'fat stains', an important group of organotropic Sudan dyes. Those that are not 'fatty' require other methods for their detection and identification. The melting point of a lipid

Table 12.1 Classification of lipids		
Class	Member	Features influencing histochemistry
NON-POLAR LIPIDS		
1. Unconjugated lipids	Fatty acids	Melting point and sudanophilia depend on number of double bonds. HYDROPHOBIC.
	Cholesterol	Melting point 144°C, therefore not sudanophilic at room temperature. Birefringent in polarized light. HYDROPHOBIC.
2. Esters	Cholesteryl esters, mono-, di-, and triglycerides	Melting point depends upon degree of saturation of constituent fatty acids. HYDROPHOBIC.
	Waxes	
POLAR LIPIDS		
1. Phospholipids		
Glycerol-based		Phospholipids contain phosphoric acid, long-chain fatty acids, polyhydric alcohols, and variable nitrogenous bases. HYDROPHILIC
	Phosphatidyl choline (lecithins)	Fatty acids linked to glycerol with an ester bond which is alkaline-labile. Contain choline. BASIC.
	Phosphatidyl serine	Ester bond. ACIDIC.
	Phosphatidyl ethanolamine (cephalins)	Ester bond. BASIC.
	Plasmalogens (mainly phosphatidyl ethanolamine-based)	Ester and ether bonds. BASIC.
Sphingosine-based	Sphingomyelins	One saturated fatty acid linked to sphingosine by an alkaline-resistant amide bond (ceramide) plus phosphoryl choline. BASIC.
2. Glycolipids	Cerebrosides	Cerebrosides contain a hexose linked to ceramide, usually glucose, but galactose in mammalian brain cerebrosides. NEUTRAL.
	Sulfatides	Sulfate esters of cerebrosides. HIGHLY ACIDIC.
	Gangliosides	Contain N-acetyl neuraminic acid (sialic acid). Water-soluble unless complexed with protein and/or phospholipids. ACIDIC.

is related inversely to the chain length of its constituent fatty acids.

Perhaps the most useful distinction from the histochemical viewpoint is between hydrophobic and hydrophilic lipids. The surface properties of lipids will determine their permeability either to aqueous reagents or to organic solvents. Phospholipids contain polar phosphoryl and basic groups which make these lipids *hydrophilic* (water-miscible). Acidic glycolipids (gangliosides and sulfatides) and neutral glycolipids (the cerebrosides) are also moderately hydrophilic. Unconjugated lipids (cholesterol and free fatty acids) and simple esters have a preponderance of non-polar groups, and these lipids are *hydrophobic*. That means that their surface tension at a lipid–water interface makes them assume a globular shape in aqueous solution. They are impermeable to aqueous reagents, but have an affinity for organotropic dyes. This important distinction between hydrophobic and hydrophilic lipids is a useful factor in several of the histochemical reactions, as well as most of the histophysical techniques to be described below.

The physical state of a lipid can be modified by admixture of other lipids. Lipid mixtures do not necessarily conform to the characteristic 'rules' of pure lipids. Much of the lipid in mammalian tissues is bound by protein or polysaccharide, or dispersed by surface-active phospholipids. Some proteins have a mainly hydrophobic composition, and behave as if they are lipids but without any lipid component. These are known as *proteolipids*. Other proteolipids have a lipid component. Lipoproteins resemble proteins but also contain a lipid which can be revealed after removal of complexed protein by proteolytic enzymes (Adams & Tuqan 1961). Such lipoprotein usually survives paraffin embedding.

Fixation

The most common method of demonstrating tissue lipids is with fresh frozen (cryostat) sections. Some degree of fixation may be necessary so that lipids and the sections themselves are able to withstand the potentially destructive or solvent effects of histochemical reagents. Ideally a fixative should protect tissues against bacterial putrefaction and autolysis without altering the reactive groups of the compounds to be demonstrated microscopically. The only reagents that truly fix lipids are osmium tetroxide and chromic acid, but both these greatly alter the chemical reactivity of the lipids. Formal calcium is the choice of fixative for lipid histochemistry and is prepared by adding 2% calcium acetate to 10% formalin. Although lipids are not strictly fixed by formaldehyde, they are better retained in a section when the supporting matrix of tissue proteins has been fixed.

Formaldehyde can chemically alter certain lipids (Brante 1949; Heslinga & Deierkauf 1961, 1962; Deierkauf & Heslinga 1962; Jones 1969), notably lecithins and plasmalogens which are slowly degraded to their water-soluble derivatives. Fortunately, the latter can be demonstrated in unfixed sections because the initial stage in the staining techniques for plasmalogens is mercuric chloride hydrolysis, and mercury salts act as fixatives in their own right. Formalin has little effect upon neutral lipids, although they may crystallize during prolonged immersion in this fixative (Hirsch & Peiffer 1957; Baker 1958) and lose their original physical characteristics.

In spite of the adverse effects of long formalin fixation, when such material is the only source available it is still worthwhile examining such a sample to determine the lipid composition. Indeed, a museum specimen of one of Richard Bright's original kidneys, removed at autopsy over 150 years ago, has been sectioned and stained successfully with Oil red O. Lipid deposits in the tubular epithelium in this, the first case of Bright's disease to be described, were clearly displayed microscopically.

Since formalin can become oxidized to formic acid during prolonged storage, it is advisable to buffer the fixative solution so that an acid medium conducive to lipid hydrolysis can be avoided. Lillie (1954) regarded calcium acetate as being as efficient as phosphate buffer in maintaining the neutrality of formalin. The calcium is a desirable additive for another reason. Baker (1944) showed that phospholipids are protected by the addition of calcium and cadmium ions by forming a lattice of complex coacervates of phospholipids with proteins or mucins. Baker used 1% calcium chloride, but Lillie's 2% calcium acetate also acts as a buffer and is recommended. Wolman and Weiner (1965) have confirmed that calcium ions reduce the solubility of myelin lipids whereas a high concentration of monovalent cations, such as sodium, actually enhances their solubility. Regular formal saline should therefore be avoided when dealing with any material which may require examination for lipids. It is important to note that calcium ions will saponify free fatty acids to acetone-insoluble soaps.

The effects of different fixatives on myelin lipids over different periods have been described (Bayliss 1972). Rat brain sections were stained with selected histochemical techniques after intervals in different fixatives. The staining intensity of myelin was compared microdensitometrically. The best general lipid fixative appeared to be Baker's calcium–cadmium–formal but the optimal fixation time varies for the different lipid classes. Unfortunately, there is no single mode of fixation for all lipids and methods. The aim is to achieve the best compromise between the maximum preservation of tissue architecture and minimum alteration in the lipids themselves.

Ideally, when any histochemistry is likely to be needed in diagnosis, fresh frozen material will give the best results, not only for enzyme and carbohydrate studies but also for lipid studies. Where fixation is helpful, postfixation of cryostat sections will suffice. The length of fixation will depend on the severity of the method and the nature of the lipid to be demonstrated. Table 12.2 gives guidelines for fixation for the various methods outlined in this chapter.

Table 12.2 Fixation protocol for lipid histochemistry

Lipid type	Method	Fixation
Fats	Oil red O*, Sudan black*	None, or short or long FC
All lipids	Bromine Sudan black (R)	None, or short or long FC
Plasmalogens (mainly phosphatidyl ethanolamine)	Plasmal reaction (R)	None
Unsaturated lipids	UV–Schiff (R)	None
Lipofuscins	Sudan black*, Autofluorescence*	None, or any
Phospholipids (including fats and fatty acids)	Nile blue sulfate (R)	None, or short FC
Phospholipids (all)	Ferric hematoxylin*, dichromate–acid hematein (R)	None, or short FC
Sphingomyelin	Ferric hematoxylin* or dichromate–acid hematein, after alkaline hydrolysis	Short or long FC
Fatty acids	Copper–rubeanic acid*, copper–pDMAB–rhodanine*	Short FC
Sulfatides	Toluidine blue/acetone*, acriflavine–DMAB (R)	Short or long FC
Gangliosides	PAS*, dilute PA–Schiff (R), borohydride–PAS (R)	None, or short or long FC
Cerebrosides	PAS*, modified PAS (R)	None, or short or long FC
Cholesterol (free)	Filipin*	None, or short or long FC
Cholesterol and/or esters	Schultz, PAN	FC, longer rather than shorter
Triglycerides	Calcium–lipase (R)	FC, longer better than shorter
Phosphoglycerides (lecithins and cephalins)	Gold hydroxamate (R)	FC, longer is better for the section, worse for the phosphoglycerides

FC, formal calcium; R, research method; *indicates preferred method; pDMAB, p-dimethylaminobenzaldehyde; PAN, perchloric acid naphthoquinone.

Microtomy

Frozen or cryostat sections are required for lipid histochemistry because routine processing for paraffin and resin sections will result in the extraction of all but a few protein-bound lipids from the tissue. Unfixed, well frozen cryostat sections will have a morphological appearance that is at least as good as that of a routine paraffin section. Cryostat sections mounted directly onto slides are treated as indicated for the techniques to be described. Formal-calcium-fixed blocks of tissue are also suitable for the cryostat but it is advisable to mount these sections onto slides that have been coated with chrome-gelatin, since the adhesive properties of the endogenous tissue proteins will have been destroyed by fixation. For some techniques, the unfixed cryostat sections may also need mounting on chrome-gelatin slides. 'Positively charged' slides also work well with frozen sections.

Control sections

Control sections are as important in lipid histochemistry as in other histochemical methods, to exclude interference from cross-reacting non-lipid compounds (negative controls) and to verify the lipidic nature of the stained material. It may be helpful to run a known 'positive' control section with all methods, if possible, particularly if the method is not used frequently. Most tissues contain some fat that could be used as an internal control.

Negative controls

De-lipidized sections should be included routinely in parallel with normal sections for all methods, particularly when the method is being set up. In normal histopathological practice, unless some most unusual reactions are found, this step is usually unnecessary. Lipids are deliberately extracted from the control section so that the reaction product under consideration in the untreated section can be attributed to lipid, or alternatively to any interfering non-lipid groups.

Delipidization

Lipids can be totally extracted with chloroform : methanol (2 : 1; v : v) if 1% hydrochloric acid is included in the solvent to release bound lipids. The addition of 4% water

is believed to facilitate the extraction of phospholipids. A general lipid solvent is composed of:

Chloroform	66 ml
Methanol	33 ml
Distilled water	4 ml
Conc. HCl	1 ml

It is used at room temperature for 1 hour.

At one time it was thought to be feasible to identify individual lipids by their differential solubilities in organic solvents (Churukin & Ciaccio 1910; Keilig 1944; Ueda 1952). However, such procedures are strictly limited; methods that can be used in the test tube are not always adaptable to tissue sections (Lison 1936; Lovern 1955), since the solubility characteristics of bound or mixed lipids do not necessarily resemble those of the pure isolated compounds. Protein-bound lipids will resist extraction until unmasked by saline (Holczinger & Bálint 1961) or proteolytic enzymes (Adams & Tuqan 1961; Adams & Bayliss 1962; Wolman 1962; Maggi & Brander 1963). Acidified solvents are used to disrupt lipoprotein bonds but the simultaneous extraction of calcium deposits should not be overlooked during techniques in which calcium salts react identically with lipids.

Any type of fixation will modify lipid extraction (Brante 1949; Edgar & Donker 1957; Pearse 1968). Prolonged exposure to formalin may induce irreversible polymerization of free fatty acids (Jones 1969). When calcium is included in the fixative, the fatty acid soaps thus formed will be insoluble in acetone and therefore require a preliminary stage of desaponification if sections are to be acetone extracted (Archibald & Orton 1970; Elleder & Lojda 1971).

Acetone extraction

Acetone has been widely used for the selective removal of hydrophobic lipids, but Elleder and Lojda (1971) showed that the water content of commercial acetone is sufficient to extract a significant amount of phosphoglycerides. They suggest treating dry sections for 20 minutes with anhydrous acetone (dried over anhydrous calcium chloride) at 48°C to selectively remove fats and cholesterol, leaving the acetone-insoluble phospholipids intact. It will be seen that this maneuver can be exploited to make certain histochemical methods selective for phospholipids. Dunnigan's (1968) modification of the Nile blue sulfate technique, for example, relies upon acetone to remove hydrophobic lipids so that staining is confined to phospholipids. Likewise the bromine–Sudan black B method can include an acetone-extracted section in which phospholipids are selectively demonstrated (Bayliss High 1981).

Positive controls

Control material for individual lipid staining methods can be obtained only rarely from known cases of the lipid storage disorders, so whenever such material does become available at biopsy or autopsy, some should be stored at −70°C for this purpose. Pure samples of most lipids are commercially available and can be applied to filter paper, which can then be treated as a tissue section in the relevant technique. This system has been used to validate the histochemical methods described in this chapter.

Alternatively, lipids can be suspended in a solution of gelatin, allowed to set, fixed, and a block prepared for the cryostat to be sectioned and treated as control material (Gillian Lewis, personal communication). Multiple sections can be conventionally prepared from a composite block, and stored at −20°C to provide a reserve of control sections containing a variety of lipid components (Table 12.3).

HISTOPHYSICAL METHODS

Differences in the physical properties of lipids allow microscopic discrimination between certain lipid classes, for example between crystalline and liquid lipids and between hydrophobic and hydrophilic types.

Birefringence of lipids

Lison (1936) pointed out that lipids cannot be identified solely by means of their optical properties. Nevertheless,

Table 12.3 Control sections	
Suggested composite block	To demonstrate
Fatty liver	Triglycerides and free fatty acids
Adrenal, atheromatous artery	Free and esterified cholesterol
Brain	Myelin phospholipids

it is always helpful to view an Oil red O-stained section in polarized light with partly crossed polars, to distinguish fatty droplets that are stained and are non-birefringent (isotropic) from crystalline lipids which remain unstained but appear anisotropic (birefringent). Clearly, the melting point of a lipid determines its appearance in polarized light, but in practice the birefringent lipids found in mammalian tissues are usually free cholesterol or its crystalline esters (Adams & Bayliss 1974).

Polarizing microscopy has also been used to distinguish between glycerol esters (the so-called neutral fats, mainly triglycerides) and cholesteryl esters. Both groups stain identically with the Sudan dyes but the cholesteryl esters in fresh tissue display, unless in crystalline form, a distinctive type of double refraction in polarized light (Hirsch & Peiffer 1957). This 'Maltese cross' birefringence (conic focal anisotropism) is due to the liquid–crystalline structure of the esters, and this physical state is usually due to the admixture of phospholipids and is influenced by temperature, fixation, and the presence of water (Weller 1967). Glycerol esters, on the other hand, never show Maltese cross birefringence; they are either liquid and isotropic, or crystalline with normal birefringence if they are more saturated lipids. However, in pathology it should be remembered that mixtures of lipids are usually present, and mixtures may not abide by the rules outlined above. It should also be kept in mind that certain non-lipid structures such as amyloid (see Chapter 15) and glove powder (starch) can also appear birefringent.

Fat stains and the Sudan dyes

Lipids that exist as fats, namely the oily and greasy hydrophobic lipids, have an affinity for the Sudan dyes. For many years a wide range of these compounds has provided almost the sole means of staining lipids, and some of these dyes are used to this day. It has been generally assumed that Sudan staining is a simple physical process, in that the dyes are more soluble in tissue fats than in their dye solvents. However, there is some evidence that staining may be by a process of adsorption (Meier 1959). The in vitro experiments of Holczinger and Bálint (1962) support this view and show that, in the case of Sudan black, the adsorbing power of fats is related to the dye concentration, temperature, and the physical state of the fats, maximal dye uptake occurring around its melting point. Therefore, only lipids that are liquid or semi-liquid at staining temperature will be stained; those in the solid or crystalline state remain unaffected.

The first Sudan dye to be introduced into histochemistry was Sudan III (Daddi 1896) but Michaelis (1901) preferred the darker staining Sudan IV. Oil red O (French 1926) is even more intensely stained and is generally preferred to the other red dyes. The most sensitive and versatile of all these dyes is Sudan black B, which was introduced by Lison and Dagnelie in 1935. In order to penetrate fats the Sudans must be dissolved in organic solvents, although the solvent vehicle should be sufficiently dilute (aqueous) to avoid extracting the lipids themselves. Various solvents have been advocated, notably isopropanol (Lillie & Ashburn 1943), triethyl phosphate (Gomori 1952), and propylene glycol (Callis et al 1951), whilst Govan (1944) prepared a colloidal suspension of the dye in an aqueous, acidified gelatin solution, to avoid the solvent action of organic reagents altogether.

For general use, 70% ethanol is an adequate solvent for Oil red O and Sudan black. For particular studies propylene glycol is preferred, since the dye can be extracted from the stained lipid by propylene glycol without dissolving the lipid, thus allowing the lipid to be re-stained. This procedure is useful where lipid mixtures are present and lipid deposition is confined to a few cells. With 70% ethanol as solvent, some neutral lipid may be lost during staining, but this loss is minor and does not affect fine localization. Unlike the other Sudan dyes, Sudan black B stains phospholipids as well as neutral fats. Lansink (1968), with chromatography and infrared spectroscopy, demonstrated two distinct fractions in this dye; the first stains neutral fats blue–black, while the second fraction, a basic dye, stains phospholipids gray. This gray reaction can be enhanced as a bronze dichroism if the section is viewed in polarized light (Diezel 1958). Lipofuscin and proteolipids are also stained gray, but show no birefringence.

Sudan black B fails to stain crystalline cholesterol, and lecithins and free fatty acids tend to be soluble in the ethanolic dye bath. These drawbacks can be overcome if bromine pre-treatment is included in the staining procedure.

Lillie (1954) had used bromine to render unsaturated lipids insoluble in organic solvents. This was applied to the Sudan black method by Bayliss and Adams (1972), who discovered that fatty acids and phosphoglycerides were retained in the tissue section during staining but free cholesterol was also sudanophilic. Bromine converts

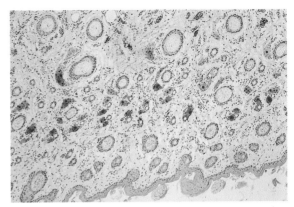

Fig. 12.1 Oil Red O method on a cryostat section of skin demonstrating lipid droplet macrophages. (Courtesy of Ms Gayle M. Callis, Montana State University, USA.)

crystalline cholesterol to derivatives that are oily at room temperature and hence permeable to the Sudan dye. The bromine–Sudan black B procedure can therefore provide a simple, sensitive method for detecting all of the main lipid classes. If a stage of acetone extraction is interposed between bromination and staining, only the acetone-resistant phospholipids remain in the section to be demonstrated by Sudan black B (Bayliss High 1981). For general localization of fats it is better to use Oil red O followed by a nuclear stain (Fig. 12.1) and, if the section can be viewed with partly crossed polars after staining with Oil red O, the distribution of unstained, birefringent cholesterol can be appreciated. Histophysical and histochemical staining methods for fats and lipids can be broadly divided into two groups: firstly those that are of general everyday use, and secondly those that are better suited to research applications. These are designated 'routine' and 'research' respectively in the methods that follow.

Oil red O in dextrin (modified by Churukian 2000)

Fixation
Fresh frozen or neutral buffered formaldehyde (NBF), rinse, frozen.

Sections
5-μm mount on SuperFrost/Plus slides, air dry.

Solutions

Oil red O solution

Oil red O	0.5 g
Absolute isopropyl alcohol	100 ml

Allow to stand overnight.

Dextrin solution

*Dextrin	1 g
Distilled water	100 ml

Working solution

Stock Oil red O	60 ml
Dextrin	40 ml

or

Oil red O solution

Oil red O	0.9 g
Absolute isopropyl alcohol	180 ml

Stir and leave overnight.

Dextrin solution

Dextrin	1.2 g
Distilled water	120 ml

Working solution

Oil red O solution	180 ml
Dextrin solution	120 ml

Allow to stand for a day or more. Stable for months, filter before use.

Method

1. Place slides directly into filtered 0.5% Oil red O in dextrin. Stain for 20 minutes, rinse with running water briefly.
2. Counterstain with Gill II hematoxylin for 20–30 seconds. Rinse with water, blue, coverslip with aqueous mounting media.

Results

Fat	brilliant red
Nuclei	blue

*Dextrin, bacteriological grade or Type III from Sigma, from corn. Dextrin is hydrolyzed corn starch. VWR (VWR Scientific) also has small quantities; must be most soluble form of dextrin.

Standard Sudan black B method for fats and phospholipids

Fixation and sections

Cryostat sections post-fixed in formal calcium; short-fixed frozen sections; unfixed cryostat sections (preferred).

Method

1. Rinse sections in 70% ethanol.
2. Stain for up to 2 hours in saturated Sudan black B in 70% ethanol.
3. Rinse in 70% ethanol to remove excess surface dye, and wash in tap water.
4. Counterstain nuclei with Kernechtrot for 2–5 minutes.
5. Wash well and mount in glycerin jelly.

Results

The standard Sudan black procedure stains unsaturated esters and triglycerides *blue–black*. Some phospholipids appear *gray* and those in myelin exhibit a *bronze* dichroism in polarized light.

Bromination enhances the reaction of these lipids and in addition stains lecithin, free fatty acids, and free cholesterol.

Note

The Sudan black solution should not be oversaturated or sections will be covered in a fine deposit. Fixation enhances the staining of phospholipids (present in all tissues) and this is unwanted in general use; thus unfixed sections are preferred.

Bromine Sudan black method for lipids
(Bayliss & Adams 1972)

Fixation and sections

Cryostat sections post-fixed for 1 hour in formal calcium; short-fixed frozen sections.

Method

1. Mount sections onto slides and allow to dry.
2. Immerse sections in 2.5% aqueous bromine for 30 minutes at room temperature, inside a fume hood.
3. Wash in water and treat with 0.5% sodium metabisulfite for 1 minute to remove excess bromine.
4. Wash thoroughly in distilled water and treat, together with an un-brominated section, for the standard Sudan black method.

Bromine–acetone–Sudan black method for phospholipids (research) (Bayliss High 1981)

1. Treat sections with 2.5% aqueous bromine for 30 minutes at room temperature inside a fume cupboard.
2. Wash well and remove excess bromine with 0.5% sodium metabisulfite for 1 minute.
3. Wash thoroughly and allow slides to dry.
4. Extract neutral lipids with anhydrous acetone for 20 minutes at 48°C.
5. Proceed with the standard Sudan black method outlined above.

Results

Phospholipids	gray
Sphingomyelin	bronze in polarized light

A major advance in lipid histochemistry was the introduction of the dye Nile blue sulfate (Smith 1908) in the first method for differentiating two lipid classes simultaneously. Lison (1936) showed that the dye comprises two components: a red *oxazone* which dissolves in neutral lipids, and a blue *oxazine* which is basic and reacts with phospholipids and free fatty acids. Although the staining of fatty acids has been reported to vary between these two colors (Adams 1965; Dunnigan 1968; Bayliss High 1970), Smith had originally demonstrated that in a concentrated dye solution the oxazone will stain fatty acids more rapidly than the blue oxazine is able to complete its reaction with their carbonyl groups; thus a red color predominates. However, if the dye solution is dilute (Cain 1947), so that the oxazone is relatively insoluble, the blue staining of fatty acids is encouraged. Lillie (1965) used the dye at pH 0.9 in order to suppress binding by phosphoric acid radicals and thereby enable fatty acids to be selectively stained. Nevertheless, on paper, some phospholipids continue to stain strongly, even under these conditions. Interference from non-lipid structures is reduced by employing an acid-hydrolyzed dye solution.

Nile blue sulfate can be used as a preliminary indicator of the type of lipid present in the tissue section. In practice, lipid mixtures tend to be stained an intermediate purple color so that a more useful application of this dye lies in Dunnigan's (1968) modification of Menschik's (1953) idea, whereby fatty acids are first extracted with acetone so the Nile blue sulfate staining will subsequently be confined to phospholipids. The acetone will fail to extract any fatty acids in this procedure if tissues have been fixed in formal calcium, since the calcium soaps of such fatty acids are insoluble and would interfere with the reaction of phospholipids, unless they have been converted into a soap beforehand.

Nile blue sulfate method for acidic and neutral lipids (after Cain 1947; Dunnigan 1968)

Fixation and sections
Cryostat sections post-fixed for 1 hour in formal calcium; short-fixed frozen sections.

Preparation of stain
Add 10 ml of 1% H_2SO_4 to 200 ml 1% Nile blue sulfate in water. Boil under reflux for 2 hours. This solution should be at pH 2 so that non-lipid reaction is minimal.

Method
1. Dry sections onto slides.
2. Stain in the Nile blue sulfate solution at 60°C for 30 minutes.
3. Differentiate sections in 1% acetic acid for 1–2 minutes.
4. Wash well and counterstain nuclei with 1% chloroform-washed methyl green for 5 minutes.
5. Wash well and mount in glycerin jelly.

Results

Unsaturated hydrophobic lipids	pink
Free fatty acids	pink to blue
Phospholipids	blue

Acetone–Nile blue sulfate method for phospholipids (Dunnigan 1968)

Fixation and sections
As in methods above.

Method
1. Mount sections onto slides and leave until dry.
2. Treat with 1 M HCl for 1 hour to convert to calcium soaps of the free fatty acids.
3. Wash and dry sections.

4. Extract with acetone at 4°C for 20 minutes.
5. Dry sections rapidly and proceed as for previous method but counterstain nuclei with Kernechtrot instead of methyl green. Compare with a delipidized control section.

Results

Phospholipids	blue

HISTOCHEMICAL METHODS

Once the presence of lipid in a specimen has been found, specific histochemical procedures to determine its identity can be applied. A technique for the identification of an unknown lipid can be used, initially using a fat stain, which can be viewed in polarized light, and acetone extraction to indicate its physical state and major category. Often there are clues about the type of lipid to expect, according to the nature of the tissue received and the clinical history of the patient.

Unlike the fat stains described above, histochemical methods involve chemical reactions with specific groups, radicals, or bonds in the lipid molecule, taking advantage of any unique configuration that enables discrimination between close members of a lipid class. The value of such methods is sometimes limited by interference from non-lipid substances, hence the importance of control sections. The validity of 60 techniques has been assessed against samples of pure lipids spotted onto filter paper, as well as lipids in tissue sections themselves. Only about half of the methods tested were found to be reliable and sufficiently selective to be recommended (Table 12.4). The methods of choice for each lipid class will be given in detail below and other relevant techniques will be mentioned briefly.

Free fatty acids

Benda's (1900) observation that free fatty acids bind heavy metal ions to form soaps led Fischler (1904) to develop a technique whereby such copper soaps could be stained with Weigert's lithium hematoxylin. Okamoto et al (1944a,b) used dimethylaminobenzylidine rhodanine for the same purpose. Neither method is as specific as Holczinger's (1959) adaptation of this principle; he visualized the copper soaps with rubeanic acid, using EDTA to remove extraneous copper. However, if Okamato's

rhodanine reagent is used to stain the soaps formed by Holczinger's copper acetate procedure, it provides an equally specific and sensitive alternative to rubeanic acid with rather less 'background' staining and is compatible with a hematoxylin nuclear stain. Calcium and iron deposits will also base exchange with copper, but can be distinguished from lipid by their persistence in a delipidized control section. Their identity can be verified by extraction with either 1% hydrochloric acid (for calcium) or 5% oxalic acid (for iron salts).

Copper rubeanic acid method for free fatty acids (Holczinger 1959)

Fixation

Cryostat sections post-fixed in formal calcium; fixed frozen sections.

Method

1. Mount duplicate sections onto slides and air dry.
2. Treat with 1 M HCl for 1 hour at room temperature to desaponify calcium soaps.
3. Wash well in distilled water and dry in air.
4. Extract free fatty acids from one section with acetone at 4°C for 20 minutes and rapidly dry in air.
5. Immerse both sections in 0.005% cupric acetate for 3 hours.
6. Wash twice for 10 seconds with 0.1% EDTA adjusted to pH 7.0 with NaOH.
7. Wash thoroughly in distilled water.
8. Treat sections for 10 minutes with 0.1% rubeanic acid (dithiooxamide) in 70% ethanol, or treat sections for 18 hours with 0.025% p-dimethylaminobenzylidine rhodanine in 70% ethanol.
9. Rinse in 70% ethanol.
10. Counterstain nuclei with Kernechtrot (for rubeanic acid) or Carazzi's hematoxylin (for p-dimethylaminobenzylidine rhodanine).
11. Wash in water and mount in glycerin jelly.

Results

Free fatty acids—dark green (rubeanic acid) or red (p-dimethylaminobenzylidine rhodanine). This reaction should be absent from the acetone-extracted control. If cryostat sections are used, the extraction is best performed before post-fixation.

Table 12.4 Combination techniques

Method	Components	Color demonstrated
1. Dichromate acid hematein	Phospholipids (myelin)	Blue
Oil red O	Fats (degenerating myelin)	Red
Methyl green	Nuclei	Green
2. Solochrome cyanin	Myelin	Blue
Oil red O	Fats (degenerating myelin)	Red
3. Copper acetate rhodamine	Fatty acids	Red
Sudan black B	Neutral fats	Blue
Polarized light	Crystalline cholesterol	Birefringent
4. PAS	Glycolipids	Pink
Sudan black B	Neutral fats and myelin	Blue
5. β-galactosidase	Lysosomes	Turquoise
Oil red O	Fats	Red
6. Succinate dehydrogenase	Mitochondria	Blue
Oil red O	Fats	Red
Methyl green	Nuclei	Green
7. Esterase	Histiocytes and macrophages	Orange
Sudan black B	Neutral fats and myelin	Blue
Methyl green	Nuclei	Green
8. Acid phosphatase	Lysosomes	Red
Sudan black B	Neutral fats and myelin	Blue

Cholesterol

In 1924 Schultz adapted the Leibermann–Burchardt reaction to demonstrate cholesterol in tissue sections. Oxidation in air with iron alum is followed by treatment with a sulfuric–acetic acid mixture to give a blue color with free and esterified cholesterol. The method was improved somewhat by Lewis and Lobban (1961) but, even so, such destructive reagents produce distorted preparations with many gas bubbles, making localization difficult. Rousssouw et al (1976) overcame some of the technical problems associated with the classical Schultz procedure by using a 'pre-mixed' reagent which is a combination of ferric chloride and acetic, sulfuric, and phosphoric acids. An iodine–sulfuric acid technique was described by Okamoto et al (1944a,b) but the color is transient and partly masked by iodine.

Adams's percholoric acid–naphthoquinone (PAN) method (1961) depends on a different principle for cho-lesterol detection and is preferred for its sensitivity, precision, and more satisfactory tissue preservation. Perchloric acid is believed to condense cholesterol to cholesta-3,5-diene, which is then converted by 1,2-naphthoquinone to a blue pigment. Free cholesterol can, in theory, be differentiated from its esters by precipitation as its digitonide, unlike esters, is insoluble in acetone and can be subsequently visualized either with the Schultz reaction (Feigin 1956; Schnabel 1964) or preferably with the PAN method (Adams & Bayliss 1974). However, unless the initial fixation of the tissue block includes digitonin, the rate of digitonin–cholesterol complexing is slower than the rate of extraction of cholesterol into the solvent, and specificity may be compromised.

It should be stressed that the above-mentioned methods are ineffective unless cholesterol has been oxidized, either chemically with ferric salts or by long exposure to atmospheric oxygen. Commercial cholesterol that has been repurified through the dibromide according to the method of Fieser (1953) is completely unreactive with all of the aforementioned methods (Adams & Bayliss High 1980).

An interesting innovation in cholesterol histochemistry is an enzymatic method (Emeis et al 1977). This is a two-stage procedure in which esterified cholesterol is firstly hydrolyzed to its free sterol by means of a cholesterol esterase, then the cholesterol is oxidized by a cholesterol oxidase, releasing hydrogen peroxide, which reacts simultaneously with diaminobenzidine to produce an insoluble brown polymer at the site of cholesterol. The free sterol alone can be visualized by omitting the initial stage of ester hydrolysis. Cholesterol esters can be selectively demonstrated after any free cholesterol has been inactivated by preliminary exposure to the oxidase enzyme alone. Esterified cholesterol has also been detected enzymically with cholesterol esterase (Morii et al 1982) in a method that resembles the calcium lipase method for triglycerides. The practical value of these techniques is somewhat limited by their cost and complexity for routine light microscopy, although they have proved to be useful at the EM level (see later).

A more recent technique uses filipin, a compound similar to digitonin, that can be used in aqueous media to complex with free cholesterol to produce a highly fluorescent compound. This has been used to detect the accumulation of free cholesterol in cultured fibroblasts from Niemann–Pick disease type C. The method can also be applied to cryostat or frozen sections (Butler et al 1987).

Percholoric acid–naphthoquinone (PAN) method for cholesterol (Adams 1961)

Fixation and sections
Formal calcium fixed frozen section; cryostat sections post-fixed in formal calcium.

Preparation of reagent

1,2-naphthoquinone-4-sulfonic acid	40 mg
Ethanol	20 ml
60% perchloric acid	10 ml
40% formaldehyde	1 ml
Distilled water	9 ml

Mix and use within 24 hours.

Method
1. Air dry sections onto slides.
2. Treat with 1% ferric chloride for 4 hours.

3. Wash well in distilled water.
4. Carefully paint the sections sparingly with the reagent using a soft camel-hair brush. (Note: wash the brush thoroughly with water after each use, and dry.) Heat them on a surface at 70°C for 1 or 2 minutes, until the color develops. The sections are kept moist by gently replenishing the reagent from time to time.
5. Place a drop of perchloric acid on a cover glass and lower section into position.

Results

Cholesterol and related steroids	blue

The insert stain is stable for several hours. Cholesterol can be distinguished from its esters by the digitonin–PAN or filipin methods.

Filipin method for free cholesterol (Kruth & Vaughan 1980)

Fixation and sections
Cryostat sections, post-fixed; frozen sections of fixed tissue.

Preparation of reagent
Stock solution
2.5 mg filipin in 1 ml dimethylformamide
Staining solution

Filipin stock solution	0.2 ml
PBS (phosphate buffered saline)	10 ml

Method
1. Wash sections in PBS.
2. Stain for 30 minutes in filipin solution.
3. Wash in PBS (×2)
4. Mount in PBS or glycerin jelly.
5. Examine by fluorescence microscopy (excitation BG12 with 515 am barrier filter).

Results
Free cholesterol shows strong silvery fluorescence.

Digitonin–PAN method for free cholesterol (research) (Adams & Bayliss 1974, after Schnabel 1964)

Fixation
As for previous method.

Method

1. Dry sections onto slides.
2. Precipitate free cholesterol with 0.5% digitonin in 40% ethanol for 2 hours at room temperature.
3. Extract cholesterol esters with acetone for 1 hour at room temperature.
4. Proceed as for the PAN technique, described above.

Results

Free cholesterol   blue

Unsaturated lipids

The reactions of double bonds (ethylene groups) in fatty acid chains can be used to distinguish between saturated and unsaturated lipids. The ethylene groups can be oxidized to Schiff-stainable aldehydes by performic acid (Pearse 1951; Lillie 1952); however, performic acid is not only destructive to tissue sections but also acts as a solvent for some lipids (Bayliss High 1972). In addition, the basis of the reaction is in doubt and it should no longer be used in lipid histochemistry. As an alternative approach, bromination followed by silver nitrate causes silver bromide to be formed at the double bond and this is subsequently reduced to visible metallic silver (Mukherji et al 1960; Norton et al 1962). Belt and Hayes (1956) used ultraviolet light to oxidize double bonds to aldehydes for subsequent Schiff staining and their method provides a useful alternative to the osmium tetroxide technique (see below) since it avoids the use of toxic and expensive osmium.

Ultraviolet–Schiff method for unsaturated lipids (Belt & Hayes 1956)

Fixation and sections

Preferably unfixed cryostat sections; otherwise use short-fixed frozen sections.

Method

1. Mount sections onto slides and expose to a source of ultraviolet light for 2 hours.
2. Treat with Schiff's reagent (see p. 171) for 15 minutes, together with a non-irradiated control section to exclude non-lipid aldehydes.

3. Rinse in distilled water and wash well in tap water.
4. Mount sections in glycerin jelly.

Result

Unsaturated lipids   magenta

Osmium tetroxide is a more sensitive and reliable detector of unsaturated lipids and possibly demonstrates the double bonds in fatty acids stoichiometrically (Adams 1965). Korn (1967) has shown that the osmium reacts with unsaturated fatty acids to form bridged bis-osmates, as suggested by Wigglesworth (1957) and Baker (1958).

Osmium tetroxide method for unsaturated lipids

Fixation and sections

Preferably unfixed cryostat sections; otherwise use short-fixed frozen sections.

Method

1. Immerse sections in 1% aqueous OsO_4 for 1 hour at room temperature.
2. Wash well in distilled water and mount in glycerin jelly.

Results

Unsaturated lipids are stained *brown to black*. Saturated lipids and free cholesterol do not react.

Note

The osmium solution must be handled inside a fume hood to avoid the effect of its toxic vapor on the cornea and mucous membranes.

Osmium demonstrates unsaturated lipids in this way because it is reduced to its black lower oxide by fatty acid ethylene bonds. The main application that osmium has in lipid histochemistry stems from an observation by Marchi in 1886 that the addition of a polar electrolyte (such as a dichromate salt) to the osmium solution prevents the staining of normal myelin, and allows only the hydrophobic cholesterol esters of degenerating myelin to appear black. The classical Marchi method for the detection of demyelination suffers the practical limitation that whole tissue slices are subjected to lengthy osmication.

Adams (1959) overcame this problem when he adapted the Marchi method for microscopy in his osmium tetroxidenaphthylamine (OTAN) procedure, which demonstrated both normal and degenerating myelin in a single section.

Although the OTAN method can successfully be used to detect myelin breakdown, cholesterol esters in other sites, such as atheroma lipid deposits, appear orange rather than black; possibly a reflection of their physical state or melting point. Studies of the method (Adams & Bayliss 1968; Elleder & Lojda 1968a,b; Bayliss High 1972; Adams & Bayliss 1974) collectively suggest that the OTAN method should no longer be used for general histochemistry. In view of the cost and toxicity of the reagents employed, a suitable alternative method is described later for the demonstration of normal and degenerating myelin: namely the dichromate acid–hematein–Oil red O combination.

Triglycerides

Triglycerides lack a unique chemical group or physical characteristic whereby they can be selectively stained, so that it is hardly surprising that this was the last group of lipids for which a specific method was devised. Adams et al (1966) used a pancreatic lipase to hydrolyze triglycerides into their constituent fatty acids. In the presence of calcium, insoluble soaps were formed that could be visualized, after conversion to lead soaps, with ammonium sulfide. Pre-existing calcium and free fatty acids will react identically, but can be detected in a non-lipase treated control section. Provided the enzyme preparation is pure, this technique is highly specific for triglycerides, and has been adapted for electron histochemistry (Adams et al 1966).

Calcium lipase method for triglycerides
(Adams et al 1966)

Fixation and sections
Cryostat sections post-fixed in formal calcium; formal calcium-fixed frozen sections.

Preparation of incubating medium
Tris buffer at pH 8.0	15 ml
2% calcium chloride	10 ml

Distilled water	25 ml
Porcine pancreatic lipase	50 mg

Warm solution to 37°C and filter before use.

Method
1. Incubate free-floating frozen or slide-mounted cryostat sections in the lipase medium at 37°C for 3 hours.
2. Wash sections well and mount onto slides.
3. Treat with 1% lead nitrate for 15 minutes.
4. Wash thoroughly in several changes of distilled water.
5. Immerse for 10 seconds in dilute ammonium sulfide (3 drops to a Coplin jar of water).
6. Wash well, counterstain with Carazzi's hematoxylin or Mayer's hematoxylin for 3 minutes.
7. Wash in tap water, followed by a rinse in distilled water.
8. Mount sections in glycerin jelly.

For control sections, start at step 3.

Results
Triglycerides	brown

Notes
a. The lipase should be shown to be uncontaminated by other lipolytic enzymes by testing it against individual lipids spotted onto paper.
b. The reaction of calcium deposits and free fatty acids is distinguished from a true reaction by inspecting the control section.
c. If fatty acids are present in large amounts they can be selectively removed by preliminary potassium hydroxide–dioxane extraction (Archibald & Orton 1970).
d. Since lipolysis is confined to the water–fat interface, only the surface of large fat globules is stained.

Glycerol-based phospholipids (phosphoglycerides)

The hydroxamic acid technique (Adams & Davison 1959; Adams et al 1963; Gallyas 1963) is recommended for the selective demonstration of phosphoglycerides (lecithins and cephalins). Alkaline hydroxylamine converts their ester bonds to hydroxamic acids which reduce silver nitrate to visible metallic silver, finally stabilized by gold 'toning'. Hydrophobic lipid esters are unstained because they are impermeable to the aqueous reagents employed in this reaction. Theoretically, they would react if present in dispersed hydrophilic form, but could be distinguished from phosphoglycerides by their solubility in anhydrous acetone. Since alkaline hydroxylamine is destructive to tissues they must be adequately fixed but, because lecithin is particularly susceptible to formalin, fixation should be minimal.

Gold hydroxamic acid method for phosphoglycerides (Adams et al 1963)

Fixation and sections

Cryostat sections post-fixed for 1 hour in formal calcium; short-fixed frozen sections.

Preparation of reagents

a. *Hydroxylamine solution*

Hydroxylamine hydrochloride	2.5 g
Sodium hydroxide	6 g
Distilled water	100 ml

b. *Silver solution*

Silver nitrate	0.1 g
Ammonium nitrate	0.2 g
Distilled water	100 ml

Adjust pH to 7.8 with dilute sodium hydroxide.

Method

1. Treat free-floating frozen sections or slide-mounted cryostat section (see Note) in the hydroxylamine solution for 20 minutes.
2. Wash the sections thoroughly in three changes of distilled water, 5 minutes each change.
3. Immerse in the silver solution for 2 hours at room temperature.
4. Wash well, rinse in 1% acetic acid and again in distilled water.
5. 'Tone' the sections for 10 minutes with 0.2% yellow gold chloride.
6. Rinse in water.
7. Remove any unreduced silver by immersing in 5% sodium thiosulfate for 5 minutes.
8. Wash well, and mount sections onto slides.
9. Counterstain nuclei with 1% methyl green for 5 minutes.
10. Mount in glycerin jelly or dehydrate, clear, and mount sections in Canada balsam or synthetic resin.

Results

Phosphoglycerides (lecithins and cephalins)   purple

Note

Cryostat sections may become detached from slides. If this happens they can be processed free-floating thereafter, using a glass 'hockey stick' to transfer them gently from one solution to the next. Alternatively, attach sections to chrome-gelatin-subbed slides.

Plasmalogen phospholipids

Feulgen and Voit (1924) used mercuric chloride to hydrolyze the unsaturated ether bonds of plasmalogens to produce a Schiff-stainable aldehyde. There has been much controversy over this and allied plasmal reactions (Verne 1929; Gérard 1935; Lison 1936; Cain 1949a,b; Hayes 1949; Elleder & Lojda 1970). Cain's explanation that two simultaneous reactions are encountered is now generally accepted: one, the specific mercuric chloride–Schiff reaction of Feulgen, and the second being merely atmospheric oxidation of double bonds to produce 'pseudoplasmal' aldehydes.

Hayes's (1949) procedure is specific for plasmalogens on paper. The extent of any non-specific reaction can be assessed by comparison with a non-hydrolyzed control section, but in practice the problem of pseudoplasmals is circumvented by using fresh frozen cryostat sections without delay. Formalin fixation not only induces a strong pseudoplasmal reaction, but also progressively destroys plasmalogen phospholipids themselves. Fortunately, unfixed cryostat sections are perfectly suitable for this method because the initial treatment with mercuric chloride effectively fixes the tissue sections.

Plasmal reaction for plasmalogen phospholipids (after Hayes 1949)

Fixation and sections

Unfixed cryostat sections, stained as soon as possible after cutting.

Method

1. Air dry duplicate sections onto separate slides.
2. Hydrolyze one section in 2% mercuric chloride for 10 minutes.

3. Wash thoroughly in distilled water, three changes.
4. Stain both sections with Schiff's reagent for 10 minutes.
5. Rinse in distilled water and wash in running tap water for 10 minutes to develop the color.
6. Counterstain nuclei with Mayer's hematoxylin for 3 minutes.
7. Wash again in tap water, rinse in distilled water, and mount sections in glycerin jelly.

Results

Plasmalogen phospholipids (mainly phosphatidyl ethanolamine)—magenta.

Note

Any pseudoplasmal reaction would also be seen in the control; if tissues are completely fresh, and have not been in contact with formalin, the control should be colorless.

Sphingomyelins

The principle of lipid chromation was introduced by Müller (1859), but Weigert's observation, that myelin had a greater affinity for hematoxylin after being treated with chromate-containing fixatives, laid the foundation for a series of methods in which metallic salts were used to mordant myelin dyes (Deitrich, Smith, Pal, Kultchitsky, for example). Baker (1946) devised the acid hematein methods with a precise schedule for fixation, chromation, and staining, which is reasonably specific for choline-containing phospholipids (Adams 1965; Bayliss High 1972) or, according to Roozemond (1971), for polar lipids that are in a particular physicochemical state. Interference from proteins can be discounted by comparison with a lipid-extracted control section. Baker's procedure was further modified by Elftman (1954) but this version compares unfavorably with the original method, with respect to lipids on paper.

Dichromate–acid hematein (DAH) method for choline-containing phospholipids (after Baker 1946)

Fixation and sections

Unfixed cryostat sections are recommended; short-fixed frozen sections can be used.

Preparation of stain

0.1% hematoxylin	50 ml
1% sodium periodate	1 ml

Heat to boiling, cool, and add 1 ml glacial acetic acid. Use on day of preparation.

Method

1. Treat sections with 5% potassium dichromate containing 1% calcium chloride for 18 hours at room temperature, followed by a further 2 hours at 37°C.
2. Wash thoroughly in distilled water for 30 minutes.
3. Stain with acid hematein solution for 2 hours at 37°C.
4. Wash well and differentiate in an aqueous solution containing 0.25% sodium tetraborate and 0.25% potassium ferricyanide, for 1 hour at 37°C.
5. Counterstain nuclei with 1% methyl green (optional).
6. Wash well and mount in glycerin jelly.

Results

Lecithins and sphingomyelin	blue–black

Notes

a. A control section, delipidized with chloroform–methanol (2 : 1), should be included to assess the extent of any protein staining.
b. Batches of hematoxylin vary in suitability.

Baker originally chromated blocks of tissue in order to preserve lecithin, a particularly soluble phosphoglyceride, but since this precludes the use of adjacent sections for other methods, it is customary to use sections throughout the procedure (Hori 1963; Adams 1965). When fresh frozen cryostat sections are directly chromated, lecithin is well preserved. The acid hematein reaction has been usefully combined with Oil red O, or a red Sudan dye, to demonstrate neutral lipids and phospholipids in the same preparation (Bourgeois & Hubbard 1965; Kanwar 1968). This dual procedure is especially valuable to demonstrate normal and degenerating myelin simultaneously in contrasting colors (Bayliss High 1983).

Similarly, the solochrome–cyanine method (Page 1965) can be used with Oil red O to stain normal (blue) and degenerating (red) myelin.

A version of the metal hematoxylin principle was introduced by Elleder and Lojda (1973). This ferric hematoxylin (FeH) method is simpler, quicker, and apparently more sensitive than the DAH technique. Although FeH may be the method of choice for sphingomyelin, staining is satisfactory only after sections have been defatted with acetone, and this precludes the application of this technique in combination with Oil red O. Furthermore, the FeH procedure causes nuclei to be stained the same dark blue as lipid; in some instances this could be a disadvantage.

Ferric hematoxylin (FeH) method for phospholipids (Elleder & Lojda 1973)

Fixation and sections
Ideally unfixed cryostat sections; otherwise short-fixed frozen sections.

Preparation of reagent

Solution a
Distilled water	298 ml
Concentrated HCl	2 ml
$FeCl_3 \cdot 6H_2O$	2.5 g
$FeSO_4 \cdot 7H_2O$	4.5 g

This solution can be stored.

Solution b
Distilled water	10 ml
Hematoxylin	0.1 g

Dissolve by gentle heat. This solution must be fresh.

Working solution
Mix three parts of (a) with one part of (b) and use within the hour.

Method
1. Treat duplicate sections as follows:
   a. Extract one section in chloroform : methanol (2 : 1) for 1 hour at room temperature.
   b. Extract the other with dry acetone at 4°C for 15 minutes.
2. Fix both sections in formal calcium for 30 minutes.
3. Rinse in distilled water.
4. Stain in the ferric hematoxylin solution for 7 minutes.
5. Wash in distilled water.
6. Dip several times in 0.2% HCl.
7. Wash in tap water.
8. Dehydrate in acetone, clear in xylene, and mount in DPX.

Results
Phospholipids	blue
Nuclei	blue

The method can be modified (Adams & Bayliss 1963) to provide a method that is specific for sphingomyelin. Preliminary alkaline hydrolysis destroys phosphoglycerides but leaves intact the alkaline-resistant phosphosphingosides, which are then selectively stained during the subsequent procedure. It is fortunate that sphingomyelin is unaffected by formaldehyde (Heslinga & Deierkauf 1961, 1962) because well-fixed material is obligatory for this technique if sections are to withstand the harsh treatment with strong alkali. Mounting on subbed or positively charged slides is also recommended.

Sodium hydroxide–ferric hematoxylin/DAH method for sphingomyelin

Fixation and sections
As above, preferably mounted on chrome-gelatin-subbed slides.

Method
1. Treat sections with 2 M sodium hydroxide for 1 hour at room temperature.
2. Wash gently but thoroughly in a large volume of water.
3. Rinse in 1% acetic acid for 5 seconds.
4. If section has become detached from the slide, remount it and proceed with the ferric hematoxylin method described above.

Results
Sphingomyelin	blue

Note
Should plasmalogens interfere, they can be excluded by treating sections with 1% mercuric chloride in 1% HCl for 10 minutes prior to alkaline hydrolysis.

Cerebrosides

These lipids can be demonstrated by reactions specific for their hexose molecules. Diezel's (1954) modification of the Molisch and Bruckner methods for carbohydrates has been used to stain glycolipids, but the procedures are too destructive to tissues to be of great use in histochemistry. Cerebrosides and related lipids are stained by the PAS method, originally designed to stain mucopolysaccharides (McManus 1946; Lillie 1947). Periodic acid converts the 1,2-glycol group in the hexose molecule to Schiff-stainable aldehyde. Other chemical configurations may react similarly; therefore a sequence of blockades was devised (Adams & Bayliss 1963) in which all interfering groups are suppressed and PAS positivity can be attributed solely to hexoses. Amino groups are converted to carbonyls by chloramine T; performic acid is used to oxidize lipid ethylene bonds to aldehydes which are then blocked with dinitrophenyl hydrazine, along with existing aldehydes; finally the PAS reaction is performed to stain hexoses. The distinction between glycolipids and non-lipid hexoses depends upon comparison with a de-lipidized control section. Although it would seem undesirable to rely upon such a 'difference' method, in practice the results are usually clear cut, except in the case of liver, when interference from PAS-positive glycogen must be excluded by removal with diastase. Personal objections to the use of performic acid (Elleder & Lojda 1970) prompted Palladini and Lauro (1970) to substitute halogenation for the performic acid oxidation in the original technique. Although theoretically a good idea, and specific for cerebroside impregnated on paper, this modification fails to detect cerebroside in myelin and so the original method will be given here.

Modified PAS reaction for cerebroside
(Adams & Bayliss 1963)

Fixation and sections
Cryostat sections post-fixed in formal calcium; fixed frozen sections.

Preparation of reagent
Performic acid
98% formic acid	45 ml
100 vol hydrogen peroxide	4.5 ml
Concentrated H_2SO_4	0.5 ml

Prepare an hour before use and stir occasionally with a glass rod, inside a fume hood, to release bubbles of gas from the solution.

Method
1. Mount duplicate sections onto separate slides and extract one of these with chloroform methanol (2 : 1 v/v) for 1 hour at room temperature.
2. Deaminate both sections in 10% aqueous chloramine T for 1 hour at 37°C.
3. Wash slides vigorously and as rapidly as possible, one at a time, in a large volume of water before transferring them immediately to performic acid for 10 minutes. The washing must be swift yet thorough, to avoid swelling and detachment of sections from slides.
4. Wash well in distilled water.
5. Treat with a filtered saturated solution of 2,4-dinitrophenyl hydrazine in M HCl at 4°C for 2 hours.
6. Wash well in water.
7. Treat with 0.5% periodic acid for 10 minutes.
8. Wash in distilled water.
9. Stain in Schiff's reagent for 15 minutes.
10. Rinse in distilled water and wash in tap water for 15 minutes to develop color.
11. Counterstain nuclei with Mayer's hematoxylin or Carazzi's hematoxylin if wished.
12. Wash in tap water, distilled water, and finally mount sections in glycerin jelly.

Results
Cerebroside   magenta

Indicated by the difference in staining intensity between the two sections.

Notes
a. Protein-bound ganglioside or related lipids may also stain.
b. In practice the routine PAS reaction is the best starting point. The method given here would only be helpful if cerebrosides were suspected, and the routine PAS reaction was positive.

Sulfatides

These sulfate esters of cerebroside are the only lipids sufficiently acidic to induce a metachromatic shift in a variety of basic aniline dyes which have been used to demonstrate the lipid deposits in sulfatide storage disease, consequently termed metachromatic leucodystrophy. With cresyl violet, for example (Hirsch & Peiffer 1957), sulfatide appears orange in contrast to the orthochromatic color of other, less acidic, myelin lipids, but trivial metachromasia may be difficult to appreciate against a strong purple background. Distinction can be improved if the stained preparation is viewed in polarized light so that the sulfatide displays a green dichroism (Dayan 1967).

Toluidine blue, the standard dye exhibiting metachromasia with acidic polymers, shows sulfatides in metachromatic leucodystrophy as yellow, brown, or purple deposits. An acetone dehydration step is used to eliminate metachromasia induced by less polar groups (Bodian & Lake 1963).

The research method of choice for sulfatide (Kahlke 1967; Pearse 1968; P. Sourander, personal communication, 1969) is Holländer's (1963) adaptation of an acriflavine staining reaction for sulfated mucopolysaccharides (Takeuchi 1961, 1962). Holländer used a reagent sufficiently acidic that only sulfatide would be stained, with the exception of mast cell granules which can be distinguished by their persistence in a chloroform–methanol-extracted control section. The acriflavine–sulfatide complex fluoresces orange in ultraviolet light, or alternatively the reaction product can be converted to a stable red pigment with p-dimethylaminobenzaldehyde, giving excellent localization of stained sulfatide against a clear ground. Another method for sulfated mucins that can be successfully adapted to frozen sections for staining sulfatide is the high iron diamine method (Spicer 1965) given in Chapter 11, when the sulfatide stains purple and the background pale blue. Among lipids the staining reaction is confined to sulfatide, and the possibility of interference from cross-reacting mucins can be excluded by comparison with a de-lipidized control section.

Toluidine blue–acetone method for sulfatide (Bodian & Lake 1963)

Fixation and sections
Post-fixed cryostat sections; formal calcium-fixed frozen sections.

Reagents
0.01% toluidine blue in phosphate–citrate buffer at pH 4.7.

Buffer solution

0.2 M Na$_2$HPO$_4$	96 ml
0.1 M citric acid	104 ml

Method
1. Mount sections onto slides.
2. Stain for 16–18 hours in buffered toluidine blue.
3. Wash in water.
4. Dehydrate with acetone for 5 minutes.
5. Mount in DPX.

Result

Sulfatide deposits	metachromatic red–brown or yellow

Acriflavine–DMAB method for sulfatide (Holländer 1963)

Fixation and sections
Post-fixed cryostat sections; formal calcium-fixed frozen sections.

Preparation of reagents
a. Acriflavine stock solution

Acriflavine	100 mg
Distilled water at 80°C	20 ml

Store in the dark at 4°C.

b. Acriflavine working solution

0.1 M citrate–HCl buffer pH 2.5	99 ml
Stock acriflavine solution	1 ml

c. DMAB solution

p-dimethylaminobenzaldehyde	0.6 g
20% hydrochloric acid	30 ml
Isopropanol	70 ml

Method
1. Mount sections onto slides.
2. Stain for 6 minutes in acriflavine solution.
3. Differentiate for 1 minute in two changes of 70% isopropanol.
4. Treat with DMAB reagent for 30–45 seconds.
5. Rinse in distilled water for 2–3 minutes.
6. Counterstain nuclei in Mayer's or Carazzi's hematoxylin.
7. Blue in tap water, rinse in distilled water and mount sections in glycerin jelly.

Results

Sulfatide   red

Notes

a. Mast cell granules appear red but resist extraction in chloroform–methanol.

b. Alternative: after stage 3 dehydrate sections in isopropanol, clear in xylene, and mount in a fluorescence-free medium.

c. Sulfatide appears orange in ultraviolet light against a green ground.

Gangliosides

Gangliosides can be distinguished from other glycolipids on account of their constituent neuraminic acid and its acyl derivatives, the sialic acids (Gottschalk 1957). The enzyme neuraminidase has been used to cleave neuraminic acid from its adjacent hexose before staining the latter with alcian blue (Spicer & Warren 1960). However, not all sialic acid residues are attacked by neuraminidase, and their position on the hexose ring determines susceptibility. Other methods (Diezel 1957; Shear & Pearse 1963, 1964) proved to be unsatisfactory until Ravetto (1964) successfully adapted the Svennerholm–Bial chromatography reagent to stain gangliosides in tissue sections. The color obtained in this way is unacceptably pale and the method is not pleasant to perform. The reagent, consisting of copper sulfate and orcinol dissolved in concentrated HCl, has to be applied in spray form so that the supposedly water-soluble gangliosides can be retained in the section. The gangliosides that accumulate intraneuronally in the metabolic storage disorders are complexed with phospholipids, cholesterol, and protein, and are not as water soluble as the free ganglioside. Since the gangliosidoses provide the major diagnostic problem for which gangliosides require to be demonstrated histochemically, the water solubility of the free glycolipid is irrelevant in this context.

In fact the conventional PAS method has proved to be the most practical and rewarding approach to ganglioside detection. Although the PAS reaction will include other glycolipids and, of course, non-lipid mucosubstances, Roberts (1977) devised a modification whereby Schiff staining could be confined to glycoproteins containing sialic acids. Sialo groups are oxidized much more rapidly than other sugar glycosides and so, by reducing the concentration of the oxidizing agent (periodate) from 1% to 0.01%, the reaction is confined to sialic acid. With slight modifications this method has been adapted to demonstrate gangliosides (the only sialolipids) within neurons in Tay–Sachs' disease (Buk & Bayliss High 1986).

Gangliosides, on account of their acidic sialic acid residues, can also be stained by the basic aniline dyes such as thionin, cresyl violet, and Nile blue sulfate, but these dyes are by no means selective and will also stain phospholipids, due to their phosphoric acids, and sulfatide on account of its sulfate radical.

As a preliminary screen, the routine PAS reaction can be first applied, and followed by the method given below for further characterization if necessary.

Borohydride–periodate–Schiff (BHPS) method

Fixation and sections

Cryostat sections post-fixed in formal calcium; frozen sections of fixed tissue.

Method

1. Destroy existing aldehyde groups (endogenous or from formalin or glutaraldehyde fixation) by reduction with 0.1 M (0.38%) sodium borohydride in 1% disodium hydrogen phosphate for 1 hour at room temperature.
2. Wash thoroughly in distilled water.
3. Oxidize with 1.2 mM (0.03%) sodium periodate for 30 minutes at room temperature.
4. Wash twice for 5 minutes each time in distilled water.
5. Stain with Schiff's reagent for 10 minutes.
6. Rinse in distilled water and wash well in tap water.
7. Counterstain with Mayer's hematoxylin or Carazzi's hematoxylin.
8. Blue in tap water, rinse in distilled, then mount sections in glycerin jelly.

Results

Gangliosides (in Tay–Sachs' disease   red
and G_m1 gangliosidosis)

Nuclei   blue

Note

A chloroform–methanol-extracted section should be used for comparison to exclude interference from non-lipid sialomucins.

Lipofuscins

These pigments will be mentioned here briefly; they have been extensively reviewed by Wolman (1964) and Pearse (1985), and their demonstration is discussed in detail in Chapter 14. The most significant lipopigments in pathology are the intraneuronal deposits encountered in Batten's disease. The storage granules appear gray with Sudan black B, may be PAS positive, may stain with Luxol fast blue and Ziehl–Neelsen, and they appear autofluorescent in ultraviolet light. The material present in at least two subtypes of the disease is a hydrophobic mitochondrial protein which has the staining properties of a lipid (proteolipid) and is similar in this respect to the lipofuscin of wear and tear pigment. On account of the variable staining reactions encountered in the different Batten subtypes, a battery of staining methods is recommended for light microscopy (Lake 1976, 1981), including acid phosphatase (see p. 411). These methods are not selective for lipofuscins and it is important to confirm the identity of the storage material by electron microscopy, when the distinctive ultrastructural patterns can be convincingly demonstrated. These are briefly discussed and illustrated in Chapter 30.

UV method for lipofuscins

Fixation and sections

Cryostat sections (5–10 μm) air-dried; frozen sections of fixed tissue; paraffin sections.

Method

1. Bring sections to xylene and mount in DPX.
2. Examine by fluorescence microscopy (dark ground transmission) or epi-illumination. Excitation filter 300–370 nm (UG5) with barrier filter at 410 nm.

Results

Lipofuscin (wear and tear pigment) has orange–yellow fluorescence.

The proteolipid in Batten's disease has yellow or silver autofluorescence.

COMBINATION TECHNIQUES

Although it is customary for histologists to use multistage polychromatic techniques to display two or more tissue elements in a single preparation with contrasting colors, histochemical methods have been conventionally applied to individual serial sections. Histochemical reactions are less likely to be compatible when applied sequentially because the first method may well inactivate or extract the component to be demonstrated afterwards. Exceptions do exist of course, for example the high iron diamine–alcian blue technique that discriminates between sulfated and carboxylated mucins, but dual techniques for lipids are comparatively rare.

Oil red O was combined with Baker's dichromate–acid hematein method (Bourgeois & Hubbard 1965; Kanwar 1968) but these workers apparently overlooked an important application of this combination, namely to demonstrate demyelination, when the blue color of normal myelin contrasts well with the red-stained fatty 'degenerate' myelin lipids within lipophages. Oil red O has also been used in conjunction with the periodic acid–silver diamine technique for glial chromatin (Bayliss et al 1970) and with orcein to demonstrate elastic fibers together with lipids in the atheromatous artery (McKinney & Riley 1967), a useful alternative to Lillie's (1954) resorcin–fuchsin–Oil red O combination.

Fat stains are also useful adjuncts to some enzyme histochemical methods, indicating the relationship between pathological lipid deposits and the cellular responses such lipids invoke. Lysosomal β-galactosidase (Lake 1974), and mitochondrial enzyme methods using nitro blue tetrazolium, have a blue end product which combines well with Oil red O. The blue color provided by Sudan black B is well suited to complement the red and orange reactions produced respectively in the red acid phosphatase and non-specific esterase techniques using hexazotized pararosanilin.

Table 12.4 (see p. 197) lists some of the dual procedures that can be used either to show two types of lipid simultaneously, or to depict fat and enzyme activity in the same section. Such combinations provide more information than can be achieved by applying the same techniques separately to adjacent tissue sections.

LIPID IMMUNOHISTOCHEMISTRY

Immunoperoxidase and immunofluorescence techniques have revolutionized most aspects of histochemistry in recent years so that tissue components can now be identified more precisely than with routine staining techniques. Lipids have received little attention from the immunologists, primarily because the majority of lipids are not antigenic. Gangliosides, which are the characteristic glycolipids of neural tissue, and galactocerebroside in myelin, have been demonstrated immunohistochemically. Antisera were raised against G_{M2} ganglioside for the immunohistochemical demonstration of gangliosides in Tay–Sachs' brain (Schwerer et al 1982), the reaction persisting even in paraffin sections. Gangliosides in the cerebral cortex were first demonstrated with immunohistochemical methods by de Baecque et al (1976), who showed that the antibodies raised (in this case against G_{M1} ganglioside) were directed against the trihexosyl moiety of the ganglioside molecule, acting as a hapten (i.e. requiring to be conjugated with a protein before it can elicit an immune response).

Further developments in this promising field can be expected. Meanwhile the conventional histochemical techniques described in this chapter presently provide the best means of localizing and identifying tissue lipids microscopically.

APPLICATIONS OF LIPID HISTOCHEMISTRY IN PATHOLOGY

Many of the methods in this chapter have been used for research projects in biology, botany, and food science, but their most valuable application would seem to be in diagnostic pathology, chiefly in disorders of the nervous system. The myelin sheath is particularly rich in lipids, being composed of compacted cell membrane, a lamellar structure of cholesterol and phospholipids, so that demyelination and the lipid storage disorders will feature in some detail below, followed by a few examples of pathological conditions outside the nervous system that can also be investigated by lipid histochemistry.

Myelin and demyelination

Primary demyelination occurs when the myelin sheath is damaged by infectious agents, toxins, or allergic influences, and in some cases the axon may remain intact; the most familiar example is multiple sclerosis. *Dysmyelination* implies a failure to myelinate properly during development. Both demyelination and dysmyelination can be demonstrated in paraffin sections by conventional

histological methods for myelin (see Chapter 19 where a further discussion on this topic can be found). To indicate active demyelination, frozen sections are preferred because the most important feature of demyelination is the transformation of normal myelin, with its distinctive hydrophilic properties due to its constituent polar phospholipids, into fatty droplets comprising cholesterol esters within macrophages, with an affinity for the Sudan dyes. Cholesterol within normal adult myelin is entirely in the free state and so these esters within lipophages are recognized as a convenient hallmark of ongoing demyelination and enable one to distinguish between active lesions and old fat-free scars. Although Luxol fast blue will demonstrate myelin (probably a protein component of myelin) in paraffin sections, its alcoholic solvent will extract the cholesterol esters, so to demonstrate both normal and degenerating myelin simultaneously frozen sections are essential. The dichromate–acid hematein–Oil red O combination is recommended because it provides a good color contrast between the blue myelin and red-stained esters within lipophages. Likewise the solochrome cyanin method (Page 1965) can also be combined with Oil red O. Established methods for normal and degenerating myelin include the osmium tetroxide–α-naphthylamine (OTAN) technique (Adams 1959), which was devised specifically for this purpose, and the PAS–Sudan red procedure of Hirsch and Peiffer (1957). A reasonable distinction can even be achieved with Sudan black B alone, because normal myelin appears gray rather than the intense blue color of the degenerating myelin lipids.

The central nervous system is also the target for Parkinson's disease and the characteristic Lewy bodies have been shown to include sphingomyelin (den Hartog Jager 1969), which can be demonstrated by the sodium hydroxide–acid hematein procedure or, more simply, with Sudan black B, viewed in polarized light to show the characteristic red birefringence attributable here to sphingomyelin. The red birefringence seen after staining with Sudan black is related to the physical organization of the lipid rather than to the identification of a particular lipid. Thus the lipid deposition in Fabry's disease (ceramide trihexoside) also shows red birefringence after Sudan black staining.

Another degenerative disorder of the CNS, Pick's presenile dementia, is reported to show ganglioside accumulation in neurons (de Groot & den Hartog Jager 1980).

Metabolic disorders affecting the nervous system

A group of rare diseases that were once believed to be degenerative in origin are now recognized as inherited disorders due to the deficiency of certain lysosomal enzymes, or their co-factors, involved with lipid catabolism. Impaired activity of the enzyme results in accumulation of the relevant lipid or its metabolites at the defective stage in their metabolic cycle. Since enzymes are not always substrate specific, the storage material may well be heterogeneous (Hers 1965). There are three major categories of storage disease: the *neurolipidoses* in which the lipids accumulate chiefly within neurons; secondly the *leucodystrophies* with lipid storage in cells of the mononuclear phagocyte series in the white matter of the brain and systemically; and thirdly the *visceral lipidoses* where storage is found predominantly in the mononuclear phagocyte system. The individual diseases have variable clinical and pathological manifestations and different ages of onset, and many are fatal during early childhood.

The most important group of storage disorders is the sphingolipidoses, and Table 12.5 indicates the enzymes responsible for these defects; the lipids that accumulate; the appropriate biopsy site, and the methods for its demonstration. Gangliosides, for example, are the lipids that are stored intraneuronally in Tay–Sachs' disease due to deficient activity of hexosaminidase A or B, and can be demonstrated with the PAS or borohydride–PAS method in rectal or appendiceal biopsy. Today, in preference to the brain biopsy procedure used formerly, suspected cases of the neurolipidoses may be routinely investigated by rectal biopsy (Bodian & Lake 1963), because ganglion cells in the gastrointestinal tract conveniently mimic the storage pattern of their CNS counterparts.

With the recognition of most of the enzyme defects in this group of disorders, diagnosis is mainly achieved by assay of the appropriate enzyme in white blood cells. Such techniques are particularly valuable to screen carriers of a defective gene and to test 'at risk' pregnancies; genetic counseling would aim to prevent further expression of the inherited defect. The most commonly occurring neurolipidosis in childhood has three main subgroups, collectively termed Batten's disease. The stored material has the staining properties of ceroid or lipofuscin, hence the alternate term ceroid lipofuscinosis.

The subgroups can best be distinguished by their ultrastructural profiles.

The leucodystrophies include metachromatic leucodystrophy (sulfatide) and Krabbe's leucodystrophy (galactocerebroside), both of which can be demonstrated histochemically with the methods indicated in Table 12.5, with the biopsy material appropriate for each condition.

Ideally the histochemical approach to these diagnostic problems should be reinforced by electron microscopy, thin layer chromatography, and enzymology where relevant, but where facilities for biochemical analyses are lacking, histochemistry may well be the sole means of diagnosis and in fact has a distinct advantage over the other techniques: namely the ability to localize metabolites within individual cells.

Cardiovascular system

Cholesterol deposition in the human arterial wall, leading to atherosclerosis, is responsible directly or indirectly for a large proportion of deaths. The extent of atheromatous involvement can be appreciated grossly by staining whole segments of aorta with Oil red O. Cholesterol is present in the atheromatous plaque in both free and ester form. A section stained with Oil red O can be viewed with partly crossed polars to show both red-stained fatty esters and the unstained birefringent crystalline cholesterol. The latter will not necessarily be free cholesterol because the typical cholesteryl ester of human atheroma lipids is oleate, which is crystalline at normal staining temperatures.

Lipid can also accumulate in the heart muscle of patients with cardiomyopathies induced by viral infections, alcohol abuse, and a variety of other toxins. In this case the lipids in question are triglycerides, which can be demonstrated by any of the fat stains and identified with the calcium–lipase method. Triglycerides are also present in the 'thrush breast' heart resulting from chronic anemia, but 'brown atrophy' in heart muscle is due to lipofuscins, which can be demonstrated by the battery of methods listed for lipopigments.

Skeletal muscle

Oil red O is routinely used to detect an excess of neutral fats in muscle biopsies. Sudan black may also be used, but if the sections are fixed frozen or post-fixed, the

Table 12.5 Lipid storage disorders (for further details see Lake 1992)

Disease	Enzyme defect	Lipid stored	Biopsy source	Histochemistry	Comments
G_{M1} gangliosidosis	β-galactosidase	G_{M1} ganglioside	Rectum Appendix	PAS, BHPS, thionin pH 3, SB, EM	Acute infantile onset. Mental retardation; short survival. Also childhood and adult forms
G_{M2} gangliosidosis (Tay–Sachs, Sandhoff)	Defective hexosaminidase activity. Many subgroups	G_{M2} ganglioside	Rectum Appendix	PAS, BHPS, SB, thionin pH 3, EM	Mental retardation and blindness. Also childhood and adult forms
Batten's disease (several subtypes)	Not known	'Ceroid-lipofuscin', a proteolipid. Subunit C of ATP synthase	Rectum Appendix Skin	SB, PAS, LFB, autofluorescence, EM	Variable survival depending on subtype
Farber's lipo-granulomatosis	Acid ceramidase	Ceramide and G_{M3} ganglioside	Skin Liver Gut	PAS, EM	Fatal during second year of life
Fabry's disease	Ceramide trihexosidase (α-galactosidase)	Ceramide trihexoside	Skin Kidney	PAS, SB, polarized light, PAN	Purple skin rash; renal failure; burning pains in extremities; X-linked; cardiomyopathy
Refsum's syndrome	Phytanic acid oxidase	Phytanic acid	Liver Nerve	Copper–rubeanic acid*	Therapy: restrict green vegetable intake
Wolman's disease	Acid esterase	Cholesteryl esters and triglycerides	Liver Lymph node WBC	PAN, SB, ORO, calcium-lipase, acid esterase	Fatal during first year. Adrenal calcification

Disease	Enzyme/defect	Lipid stored	Tissue	Staining methods	Clinical features
Cholesteryl ester storage disease	Acid esterase	Cholesteryl esters and triglycerides	Liver, Lymph node, WBC	PAN, SB, ORO, calcium-lipase, acid esterase	Benign; compatible with survival to adulthood
Tangier disease	Impaired synthesis of apoprotein A	Cholesteryl esters	Tonsils	PAN*, PAN + digitonin	Follows a fairly benign course
Niemann–Pick disease types A + B	Sphingomyelinase	Sphingomyelin and cholesterol	Bone marrow, Liver, Rectum	SB-polarized light, NaOH–DAH/FeH, PAN, EM	Hepatosplenomegaly and mental retardation Type B, no neurological involvement
Niemann–Pick disease type C	Not known. Defect of cholesterol esterification	Cholesterol; phospholipids; hexosides; sphingomyelin in spleen	Rectum, Bone marrow, Liver	PAS, SB, NaOH–DAH/FeH, EM	Neonatal hepatitis in 60%; ataxia; retardation; hepatosplenomegaly
Gaucher's disease (three forms)	Glucocerebrosidase	Glucocerebrosidase	Bone marrow, Liver	PAS, modified PAS	Hepatosplenomegaly; mental retardation
Krabbe's leucodystrophy	Galactocerebroside β-galactosidase	Galactocerebroside	Brain	PAS, modified PAS	Multinucleate 'globoid' cells around vessels; mental retardation
Metachromatic leucodystrophy	Arylsulfatase A	Sulfatide	Urine deposit, Sural nerve	Toluidine blue–acetone, Acriflavine–DMAB, High iron diamine	Loss of myelin; mental retardation; fatal during first decade

ATP, Adenosine triphosphate; BHPS, borohydride–periodate–Schiff; EM, electron microscopy; LFB, luxol fast blue; NaOH-DAH/FeH, Sodium hydroxide-dichromate-acid hematein/ferric hematoxylin; ORO, oil red O; PAS, periodic acid–Schiff; PAN, perchloric acid naphthoquinone; SB, Sudan black; WBC, white blood cells. * Predicted but not tested.

phospholipids in mitochondria are also demonstrated, and this might cause interpretative difficulties. Excess lipid occurs in primary and secondary lipid storage myopathies, which include carnitine palmitoyl transferase deficiency, the acyl coenzyme A dehydrogenase deficiencies and disorders of the respiratory chain.

Acknowledgment

Olga Bayliss High contributed this chapter for the first three editions, and Brian Lake updated the text for the fourth edition. Our acknowledgments are due to them for their contributions.

REFERENCES

Adams C.W.M. (1959) A histochemical method for the simultaneous demonstration of normal and degenerating myelin. Journal of Pathology and Bacteriology 77:648.

Adams C.W.M. (1961) A perchloric acid–naphthoquinone method for the histochemical localization of cholesterol. Nature (London) 193:331.

Adams C.W.M. (1965) Neurohistochemistry. Amsterdam: Elsevier, p. 16.

Adams C.W.M., Bayliss O.B. (1962) The release of protein, lipid and polysaccharide components of the arterial elastica by proteolytic enzymes and lipid solvents. Journal of Histochemistry and Cytochemistry 10:222.

Adams C.W.M., Bayliss, O.B. (1963) Histochemical observations on the localization and origin of sphingomyelin, cerebroside and cholesterol in normal and atherosclerotic human artery. Journal of Pathology and Bacteriology 85:113.

Adams C.W.M., Bayliss O.B. (1968) Reappraisal of osmium tetroxide and OTAN histochemical reactions. Histochemie 16:162.

Adams C.W.M., Bayliss O.B. (1974) Lipid histochemistry. In: Glick D., Rosenbaum R.M., eds. Techniques of biochemical and biophysical morphology. New York: Wiley-Interscience, Vol. 2, pp. 99–156.

Adams C.W.M., Bayliss High O.B. (1980) Preliminary oxidation in histochemical staining methods for cholesterol. Journal of Microscopy 119:427.

Adams C.W.M., Davison A.N. (1959) The histochemical identification of myelin phosphoglycerides by their ferric hydroxamates. Journal of Neurochemistry 3:347.

Adams C.W.M., Tuqan N.A. (1961) Elastic degeneration as a source of lipids in the early lesion of atherosclerosis. Journal of Pathology and Bacteriology 82:131.

Adams C.W.M., Bayliss, O.B., Ibrahim M.Z.M. (1963) Modifications to histochemical methods for phosphoglyceride and cerebroside. Journal of Histochemistry and Cytochemistry 11:560.

Adams C.W.M., Abdulla Y.H., Bayliss O.B., Weller R.O. (1966) Histochemical detection of triglyceride esters with specific lipases and a calcium lead sulphide technique. Journal of Histochemistry and Cytochemistry 14:385.

Archibald R.W.R., Orton C.C. (1970) Specific identification of free and esterified fatty acids in tissue sections. Histochemical Journal 2:411.

Baker J.R. (1944) Structure and chemical composition of the Golgi element. Quarterly Journal of Microscopical Science 85:1.

Baker J.R. (1946) The histochemical recognition of lipine. Quarterly Journal of Microscopical Science 87:441.

Baker J.R. (1958) Fixation in cytochemistry and electron-microscopy. Journal of Histochemistry and Cytochemistry 6:303.

Bayliss O.B. (1972) Fixation of tissues for lipid histochemistry. Proceedings of the Royal Microscopical Society 7:47.

Bayliss O.B., Adams C.W.M. (1972) Bromine Sudan black (BSB). A general stain for tissue lipids including free cholesterol. Histochemical Journal 4:505.

Bayliss O.B., Adams C.W.M., Hallpike J.F. (1970) The PASDORO method for simultaneously demonstrating DNA and lipids in brain. Histochemical Journal 2:87.

Bayliss High O.B. (1970) The validity of histochemical lipid techniques. F.I.M.L.T. Thesis. London.

Bayliss High O.B. (1972) Lipid histochemistry: validity of techniques. M. Phil. Thesis: London.

Bayliss High O.B. (1981) The histochemical versatility of Sudan black B. Acta Histochemica. Supplementband 24:247.

Bayliss High O.B. (1983) Degenerative diseases of the central and peripheral nervous system. In: Filipe I.M., Lake B.D., eds. Histochemistry in pathology. Edinburgh: Churchill Livingstone, p. 48.

Belt W.D., Hayes E.R. (1956) An ultraviolet–Schiff reaction for unsaturated lipids. Stain Technology 31:117.

Benda C. (1900) Eine makro- und mikrochemisch Reaction der Fett Gewebsnekrose. Virchow's Archiv fur Pathologische Anatomie und Physiologie und fur Klinische Medizin 161.

Bodian M., Lake B.D. (1963) The rectal approach to neuropathology. British Journal of Surgery 50:702.

Bourgeois C., Hubbard B. (1965) A method for simultaneous demonstration of choline-containing phospholipids and neutral lipids in tissue sections. Journal of Histochemistry and Cytochemistry 13:571.

Brante G. (1949) Studies on lipids in the nervous system. Acta Physiologica Scandinavica. Supplement 18:63.

Buk S.J.A., Bayliss High O.B. (1986) Periodate oxidation of glycolipids, a borohydride–periodate–Schiff method for gangliosides in tissue sections. Histochemical Journal 18:22–23.

Butler J. De B., Comly M.E., Kruth H.S. et al. (1987) Niemann–Pick variant disorders: comparison of errors of cellular cholesterol homeostasis in Group D and Group C fibroblasts. Proceedings of the National Academy of Sciences of the USA 84:556–560.

Cain A.J. (1947) Use of Nile Blue in the examination of lipoids. Quarterly Journal of Microscopical Science 88:383.

Cain A.J. (1949a) On the significance of the plasmal reaction. Quarterly Journal of Microscopical Science 90:75.

Cain A.J. (1949b) A critique of the plasmal reaction, with remarks on recently proposed techniques. Quarterly Journal of Microscopical Science 90:411.

Callis G., Chiffelle T.L., Putt F.A. (1951) Propylene and ethylene glycol as solvents for Sudan IV and Sudan Black B. Stain Technology 26:51.

Churukian C.J. (2000) Manual of the special stains laboratory, 8th edn. Rochester, NY: University of Rochester.

Churukin C., Ciaccio C. (1910) Contributo alla conoscenza dei lipoidi cellulari. Anatomischer Anzeiger 35:17.

Daddi L. (1896) Nouvelle méthode pour colorer la graisse dans les tissues. Archives Italiennes de Biologie 26:143.

Dayan A.D. (1967) Dichroism of cresyl violet-stained cerebroside sulfate (sulfatide). Journal of Histochemistry and Cytochemistry 15:421.

de Beacque C., Johnson A.B., Naiki M. et al. (1976) Ganglioside localization in cerebeller cortex: an immunoperoxidase study with antibody to GG_{M1} ganglioside. Brain Research 114(11):7.

de Groot P.A., den Hartog Jager W.A. (1980) A storage product in Pick's presenile dementia. Abstracts 6th International Histochemistry and Cytochemistry Congress, Royal Microscopical Society, 151.

Deierkauf F.A., Heslinga F.J.M. (1962) The action of formaldehyde on rat brain lipids. Journal of Histochemistry and Cytochemistry 10:79.

den Hartog Jager W.A. (1969) Sphingomyelin in Lewy inclusion bodies in Parkinson's disease. Archives of Neurology 21:615.

Diezel P.B. (1954) Histochemische Untersuchungen an primären Lipoidosen: Amaurotische Idiotie, Gargoylismus, Niemann-Picksche Krankheit, Gauchersche Krankheit, mit besonderer Berücksichtigung des zentral nerven Systems. Virchow's Archiv fur Pathologische Anatomie und Physiologie und fur Klinische Medizin 326:89.

Diezel P.B. (1957) Histochemical studies of primary lipidoses. In: Cumings J.N., ed. Cerebral lipidoses. Oxford: Blackwell, pp. 11–29.

Diezel P.B. (1958) Die Metachromasie mit verschiedenen Farbstoffen im Mischlicht und im polarisierten Licht. Acta Histochemica. Supplementband 1:134.

Dunnigan M.G. (1968) The use of Nile blue sulphate in the histochemical identification of phospholipids. Stain Technology 43:249.

Edgar G.W.F., Donker C.H.M. (1957) Influence of lipid solvents on sphingolipids (sphingomyelins, cerebrosides, gangliosides) in tissue sections. Acta Neurologica et Psychiatrica Belgica 5:451.

Elftman H. (1954) Controlled chromation. Journal of Histochemistry and Cytochemistry 2:1.

Elleder M., Lojda Z. (1968a) Remarks on the detection of osmium derivatives in tissue sections. Histochemie 13:276.

Elleder M., Lojda Z. (1968b) Remarks on the 'OTAN' reaction. Histochemie 14:47.

Elleder M., Lojda Z. (1970) Studies in lipid histochemistry III. Reaction of Schiff's reagent with plasmalogens. Histochemie 24:328.

Elleder M., Lojda Z. (1971) Studies in lipid histochemistry VI. Problems of extraction with acetone in lipid histochemistry. Histochemie 28:68.

Elleder M., Lojda Z. (1973) New, rapid, simple and selective method for the demonstration of phospholipids. Histochemie 36:149.

Emeis J.J., Van Gent C.M., Van Sabben C.M. (1977) An enzymatic method for the histochemical localization of free and esterified cholesterol separately. Histochemical Journal 9:197.

Feigin I. (1956) A method for the histochemical differentiation of cholesterol and its esters. Journal of Biophysical and Biochemical Cytology 2:213.

Feulgen R., Voit K. (1924) Ueber einen Weitverbreiteten festen Aldehyd seine Entstehung aus einer Varstufe, sein mikrochemischer Nachweis und die Wege zu seiner proparativen Darstellung. Pflügers Archiv für die gesamte Physiologie des Menschen und der Tiere 206:389.

Fieser L.F. (1953) Cholesterol and companions. VII. Steroid dibromides. Journal of the American Chemical Society 75:5421.

Fischler F.J. (1904) Über die Unterscheidung von Neutralfetten, Fettsäuren und Sefein in Gewebe. Zentralblatt für allgemeine Pathologie und Pathologische Anatomie 15:913.

French R.W. (1926) Azure C as tissue stain. Stain Technology 1:79.

Gallyas F. (1963) The histochemical identification of phosphoglycerides in myelin. Journal of Neurochemistry 10:125.

Gérard P. (1935) Sur la reaction plasmale. Bulletin d'Histologie Appliquée à Physiologie et à la Pathologie et de Technique Microscopique 12:274.

Gomori G. (1952) Microscopic histochemistry. Chicago: Chicago University Press.

Gottschalk A. (1957) Neuraminidase: the specific enzyme of influenza virus and Vibrio cholerae. Biochimica et Biophysica Acta 23:645.

Govan A.D.T. (1944) Fat-staining by Sudan dyes suspended in watery media. Journal of Pathology and Bacteriology 56:262.

Hayes B.R. (1949) A rigorous re-definition of the plasmal reaction. Stain Technology 24:19.

Hers H.G. (1965) Inborn lysosomal disorders. Gastroenterology 48:625.

Heslinga F.J.M., Deierkauf F.A. (1961) The action of histological fixatives on tissue lipids. Comparison of the action of several fixatives using paper chromatography. Journal of Histochemistry and Cytochemistry 9:572.

Heslinga F.J.M., Deierkauf F.A. (1962) The action of formaldehyde solutions on human brain lipids. Journal of Histochemistry and Cytochemistry 10:704.

Hirsch T., Peiffer J. (1957) In: Cumings J.N., ed. Cerebral lipidoses. Oxford: Blackwell, p. 68.

Holczinger L. (1959) Histochemischer Nachweis freier Fattsäuren. Acta Histochemica 8:167.

Holczinger L., Bálint S. (1962) Experimental data to the theory of fat staining. Histochemie 2:389.

Holczinger L., Bálint, Z. (1961) The staining properties of masked lipids. Acta Histochemica 11:284.

Holländer H. (1963) A staining method for cerebroside-sulphuric-esters in brain tissue. Journal of Histochemistry and Cytochemistry 11:118.

Hori S.H. (1963) A simplified acid hematein test for phospholipids. Stain Technology 38:221.

Jones D. (1969) The reactions of formaldehyde with unsaturated fatty acids during histological fixation. Histochemical Journal 1:459.

Kahlke W. (1967) In: Schetter G., ed. Lipids and lipidoses. Berlin: Springer, p. 310.

Kanwar K.C. (1968) Differential staining of phospholipids and fats in gelatin-embedded frozen sections. Stain Technology 43:119.

Keilig I. (1944) Uber Specifitätsbreite und Grundlagen der Markscheiden färbungen. Virchow's Archiv fur Pathologishe Anatomie und Physiologie und fur Klinische Medizin 312:404.

Korn E.D. (1967) A chromatographic and spectrophotometric study of the products of the reaction of osmium tetroxide with unsaturated lipids. Journal of Cell Biology 34:627.

Kruth H.S., Vaughan M. (1980) Quantification of low density lipoprotein binding and cholesterol accumulation by single human fibroblasts using fluorescence microscopy. Journal of Lipid Research 21: 123–130.

Lake B.D. (1974) An improved method for the detection of β–galactosidase activity and its application to G_{M1}-gangliosidosis and mucopolysaccharidosis. Histochemical Journal 6:211.

Lake B.D. (1976) The differential diagnosis of the various forms of Batten disease by rectal biopsy. Birth Defects XII(3):455.

Lake B.D. (1981) Metabolic disorders: general considerations. In: Berry C.L., ed. Paediatric pathology. Berlin: Springer, p. 617.

Lake B.D. (1992) Lysosomal and peroxisomal disorders. In: Hume Adams J., Duchen W., eds. Greenfield's neuropathology, 5th edn. London: Arnold, p. 709.

Lansink A.G.W. (1968) Thin layer chromatography and histochemistry of Sudan Black B. Histochemie 16:68.

Lewis P.R., Lobban M.C. (1961) The chemical specificity of the Schultz test for steroids. Journal of Histochemistry and Cytochemistry 9:2.

Lillie R.D. (1947) PAS techniques. Journal of Laboratory and Clinical Medicine 32:910.

Lillie R.D. (1952) Ethylenic reaction of ceroid with performic acid and Schiff reagent. Stain Technology 27:37.

Lillie R.D. (1954) In: Histopathologic technic and practical histochemistry, 2nd edn. New York: Blakiston, p. 312.

Lillie R.D. (1965) In: Histopathologic technic and practical histochemistry, 3rd edn. New York: Blakiston.

Lillie R.D., Ashburn L.L. (1943) Supersaturated solutions of fat stains in dilute isopropanol for demonstration of acute fatty degeneration not shown by Herxheimer's technic. Archives of Pathology 36:432.

Lison L. (1936) Histochemie animale. Paris: Gauthier-Villars.

Lison L., Dagnelie J. (1935) Methods nouvelles de coloration de la myéline. Bulletin d' Histologie Appliquée à la Physiologie et à la Pathologie et de Technique Microscopique 12:85.

Lovern J.A. (1955) The chemistry of lipids of biochemical significance. London: Methuen, Ch. 1.

Maggi V., Brander W. (1963) A histochemical study of bound lipids of the arterial wall. Biochemical Journal 89:28P.

Marchi V. (1886) Sulle degenerazioni consecutive all Estirpazione totale e parziale del cervelletto. Rivista Sperimentale di'Freniatriae Medicina Legale delle Alienaziomi Mentali 12:50.

McKinney B., Riley M. (1967) An orcein–Oil red O stain for concomitant demonstration of elastic tissue and lipid. Stain Technology 42:245.

McManus J.F.A. (1946) Histological demonstration of mucin after periodic acid. Nature (London) 158:202.

Meier W. (1959) Untersuchungen zur Theorie de Fettfärbung. Zeitschrift fur Wissenschaftliche Mikroskopie und Mikroskopische Technik 64:193.

Menschik Z. (1953) Nile Blue histochemical method for phospholipids. Stain Technology 28:13.

Michaelis L. (1901) Ueber Fett-Farbstoffe. Virchow's Archiv fur Pathologische Anatomie und Physiologie und fur Klinische Medizin 164:263.

Morii S., Takigami S., Kaneda Y., Shikata N. (1982) Ultracytochemical analysis of cytoplasmic lipids by enzymic digestive methods. Acta Histochimica et Cytochemica 15:185.

Mukherji M., Deb C., Sen P.B. (1960) Histochemical demonstration of unsaturated lipids by bromine silver method. Journal of Histochemistry and Cytochemistry 8:189.

Müller H. (1859) Ueber glatte Muskeln und Nervenge flechte de Chorioidea un menschliche Auge. Verhandlungen der Physikalisch-Medizinischen Gesellschaft Zu Würzburg 10:179.

Norton W.T., Korey S.R., Brotz M. (1962) Histochemical demonstration of unsaturated lipids by a bromine–silver method. Journal of Histochemistry and Cytochemistry 10:83.

Okamoto K., Shimamoto H., Sonoda H. (1944a) (Cited by Pearse 1968). Japanese Journal of Constitutional Medicine 13:113.

Okamoto K., Ueda M., Kato A. (1944b) (Cited by Pearse 1968), Japanese Journal of Constitutional Medicine 13:102.

Page K. (1965) A stain for myelin using solochrome cyanin. Journal of Medical Laboratory Technology 22:224.

Palladini G., Lauro G. (1970) Histochemistry of complex lipids. I. Demonstration of vic-glycol groups. Histochemie 21:117.

Pearse A.G.E. (1951) A review of modern methods in histochemistry. Journal of Clinical Pathology 4:1.

Pearse A.G.E. (1968) Histochemistry, theoretical and applied. London: Churchill Livingstone.

Pearse A.G.E. (1985) Histochemistry: theoretical and applied, 4th edn. Edinburgh: Churchill Livingstone, Vol. 2, Ch. 16.

Ravetto C. (1964) Histochemical identification of sialic (neuraminic) acids. Journal of Histochemistry and Cytochemistry 12:306.

Roberts G.P. (1977) Histochemical detection of sialic acid residues using periodate oxidation. Histochemical Journal 9:97.

Roozemond R.C. (1971) The staining and chromium binding of rat brain tissue and of lipids in model systems subjected to Baker's acid hematein technique. Journal of Histochemistry and Cytochemistry 19:244.

Roussouw D.J., Chase C.C., Raath I., Engelbrecht F.H. (1976) The histochemical localization of cholesterol in formalin-fixed and fresh frozen sections. Stain Technology 51:143.

Schnabel R. (1964) Eine topochemische Methode zur Differenzierung des freien und veresterten Cholesterins. Acta Histochimica 18:161.

Schultz A. (1924) Eine Methode des mikrochemischen Cholesterin-nachweises an Gewebsschnitt. Zentralblatt fur allgemeine Pathologische Anatomie 35:314.

Schwerer B., Lassman H., Bernheimer, H. (1982) Antisera against ganglioside GM₂: immunochemical and immunohistological studies. Neuropathology and Applied Neurobiology 8:217.

Shear M., Pearse A.G.E. (1963) A direct histochemical method for the determination of sialic acid. Nature (London) 198:1273.

Shear M., Pearse A.G.E. (1964) Shear and Pearse method for direct histochemical demonstration of sialic acid. Nature (London) 201:630.

Smith J.L. (1908) On the simultaneous staining of neutral fat and fatty acid by oxazine dyes. Journal of Pathology and Bacteriology 12:1.

Spicer S.S. (1965) Diamine methods for differentiating mucosubstances histochemically. Journal of Histochemistry and Cytochemistry 13:211.

Spicer S.S., Warren L. (1960) Histochemistry of sialic acid-containing mucoproteins. Journal of Histochemistry and Cytochemistry 8:135.

Takeuchi J. (1961) Staining of sulphated MPS on filter paper by means of acriflavine. Stain Technology 36:159.

Takeuchi J. (1962) Staining of sulphated mucopolysaccharides in sections by means of acriflavine. Stain Technology 37:105.

Ueda M. (cited by Pearse 1985) In: Histochemistry: theoretical and applied, 4th edn. Edinburgh: Churchill Livingstone, Vol. 2, Ch. 16.

Verne J. (1929) Etude histochemique des substances aldéhydiques formées au cours du metabolisme des corps gras. Annales de Physiologie 5:245.

Weller R.O. (1967) Cytochemistry of lipids in atherosclerosis. Journal of Pathology and Bacteriology 94:171.

Wigglesworth V.B. (1957) The use of osmium in the fixation and staining of tissues. Proceedings of the Royal Society (London) B147:185.

Wolman M. (1962) Extraction of complexes from central and peripheral myelin in man. Journal of Neurochemistry 9:59.

Wolman M. (1964) Histochemistry of lipids in pathology. In: Handbuch der Histochemie. Stuttgart: Fischer, Vol. 5.

Wolman M., Weiner H. (1965) Structure of the myelin sheath as a function of concentration of ions. Biochimica et Biophysica Acta 102:269.

FURTHER READING

Angermüller S., Fahimi H.D. (1982) Imidazole–buffered osmium tetroxide: an excellent stain for visualization of lipids in transmission electronmicroscopy. Histochemical Journal 14:823.

13

Proteins and Nucleic Acids

Jerry L. Fredenburgh, John D. Bancroft, William E. Grizzle
and Russell B. Myers

INTRODUCTION

Proteins and nucleic acids are major cell and tissue constituents. Proteins are highly organized complex macromolecules that are made up of twenty common amino acids linked together by peptide bonds which occur in cells and tissues as simple and conjugated proteins. Simple proteins are made up of amino acids only, e.g. albumins, globulins, fibrous structural proteins, and enzymes. Fibrous proteins and enzymes are discussed in Chapters 10 and 20 respectively. Conjugated proteins are amino acid complexes that are conjugated to other substances by covalent bonds, e.g. lipoproteins and mucoproteins. The identification of lipoproteins and mucoproteins in tissues is usually based on the demonstration of the mucopolysaccharide and lipid components respectively; these techniques are discussed in Chapters 11 and 12. Specific mucoproteins and lipoproteins may be identified by immunohistochemistry techniques (see Chapters 20 and 21).

Nucleic acids can be divided into two major classes: deoxyribonucleic acid (DNA) and ribonucleic acid (RNA). They are amino acid complexes of purines, pyrimidines, carbohydrates, and phosphoric acid. Histochemical techniques for the demonstration of nucleic acids in tissue are based on all their constituents. However, DNA and RNA can be localized in cells by the affinity of their negatively charged phosphate ester groups for almost any basic dye, particularly hematoxylin or methyl green and pyronine (Spicer 1987). RNA is usually evident only in cells whose cytoplasm is particularly rich in this nucleic acid (e.g. plasma cells and serous acinar cells). Hematoxylin is by no means specific for DNA and RNA,

and it will also stain glycosaminoglycans and other anionic complexes.

The value of identification of protein and nucleic acid by histochemical methods for research and diagnostic purposes is limited in the present-day histology laboratory. This is due to the lack of specificity of the methods available and the advances in immunohistochemistry, in situ hybridization, and proteomics. Fixation also plays an important part in the ability to demonstrate proteins and nucleic acids. The denaturation and cross-linking effect of different fixatives have a great impact on the molecular structure of proteins. All cross-linking fixatives react with specific amino acid side chains, and these same chains are the sites where the majority of cross-linking occurs. The effects of fixation on proteins are covered in depth in Chapter 4.

This chapter concentrates on simple protein identification by histochemical methods that identify the functional groups of amino acids that form side chains. Nucleic acid identification is limited to histochemical techniques but includes a chart listing antibodies specific to selected nuclear proteins. In situ hybridization is discussed in Chapter 26. This chapter does not cover all the histochemical methods for proteins and nucleic acids; for a complete review see Pearse (1968) and Kiernan (1999).

PROTEINS

All amino acids have a common structure of a central carbon atom to which an amino group, a carboxylic acid group, a hydrogen atom, and side chains are covalently

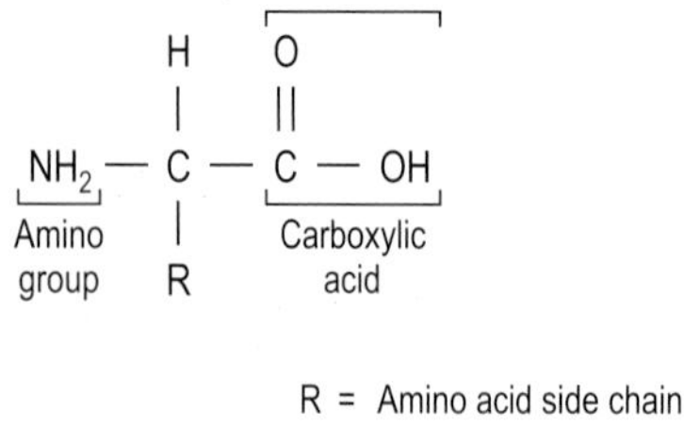

R = Amino acid side chain

Fig. 13.1 Basic structure of an amino acid.

bonded. They differ from each other only by their side chains (Fig. 13.1).

Most if not all of the histochemical methods for proteins rely on the presence of a small number of functional groups located on the side chains of amino acids or on techniques that create functional groups on these side chains. These groups react with specific reagents to produce a chromogenic reaction. Figure 13.2 represents amino acids with functional groups that are utilized in histochemical staining methods given in this chapter. The ninhydrin–Schiff method for amino groups is an exception to side chain functional group histochemistry; this method demonstrates all protein-bound amino groups by the reaction of ninhydrin with the amino group to produce aldehydes that are then made visible by the Schiff reaction. Most often, the chromogenic reaction with the amino acid functional group is not specific and blocking techniques must be employed.

Blocking techniques

Blocking techniques chemically alter functional groups so they can no longer take part in a reaction that pro-duces a chromophore. Many of the blocking techniques are not specific and on occasion it is necessary to employ more than one blocking method to discover the site or presence of a single functional group by the process of elimination. For a comprehensive review see Kiernan (1999).

Amino acid histochemical methods

Protein-bound amino groups

These can be demonstrated by the ninhydrin–Schiff reaction. At neutral pH and 37°C, ninhydrin reacts with α-amino groups to produce aldehydes which can then be demonstrated using Schiff's reagent.

Ninhydrin–Schiff method for amino groups (Yasuma & Itchikawa 1953)

Fixation
Neutral buffered formalin; formaldehyde vapor (for freeze-dried tissue).

Sections
Paraffin, cryostat, or freeze dried.

Solutions
0.5% ninhydrin in absolute alcohol
Schiff's reagent (see p. 171).

Method
1. Take sections to 70% alcohol.
2. Treat with ninhydrin solution at 37°C overnight.

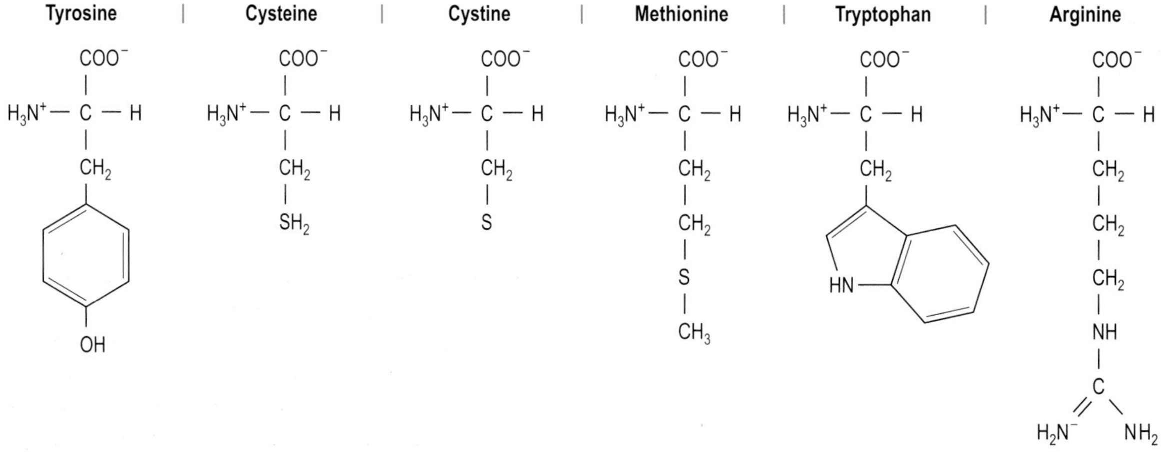

Fig. 13.2 Example of amino acid functional groups.

3. Wash in running tap water.
4. Treat in Schiff's reagent for 45 min.
5. Wash in running tap water.
6. Counterstain with an alum hematoxylin.
7. Wash in tap water; dehydrate through alcohols, clear in xylene, and mount in xylene-miscible mounting media.

Results

Amino groups   pinkish-purple

Notes

a. Control sections should be used to exclude other PAS-positive material.
b. Amino groups may also be demonstrated by the hydroxynaphthaldehyde method of Weiss et al (1954), although a non-formalin fixative is preferable for this technique.

Phenyl groups

These can be demonstrated by a modification of the well-known biochemical test, the Millon reaction (Baker 1956). A red or pinkish color develops at the site of tyrosine-containing proteins when the section is treated with a hot mercuric sulfate–sulfuric acid–sodium nitrite mixture. Tyrosine is the only amino acid that contains the hydroxyphenyl group in a form which can be demonstrated histochemically. The method can therefore be regarded as specific for tyrosine, but since tyrosine is an almost invariable constituent of all tissue proteins, the Millon reaction is a suitable general protein method. The color reaction of the Millon reaction is rarely strong and there may be difficulty encountered in keeping the sections on the slide. A less well-known, but more reliable, technique is the diazotization-coupling method (Glenner & Lillie 1959).

Solutions

Solution a

10 g of mercuric sulfate is added to a mixture of 90 ml distilled water and 10 ml of concentrated sulfuric acid, and is dissolved by heating. After cooling to room temperature, 100 ml of distilled water is added.

Solution b

250 mg of sodium nitrite is dissolved in 10 ml of distilled water.

Staining solution

5 ml of solution b is added to 50 ml of solution a.

Method

1. Take sections to water.
2. Immerse sections in staining solution in a small beaker and gently bring to boil; simmer for 2 min.
3. Allow to cool to room temperature.
4. Wash in three changes of distilled water, 2 min each.
5. Dehydrate through alcohols, clear in xylene, and mount.

Result

Tyrosine-containing proteins   red or pink

Note

a. A suitable positive control tissue is pancreas.
b. Mercury-containing reagents must be disposed of according to law.
c. Caution should be used when diluting sulfuric acid with water.

Millon reaction for tyrosine (Baker 1956)

Fixation

Neutral buffered formalin; formaldehyde vapor (for freeze-dried tissue).

Sections

Paraffin, fixed cryostat, freeze dried, or celloidin.

Diazotization-coupling method for tyrosine

This method employs 8-amino-1-naphthol-5-sulfonic acid as a coupling amine for the diazonium nitrites produced by nitrozation of tyrosine. It is necessary to carry out both incubation stages in the dark and at a low temperature. In our hands, this gives better and stronger results than the previous technique.

Diazotization-coupling method for tyrosine (Glenner & Lillie 1959)

Solutions

Incubating solution a

Sodium nitrite	3.5 g
Concentrated acetic acid	4.4 ml
Distilled water	47 ml

Incubating solution b

8-amino-1-naphthol-5-sulfonic acid	0.5 g
Potassium hydroxide	0.5 g
Ammonium sulfamate	0.5 g
70% alcohol	50 ml

Technique

1. Bring sections to water.
2. Place sections in incubating solution (a) at 4°C for 24 hours in the dark.
3. Rinse in four changes of distilled water at 4°C.
4. Transfer sections to incubating solution (b) at 4°C for 1 hour in the dark.
5. Wash in three changes of 0.1 M HCl, 5 min each.
6. Rinse in running tap water for 10 min.
7. Counterstain if required.
8. Dehydrate through alcohols to xylene, and mount.

Results

Tyrosine-containing proteins—purple and red.

Disulfide and sulfhydryl linkages

These are found in the amino acids cysteine and methionine, and in the derived amino acid cystine. The disulfide linkage occurs between two sulfur atoms (—S—S—) and the sulfhydryl grouping is found between a sulfur atom and a hydrogen atom (—S—H). The sulfhydryl group can be produced by reduction of a disulfide link. A number of reactions, for example the Schmorl ferricyanide technique (see p. 243), can demonstrate both these sulfur-containing groups histochemically. The method given below is consistent and uses common reagents. To confirm that a positive reaction is due to the presence of sulfhydryl groups, a duplicate section should be treated with saturated aqueous mercuric chloride solution for 24 hours at room temperature prior to the technique. Mercury condenses specifically with sulfhydryl groups and will provide a reliable negative control.

Performic acid–alcian blue method (Adams & Sloper 1955)

Fixation

Neutral buffered formalin; formaldehyde vapor (for freeze-dried tissue).

Sections

Paraffin, freeze-dried, frozen cryostat sections.

Solutions

Performic acid solution

Concentrated formic acid	40 ml
30% hydrogen peroxide	4 ml
Concentrated sulfuric acid	0.5 ml

Alcian blue solution

Alcian blue	1 g
Concentrated sulfuric acid	2.7 ml
Distilled water	47.2 ml

Method

1. Take sections to water; blot to remove surplus water.
2. Emerge sections in performic acid solution (see Note a), 5 min.
3. Wash well in tap water (see Note b), 10 min.
4. Dry in 60°C oven until just dry.
5. Rinse in tap water.
6. Stain in alcian blue solution at room temperature, 1 hour.
7. Wash in running tap water.
8. Counterstain (e.g. neutral red) if required.
9. Wash in tap water.
10. Dehydrate through alcohols, clear in xylene, and mount.

Result

Disulfides	blue

The intensity of the blue color will depend on the amount of disulfide present.

Notes

a. The performic acid solution should be prepared fresh and allowed to stand for 1 hour before use.
b. The section should be washed adequately but carefully; it may lift off if the washing is too vigorous following treatment in performic acid. The drying stage reduces the risk of section loss.
c. Keratin contains abundant disulfide-containing amino acids, so hair-bearing skin makes a suitable

positive control. The pituitary is another useful control tissue as some of the basophil cells will be positive.

Indole groups

These can be demonstrated by the histochemical reaction of the amino acids tryptamine and tryptophan. The most reliable method is the DMAB–nitrite method of Adams (1957) (Fig. 13.3). The best results (i.e. most intense coloration and most precise localization) are obtained with freeze-dried sections, but satisfactory results are obtainable with paraffin sections. The principle of the method is that tryptophan reacts with DMAB (p-dimethylaminobenzaldehyde) to produce a substance known as β-carboline, which is then oxidized by the nitrite solution to produce a deep blue pigment.

DMAB–nitrite method for tryptophan
(Adams 1957)

Fixation
Neutral buffered formalin; formaldehyde vapor (for freeze-dried tissue).

Sections
Paraffin, freeze-dried, frozen cryostat sections.

Solutions

DMAB solution
5 g of p-dimethylaminobenzaldehyde is dissolved in 100 ml of concentrated hydrochloric acid.

Nitrite solution
1 g of sodium nitrite is dissolved in 100 ml of concentrated hydrochloric acid.

Method
1. Take sections to absolute ethanol.
2. Celloidinize in 0.5% celloidin.
3. Place sections in DMAB solution for 1 min.
4. Transfer sections to nitrite solution for 1–2 min.
5. Wash gently in tap water for 30 s.
6. Rinse in acid alcohol for 15 s.
7. Wash in water and optionally counterstain in 1% aqueous neutral red for 5 min.
8. Dehydrate through ethanols, clear in xylene, and mount.

Results
Tryptophan	dark blue
Nuclei	red

Notes
a. Pancreas is an excellent positive control tissue.
b. This is one of the most satisfactory and rewarding of amino acid histochemical methods.
c. The reagents give off toxic fumes and should be prepared (and used if possible) in a fume hood.

Guanidyl groups

These can be demonstrated in tissues by a histochemical method based on the Sakaguchi reaction. In this method an orange–red color develops when arginine reacts with α-naphthol and an alkaline hypochlorite solution. The color fades rapidly and the section must be examined immediately after the staining procedure. Arginine is the only amino acid that can be demonstrated histochemically by this reaction because it is the only amino acid that contains the guanidyl group.

The modified Sakaguchi reaction for arginine (Baker 1947)

Fixation
Neutral buffered formalin; formaldehyde vapor (for freeze-dried tissue).
Formaldehyde mixtures.

Sections
(See Note a). Paraffin, freeze dried, fixed cryostat.

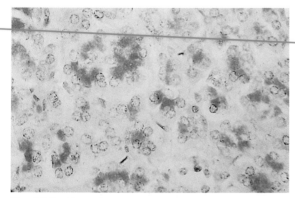

Fig. 13.3 Normal exocrine pancreas showing cytoplasmic tryptophan dark blue, cell nuclei red. DMAB–nitrite technique with neutral red counterstain.

Incubating solution

1% sodium hydroxide	2 ml
1% α-naphthol in 70% ethanol	2 drops
1% sodium hypochlorite	4 drops in distilled water

Pyridine–chloroform solution

Pyridine	30 ml
Chloroform	10 ml

Method

1. Take sections to water.
2. Rinse in 70% ethanol.
3. Flood slide with incubating solution for 15 min.
4. Drain and gently blot dry.
5. Immerse in pyridine–chloroform solution, 2 min.
6. Mount in fresh pyridine–chloroform solution and ring coverslip with clear nail polish to seal.

Result

Arginine	orange–red

Notes

a. The best results are obtained with sections that are about 12–15 mm thick.
b. Use silane-coated slides.
c. The color reaction is often weak.
d. Testis contains abundant arginine and is the most suitable positive control.
e. It is vital to examine the section as soon as possible due to the rapid fading of the color.
f. The method is capricious.

General comments on amino acid histochemistry

Currently, it is unusual to use any of these methods to demonstrate specific amino acids in tissue. Thus, in the preceding account, only one method has been given for each type of group or linkage, except for phenyl groups. In general, the methods presented are the simplest and have proved the most reliable in our hands, although not always specific. Many other methods exist, although they are usually more complicated than those given above. For further details of these methods, the reader is referred to Pearse (1968), Bancroft (1975), and James and Tas (1984). In our experience, the best results with amino acid histochemical methods are obtained using freeze-dried sections; the color intensity is usually greater and the localization is more accurate. This is so even though the warm formaldehyde vapor, essential in the fixation of freeze-dried tissues, is generally regarded as being more likely to destroy the reactive groups than formaldehyde-based solutions. These methods are included to provide a historical basis for localizing subtypes of proteins. Current technology using immuno-histochemistry and proteomics can provide a much better localization of proteins specifically as well as protein/peptide subtypes.

Immunohistochemical methods for the identification of proteins

Identification of proteins/peptides in tissues has evolved from non-specific staining to more specific methods incorporated under the term 'protein assays' such as immunohistochemistry. Immunohistochemical methods provide specific identification and localization of specific proteins such as immunoglobulins, enzymes, and hormones. This type of technique offers accurate identification and localization of specific proteins and polypeptides. The principles and methods of immunohistochemistry are discussed in detail in Chapter 21.

Proteomics/genomics

The 'proteome' is the sum total of proteins in a cell or tissue and proteomics is the study of part or all of the proteome. Specifically, tissue can be extracted biochemically for various types of molecules. Tissue extracts can be run on electrophoretic gel matrices and transferred from the gels electrolytically (blotted) to membranes. These membranes can be stained with general stains for proteins (e.g. silver stains) or antibodies to demonstrate proteins more specifically (Western blots). Tissue extracts can also be run on a two-dimensional gel electrophoresis system stained ether non-specifically for proteins or with antibodies to classes of proteins (phosphoproteins). Uses include comparing the 2-D gel electrophoresis pattern from a normal tissue with one from a diseased tissue to identify proteins/peptides associated only with that disease. Similarly, the extract of tissues/cells can be analyzed for multiple proteins using multiplex immunoassays, antibody arrays, or MALDI or SELDI (matrix-assisted/surface-enhanced laser desorption/ionization) time of flight mass spectroscopy (Grizzle et al 2005). Simultaneously, change in gene expression can be compared with levels of proteins for these same genes. The recent development of multiplex immunoassays and multiplex RT-PCR (reverse transcriptase–polymerase chain reaction) permits a simultaneous analysis of many proteins/mRNA species (up to 100) in just two assays (Steg et al 2006). Tissue extraction regimens are improving rapidly, including methods that are applicable to the extraction of proteins and mRNA from paraffin-embedded tissues (Hood et al 2005). These recent advances in methodology make many histochemical approaches to identify general categories of proteins obsolete.

NUCLEIC ACIDS

Nucleoproteins are combinations of basic proteins (protamines and histones) and nucleic acids. The two nucleic acids are deoxyribonucleic acid (DNA), which is mainly found in the nucleus of the cell, and ribonucleic acid (RNA), which is located in the cytoplasm of cells, mainly in the ribosomes. Both the DNA and RNA molecules consist of alternate sugar and phosphate groups with a nitrogenous base being attached to each sugar group. The sugar in DNA is the five-carbon sugar deoxyribose; in RNA it is ribose.

There are usually four nitrogenous bases in DNA, the purines, adenine and guanine, and the pyrimidines, thymine and cytosine, while in RNA the purines adenine and guanine are present but the pyrimidines are uracil and cytosine. On hydrolysis, the nucleic acids will yield (1) phosphate groups, (2) sugars, and (3) nitrogenous bases. The demonstration of nucleic acid depends upon either the reaction of dyes with the phosphate groups or the production of aldehydes from the sugar deoxyribose. No histochemical methods are available to demonstrate the nitrogenous bases.

The basic proteins are readily and selectively demonstrated by staining with such dyes as Biebrich scarlet or fast green at a high pH (9.5). This is rarely called for in routine diagnostic work.

Demonstration of nucleic acids

Fixation

In general terms, the nucleic acids are best preserved in alcoholic and acidic fixatives, a good example being Carnoy's fluid which contains both alcohol and glacial acetic acid. Formalin has only a limited reaction with DNA and RNA, but for routine work gives acceptable results. Low (4°C) temperature fixation in neutral buffered formalin has been shown to prevent DNA degrada-

tion by cell nucleases, which is of some importance when carrying out molecular biology studies (Tokuda et al 1990).

Decalcification

Treatment of tissue with strong inorganic acids such as nitric or hydrochloric and Bouin's fixative is to be avoided, as nucleic acids are progressively extracted. Using an organic acid for short periods of time to decalcify tissue will normally permit acceptable results with the standard special stains; for example, by treating a trephine bone biopsy for around 8 hours in 5% formic acid, acceptable methyl green–pyronin staining should be possible. EDTA decalcification gives the best results but, used alone, is much slower in action. One of the most noticeable effects of over-decalcification using an acid is that cell nuclei become pyroninophilic with the methyl green–pyronin stain. In other words, denatured DNA stains red rather than the usual green coloration of cell nuclei.

Basophilia

DNA and RNA both stain strongly with most cationic dyes. Selectivity of staining can be achieved by using, for example, methylene blue at a pH range of 3.0–4.0. A distinction has been drawn between the link formed by simple cationic dyes such as neutral red and methylene blue and nucleic acid, and the nuclear stain formed by metal complex dyes such as alum hematoxylin (Marshall & Horobin 1973). The former type of staining can be markedly reduced by prior treatment with acids, and is considered to be largely coulombic (electrostatic) in nature. Alum hematoxylin staining of cellular nuclei is much less affected by prior acid treatment. This partly acid-fast effect is attributed to the metal–dye complex also forming non-electrostatic bonding interactions, such as hydrophobic bonding and van der Waals' attraction forces, with nucleic acids. Interestingly, whilst nucleic acids exhibit strong basophilia, they do not usually exhibit metachromasia with the standard metachromatic dyes such as toluidine blue or azure A.

Deoxyribonucleic acid (DNA)

The typical demonstration of DNA is by either the Feulgen technique, which will demonstrate the sugar deoxyribose, or the methyl green–pyronin technique in which the phosphates combine with the basic dye methyl green at an acid pH. DNA can also be demonstrated by fluorescent methods using acridine orange, although the reliability of this type of method is less than that of the previous methods. Both DNA and RNA can be demonstrated by the gallocyanin–chrome alum method; the method does not separate the two nucleic acids and suitable extraction techniques must be used. The definitive, most sensitive technique for identifying DNA is that of in situ hybridization (see Chapter 26).

Feulgen reaction

The method of Feulgen and Rossenbeck (1924) is the standard technique for demonstrating deoxyribose. Mild acid hydrolysis, employing 1 M hydrochloric acid at 60°C, is used to break the purine–deoxyribose bond; the resulting 'exposed' aldehydes are then demonstrated by the use of Schiff's reagent. Elements containing DNA are stained a red–purple color. The ribose–purine bond is unaffected by the hydrolysis and RNA is not demonstrated (Fig. 13.4).

The hydrolysis is the critical part of the method; an increasingly stronger reaction is obtained as the hydrolysis time is increased until the optimum is reached. Beyond this the reaction becomes weaker, and if the hydrolysis is continued the reaction may fail completely. An important consideration in selecting the correct hydrolysis time is the fixative used. Bouin's fixative is not suitable as it causes over-hydrolysis of the nucleic acid during fixation. Bauer (1932) discussed the times of hydrolysis for various fixatives; some of these are reproduced in Table 13.1.

Table 13.1   Hydrolysis times in pre-warmed 1 M HCl at 60°C

Fixative	Time (minutes)
Bouin	Unsuitable
Carnoy 6.3.1	8
Chrome acetic	14
Flemming	16
Formaldehyde vapour	30–60
Formalin	8
Formal sublimate	8
Helly	8
Newcomer	20
Regaud	14
Regaud sublimate	8
Susa	18
Zenker	5
Zenker formal	5

Feulgen nuclear reaction for DNA (Feulgen & Rossenbeck 1924)

Fixation

Not critical but not Bouin's (see Table 13.1).

Solutions

a. *1 M hydrochloric acid*

Hydrochloric acid (conc.)	8.5 ml
Distilled water	91.5 ml

b. *Schiff reagent*
(See p. 171).

c. *Bisulfite solution*

10% potassium metabisulfite	5 ml
1 M hydrochloric acid	5 ml
Distilled water	90 ml

Method

1. Bring all sections to water.
2. Rinse sections in 1 M HCl at room temperature.
3. Place sections in 1 M HCl at 60°C (see Table 13.1).
4. Rinse in 1 M HCl at room temperature, 1 min.
5. Transfer sections to Schiff's reagent, 45 min.
6. Rinse sections in bisulfite solution, 2 min.
7. Repeat wash in bisulfite solution, 2 min.
8. Repeat wash in bisulfite solution, 2 min.
9. Rinse well in distilled water.

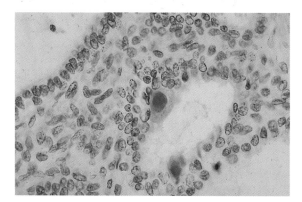

Fig. 13.4 Nuclear cytomegalovirus inclusion bodies magenta but smaller in size. Feulgen technique with light green counterstain.

10. Counterstain if required in 1% light green, 2 min.
11. Wash in water.
12. Dehydrate through alcohols to xylene and mount.

Results

DNA	red–purple
Cytoplasm	green

Notes

a. The hydrolysis time is important (see Table 13.1), and the correct time for the fixative should be used.
b. The 1 M HCl should be preheated to 60°C.
c. Elias et al (1972) use 5 M HCl at room temperature for hydrolysis. The hydrolysis time needs to be longer than at 60°C.
d. The post-Schiff bisulfite solution washing is optional and, in our experience, can be safely omitted.

Naphthoic acid hydrazide–Feulgen (NAH) method

This technique can be used as a control method for the standard Feulgen reaction. The sections are hydrolyzed in 1 M hydrochloric acid as in the Feulgen technique. The aldehydes produced by this hydrolysis are coupled with 2-hydroxy-3-naphthoic acid, which in turn is coupled to the diazonium salt, fast blue B. The results with this technique are identical to the true Feulgen reaction.

Naphthoic acid hydrazide–Feulgen method for DNA (Pearse 1951)

Fixation
Not critical.

Solutions

a. 1 M hydrochloric acid

Concentrated hydrochloric acid	8.5 ml
Distilled water	91.5 ml

b. NAH solution

2-Hydroxy-3-naphthoic acid hydrazide	50 mg
Absolute alcohol	47 ml
Acetic acid (conc.)	3 ml

c. Fast blue B solution

Fast blue B	50 mg
Veronal acetate buffer, pH 7.4 (see Appendix III)	50 ml

This solution must be freshly prepared.

Method

1. Bring all sections to water.
2. Rinse briefly in 1 M HCl.
3. Place sections in 1 M HCl at 60°C (see Table 13.1).
4. Rinse sections in 1 M HCl at room temperature, 1 min.
5. Rinse sections in distilled water, 1 min.
6. Rinse sections in 50% ethanol, 1 min.
7. Place sections in NAH solution at room temperature, 3–6 hours.
8. Rinse sections in 50% ethanol, 10 min.
9. Rinse sections in 50% ethanol, 10 min.
10. Rinse sections in 50% ethanol, 10 min.
11. Rinse sections in distilled water, 1 min.
12. Place sections in fresh fast blue B solution, 3 min.
13. Dehydrate through ethanols to xylene, and mount.

Result

DNA	blue to bluish-purple
Protein material possibly	purplish-red

Blue thionin–Feulgen reaction for DNA ploidy studies

While the Feulgen reaction has only a limited diagnostic role, it is commonly used in conjunction with microdensitometry to study cancer cell nuclear morphology and ploidy (Poulin et al 2003). The Feulgen reaction is useful for ploidy studies because it has reproducible stoichiometry with DNA. In the reaction, parameters are changed such that nuclei are stained a pure blue without any of the 'red' elements in the spectrum. This is important because instrumentation relies on a complete separation of red–blue spectrum components. For example, it has been employed as such to show an inverse relationship between DNA content of certain lymphoma cells and the tumor prognosis (Vuckovic et al 1990).

Blue thionin–Feulgen reaction for DNA

Fixation
Formalin.
Post fixation in Boehm–Sprenger fixative.

Preparation of solutions

a. *Boehm–Sprenger fixative*

Methanol	80 ml
Formaldehyde (37%)	15 ml
Acetic acid (glacial)	5 ml

b. *5 N hydrochloric acid*

5 N hydrochloric (conc.)	41.7 ml
Distilled water	58.3 ml

c. *1 N hydrochloric acid*

Hydrochloric acid (conc)	8.5 ml
Distilled water	91.5 ml

d. *Thionin (blue) Schiff reagent*

Thionin	0.25 g
Distilled water	220 ml

Dissolve the thionin and boil for 5 minutes. Cool until lukewarm then add:

Tertiary butanol	220 ml
1 N hydrochloric acid	65 ml
Sodium bisulfite	4.3 g

Stir for 1.5 hours and let sit for at least 20 hours at room temperature.
Filter before use.

e. *Sodium bisulfite differentiating solution*

Sodium bisulfite	1.5 g
Distilled water	285 ml
1 N HCl	15 ml

Method
1. Bring sections to water.
2. Post-fix specimen in Boehm–Sprenger fixative for 10 min.
3. Rinse sections briefly in distilled water.
4. Hydrolyze specimen in 5 N HCl for 60 min.
5. Transfer sections to thionin Schiff's reagent for 60 min.
6. Rinse in three changes of sodium bisulfite differentiating solution for a total of 10 min.
7. Rinse in two changes of distilled water.
8. Dehydrate through alcohols to xylene, and mount.

Results

DNA	blue
Cytoplasm	unstained

Ribonucleic acid (RNA)

The method of choice for demonstrating RNA is the methyl green–pyronin technique. RNA can also be demonstrated by acridine orange and by the gallocyanin–chrome alum technique, along with DNA, with suitable extraction procedures.

Methyl green–pyronin

This will demonstrate both DNA and RNA and was first published by Pappenheim (1899), and later modified by Unna (1902). Since then there has been considerable debate and many modifications of the original technique. Methyl green is an impure dye containing methyl violet. When the methyl violet has been removed by washing with chloroform, the pure methyl green (when used at a slightly acid pH) appears to be specific for DNA.

The rationale of the technique is that both dyes are cationic; when used in combination methyl green binds preferentially and specifically to DNA, and the pyronin binds RNA (Fig. 13.5). The methyl green-specific reactivity is attributed to the spatial alignment of the NH_2 groups of the dye to phosphate radicals on the DNA double helix. Pyronin staining, on the other hand, does not show this spatial affinity and any negatively charged tissue constituent will stain red. In practice, not only RNA stains: acid mucins present in epithelium and cartilage will also stain.

Carefully controlled conditions have to be employed; the pH of the staining solution is critical as well as the concentration of the two dyes. The final dehydration is also important. In most methods washing in water after

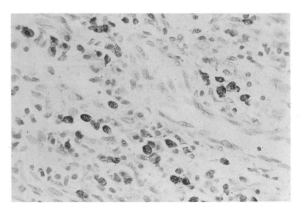

Fig. 13.5 Normal plasma cells showing nuclear DNA green, cytoplasmic RNA red. Combined methyl green–pyronin technique employing a final wash in 93% alcohol.

staining is avoided. Dehydration in 93% ethanol after staining will give a greener nuclear staining effect. Elias (1969) claims that better results are obtained by first washing in ice-cold water, followed by further differentiation in tertiary butanol. Good results have been obtained with the method given below, along with a standard method, taken from Bancroft and Cook (1994). For further discussion of this method, the reader is referred to Horobin (1988).

Methyl green–pyronin method (Pappenheim 1899; Unna 1902 from Bancroft & Cook 1994)

Fixation
Carnoy preferred, but formalin acceptable.

Solution

Methyl green pyronin Y

2% methyl green in distilled water (chloroform washed)	9 ml
2% pyronin Y in distilled water	4 ml
Acetate buffer pH 4.8	23 ml
Glycerol	14 ml

Mix well before use.

Method
1. Take sections down to water.
2. Rinse in acetate buffer pH 4.8.
3. Place in methyl green–pyronin Y solution for 25 min.
4. Rinse in buffer.
5. Blot dry.
6. Rinse in 93% ethanol, then in absolute ethanol.
7. Rinse in xylene and mount.

Results
DNA	green–blue
RNA	red

Notes
a. Some mucous cells may be stained by the pyronin.
b. Although acid decalcification, e.g. of bone, is said to interfere with the methyl green–pyronin Y method (see earlier discussion on the effect of decalcification), satisfactory results have been obtained by adjusting the proportions of the two dyes. In general, the methyl green needs to be increased and the pyronin Y decreased.

Methyl green–pyronin Y alternative method (Pappenheim 1899; Unna 1902; Elias 1969)

Solutions

Methyl green solution

Methyl green	1 g
Acetate buffer pH 4.1 (see Appendix III, buffer table)	200 ml

Wash in chloroform until completely free of traces of methyl violet.

Staining solution

Methyl green solution	100 ml
Pyronin Y	200 mg

The solution is well stirred and stored at 4°C, and filtered before use.

Method
1. Bring sections down to distilled water.
2. Place in staining solution at 37°C for 1 hour.
3. Rinse in distilled water at 1°C for 2 s.
4. Blot sections dry.
5. Rinse in *tert*-butanol.
6. Dehydrate in two changes of *tert*-butanol, 5 min.
7. Clear xylene and mount.

Results
DNA	green–blue
RNA	red

Note
The temperature of the distilled water wash is critical.

Other techniques

Gallocyanin–chrome alum

This technique relies upon the combination of the phosphoric acid residue of the nucleic acids with gallocyanin at an acid pH. Extraction techniques can be used to identify either DNA or RNA if required (see below).

Gallocyanin–chrome alum method for RNA and DNA (Einarson 1932, 1951)

Staining solution

Chrome alum	5 g
Distilled water	100 ml
Gallocyanin 1	50 mg

The chrome alum is dissolved in the distilled water, the gallocyanin added, and the solution slowly heated until it boils. It is allowed to boil for 5 min. When the solution has cooled to room temperature, the volume is adjusted to 100 ml. The solution is filtered before use.

Method

1. Bring sections down to water.
2. Stain in gallocyanin–chrome alum solution for 18–48 hours.
3. Wash in tap water.
4. Dehydrate through alcohols and mount.

Results

RNA, DNA	blue

Note

This method does not distinguish between RNA and DNA but appears specific for nucleic acids if used at a pH of 1.0 (Pearse 1968). Used at the standard pH of 1.64, it has been shown that gallocyanin will also stain non-nucleic acid material in the nuclear karyoplasm of cells (Clark 1969).

Digestion methods for nucleic acids

Specific enzymes can be used to digest DNA and RNA in tissue sections. Pure deoxyribonuclease will remove DNA, while ribonuclease will digest RNA. In a pure state, the enzymes will not affect the other nucleic acid.

Enzyme extraction of DNA (Brachet 1940)

Fixation

Potassium dichromate will inhibit digestion, and should be avoided.

Digestion solution

Deoxyribonuclease	10 mg
0.2 M Tris buffer, pH 7.6	10 ml
Distilled water	50 ml

Method

1. Bring both test and control sections to water.
2. Place test section in extraction solution, control in Tris buffer, pH 7.6; incubate both test and control section at 37°C, for 4 hours.
3. Wash in running tap water.
4. Stain both sections by the Feulgen method.

Results

Test section	DNA negative
Control section	DNA red

Enzyme extraction of RNA (Brachet 1940)

Fixation

Potassium dichromate and mercuric chloride should be avoided, as digestion is inhibited.

Digestion solution

Ribonuclease	8 mg
Distilled water	10 ml

Method

1. Bring both test and control slides to water.
2. Place test slide in ribonuclease solution, and control slide in distilled water; incubate both test and control sections at 37°C for 1 hour.
3. Wash in distilled water.
4. Apply methyl green–pyronin method.

Results

Test slide	RNA negative, DNA green
Control slide	RNA red, DNA green

Chemical extraction methods of nucleic acids

A considerably cheaper but non-specific removal of nucleic acids is achieved with perchloric acid.

Extraction of nucleic acids with perchloric acid

Solutions

Solution a

Perchloric acid	2.5 ml
Distilled water	47.5 ml

Solution b

Perchloric acid	5 ml
Distilled water	45 ml

Solution c

Sodium carbonate	1 g
Distilled water	100 ml

Method

To remove RNA only:

1. Bring sections down to water.
2. Place sections in 10% perchloric acid (solution b) at 4°C overnight.
3. Briefly rinse in distilled water.
4. Transfer to the sodium carbonate (solution c), 5 min.
5. Wash in tap water.
6. Employ nucleic acid method.

To remove both RNA and DNA, place sections in 5% perchloric acid (solution a) at 60°C for 30 min at stage 2, then continue method.

Trichloroacetic acid extraction of nucleic acids

Bring sections to water and treat with 4% trichloroacetic acid at exactly 90°C for 15 min. Wash and stain with toluidine blue. Both types of nucleic acid are extracted by this procedure.

Hydrochloric acid extraction of nucleic acids

Bring sections to water and treat with 1 M HCl for 3 hours at 37°C. Wash and stain with dilute methylene blue at pH 5.7 for 12–24 hours, or with any other suitable basic dye for shorter periods. This method removes both types of nucleic acid.

Fluorescent methods for DNA and RNA

Fluorescent methods have been developed for the demonstration of nucleic acids; the most used is the acridine orange technique (Bertalanffy & Von Nagy 1962) where DNA is stained yellow–green and RNA red (Fig. 13.6). The results are not permanent and the technique cannot

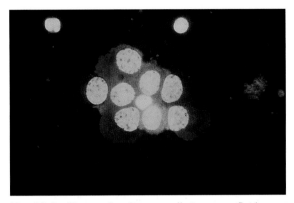

Fig. 13.6 Clump of malignant cells in serous fluid showing increased RNA content red, nuclear DNA yellow. Acridine orange fluorescence.

be successfully applied to formalin-fixed tissues. It is therefore of little value for general purposes, although it has been used in exfoliative cytology and with alcohol-fixed tissues. Newer methods utilize fluorescent methods to analyze nuclear morphometry and/or cellular ploidy in three dimensions (Huisman et al 2005).

Another fluorochrome, which can be employed in the study of nucleic acids, is acriflavine. It is used either as 0.01% alcoholic solution preceded by acid hydrolysis (Levinson et al 1977), or as an alternative to basic fuchsin in Schiff's reagent, again preceded by acid hydrolysis. DNA is stained by a fluorescent yellow color in both of these Feulgen-type reactions, the latter of which is of acceptable specificity (Tanke & Van Ingen 1980).

Immunohistochemical methods for the identification of nuclear proteins

These techniques are specific and show accurate identification and localization of nuclear proteins. The principles and methods of immunohistochemistry are discussed in Chapter 21.

Acknowledgment

John Bancroft and Alan Stevens wrote this chapter for the first three editions, and Harry Cook and John Bancroft updated the text for the fourth edition, and John Bancroft for the fifth. Our thanks are due to them for their contributions.

REFERENCES

Adams C.W.M. (1957) A *p*-dimethylaminobenzaldehyde–nitrite method for the histochemical demonstration of tryptophane and related compounds. Journal of Clinical Pathology 10:56.

Adams C.W.M., Sloper J.C. (1955) Technique for demonstrating neurosecretory material in the human hypothalamus. Lancet i:651.

Baker J.R. (1947) The histochemical recognition of certain guanidine derivatives. Quarterly Journal of Microscopical Science 88:115.

Baker J.R. (1956) The histochemical recognition of phenols, especially tyrosine. Quarterly Journal of Microscopical Science 97:161.

Bancroft J.D. (1975) Histochemical techniques, 2nd edn. London: Butterworths.

Bancroft J.D., Cook H.C. (1994) Manual of histological techniques and their diagnostic application. Edinburgh: Churchill Livingstone.

Bauer H. (1932) Die Feulgensche Nuklealfärbung in ihrer Anwendung auf cytologische Untersuchungen. Zeitschrift für Zellforschung und Mikroskopische Anatomie 15:225.

Bertalanffy F.D., Von Nagy K.P. (1962) Fluorescence microscopy and photomicrography with acridine orange. Medical Radiography and Photography 38:82.

Brachet J. (1940) La détection histochemique des acides pentose-nucléiques. Comptes Rendus des Séances de la Société de Biologie et de ses Filiales 133:88.

Clark G. (1969) Neuron staining by basic dyes versus basic metal–dye complexes: differences shown by histochemical blocking reactions. Stain Technology 44:15.

Einarson L. (1932) A method for progressive selective staining of Nissl and nuclear substances in nerve cells. American Journal of Pathology 8:295.

Einarson L. (1951) On the theory of gallocyanin–chromalum staining and its application for quantitative estimation of basophilia. Acta Pathologica et Microbiologica Scandinavica 81:256.

Elias J.M. (1969) Effects of temperature, poststaining rinses and ethanol–butanol dehydrating mixtures on methyl green pyronin staining. Stain Technology 44:201.

Elias J.M., Conkling K., Makar M. (1972) Cold feulgen hydrolysis: its effect on displacement of tritiated thymidine. Acta Histochemica et Cytochemica 5:125.

Feulgen R., Rossenbeck H. (1924) Mikroskopischchemischer Nachweis einen Nucleinsaure von Typus der Thymonucleinsaure und die darauf berhende elektive Färbung von Zellkernen in microskopischen Präparaten. Zeitschrift fur Physiologische Chemie 135:203.

Glenner G., Lillie R.D. (1959) Observations on the diazotization-coupling reaction for the histochemical demonstration of tyrosine: metal chelation and formazan variants. Journal of Histochemistry and Cytochemistry 7:416.

Grizzle W.E., Semmes O.J., Bigbee W. et al. (2005) The need for review and understanding of SELDI/MALDI mass spectroscopy data to analysis. Cancer Informatics 1(1):86–97.

Hood B.L., Darfler MM., Guiel T.G. et al. (2005) Proteomic analysis of formalin-fixed prostate cancer tissue. Molecular and Cellular Proteomics 4:1741–1753.

Horobin R.W. (1988) Understanding histochemistry. Chichester: Horwood.

Huisman A., Ploeger L.S., Dullens H.F. et al. (2005) Development of 3-D chromatin texture analysis using confocal laser scanning microscope. Cell Oncology 27(5–6):335–345.

James J., Tas J. (1984) Histochemical protein methods. RMS Handbook D4. London: Oxford University Press.

Kiernan J.A. (1999) Histological and histochemical methods: theory and practice, 3rd edn. Oxford, UK: Butterworth-Heinemann.

Levinson J.J., Retzel S., McCormick J.J. (1977) An improved acriflavine–feulgen method. Journal of Histochemistry and Cytochemistry 25:355.

Marshall P.N., Horobin R.W. (1973) The mechanism of action of 'mordant' dyes—a study using preformed metal complexes. Histochemie 35:361–371.

Pappenheim A. (1899) Vergleichende Untersuchungen über die elementare Zusammensetzung des rothen Knockenmarkes einiger Säugenthiere. Virchows Archiv für Pathologische Anatomie und Physiologie 157:19.

Pearse A.G.E. (1951) Review of modern methods in histochemistry. Quarterly Journal of Microscopical Science 92:393.

Pearse A.G.E. (1968) Histochemistry, theoretical and applied. London: Churchill Livingstone.

Poulin N., Frost A., Carraro A. et al. (2003) Risk biomarker assessments for breast cancer progression: replication precision of nuclear morphometry. Analytic Cellular Pathology 25(3):129–38.

Spicer S.S. (1987) Histochemistry in pathologic diagnosis. Oxford: Marcel Dekker.

Steg A., Wang W., Blanquicett C. et al. (2006) Multiple gene expression analyses in paraffin-embedded tissue by TaqMan low-density array: application to hedgehog and Wnt pathway analysis in ovarian endometrioid adenocarcinoma. Journal of Molecular Diagnostics 8(1):76–83.

Tanke H.J., Van Ingen E.M. (1980) A reliable Feulgen–acriflavine–SO2 staining procedure for quantitative DNA measurements. Journal of Histochemistry and Cytochemistry 28:1007.

Tokuda Y., Nakamura T., Satonaka K. et al. (1990) Fundamental study on the mechanism of DNA degradation in tissues fixed in formaldehyde. Journal of Clinical Pathology 43:748–751.

Unna P.G. (1902) Eine Modifikation der Pappenheimschen Färbung auf Granoplasma. Monatshefte für Praktische Dermatologie 35:76.

Vuckovic J., Dubravcic M., Matthews J.M. et al. (1990) Prognostic value of cytophotometric analysis of DNA in lymph node aspirates from patients with non-Hodgkin's lymphoma. Journal of Clinical Pathology 43:626–629.

Weiss L.P., Tsou K.C., Seligman A.M. (1954) Histochemical demonstration of protein-bound amino groups. Journal of Histochemistry and Cytochemistry 2:29.

Yasuma A., Itchikawa T. (1953) Ninhydrin–Schiff and alloxan–Schiff staining. Journal of Laboratory and Clinical Medicine 41:296.

14

Pigments and Minerals

Charles J. Churukian

INTRODUCTION

In biology, pigments are defined as substances occurring in living matter that absorb visible light. Therefore, various pigments may greatly differ in origin, chemical constitution, and biological significance. The reason that they are grouped together is because they all absorb electromagnetic energy within a narrow band that lies approximately between 400 and 800 nm. They can be either organic or inorganic compounds that remain insoluble in most solvents. Pigments can be classified under the following headings.

1. Endogenous pigments

These substances are produced either within tissues and serve a physiological function, or are by-products of normal metabolic processes. They can be further subdivided into:

- hematogenous (blood-derived) pigments
- non-hematogenous pigments
- endogenous minerals.

2. Artifact pigments

These are deposits of artifactually produced material caused by the interactions between certain tissue components and some chemical substances, such as the fixative formalin. Certain of these pigments, e.g formalin and malaria, are sometimes classified as a subdivision of endogenous pigments.

3. Exogenous pigments and minerals

These substances gain access to the body accidentally and serve no physiological function. Entry is gained either by inhalation into the lungs or by implantation into the skin. Most exogenous pigments are minerals, few of which are pigmented.

The above classification, although not scientifically precise, is used as a convenient aid in the identification of pigments. It is important to bear in mind that the same pigment may present itself in tissue sections in a variety of ways. Iron, for example, may be present as an endogenous pigment in liver sections in an iron overload condition and as an exogenous pigment in the case of a shrapnel wound. Furthermore, it is advisable to note a pigment's morphology, tissue site, and relevant clinical data before carrying out the various stains and histochemical reactions available in order that a pigment can be identified.

ENDOGENOUS PIGMENTS

Hematogenous

This group contains the following blood-derived pigments:

- hemosiderins
- hemoglobin
- bile pigments
- porphyrins.

Hemosiderins

Hemosiderin pigments are seen as yellow to brown granules and normally appear intracellularly. They contain iron in the form of ferric hydroxide that is bound to a protein framework and is unmasked by various chemicals. Iron is a vital component of the human body as it is an essential constituent of the oxygen-carrying

233

hemoglobin found in the red cells, where 60% of the body's total iron content resides. It also occurs in myoglobin and certain enzymes such as cytochrome oxidase and the peroxidases.

Normal and abnormal iron metabolism

Dietary iron is absorbed in the small intestine and attached to a protein molecule for transfer to the sites in the body where it is to be utilized or stored. Approximately 30% is stored within the reticuloendothelial system, especially the bone marrow. The bone marrow is also the main site of iron utilization in the body, where it is incorporated into the hemoglobin molecule during red cell formation. The normal breakdown of worn-out red cells results in the release of iron that is recirculated back into the various areas of iron storage for further utilization. Under normal conditions, this efficient system of recycling usually means that iron deficiency rarely occurs. There is a minimal loss of iron by the way of epithelial desquamation, hair loss, and sweating. The main reason for loss of iron from the body is hemorrhage in the form of either chronic bleeding, e.g. a peptic ulcer, carcinoma of the stomach or colon, or in the female by menstruation, with approximately 25% of females being iron deficient. The small intestine normally only absorbs sufficient iron from the excess iron in the diet to counteract any losses, but in excessive blood loss the dietary content may be relatively inadequate for the need, and even though the absorption mechanism is working at full efficiency, a state of clinical iron deficiency occurs. In iron deficiency, the iron stores in the bone marrow become depleted, insufficient hemoglobin is produced because of the lack of iron, and anemia develops in which the red cells contain inadequate amounts of hemoglobin. The iron deficiency is demonstrated by the absence of stainable iron in the bone marrow.

There is no active method of iron excretion from the body. Iron excess is a much less common condition, because under normal conditions the intestine will not absorb iron from the diet when there is already a surplus within the body. However, this controlling mechanism may be bypassed when iron is given therapeutically, in the form of either iron injections or blood transfusion. If excess iron is given this way, the iron stores may become overloaded, and excessive amounts of hemosiderin be deposited in the organs with a prominent reticuloendothelial component (e.g. spleen, bone marrow, liver). This condition is called *hemosiderosis*. A rarer cause of iron

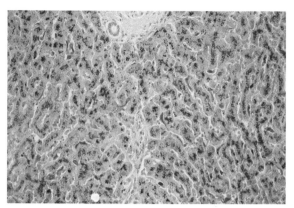

Fig. 14.1   A section of liver from a patient with hemochromatosis stained for ferric iron with Perls' method. Ferric iron is stained blue. Original magnification ×100.

overload is the disease *hemochromatosis*, in which the controlling mechanism at the small intestine absorption stage becomes impaired, and the iron is absorbed indiscriminately in amounts irrelevant to the state of the body's iron stores. In this disorder large quantities of hemosiderin are deposited in many of the organs, often interfering with the organs' structure and function.

Demonstration of hemosiderin and iron

In unfixed tissue, hemosiderin is insoluble in alkalis but freely soluble in strong acid solutions; after fixation in formalin, it is slowly soluble in dilute acids, especially oxalic acid. Fixatives that contain acids but no formalin can remove hemosiderin or alter it in such a way that reactions for iron are negative. Certain types of iron found in tissues are not demonstrable using traditional techniques. This is because the iron is tightly bound within a protein complex. Both hemoglobin and myoglobin are examples of such protein complexes and, if treated with hydrogen peroxide (100 vol), the iron is released and can then be demonstrated using Perls' Prussian blue reaction (Fig. 14.1). A similar result is obtained if the acid ferrocyanide solution is heated to 60°C in a water bath, oven, or microwave oven. However, the use of heat will sometimes cause a fine blue precipitate to form on both the tissue section and slide. This precipitate will not occur when the slides are stained at room temperature. Metallic iron deposits, or inert iron oxide seen in tissues because of industrial exposure, are

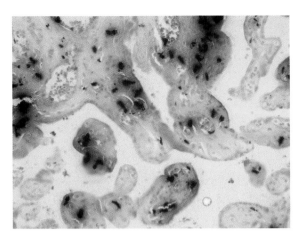

Fig. 14.2 A section of placenta treated with ferrous sulfate and stained with Lillie's method for ferrous iron. Ferrous iron is stained dark blue. Original magnification ×200.

not positive when treated with acid ferrocyanide solutions. Because of the tissue response, various mechanisms release some of the iron in a demonstrable form, and such deposits are almost invariably surrounded by hemosiderin. In almost all the instances where demonstrable iron appears in tissues, it does so in the form of a ferric salt. On those rare occasions that iron appears in its reduced state as the ferrous salt, then the use of Lillie's (1965) method may be used to achieve the Turnbull's blue reaction to visualize its presence in tissue sections (Fig. 14.2).

An interesting and sometimes useful modification of a serum iron technique was introduced by Hukill and Putt (1962) to demonstrate both ferrous and ferric iron in tissue sections. This method was claimed to be a more sensitive demonstration for the detection of both ferric and ferrous salts, but has not succeeded in replacing the more traditional method for the demonstration of iron. The method uses bathophenanthroline, and the resultant color of any iron present in tissues is bright red.

Perls' Prussian blue reaction for ferric iron
(Perls 1867)

This method is considered to be the first classical histochemical reaction. Treatment with an acid ferrocyanide solution will result in the unmasking of ferric iron in the form of the hydroxide, $Fe(OH)_3$, by dilute hydrochloric acid. The ferric iron then reacts with a dilute potassium ferrocyanide solution to produce an insoluble blue compound, ferric ferrocyanide (Prussian blue).

Fixation
Avoid the use of acid fixatives. Chromates will also interfere with the preservation of iron.

Sections
Works well on all types of section, including resin.

Ferrocyanide solution
1% aqueous potassium ferrocyanide	20 ml
2% aqueous hydrochloric acid	20 ml

Preferably freshly prepared just before use.

Method
1. Take a test and control section to water.
2. Treat sections with the freshly prepared acid ferrocyanide solution for 10–30 minutes (see Note a below).
3. Wash well in distilled water.
4. Lightly stain the nuclei with 0.5% aqueous neutral red or 0.1% nuclear fast red.
5. Wash rapidly in distilled water.
6. Dehydrate, clear, and mount in synthetic resin.

Results
Ferric iron	blue
Nuclei	red

Notes
a. Depending on the amount of ferric iron present, it may be necessary to vary the staining times.
b. Some laboratories keep the two stock solutions made up separately and stored in the refrigerator. The two solutions must not be stored for prolonged periods; this precaution will ensure that the solutions retain their viability.
c. It is essential that a positive control is used with all test sections. The choice of material that is most suitable as a control specimen is important. A useful control would be postmortem lung tissue that contains a reasonable number of iron-positive macrophages (heart failure cells). Freshly formed deposits of iron may be dissolved in the hydrochloric acid.

Lillie's method for ferric and ferrous iron
(Lillie & Geer 1965)

Fixation
Avoid the use of acid fixatives. Chromates will also interfere with the preservation of iron.

Sections
Paraffin, frozen, and resin.

Method
1. Take test and control sections to distilled water.
2. Dissolve 400 mg of potassium ferrocyanide in 40 ml of 0.5% hydrochloric acid when testing for ferric iron. For testing ferrous iron substitute, 400 mg of potassium ferricyanide. Prepare just before use. Expose sections for 30 minutes.
3. Wash well in distilled water.
4. Stain nuclei with 0.1% aqueous nuclear fast red for 5 minutes.
5. Rinse in distilled water.
6. Dehydrate, clear, and mount in synthetic resin.

Results
Ferric iron	dark Prussian blue
Ferrous iron	dark Turnbull's blue
Nuclei	red

Hukill and Putt's method for ferrous and ferric iron (Hukill & Putt 1962)

Fixation
Not critical but avoid prolonged exposure in acid fixatives.

Sections
All types of tissue section may be used including resin.

Solution
Bathophenanthroline (4,7-diphenyl-1, 10-phenanthroline)	100 mg
3% aqueous acetic acid	100 ml

Place in oven at 60°C for 24 hours, agitating at regular intervals. Cool to room temperature and filter. This solution is stable for about 4 weeks. Before use add thioglycolic acid to a concentration of 0.5% (this should be replenished each time before use as it rapidly undergoes oxidation on exposure to air).

Method
1. Take test and control sections to distilled water.
2. Stain sections in bathophenanthroline solution for 2 hours at room temperature.
3. Rinse well in distilled water.
4. Counterstain in 0.5% aqueous methylene blue for 2 minutes.
5. Rinse well in distilled water.
6. Stand slides on end until completely dry.
7. Dip slides in xylene and mount in synthetic resin.

Results
Ferrous iron	red
Nuclei	blue

Notes
a. It is important that the bathophenanthroline is completely dissolved prior to use.
b. Dehydration with alcohol will remove the resultant red coloration.

Hemoglobin

Hemoglobin is a basic conjugated protein that is responsible for the transportation of oxygen and carbon dioxide within the bloodstream. It is composed of a colorless protein, globin, and a red pigmented component, heme. Four molecules of heme are attached to each molecule of globin.

Heme is composed of protoporphyrin, a substance built up from pyrrole rings and combined with ferrous iron. Histochemical demonstration of the ferrous iron is possible only if the close binding in the heme molecules is cleaved. This can be achieved by treatment with hydrogen peroxide, but this has no practical use. As hemoglobin appears normally within red blood cells its histological demonstration is not usually necessary. The need to demonstrate the pigment may arise in certain pathological conditions such as casts in the lumen of renal tubules in cases of hemoglobinuria or active glomerulonephritis.

Demonstration of hemoglobin
Two types of demonstration method can be used to stain hemoglobin in tissue sections. The first demonstrates the enzyme, hemoglobin peroxidase, which is reasonably stable and withstands short fixation and paraffin processing. This peroxidase activity was originally

demonstrated by the benzidine–nitroprusside methods, but because of the carcinogenicity of benzidine these methods are not recommended and are no longer used. Lison (1938) introduced the Patent blue method that was later modified by Dunn and Thompson (1946) (Fig. 14.3). Tinctorial methods have also been used for the demonstration of hemoglobin; the Amido black technique (Puchtler & Sweat 1962) and the Kiton red–Almond green technique (Lendrum 1949) are worth noting.

Leuco Patent blue V method for hemoglobin (Dunn & Thompson 1946)

Fixation

Formalin or formal mercury. Poor preservation with Heidenhain's Susa has been noted by Drury and Wallington (1980).

Solutions

Stock solution

1% aqueous Patent blue V (CI 42045)	25 ml
Powdered zinc	2.5 g
Glacial acetic acid	0.5 ml

Mix well on a magnetic stirrer. The solution will become pale green–blue. Filter and store in a refrigerator at 3–6°C. The solution is stable for about 1 week.

Working solution

Stock solution	10 ml
Glacial acetic acid	2 ml
3% hydrogen peroxide	1 ml

Prepare immediately before use.

Method

1. Take test and control sections to distilled water.
2. Stain in Patent blue solution for 5 minutes at room temperature.
3. Rinse in distilled water.
4. Lightly counterstain in 0.5% aqueous neutral red or 0.1% aqueous nuclear fast red for 1 minute.
5. Rinse in distilled water.
6. Dehydrate, clear, and mount in synthetic resin.

Results

Hemoglobin peroxidase (red blood cells and neutrophils)	dark blue
Nuclei	red

Notes

a. Experience has shown that the hemoglobin demonstrated by this method tends to be more of a greenish-blue color.
b. In some instances, if the staining solution is left on the section for too long, it may start to decolorize a positive reaction.
c. Fixation in excess of 36 hours may give rise to unreliable results.
d. This method demonstrates peroxidase activity, including the peroxidases in other blood cells, particularly in the lysosomes of polymorphonuclear leucocytes and their precursors. Tissue peroxidases are also demonstrated.

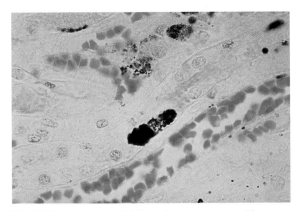

Fig. 14.3 A section of kidney from a patient with hemoglobinuria stained for hemoglobin with Lison's method. Hemoglobin is stained blue. Original magnification ×400.

Bile pigments

Red blood cells are broken down in the reticuloendothelial system when they have reached the end of their useful life, usually after 120 days. Hemoglobin is released after the red cell membrane has been ruptured. The protein, globin, and iron components are released for recycling within the body after the hemoglobin has been broken down. After the heme portion has been split from the globin, the tetra-pyrrole ring of the heme molecule is cleaved and opened out into a chain composed of four linked pyrrole groups. With the opening out of the tetra-pyrrole ring, the iron component is removed to be stored in those tissues that specialize in iron storage; this iron component is now free to be incorporated into the hemoglobin molecule during red cell formation. The opened tetra-pyrrole ring, which has had its iron component removed, is known as biliverdin. This residue is formed in the phagocytic cells that populate the reticulo-endothelial system, particularly the bone marrow and spleen. Biliverdin is transported to the liver where it is reduced to form bilirubin. In this form, the bilirubin is insoluble in water, but after conjugation with glucuronic acid it forms a water-soluble compound, bilirubin–glucuronide. This process takes place in liver hepatocytes due to the activity of the enzyme glucuronyl transferase. The conjugated bilirubin passes from the hepatocytes into the bile canaliculi, and then via the hepatic ducts into the gallbladder, which acts as a reservoir. The bilirubin passes along the common bile duct to be released into the duodenum via the ampulla of Vater.

The term *bile pigments* used by many authors when discussing the various staining techniques can be applied to all bile pigments. In using this terminology, it is implied that all bile pigments react in an identical manner, but this is not the case. Contained within the group 'bile pigments' are both conjugated and unconjugated bilirubin, biliverdin, and hematoidin, all of which are chemically distinct and show different physical properties, particularly with regard to their solubility in water and alcohol. Microscopical examination of any liver section that contains 'bile pigments' will almost certainly reveal a mixture of biliverdin and both conjugated and unconjugated bilirubin. This is particularly likely when the liver contains an excess of bile pigments, either through bile duct obstruction, e.g. due to a stone or tumor, an abnormality of biliverdin–bilirubin metabolism in the rare congenital enzyme disorders, or where there is extensive liver cell death or degeneration. The non-specific term *bile* will be used to include biliverdin and both conjugated and unconjugated bilirubin in the following text.

In a hematoxylin and eosin (H&E) stained section of liver, bile, if present, is most commonly seen in the hepatocytes in the early stages as small yellow–brown globules and then subsequently within the bile canaliculi as larger, smooth, round-ended rods or globules sometimes referred to as *bile thrombi* (a term considered inaccurate by most pathologists). The latter, if present, in liver sections is a histopathological indication that the patient has obstructive jaundice due to a blockage in the normal flow of bile from the liver into the gallbladder and subsequently into the bowel, probably because of gallstones or a carcinoma of the head of pancreas. Masses of bile in the canaliculi of liver sections are easily distinguished microscopically because of their characteristic morphology and their situation. Bile in hepatocytes must be distinguished from the lipofuscins that are also commonly seen within these cells and can appear as small yellow–brown globules. The need to distinguish between bile and lipofuscin in hepatocytes is particularly important in liver biopsies taken from liver transplant patients where sepsis is suspected. It is important to note that both bile and lipofuscin can be positive with Schmorl's ferric ferricyanide reduction test (Golodetz & Unna 1909). Bile is also seen in H&E-stained sections in the gallbladder where it can appear as amorphous, yellow–brown masses adherent to the mucosa or included as yellow–brown globules within the epithelial-lined Aschoff–Rokitansky sinuses in the gallbladder. Bile is also present, together with cholesterol, in gallstones.

Virchow (1847) first described extracellular yellow–brown crystals and amorphous masses within old hemorrhagic areas, which he called hematoidin. Pearse (1985) reviewed the histochemistry of bile pigments. Microscopically, *hematoidin* frequently appears as a bright yellow pigment in old splenic infarcts, where it contrasts well against the pale gray of the infarcted tissue. Hematoidin can also be found in old hemorrhagic areas in the brain. Bearing in mind the differences discussed above, it is almost certain that hematoidin is related to both bilirubin and biliverdin, even though it differs from them both morphologically and chemically. It is thought that heme has undergone a chemical change within these areas which has led to it being trapped, thus preventing it from being transported to the liver to be processed into bilirubin.

Demonstration of bile pigments and hematoidin

The need to identify bile pigments arises mainly in the histological examination of the liver, where distinguishing bile pigment from lipofuscin may be of significant importance. Both appear yellow–brown in H&E-stained paraffin sections, and it is worth remembering that the green color of biliverdin is often masked by eosin. In such cases, unstained paraffin or frozen sections, lightly counterstained with a suitable hematoxylin (e.g. Mayer), will prove of value. Bile pigments are not autofluorescent and fail to rotate the plane of polarized light (monorefringent), whereas lipofuscin is autofluorescent. The most

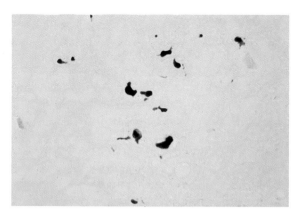

Fig. 14.4   Bile in a section of liver stained with Hall's method for bilirubin. Bilirubin is stained emerald green. Original magnification ×100.

commonly used routine method for the demonstration of bile pigments is the modified Fouchet technique (Hall 1960), in which the pigment is converted to the green color of biliverdin and blue cholecyanin by the oxidative action of the ferric chloride in the presence of trichloracetic acid (Fig. 14.4). The Fouchet technique is quick and simple to carry out, and when counterstained with van Gieson's solution the green color is accentuated.

Modified Fouchet's technique for liver bile pigments (Hall 1960)

Fixation
Any fixative appears suitable.

Sections
Any.

Solutions
Fouchet's solution

25% aqueous trichloracetic acid	36 ml
10% aqueous ferric chloride	4 ml

Freshly prepared before use.

Van Gieson stain

Dissolve 100 mg of acid fuchsin (CI 42685) in 100 ml of saturated aqueous picric acid (see Note c below).

Method
1. Take test and control sections to distilled water.
2. Treat with the freshly prepared Fouchet's solution for 10 minutes.

3. Wash well in running tap water for 1 minute.
4. Rinse in distilled water.
5. Counterstain with van Gieson solution for 2 minutes.
6. Dehydrate, clear, and mount in synthetic resin.

Results

Bile pigments	emerald to blue–green
Muscle	yellow
Collagen	red

Notes
a. Two control sections are stained with the test section, one stained with Fouchet's reagent and van Gieson, and the other with Fouchet's reagent alone.
b. Although the solutions used in Fouchet's reagent have a reasonable shelf life, experience has shown that a freshly prepared solution gives a more reliable result.
c. Bile that may be present in situations outside the liver such as that seen in the Aschoff–Rokitansky sinuses or in hemorrhagic and infarcted areas is likely to show no color change with this method. This type of pigment can be shown using the Gmelin (see below) or the Stein technique. Sirus Red F3B (CI 35780) may be substituted for acid fuchsin. Bile is a reducing substance and therefore will stain with the Masson–Fontana and Schmorl techniques.

Gmelin technique (Tiedermann & Gmelin 1826)

This technique is the only method that shows an identical result with liver bile, gallbladder bile, and hematoidin. The method tends to be messy, capricious, and gives impermanent results. Deparaffinized sections of tissue containing bile pigments are treated with nitric acid, and a changing color spectrum is produced. Because it can be unreliable, it is advisable to repeat the test at least three times before a negative result is acceptable. A popular modification of this technique is that of Lillie and Pizzolato (1967), in which bromine in carbon tetrachloride is used as an oxidant.

Sections
Paraffin.

Method
1. Sections to distilled water and mount in distilled water.
2. Place mounted section under the microscope using an objective with reasonable working distance.
3. Place 2–3 drops of concentrated nitric acid to one side of the coverglass and draw under the coverglass by means of a piece of blotting paper on the opposite side.
4. Remove excess solution and observe pigment for color changes.

Results
Bile pigments will gradually produce the following spectrum of color change: yellow–green–blue–purple–red.

Notes
a. This method is impermanent, thus preventing storage of sections.
b. The reaction can occur rapidly, but by using a 50–70% solution of nitric acid it can be slowed down.
c. Sulfuric acid can also be used in this method.

Oxidation methods aim to demonstrate bilirubin by converting it to green biliverdin. In practice they fail to produce the bright blue–green color seen in the more popular Fouchet technique and tend to be a dull olive green color. These oxidation methods are of little value in routine surgical pathology and are rarely used. Another group of methods that has been used to demonstrate bile pigments is the diazo methods that are based on a well-known technique previously used in chemical pathology, namely the van den Burgh test for bilirubin in blood. The method is based on the reaction between bilirubin and diazotized sulfanilic acid. Raia (1965, 1967) modified the method for use on cryostat sections but the reagents are complex to make up and section loss may be high, therefore its use is limited.

Porphyrin pigments

These substances normally occur in tissues in only small amounts. They are considered to be precursors of the heme portion of hemoglobin. The porphyrias are rare pathological conditions that are disorders of the biosynthesis of porphyrins and heme.

In erythropoietic protoporphyria, porphyrin pigment can be seen as focal deposits in liver sections. The pigment appears as a dense dark brown pigment and in fresh frozen sections exhibits a brilliant red fluorescence that rapidly fades with exposure to ultraviolet light. The pigment, when seen in paraffin sections and viewed using polarized light, shows as bright red in color with a centrally located, dark Maltese cross.

Non-hematogenous endogenous pigments

This group contains the following:

- melanins
- lipofuscins
- chromaffin
- pseudomelanosis (melanosis coli)
- Dubin–Johnson pigment
- ceroid-type lipofuscins
- Hamazaki–Weisenberg bodies.

Melanins

Melanins are a group of pigments whose color varies from light brown to black. The pigment is normally found in the skin, eye, substantia nigra of the brain, and hair follicles. (A fuller account of these sites is given later.) Under pathological conditions, it is found in benign nevus cell tumors and malignant melanomas. The chemical structure of the melanins is complex and varies from one type to another. Melanin production is not fully understood but the generally accepted view is that melanins are produced from tyrosine by the action of an enzyme tyrosinase (syn. DOPA oxidase). This enzyme acts on the tyrosine slowly to produce the substance known as DOPA (dihydroxyphenylalanine) which is subsequently rapidly acted upon by the same enzyme to produce an intermediate pigment which then polymerizes to produce melanin. The later stages of melanogenesis remain largely speculative and it is beyond the scope of this chapter to evaluate the many studies relating to melanin biosynthesis that have been carried out recently. Pearse (1985) gives a more detailed account of melanin production.

The melanins are bound to proteins, and these complexes are localized in the cytoplasm of cells within so-called 'melanin granules'. Ghadially (1982) described these granules as the end stage of the development of the melanosome as seen at ultrastructural level. The stages are as follows:

1. Tyrosine is synthesized in the Golgi lamellae and pinched off into vesicles with no melanin present.
2. The characteristic lattice-like appearance becomes evident at this stage.
3. Melanin deposition is first observed.
4. The fully mature granule has its structure obscured by melanin pigment.

The enzyme tyrosinase cannot be demonstrated in the mature granule.

The most common sites where melanin can be found are:

1. *Skin*, where it is produced by cells called melanocytes that are usually scattered within the basal layer of the epidermis. In certain inflammatory skin diseases melanin may also be found in phagocytic cells ('melanophages') in the upper dermis. The melanophages may also phagocytize other material such as lipofuscins and lipoproteins, thus producing a mixture that after denaturation may give unexpected staining results. Pathological deposition of melanin occurs in a benign lesion called a nevus or 'mole'. The malignant counterpart to the nevus is the malignant melanoma; it is in the diagnosis of this important tumor, and its metastases, that histological demonstration of melanin finds its most important practical application (Fig. 14.5). Melanin is also found in the hair follicles of dark-haired people.
2. *Eye*, where it is found normally in the choroid, ciliary body, and iris. Similar brown–black pigment is found in the retinal epithelium but its identity with melanin is uncertain. Melanomas can occur in the eye but these tumors are rare.
3. *Brain*, where it is found particularly in the substantia nigra, in such quantities that this structure is macroscopically visible as a black streak on both sides of the mesencephalon. In patients with long-standing Parkinson's disease this area is markedly reduced. Black melanin is also found in patches in the arachnoid covering some human brains, and has been described as having a 'sooty' appearance.

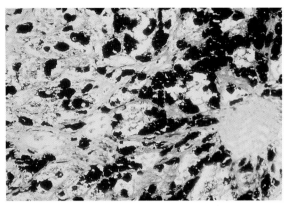

Fig. 14.5 A section of liver from a patient with malignant metastatic melanoma stained with Churukian's method for melanin. Melanin is stained black. Original magnification ×400.

A number of methods can be used for the identification of melanin and melanin-producing cells. The most reliable of these are:

1. Reducing methods such as the Masson–Fontana silver technique and Schmorl's ferric–ferricyanide reduction test.
2. Enzyme methods (e.g. DOPA reaction).
3. Solubility and bleaching characteristics.
4. Fluorescent methods.
5. Immunohistochemistry.

Melanin and melanin precursors are capable of reducing both silver and acid ferricyanide solutions. It also shows the marked physical property of being completely insoluble in most organic solvents, which is almost certainly due to the fact that formed melanin is tightly bound to protein within the melanosome. The other physical characteristic shown by melanin is its ability to be bleached by strong oxidizing agents, although the process is slow. These two physical characteristics relate to formed melanin and not to melanin precursors.

The enzyme tyrosinase can be demonstrated by the DOPA reaction and is therefore demonstrable in any cell capable of synthesizing melanin. Cells that have produced an abundance of melanin, and in which the melanosomes are filled with pigment, are said no longer to show tyrosinase activity, but some workers have found that tyrosinase is active in most cells, even though melanin may be present in large quantities.

The fluorescent method depends upon the ability of certain biogenic amines, including DOPA and dopamine, to show fluorescence after exposure to formaldehyde (formalin-induced fluorescence). This method therefore demonstrates melanin precursors rather than formed melanin. Recent advances in antibody production have made better markers in immunohistochemistry available for the identification of melanocytic lesions.

Reducing methods for melanin

Melanin is a powerful reducing agent and this property is used to demonstrate melanin in two ways:

1. The reduction of ammoniacal silver solutions to form metallic silver without the use of an extraneous reducer is known as the argentaffin reaction. Masson's (1914) method (using Fontana's silver solution) and its various modifications, which also rely on melanin's argentaffin properties, are now widely used for routine purposes. Melanins are blackened by acid silver nitrate solutions. Melanin is also argyrophilic, meaning that melanin is colored black by silver impregnation methods that use an extraneous reducer. This is not a property considered to be of diagnostic value.

2. Melanin will reduce ferricyanide to ferrocyanide with the production of Prussian blue in the presence of ferric salts (the Schmorl reaction). This type of reaction is also seen with certain other pigments (e.g. some lipofuscins, bile, and neuroendocrine cell granules).

3. Other methods for demonstrating melanin are Lillie's ferrous ion uptake (described in Lillie & Fullmer 1976) and Lillie's Nile blue A (1956).

Masson–Fontana method for melanin
(Fontana 1912; Masson 1914)

Fixation
Formalin is best; chromate and mercuric chloride should be avoided.

Sections
Works on all types of section, although some adjustment may be necessary for resin sections.

Preparation of silver solution (after Fontana)
Place 20 ml of a 10% aqueous silver nitrate solution in a glass flask. Using a fine-pointed dropper pipette, add concentrated ammonia drop by drop, constantly agitating the flask until the formed precipitate *almost* dissolves. This titration is critical if the method is to

work consistently well. The end point of the titration is seen when a faint opalescence is present, and is best viewed using reflected light against a black background. If too much ammonia is inadvertently added then the addition of a few drops of 10% silver nitrate will restore the opalescence. To this correctly titrated solution add 20 ml triple distilled water and then filter into a dark bottle. Store the solution in the refrigerator and use within 4 weeks. Ammoniacal silver solutions are potentially explosive if stored incorrectly.

Method
1. Take test and control sections to distilled water.
2. Treat with the ammoniacal silver solution in a Coplin jar that has been covered with aluminum foil, for 30–40 minutes at 56°C or overnight at room temperature.
3. Wash well in several changes of distilled water.
4. Treat sections with 5% aqueous sodium thiosulfate (hypo) for 1 minute.
5. Wash well in running tap water for 2–3 minutes.
6. Lightly counterstain in 0.5% aqueous neutral red or 0.1% aqueous nuclear fast red for 5 minutes.
7. Rinse in distilled water.
8. Dehydrate, clear, and mount in a synthetic resin.

Results
Melanin, argentaffin, chromaffin and some black lipofuscins
Nuclei   red

Notes
a. Only use thoroughly clean glassware, as the silver solution will react with any residual contaminant left on glassware.
b. Prolonged exposure to 56°C may give rise to a fine deposit over the section.
c. Friable material may need to be coated with celloidin as the ammonia in the silver solution could lead to sections lifting off the slide.

Microwave ammoniacal silver method for argentaffin and melanin (Churukian 2005)

See Figure 14.5.

Fixation
10% buffered neutral formalin.

Sections
Paraffin.

Preparation of solutions

Ammoniacal silver

To 10 ml of 2% silver nitrate add 5 ml of 0.8% lithium hydroxide monohydrate. Then add 28% ammonium hydroxide, drop by drop with constant shaking, until the precipitate almost dissolves. Make up the solution to 200 ml with distilled water and store in a refrigerator at 3–6°C. The solution is stable for at least 1 month.

0.2% aqueous gold chloride

2% aqueous sodium thiosulfate

Method

1. Take slides to distilled water.
2. Place slides in 40 ml of refrigerated cold ammoniacal silver solution in a plastic Coplin jar and microwave at power setting 6 (360 W) for 35 seconds. Gently agitate the Coplin jar for about 15 seconds. Microwave again at power setting 6 for 35 seconds. Gently agitate the Coplin jar for about 15 seconds. Allow the slides to remain in the hot solution (approximately 80°C) for 2–3 minutes or until the sections appear a light brown.
4. Rinse in four changes of distilled water.
5. Place slides in 0.2% aqueous gold chloride for 1 minute.
6. Rinse in two changes of distilled water.
7. Place slides in 2% aqueous sodium thiosulfate for 1 minute.
8. Rinse in four changes of distilled water.
9. Counterstain with 0.1% aqueous nuclear fast red for 3 minutes.
10. Rinse in three changes of distilled water.
11. Dehydrate, clear, and mount in synthetic resin.

Results

Melanin, argentaffin, chromaffin, lipofuscin and other silver reducing substances	black
Nuclei	red

Notes

The results obtained with this method are similar to those obtained with the Masson–Fontana technique.

a. When preparing the ammoniacal silver solution, care must be taken not to add too much ammonium hydroxide. Add just enough almost to dissolve the precipitate.

b. The microwave oven used in this method had a maximum output of 600 watts with multiple power settings. Microwave ovens of higher or lower wattage may be used for this method by varying the microwave exposure times.

Schmorl's reaction (taken from Lillie 1954)

See Figure 14.6.

Fixation

10% buffered neutral formalin.

Solution

Freshly prepared 0.4% aqueous potassium ferricyanide	4 ml
Freshly prepared 1% aqueous ferric chloride (or 1% ferric sulfate)	30 ml

N.B. Use this solution soon after mixing.

Method

1. Take test and control sections to distilled water.
2. Treat sections with the ferric–ferricyanide solution for 5–10 minutes.
3. Wash well in running tap water for several minutes to ensure that all residual ferricyanide is completely removed from the section.
4. Lightly counterstain with 0.5% aqueous neutral red or 0.1% aqueous nuclear fast red for 5 minutes.
5. Dehydrate, clear, and mount in synthetic resin.

Results

Melanin, argentaffin cells, chromaffin, some lipofuscins, thyroid colloid and bile	dark blue
Nuclei	red

Notes

a. This modification is preferred to the more traditional method because it is easier to control and gives less background staining.

b. The time for the reaction to take place depends on the substance to be demonstrated, with melanin generally reacting more quickly than lipofuscin. This fact should not be taken as a definitive diagnostic pointer but only as a general guideline.

c. When choosing a control section it is important to remember that melanin reduces the ferric–

ferricyanide more quickly than other reducing substances. Therefore control sections should always match the test sections so that a lipofuscin control should not be used if the test pigment is thought to be melanin.

Enzyme methods

Cells that are capable of producing melanin can be demonstrated by the DOPA (dihydroxyphenylalanine) method. The enzyme tyrosinase that is localized within these cells will oxidize DOPA to form an insoluble brown–black pigment. The best results are obtained when using post-fixed cryostat sections, although a useful but less reliable method is that which uses freshly fixed blocks of tissue.

In the past, cells that are capable of producing melanin have been demonstrated by the DOPA oxidase methods. The enzyme tyrosinase that is located within these cells will oxidize DOPA to form an insoluble brown–black pigment. These methods are those of Bloch (1917) and Laidlaw and Blackberg (1932) for tissue sections, and Bloch (1917) and Rodriguez and McGavran (1969) for tissue blocks. Though previously included in the fifth edition of this book, these methods are currently not in use.

Solubility and bleaching methods

Melanins are insoluble in most organic solvents or in anything that will significantly destroy the tissue that contains them. The insolubility shown by melanin is due to the tight bond it has with its protein component. Use of strong oxidizing agents, such as permanganate, chlorate, chromic acid, peroxide, and peracetic acid, will bleach melanin, although the process is slow, taking 16 hours. The blacker the melanin, the longer the bleach takes to decolorize the pigment. Lipofuscin tends to take longer to be bleached from paraffin sections than melanin. The method of choice is peracetic acid but treatment with 0.25% potassium permanganate followed by 2% oxalic acid also works well.

Formalin-induced fluorescence (FIF)

Certain aromatic amines such as 5-hydroxytryptamine, dopamine, epinephrine (adrenaline), norepinephrine (noradrenaline), and histamine, when exposed to formaldehyde, show a yellow primary fluorescence. This is particularly useful when demonstrating amelanotic melanoma, because these tumors can be difficult to diagnose using conventional methods due to their lack of pigment. Any melanin precursors present will form a product of isocarboline derivatives that are dehydrogenated and will show yellow fluorescence. The best results are seen when using tissue that has been freeze-dried (see Chapter 7) and then fixed using paraformaldehyde vapor. Formalin-fixed frozen sections will give acceptable results. Paraffin-processed tissue can also be used but shows weak fluorescence that is difficult to visualize.

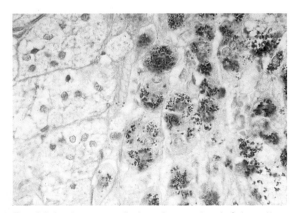

Fig. 14.6 A section of adrenal stained with Schmorl's method for reducing substances. Chromaffin is stained blue. Original magnification ×400.

Formaldehyde-induced fluorescence method for melanin precursor cells
(Eranko 1955)

Fixation
10% buffered neutral formalin.

Sections
Cryostat, or 5-μm paraffin sections.

Method
1. Deparaffinize sections in xylene. Fix frozen sections in 10% buffered formalin for 5 minutes, dehydrate, and place in xylene.
2. Rinse in fresh xylene.
3. Mount in a medium that is fluorescence free.
4. Examine using a fluorescence microscope with BG38, UG1, and a barrier filter.

Results
Melanin precursor cells   weak yellow fluorescence

Notes

a. A brighter image will be seen if epi-illumination is used.

b. Some commercially produced mountants are unsuitable as they fluoresce and will confuse the result.

c. One of the claims originally made about FIF was that archived paraffin-processed material could be examined to see if there was evidence of melanin precursor cells, but because of the indifferent results it is not widely used.

Other methods for melanin

Ferrous ion uptake reaction for melanin
(Lillie & Fullmer 1976)

See Figure 14.7.

Fixation
Formalin is best: avoid all chromate fixatives.

Sections
Paraffin.

Solutions
2.5% ferrous sulfate
1% potassium ferricyanide in 1% acetic acid

Method
1. Take test and control sections to distilled water.
2. Place in 2.5% ferrous sulfate for 1 hour.
3. Wash with six changes of distilled water.
4. Place in 1% potassium ferricyanide in 1% acetic acid for 30 minutes
5. Wash with four changes of distilled water.
6. Counterstain with 0.5% aqueous neutral red or 0.1% nuclear fast red.
7. Rinse in two changes of distilled water.
8. Dehydrate, clear, and mount in synthetic resin.

Results

Melanins of skin, eye, pina, and neuromelanin	dark green
Nuclei	red

Notes

a. According to Lillie, this method is specific for melanin.

b. Ferric iron and lipofuscins do not stain with the method.

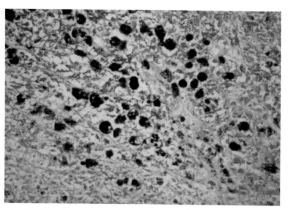

Fig. 14.7   A section of liver from a patient with malignant melanoma stained with Lillie's ferrous ion uptake method for melanin. Melanin is stained black. Original magnification ×200.

Nile blue method for melanin and lipofuscin (Lillie 1956)

See Figures 14.8 and 14.9.

Fixation
10% buffered neutral formalin.

Sections
Paraffin.

Solution
Dissolve 0.05 g Nile blue (CI 51180) in 99 ml of distilled water and then add 1.0 ml of sulfuric acid.

Method
1. Take test and control sections to distilled water.
2. Place in Nile blue solution for 20 minutes.
3. Wash with four changes of distilled water.
4. Mount in an aqueous mountant (e.g. glycerin jelly).

Results

Melanin	dark blue
Lipofuscin	dark blue
Nuclei	blue or unstained

Notes

a. Some samples of Nile blue may not yield satisfactory results with this method.

b. Using frozen sections, this method will stain neutral lipids (triglycerides, cholesterol esters, and steroids) red to pink. Acidic lipids (fatty acids and phospholipids) stain blue.

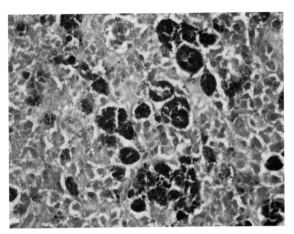

Fig. 14.8 A section of liver from a patient with malignant melanoma stained with Lillie's Nile blue method for melanin. Melanin is stained dark blue. Original magnification ×200.

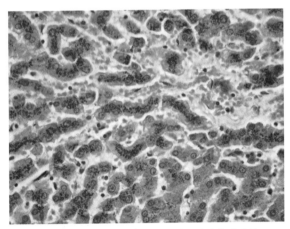

Fig. 14.9 A section of liver stained with Lillie's Nile blue method for lipofuscin. Lipofuscin within the hepatocytes is stained dark blue. Original magnification ×200.

Immunohistochemistry

There are a few antibodies that can be used to demonstrate melanocytic lesions, none of which is absolutely specific. The more widely used antibodies are S100, HMB-45, melanin A, and to a lesser extent PGP 9.5. HMB-45 is said to demonstrate melanosome formation and therefore melanocytic differentiation. It is a melanocytic antigen and not a melanoma antigen (Skelton et al 1991).

Lipofuscins

These yellow–brown to reddish-brown pigments occur widely throughout the body and are thought to be produced by an oxidation process of lipids and lipoproteins. The oxidation process occurs slowly and progressively, and therefore the pigments exhibit variable staining reactions, different colors, and variation in shape and size, which appears to be dependent upon their situation. This type of pigment is found in the following sites:

- Hepatocytes, sometimes as a mixture with other types of pigment.
- Cardiac muscle cells, particularly around the nucleus. Large amounts of pigment are found in the small brown hearts of elderly debilitated people, a condition known as 'brown atrophy of the heart'.
- Inner reticular layer of the normal adrenal cortex, where the pigment imparts a brown color, is particularly prominent in patients dying after a long and stressful illness.
- Testis, particularly in the interstitial cells of Leydig; it is responsible for giving testicular tissue its brown color.
- Ovary, in the walls of involuting corpora lutea and in some macrophages around the corpora lutea. Hemosiderin tends to be seen more commonly in this situation.
- Cytoplasmic inclusions in the neurons of the brain, spinal cord, and ganglia.
- The edge of a cerebral hemorrhage or infarct.
- Some lipid storage disorders such as Batten's disease.
- Other tissues such as bone marrow, involuntary muscle, cervix, and kidney.

Demonstration of lipofuscins

It is important to bear in mind that because lipofuscin is formed by a slow progressive oxidation process of lipids and lipoproteins, histochemical reactions will vary according to the degree of oxidation present in the pigment when the demonstration techniques are applied. Therefore, it is advisable to carry out a variety of techniques in order to be sure whether the pigment is lipofuscin. The lipofuscins react with a variety of histochemical and tinctorial staining methods, the most common and useful being:

- Periodic acid–Schiff method (see p. 171)
- Schmorl's ferric–ferricyanide reduction test (see above)
- Long Ziehl–Neelsen method (see below)

- Sudan black B method
- Gomori's aldehyde fuchsin technique (see Fig. 14.10)
- Masson–Fontana silver method (see above)
- Basophilia, using methyl green
- Churukian's silver metho
- Lillie's Nile blue sulfate method.

Long Ziehl–Neelsen method (Pearse 1953)

Fixation
Any fixative.

Sections
Works well on all types of tissue section.

Method
1. Slides to distilled water.
2. Stain in a Coplin jar with filtered carbol fuchsin (see p. 314) using a 60°C water bath for 3 hours, or overnight at room temperature.
3. Wash well in running water.
4. Differentiate in 1% acid alcohol until the background staining is removed.
5. Wash well in running tap water.
6. Counterstain nuclei with 0.25% aqueous methylene blue in 1% aqueous acetic acid for 1 minute.
7. Dehydrate, clear, and mount in synthetic resin.

Results
Lipofuscin	magenta
Ceroid	magenta
Nuclei	blue
Background	pale magenta to pale blue

Notes
a. Experience has shown that a more reliable result is obtained if the staining is carried out using a thermostatically controlled water bath.
b. A useful variant of this method is cited by Lillie (1954), in which the staining solution is modified so that Victoria blue is substituted for basic fuchsin. It is sometimes difficult to distinguish between the red of the fuchsin and the reddish-brown of the pigment, whereas the blue color of lipofuscin with the Victoria blue may be more convincing.

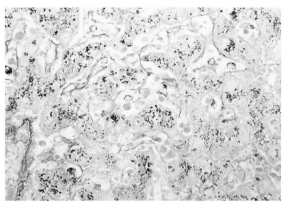

Fig. 14.10 A section of liver stained with Gomori's aldehyde fuchsin. Lipofuscin is stained purple. Original magnification ×400.

Aldehyde fuchsin technique (Gomori 1950)

See Figure 14.10.

Fixative
10% buffered neutral formalin.

Sections
Paraffin.

Solutions
Acidified potassium permanganate solution (0.25% aqueous potassium permanganate in 0.1% sulfuric acid)
2% aqueous oxalic acid

Aldehyde fuchsin
Dissolve 1 g pararosanilin (CI 42500) in 100 ml aqueous 70% ethanol. Add 1 ml concentrated hydrochloric acid and 2 ml paraldehyde or acetylaldehyde, shaking the mixture thoroughly. Stand for 3–5 days at room temperature or preferably longer, near natural light, to allow the solution to blue. Store solution at 4°C. The solution will remain viable for approximately 2 months. Any increase in the background staining will indicate deterioration of the staining solution.

Method
1. Sections to distilled water.
2. Treat with acidified potassium permanganate solution for 5 minutes.
3. Wash well in distilled water and treat for 2 minutes with oxalic acid solution to bleach section.

4. Wash well in distilled water.

5. Rinse in 70% ethyl alcohol.

6. Stain section in aldehyde fuchsin for 5 minutes. Longer staining times will be needed as the solution ages.

7. Rinse in 70% ethyl alcohol followed by a rinse in three changes of distilled water.

8. Dehydrate, clear, and mount in synthetic resin.

Results

Lipofuscin	purple
Elastic	purple

Notes

a. Paraldehyde should be freshly opened (Moment 1969). It keeps well when stored in the freezing compartment of a refrigerator. If paraldehyde is not available, acetaldehyde may be used and need not be refrigerated.

b. Other tissue constituents, such as beta cells of the pancreas and pituitary, elastin, sulfated mucins, gastric chief cells, and neurosecretory granules, will stain with this method.

c. The basic fuchsins rosanilin and new fuchsin are closely related to pararosanilin. Only pararosanilin will give satisfactory staining results in this procedure.

Chromaffin

This pigment is normally found in the cells of the adrenal medulla as dark brown, granular material. It may occur in tumors of the adrenal medulla (pheochromocytomas).

Fixation in formalin is not recommended, and fixatives containing alcohol, mercury bichloride, or acetic acid should be avoided. Orth's or other dichromate-containing fixatives are recommended. Chromaffin may be demonstrated by Schmorl's reaction, Lillie's Nile blue A, the Masson–Fontana, Churukian's microwave ammoniacal silver method, and the periodic acid–Schiff (PAS) technique.

Pseudomelanosis pigment (melanosis coli)

This pigment is sometimes seen in macrophages in the lamina propria of the large intestine and appendix. Various theories have been put forward as to its nature. The current view is that it is an endogenous lipopigment whose reactions are those of a typical ceroid-type lipofuscin. It appears to be strongly associated with anthra-quinone purgatives ('cascara sagrada'). Its distinction from melanin may occasionally be important. Pseudomelanosis will, in general, stain with those methods that are used to demonstrate lipofuscin, such as Masson–Fontana and Schmorl.

Dubin–Johnson pigment

This pigment is found in the liver of patients with Dubin–Johnson syndrome and is due to defective canalicular transport of bilirubin. It is characterized by the presence of a brownish-black, granular, intracellular pigment situated in the centrilobular hepatocytes. The true nature of the pigment has yet to be established, but histochemically it is similar to lipofuscin, though there are ultrastructural differences.

Ceroid-type lipofuscins

Lillie et al (1941, 1942) were the first to describe ceroid in the cirrhotic livers of animals maintained on inadequate diets. Lillie thought that ceroid was different from lipofuscin because it failed to stain with the ferric–ferricyanide reaction. Pearse (1985) states that ceroid is in fact a lipofuscin at an early stage of oxidation. Further oxidation would produce lipofuscin proper.

Hamazaki–Weisenberg bodies

These small, yellow–brown spindle-shaped structures are found mainly in the sinuses of lymph nodes, either lying free or as cytoplasmic inclusions, and their significance is unknown. First described by Hamazaki (1938), they have been described as being present in lymph nodes from patients with sarcoidosis (Weisenberg 1966). Further studies have shown them to be present in a number of conditions (Boyd & Valentine 1970). Hall and Eusebi (1978) have reported their presence in association with melanosis coli. Histochemically they are similar to lipofuscin, and at ultrastructural level have an appearance that suggests that they are probably giant lysosomal residual bodies (Doyle et al 1973).

Endogenous minerals

Iron is discussed under the heading 'Hematogenous pigments' on p. 233.

Calcium

Insoluble inorganic calcium salts are a normal constituent of bones and teeth, and their demonstration is well covered in Chapter 18. From a histochemical viewpoint,

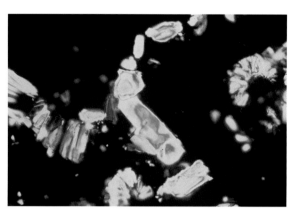

Fig. 14.11 A section of kidney with calcium oxalate crystals as seen with polarization microscopy. Original magnification ×400.

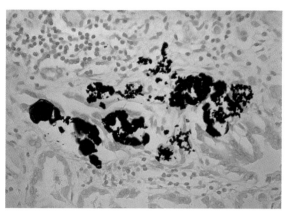

Fig. 14.12 A section of kidney stained with von Kossa's silver nitrate method for calcium. An ultraviolet lamp was used to perform the method. Calcium is stained black. Original magnification ×400.

the free ionic form of calcium, found in the blood, cannot be demonstrated. Abnormal depositions of calcium can be found in necrotic areas of tissue associated with tuberculosis, infarction (Gandy–Gamna bodies), atheroma in blood vessels, and malakoplakia of the bladder (Michaelis–Gutman bodies). The most common forms of calcium salts occurring in these conditions are phosphates and carbonates. Calcium salts are usually monorefringent but calcium oxalate is birefringent. (See Figure 14.11.) Calcium usually stains purple blue with H&E.

The use of various dyes that act by forming chelate complexes with calcium has been practiced by many workers. These dyes include alizarin red S, purpurin, naphthochrome green B, and nuclear fast red. In general, these dyes demonstrate medium to large amounts of calcium better than particulate deposits that stain weakly, the exception being alizarin red S, which tends to give more reliable results with small deposits. None of these dyes is specific for calcium salts, although alizarin red S when used at pH 4.2 is said to be. The classic method of von Kossa (1901), which uses silver nitrate, is preferred for routine demonstration purposes on paraffin sections (Fig. 14.12).

It demonstrates only phosphate and carbonate radicals, giving good results with both large and small deposits of calcium. The method is not specific, as melanin will also reduce silver to give a black deposit. As a general rule, fixation of tissue containing calcium deposits is best when using non-acidic fixatives such as buffered neutral formalin, formal alcohol, or alcohol.

Alizarin red S method for calcium (Dahl 1952; McGee-Russell 1958; Luna 1968)

Fixation
Buffered neutral formalin, formal alcohol, and alcohol.

Sections
Paraffin or frozen.

Solutions
1% aqueous alizarin red S (CI 58005) adjusted to pH 4.2 or 6.3–6.5 (see Note c) with 10% ammonium hydroxide.
0.05% fast green FCF (CI 42053) in 0.2% acetic acid.

Method
1. Sections to 95% alcohol.
2. Stand slides on end and thoroughly air dry.
3. Place sections in a Coplin jar filled with the alizarin red S solution for 5 minutes (see Notes below).
4. Rinse quickly in distilled water.
5. Counterstain with fast green for 1 minute.
6. Rinse in three changes of distilled water.
7. Dehydrate, clear, and mount in synthetic resin.

Results
Calcium deposits	orange–red
Background	green

Notes

a. The staining time is dependent on the amount of calcium present.

b. Calcium deposits are birefringent after staining with alizarin red S.

c. McGee-Russell recommends using the alizarin red S at pH 4.2. Dahl indicated that it be used at pH 6.36 to pH 6.4. Churukian is in agreement with Dahl as to the higher pH and has observed that a pH as high as 7.0 produces good results.

d. This method is particularly useful in the identification and detection of small amounts of calcium like those seen in heterotropic calcification in the kidney (hypercalcinosis). This type of tissue also makes excellent control material.

Copper

Many enzymes in the body would fail to function without the presence of copper, although copper deficiency is extremely rare. Copper accumulation is associated with Wilson's disease, the most important disorder of copper metabolism. This disease is a rare, inherited, autosomal recessive condition which gives rise to copper deposition in the liver, basal ganglia of the brain, and eyes. In the eye, the Kayser–Fleischer ring, a brown ring of deposited copper, may be seen in the cornea (Descemet's membrane), and is diagnostic of this condition. Copper deposition in the liver is also associated with primary biliary cirrhosis and certain other hepatic disorders.

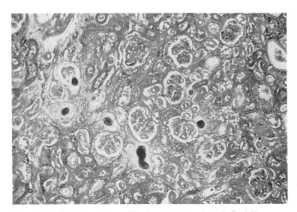

Fig. 14.13 A section of kidney stained with Dahl's alizarin red S method at pH 6.4. Calcium is stained orange–red. Original magnification ×100.

Copper, like many metallic cations, is capable of forming a blue dye lake using Mallory's unripened hematoxylin. Uzman (1956) modified the Okamoto–Utamura rubeanate method (1938) and obtained excellent results on formalin-fixed tissue. The rhodanine method (Lindquist 1969) has also been used to demonstrate copper and copper-associated protein (CAP). Although the quality of the reagent, dimethylaminobenzylidine rhodanine (DMABR), varies considerably, it is considered to be the method of choice. The CAP is also well demonstrated by the Shikata orcein method (Shikata et al 1974).

Rubeanic acid method for copper
(Okamoto & Utamura 1938; Uzman 1956)

Fixative
10% buffered neutral formalin.

Solution

0.1% rubeanic acid (dithio-oxamide) in absolute ethyl alcohol	5 ml
10% aqueous sodium acetate	100 ml

Prepare fresh before use.

Method

1. Take the test section, together with a known positive control section, to distilled water.
2. Place sections in a Coplin jar filled with rubeanic–acetate solution for at least 16 hours at 37°C. Times may need to be extended and the method is best carried out in a water bath.
3. Wash in 70% ethyl alcohol.
4. Rinse briefly in distilled water.
5. Drain section and blot dry.
6. Lightly counterstain with 0.5% aqueous neutral red or 0.1% aqueous nuclear fast red for 1 minute.
7. Rinse in distilled water.
8. Dehydrate, clear, and mount in synthetic resin.

Results

Copper	greenish black
Nuclei	pale red

Notes

a. Correct choice of fixative is essential. Buffered neutral formalin is acceptable, but avoid the use of acid formalin and fixatives containing mercury and chromium salts.

b. To demonstrate any copper that is bound to CAP, deparaffinized sections are placed downwards over a beaker of concentrated hydrochloric acid for 15 minutes. The sections are washed well in absolute alcohol and then transferred to the rubeanic–acetate solution.

c. The method is best carried out using a thermostatically controlled water bath.

Modified rhodanine technique
(Lindquist 1969)

Fixative
10% buffered neutral formalin.

Sections
Paraffin.

Solutions

Rhodanine stock solution
5-p-Dimethylaminobenzylidene-rhodanine	0.05 g
Absolute ethanol	25 ml

Prepare fresh and filter prior to use.

Working solution
Take 5 ml of the stock rhodanine solution and add to 45 ml of 2% sodium acetate trihydrate.

Borax solution
Disodium tetraborate	0.5 g
Distilled water	100 ml

Method
1. Take test and control sections to water.
2. Incubate in the rhodanine working solution at 56°C for 3 hours or overnight in a 37°C oven.
3. Rinse in several changes of distilled water for 3 minutes.
4. Stain in acidified Lillie–Mayer or other alum hematoxylin for 10 seconds.
5. Briefly rinse in distilled water and place immediately in borax solution for 15 seconds.
7. Rinse well in distilled water.
8. Mount with Apathy's mounting media.

Results
Copper and copper associated protein	red to orange–red
Nuclei	blue
Bile	green

Notes
a. Certain synthetic mountants will cause fading of the copper and CAP in archived material. No fading occurs when sections are mounted with Apathy's media. This method will give the most consistent results when in the hands of an experienced practitioner.

c. Results help distinguish between bile and iron pigments (Irons et al 1977).

d. Analytical grade reagents and triple distilled water are recommended when performing this technique.

e. Control material is best obtained from livers of patients suffering from Wilson's disease, primary biliary cirrhosis, or other forms of chronic cholestasis. Fetal liver of the third trimester (Fig. 14.14) fixed in buffered neutral formalin for not more than 36 hours makes a good positive control.

Uric acid and urates

Uric acid is a breakdown product of the body's purine (nucleic acid) metabolism, but a small proportion is obtained from the diet. Most, but not all, uric acid is excreted by the kidneys. The uric acid circulating in the blood is in the form of monosodium urate, which in patients with gout may be high, forming a supersaturated solution. These high levels may result in urate

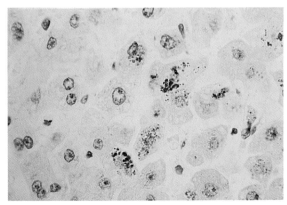

Fig. 14.14 A section of fetal liver of the third trimester stained with Lindquist's method for copper. Copper is stained red to orange–red. Original magnification ×400.

depositions, which are water soluble in tissues, causing:

- subcutaneous nodular deposits of urate crystals ('tophi')
- synovitis and arthritis
- renal disease and calculi.

Another condition that occasionally can mimic gout is known as *pseudogout* or *chondrocalcinosis*, and is a pyrophosphate arthropathy. This results in calcium pyrophosphate crystals being deposited in joint cartilage. The cause of this deposition is unknown and is more common in the elderly, affecting mainly the large joints, such as the knee. It is important that gout and pseudogout are distinguishable. To aid the diagnosis, a polarizing microscope fitted with a quartz first-order red compensator will prove useful. While pyrophosphate crystals exibit a positive birefringence, urate crystals show a negative birefringence. Urates can be extracted by saturated aqueous lithium carbonate solution (Gomori 1951), while pyrophosphate crystals are unaffected by it. If this extraction sequence is used in combination with Grocott's modification of Gomori's hexamine silver technique, both types of crystal can usually be identified.

Lithium carbonate extraction-hexamine silver technique (Gomori 1936, 1951; Grocott 1955)

Fixation
Urate crystals are water soluble, therefore fixation in alcohol will give a more specific reaction.

Sections
Paraffin, frozen, or celloidin.

Solutions
Grocott's hexamine silver solution
Saturated aqueous lithium carbonate solution
2% aqueous sodium thiosulfate (hypo)
0.05% aqueous fast green (CI 42053) in 0.2% acetic acid

Method
1. Take two test sections and two control sections to 70% ethyl alcohol.
2. Place one section from each pair in saturated aqueous lithium carbonate solution for 30 min.
3. Rinse all sections in distilled water.
4. Place all sections in a Coplin jar filled with hexamine silver solution for 1 hour at 45°C.
5. Wash sections in distilled water.
6. Treat sections with hypo for 30 seconds.
7. Counterstain with fast green solution for 1 minute.
8. Wash in water, dehydrate, clear, and mount in synthetic resin.

Results

Extracted sections	urates only are extracted
Unextracted sections	urates and possibly pyrophosphates are blackened
Background	green

Notes
a. The urates reduce the silver solution due to their argentaffin properties.
b. More accurate control of incubation temperature is achievable using a thermostatically controlled water bath.

ARTIFACT PIGMENTS

This group of pigments comprises:

- formalin
- malaria
- schistosome
- mercury
- chromic oxide
- starch.

Formalin pigment

This pigment is seen as a brown or brownish-black deposit in tissues that have been fixed in acidic formalin. The deposit is usually present in blood-rich tissues such as spleen, hemorrhagic lesions, and large blood vessels filled with blood. The morphology of the pigment can vary but is commonly seen as a microcrystalline deposit that is anisotropic (birefringent). It is related to the acid hematins, but is spectroscopically distinct from hydrochloric acid and acetic acid hematins (Herschberger & Lillie 1947).

One way of removing this pigment from tissue sections is by treating unstained tissue sections with saturated alcoholic picric acid. Alcoholic solutions of both sodium and potassium hydroxide will also remove the pigment but these may have deleterious effects on subsequent staining techniques. Treatment with 10% ammonium hydroxide in 70% alcohol for 5–15 minutes will remove this pigment and is less harmful to tissue sections than the other hydroxides. The use of buffered neutral formalin will help to minimize the problem of formalin pigment deposition. Fixation of large blood-rich organs, such as spleen, for a long period will tend to increase the amount of formalin pigment formed. Under these conditions it is advisable to change the fixative on a regular basis.

Malarial pigment

This pigment is morphologically similar to formalin pigment and occasionally may be identical, even though it is produced in a slightly different manner. It is formed within, or in the region of, red blood cells that contain the malarial parasite. In cases of cerebral malaria, due to infection with *Plasmodium falciparum*, malarial pigment can be seen in or over the red blood cells within the tiny blood capillaries of the brain. The pigment may, on occasion, be so heavily deposited that it obscures the visualization of the malarial parasite. Malarial pigment may also be present within phagocytic cells that have ingested infected red cells, therefore one should carefully examine the Kupffer cells of the liver, the sinus lining cells of lymph nodes and spleen, and within phagocytic cells in the bone marrow. Malarial pigment, like formalin pigment, exhibits birefringence and can be removed from tissue sections with saturated alcoholic picric acid, but usually requires 12–24 hours' treatment for complete removal.

Much less time is required to remove the pigment by using 10% ammonium hydroxide, as described above.

Extraction method for formalin and malarial pigment

Solutions
10% ammonium hydroxide in 70% ethyl alcohol.

Method
1. Sections to 70% ethyl alcohol.
2. Place sections to a Coplin jar containing ammonium hydroxide alcohol for 5–15 minutes.
3. Wash well in distilled water.
4. Apply staining method desired.

Notes
a. The time necessary for the removal of formalin pigment will vary, depending on the amount of pigment present.
b. Malarial pigment usually requires treatment for at least 15 minutes or longer.

Schistosome pigment

This pigment is occasionally seen in tissue sections where infestation with *Schistosoma* can be seen; the pigment, which tends to be chunky, shows similar properties to those of both formalin and malaria pigments.

Mercury pigment

This pigment is seen in tissues that have been fixed in mercury-containing fixatives, although it is rarely seen in tissue fixed in Heidenhain's Susa. Mercury pigment varies in its appearance but it is usually seen as a brownish-black, extracellular crystal. Although usually seen as monorefringent, occasionally it is birefringent, particularly when formalin-fixed tissue has been secondarily fixed in formal mercury.

A little-known but unusual finding is that prolonged storage of stained sections that contain mercury pigment can bring about a change in the structure of the pigment. The pigment changes from a crystalline form to a globular one (H.C. Cook, personal communication). The reason for this is unclear but it may be caused by interaction between the pigment and the mounting medium. Furthermore, the globular form exhibits a Maltese cross birefringence.

Treatment of sections with iodine solutions, such as Lugol's iodine, is the classical method of removing the pigment. Subsequent bleaching with a weak sodium thiosulfate (hypo) solution completes the treatment.

It is advisable *not* to remove mercury pigment with iodine solutions prior to staining with Gram's method. The effect is such that connective tissue will take up the crystal violet and then resist acetone decolorization. Staining methods such as phosphotungstic acid hematoxylin may be impaired if 'hypo' is used before staining.

Chromic oxide

This pigment is rarely seen in tissue sections and is extremely difficult to produce intentionally. When seen, it presents as a fine yellow–brown particulate deposit in tissues, as a result of not washing in water, tissues that have been fixed in chromic acid or dichromate-containing fixatives. Subsequent treatment of tissues with graded alcohols, as used in tissue processors, may result in the reduction of chrome salts to the chromic oxides, which are insoluble in alcohol. The pigment is monorefringent and extracellular. It can be removed from sections by treatment with 1% acid alcohol.

Starch

This pigment is introduced by talcum powder from the gloves of surgeons, nurses, or pathologists. It is PAS and Gomori methenamine silver (GMS) positive and can be easily identified by its characteristic appearance and because when polarized it will produce a Maltese cross configuration.

EXOGENOUS PIGMENTS AND MINERALS

Although often listed as being exogenous pigments, the majority of the following substances are, in fact, colorless. Some of these substances are inert and unreactive, while other materials can be visualized in tissue sections using various histochemical methods that are often capricious and unreliable. Most routine surgical pathology laboratories rarely see this type of material. Certain types of mineral gain access to the body by inhalation, ingestion, or skin implantation, commonly as a result of industrial exposure. Some minerals, in the form of dye complexes, can be seen in the skin and adjacent lymph nodes as a result of tattooing. Occasionally mineral deposition may occur due to medication or wound dressing. Where there is a need to identify one of these substances, for example with an industrial injury insurance claim, then use of the electron probe micro analyzer (EDAX) will prove to be the most reliable method. This specialized piece of equipment can usually be found in teaching and research laboratories.

The most common minerals seen in tissue sections are carbon, silica, and asbestos. Other less common minerals that may be present in tissues are lead, beryllium, aluminum, mercury, silver, and bismuth.

Tattoo pigment

This is associated with skin and any adjacent lymphoid areas. If viewed using reflected light, the various colors of the dye pigments used to create the tattoo can be seen.

Amalgam tattoo

Brown–black areas of pigmentation in the mouth may result from traumatic introduction of mercury and silver from dental amalgam during dental procedures. Histologically, brown granules are deposited in collagen, basement membranes, nerve sheath, blood vessel walls, and elastic fibers. The pattern of distribution is similar to that seen in the skin in argyria (see p. 257).

Carbon

This exogenous substance is the most commonly seen mineral in tissues and is easily recognized in stained tissue sections. Commonly found in the lung and adjacent lymph nodes of urban dwellers and tobacco smokers, the main sources of this mineral are car exhausts and smoke from domestic and industrial chimneys. Tobacco smokers inhale particulate carbon, and also give passers-by a dilute sample. Inhaled carbon particles generally are trapped by the thin film of mucus in the nose, pharynx, trachea, and bronchi. A small amount will find its way into the alveoli of the lung, where it is phagocytized by alveolar macrophages. Some carbon particles will also find their way into the peribronchiolar lymphatics and lymph nodes draining the lungs.

Black pigmentation of the lung (anthracosis) is seen as a result of massive deposition of carbon in coal workers and some city dwellers. There is, at present, no evidence that carbon causes tissue damage. Coal miners inhale the largest amounts of carbon and the lungs, when examined macroscopically, appear almost black. The lung disease known as coal workers' pneumoconiosis is caused by the inhalation of silica, which is found in association with coal and other mined ores. Coal workers are also prone to cuts and abrasions while working and carbon deposition is fairly common in the skin.

Carbon is extremely inert and unreactive and fails to be demonstrated with conventional histological stains and histochemical methods. The site and nature of the carbon deposits make identification relatively easy. It may be confused with melanin deposition but treatment with bleaching agents will show carbon unaffected, whereas melanin will be dissolved.

Silica

Silica in the form of silicates is associated with the majority of all mined ores because they are found in or near rocks that contain silica. Mine workers inhale large quantities of silica that can give rise to the disease silicosis. This disease presents as a progressive pulmonary fibrotic condition which gives rise to impaired lung capacity and in some cases extreme disability. Silicates are also abundant in stone and sand, and any industrial worker involved in grinding stone or sand blasting will be at risk from silicosis. Silica is unreactive, and is thus not demonstrated by histological stains and histochemical methods. It is anisotropic (birefringent) when examined using polarized light.

Asbestos

Asbestos, which is a special form of silica, has been used for many years as a fire-resistant and insulating material. It is widely used in the motor industry as a brake lining. There are several types of asbestos, and the fibers that cause pulmonary disease in humans are called amphiboles. The most dangerous type is crocidolite (Cape blue asbestos). The fibers are 5–100 μm long and only 0.25–0.5 μm in diameter, and can collect in the alveoli at the periphery of the lung. These fibers are anisotropic but fail to show birefringence when they appear as an asbestos body, because of the protein coat covering the fiber. The characteristic appearance of the asbestos body is as a beaded, yellow–brown, dumb-bell shape in lung sections. The proteinaceous coat contains hemosiderin and is positive with Perls' Prussian blue. Micro-incineration techniques have been used in the past to demonstrate asbestos fibers, as they withstand the high temperatures produced by the oven. In cases where asbestosis is suspected but no asbestos fibers or bodies are readily demonstrable, lung tissue from the lower lobes can be digested with 40% sodium hydroxide. The resultant tissue sludge is then centrifuged and washed in water. Smears from the deposit are made and examined using polarized light. This method has proved to be reliable when detecting asbestos fibers and bodies. Alternatively, thick paraffin sections (20 μm) of lung tissue are mounted on glass slides coated with an adhesive. The sections are dewaxed and mounted unstained, then examined using polarized light. Many thick sections may be needed before a positive result is seen.

Lead

Environmental pollution due to lead has been greatly reduced in recent times. Lead pipes that carried much of the domestic water supply have been replaced by alternative materials. Lead in paint, batteries, and gasoline

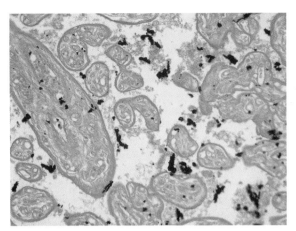

Fig. 14.15   A section of placenta that was treated with lead nitrate stained with Lillie's rhodizonate method for lead. Lead is stained black. Original magnification ×200.

has been reduced by the various manufacturers. Cases of lead poisoning are rare and are usually diagnosed biochemically using the serum from suspected cases. In chronic lead poisoning, excessive amounts can be deposited within many tissues, particularly bone and kidney tubules. For many years various methods have been used to demonstrate lead in tissue sections; the most popular method is the rhodizonate method (Lillie 1954) (Fig. 14.15). Other methods for lead include the sulfide–silver of Timm (1958) and the unripened hematoxylin technique of Mallory and Parker (1939), but neither of these is specific for lead.

Rhodizonate method for lead salts
(Lillie 1954)

Fixation
Avoid the use of mercury-containing fixatives. Bones containing lead salts can be decalcified in 5–10% sulfuric acid containing 5–10% sodium sulfate. This procedure should convert lead deposits into insoluble lead sulfate.

Sections
Paraffin.

Solutions
Sodium rhodizonate	100 mg
Distilled water	50 ml
Glacial acetic acid	0.5 ml

0.05% fast green FCF (42053) in 0.02% acetic acid

Method
1. Sections to distilled water.
2. Place in rhodizonate solution for 1 hour.
3. Rinse well in distilled water.
4. Counterstain in 0.05% aqueous fast green in 0.2% acetic acid for 1 minute.
5. Rinse in three changes of distilled water.
6. Dehydrate, clear, and mount in synthetic resin.

Results
Lead salts	black
Background	green

Notes
a. This method relies on any lead salts present forming a red chelated compound when treated with the chelating agent sodium rhodizonate.
b. This method can be performed using a microwave oven by heating the solution to 60–65°C and allowing the slides to remain in the heated solution for 5 minutes.

Beryllium and aluminum

The same methods are used to demonstrate both of these metals. It is therefore convenient to consider both together. Beryllium is used in the manufacture of fluorescent light tubes and gains access to the body by inhalation or traumatization of the skin. A foreign body granuloma is formed, often resembling the appearance of sarcoidosis. Conchoidal (shell-like) bodies can also be found, which are typical of, but not specific to, beryllium. These bodies usually give a positive reaction with Perls' Prussian blue. Aluminum is rarely seen in tissues but gains access to the body in a similar way to beryllium. It can also be found in bone biopsies from patients with encephalopathy on regular hemodialysis for chronic renal failure. Prolonged dialysis can cause osteodystrophy in the present era. It can develop insidiously and may present with a non-specific ache. The most severe pain occurs with osteomalacia particularly when it is associated with aluminum deposition (Brenner 2004). Beryllium and aluminum can both be demonstrated by solochrome azurine that forms a deep blue chelate. Aluminum is also positive with the fluorescent Morin method (Pearse 1985), together with other minerals such as calcium, barium, and zirconium. Naphthochrome green can also be used to demonstrate beryllium and aluminum, but is less specific than the solochrome azurine method as other metallic dye lakes can be formed.

Solochrome azurine method for beryllium and aluminum (Pearse 1957)

Fixation
Not critical.

Sections
Paraffin or frozen.

Preparation of solutions
a. 0.2% solochrome azurine (syn. Pure blue B).
b. 0.2% solochrome azurine in normal sodium hydroxide.

Method
1. Take two test sections to distilled water.
2. Stain one section in solution a and one in solution b for 20 min.
3. Wash in distilled water.
4. Lightly counterstain in 0.5% aqueous neutral red or 0.1% aqueous nuclear fast red for 5 min.
5. Wash in distilled water and mount in synthetic resin.

Results
Solution A: aluminum and beryllium	blue
Solution B: beryllium only	blue–black
Nuclei	red

Notes
a. This method is reliable and will give consistent results.
b. Control sections should always be used if readily available.
c. Aluminum will fail to react at an alkaline pH.
d. A modification of this method applicable to resin sections of undecalcified bone is given on p. 353.

Aluminon method for aluminum (Lillie & Fullmer 1976)

Sections
Undecalcified glycol methacrylate or paraffin sections cut at 5 μm.

Solutions
pH buffer 5.2. Dissolve 40 g ammonium acetate and 28 g ammonium chloride in 210 ml distilled water.

Add 27 ml 6 M (50%) hydrochloric acid. Adjust to pH 5.2 with hydrochloric acid or 28% ammonium hydroxide. Store in refrigerator at 3–6°C.

Aluminon solution
Dissolve 0.8 g aluminon (aurine tricarboxylic acid) in 40 ml pH buffer 5.2 with the aid of heat to 80–85°C. Prepare just before use.

Decolorizing solution
To 22 ml buffer pH 5.2 add 8 ml 1.6 M ammonium carbonate that consists of 15.4 g ammonium carbonate in distilled water to make a total of 100 ml.

Fast green counterstain
Dissolve 0.05 g fast green FCF (CI 42053) in 100 ml 0.2% acetic acid

Method
1. Sections to distilled water.
2. Pour freshly prepared aluminon solution that is heated to 80–85°C in a plastic Coplin jar. Place slides in this solution.
3. Place Coplin jar in a 600-W microwave oven and microwave at power setting 2 (120 W) for 30 seconds. Allow the slides to remain in the solution for 10 minutes.
4. Rinse in three changes of distilled water.
5. Place in freshly prepared decolorizing solution for 5 seconds.
6. Rinse in three changes of distilled water.
7. Counterstain with fast green solution for 3 minutes.
8. Rinse in three changes of distilled water.
9. Stand slides on end and allow slides to air dry.
10. Dip in xylene and mount with synthetic resin.

Results
Aluminum	red
Background	green

Notes
a. Currently available microwave ovens have a maximum wattage of 900–1500 W. Therefore, when using a microwave oven greater than 600 W, the time of exposure to microwaves should be reduced in step 3.
b. Another counterstain that may be used in this method is methylene blue as it contrasts well with the red positive stain (Fig. 14.16), like the fast green.

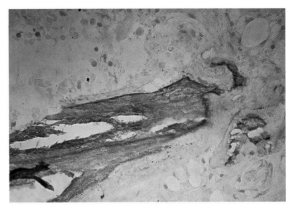

Fig. 14.16 An undecalcified plastic section of bone stained with Lillie's aluminon method for aluminum. Aluminum is stained red. Original magnification ×400.

Silver

Silver is rarely found in the skin of silver workers as a result of industrial exposure. It is now more commonly seen as a localized change in the mouth (amalgam tattoo, see p. 254) or in association with silver earrings in ineptly pierced lobes. The resultant permanent blue–gray pigmentation is called argyria and is most marked in those areas exposed to sunlight. In unstained and H&E-stained sections the silver appears as fine dark brown or black granules, particularly in basement membranes and sweat glands. The method of Okamoto and Utamura (1938), a metal chelating method that utilizes dimethylaminobenzylidene-rhodanine, will demonstrate silver. The method tends to be capricious and may give rise to the diffusion of chelate complex. The best results are obtained using frozen sections.

Rhodanine method for silver (Okamoto & Utamura 1938)

Fixation
Not critical but avoid the use of mercury-containing fixatives.

Sections
Paraffin; frozen (see Note a below).

Incubating solution
p-Dimethylaminobenzylidene-rhodanine (saturated solution in 90%)	3.5 ml
M-nitric acid	3 ml
Distilled water	93.5 ml

Method

1. Paraffin sections to distilled water.
2. Incubate sections in rhodanine solution at 37°C for 24 hours.
3. Wash well in distilled water.
4. Mount in glycerin jelly.

Results

Silver deposits   reddish-brown

Notes

a. Better results are obtained on free-floating frozen sections using a 0.2% rhodanine solution in 0.1% nitric acid for 2 hours at 37°C.
b. The reaction product is not completely insoluble and some diffusion occurs, so sections should be examined immediately. Long incubation times will give poor localization.

Acknowledgments

Alan Stevens wrote this chapter for the first three editions; he and Brian Chalk updated the text for the fourth edition. Our acknowledgments are due to them for their contributions.

REFERENCES

Bloch B. (1917) Des Problem Pigmentbildung in der Haut. Archives Dermato-Syphiligraphiques 124:129.

Boyd J.F., Valentine J.C. (1970) Unidentified yellow bodies in human lymph-nodes. Journal of Pathology 102:58–60.

Brenner B.M., ed. (2004) Brenner and Rector's the kidney, 7th edn. Philadelphia: Saunders.

Churukian C.J. (2005) Manual of the special stains laboratory, 10th edn. Rochester: University of Rochester, pp. 101, 102.

Dahl L.K. (1952) A simple and sensitive histochemical method for calcium. Journal of Experimental Medicine 95:474–479.

Doyle W.F., Braham H.D., Burgess J.H. (1973) The nature of yellow–brown bodies in peritoneal lymph nodes. Histochemical and electron microscopic evaluation of these bodies in a case of sarcoidosis. Archives of Pathology 96:320–326.

Drury R.A.B., Wallington E.A. (1980) Carleton's histological technique, 5th edn. Oxford: Oxford University Press.

Dunn R.C., Thompson E.C. (1946) A simplified stain for hemoglobin in tissue and smears using patent blue. Stain Technology 21:65.

Eranko O. (1955) Distribution of adrenalin and noradrenalin in the adrenal medulla. Nature 175:88.

Fontana A. (1912) Verfahren zur intensiven und raschen Färbung des Treponema pallidum und anderer Spirochaten. Dermatologische Wochenshrift 55:1003.

Ghadially F.N. (1982) Ultrastructural pathology of the cell and matrix. London: Butterworth, 602.

Golodetz L., Unna P.C. (1909) Zur Chemie der Haut III. Das Reduktionsvermogen der histologischen Elemente der Haut. Mh. Prakt. Dermatogie 48:149.

Gomori G. (1936) Microchemical demonstration of iron. American Journal of Pathology 13:655.

Gomori G. (1950) Aldehyde fuchsin: a new stain for elastic tissues. American Journal of Clinical Pathology 20:665.

Gomori G. (1951) Methods in Medical Research 4:3.

Grocott R.G. (1955) A stain for fungi in tissue sections and smears. American Journal of Clinical Pathology 25:975.

Hall M., Eusebi V. (1978) Yellow–brown spindle bodies in mesenteric lymph nodes: a possible relationship with melanosis coli. Histopathology 2:47–52.

Hall M.J. (1960) A staining reaction for bilirubin in tissue sections. American Journal of Clinical Pathology 34:313.

Hamazaki Y. (1938) Uber eine neues, saurefeste Substanz führendes Spindelkörperchen der menschlichen Lymphdrusen. Virchows Archiv fur Pathologische Anatomie und Physiologie 301:490–522.

Herschberger L.R., Lillie R.D. (1947) Physical properties of acid formalin hematin, or formalin pigment. Journal of Technical Methods and Bulletin of the International Association of Medical Museums 27:162.

Hukill P.B., Putt, F.A. (1962) A specific stain for iron using 4,7-diphenyl-1,10-phenanthroline. Journal of Histochemistry 10:490.

Irons R.D., Schenk E.A., Lee J.C.K. (1977) Cytochemical methods for copper semiquantitation screening procedure for identification of abnormal copper levels in liver. Archives of Pathology and Laboratory Medicine 101:298.

Laidlaw G.F., Blackberg S.N. (1932) Melanoma studies; DOPA reaction in normal histology. American Journal of Pathology 8:491.

Lendrum A.C. (1949) Staining of erythrocytes in tissue sections; a new method and observations on some of the modified Mallory connective tissue stains. Journal of Pathology and Bacteriology 61:443.

Lillie R.D. (1954) Histopathologic technic and practical histochemistry. New York: Blakiston.

Lillie R.D. (1956) A Nile blue staining technic for the differentiation of melanin and lipofuscin. Stain Technology 31:151.

Lillie R.D. (1965) Histopathologic technic and practical histochemistry, 3rd edn. New York: McGraw-Hill.

Lillie R.D., Fullmer H.M. (1976) Histopathologic technic and practical histochemistry, 4th edn. New York: McGraw-Hill, pp. 526–527.

Lillie R.D., Geer J.C. (1965) On the relation of enterosiderosis pigments of man and guinea pig, melanosis and pseudomelanosis of colon and villi and the intestinal iron uptake and storage mechanism. American Journal of Pathology 47:965–1007.

Lillie R.D., Pizzolato P. (1967) A stable histochemical Gmelin reaction of bile pigments with dry bromine carbon tetrachloride solution. Journal of Histochemistry and Cytochemistry 15:600.

Lillie R.D., Daft F.S., Sebrell W.N.J. (1941) Cirrhosis of liver in rats on deficient diet and effect of alcohol. Public Health Reports 56:1255.

Lillie R.D., Ashburn L.L., Sebrell W.H.J. et al. (1942) Histogenesis and repair of hepatic cirrhosis in rats produced on low protein diets and preventable with choline. Public Health Reports 57:502.

Lindquist R.R. (1969) Studies on the pathogenesis of hepatolenticular degeneration. II: Cytochemical methods for the localisation of copper. Archives of Pathology 87:370.

Lison L. (1938) Zur Frage der Ausscheidung und Speicherung des Hämoglobins in der Amphibienniere. Beitrage zur Pathologischen Anatomie und zur Allgemeinen Pathologie 101:94.

Luna L.G. (1968) Manual of histologic staining methods of the armed forces institute of pathology, 3rd edn. New York: McGraw-Hill, pp. 175–176.

Mallory F.B., Parker F. (1939) Fixing and staining methods for lead and copper in tissues. American Journal of Pathology 16:517.

Masson P. (1914) La glande endocrine de l'intestine chez l'homme. Comptes Rendus Hebdomadaires des Séances de l'Académie des Sciences 158:59.

McGee-Russell S.M. (1958) Histochemical methods for calcium. Journal of Histochemistry and Cytochemistry 6:22.

Moment G.B. (1969) Deteriorated paraldehyde: an insidious cause of failure in aldehyde fuchsin staining. Stain Technology 44:52–53.

Okamoto K., Utamura M. (1938) Biologische Untersuchen des Kupfers über die histochemische Kupfernachweiss Methode. Acta Scholae Medicinalis Universitatis Imperialis in Kisto 20:573.

Pearse A.G.E. (1953) Histochemistry, theoretical and applied. London: Churchill.

Pearse A.G.E. (1957) Solochrome dyes in histochemistry with particular reference to nuclear staining. Acta Histochimica 4:95.

Pearse A.G.E. (1960) Histochemistry, theoretical and applied. London: Churchill.

Pearse A.G.E. (1985) Histochemistry: theoretical and applied, Vol. 2. Edinburgh: Churchill Livingstone.

Perls M. (1867) Nachweis von Eisenoxyd in geweissen Pigmentation. Virchows Archiv fur Pathologische Anatomie und Physiologie und fur Klinische Medizin 39:42.

Puchtler H., Sweat F. (1962) Amido black as a stain for hemoglobin. Archives of Pathology 73:245.

Raia S. (1965) Histochemical demonstration of conjugated and unconjugated bilirubin using a modified diazoreagent. Nature (London) 205:304.

Raia S. (1967) PhD Thesis. London: University of London.

Rodriguez H.A., McGavran M.H. (1969) A modified DOPA reaction for the diagnosis and investigation of pigment cells. American Journal of Clinical Pathology 52:219.

Shikata T., Uzawa T., Yoshiwara N. et al. (1974) Staining methods for Australia antigen in paraffin sections—detection of cytoplasmic inclusion bodies. Japanese Journal of Experimental Medicine 44:25.

Skelton H.G., Smith K.J., Barrett T.L. et al. (1991) HMB-45 staining in benign and malignant melanocytic lesions. American Journal of Dermatopathology 13(6):543.

Tiedermann F., Gmelin L. (1826) Die Verdauung nach Versuchen. Heidelberg: K. Gross, Vol. 1, p. 89.

Timm F. (1958) Zur Histochemie der Schwermetalle; das Sulfid-silberverfahren. Deutsche Zeitschrift für die Gesampte Gerichtliche Medizin 46:706.

Uzman L.L. (1956) Histochemical localisation of copper with rubeanic acid. Laboratory Investigations 5:299.

Virchow R. (1847) Die pathologischen pigmente. Archiv fur Pathologische Anatomie und Physiologie Kinische Medizin 379.

von Kossa J. (1901) Ueber die im Organismus kuenstlich erzeugbaren Verkakung. Beiträge zur Pathologischen Anatomie und zur Allgemeinen Pathologie 29:163.

Weisenberg W. (1966) Über saurefeste 'Spindelkorper Hamazaki' bei Sarkoikose der Lymphknoten und über doppellichtbrechende Zelleinschlusse bei Sarkoidose der Lungen. Archiv für Klinische und Experimentelle Dermatologie 227:101–107.

15

Amyloid

Geoffrey H. Vowles

INTRODUCTION

Amyloid is an amorphous, extracellular, eosinophilic material deposited in various body tissues and organs giving the disease known as amyloidosis. Amyloid may be present as microscopic deposits, as plaques, or as confluent masses that may progressively replace the parenchyma of affected organs, which may become enlarged, firm, and pale in macroscopic appearance, with progressive loss of function leading to eventual organ failure and death. Such affected organs may show a 'waxy' texture to their cut surface, a feature that led early pathologists to refer to this condition as 'waxy degeneration' or 'lardaceous disease' (Von Rokitansky 1842). During the nineteenth century this appearance was a frequent postmortem finding in those suffering from the prevalent chronic inflammatory diseases such as tuberculosis but amyloidosis itself was rarely diagnosed during the patient's lifetime. Early attempts to define the nature of the waxy substance were limited by the technology of the day. Virchow (1853) used an iodine reaction on affected organs, obtaining a violet coloration, and used the name amyloid, a term then in use for similar appearing carbohydrate substances in botany. Soon after it was reported that 'amyloid livers and spleens yield such a high proportion of nitrogen that we have come to the conclusion that amyloid is of an albuminous nature', that is, composed of protein (Friedrich & Kékulé 1859). Further attempts to discover the composition of amyloid over the following hundred years were hampered by the inability to obtain suitably pure samples, with the result that analyses were confusing and frequently contradictory. As techniques improved during the twentieth century a consensus was arrived at that amyloid was largely composed of protein

with a variable amount, about 1–5%, of various mucopolysaccharides.

Various techniques for the histological demonstration of amyloid were devised including the early use of crystal violet and later the dye Congo red, initially for gross demonstration, then for histological use (Bennhold 1922), with the subsequent discovery of an apparently unique optical activity of Congo red-stained amyloid to give 'apple green' birefringence when viewed under polarized light (Divery & Florkin 1927).

The use of electron microscopy in the 1950s and 1960s showed that all amyloid has a unique fibrillary ultrastructure, which appeared to be independent of anatomical site, mode of production or generic origin, and quite different to any other ultrastructural fibrils described before or since.

In the 1960s X-ray diffraction of amyloid extracts was used to show that the protein within fibrils was arranged in an anti-parallel β-pleated sheet conformation (Eanes & Glenner 1968). All amyloid deposits have been shown to share this conformation and after it was demonstrated that if the integrity of the β-pleated structure was broken then the traditional properties of amyloid were lost (Harada et al 1971), a consensus as to a definition of amyloid emerged.

Amyloid:

- is an extracellular, usually amorphous eosinophilic material
- gives an 'apple green' positive birefringence with polarized light after staining with Congo red dye
- has a characteristic unique ultrastructural fibrillary structure
- is predominantly composed of protein in a β-pleated sheet conformation.

261

Amyloid and amyloidosis remain important in modern medical practice. Although the inflammatory disease-associated amyloid of the nineteenth century is now rarely seen, amyloid is widely encountered in other conditions such as rheumatoid arthritis, diabetes and, as the commonest amyloid seen in modern pathological practice, Alzheimer's disease (Glenner 1983). Indeed, as amyloids form an integral, if not causal, part of several such high-profile conditions, the study of amyloid and its formation has never been more intense.

Composition

With the development of suitable extraction techniques (Pras et al 1968; Glenner et al 1972) it became clear that the bulk of amyloid deposits were composed of protein, and X-ray diffraction techniques showed that the protein was predominantly arranged in an anti-parallel β-pleated sheet conformation (Eanes & Glenner 1968).

There were many attempts to identify amyloid protein that led in 1970 to the identification of a homology between what was then known as 'primary amyloid' with immunoglobulin light chain (Glenner et al 1970). Sequencing of the amyloid found in secondary amyloidosis revealed a protein named as amyloid A component; subsequently a homologous serum protein was identified and named serum amyloid A (Husby et al 1973a). Since then some 25 normal human proteins have been identified as forming amyloid deposits (Table 15.1). With the exception of a group of the apolipoproteins there is little obvious connection between most of these proteins, beyond their ability to form amyloid fibrils.

Amyloid deposits also always contain up to 15% of a non-fibrillary glycoprotein known as amyloid P component (AP) that is identical to a circulating plasma protein, serum amyloid P (SAP). SAP is a calcium-dependent ligand binding protein that forms a normal component of basement membranes and elastin fibrils, and may have a function related to its binding reactions to glycosaminoglycans (GAGs), fibronectin, and other cellular and extracellular components (Pepys & Baltz 1983; Pepys 1992). SAP belongs to a family of plasma proteins called the pentaxins that are characterized by their pentameric quaternary structure, although SAP is decameric in that two identical pentameric rings are bound to each other (Gewurz et al 1995). Why SAP is found in amyloid deposits is not known although it has been postulated that it binds to the GAGs also always present in amyloid

(Pepys 1992) or that it forms an integral part of amyloid fibrils (Holck et al 1979; Inoue & Kisilevsky 1996).

Early extraction techniques led to rather variable analyses of other components of amyloid, although it was established that GAGs were invariably present (Hass 1942). These GAGs were further identified as including heparin sulfate, chondroitin sulfate, and dermatan sulfate (Bitter & Muir 1966; Muir & Cohen 1968). There is an intimate association between GAGs and amyloid fibril proteins at the ultrastructural level (Snow et al 1987) and the possibility that GAGs may be involved in amyloidogenesis continues to be actively investigated (Ancsin 2003). The presence of the carbohydrate moieties of GAGs provides a possible explanation for the staining reaction in some of the histological methods used for amyloid detection.

ULTRASTRUCTURE

Electron microscopic studies of amyloid have shown that all amyloid deposits display a unique fibrillary arrangement. In pathological material routinely prepared for electron microscopy, amyloid deposits appear as masses of extracellular, unbranched filaments, usually in a random orientation, occasionally in parallel arrays of a few fibres. Each fibril consists of two electron-dense filaments 2.5–3.5 nm in diameter, separated by a 2.5-nm space giving a total diameter of 8–10 nm with a variable length of up to several millimicrons (Cohen & Calkins 1959; Glenner 1981).

This conformation has been seen in all amyloid deposits studied leading to the question of why apparently unrelated proteins of different sizes and properties form fibrils that appear identical in size and appearance (Snow et al 1987). The involvement of certain GAGs and of AP component in most amyloid fibrils studied suggests that the fibrils may have a complicated structural organization (Holck et al 1979; Kisilevsky 1990).

Modern methods of fibril preparation have allowed refinement of the basic fibril model, but there is no current consensus as to amyloid fibril structure. Experimentally induced amyloid fibrils in mice are apparently composed of a fibril core of SAP that is then surrounded by a helix of chondroitin sulfate proteoglycan, a further coat of heparan sulfate proteoglycan, and with β-pleated sheet polymers of AA protein arrayed on their surface (Inoue & Kisilevsky 1996). In an in vitro study of an experimentally produced SH3 amyloid, the fibril is

Table 15.1 Amyloid proteins

Abbreviation	Protein precursor	Associated illnesses
AA	Serum amyloid A	Reactive secondary amyloidosis Familial Mediterranean fever
AL	Immunoglobulin light chain	Primary amyloidosis Myeloma-associated amyloidosis
AH	Immunoglobulin heavy chain	Primary and myeloma associated-amyloidosis
ATTR	Transthyretin (prealbumin)	Senile cardiac amyloid Familial polyneuropathies—Portuguese and Danish types
AApoAI	Apolipoprotein AI	Familial polyneuropathy—Iowa type Isolated amyloid of aorta
AApoAII	Apolipoprotein AII	Familial amyloidosis
AApoAIV	Apolipoprotein AIV	Sporadic aging amyloidosis
AGel	Gelsolin	Familial amyloidosis—Finnish type
ACys	Cystatin C	Familial CAA—Icelandic type
$A\beta$	Amyloid β-protein precursor—AβPP (or βAPP)	Alzheimer's disease, CAA Down's syndrome
$A\beta_2M$	β_2 microglobulin	Dialysis-associated amyloidosis
APrP	Prion protein	Prion diseases, CJD
ACal	Calcitonin	Medullary carcinoma of thyroid-associated amyloid
AANF	Atrial natriuretic factor	Senile amyloid of atria of heart
AIAPP	Amylin	Type II diabetes amyloid, insulinoma
AFib	Fibrinogen α-chain	Hereditary renal amyloidosis
ALys	Lysozyme	Familial amyloidosis, Ostertag type
APro	Prolactin	Aging pituitary prolactinoma
AIns	Insulin	Iatrogenic
ABri	ABriPP	Familial CAA—British type
ADan	ADanPP	Familial CAA—Danish type
AMed	Lactadherin	Aging amyloid of arteries
ALac	Lactoferrin	Corneal amyloidosis
AKer	Kerato-epithelin	Familial corneal amyloidosis
APin*	Unknown	Pindborg odontogenic tumors

Known amyloid proteins as at March 2005. CAA, cerebral amyloid angiopathy; CJD, Creutzfeldt–Jakob disease. ADan and ABri are derived from the same gene.

*Preliminary designation. Awaiting confirmation by Nomenclature Committee of the International Amyloidosis Society. References for the discovery and reviews of these amyloidogenic proteins can be found in 'Amyloid Proteins' (Sipe 2005).

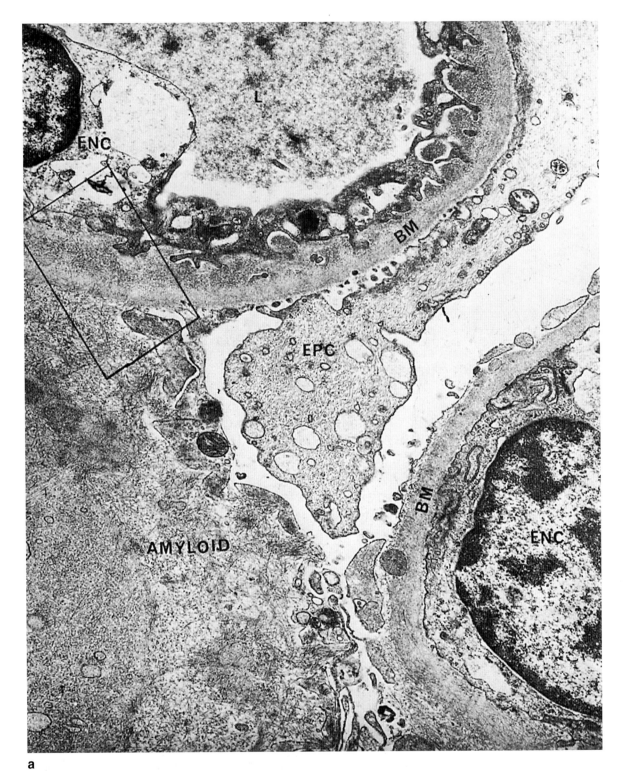

a

Fig. 15.1 (a) An electron micrograph of kidney from a case of amyloidosis with renal involvement. Two glomerular capillary loops can be seen which include capillary basement membrane (BM), endothelial cell (ENC), and capillary lumen (L). An elongated mass of epithelial cell cytoplasm (EPC) extends from one side of the photograph and its foot processes rest on one of the basement membranes. Tangled masses of amyloid fibrils are present in the urinary space. (Glutaraldehyde/osmium fixed, stained with uranyl acetate and lead citrate.)

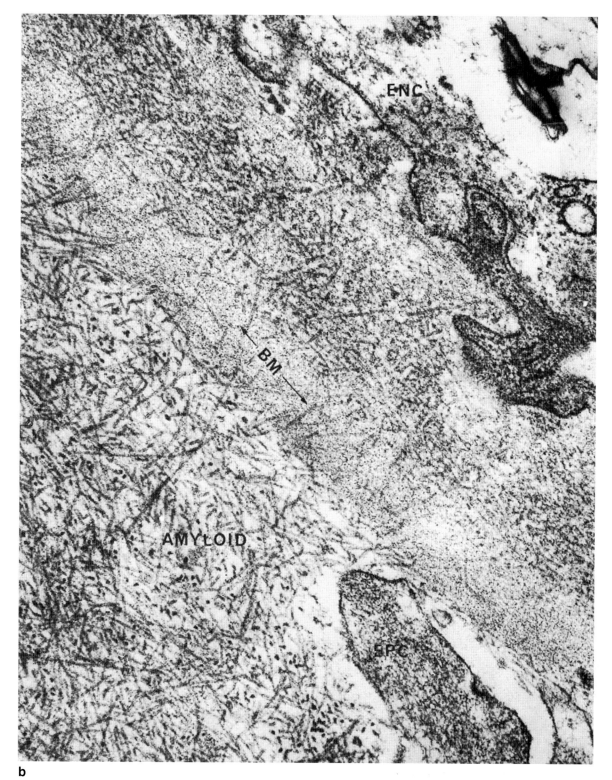

b

Fig. 15.1 (*continued*) (b) A higher magnification (×54,000) taken from the area within the rectangle. Amyloid fibrils can clearly be seen on both epithelial and endothelial sides of the capillary basement membrane (BM), which runs diagonally across the field. Fibrils appear to be passing through the basement membrane. The double filament structure of the fibril may be seen in some places.

Fibril aggregate

A tangled mass of amyloid fibrils of random orientation

Occasional parallel bundles are seen, predominantly extracellular

The amyloid fibril

A double helix of 1000 Å periodicity consisting of two pleated sheet micelles in the form of twin filaments separated by a clear interspace

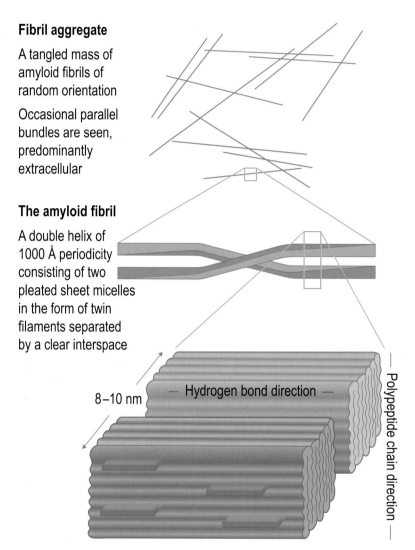

8–10 nm

— Hydrogen bond direction —

Polypeptide chain direction

The amyloid filament

Lozenge-shaped Congo red or toluidine blue dye molecules retained in grooved face of β-pleated sheet protein by hydrogen bonds

Fig. 15.2 Schematic diagram of amyloid structure.

composed of four protofilaments that appear to be β-pleated—strands arranged perpendicular to, and β-sheets parallel with, the fibril axis, arrayed around a hollow core (Jimenez et al 1999). This is a pattern that conforms with recent modern X-ray fiber diffraction studies (Sunde et al 1997).

CLASSIFICATION

It was apparent to early pathologists that amyloid was frequently associated with a predisposing disease and had a localized or systemic distribution. This led to early classification schemes such as that of Wilks in 1856 which recognized both idiopathic amyloidosis and a class that was 'connected with syphilis, rheumatism, etc.' (referred to by Husby 1994).

The main classification scheme for amyloid used until the 1980s was that of Reimann et al (1935) which divided amyloid types into four categories:

1. Primary amyloid occurring spontaneously in the absence of apparent predisposing illness and frequently affecting tissue of mesodermal origin such as muscle, heart, skin, and tongue often with localized deposits. The spleen, liver, and kidneys are infrequently affected in this type of amyloidosis.
2. Secondary amyloid occurring in association with a wide range of predisposing or coexistent pathology. In the past these were often chronic infective diseases such as syphilis or tuberculosis, but nowadays inflammatory conditions such as rheumatoid arthritis are more common. The distribution of the amyloid deposits is typically systemic, being found in the liver, spleen, kidneys, and adrenal glands.
3. Tumor-associated amyloids.
4. Myeloma-associated amyloid, found in a proportion of patients with plasma cell diseases such as multiple myeloma.

Subsequent discoveries suggested that there were other categories of amyloidosis such as endocrine-associated amyloid, familial amyloid, and amyloid associated with aging; moreover, once the constituent proteins of amyloid fibrils had been identified, it became clear that traditional classification schemes were unsatisfactory and a classification according to the amyloid fibril protein subunit was proposed (Husby 1980). By 1990 several other proteins that formed amyloid deposits had been identified leading to proposals for an expanded scheme

(Husby et al 1990; Husby 1992). This scheme was adopted by the World Health Organization–International Union of Immunological Societies (WHO–IUIS) Nomenclature Subcommittee in 1993 (Kazatchkine et al 1993) and is currently universally accepted for the classification of amyloid. Amyloids are identified by an abbreviation of their originating protein preceded by a capital A. Table 15.1 gives the 25 currently known human amyloids, their abbreviation, their protein precursor, and the conditions most commonly associated with them. This scheme is currently administered by the Nomenclature Committee of the International Society of Amyloidosis and is periodically reviewed in the journal *Amyloid* (Westermark et al 2002, 2005).

PATHOGENESIS

What causes those proteins involved in amyloid formation to convert from being normal functioning proteins into inert amyloid deposits is the focus of much research. There is little to connect the proteins involved; whilst several contain large amounts of β-pleated sheet conformation in their native form, one, prion protein, contains none and the formation of β-pleated sheets de novo is the pathological event of the prion diseases. In other amyloidoses the whole parent protein may be involved as with serum amyloid A, or there may be proteolysis of the parent protein with liberation of a smaller amyloidogenic fragment as with AβPP. In transthyretin amyloidosis the native protein is a tetramer and the pathological event appears to be the release of the monomer. The pathogenesis of amyloid has been recently reviewed (Sipe 2005).

'Conformational disease' or 'protein folding disorders'

Professor Robin Carrell has commented that the key feature of not only amyloidosis but several other conditions is a post-translational change in the conformation of the protein concerned and suggested a broader concept of 'conformational disease'. Conformational diseases involve the self-aggregation or polymerization of protein after some precipitating event due to the presence of a large proportion of β-pleated sheet secondary conformation. It is argued that such a grouping helps provide an understanding of the etiology of, and an explanation for, the often late or episodic onset of these diseases and opens the prospect for common approaches to therapeutic stratagems in the same way, say, that recognition of bacteria as the causative agents of many infections allowed the idea of antibiotics being useful in all such conditions or of steroid therapy being of potential use for all inflammatory conditions (Carrell & Lomas 1997; Carrell & Gooptu 1998). In this context it is interesting to note the development of 'designer' peptides that bind to Aβ and to prion protein preventing and even reversing the conformational change responsible for the respective disease processes (Soto et al 2000). This concept is increasingly accepted and it is becoming evident that amyloid is but one, albeit definable, subgroup within a larger group of misfolded or altered protein deposits associated with human disease. See Table 15.2.

DIAGNOSIS

Whilst there may be strong clinical grounds for suspecting amyloidosis there is general agreement that definitive diagnosis depends on demonstration of amyloid in a tissue biopsy (Westermark 1995; Buxbaum 1996; Falk et al 1997). Biopsy of an obviously affected organ is likely to offer the best chance of a positive result, for example of the kidney in dialysis, or diabetic patients with a suspicion of amyloidosis, or of sural nerve in familial polyneuropathies, but this approach may be unacceptably invasive in the case of, for example, brain or cardiac disease. Many anatomical sites have been compared for optimal identification of amyloid. Such studies have

Table 15.2 Protein conformation diseases

Conditions	Affected proteins	Associated diseases
Amyloidosis	25 known in humans—see Table 15.1	
Serpinopathies	α1-Antitrypsin Neuroserpin	αl-Antitrypsin storage disease
Hemoglobinopathies	Hemoglobulin	Sickle cell anemia Drug and aging induced inclusion body hemolysis
Lewy body diseases	α-Synuclein	Parkinson's disease
Neuronal inclusion bodies	Tau	Alzheimer's disease
		Pick's disease
		Progressive supranuclear palsy
	Superoxide dismutase	Motor neuron disease, AML
	Ferritin	Familial neurodegenerative disorder
Hirano bodies	Actin	Alzheimer's disease
Polyglutamine repeats	Huntingtin	Huntington's disease
	Ataxin	Spinocerebellar ataxias
	Androgen receptor	Spinomuscular atrophies
Prion diseases	Prion protein	Creutzfeldt–Jacob disease (CJD) Variant CJD
		Gerstmann–Straussler–Scheinker
		Kuru
		Fatal familial insomnia
		Japanese CAA

shown that in systemic amyloidosis renal biopsy allows the greatest detection rate; however, the less invasive technique of rectal biopsy also allows a high rate of detection (Fentem et al 1962; Tribe 1966; Delgado & Mosqueda 1989). Other methods include fine-needle aspiration of abdominal subcutaneous fat (Westermark & Stenkvist 1973). Amyloid is present in more than 90% of rectal and/or subcutaneous fat biopsies in systemic AA or AL amyloidosis (Pepys 1992), whereas skin and gingival biopsies have been shown to give poorer results (Kyle & Greipp 1983). With rectal biopsies it is important to obtain a full thickness of the muscularis as amyloid deposits are usually to be found in the walls of small submucosal vessels. A negative result does not exclude the possibility of amyloidosis due to the unavoidable problem of sampling error and the variability of amyloid deposition between sites.

Isotope-labeled SAP has recently been introduced as a specific tracer for amyloid as a method of in vivo diagnosis (Hawkins et al 1990). Using this technique important in vivo observations of amyloid have been made that have allowed an improved understanding of the distribution of amyloid in different forms of the disease. Direct evidence of the progression and regression of amyloid deposition is possible using such imaging, allowing the monitoring of treatment regimes (Pepys 1992; Hawkins et al 1993; Hawkins 1994). This technique remains restricted in its availability.

DEMONSTRATION

Most amyloid-containing material will have been routinely formalin fixed and paraffin embedded, and no special fixation or processing regimes are necessary; however, after prolonged formalin fixation many staining reactions become progressively less intense. It is important to use a known positive control section to confirm the reactivity of staining solutions when demonstrating amyloid. Such control sections should be relatively freshly cut as they tend to lose their reactivity if stored for long periods. Tissues containing massive deposits, presumably of long standing, give less intense histochemical reactions than small, newly formed deposits.

Amyloid appears in H&E-stained sections as an amorphous, eosinophilic, extracellular, faintly refractile substance. It is variably periodic acid–Schiff positive and weakly birefringent using a powerful light source. None of these methods is of use in the differential detection of amyloid, and while large deposits may be easily recognized in H&E-stained sections, small deposits are often missed and differentiation between amyloid and other amorphous eosinophilic substances such as hyaline and fibrinoid is difficult.

The earliest 'special stain' used for amyloid demonstration was that of iodine by Virchow; it is rarely used nowadays and interested parties should refer to the method and discussion given in earlier editions of this book.

Methyl or crystal violet metachromasia

The triphenylmethane dye, methyl violet, was the first synthetic dye used for the demonstration of amyloid (Cornil 1875). The rationale of the staining reaction remains unexplained. It was long assumed that the mucopolysaccharide content of amyloid was responsible for the staining reaction, but this is now thought unlikely.

Methyl violet is a mixture of tetra-, penta-, and hexamethyl pararosaniline, and the staining of amyloid is probably by selective affinity for one of these colored fractions; hence polychromasia rather then metachromasia would be a more likely explanation of this reaction (Windrum & Kramer 1957). The staining of amyloid is far from specific and because of the lack of a marked color variation from other tissue components minimal amyloid deposits may be missed, especially in rectal biopsies, since mucins give a similar red–purple color. It is necessary to mount methyl violet-stained sections in an aqueous mountant as dehydration partially destroys the red polychromasia, and the examination of wet sections prior to mounting is recommended. The amyloid from some primary amyloidosis fails to give a positive reaction. Because of this low sensitivity and lack of specificity this method is not nowadays recommended for amyloid detection and diagnosis (Westermark et al 1999).

Crystal violet method (Hucker & Conn 1928)

Either methyl or crystal violet can be used in this method. Ammonium oxalate is said to accentuate the polychromatic effect. Apathy's mountant is preferred to glycerine jelly to minimize the marked diffusion of dye that occurs with the latter.

Preparation of solution

Dissolve 2 g of crystal violet in 20 ml of 95% alcohol. Add 80 ml of 1% aqueous ammonium oxalate. Dissolve using a minimum of heat. Cool and filter.

Method

1. Sections to water, removing pigment where necessary.
2. Stain in crystal violet solution, 5 minutes.
3. Wash and differentiate in 0.2% aqueous acetic acid, controlling the differentiation microscopically, stopping differentiation in water, and repeating until good contrast is obtained between amyloid and the background.
4. Wash and mount in modified Apathy's medium (see Highman's modification in Appendix V, p. 693).

Results

Amyloid, mucin, renal hyaline	red–purple
Background	blue

Note

1. For critical work involving minimal deposits, sections should be examined wet before mounting in Apathy's medium.
2. In a modified formic acid–crystal violet method the polychromatic effect is accentuated by the presence of formic acid in both the staining and differentiation solutions (Fernando 1961).

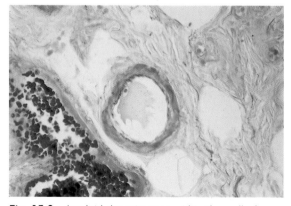

Fig. 15.3 Amyloid deposits seen within the wall of an arteriole in a rectal biopsy from a patient suffering from systemic amyloidosis stained with Hucker and Conn's crystal violet method showing red–purple metachromasia of the amyloid. Original magnification ×217.

Congo red

Since its introduction by Bennhold in 1922, the highly selective affinity of the dye Congo red for amyloid, and the subsequent green birefringence when viewed using polarizing microscopy, has been the method of choice for amyloid demonstration; indeed these properties form part of the accepted definition of amyloid. It was first introduced as a diagnostic test for amyloid in vivo and then, in the same year, to tissue sections (Bennhold 1922). First introduced as a colorant for the cotton industry in 1884, Congo red is an acidic diazo dye that is comprised of two identical halves each composed of a phenyl ring bound to a naphthalene moiety by a diazo group. The two phenyl groups are bound together by a diphenyl bond linked so as to give a linear molecule that is largely hydrophobic (Turnell & Finch 1992).

For many years the rationale of the reaction was unknown but it has been shown that staining of amyloid by Congo red is through hydrogen bonding as opposed to the electrochemical bonds formed between the dye and most other tissue components. In aqueous solution Congo red stains many tissue components, although there is always a greater affinity for amyloid. In retrospect, many of the early modifications to Bennhold's aqueous method, e.g. using alkaline alcoholic solvents (Highman 1946), or using competitive inhibition by salt solutions (Puchtler et al 1964), had the effect of suppressing the electrochemical staining of other tissue components, enhancing hydrogen bonding, and so improving selectivity for amyloid. Experiments on purified extracts of amyloid show that the uptake is stoichiometric and can be used as a quantitative test for the fibrils (Pras et al 1968).

Two factors are important to the Congo red–amyloid reaction: the linearity of the dye molecule and the β-pleated sheet configuration. If the spatial configuration of either is altered, even though the chemical groupings are left intact, the reaction fails. Furthermore the Congo red-mediated positive birefringence of amyloid implies that the dye molecules are arranged in parallel fashion (Romhanyi 1971). Recent work confirms the long-held belief that the Congo red molecule intercalates between two protein moieties at the interface between two adjacent antiparallel β-pleated sheets by disrupting the hydrogen bonds that are responsible for maintaining the β-sheet polymer, yet allowing maintenance of the integrity of the structure by the formation of new hydrogen bonds between protein and dye (Carter & Chou 1998).

As previously noted prolonged formalin fixation may diminish Congo red staining intensity. A method using Mesitol WLS and Congo red was devised to circumvent this problem when staining archival material although the method was not tested on material fixed for longer than a year (Meloan & Puchtler 1978).

A variety of the other cotton dyes used in the textile industry have been tested and compared with Congo red, some favorably, in particular Sirius red (Puchtler et al 1964; Sweat & Puchtler 1965). The authors claim that the dye gave a more intense staining reaction than Congo red, but it has not gained wide acceptance because any advantages over Congo red are marginal and, unlike Congo red, it has no fluorochromic properties which can be used to accentuate equivocally weak staining with the latter dye (Puchtler & Sweat 1965; Cohen 1967).

Recent comparison of several Congo red staining methods made during a run of the UK NEQUAS histology external quality control scheme found that the method of Stokes (1976) gave the highest scores.

Highman's Congo red technique
(Highman 1946)

This simple method has found wide application. The solutions are relatively stable and the method affords a high degree of selectivity in practiced hands.

Fixation
Not critical; formal saline gives satisfactory results.

Solutions
0.5% Congo red in 50% alcohol
0.2% potassium hydroxide in 80% alcohol

Method
1. Sections to water, removing pigment where necessary.
2. Stain in Congo red solution, 5 minutes.
3. Differentiate with the alcoholic potassium hydroxide solution, 3–10 seconds.
4. Wash in water, stain nuclei in alum hematoxylin, differentiate, and blue.
5. Dehydrate, clear, and mount.

Results
Amyloid, elastic fibres, eosinophil granules   red
Nuclei   blue

Note
Differentiation in step 3 can be arrested in water and resumed if necessary. Over-differentiation can occur.

Alkaline Congo red technique (Puchtler et al 1962)

The method obviates the need for a differentiation step by the inclusion of a high concentration of sodium chloride; this reduces background electrochemical staining whilst enhancing hydrogen bonding of Congo red to amyloid, resulting in a progressive and highly selective technique. The solutions should be freshly made.

Fixation
Not critical.

Stock solutions

Stock solution A
Saturated sodium chloride in 80% ethanol.

Stock solution B
Saturated Congo red in 80% ethanol saturated with sodium chloride.
1% aqueous sodium hydroxide.

Working solutions
To 100 ml of stock solution A add 1 ml of 1% aqueous sodium hydroxide and filter.
To 100 ml of stock solution B add 1 ml of 1% aqueous sodium hydroxide and filter.

Method
1. Sections to water, removing pigment where necessary.
2. Stain nuclei in alum hematoxylin, differentiate, and blue.
3. Immerse in alkaline sodium chloride solution for 20 minutes.
4. Transfer directly to the alkaline Congo red solution for 20 minutes.
5. Rinse briefly in alcohol, clear, and mount.

Congo red technique (Stokes 1976)

In this method there is no differentiation step as Congo red is applied in an alkaline alcoholic solution. Harris's hematoxylin was originally used as a counterstain but any alum hematoxylin will suffice.

Fixation
Not critical.

Preparation of solutions
Staining solution
Dissolve 0.5 g potassium hydroxide in 50 ml distilled water, add 200 ml absolute alcohol and add Congo red until saturated (about 3 g). Stand overnight before use and discard after 3 months

Method
1. Sections to water, removing pigment where necessary.
2. Stain in filtered Congo red solution, 25 minutes.
3. Wash in distilled water then running tap water, 5 minutes
4. Counterstain nuclei in Harris's hematoxylin, 1 minute.
5. Blue, differentiate, hematoxylin if necessary, blue.
6. Dehydrate, clear, and mount.

Results
Amyloid, elastic tissue, eosinophil granules   red
Nuclei   blue

Sirius red technique (Llewellyn 1970)

This method, a modification of Sweat's, uses the direct cotton dye Sirius red F3B which, according to the authors, compares favorably with Congo red as a method for the detection of amyloid. The mechanism of staining is probably similar to that of Congo red. Although this modification is considerably simpler than the original technique, the staining solution does not keep well and is liable to precipitate out during preparation.

Fixation
Not critical.

Preparation of solution
Dissolve 0.5 g Sirius red F3B in 45 ml distilled water. Add 50 ml absolute alcohol and 1 ml 1% sodium hydroxide. Stirring the solution vigorously, slowly add just sufficient 20% sodium chloride (c. 4 ml) to produce a fine precipitate when viewed against strong backlighting. Leave to stand overnight and filter.

Method
1. Sections to water, removing pigment where necessary.
2. Stain nuclei in alum hematoxylin, differentiate, and blue.
3. Rinse in water and then 70% ethanol.
4. Treat with Sirius red solution for 1 hour.
5. Wash in tap water for 10 minutes.
6. Dehydrate, clear, and mount.

Results
Amyloid, elastic, eosinophil, and Paneth   red
cell granules
Nuclei   blue

Note
The staining solution is liable to precipitation, especially if excess 20% sodium chloride is added during preparation.

POLARIZING MICROSCOPY AND CONGO RED

When viewed using polarized light and an analyzing polarizing filter, Congo red-stained amyloid exhibits a

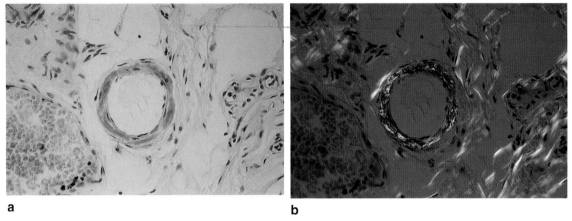

a   b

Fig. 15.4 (a) The same vessel as Figure 15.3 stained with Puchtler and Sweat's Congo red method showing congophilic amyloid deposits within the wall of the arteriole. (b) The same preparation photographed by polarized light, showing the 'apple-green' birefringence that is characteristic of amyloid deposits. Original magnification ×217.

characteristic bright green birefringence, usually termed 'apple-green birefringence' (see Figure 15.4b). This property is shared by other β-pleated sheet proteins and appears to be specific to that conformation.

Birefringence is an optical property of anisotropic substances, that is, substances that have different physical properties in different directions. It is observed in crystals and is widely used in mineralogy as a qualitative test for the identification of various minerals. Such an optically active substance will have two differing refractive indices (RI) so that two rays of light vibrating in perpendicular planes will travel at different velocities through the substance, producing a faster ray and a slower ray. The substance is said to show positive birefringence if the plane of vibration of the slow ray (greater RI) is parallel to the length of the fiber or crystal, or negative if the plane of vibration of the slow ray is perpendicular to the length of the fiber. Normally birefringent substances appear colorless (white) against a dark background viewed through crossed polarizing filters, but where the thickness of the crystal or fibre is uniform, interference colors may be produced when the two rays are reunited in the analyzer. Such colors are characteristic of and can thus be used to identify the substance being viewed. Practical details of polarizing microscopy and birefringence are given in Chapter 3.

Amyloid in unstained sections can be seen to be weakly birefringent when using a strong light source;

weak birefringence may also often be seen following methyl violet, toluidine blue, and eosin staining. Such birefringence is usually faint, unreliable, and non-specific, and is therefore of little diagnostic use. In contrast, the bright apple-green birefringence of amyloid following Congo red staining is easily visualized, highly selective, and thought by many to be the most reliable diagnostic characteristic of amyloid in current use (Missmahl & Hartwig 1953; Cohen 1967; Pearse 1968). This green birefringence, first noticed by Divery and Florkin (1927), is an intrinsic property of the amyloid fibril–Congo red complex. The thickness of section is critical; 8–10 μm is ideal (Wolman & Bubis 1965). Too-thin sections may show faint red colors, while yellow birefringent colors can be seen if the section is too thick, if there is strain birefringence in the optical system, or if the direction of the fibrils is oblique to the direction of the polarizer.

The use of a good microscope of high optical quality with color-corrected optics is essential to visualize faint birefringence. A revolving stage and subdued background lighting are also advisable. The strongest possible light source should be used; in our experience most laboratory microscopes do not have strong enough light sources and sections should preferentially be viewed using a modern photomicroscope, most of which are equipped both with essentially perfect optics and with powerful lamps. Only by using such a setup can the smallest of amyloid deposits be appreciated.

Apple-green birefringence is also given by certain other filamentous structures, most notably the neuro-fibrillary tangles characteristic of Alzheimer's disease and certain other degenerative brain diseases, as well as the intracellular inclusions seen in adrenal cortical cells (Eriksson & Westermark 1990). Whilst these structures fulfill many of the characteristics of amyloid, they are not currently considered to be so, although the matter remains under debate (Westermark et al 2005). Green birefringence is also given by cellulose and chitin, both of which avidly bind Congo red. They are easily distinguished from amyloid on morphological grounds. Occasionally other structures may appear to give green birefringence, most commonly dense collagen. This can usually be distinguished from amyloid by its whiter color, and the difference can be emphasized by the use of sections cut at the recommended thickness.

Congo red is a fluorescent dye, and provided that sections have been mounted in a non-fluorescent mountant this property can be used to detect small amyloid deposits. The fluorescence should not be considered as specific for amyloid as is the apple-green birefringence seen with polarizing microscopy (Puchtler & Sweat 1965; Westermark et al 1999).

Differentiation between different amyloids

With the recognition that different diseases were associated with different amyloids came a desire to identify particular deposits histologically. Methods of section pretreatment using trypsin or potassium permanganate before Congo red staining were devised (Wright et al 1976, 1977). After such pretreatment some amyloids lose their affinity for Congo red, most notably AA amyloid, whereas AL amyloid is resistant. These methods were always equivocal in practice and have been rendered obsolete by the use of immunohistochemistry to identify specifically and reliably the particular proteins involved.

Acquired fluorescence methods

The ability of amyloid to fluoresce following treatment with fluorochromic dyes was discovered by Chiari (1947), although little use was made of this property until Vassar and Culling (1959) recommended the basic fluorochrome dye thioflavine T. The method has the advantage of not requiring microscopical differentiation, and, save for staining of renal tubular myeloma casts and mast cell granules, specificity for amyloid was claimed.

Thioflavine T staining has enjoyed considerable popularity as a screening method for amyloid as the intensity of fluorescence allows good visualization of minimal deposits. It has become evident that the specificity originally claimed for the method was overstated and that many other tissue components including fibrinoid, arteriolar hyaline, keratin, intestinal muciphages, Paneth cells, and zymogen granules also have an affinity for the dye.

The addition of 0.4 M magnesium chloride to a 0.1% thioflavine T solution at pH 5.7 is claimed to improve selectivity by competitive ionic inhibition (Mowry & Scott 1967). Similar results are obtained by using thioflavine T at pH 1.4, favoring the reaction of the blue fluorescing dye component responsible for fluorescence of amyloid (Burns et al 1967).

The mechanism of binding of thioflavine T to amyloid is not known but in vitro studies of binding to purified amyloid fibrils and synthetic amyloids show that the dye interacts with the quaternary structure of the β-pleated sheet rather than with protein moieties, and so the binding is not dependent on any amino acid sequence (LeVine 1995).

A related fluorochrome, thioflavine S, has been widely used for the demonstration of amyloid (Schwartz 1970); however it is considered to be non-specific and is not recommended (Puchtler et al 1985).

Thioflavine T method (Vassar & Culling 1959)

Fixation
Not critical.

Preparation of solution
1% aqueous thioflavine T.

Method
1. Sections to water, removing pigment where necessary.
2. Treat with alum hematoxylin solution, 2 minutes.

3. Wash in water and stain in thioflavine T solution, 3 minutes.
4. Rinse in water and differentiate excess fluorochrome from background in 1% acetic acid, 20 minutes.
5. Wash well in water, dehydrate, clear, and mount in a non-fluorescent mountant.

Results (see Fig. 15.5)

Using a UV light source (mercury vapor lamp), UG1 Exciter filter, BG38 red suppression filter, and K430 barrier filter: amyloid, elastic tissue, etc.—silver–blue fluorescence

Using blue light fluorescence quartz–iodine or mercury vapor lamp with BG12 exciter filter and K530 barrier filter: amyloid, elastic tissue, etc.—yellow fluorescence.

Notes

a. Step 2 quenches nuclear autofluorescence.
b. The mountant must be non-fluorescent such as glycerine–saline (1 : 9 parts) or DPX. Avoid Canada balsam, which autofluoresces.

c. Thioflavine T deteriorates, especially if kept in sunlight, as do the stained sections on prolonged storage.

pH 1.4 thioflavine T (Burns et al 1967)

Acid pH increases the selectivity by favoring the fluorochromic fraction binding to amyloid while depressing non-amyloid fluorochrome staining.

Method

As above but use a freshly prepared solution of 0.5% thioflavine T in 0.1 M hydrochloric acid.

Results

Amyloid, Paneth cells, and oxyntic cells—silver–blue or yellow fluorescence according to filters used.

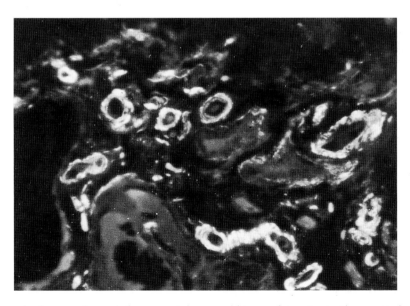

Fig. 15.5 A group of submucosal vessels from a rectal mucosal biopsy of a patient with suspected amyloidosis, secondary to rheumatoid arthritis. Thioflavine T fluorescence of the amyloid contained within these vessel walls is striking, even at low power.

MISCELLANEOUS METHODS

Many dyes, notably alcian blue and toluidine blue, commonly used for the identification of mucopolysaccharides, have been used on amyloid-containing tissue sections to substantiate histochemically the mucopolysaccharides frequently found in biochemical assays of amyloid tissue extracts. In most instances results have been disappointing; uptake of these dyes is poor and variable. Differing electrolyte concentrations (Mowry & Scott 1967) and partial pepsin digestion (Windrum & Kramer 1957) may enhance alcian blue uptake and toluidine blue metachromasia respectively, but staining is never strong and interpretation difficult. The variable periodic acid–Schiff's staining of amyloid, which is often intense, was thought to indicate the presence of carbohydrate within amyloid fibrils, but this has been disproved; the glycoprotein AP component is now thought to be the origin of this positivity.

Alcian blue–borax, with a celestine blue–hemalum and van Gieson counterstain, elegantly demonstrates some amyloid, but the method is not specific (Lendrum et al 1972).

There are several silver impregnation methods that have been used for the demonstration of amyloid, such as that of King (1948). There are several silver methods used on central nervous system tissue for the detection of amyloid-containing plaques (and neurofibrillary tangles) in Alzheimer's disease. There have been several reviews of these methods (Lamy et al 1989; Wisniewski et al 1989; Wilcock et al 1990; Vallet et al 1992), and the methenamine silver method of Haga is given in Chapter 19 on the nervous system.

IMMUNOHISTOCHEMISTRY FOR AMYLOID

Given that the major components of all amyloid fibrils are proteins it might be expected that immunohistochemistry would have been used for the specific identification of individual amyloid deposits from early after its introduction as a mainstream histological technique in the 1970s. That this was not the case is due to the altered conformation of these proteins within amyloid fibrils presumably obscuring many antigenic sites. It would seem that the β-pleated conformation in itself 'hides' antigenic sites on many of the amyloid proteins rather than any non-antigenicity being due to cross-linking of amino acid side groups by fixation. Thus the conventional cross-link breaking techniques of enzymatic digestion and heat treatment may not in themselves be sufficient to reveal antigenic sites in amyloid deposits, even if such antigen recovery is perfectly effective for the same protein and antibody in non-amyloid demonstration.

It was always hoped that a single protein that could be used to identify all amyloid deposits would be found. Amyloid P component, AP, has been shown to fulfill this function. AP is found in variable proportion in all amyloids; it is a non-fibrillar component that does not have a β-pleated conformation and is moderately antigenic. SAP is found naturally bound to various other tissue components such as basement membranes so that, although antiserum to AP is readily available and can be used to identify amyloid deposits immunohistochemically, care should be taken in interpretation. Most laboratories still use Congo red with polarizing microscopy as the method of choice for amyloid detection, using AP immunohistochemistry as an adjunct.

Once it was realized that amyloids were derived from different proteins and laid down in different diseases it became important to be able further to identify individual deposits in order to characterize the causal disease.

Early attempts to use immunohistochemistry to identify individual amyloid deposits had varied success due to variable antigenicity (Fujihara et al 1980; Livni et al 1980; Shirahama et al 1981). Trypsin and pronase were ineffective as antigen recovery methods for transthyretin-derived amyloid whereas protein denaturing agents such as high molarity urea and guanidine were successful (Costa et al 1986). Concentrated formic acid was used to reveal antigenicity in Aβ, AA, APrP, and ATTR (Kitamoto et al 1987), whereas microwave heating was used for Aβ and APrP with good results (Sherriff et al 1994; Liberski et al 1996). Since each antibody differs in the epitope that it recognizes, it is important to try the whole range of available antigen recovery methods for each antiserum and each amyloid tried. Antisera have become commercially available to almost all 25 of the amyloid-forming proteins. It would be uneconomical to carry all such antisera in routine laboratories; however several amyloid related diseases are commoner than others and are of importance in the context of routine hospital work (Fig. 15.6). The identification of inflammation-related amyloid AA and of myeloma-

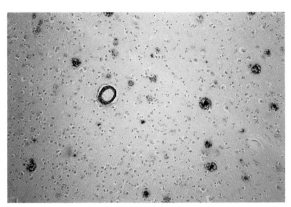

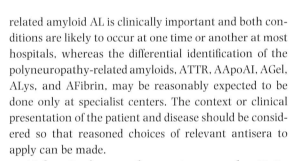

Fig. 15.6 Immunoperoxidase–DAB stain using Aβ antiserum with formic acid antigen recovery in brain section from a patient with Alzheimer's disease. Plaques typical of Alzheimer's disease and concomitant cerebral amyloid angiopathy can be seen. Original magnification ×87.

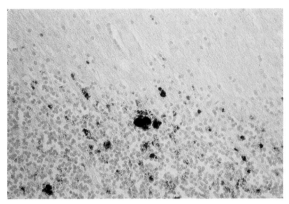

Fig. 15.7 Immunoperoxidase–DAB stain using the prion protein antiserum KG9 with combined autoclaving/formic acid/4 M guanidine thiocyanide antigen recovery on a section of cerebellum from a patient with Creutzfeldt–Jakob disease. ×87.

related amyloid AL is clinically important and both conditions are likely to occur at one time or another at most hospitals, whereas the differential identification of the polyneuropathy-related amyloids, ATTR, AApoAI, AGel, ALys, and AFibrin, may be reasonably expected to be done only at specialist centers. The context or clinical presentation of the patient and disease should be considered so that reasoned choices of relevant antisera to apply can be made.

AL deposits show a rather greater range of positivity regardless of the antigen recovery methods tried; only about half of such deposits are demonstrable using κ and λ antisera. This is thought to be because AL deposits are formed from the variable light chain fragment of the immunoglobulin molecule which is largely unique for each monoclonal protein (Pepys 1992).

The demonstration of prion-derived amyloid deposits, APrP, has been particularly difficult. In our laboratory we follow the consensus criteria from the Creutzfeldt–Jakob Disease Surveillance Unit and obtain consistently good results (Bell et al 1997; see Fig. 15.7). It is important to follow these criteria so as to avoid false-positive interference from normal prion protein and it should be noted that the proteins within all amyloid deposits differ from the normal precursor proteins largely by alteration of conformation rather than any antigenically determinable character.

The possibility of the presence of small quantities of AA amyloid within deposits of, for example, AL amyloid

has been raised and such deposits have been immunohistochemically detected (Husby et al 1973b). They should not obscure the primary nature of the amyloid.

EVALUATION OF METHODS

The accepted standard for amyloid detection remains the use of Congo red staining, with positivity being judged on the presence of 'apple-green' birefringence. The Congo red method of Stokes is preferred. False positives and false negatives may occur, but attention to the details given herein, especially to the use of a powerful light microscope for polarizing microscopy, should reduce their occurrence. Sirius red remains a viable alternative dye, but since the definition of amyloid is by positivity with Congo red staining this remains the dye of choice. Thioflavine T and other fluorescent dyes may offer greater sensitivity in the detection of amyloid; however they may be less selective than Congo red as both hyaline and fibrinoids also give positive results (Cooper 1969).

Immunohistochemistry with AP antisera should be used in conjunction with Congo red staining rather than as a substitute for the detection of amyloid. It is imperative to attempt further to characterize each amyloid deposit immunohistochemically. If the causal disease is not known then there will be a clinical need to discover it. The choice and success of treatment may well depend upon such identification. If a laboratory is unable to undertake such identification, referral to a specialist amyloid center should be considered.

Acknowledgment

Robert Francis contributed this chapter for the first four editions and co-authored it for the fifth edition. Our thanks are due to him.

REFERENCES

Ancsin J.B. (2003) Amyloidogenesis: historical and modern observations point to heparin sulfate proteoglycans as a major culprit. Amyloid: Journal of Protein Folding Disorders 10:67–79.

Bell J.E., Gentleman S.M, Ironside J.W. et al. (1997) Prion protein immunocytochemistry—UK five centre consensus report. Neuropathology and Applied Neurobiology 23(1):26–35.

Bennhold H. (1922) Eine specifische amyloid-färbung mit kangorot. Münchener Medizinische Wochenschrift 33:1537–1541.

Bitter T., Muir H. (1966) Mucopolysaccharides of whole human spleens in generalised amyloidosis. Journal of Clinical Investigation 45:963.

Burns J., Pennock C.A., Stoward P.J. (1967) The specificity of the staining of amyloid deposits with thioflavine T. Journal of Pathology and Bacteriology 94:337–344.

Buxbaum J. (1996) The amyloidoses. Mount Sinai Journal of Medicine 63(1):16–23.

Carrell R.W., Gooptu B. (1998) Conformational changes and disease—serpins, prions and Alzheimer's. Current Opinion in Structural Biology 8(6):799–809.

Carrell R.W., Lomas D.A. (1997) Conformational disease. Lancet 350(9071):134–138.

Carter D.B., Chou K.C. (1998) A model for structure-dependent binding of Congo red to Alzheimer beta-amyloid fibrils. Neurobiology of Aging 19(1):37–40.

Chiari H. (1947) Ein Beitrag zue sekundaren fluorezenzdesogen localen Amyloids. Mikroscopie 2:79.

Cohen A.S. (1967) Amyloidosis. New England Journal of Medicine 277:522–530.

Cohen A.S., Calkins E. (1959) Electron microscopic observations on a fibrous component in amyloid of diverse origins. Nature 183:1202–1203.

Cooper J.H. (1969) An evaluation of current methods for the diagnostic histochemistry of amyloid. Journal of Clinical Pathology 22(4):410–413.

Cornil V. (1875) Cited by Cohen A.S. (1965) CR (Paris) 80:1288.

Costa P.P, Jacobsson B., Collin V.P. et al. (1986) Unmasking antigen determinants in amyloid. Journal of Histochemistry and Cytochemistry 34(12):1683–1685.

Delgado W.A., Mosqueda A. (1989) A highly sensitive method for diagnosis of secondary amyloidosis by labial salivary gland biopsy. Journal of Oral Pathology and Medicine 18(5):310–314.

Divery P., Florkin M. (1927) Sur les propriétés optiques de l'amyloide. Comptes Rendus des Séances de la Société de Biologie et des Filiales 97:1808–1810.

Eanes E.D., Glenner G.G. (1968) X-ray diffraction studies on amyloid filaments. Journal of Histochemistry and Cytochemistry 16:673–677.

Eriksson L., Westermark P. (1990) Age-related accumulation of amyloid inclusions in adrenal cortical cells. American Journal of Pathology 136(2):461–466.

Falk R.H., Comenzo R.L., Skinner M. (1997) The systemic amyloidoses [see comments]. New England Journal of Medicine 337(13):898–909.

Fentem P.H., Turnberg L.A., Wormsley K.G. (1962) Biopsy of the rectum as an aid in the diagnosis of amyloid. British Medical Journal 1:364.

Fernando J.C. (1961) A durable method of demonstrating amyloid in paraffin sections. Journal of the Institute of Science Technology 7:40.

Friedrich N., Kékulé A. (1859) Zur Amyloidfrage. Virchows Archiv fur Pathologische Anatomie und Physiologie und fur Klinische Medizin 16:50.

Fujihara S., Balow J.E., Costa J.C. et al. (1980) Identification and classification of amyloid in formalin-fixed, paraffin-embedded tissue sections by the unlabeled immunoperoxidase method. Laboratory Investigation 43(4):358–365.

Gewurz H., Zhang X.H., Lint T.F. (1995) Structure and function of the pentraxins. Current Opinion in Immunology 7(1):54–64.

Glenner G.G. (1981) The bases of the staining of amyloid fibers: their physico-chemical nature and the mechanism of their dye–substrate interaction. Progress in Histochemistry and Cytochemistry 13(3):1–37.

Glenner G.G. (1983) Alzheimer's disease. The commonest form of amyloidosis. Archives of Pathology and Laboratory Medicine 107(6):281–282.

Glenner G.G., Harbaugh J., Ohma J.I. (1970) An amyloid protein: the amino-terminal variable fragment of an immunoglobulin light chain. Biochemistry and Biophysical Research Communications 41(5):1287–1289.

Glenner G.G., Terry W., Harada M. (1971) Amyloid fibril proteins: proof of homology with immunoglobulin light chains by sequence analyses. Science 172(988):1150–1151.

Glenner G.G., Harada M., Isersky C. (1972) The purification of amyloid fibril proteins. Preparative Biochemistry 2(1):39–51.

Harada M., Isersky C., Cuatrecasas P. et al. (1971) Human amyloid protein: chemical variability and homogeneity. Journal of Histochemistry and Cytochemistry 19:1.

Hass G. (1942) Studies on amyloid. II. The isolation of a polysaccharide from amyloid-bearing tissues. Archives of Pathology 34:92–105.

Hawkins P.N. (1994) Studies with radiolabelled serum amyloid P component provide evidence for turnover and regression of amyloid deposits in vivo. Clinical Science (Colch) 87(3):289–295.

Hawkins P.N., Lavender J.P., Pepys M.B. (1990) Evaluation of systemic amyloidosis by scintigraphy with ^{123}I-labeled serum amyloid P component. New England Journal of Medicine 323(8):508–513.

Hawkins P.N., Richardson S., Vigushin D.M. et al. (1993) Serum amyloid P component scintigraphy and turnover studies for diagnosis and quantitative monitoring of AA amyloidosis in juvenile rheumatoid arthritis. Arthritis and Rheumatism 36(6):842–851.

Highman B. (1946) Improved methods for demonstrating amyloid in paraffin sections. Archives of Pathology 41:559.

Holck M., Husby G., Sletten K. et al. (1979) The amyloid P-component (protein AP): an integral part of the amyloid substance? Scandanavian Journal of Immunology 10(1):55–60.

Hucker G.J., Conn H.J. (1928) Gram stain. I. A quick method for staining Gram-positive organisms in the tissues. Archives of Pathology 5:828.

Husby G. (1980) A chemical classification of amyloid. Correlation with different clinical types of amyloidosis. Scandanavian Journal of Rheumatology 9(1):60–64.

Husby G. (1992) Nomenclature and classification of amyloid and amyloidoses. Journal of International Medical Research 232(6):511–512.

Husby G. (1994) Classification of amyloidosis. Baillieres Clinical Rheumatology 8(3):503–511.

Husby G., Blomhoff J.P., Skrede S. et al. (1973a) Detection of immunoglobulins in paraffin-embedded liver biopsies. Studies in 100 patients with special regard to immunological findings in active chronic hepatitis. Scandanavian Journal of Gastroenterology 8(7):621–629.

Husby G., Natvig J.B., Michaelsen T.E. et al. (1973b) Unique amyloid protein subunit common to different types of amyloid fibril. Nature 244(5415):362–364.

Husby G., Araki S., Benditt E.P. et al. (1990) The 1990 guidelines for the nomenclature and classification of amyloid and amyloidosis. In: Natvig J., Forre O., Husby G., eds. Amyloid and amyloidosis. Dordrecht: Kluwer Academic Publishers, pp. 7–11.

Inoue S., Kisilevsky R. (1996) A high resolution ultrastructural study of experimental murine AA amyloid. Laboratory Investigation 74(3):670–683.

Jimenez J.L., Guijarro J.I., Orlova E. et al. (1999) Cryo-electron microscopy structure of an SH3 amyloid fibril and model of the molecular packing. EMBO Journal 18(4):815–821.

Kazatchkine M.D., Husby G., Araki S. et al. (1993) Nomenclature of amyloid and amyloidosis. Bulletin of the World Health Organization 71(1):105–108.

King L.S. (1948) Atypical amyloid disease, with observations on a new silver stain for amyloid. 45th Annual Meeting of the American Association of Pathologists and Bacteriologists. Philadelphia: AAPB.

Kisilevsky R. (1990) Heparan sulphate proteoglycans in amyloidosis: an epiphenomenon, a unique factor, or the tip of a more fundamental process? Laboratory Investigation 63(5):589–591.

Kitamoto T., Ogomori K., Tateishi J. et al. (1987) Formic acid pretreatment enhances immunostaining of cerebral and systemic amyloids. Laboratory Investigation 57(2):230–236.

Kyle R.A., Greipp P.R. (1983) Amyloidosis (AL). Clinical and laboratory features in 229 cases. Mayo Clinic Proceedings 58(10):665–683.

Lamy C., Duyckaerts C., Delaere P. et al. (1989) Comparison of seven staining methods for senile plaques and neurofibrillary tangles in a prospective series of 15 elderly patients. Neuropathology and Applied Neurobiology 15(6):563–578.

Lendrum A.C., Slidders W., Fraser D.S. (1972) Renal hyaline. A study of amyloidosis and diabetic vasculosis with new staining methods. Journal of Clinical Pathology 25:373.

LeVine H.I. (1995) Thioflavin T interaction with amyloid β-sheet structures. Amyloid 2(7):6.

Liberski P.P., Yanagihara R., Brown P. et al. (1996) Microwave treatment enhances the immunostaining of amyloid deposits in both the transmissible and non-transmissible brain amyloidoses. Neurodegeneration 5(1):95–99.

Livni N., Laufer A., Levo Y. (1980) Demonstration of amyloid in murine and human secondary amyloidosis by the immunoperoxidase technique. Journal of Pathology 132(4):343–348.

Llewellyn B.D. (1970) An improved Sirius red method for amyloid. Journal of Medical Laboratory Technology 27:308.

Meloan S.N., Puchtler H. (1978) Demonstration of amyloid with Mesitol WLS–Congo Red: application of a textile auxiliary to histochemistry. Histochemistry 58(3):163–166.

Missmahl H.P., Hartwig H. (1953) Polarisation-optische untersuchungen an der amyloidsubstanz. Virchows Archiv fur Pathologische Anatomie und Physiologie und fur Klinische Medizin 324:489.

Mowry R.W., Scott J.E. (1967) Observations on the basophilia of amyloids. Histochemie 10:8.

Muir H., Cohen A.S. (1968) Symposium on amyloidosis, Amsterdam: Excerpta Medica.

Pearse A.G.E. (1968) Histochemistry: theoretical and applied. Edinburgh: Churchill Livingstone.

Pepys M.B. (1992) Amyloid P component and the diagnosis of amyloidosis. Journal of International Medical Research 232(6):519–521.

Pepys M.B., Baltz M.L. (1983) Acute phase proteins with special reference to C-reactive protein and related proteins (pentaxins) and serum amyloid A protein. Advances in Immunology 34:141.

Pras M., Schubert M., Zucker-Franklin D. et al. (1968) The characterization of soluble amyloid prepared in water. Journal of Clinical Investigation 47(4):924–933.

Puchtler H., Sweat F. (1965) Congo red as a stain for fluorescence microscopy of amyloid. Journal of Histochemistry and Cytochemistry 13(8):693–694.

Puchtler H., Sweat F. (1966) A review of early concepts of amyloid in context with contempory chemical literature from 1839 to 1859. Journal of Histochemistry and Cytochemistry 14:123.

Puchtler H., Sweat F., Levine M. (1962) On the binding of Congo red by amyloid. Journal of Histochemistry and Cytochemistry 10:355.

Puchtler H., Sweat F., Kuhns J.G. (1964) On the binding of direct cotton dyes by amyloid. Journal of Histochemistry and Cytochemistry 12:900.

Puchtler H., Sweat Waldrop F., Meloan S.N. (1983) Application of thiazole dyes to amyloid under conditions of direct cotton dyeing: correlation of histochemical and chemical data. Histochemistry 77(4):431–445.

Puchtler H., Sweat Waldrop F., Meloan S.N. (1985) A review of light, polarization and fluorescence microscopic methods for amyloid. Applied Pathology 3(1–2):5–17.

Reimann H.A., Koucky R.F., Eklund C.M. (1935) Primary amyloidosis limited to tissue of mesodermal origin. American Journal of Pathology 11:977.

Romhanyi G. (1971) Selective differentiation between amyloid and connective tissue structures based on the collagen specific topo-optical staining reaction with Congo red. Virchows Archiv. A: Pathology. Pathologische Anatomie 354(3):209–222.

Schwartz P. (1970) Amyloidosis: cause and manifestation of senile deterioration. Springfield, IL: Charles C. Thomas.

Sherriff F.E., Bridges L.R., Jackson P. (1994) Microwave antigen retrieval of beta-amyloid precursor protein immunoreactivity. Neuroreport 5(9):1085–1088.

Shirahama T., Skinner M., Cohen A.S. (1981) Immunocytochemical identification of amyloid in formalin-fixed paraffin sections. Histochemistry 72(2):161–171.

Sipe J.D., ed. (2005) Amyloid proteins. The beta sheet conformation and disease. Weinheim: Wiley-VCH.

Snow A.D., Willmer J., Kisilevsky R. (1987) Sulfated glycosaminoglycans: a common constituent of all amyloids? Laboratory Investigation 56(1):120–123.

Soto C., Kascsak R.J., Saborio G.P. et al. (2000) Reversion of prion protein conformational changes by synthetic beta-sheet breaker peptides. Lancet 355(9199):192–197.

Stokes G. (1976) An improved Congo red method for amyloid. Medical Laboratory Sciences 33:79.

Sunde M., Serpell L.C., Bartlam M. et al. (1997) Common core structure of amyloid fibrils by synchrotron X-ray diffraction. Journal of Molecular Biology 273(3): 729–739.

Sweat F., Puchtler H. (1965) Demonstration of amyloid with direct cotton dyes. Experiences with a new method for the selective staining of amyloid by Sirius red F3BA and Sirius supra scarlet GG-CF. Archives of Pathology 80(6):613–620.

Tribe C.R. (1966) Modern trends in rheumatology. London: Butterworth.

Turnell W.G., Finch J.T. (1992) Binding of the dye Congo red to the amyloid protein pig insulin reveals a novel homology amongst amyloid-forming peptide sequences. Journal of Molecular Biology 227(4):1205–1223.

Vallet P.G., Guntern R., Hof P.R. et al. (1992) A comparative study of histological and immunohistochemical methods for neurofibrillary tangles and senile plaques in Alzheimer's disease. Acta Neuropathologica 83(2): 170–178.

Vassar P.S., Culling F.A. (1959) Fluorescent stains with special reference to amyloid and connective tissue. Archives of Pathology 68:487.

Virchow R. (1853) Weitere mittheilungen über das vorkommen der planzlichen cellulose beim menschen. Virchows Archiv für Pathologische Anatomie und Physiologie und für Klinische Medizin 6(246).

Von Rokitansky C.F. (1842) On the abnormalities of the liver. Vienna: Braumuller Seidel.

Westermark G.T., Johnson K.H., Westermark P. (1999) Staining methods for identification of amyloid in tissue. Methods in Enzymology 309:3–25.

Westermark P. (1995) Diagnosing amyloidosis. Scandinavian Journal of Rheumatology 24(6):327–329.

Westermark P., Stenkvist B. (1973) A new method for the diagnosis of systemic amyloidosis. Archives of Internal Medicine 132(4):522–523.

Westermark P., Benson M.D., Buxbaum J.N. et al. (2002) Amyloid fibril protein nomenclature. Amyloid: Journal of Protein Folding Disorders 9:197–200.

Westermark P., Benson M.D., Buxbaum J.N. et al. (2005) Amyloid: towards terminology clarification. Report from the Nomenclature Committee of the International Society of Amyloidosis. Amyloid 12(1):1–4.

Wilcock G.K., Matthews S.M., Moss T. (1990) Comparison of three silver stains for demonstrating neurofibrillary tangles and neuritic plaques in brain tissue stored for long periods. Acta Neuropathologica 79(5):566–568.

Windrum G.M., Kramer H. (1957) Fluorescence microscopy of amyloid. Archives of Pathology 63:373.

Wisniewski H.M., Wen G.Y., Kim K.S. (1989) Comparison of four staining methods on the detection of neuritic plaques. Acta Neuropathologica 78(1):22–27.

Wolman M., Bubis J.J. (1965) The cause of the green polarization color of amyloid stained with Congo red. Histochemie 4(5):351–356.

Wright J.R., Humphrey R.L. Calkins E. et al. (1976) Different molecular forms of amyloid histologically distinguished by susceptibility or resistance to trypsin digestion. Amyloidosis: Proceedings of the Fifth Sigrid Fuselius Foundation Symposium. London: Academic Press.

Wright J.R., Calkins E., Humphrey R.L. (1977) Potassium permanganate reaction in amyloidosis. A histologic method to assist in differentiating forms of this disease. Laboratory Investigation 36(3):274–281.

16

The Dispersed Neuroendocrine System, Cytoplasmic Granules, and other Organelles

William E. Grizzle and John D. Bancroft

THE NEUROENDOCRINE SYSTEM

Introduction

The evolution of complex animals resulted in the development of multiple forms of communication between cells, tissues, and multicellular organs and tissues. These included a local system acting primarily via soluble peptide/proteins providing local signals between the same types of cell (autocrine communication) and between different types of cell (paracrine communication). Communication also developed between distant cells and tissues via an endocrine system in which primarily steroids, amines, and peptide/proteins are transported by the blood–vascular system to distant sites of action. In addition, a nervous system developed in which electrical impulses were transferred along a network of cells with long processes (e.g. axons) allowing information to travel back and forth between the brain and distant neural cells. In this system, signals are passed between the close processes of neural cells via chemicals similar to amines and peptides. Staining of the nervous system is described in detail in Chapter 19.

The concept of a group of related intercommunicative cells distributed throughout the body arose from histological and physiological studies reported early in the last century. Feyrter (1938) originally proposed that the argentaffin, argyrophil, and chromaffin cells of the bronchial tree, gastrointestinal (GI) tract, and other organs should be considered components of a diffuse epithelial endocrine system. Subsequently, the descriptions of neurohormonal control of pituitary function led to the expansion of this concept to include neurohormonal cells in general. Pearse and colleagues proposed that the cells of these systems had a common biochemistry, specifically the ability to take up precursors of biological amines and to decarboxylate them to form indoleamines, including catecholamines and related molecules. Pearse designated these cells as a part of the 'amine precursor uptake and decarboxylase' (APUD) system (Pearse 1966, 1968, 1969, 1977; Pearse et al 1970). Studies failed to confirm the originally proposed common embryological origin of APUD cells, especially an origin from the neural crest area. Even without a common embryological origin, the consideration of these cells as an inter-related group led to the expansion of the biochemical characteristics, which include the ability to synthesize and release regulatory peptides or neurotransmitters. To maintain a linkage due to these similarities, these cells frequently are designated as components of the dispersed neuroendocrine system (Pearse 1977; Tischler 1989).

THE DISPERSED NEUROENDOCRINE SYSTEM (DNS)

The cellular components and organs of the DNS are listed in Table 16.1 and their biochemical and biomarker characteristics in Table 16.2. Many, but not all, of these cells stain histochemically with argyrophil

Table 16.1   Components of the dispersed neuroendocrine system

1. Cells of the ganglia of the sympathetic and parasympathetic nervous system including the adrenal medulla; tumors arising from the sympathetic or parasympathetic nervous system including pheochromocytomas/paragangliomas, neuroblastomas, ganglioneuroblastomas, gangliomas, and mixed tumors with more than one of the above elements. These cells arise embryologically from the neural crest area.
2. Cells of the endocrine pancreas and islet cell tumors/pancreatic carcinoids; glucagon-producing cells (α-cells) and glucagonomas; insulin-producing cells (β-cells) and insulinomas, other islet cells producing hormones and their associated tumors such as somatostatinomas.
3. Cells of the anterior pituitary and pituitary adenomas.
4. Cells of the parathyroid glands and tumors/hyperplasias of the parathyroid glands.
5. Thyroid C-cells and medullary carcinomas of the thyroid.
6. Neuroendocrine cells of the gastrointestinal tract and neuroendocrine tumors of the gastrointestinal tract, including carcinoids, gastrinomas, and gastrointestinal autonomic nervous system tumors (plexosarcomas) (Herrera et al 1984).
7. Neuroendocrine cells of the bronchopulmonary tree and bronchopulmonary neuroendocrine tumors, including bronchial carcinoids, neuroendocrine carcinomas, and small cell undifferentiated carcinomas/oat cell carcinomas.
8. Sensory neuronal cells—retinal visual cells, hair cells of the inner ear, olfactory cells, sensory cells of taste bud.
9. Neuroendocrine cells of the urogenital tract and small cell undifferentiated tumors of the prostate, cervix, bladder, and ovary/testis (Turbat-Herrera et al 1988).
10. Pinealocytes and pinealomas.
11. Merkel cells and Merkel cell tumors of the skin.

Information from (Pearse 1966, 1968, 1969, 1977; Pearse et al 1970; Woodti & Hedinger 1976; Polak & Bloom 1980; Smith & Haggitt 1983; Tischler 1989; DeLellis & Dayal 1991; Grizzle 1996)

methods. Similarly, the tumors arising from these DNS cells are related morphologically, functionally, and biochemically, and have similar staining characteristics with argyrophil methods (Pearse 1966, 1968, 1969, 1977; Pearse et al 1970; Woodti & Hedinger 1976; Polak & Bloom 1980; Smith & Haggitt 1983; Tischler 1989; DeLellis & Dayal 1991; Grizzle 1996). Until the widespread use of immunostaining, argyrophil and argentaffin staining methods were used as screening methods to identify cells and tumors of the DNS (Grizzle 1996). Tumors arising from the DNS are frequently well differentiated and have similar phenotypic features to the cells from which they arise.

The cells of the DNS do not share a common embryological origin, but there are reasons for considering the cellular components of the dispersed neuroendocrine system as an inter-related group rather than splitting them into multiple related groups. Some of these common cellular features are listed in Table 16.2. Examples of

familial tumor syndromes that link tumors of the DNS are listed in Table 16.3.

Morphology and ultrastructure of the DNS

The appearance on H&E staining of neuroendocrine cells of the DNS is characteristic, as they are oriented so that they can release their contents into capillaries, interstitial fluids, or tissues. This usually results in cells with a pear shape in which a broad base of a cell abuts capillaries, and the cytoplasm at the cellular base contains numerous membrane-bound secretory granules. Some of these cells may have narrow, limited access to a luminal surface, 'open type', while the 'closed type' have only a basal outlet and no contact with the luminal surface. In addition, because of their function, each cell has abundant cytoplasm. Most neuroendocrine cells stain with argyrophil techniques (Grizzle 1996), but as most

Table 16.2. Common, but not required, features of cells of the dispersed neuroendocrine system

Stain with argyrophil/argentaffin silver stains

Express biomarkers including:
Neuron-specific enolase
Chromogranin A
Synaptophysin
Neurofilaments
Lymphoreticular antigens (Thy-1, Leu-7)
Other characteristic antigens: protein gene product 9.5

Biochemical characteristics:
Synthesis of regulatory peptides (e.g. hormones)
APUD (express aromatic amino acid decarboxylase)
α-Glycerophosphate dehydrogenase
Contain formalin-induced amine fluorescence before or after exposure to amine precursors
Cytochrome a561
Tetanus toxin binding sites
Non-specific esterase or cholinesterase

Other characteristics:
Voltage-dependent calcium or sodium channels
Electrical excitability

Information from (Pearse 1966, 1968, 1969, 1977; Pearse et al 1970; Woodti & Hedinger 1976; Polak & Bloom 1980; Smith & Haggitt 1983; Tischler 1989; DeLellis & Dayal 1991; Grizzle 1996)

neurohormonal cell types produce specific hormones, and neuroendocrine cells in general produce some of the same molecules across the neurohormonal cell spectrum (see Table 16.2), immunohistochemical staining is also useful for detecting cellular components of this group of cells. Ultrastructurally, the characteristic feature of neurohormonal cells is the presence of numerous membrane-bound neurosecretory cytoplasmic granules in which hormonal products are packaged. These neurosecretory granules have characteristic shapes which may be associated with the specific hormones and/or molecules that each contains. These granules typically contain one or more hormones (e.g. calcitonin in cells of thyroid), regulatory peptides (e.g. ACTH in basophil cells of pituitary), or neurotransmitters (e.g. norepinephrine in medullary cells of adrenal), and their contents are secreted into the blood or interstitial fluids. The granules also contain, or are associated with, specific peptides/proteins such as chromogranin A and synaptophysin. Some of the cells express proteins/peptides that are found characteristically in neurons (e.g. neurofilaments or neuron specific enolase). Neuroendocrine tumors usually have the same cytological, ultrastructural, and immunological features as the neurohormonal cells from which they develop. Familial forms are associated with specific genetic abnormalities, reviewed in Maitra and Abbas (2005).

Table 16.3 Familial tumor syndromes linking tumors of the dispersed neuroendocrine system

| Multiple endocrine neoplasia | | | Von Recklinghausen's disease (neurofibromatosis) |
Type I	Type II	Type III (IIb)	
Pituitary adenomas	Medullary carcinoma of thyroid	Medullary carcinoma of thyroid	Neurofibromas
Pancreatic islet tumors	Pheochromocytoma	Pheochromocytoma/ paraganglioma	Pheochromocytomas/ paragangliomas
Parathyroid islet hyperplasia	Parathyroid hyperplasia	Mucosal neuromas	Neurofibrosarcomas
Associated with carcinoids		Less commonly parathyroid hyperplasia	Malignant peripheral nerve sheath tumors

Cells of the endocrine pancreas

The islets of Langerhans make up the neuroendocrine portion of the pancreas and are composed primarily of four types of cell: α-cells (A cells) producing glucagon and the β-cells (B cells) producing insulin are the two most common. These two cell types are present in a ratio of approximately 1α to 4β in islets of the tail, body, and anterior head of the pancreas as demonstrated in Figure 16.1, a and b. Alpha cells are located at the periphery of the islets and stain with argyrophil stains. β-Cells are found central to the α-cells and stain with aldehyde pararosaniline but not argyrophil stains. Immunohistochemical stains for glucagon or insulin demonstrate clearly these patterns (Fig. 16.1). The posterior portion of the head of the pancreas contains islets cells that secrete pancreatic polypeptide (PP cells) instead of glucagon. PP cells also stain with argyrophil methods (Bloodworth & Greider 1982; Bordi 1987). The fourth type of cell is the δ-cell (D cell), which contains somatostatin; these cells do not stain with argyrophil, argentaffin, or aldehyde pararosaniline but can be detected immunohistochemically (Fig. 16.1c). Rare cells containing gastrointestinal hormones can be detected in some apparently normal islets of the pancreas. Islets also produce numerous peptide/proteins including survivin, clusterin, and the TRAIL death receptors DR-4 and DR-5 (Fig. 16.1f).

Islet cell tumors may in addition produce one or more of the primary pancreatic hormones, gastrin, vasoactive intestinal peptide (VIP), serotonin, and, rarely, other peptides such as adrenocorticotropic hormone (ACTH) and growth hormone-releasing hormone. Multiple hormones can be identified by immunohistochemistry in some islet cell tumors. These tumor names are based either on the characteristic symptoms produced or according to the major hormone identified within the tumor. The clinical symptoms and predominant hormone associated with islet cell tumors are of importance in determining prognosis. The typical features of islet cell tumors are summarized in Table 16.4. Non-functional islet cell tumors that develop in the pancreas are sometimes called pancreatic carcinoids.

Ganglia of the autonomic nervous system and the adrenal medulla

The ganglia of the sympathetic and parasympathetic nervous systems are located throughout the body, including the sympathetic chain, aortic arch (e.g. aortic body), cranial ganglia (e.g. carotid body), organ of Zuckerkandl (located around the inferior mesenteric artery), and the pericystic area of the bladder (Carney 1997; Tischler 1997). The adrenal medulla is part of the sympathetic nervous system and is analogous to a sympathetic ganglion. The adrenal medullary cells and neurons of the sympathetic and parasympathetic ganglia stain with argyrophil techniques.

The adrenal medulla consists primarily of pheochromocytes, but also contains sustenacular and scattered ganglion cells. The pheochromocytes and ganglion cells stain with argyrophil techniques by immunohistochemistry techniques using antibodies for chromogranin A, synaptophysin, neuron specific enolase (NSE), and neurofilaments. The sustentacular cells stain with S100 (Carney 1997; Tischler 1997).

Tumors of the sympathetic and parasympathetic nervous system and adrenal medulla, which occur primarily in children, include neuroblastomas and ganglioneuroblastomas. A related benign tumor, the ganglioma, is found in children and adults. The cells of these tumors stain with argyrophil techniques and with related immunohistochemical stains, e.g. NSE and chromogranin A. In adults, tumors of the sympathetic and parasympathetic nervous system and adrenal medulla are typically paragangliomas. An intra-adrenal paraganglioma is usually called a pheochromocytoma. Paragangliomas stain with argyrophil techniques and with general neuroendocrine immunohistochemical stains including NSE, chromogranin A, and synaptophysin (Glenner & Grimley 1974; Gould & Summers 1982; Sano & Saito 1990; Carney 1997; Tischler 1997). More rarely, gangliomas, neurofibromas, and neurilemmomas may be found in the area of the adrenal in locations that reflect the locations of the ganglia and paraganglia of the sympathetic and parasympathetic nervous system (Carney 1997; Tischler 1997).

Carcinoid tumors of the gastrointestinal tract

The term carcinoid tumor is applied to four broad categories of neuroendocrine/neuroectodermal tumors, including those of the foregut, midgut and hindgut, and 'other' categories including lung and pancreas (Table 16.5). Carcinoids of the GI system most likely arise from neuroendocrine cells scattered through the epithelium of the gastrointestinal tract. More than

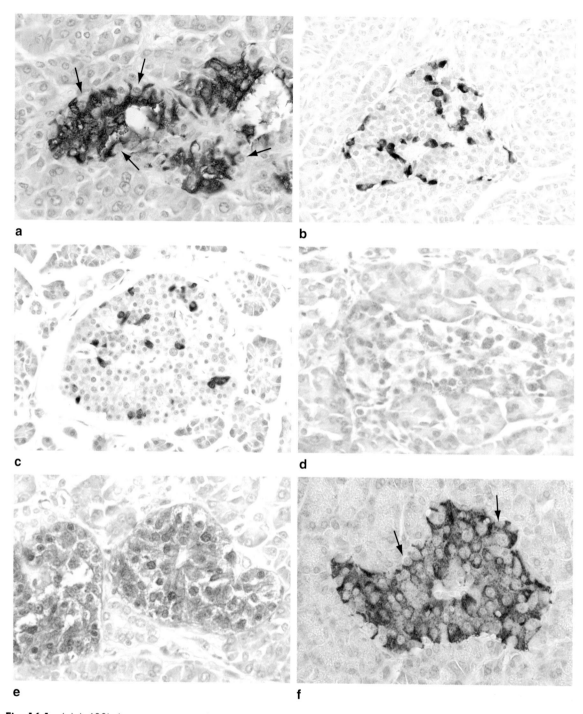

Fig. 16.1 (a) (×600) demonstrates an islet stained immunohistochemically for insulin. Note: cells staining for insulin are in the more central portion of the islet but there are peripheral islet cells (arrows) which do not stain. These are likely α-cells. (b) (×400) is an islet stained immunohistochemically for glucagons. Note α-cells staining around the periphery. (c) (×400) is an islet stained immunohistochemically for somatostatin cells (δ-cells). (d) (×600) demonstrates an islet stained for somatostatin receptor. (e) (×600) is an islet stained for neuron specific enolase. (f) (×600) is stained with an antibody to death receptor 5 of the TRAIL system. Note peripheral cells (arrows) that do not stain.

Table 16.4 Pancreatic or gastrointestinal hormones in islet tumors (Bloodworth & Greider 1982; Bordi 1987; Klimstra 1997)

Hormone (tumor designation)	Predominant cell and proportion of most cases	Argyrophil staining pattern of predominant cell	Granule type	Biological behavior	Classic clinical symptoms
Insulin (insulinoma)	β (70%)	Negative	Variable; many with a wide halo with crystalline core	Most benign	Hypoglycemia
Gastrin (gastrinoma)	G (20%)	Positive		Low-grade malignancy	Severe peptic ulcer disease; tumors frequently multiple so removal of one tumor may not relieve symptoms
Vasoactive intestinal peptide (VIPoma)	VIP (3–5%)	Positive		Low-grade malignancy	Severe watery diarrhea and hypochloremic acidosis (WDHA syndrome)
Pancreatic polypeptide (PPoma)	PP (1%)	Positive	Relatively small; round with very dense core	Usually benign	Mild diarrhea; otherwise asymptomatic
Glucagon (glucagonoma)	α (<1%)	Positive	Variable size; round with eccentric dense core	If symptomatic, low-grade malignancy	Stomatitis, necrolytic skin rash, glucose intolerance, weight loss, anemia, hypoglycemia
Somatostatin (somato-statinoma)	δ (<1%)	Negative	Round, thin halo, core less dense than α- or δ-cells	If symptomatic, low-grade malignancy	Glucose intolerance, gallstones, anemia, diarrhea
Serotonin (carcinoid)	Enterochromaffin cell (<1%)	Positive		Low-grade malignancy	Carcinoid syndrome— flushing, diarrhea, shortness of breath, abdominal pain, bronchial constriction

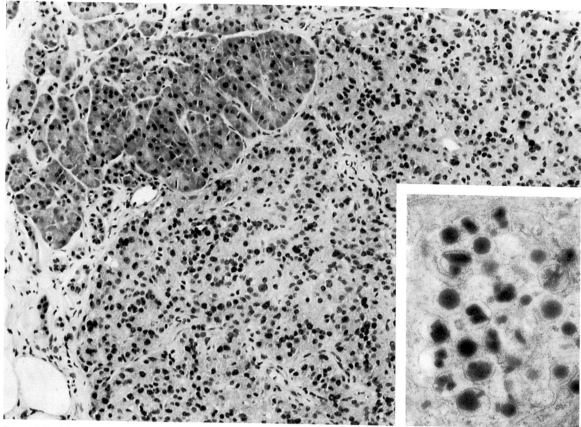

Fig. 16.2 Islet cell tumor of the pancreas showing closely packed trabeculae of moderately pleomorphic tumor cells; residual pancreatic acini are present in the upper left of the picture; H&E. Inset: Transmission electron micrograph of the same tumor showing vesicular neurosecretory granules (average size 300 nm) that have variably dense angular cores. These are characteristic of insulin-containing granules. Clinically the patient had hypoglycemic attacks as a result of inappropriately excessive insulin secretion.

Table 16.5 **Characteristics of carcinoid tumors** (Glenner & Grimley 1974; Gould & Summers 1982; Sano & Saito 1990)

	Foregut	Midgut	Hindgut
Argyrophil stain	Positive	Positive	Positive; sometimes weakly positive or negative
Argentaffin stain	Usually negative	Positive	Often negative
Neuron-specific enolase	Positive	Positive	Positive
5-Hydroxytryptamine (serotonin)	Low	High	Rarely detected
5-Hydroxytryptophan secretion	Frequent	Rare	Very rare
Urinary 5-hydroxyindole acetic acid	High	High	Usually normal
Metastases of liver	Common	Common	Common
Metastases to bone and skin	Common	Rare	Common
Carcinoid syndrome	10% of cases	10% of cases	Very rarely

twenty hormones including somatostatin and gastrin have been identified as being present in these cells, which have been subdivided into more than nineteen cellular types.

GI carcinoid tumors may produce ectopic hormones, especially peptide hormones such as ACTH and met-enkephalin. As with most components of the DNS, immunoperoxidase staining can be used to identify DNS markers. Some immunoperoxidase methods identify each peptide/protein separately, e.g. ACTH, while others such as NSE identify a wide range of neuroendocrine cells. The Grimelius stain or rapid argyrophil silver stain and general immunoperoxidase stains, such as neuron specific enolase, are more useful in generalized screening as many neuroendocrine granules and neuroendocrine cells stain by these procedures (Lechago 1982; Kameya 1990; Ulich & Lewin 1990).

In general pulmonary, pancreatic, gastric, and rectal carcinoids are argyrophil positive and argentaffin negative. Carcinoids of the midgut area of the gastrointestinal tract contain unidentified substances that can reduce silver, as well as secretory granules that stain similarly to enterochromaffin cells of the gastrointestinal tract; thus, some investigators consider that these gastrointestinal carcinoid tumors arise from enterochromaffin cells. These tumors of the small bowel and appendix are classified as argentaffin-positive tumors and stain by argyrophil methods, because silver ions are reduced and elemental silver is deposited as soon as the ionic silver solution is applied. Subsequently, the rest of the argyrophil procedure does not remove elemental silver.

Neuroendocrine cells of the respiratory system

Neuroendocrine cells of the lung are distributed as single cells or groups of cells (neuroepithelial aggregates). The individual neuroendocrine cells are either closed or open types as in the GI system. The neuroepithelial aggregates and single cells may contain bombesin/gastrin releasing peptide, calcitonin, and/or serotonin while single cells are more likely to contain leu-enkephalin (DeLellis & Dayal 1997).

Neuroendocrine tumors that develop in the lung most likely develop from these cells of the DNS. They include carcinoid tumors, neuroendocrine carcinomas, and small cell undifferentiated carcinomas (oat cell tumors).

During the development of dysplasia and/or tumors, the neoplastic neuroendocrine cells may begin to produce somatostatin, ACTH, and vasoactive intestinal peptides. ACTH production is the most common feature of neoplastic neuroendocrine cells of the lung probably because this is a clinically potent peptide typically causing Cushing's syndrome. In general, staining of the normal neuroendocrine and neoplastic neuroendocrine cells of the lung is similar to that of the neuroendocrine cells of the GI system.

Parathyroid gland

The parathyroid glands control calcium levels by secreting parathyroid hormone (PTH). Ninety per cent of humans have four parathyroid glands; rare individuals have two to twelve. There are primarily three types of cell in the parathyroid gland: the chief cell, which has clear to amphophilic cytoplasm, the oxyphil, which has strongly eosinophilic cytoplasm, and mature fat cells. Ultrastructurally secretory granules can be observed in the chief cells. The chief cells stain with chromogranin A and with argyrophil stains, and are thought to produce and secrete PTH. In contrast, the cytoplasm of the oxyphil cell is packed with mitochondria, has few secretory granules, is thought to be hormonally inactive in most cases, and does not stain for chromogranin A or with argyrophil stains (Golden & Kerwin 1982 ; Roth & Abu-Jawdeh 1997).

Adenomas and hyperplasia of the parathyroid gland typically have nodules of oxyphil and chief cells, and reduced or absent fat cells. They stain by argyrophil methods in areas of chief cells, but do not stain in areas with nodules of oxyphil-type cells.

Parafollicular cells of the thyroid

The C cells (parafollicular cells) of the thyroid typically occur in small groups (3–5 cells) that are sparsely distributed (0.1% of gland) within the interfollicular stroma of the thyroid gland; however they can occasionally be identified between follicular cells. C cells appear larger than follicular cells, and their cytoplasm is frequently granular and pale staining (Mendelsohn 1987; LiVolsi 1991). C cells characteristically produce calcitonin, a weak hormone of the calcium regulatory pathway. Immunohistochemical stains for calcitonin as well as for NSE and argyrophil stains can be used to detect these cells.

Medullary carcinoma of the thyroid (MCT) develops from the parafollicular cells of the thyroid. These tumors may occur sporadically or in familial patterns secondary to mutation of the *Ret* oncogene including MEN-II and MEN-III (DeLellis et al 1986; see Table 16.3). Like C cells, the cells of MCT characteristically stain with argyrophil stains and produce and secrete calcitonin. Thus, both argyrophil stains and immunohistochemical stains for calcitonin can be used to separate MCT from follicular and other neoplastic lesions of the thyroid and head and neck area. The cells of MCT also may produce and secrete 'ectopic' hormones, including ACTH (Mendelsohn 1987; LiVolsi 1991).

Anterior pituitary

The anterior pituitary gland contains several cell types each of which secretes a different peptide hormone such as growth hormone (GH), prolactin (P), thyroid stimulating hormone (TSH), or the pro-opiomelanocortin-related hormones, including ACTH. One type of cell, the gonadotroph, secretes follicular stimulating hormone (FSH) and/or luteinizing hormone (LH).

Multiple special stains have been utilized to identify the distribution of the cell types within the pituitary gland and to characterize pituitary tumors. Cells secreting growth hormone and prolactin typically stain acidophilic with hematoxylin and eosin (H&E), and stain with orange G or light green, whereas TSH, FSH/LH, and ACTH cells typically stain basophilic with H&E and stain with the periodic–acid Schiff (PAS) stain. Any of the cell types may stain poorly with the H&E stain and such cells are classified as chromophobic cells. These cells are thought to correspond to cells with decreased numbers of secretory granules (Table 16.6). The development of immunohistochemical and immunofluorescent staining made further development of histochemical stains to subcategorize pituitary cells mostly redundant (Ezrin et al 1982; McKeever & Spicer 1987; Pernicone et al 1997). This chapter, however, includes several of the classic histochemical stains which were once used to subtype cells of the anterior pituitary.

Corticotrophs and the tumors arising from them are argyrophil positive. It is possible that PAS-positive cells may be identified by oxidation–reduction silver stains if the conditions are properly selected. Silver stains do not provide additional information to that seen with H&E, PAS, aldehyde thionin–PAS–orange G, and other special histochemical stains (Ezrin et al 1982; McKeever & Spicer 1987; Pernicone et al 1997).

ARGYROPHIL AND ARGENTAFFIN STAINING PROCEDURES

Argyrophil and argentaffin staining techniques in the past have been useful in identifying some of the types of cell in the DNS as well as tumors arising from them. The argyrophil stain relies on the absorption of silver salts from basic solutions by cellular organelles. Silver salts that are not 'bound/absorbed' are washed away. Adding a reducing agent reduces the bound/absorbed silver ions

Table 16.6 Main staining reactions of the adenohypophyseal cells

Cell	Granules	Acid dye (e.g. eosin)	Carmoisine erythrocin	PAS basophile	Bromine alcian blue	Immuno-histochemistry
Somatotroph	Dense	++	–	–	–	GH
	Sparse	–	–	–	–	GH
Lactotroph	Dense	++	++	–	–	PRL
	Sparse	–	–	–	–	PRL
Corticotroph	Dense	–	–	+	++	ACTH
	Sparse	–	–	–	–	ACTH
Gonadotroph	Usually sparse	–	–	+/–	–	FSH, LH

(Ag^{+1}) to metallic silver (Ag^0) which is deposited at the sites of absorption. In the case of argentaffin staining, sites in cells which have active reducing groups, such as aldehyde groups, reduce silver ions and are stained by the metallic silver deposited. The cells staining by argentaffin methods reduce silver ions to metallic silver as soon as the silver solution enters the cell; silver is deposited at these reducing sites and the non-reduced silver ions are washed away. No exogeneous reducing agent is necessary. If a cell stains with argentaffin stains, it also stains with argyrophil stains (Grizzle 1996), but is classified as argentaffin because the argentaffin reaction is actually causing the staining.

The key to the successful performance of argyrophil and argentaffin stains is the use of appropriate positive and negative controls (Table 16.7) and the attention to detail. Pure water should be used to prepare fresh stains and in washing. Utensils must be thoroughly cleaned. The control and use of high temperatures (Grizzle 1996) is especially important, making the staining time shorter and thus more consistent.

Argyrophil granules were initially demonstrated by silver impregnation techniques used in staining neural tissues (Van Campenhout 1933; Dawson & Barnett 1944; Gorgas & Bock 1976). Subsequently more effective argyrophil methods were developed. The most commonly used are based on the techniques of Hellerström and Hellman (1960), Singh (1964), and Grimelius (1968a), but the method of Grimelius became the most frequently used (Grimelius 1968a, 1968b; Grimelius & Wilander 1980). Modifications proposed by Pascual (1976), Lack and Mercer (1977), and Churukian and Schenk (1979) improved the reproducibility of the procedure by modifying the concentrations of silver and by inclusion of a double impregnation step. Subsequently, Brinn (1983) and others reduced non-specific silver precipitation and section detachment from slides by reducing the staining time through increasing the temperature of staining solutions using a microwave (Sheehan & Hrapchak 1980; Koski 1981; Pickett & Roggli 1982; Staples & Grizzle 1986, 1987; Staples & Clark 1990). Microwaves are not required as excellent argyrophil staining can be obtained rapidly (10 min) with low concentrations of silver, if the silver solutions are made with freshly boiled distilled water after the water cools below 70°C (Staples & Grizzle 1987).

With the rapid argyrophil methods using low (< 1%) silver concentrations, both reliable and reproducible argyrophil staining can be obtained. Counterstains such as methyl green that contrast with the brown–black colors produced by argyrophil procedures are also useful (Staples & Grizzle 1986).

Table 16.7 Controls for argyrophil stains

Normal cells (argyropilic)	Selected cells of islet of pancreas, adrenal medulla, and ganglia
Small bowel	Carcinoid tumors (argyrophilic)
Pancreas	Islet tumors (insulinomas, gastrinomas, glucagonomas, pancreatic polypeptides)
Appendix	Carcinoid tumors of bowel
Thyroid	Medullary carcinoma of the thyroid
Stomach (pyloric area)	Gastrinomas
Bronchus	Bronchial carcinoids, endocrine carcinomas, undifferentiated small cell carcinoma (oat cell)
Pituitary	Pituitary adenoma
Adrenal gland	Paragangliomas/pheochromocytomas, neuroblastomas, ganglioneuroblastomas, gangliomas, peripheral neural sheath tumors

Rapid argyrophil procedure for neurosecretory granules (Staples & Grizzle 1987; Staples & Clark 1990)

Fixation

10% buffered neutral formalin is preferred; controls should match the tissue to be stained.

Solutions

2% silver nitrate solution

Silver nitrate crystals	2 g
Distilled water	100 ml

Working silver solution

2% silver nitrate solution	2 ml
Distilled water	50 ml

Prepare immediately before use. Bring the distilled water to a boil using a hot plate or microwave oven. Pour water into a plastic Coplin jar and allow the water to cool to 70°C; then add the silver solution.

Reducing solution

Sodium sulfite	2.5 g
Hydroquinone	0.5 g
Distilled water	50 ml

Prepare immediately before use. Bring distilled water to a boil using a hot plate or microwave oven. Pour water into a plastic Coplin jar and allow the water to cool to 70°C. Add sodium sulfite, and mix well to dissolve crystals thoroughly. Add hydroquinone and mix well.

1% acidified methyl green

Methyl green (C.I. 42590)	1 g
Distilled water	99 ml
Glacial acetic acid	1 ml

Combine the distilled water, acetic acid, and methyl green. Mix well and filter the solution through rapid filter paper. The solution is stable for several months.

Method

1. Deparaffinize and hydrate slides to distilled water.
2. Place sections in working silver solution (60–70°C) for 2 min.
3. Rinse slides quickly in distilled water.
4. Place sections in reducing solution (60–70°C) for 1 min.
5. Wash thoroughly in several changes of distilled water.
6. Return sections to original silver solution for 1 min.
7. Rinse briefly in distilled water and place section in original reducing solutions.
8. Wash sections in running water.
9. Counterstain for 1 minute in acidulated methyl green (Staples & Grizzle 1986).
10. Rinse sections in water.
11. Dehydrate rapidly through graded alcohols to absolute alcohol, clear in xylene, and mount using a synthetic medium.

Results

Neurosecretory granules	brown to black
Nuclei	blue–green
Background	light green

Fontana–Masson argentaffin reaction

Control

Use normal appendix, skin, or intestine from adult (not infant or child). Melanoma, with and without bleaching, must be used for melanoma cases.

Fixation

10% neutral buffered formalin.

Note

Avoid alcoholic fixatives, as they will dissolve the argentaffin granules.

Solutions

Stock silver nitrate solution

Dissolve 1 g silver nitrate crystals in 100 ml distilled water. To 95 ml of this solution, add concentrated ammonium hydroxide until a clear solution with no precipitate is obtained. Add, drop by drop, enough of the remaining 5 ml silver nitrate solution to cause the solution to become cloudy. The solution may be used immediately, but it improves if allowed to stand overnight. Store solution in the dark at room temperature; it is stable for approximately 1 month.

Working silver solution

Just before use, dilute 12.5 ml stock silver nitrate solution with 38.5 ml distilled water

0.2% gold chloride

1% stock aqueous gold chloride	10 ml
Distilled water	40 ml

5% aqueous sodium thiosulfate

Nuclear fast red (Kernechtrot) solution

Method

1. Deparaffinize slides and hydrate to distilled water.
2. Preheat working silver solution in microwave oven (400 W) for 45 s on HI or on hot plate to 60–70°C. The temperature of the solution should be 60–75°C. Immerse slides in the preheated solution for 5 min. Alternately, the slides may be immersed in the silver nitrate solution for 2 hours at room temperature. Check slides microscopically for impregnation of the silver before proceeding to the next step.
3. Rinse sections in distilled water.
4. Tone section in 0.2% gold chloride solution for 10 s.
5. Rinse sections in distilled water.
6. Immerse sections in 5% sodium thiosulfate for 1 min.
7. Rinse sections in distilled water.
8. Counterstain in nuclear fast red for 5 min.
9. Rinse sections in distilled water, dehydrate in ethanols, clear, and mount in a synthetic medium.

Results

Argentaffin cell granules	black
Nuclei	pink–red
Cytoplasm	pale pink

Singh's modification of the Masson–Hamperl argentaffin technique

(Singh 1964)

Fixation

Formaldehyde, glutaraldehyde, or picric alcohol.

Section

Paraffin.

Preparation of silver solution

To 10 ml of 10% aqueous silver nitrate add concentrated ammonia drop by drop until the precipitate formed just dissolves. To this clear solution, add 10% aqueous silver nitrate drop by drop until a faint opalescence is seen. For use, dilute the silver solution 1 in 10 with distilled water. This solution is best when freshly prepared.

Method

1. Remove paraffin with xylene; remove xylene with absolute ethanol. Rehydrate sections through graded ethanols to distilled water.
2. Place sections in preheated silver solution at 60°C for 15–30 min. Examine sections at 5-min intervals until they are light brown in color; then remove them.
3. Wash well in distilled water.
4. Immerse in 1% aqueous sodium thiosulfate for 1 min.
5. Wash well in tap water.
6. Lightly counterstain with 0.5% aqueous neutral red.
7. Wash in tap water.
8. Dehydrate with graded alcohols, clear with xylene, and mount in a resinous mountant.

Results

Argentaffin granules	black
Nuclei	red

Notes

When making up the silver solutions, use chemically clean glassware. When titrating the silver solution use fine-capillary Pasteur pipettes for more accurate control. If possible, use a water bath for the silver impregnation, as this will give better temperature control.

ADDITIONAL TECHNIQUES FOR THE DEMONSTRATION OF NEUROENDOCRINE CELLS

Prior to the impact of immunohistochemistry, the demonstration of neuroendocrine cells used a number of well-established methods that were developed empirically. Their rationales remain largely unknown but most are thought to depend on the presence of certain amine and peptide residues produced by neuroendocrine cells. Below we describe various methods and give examples of technical protocols that we find the most useful. No single technique will demonstrate every neuroendocrine cell and the demonstration of neuroendocrine characteristics may be difficult in poorly differentiated tumors.

Fluorescent histochemical methods

These largely historical methods identify monoamines (e.g. catecholamines, 5-hydroxtryptamine; 5-HT) and specific residues on peptides by the induction of fluorescence with ultraviolet illumination. As most bioactive amines diffuse rapidly from the neuroendocrine granules in their cell of origin, rapid freeze drying and vapor fixation are required to preserve them; 5-HT diffuses more slowly than most and reacts better with paraformaldehyde or formaldehyde to give β-carboline (Barter & Pearse 1955). This compound produces a bright yellow fluorescence (absorption peak 410 nm; emission peak 525 nm) when viewed with ultraviolet light.

Formaldehyde-induced fluorescence (Falck & Owman 1965)

Fixation
Freeze-dried tissue is transferred to a closed box of 1-liter capacity, containing 5 g paraformaldehyde powder. Seal the lid tightly, and place in an oven at 60°C for 1–3 hours.

Sections
After fixation, remove the tissue from the container and vacuum-embed in paraffin; some workers prefer to use paraffin with the addition of high concentration of plastic polymer as an aid to thin sectioning. Sections are cut and mounted on clean slides.

Method
After drying the sections in the 60°C oven, de-wax the sections in xylene and mount in a suitable mounting medium. Examine sections with the fluorescent microscope using BG38, UG1, and barrier filters.

Results
Bioactive amines   bright yellow fluorescence

Empirical dye methods for demonstrating neuroendocrine cells

Many stains have been developed over the years that will demonstrate different cells in the neuroendocrine system. These are empirical dye methods and are not specific for endocrine cells or their peptide products. They have been particularly useful in the demonstration of pituitary and pancreatic cells, and are still useful in the routine laboratory. The following are recommended:

Periodic acid–Schiff–orange G technique (TRIPAS) (Hotchkiss 1948)

Fixation
Most types of fixative.

Sections
Paraffin or frozen sections are suitable.

Solutions
Periodic acid solution

Periodic acid	0.4 g
Ethanol	35 ml
Distilled water	10 ml

0.2 M sodium acetate solution
(2.72 g of hydrated sodium acetate in 100 ml of distilled water)
To 45 ml of periodic acid solution, add 5 ml of 0.2 M sodium acetate solution. Store in dark at 0°C, but use at room temperature. Discard if a brown color develops.

Reducing solution

Potassium iodide	1 g
Sodium thiosulfate	1 g
Absolute ethanol	30 ml
Distilled water	20 ml
20% aqueous hydrochloric acid	20 ml

Dissolve potassium iodide and sodium thiosulfate in the mixed ethanol and distilled water. Add the hydrochloric acid and store at 0°C until use. Discard after 14 days. Ignore any precipitate.

Orange G solution

Orange G	2 g
5% phosphotungstic acid	100 ml

Mix and allow to stand for 24 hours; filter before use.

Schiff's reagent (see p. 171)

Method
1. Remove paraffin and hydrate via graded ethanols.
2. Take sections to distilled water.

3. Wash well in 70% ethanol.
4. Treat sections with periodic acid solution for 5 min.
5. Rinse in 70% ethanol.
6. Treat with reducing solution for 3–5 min, changing the solution at least twice.
7. Rinse well in 70% alcohol.
8. Treat with Schiff's reagent for 6 min.
9. Wash in running tap water for 10 min.
10. Stain nuclei in an iron hematoxylin, differentiate, and 'blue' section in tap water.
11. Stain in orange G solution for 10 seconds.
12. Differentiate in tap water for about 30 seconds until the acidophil cells are red and only blood cells are yellow.
13. Dehydrate, clear, and mount in non-aqueous medium.

Results

Colloid of mid-pituitary vesicle and basophil cells	magenta
Nuclei	blue–black
Red blood cells and acidophil cells	yellow
Chromophobes	pale blue–grey

Notes

This method is recommended for the demonstration of cells of the adenohypophysis, but not as a demonstrational method for glycogen and other PAS-positive substances. The reducing solution has the advantage of preventing reactions in such structures as collagen, giving a cleaner background.

OFG method for the anterior pituitary
(Slidders 1961)

Fixation

Sublimate preferred: formaldehyde; Helly's and Bouin's acceptable.

Sections

Paraffin (thin, 3–4 g).

Preparation of solutions

Orange G

Orange G	500 mg
Phosphotungstic acid	2 g
Absolute ethanol	95 ml
Distilled water	5 ml

Acid fuchsin

Acid fuchsin	500 mg
Glacial acetic acid	0.5 ml
Distilled water	99.5 ml

Celestine blue solution

Celestine blue B	2.5 g
Ferric ammonium sulfate	2.5 g
Glycerin	70 ml
Distilled water	500 ml

Ferric ammonium sulfate is dissolved in cold distilled water. The celestine blue B is added and the mixture is boiled for a few minutes. After the solution cools, filter and add glycerin.

Method

1. Take sections to tap water.
2. Stain nuclei with celestine blue for 5 minutes.
3. Rinse in distilled water.
4. Stain in alum hematoxylin (e.g. Mayer's or Cole's) for 5 min.
5. Wash in tap water.
6. Differentiate in acid alcohol.
7. Wash in running top water.
8. Rinse in 95% alcohol.
9. Stain in orange G solution, 2 min.
10. Rinse in distilled water.
11. Stain in acid fuchsin solution, 2–5 min; the basophil cells are strongly colored.
12. Rinse in tap water.
13. Treat with 1% phosphotungstic acid (aqueous), 5 min.
14. Rinse in tap water.
15. Stain in 1.5% light green in 1.5% acetic acid, 1 min.
16. Rinse in tap water to remove excess stain.
17. Flood with absolute alcohol.
18. Clear in xylene.
19. Mount in non-aqueous medium.

Results

Acidophils	orange–yellow
Basophils	magenta–red
Chromophobes	pale grayish-green
RBCs	yellow
Nuclei	blue–black

Notes

This method requires a certain amount of expertise to obtain good results. The method works particularly well after formal mercury fixation.

AB–OFG method for the anterior pituitary
(Slidders 1961)

Fixation
Any.

Sections
Paraffin 3–4 µm.

Preparation of solutions
Bromine water
10% hydrobromic acid (aqueous)	45 ml
2.5% potassium permanganate (aqueous)	5 ml

Alcian blue
Alcian blue	100 mg
Sulfuric acid (concentrated)	1 ml
Glacial acetic acid	9 ml
Distilled water	90 ml

Carefully mix the dye by slowly adding the sulfuric acid; stir with a glass rod. Slowly add the glacial acetic acid. Stir again. Add the acid–dye mixture slowly and carefully to distilled water. Make up to 100 ml and filter.

Method
1. Take sections to water.
2. Treat with bromine water, 5 min.
3. Wash in running tap water, 5 min.
4. Rinse in distilled water.
5. Stain in alcian blue solution, 1 hour.
6. Wash well in tap water.
7. Proceed with the OFG method (p. 296).

Results
Acidophils	orange–yellow
Basophil cells (S)	dark green–blue
Basophil cells (I)	magenta–red
Chromophobe cells	pale gray–green
Nuclei	gray–blue
Red blood cells	yellow

Carmoisine–orange G–wool green technique for differentiating acidophil cells
(Brookes 1968)

Solutions
1% carmoisine L in 1% acetic acid
Saturated orange G in 2% phosphotungstic acid, in 95% ethanol
0.5% wool green S, in 0.5% acetic acid

Method
1. Take sections to water.
2. Place in 10% aqueous copper sulfate for 2 hours at 44°C.
3. Wash well in tap water for 10–20 min, then in distilled water.
4. Stain with the carmoisine solution for 30 min.
5. Wash in distilled water.
6. Wash in 95% alcohol.
7. Stain with the orange G solution for 5–30 min. Replacement of the carmoisine by the orange G in the somatotrophic cells will take place; this should be controlled by washing the slide at intervals in 2% phosphotungstic acid 95% ethanol and examining microscopically.
8. Rinse well in distilled water.
9. Re-stain in the carmoisine solution for 5 min.
10. Rinse in distilled water and counterstain in wool green solution for 10 min.
11. Rinse in distilled water, then treat with 1% acetic acid for 2 min to remove excess wool green.
12. Dehydrate, clear, and mount in a resinous mountant.

Results
Somatotropes	yellow
Lactotropes	red
Red blood cells	red
Basophils	green

Note
The technique is capable of giving good results but requires some degree of expertise in order to obtain clear-cut color differentiation of somatotrophic from lactotrophic pituitary acidophil cells.

Chrome alum hematoxylin–phloxine stain
(Gomori 1941)

Fixation
Thin slices of tissue primarily fixed in Bouin's or Helly's are preferable, although good results can be obtained by secondary treatment after initial fixation in 10% NBF.

Sections
Paraffin sections.

Preparation of solutions

Chrome alum hematoxylin

Hematoxylin	500 mg
Chromium alum	1.5 g
5% potassium dichromate	2 ml
0.5 M sulfuric acid	2 ml
Distilled water	100 ml

The mixture is ripe in 48 hours and may be used when a film with a metallic luster continues to form on the surface of the mixture that has stood in a Coplin jar for 24 hours. The solution lasts 4–8 weeks. Filter each time before use.

Method

1. Take sections to water.
2. Place in Bouin's fluid for 16–24 hours.
3. Wash sections thoroughly in tap water to remove picric acid.
4. Treat sections for 1 min with an equal parts mixture of 0.3% potassium permanganate and 0.3% sulfuric acid.
5. Decolorize with a 5% solution of sodium bisulfite.
6. Wash well in running tap water.
7. Stain in the chrome hematoxylin solution for 10 min until microscopic examination shows β-cells to be deep blue.
8. Rinse in water and differentiate in 1% acid ethanol for 1 min to remove background staining.
9. Wash in running tap water until the section is a clear blue.
10. Stain in 0.5% aqueous phloxine for 5 min.
11. Rinse in water and treat with 5% phosphotungstic acid, 1 min.
12. Wash in running tap water for 5 min, when the section should regain its red color.
13. Differentiate in 95% ethanol. If the section is too red and α-cells are not clear, rinse for 10–20 seconds in 80% ethanol.
14. Dehydrate with absolute ethanol, clear in xylene, and mount in a non-aqueous mountant.

Results

B cells	blue
A cells	red
D cells	pink to red

Modified aldehyde fuchsin stain
(Halami 1952)

Fixation

Formal saline or Bouin's fluid.

Sections

Thin paraffin sections.

Preparation of solutions

Aldehyde fuchsin (see p. 154)

Counterstain

Light green	200 mg
Orange G	1 g
Phosphotungstic acid	500 mg
Glacial acetic acid	1 ml
Distilled water	100 ml

This is a stable solution.

Method

1. Take sections to water.
2. Oxidize with Lugol's iodine, 10 min.
3. Rinse in tap water and bleach with 2.5% sodium thiosulfate.
4. Wash in tap water followed by 70% ethanol.
5. Stain in aldehyde fuchsin stain for 15–30 min.
6. Wash in 95% alcohol followed by water.
7. Stain nuclei with celestine blue and hemalum (p. 125)
8. Wash in water, differentiate briefly in acid ethanol, and wash well in tap water.
9. Rinse with distilled water and counterstain with orange G–light green solution, 45 seconds.
10. Rinse briefly with 0.2% acetic acid followed by 95% ethanol.
11. Dehydrate in absolute ethanol, clear in xylene, and mount in a resinous mountant.

Results

B cells	purple–violet
A cells	yellow
D cells	green
Nuclei	blue

Masked metachromasia

Many neuroendocrine cells exhibit masked metachromasia. This tinctorial characteristic can be unmasked by prior treatment of tissue sections by hot acid hydrolysis. This releases carboxyl groups from polypeptides which are then free to react with and change the color of basic dyes such as toluidine blue and azure A.

Masked metachromasia method (Solcia et al 1968)

Fixation
Formalin, paraformaldehyde, glutaraldehyde, Bouin's or Helly's solution.

Sections
Paraffin.

Preparation of solutions

Azure A solution
0.005% azure A in distilled water.

Toluidine blue solution
0.01% toluidine blue in 20 mM McIlvaine's buffer (pH 5.0)

Acid solution for hydrolysis
0.2 M hydrochloric acid

Method
1. Take paraffin sections to distilled water.
2. Hydrolyze in the 0.2 M HCl for 3–4 hours at 60°C (formalin, paraformaldehyde, Bouin's-fixed material) or 12 hours at 60–65°C (glutaraldehyde or Helly-fixed material).
3. Wash well in distilled water.
4. Stain in either azure A or toluidine blue solution for 6 hours.
5. Wash well in distilled water.
6. Either mount in glycerin jelly, or blot dry, soak in absolute isopropanol for 1 minute, clear in xylene, and mount in a resinous mountant.

Results
Endocrine cell granules   purple–red

Lead hematoxylin

MacConaill's lead hematoxylin technique, modified by Solcia et al (1969), has enjoyed wide popularity. In experienced hands it reliably demonstrates many neuroendocrine cells. Similar to the masked metachromasia method, it probably works by reacting with carboxyl groups. In this technique the carboxyl groups do not require unmasking.

Lead hematoxylin method (Solcia et al 1969)

Fixation
10% NBF, glutaraldehyde, or glutaraldehyde with picric acid.

Sections
Paraffin.

Preparation of solutions

Stabilized lead solution
5% aqueous lead nitrate	50 ml
Saturated aqueous ammonium acetate	50 ml

Mix well, filter, then add 2 ml of formaldehyde (37%).

Lead hematoxylin staining solution
Stabilized lead solution	10 ml
0.2 g hematoxylin in 95% ethanol	1.4 ml
Distilled water	10 ml

Mix well and add in the above order, stirring repeatedly. Allow mixture to stand for 30 min then filter. Mix the filtrate in 75 ml distilled water.

Method
1. Rehydrate sections through graded alcohols to distilled water.
2. Stain in lead hematoxylin solution for 2–3 hours at 37°C, or for 1–2 hours at 45°C.
3. Wash in distilled water, dehydrate, clear, and mount in a resinous mountant.

Results
Endocrine cell granules	dark blue–black
Muscle, neurons, and other tissue structures also may stain	blue–black

Notes
a. The saturation point of ammonium acetate is high (>100 g/100 ml).
b. Do not use old batches of formaldehyde in the stabilized lead solution, as this can give rise to poor results.
c. Old batches of hematoxylin powder (dark brown in color) must not be used. Best results are seen with the buff-colored powder.
d. Staining times will need to be increased if tissues have been fixed in paraformaldehyde or Helly's fluid.

e. Although the stabilized lead solution may be used for several weeks, better results are seen with a freshly prepared solution.

f. The use of acid hydrolysis prior to staining, as detailed in the masked metachromasia method, may give a better result.

Alkaline diazo

The diazo methods are used to demonstrate cells rich in 5-HT. As has been mentioned, certain fixatives (formaldehyde, paraformaldehyde) produce β-carboline from 5-HT. This reducing agent will react with diazonium salts to produce an insoluble azo dye, the color of which depends on the diazonium salt used.

Alkaline diazo method (Gomori 1952)

Fixation
Formaldehyde, paraformaldehyde.

Sections
Paraffin.

Preparation of solution
Diazonium solution

1% aqueous fast red B salt	5 ml
Saturated aqueous lithium carbonate	2 ml

Prepare solutions just before use and cool to 4°C.
   Mix the solutions just prior to staining, filter, and use immediately.

Method
1. Rehydrate sections through graded ethanols to distilled water.
2. Place sections in the diazonium solution for 1 min at 4°C.
3. Wash well in distilled water at 4°C.
4. Lightly stain nuclei in Mayer's hematoxylin.
5. Wash well in tap water.
6. Dehydrate, clear, and mount in a resinous mountant.

Results

Argentaffin granules	orange–red
Nuclei	blue
Background	yellow

Notes
The method needs to be carried out at 4°C. If the reaction is carried out at room temperature the background becomes over-stained and positive results may be difficult to see. Best results are obtained with freshly fixed surgical material. The method rarely works on postmortem tissue. Other diazonium salts may be used, e.g. fast garnet GBC. Over-staining with hematoxylin will easily mask a positive reaction.

CELLULAR ORGANELLES

These include mitochondria and lysosomes found in most cells as well as specific cellular features that are characteristic of specific cells, diseases, or conditions. The expression of large numbers of organelles or enlarged organelles may change the appearance of the cell. For example, oncocytic changes or oncocytes (i.e. cells with bright red cytoplasm) occur in several situations including parathyroid hyperplasia (adenomas), Hürtle cell tumors of the thyroid, oncocytomas of the kidney, and oncocytic changes in follicular cells of the thyroid in Hashimoto's thyroiditis. In these cases the eosinophilia of the cytoplasm is secondary to the accumulation of large numbers of mitochondria in the cytoplasm. Similar eosinophilic changes occur when lysosomes accumulate in the cytoplasm.

Mitochondria

Mitochondria are the source of most of the energy by which cells operate. They vary greatly in shape (e.g. rod-shaped to round) and in size with smaller types of mitochondria visible only using an electron microscope. They contain inherited maternal DNA. The number, size, and shape of mitochondria are specific for types of animal cells. Mitochondria have two membranous walls, the inner of which is thrown up into folds (cristae) that protrude into the center of the mitochondrion. The folds contain organized enzymes which participate in oxidative phosphorylation and the Krebs cycle. Mitochondria are also an important component of an apoptotic pathway.

   Mitochondria are best visualized by electron microscopy (Fig. 16.3). Histopathological methods such as Altmann's technique for mitochondria (Piva et al 2003)

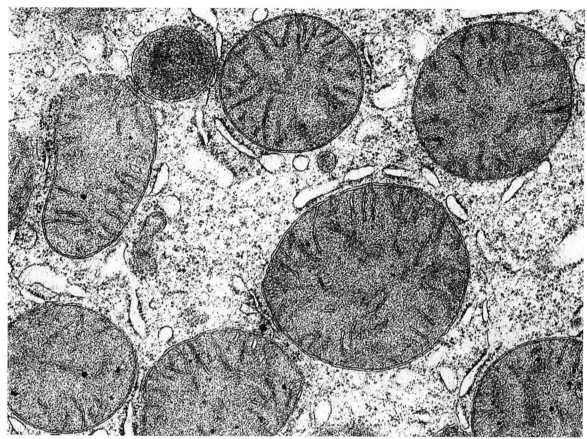

Fig. 16.3 Electron micrograph of mitochondria from the liver cell of a rat. Note the round-to-oval shape, the double membrane, and the cristae. Such numerous prominent mitochondria may well be detectable by histological staining methods (see below).

are useful but immunohistochemistry has replaced histochemical and enzymatic methods such as succinate dehydrogenase (see Chapter 20). An antibody to cytochrome C (Clone CTC05) is particularly useful in detecting mitochondria in human and mouse. Multiple other immunohistochemical markers of mitochondria are available.

Successful histological demonstration of mitochondria is dependent on several factors: tissues must be freshly fixed, and the sections must be thin, 2–3 μm. Rapid fixation is vital, because mitochondria are among the first cytoplasmic organelles to show degenerative changes after cell anoxia or death. Suitable staining methods include the Champy–Kull method which may give the best results but is technically difficult, the Altmann acid fuchsin–picric acid method which is

simpler, and Heidenhain's iron hematoxylin which requires accurate differentiation.

Altmann's technique for mitochondria (Altmann 1894)

Fixation
Champy's fluid is usually recommended; Helly's fluid works equally well.

Sections
Thin paraffin sections (3 μm).

Preparation of solutions
Aniline–acid fuchsin
This is a saturated solution of acid fuchsin in 5% aniline in distilled water. For this method to work well

it is important to have the maximum amount of acid fuchsin in solution. Saturation appears to be about 15%. Acid fuchsin is added slowly over a period of 24 hours. This solution should be filtered before use.

Differentiator 1

Saturated ethanolic picric acid	10 ml
30% alcohol	40 ml

Differentiator 2

Saturated ethanolic picric acid	5 ml
30% alcohol	40 ml

Method

1. Take sections down to water.
2. Flood sections with aniline–acid fuchsin solution.
3. Gently heat the slide until steam rises and leave for 5 min.
4. Rinse in tap water.
5. Differentiate in solution 1 until the excess red stain is removed.
6. Complete differentiation in solution 2, controlling microscopically.
7. Dehydrate rapidly in two changes of absolute ethanol.
8. Clear in xylene and mount in a non-aqueous mounting medium.

Results

Mitochondria	red
RBC and nuclei	red
Background tissue	yellow

Note

Care should be taken to avoid losing the yellow background staining.

Lysosomes/Ectosomes

Lysosomes are membrane-bound cytoplasmic organelles that function in the enzymatic breakdown of phagocytosed material and of degenerate cellular organelles. The autophagic destruction of cellular organelles frequently results in lipofuscin granules and residual bodies that are lysosomal remnants. Lysosomes can be identified by the enzymes they contain, especially acid phosphatase (see Chapter 20). New immunohistochemical methods to identify lysosomes rely on demonstrating proteins such as lysosome-associated membrane proteins (e.g. LAMP1 and LAMP2). Similar to lysosomes are exosomes, which are membrane-bound vesicles (up to 100 nM) that are released from cells and may function in cell to cell signaling (Liu et al 2006).

Russell Bodies

These are smooth rounded bodies which occur in the cytoplasm of plasma cells, particularly in chronically inflamed tissues and in the plasma cell neoplasms, multiple myeloma or plasmacytoma. They may number two or three per cell and may become so big that the cell size is increased and the nucleus is virtually invisible, giving the appearance of an extracellular body. They stain bright orange–red with eosin and are almost invariably strongly PAS positive. They are predominantly protein in nature and therefore give a positive Millon reaction. Since they occur in plasma cell cytoplasm they inevitably have some RNA within them, so they are variably pyroninophilic. These and other staining reactions are shown in Table 16.8.

HAIR, KERATIN, AND KERATOHYALINE

Hair and superficial keratin of the skin are composed of insoluble proteins composed of many amino acids with a high sulfhydryl and disulfide content. Keratohyaline is found as basophilic granules within the cytoplasm of the cells of the stratum granulosum of the epidermis. Hair and keratin stain red with H&E, while keratohyaline stains deep blue. Because of their high sulfur content both hair and keratin can be demonstrated by the amino acid histochemical methods for disulfide and sulfhydryl groups such as the performic acid–alcian blue technique. Keratin retains the red phloxine stain avidly, so

Table 16.8 Staining reactions of Russell bodies

Method	Results	Page no.
PAS	Positive	171
Gram	Positive*	312
Ziehl–Neelsen	Variable	314
Millon reaction	Positive	219
Phloxine–tartrazine	Positive	325

*Unless acetone is used as the differentiator.

Lendrum's phloxine–tartrazine technique is a suitable method for its demonstration (see p. 325). Hair and keratohyaline are usually Gram-positive, but keratin only weakly so. Hair stains purple with the periodic acid–Schiff reaction, but keratin and keratohyaline are negative.

The keratins found in skin typically are of high molecular weight while those of non-stratified epithelia (e.g. glands of the breast) tend to be of low molecular weight. Keratins can be divided into over twenty subtypes. Keratin subtypes have proven to be useful as biomarkers and their detection has been useful in characterizing tumors (see Immunohistochemical techniques, Chapter 21).

ALCOHOLIC HYALINE

This is an unusual protein substance whose precise chemical nature is unknown. It is said to occur within the cytoplasm of liver cells in certain patients who have liver disease due to excess consumption of ethanol. The material is in the form of a perinuclear pale-staining, often grayish, zone in the liver cell. The material can be demonstrated more prominently by Mallory's phloxine method or by Laqueur's modified Altmann method (Lillie 1965).

NUCLEOLAR ORGANIZER REGIONS (NORs)

These regions are segments of chromosomes encoded for ribosomal RNA, and are present on specific loops of DNA that project into the nucleoli where they can be seen by electron microscopy as ill-defined pale-staining regions within the more electron-dense areas. Some of the nucleolar organizer regions can be identified in histological sections by the use of a silver nitrate method, which demonstrates an acidic protein with which some of these sites are associated. It is important to realize that these silver-staining NOR-associated protein (AgNOR) sites represent only some of the nucleolar organizer regions present in each nucleolus. Furthermore, the spot-like silver reactions seen within the nucleoli in paraffin sections may each represent more than one AgNOR site since they tend to be closely aggregated in the nucleoli of normal or benign cells. The study of AgNORs once enjoyed a vogue in diagnostic tumor pathology in the belief that increased numbers of AgNOR sites correlated with increased cellular proliferation. It was thought that the method was of value in distinguishing between benign and malignant cells.

Silver nitrate method for AgNOR protein sites (after Ploton et al 1986)

Sections
Formalin-fixed, 2–3-μm paraffin sections.

Solutions
50% silver nitrate solution

Silver nitrate	50 g
Distilled water	100 ml

Gelatin solution

Gelatin	2 g
Formic acid	1 ml
Distilled water	100 ml

Working solution

Silver nitrate solution	2 parts by volume
Gelatin solution	1 part by volume

Mix in above proportion immediately before use; the volume of working solution used depends on the number of slides to be stained.

Method
1. Dewax sections in xylene, hydrate through ethanols to water.
2. Rinse sections in distilled water.
3. Incubate in freshly prepared working solution for 45 min at room temperature.
4. Wash in distilled water for 1 min.
5. Dehydrate, clear, and mount in non-aqueous mounting medium.

Results

AgNOR sites	intranuclear black dots
Background	pale yellow

Notes
Sections may be lightly counterstained with neutral red or carmalum. Heavy counterstaining may obscure some AgNOR sites. Sections may be toned using 1% gold chloride. The working solution deteriorates rapidly on standing so must be used immediately after mixing. The silver nitrate solution is expensive, so a minimum amount of working solution should be prepared, and batch staining of slides is more economical.

Table 16.9 *Staining reactions of mast cells*

Method	Results	Page no.
Toluidine blue	Purple	
Azure A	Red	179
Thionin	Blue or red according to age	
Csaba's alcian blue safranin	Purple to red	
Aldehyde fuchsin	Yellow to brown	298
PAS	Variable	171
Gram	Negative	312
Schmorl	Negative	243
ZN	Negative	314
Chloroacetate esterase (fast blue RR)	Dark blue	427
Chloracetate esterase (pararosanilin)	Deep pink to red	428

MAST CELLS

Although distributed throughout the body, mast cells are predominantly located near blood vessels, nerves, and subepithelial areas especially in skin. They contain membrane-bound secretory granules containing histamine, proteases, and cytokines. Mast cells also contain heparin as well as biotin. They sometimes accumulate in the skin, especially in children (mastocytosis). Mast cell tumors are the most common cutaneous tumor in the dog, where they have been identified using a modified silver method (Piva et al 2003). Several methods demonstrate mast cells, including treating tissues with a biotin–avidin–peroxidase complex followed by diaminobenzidine (DAB), a microwave version of Del Rio Hortega's carbonate method modified by excluding 1% formalin reduction, the acidified toluidine blue method, and the alcian blue stain (Cook 1961; Csaba 1969; Churukian & Schenk 1981; Duffy et al 1998; Churukian et al 2000; Henwood 2002). Antibodies against mast cell tryptase for human mast cells or mast cell protease 6 for mast cells in mice have proven useful in detection by immunohistochemistry. Classical methods to detect mast cells are reviewed in Table 16.9.

PANETH CELLS

Paneth cells are pyramidal shaped cells whose apex points toward the lumen of the bowel and whose supra-nuclear cytoplasm is packed with large eosinophilic granules easily visible on H&E staining. They comprise the majority of cells at the base of crypts of the small bowel and are scattered through the ascending colon and appendix. The granules of Paneth cells contain lysosomes, immunoglobulins, and a high content of zinc. Picric acid and other acid fixatives (Hollande's and Bouin's) interfere with visualization by H&E because they tend to destroy the granules. The phloxine–tartrazine technique of Lendrum (1947) or Masson's trichrome works well to demonstrate Paneth cells.

Acknowledgments

This chapter is a merging of two chapters from the previous edition. John Bancroft and Alan Stevens wrote Cytoplasmic granules, organelles and special tissues for editions one to four. Ian Dawson contributed the APUD system to the second edition, and Philip Wilson and Brian Chalk for the third and fourth editions contributed the Neuroendocrine chapter. Our acknowledgments are due to them for their contributions.

REFERENCES

Altmann R. (1894) Die Elementaroganismen und ihre Beziehunger zu den Zellen, 2nd edn. Leipzig: Veit.

Barter R., Pearse A.G.E. (1955) Mammalian enterochromaffin cells as the source of serotonin (5-hydroxytryptamine). Journal of Pathology and Bacteriology 69: 25–31.

Bloodworth J.M.B., Greider M.H. (1982) The endocrine pancreas and diabetes mellitus. In: Bloodworth J.M.B., ed. Endocrine pathology—general and surgical. Baltimore, MD: Williams and Wilkins, pp. 556–721.

Bordi C. (1987) Endocrine pancreas. In: Spicer S.S., ed. Histochemistry in pathologic diagnosis. New York: Marcel Dekker, pp. 457–479.

Brinn N.T. (1983) Rapid metallic histological staining using the microwave oven. Journal of Histotechnology 6:125–129.

Brookes L.D. (1968) A stain for differentiating two types of acidophil cells in the rat pituitary. Stain Technology 43:41–42.

Carney J.A. (1997) Adrenal gland. In: Sternberg S.S., ed. Histology for pathologists, 2nd edn. New York: Lippincott-Raven Press, pp. 1107–1131.

Churukian C.T., Schenk E.A. (1979) A modification of Pascual's at gyrophil method. Journal of Histotechnology 2:102–103.

Churukian C.J., Schenk E.A. (1981) A toluidine blue method for demonstrating mast cells. Journal of Histotechnology 4:85–86.

Churukian C.J., Frank M., Horobin RW. (2000) Alcian blue pyridine variant—a superior alternative to alcian blue 8GX: staining performance and stability. Biotechnic and Histochemistry 75:147–150.

Cook H.C. (1961) A modified thionin technique for mast cells in tissue sections. Journal of Medical Laboratory Technology 18:188.

Csaba G. (1969) Mechanism of the formation of mast cell granules. Acta Biologica Academiae Scientiarum Hungaricae 20:205.

Dawson A.B., Barnett J. (1944) Bodian's protargol method as applied to other than neurological preparations. Stain Technology 19:115–118.

DeLellis R.A., Dayal Y. (1991) Neuroendocrine system. In: Sternberg S.S., ed. Histology for pathologists. New York: Raven Press, pp. 347–362.

DeLellis R.A., Dayal Y. (1997) Neuroendocrine system. In: Sternberg S.S., ed. Histology for pathologists, 2nd edn. Philadelphia, PA: Lippincott-Raven Press, pp. 1133–1151.

DeLellis R.A., Dayal Y., Tischler A.S. et al. (1986) Multiple endocrine neoplasia syndromes: cellular origins and interrelationships. International Review of Experimental Pathology 28:163–215.

Duffy J.P., Smith P.J., Darton S.J. et al. (1998) Combination of specific histochemical staining of eosinophils and mast cells with immunohistochemical demonstration of neural antigens. Journal of Histotechnology 21(1):29–31.

Ezrin C., Kovacs K., Horvath E. (1982) Pathology of the adenohypophysis. In: Bloodworth J.M.B., ed. Endocrine pathology—general and surgical. Baltimore, MD: Williams and Wilkins, pp. 101–132.

Falck B., Owman C.A. (1965) A detailed methodological description of the fluorescence method for the cellular distribution of biogenic monoamines. Acta Universitatis Lundensis 7(sect 11):5–23.

Feyrter F. (1938) Uber Diffuse Endokrine Epithaliale Organe. Leipzig: Barth.

Glenner G.G., Grimley P.M. (1974) Tumors of the extra-adrenal paraganglion system (including chemoreceptors). In: Firrninger H.I., ed. Atlas of tumor pathology. Washington, DC: Armed Forces Institute of Pathology.

Golden A., Kerwin D.M. (1982) The parathyroid glands. In: Bloodworth J.M.B., ed. Endocrine pathology—general and surgical. Baltimore, MD: Williams and Wilkins, pp. 205–220.

Gomori G. (1941) Observations with differential stains on human islets of Langerhans. American Journal of Pathology 17:395.

Gomori G. (1952) Microscopic histochemistry. Chicago: Chicago University Press.

Gorgas K., Bock P. (1976) Improved methods for the light microscopic study of enterochromaffin cells, in endocrine, gut and pancreas. In: Fujita T., ed. Endocrine gut and pancreas. Amsterdam: Elsevier Scientific, pp. 1–11.

Gould V.E., Summers S.C. (1982) Adrenal medulla and paraganglia. In: Bloodworth J.M.B., ed. Endocrine pathology—general and surgical. Baltimore, MD: Williams and Wilkins, pp. 473–511.

Grimelius L. (1968a) A silver nitrate stain for α-2 cells in human pancreatic islets. Acta Societatis Medicorum Upsaliensis 73:243–270.

Grimelius L. (1968b) The argyrophil reaction in islet cells of adult human pancreas studied with a new silver nitrate procedure. Acta Societatis Medicorum Upsaliensis 73:271–294.

Grimelius L., Wilander E.D. (1980) Silver stains in the study of endocrine cells of the gut and pancreas. Investigative and Cell Pathology 3:3–12.

Grizzle W.E. (1996) Silver staining methods to identify cells of the dispersed neuroendocrine system. Journal of Histotechnology 19(3):225–234.

Halami N.S. (1952) Differentiation of the two types of basophils in an adenophpophysis of the rat and the mouse. Stain Technology 27:61.

Hellerström C., Hellman B. (1960) Some aspects of silver impregnation of the islets of Langerhans in the rat. Acta Endocrinologica 35:518–532.

Henwood A. (2002) Improved demonstration of mast cells using alcian blue tetrakis (methylpyridium) chloride. Biotechnic and Histochemistry 77(2):93–94.

Herrera G.A., De Moraes H.P., Grizzle W.E., Han S.G. (1984) Malignant small bowel neoplasm of enteric plexus derivation (plexosarcoma). Light and electron microscopic study confirming the origin of the neoplasm. Digestive Diseases and Sciences 29(3):275–284.

Hotchkiss R.D. (1948) A microchemical reaction resulting in the staining of polysaccharide structures in fixed tissue preparations. Archives of Biochemistry 16:131.

Kameya T. (1990) Spectrum of neuroendocrine marker substance production in carcinoid tumors revealed by immunohistochemistry. In: Lechago J., Kameya T., eds. Endocrine pathology update. (distributed by WW Norton & Co, New York) Field and Wood, Medical Publishers, pp. 151–169.

Klimstra D.S. (1997) Pancreas. In: Sternberg S.S., ed. Histology for pathologists. Philadelphia, PA: Lippincott, Williams & Wilkins, pp. 613–647.

Koski J.P. (1981) Silver–methenarnine borate (SMB): cost reduction with technical improvements in silver nitrate–gold chloride impregnations. Journal of Histotechnology 4:115–120.

Lack E.R., Mercer L. (1977) A modified Grimelius argyrophil technique for neurosecretory granules. American Journal of Surgical Pathology 77:275–277.

Lechago J. (1982) The endocrine cells of the digestive and respiratory systems and their pathology. In: Bloodworth J.M.B., ed. Endocrine pathology—general and surgical. Baltimore, MD: Williams and Wilkins, pp. 513–555.

Lendrum A.C. (1947) The phloxine–tartrazine method as a histological stain and for the demonstration of inclusion bodies. Journal of Pathology and Bacteriology 59:399.

Lillie R.D. (1965) Histopathologic technique and practical histochemistry, 3rd edn. New York: McGraw-Hill.

Liu C., Yu S., Zinn K. et al. (2006) Murine mammary carcinoma exosomes promote tumor growth by suppression of NK cell function. Journal of Immunology 176(3): 1375–1385.

LiVolsi V.A. (1991) Thyroid. In: Sternberg S.S., ed. Histology for pathologists. New York: Raven Press, pp. 301–310.

Maitra A., Abbas A.K. (2005) The endocrine system. In: Robbins and Cotran pathologic basis of disease, 7th edn. Philadelphia, PA: Elsevier-Saunders.

McKeever P.E., Spicer S.S. (1987) The pituitary: contributions of cytochemistry to pathological diagnosis. In: Spicer S.S., ed. Histochemistry in pathologic diagnosis. New York: Marcel Dekker, pp. 603–645.

Mendelsohn G. (1987) Diagnostic histochemistry and immunohistochemistry of the thyroid, parathyroid, and adrenal glands. In: Spicer S.S., ed. Histochemistry in pathologic diagnosis. New York: Marcel Dekker, pp. 647–664.

Pascual J.S.F. (1976) A new method for easy demonstration of argyrophil cells. Stain Technology 51:231–235.

Pearse A.G.E. (1966) Common cytochemical and ultrastructural characteristics of cell producing polypeptide hormones, with particular reference to calcitonin and the thyroid C cells. Veterinary Record 79:587–590.

Pearse A.G.E. (1968) Common cytochemical and ultrastructural characteristics of cells producing polypeptide hormones (the APUD series I) and their relevance to thyroid and ultimobranchial C cells and calcitonin. Proceedings of the Royal Society B 170:71–80.

Pearse A.G.E. (1969) The cytochemistry and ultrastructure of polypeptide hormone-producing cells of the APUD series and the embryologic, physiologic, and pathologic implications of the concept. Journal of Histochemistry and Cytochemistry 17:303–313.

Pearse A.G.E. (1977) The diffuse neuroendocrine system and the APUD concept: related endocrine peptides in brain, intestine, pituitary, placenta and anuran cutaneous glands. Medical Biology 55:115–125.

Pearse A.G.E., Coulling I., Weavers B., Friesen S. (1970) The endocrine polypeptide cells of the human stomach, duodenum and jejunum. Gut 11:649–658.

Pernicone P.T., Scheithauer B.W., Horvath E., Kovacs K. (1997) Pituitary and sellar region. In: Sternberg S.S., ed. Histology for pathologists. Philadelphia, PA: Lippincott-Raven, pp. 1053–1074.

Pickett J.P., Roggli C.V. (1982) Rapid histological staining procedures for materials from immune-suppressed patients. American Journal of Medical Technology 48:893–902.

Piva J.R., Canal A.M., Piva C.E. et al. (2003) Microwave-assisted silver-stain method in the diagnosis of canine mast cell tumors: correlation with traditional methods by digital image analysis. Journal of Histotechnology 26(1):31–35.

Ploton D., Menager M., Jameson P. et al. (1986) Improvement in the staining and visualization of the argyrophilic proteins of the nucleolar organizer region at the optical level. Histochemical Journal 18:5.

Polak J.M., Bloom S.R. (1980) Peripheral localization of regulatory peptides as a clue to their function. Journal of Histochemistry and Cytochemistry 28:918–924.

Roth S.I., Abu-Jawdeh G.M. (1997) Parathyroid glands. In: Sternberg S.S., ed. Histology for pathologists, 2nd edn. Philadelphia, PA: Lippincott-Raven, pp. 1093–1105.

Sano T., Saito H. (1990) Peptide hormones in pheochromocytoma. In: Lechago J., Kameya T., eds. Endocrine pathology update. (Distributed by WW Norton & Co. New York), Field and Wood, Medical Publishers, pp. 119–131.

Sheehan D.C., Hrapchak B.D. (1980) Theory and practice of histotechnology, 2nd edn. St. Louis, MO: C.V. Mosby, p. 277.

Singh I. (1964) A modification of the Masson–Hamperl method for staining argentaffin cells. Anatomischer Anzeiger 115.

Slidders W. (1961) The OFG and BrAB-OFG methods for staining the adenohypophysis. Journal of Pathology and Bacteriology 82:532.

Smith D.M. Jr., Haggitt R.C. (1983) A comparative study of generic stains for carcinoid secretory granules. American Journal of Surgical Pathology 7:61–68.

Solcia E., Vassallo G., Capella C. (1968) Selective staining of endocrine cells by basic dyes after acid hydrolysis. Stain Technology 43.

Solcia E., Capella C., Vassalo G. (1969) Lead haematoxylin as a stain for endocrine cells. Significance of staining and comparison with other selective methods. Histochemie 20:116.

Staples T.C., Clark L. (1990) Dilute ammoniacal silver solutions for the demonstration of reticulum and argentaffin granules. Journal of Histotechnology 13:137–139.

Staples T.C., Grizzle W.E. (1986) A methyl green nuclear stain for argyrophil procedures. Laboratory Medicine 17:532–534.

Staples T.C., Grizzle W.E. (1987) Effect of temperature on argyrophil impregnation: development of a high temperature rapid argyrophil procedure. Stain Technology 62:41–49.

Tischler A.S. (1989) The dispersed neuroendocrine cells: the structure, function, regulation and effects of xenobiotics on this system. Toxicology and Pathology 17:307–316.

Tischler A.S. (1997) Paraganglia. In: Sternberg S.S., ed. Histology for pathologists, 2nd edn. New York: Lippincott-Raven, pp. 1153–1172.

Turbat-Herrera E.A., Herrera G.A., Gore L. et al. (1988) Neuroendocrine differentiation in prostatic carcinomas. Archives of Pathology and Laboratory Medicine 112:1100–1105.

Ulich T.R., Lewin J.K. (1990) The carcinoma–carcinoid spectrum. In: Lechago J., Kameya T., eds. Endocrine pathology update. (Distributed by WW Norton & Co. New York), Field and Wood, Medical Publishers, pp. 133–150.

Van Campenhout E. (1933) Argentaffinic cells of the pancreas. Proceedings of the Society of Experimental Biology and Medicine 30:617–618.

Woodtli W., Hedinger C. (1976) Histologic characteristics of insulinomas and gastrinomas: value of argyrophilia, metachromasia, immunohistology, and electron microscopy for the identification of gastrointestinal and pancreatic endocrine cells and their tumors. Virchows Archiv. A: Pathological Anatomy and Histology 371:331–350.

FURTHER READING

Grizzle W.E. (1996) Theory and practice of silver staining in histopathology. Journal of Histotechnology 19(3):183–195.

Singh I. (1964) A new argyrophile method for the rapid staining of enterochromaffin cells in paraffin sections. Acta Anatomica 59:290–296.

17

Microorganisms

Jeanine H. Bartlett

INTRODUCTION

We have all heard the expression, 'The world is getting smaller.' Nowhere is that statement truer than in the world of microorganisms. Microorganisms (also called microbes) are organisms which share the property of being sub-microscopic. Most do not normally cause disease in humans, existing in a state of commensalism, where there is little or no benefit to the person, or mutualism, where there is some benefit to both parties. Pathogens are agents that cause disease. These fall into five main groups (Microbiology at Leicester website):

- Viruses
- Bacteria
- Fungi
- Protozoa
- Helminths.

With the advent of new and more powerful antibiotics, improved environmental hygiene, and advances in microbiological technique, it was widely expected that the need for diagnosis of infectious agents in tissue would diminish in importance. This assumption underestimated the infinite capacity of infectious agents for genomic variation, enabling them to exploit new opportunities to spread infections that are created when host defenses become diminished and inadequate. The following are currently the most important factors influencing the presentation of infectious diseases:

- Increased mobility of the world's population through tourism, immigration, and international commerce has distorted natural geographic boundaries to infection, exposing weaknesses in host defenses, and in knowledge. Some, such as Ebola, have been around for many years but the first human outbreaks were not recorded until 1976. Previous outbreaks would flare up and then burn themselves out, undetected and confined before deforestation and the like altered this state.
- Immunodeficiency states occurring either as part of a natural disease, such as acquired immune deficiency syndrome (AIDS), or as an iatrogenic disease. As treatment becomes more aggressive, depression of the host's immunity often occurs, enabling organisms of low virulence to become life-threatening, and allows latent infections accrued throughout life to reactivate and spread unchecked.
- Emerging, re-emerging, and antibiotic-resistant organisms such as the tubercle bacillus and staphylococcus are a constant concern.
- Adaptive mutation occurring in microorganisms, which allows them to jump barriers of species and explore new physical environments, evading host defenses, and resisting agents of treatment.
- Bioterrorism has become a major concern since September 11, 2001. The world public health systems and primary healthcare providers must be prepared to address varied biological agents, including pathogens that are rarely seen in the developed countries. High-priority agents include organisms that pose a risk to national security because they:
  - Can be easily disseminated or transmitted from person to person
  - Cause high mortality, with potential for a major public health impact
  - Might cause public panic and social disruption, and require special action for public health preparedness.

The following are listed by the Centers for Disease Control and Prevention (CDC) in the United States as high-risk biological agents:

- Anthrax
- Smallpox
- Botulism
- Tularemia
- Viral hemorrhagic fever.

These factors, acting singly or together, provide an ever-changing picture of infectious disease where clinical presentation may involve multiple pathological processes, unfamiliar organisms, and modification of the host response by a diminished immune status.

Size

The term 'microorganism' has been interpreted liberally in this chapter. Space limitation precludes a comprehensive approach to the subject; the reader is referred to additional texts such as that of von Lichtenberg (1991) for greater depth. The organisms in Table 17.1 are discussed, with techniques for their demonstration described.

Safety

Most infectious agents are rendered harmless by direct exposure to formal saline. Standard fixation procedures should be sufficient to kill microorganisms, one exception being material from patients with Creutzfeldt–Jakob disease (CJD). It has been shown that well-fixed tissue, paraffin-processed blocks, and stained slides from CJD remain infectious when introduced into susceptible animals. Treatment of fixed tissue or slides in 96% formic

Table 17.1	Size of organisms
Organisms	**Size**
Viruses	20–300 nm
Mycoplasms	125–350 nm
Chlamydia	200–1000 nm
Rickettsia	300–1200 nm
Bacteria	1–14 μm
Fungi	2–200 μm
Protozoa	1–50 μm
Metazoans	3–10 mm

acid for 1 hour followed by copious washing inactivates this infectious agent without adversely affecting section quality (Brown et al 1990). Laboratory safety protocols should cover infection containment in all laboratory areas, and the mortuary, or necropsy area, where handling unfixed material is unavoidable. When available, unfixed tissue samples should be sent for microbiological culture as this offers the best chance for rapid and specific identification of etiological agents, even when heavy bacterial contamination may have occurred.

DETECTION AND IDENTIFICATION

The diagnosis of illness from infectious disease starts with clinical presentation of the patient, and in most cases a diagnosis is made without a tissue sample being taken. Specimens submitted to the laboratory range from autopsy specimens, where material is plentiful and sampling error presents little problem, to cervical smears where cellular material is often scarce and lesions may easily be missed. A full clinical history is important, especially details of the patient's ethnic origin, immune status, any recent history of foreign travel, and current medication. The macroscopic appearance of tissue, such as abscesses and pus formation, cavitations, hyperkeratosis, demyelination, pseudo-membrane or fibrin formation, focal necrosis, and granulomas can provide evidence of infection. These appearances are often non-specific but occasionally in hydatid cyst disease or some helminth infestations the appearances are diagnostic. The microscopic appearance of routine stains at low-power magnification often reveals indirect evidence of the presence of infection, such as neutrophil or lymphocytic infiltrates, granulomata, micro-abscesses, eosinophilic aggregates, Charcot–Leyden crystals, and caseous necrosis. Some of these appearances may be sufficiently reliable to provide an initial, or provisional, diagnosis and allow treatment to be started even if the precise nature of the suspect organism is never identified, particularly in the case of tuberculosis.

At the cellular level the presence of giant cells, such as Warthin–Finkeldy, or Langhans' giant cells, likely indicates measles and tuberculosis, respectively. Other cellular changes include intracytoplasmic edema of koilocytes, acantholysis, spongiform degeneration of brain, margination of chromatin, syncytial nuclear appearance, 'ground-glass' changes in the nucleus or cytoplasm, or inclusion bodies, and can indicate infectious etiology. At some stage in these processes, suspect organisms may be visualized. A well-performed hematoxylin and eosin (H&E) method will stain many organisms. Papanicolaou stain and Romanowsky stains, such as Giemsa, will also stain many organisms together with their cellular environment. Other infectious agents are poorly visualized by routine stains and require special techniques to demonstrate their presence. This may be due to the small size of the organism, as in the case of viruses where electron microscopy is needed. Alternatively, the organism may be hydrophobic, or weakly charged, as with mycobacteria, spirochetes, and cryptococci, in which case the use of specific histochemical methods is required for their detection. When organisms are few in number, fluorochromes may be used to increase microscopic sensitivity of a technique. Finally, there are two techniques that offer the possibility of specific identification of microorganisms that extend to the appropriate strain level. There is a growing catalog of *biotinylated antisera* against organism-specific proteins that can be demonstrated immunohistochemically. To date, those developed for protozoan, chlamydial, and viral organisms have been most widely used diagnostically in histopathology; however, this will undoubtedly change in the future.

In situ hybridization has even greater potential for microbial detection. The use of single-stranded nucleic acid probes offers even greater possibilities by identifying latent viral genomic footprints in cells, which may have relevance to extending our knowledge of disease, AIDS and HIV being good examples. The polymerase chain reaction technique, to increase sensitivity and make use of stored blocks and slides to study evolutionary aspects of infectious disease, is being used increasingly in research. Future demonstration methods for infectious diseases may lie with these techniques. While modern advances in technique are important, emphasis is also placed upon the ability of the microscopist to interpret suspicious signs from a good H&E stain. The growing number of patients whose immune status is compromised, and who can mount only a minimal or inappropriate response to infection, further complicates the picture, justifying speculative use of special stains such as those for mycobacteria and fungi on tissue from AIDS patients. It should be remembered that, for a variety of reasons, negative results for the identification of an infectious agent do not exclude its presence. For instance, administration of antibiotics to the patient before a biopsy might be the reason for failure to detect a causal microorganism in tissue.

Detection and identification of bacteria

When bacteria are present in large numbers in an abscess or in vegetation on a heart valve, they appear as blue–gray granular masses with an H&E stain; often organisms are invisible or obscured by cellular debris. The reaction of pyogenic bacteria to the Gram stain, together with their morphological appearance, i.e. cocci or bacilli, provides the basis for a simple classification: see Table 17.2.

Table 17.2 A simplified classification of important bacteria

Gram-positive		Gram-negative		
Cocci	Bacilli	Cocci	Bacilli	Coccobacilli
Staphylococcus sp.	*Bacillus*	*Neisseria*	*Escherichia*	*Brucella*
Streptococcus sp. (inc. *Pneumococcus*)	*Clostridium*		*Klebsiella*	*Bordetella*
	Corynebacterium		*Salmonella*	*Hemophilus*
	Mycobacteria (weak+)		*Shigella*	
	Lactobacillus (commensal)		*Proteus*	
	Listeria		*Pseudomonas*	
			Vibrio	
			Pasteurella	

Use of control sections

The use of known positive control sections with all special stain methods for demonstrating microorganisms is essential. Results are unsafe in the absence of positive controls, and should not be considered valid. The control section should be appropriate, where possible, for the suspected organism. A pneumocystis-containing control, for instance, should be used for demonstrating *Pneumocystis carinii*. A Gram control should contain both Gram-positive and Gram-negative organisms. Postmortem tissues can often be a good source of control material or, as a last resort, a suspension of Gram-positive and Gram-negative organisms can be injected into the thigh muscle of a rat shortly before it is sacrificed for some other purpose. Gram-positive and Gram-negative organisms can also be harvested from microbiological plates, suspended in 10% neutral buffered formalin (NBF), centrifuged, and small amounts mixed with minced normal kidney, then chemically processed along with other tissue blocks (Swisher & Nicholson 1989).

THE GRAM STAIN

In spite of more than a century having passed since Gram described his technique in 1884, its chemical rationale is still obscure. It is probably due to a mixture of factors, the most important being increased thickness, chemical composition, and the functional integrity of cell walls of Gram-positive bacteria. When these bacteria die, they become Gram negative. The following procedure is only suitable for the demonstration of bacteria in smears of pus and sputum. It may be of value to the pathologist in the necropsy room where a quick technique such as this may enable rapid identification of the organism causing a lung abscess, wound infection, septicemic abscesses, or meningitis.

Gram method for bacteria in smears

Method

1. Fix dry film by passing it three times through a flame or placing on a heat block.
2. Stain for 15 seconds in 1% crystal violet or methyl violet, then pour off excess.
3. Flood for 30 seconds with Lugol's iodine, pour off excess.
4. Flood with acetone for not more than 2–5 seconds; wash with water immediately.
5. Alternatively decolorize with alcohol until no more stain comes out. Wash with water.
6. Counterstain for 20 s with dilute carbol fuchsin, or freshly filtered neutral red for 1–2 min.
7. Wash with water and carefully blot section until it is dry.

Results

Gram-positive organisms	blue–black
Gram-negative organisms	red

Modified Brown–Brenn method for Gram-positive and Gram-negative bacteria in paraffin sections (Churukian & Schenk 1982)

Sections

Formalin-fixed, 4–5 micron, paraffin-embedded sections.

Solutions

Crystal violet solution (commercially available)

Crystal violet, 10% alcoholic	2 ml
Distilled water	18 ml
Ammonium oxalate, 1%	80 ml

Mix and store; always filter before use.

Modified Gram's iodine commercially available, or

Iodine	2 g
Potassium iodide	4 g
Distilled water	400 ml

Dissolve potassium iodide in a small amount of the distilled water, add iodine and dissolve; add remainder of distilled water.

Ethyl alcohol–acetone solution

Ethyl alcohol, absolute	50 ml
Acetone	50 ml

0.5% basic fuchsin solution (stock) commercially available, or

Basic fuchsin or pararosaniline	0.5 g
Distilled water	100 ml

Dissolve with aid of heat and a magnetic stirrer.

Basic fuchsin solution (working)

Basic fuchsin solution (stock)	10 ml
Distilled water	40 ml

Picric acid–acetone

Picric acid	0.1 g
Acetone	100 ml

Note

With concerns over the explosiveness of dry picric acid in the lab, it is recommended that you purchase the picric acid–acetone solution pre-made. It is available through most histology vendors.

Acetone–xylene solution

Acetone	50 ml
Xylene	50 ml

Staining method

1. Deparaffinize and rehydrate through graded alcohols to distilled water.
2. Stain with filtered crystal violet solution, 1 min.
3. Rinse well in distilled water.
4. Iodine solution, 1 min.
5. Rinse in distilled water, blot slide but NOT the tissue section.
6. Decolorize by dipping in alcohol–acetone solution until the blue color stops running. (One to two dips only!)
7. Counterstain in working basic fuchsin for 1 min. Be sure to agitate the slides well in the basic fuchsin before starting the timer.
8. Rinse in distilled water and blot slide but not section.
9. Dip in acetone, one dip.
10. Dip in picric acid–acetone until the sections have a yellowish-pink color.
11. Dip several times in acetone–xylene solution. At this point, check the control for proper differentiation. (Go back to picric acid–acetone if you need more differentiation.)
12. Clear in xylene and mount.

Results

Gram-positive organisms, fibrin, some fungi, Paneth cells granules, keratohyalin, and keratin	blue
Gram-negative organisms	red
Nuclei	red
Other tissue elements	yellow

Be sure you do not allow the tissue sections to dry at any point in the staining process. If this occurs after treatment with iodine, decolorization will be difficult and uneven.

Gram–Twort stain (Twort 1924; Ollet 1947)

Sections

Formalin fixed, paraffin.

Solutions

Crystal violet solution (see previous method)

Gram's iodine (see previous solution)

Twort's stain

1% neutral red in ethanol	9 ml
0.2% fast green in ethanol	1 ml
Distilled water	30 ml

Mix immediately before use.

Method

1. Deparaffinize and rehydrate through graded alcohols to distilled water.
2. Stain in crystal violet solution, 3 min.
3. Rinse in gently running tap water.
4. Treat with Gram's iodine, 3 min.
5. Rinse in tap water, blot dry, and complete drying in a warm place.
6. Differentiate in preheated acetic alcohol until no more color washes out (2% acetic acid in absolute alcohol, pre-heated to 56°C). This may take 15–20 min; the section should be light brown or straw colored.
7. Rinse briefly in distilled water.
8. Stain in Twort's, 5 min.
9. Wash in distilled water.
10. Rinse in acetic alcohol until no more red runs out of the section; this takes only a few seconds.
11. Rinse in fresh absolute alcohol, clear, and mount.

Results

Gram-positive organisms	blue–black
Gram-negative organisms	pink–red
Nuclei	red
Red blood cells and most cytoplasmic structures	green
Elastic fibers	black

TECHNIQUES FOR MYCOBACTERIA

These organisms are difficult to demonstrate by the Gram technique because they possess a capsule containing a long-chain fatty acid (mycolic acid) that makes them hydrophobic. The fatty capsule influences the penetration and resistance to removal of the stain by acid and alcohol (acid-and alcohol-fastness), and is variably robust between the various species that make up this group. Phenolic acid, and frequently heat, are used to reduce surface tension and increase porosity, thus forcing dyes to penetrate this capsule. The speed with which the primary dye is removed by differentiation with acid alcohol is proportional to the extent of the fatty coat. The avoidance of defatting agents, or solvents, such as alcohol and xylene, in methods for *Mycobacterium leprae*, is an attempt to conserve this fragile fatty capsule.

Mycobacteria are PAS positive due to the carbohydrate content of their cell walls; however, this positivity is evident only when large concentrations of the microorganisms are present. When these organisms die, they lose their fatty capsule and consequently their carbol fuchsin positivity. The carbohydrate can still be demonstrated by Grocott's methenamine silver reaction, which may prove useful when acid-fast procedures fail, particularly if the patient is already receiving therapy for tuberculosis.

A possible source of acid-fast contamination may be found growing in viscous material sometimes lining water taps and any rubber tubing connected to them. These organisms are acid- and alcohol-fast but are usually easily identified as contaminants by their appearance as clumps, or floaters, above the microscopic focal plane of the section.

Ziehl–Neelsen (ZN) stain for *Mycobacterium* bacilli (Kinyoun 1915)

Sections
Formalin or fixative other than Carnoy's, paraffin.

Solutions

Carbol fuchsin commercially available, or

Basic fuchsin	0.5 g
Absolute alcohol	5 ml
5% aqueous phenol	100 ml

Mix well and filter before use.

Acid alcohol

Hydrochloric acid	10 ml
70% alcohol	1000 ml

Methylene blue solution (stock) commercially available, or

Methylene blue	1.4 g
95% alcohol	100 ml

Methylene blue solution (working)

Methylene blue (stock)	10 ml
Tap water	90 ml

Method
1. Deparaffinize and rehydrate through graded alcohols to distilled water.
2. Carbol fuchsin solution, 30 min.
3. Wash well in tap water.
4. Differentiate in acid alcohol until solutions are pale pink. (This usually only takes 2–5 dips.)
5. Wash in tap water for 8 minutes then dip in distilled water.
6. Counterstain in working methylene blue solution until sections are pale blue.
7. Rinse in tap water then dip in distilled water.
8. Dehydrate, clear, and mount.

Results

Mycobacteria, hair shafts, Russell bodies, Splendore–Hoeppli immunoglobulins around actinomyces, and some fungal organisms	red
Background	pale blue

Notes
a. The blue counterstain may be patchy if extensive caseation is present. Care should be taken to avoid over-counterstaining as scant organisms can easily be obscured.
b. Decalcification using strong acids can destroy acid-fastness; formic acid is recommended.
c. Victoria blue can be substituted for carbol fuchsin and picric acid for the counterstain if color blindness causes a recognition problem.

Fluorescent method for *Mycobacterium bacilli* (Kuper & May 1960)

Sections
Formalin fixed, paraffin.

Solution
Auramine O	1.5 g
Rhodamine B	0.75 g
Glycerol	75 ml
Phenol crystals (liquified at 50°C)	10 ml
Distilled water	50 ml

Method
1. Deparaffinize (1 part groundnut oil and 2 parts xylene for M. *leprae*).
2. Pour on pre-heated (60°C), filtered staining solution, 10 min.
3. Wash in tap water.
4. Differentiate in 0.5% hydrochloric acid in alcohol for M. *tuberculosis*, or 0.5% aqueous hydrochloric acid for M. *leprae*.
5. Wash in tap water, 2 min.
6. Eliminate background fluorescence in 0.5% potassium permanganate, 2 min.
7. Wash in tap water and blot dry.
8. Dehydrate (not for M. *leprae*), clear, and mount in a fluorescence-free mountant.

Results
Mycobacteria	golden yellow (using blue light fluorescence below 530 nm)
Background	dark green

Notes
The advantage of increased sensitivity of this technique is offset by the inconvenience of setting up the fluorescence microscope. Preparations fade over time, as a result of their exposure to UV light.

Modified Fite method for M. *leprae* and *Nocardia*

Fixation
10% neutral buffered formalin (NBF).

Sections
Paraffin sections at 4–5 μm.

Solutions
Carbol fuchsin solution commercially available, or
0.5 g basic fuchsin dissolved in 5 ml of absolute alcohol; add 100 ml of 5% aqueous phenol. Mix well and filter before use. Filter before each use with #1 filter paper.

5% sulfuric acid in 25% alcohol
25% ethanol	95 ml
Sulfuric acid, concentrated	5 ml

Methylene blue (stock) *commercially available, or*
Methylene blue	1.4 g
95% alcohol	100 ml

Methylene blue, working
Stock methylene blue	5 ml
Tap water	45 ml
Xylene–peanut oil	1 part oil : 2 parts xylene

Method
1. Deparaffinize in two changes of xylene–peanut oil, 6 minutes each.
2. Drain slides vertically on paper towel and wash in warm, running tap water for 3 minutes. (The residual oil preserves the sections and helps accentuate the acid fastness of the bacilli.)
3. Stain in carbol fuchsin at room temperature for 25 minutes. (Solution may be poured back into bottle and reused.)
4. Wash in warm, running tap water for 3 minutes.
5. Drain excess water from slides vertically on paper towel.
6. Decolorize with 5% sulfuric acid in 25 % alcohol, two changes of 1.5 minutes each. (Sections should be pale pink.)
7. Wash in warm, running tap water for 5 minutes.
8. Counterstain in working methylene blue, one quick dip. (Sections should be pale blue.)
9. Wash in warm, running tap water for 5 minutes.
10. Blot sections and dry in 50–55°C oven for 5 minutes.
11. Once dry, one quick dip in xylene.
12. Mount with permanent mountant.

Results *(Fig. 17.1)*

Acid-fast bacilli including M. *leprae*	bright red
Nuclei and other tissue elements	pale blue

Quality control/notes

Be careful not to over-stain with methylene blue and do not allow sections to dry between carbol fuchsin and acid alcohol.

Cresyl violet acetate method for *Helicobacter* sp.

Sections

Formalin fixed, paraffin.

Method

1. Deparaffinize and rehydrate through graded alcohols to distilled water.
2. Filter 0.1% cresyl violet acetate onto slide or into Coplin jar, 5 min.
3. Rinse in distilled water.
4. Blot, dehydrate rapidly in alcohol, clear, and mount.

Results

Helicobacter and nuclei	blue–violet
Background	shades of blue–violet

Notes

This simple method allows for good differentiation of *Helicobacter* sp. from other organisms.

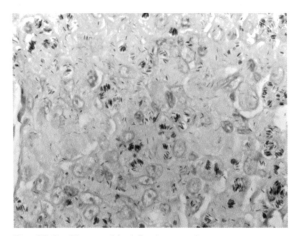

Fig. 17.1 The modified Fite's procedure is necessary to demonstrate *Mycobacterium leprae* due to the organism's fragile, fatty capsule (×63).

Gimenez method for *Helicobacter pylori*
(Gimenez 1964; McMullen et al 1987)

Sections

Formalin fixed, paraffin.

Solutions

Buffer solution *(phosphate buffer at pH 7.5, or 0.1 M)*

0.1 M sodium dihydrogen orthophosphate	3.5 ml
0.1 M disodium hydrogen orthophosphate	15.5 ml

Stock carbol fuchsin

Commercial cold acid-fast bacilli stain, or

Basic fuchsin	1 g
Absolute alcohol	10 ml
5% aqueous phenol	10 ml

Filter before use.

Working carbol fuchsin

Phosphate buffer	10 ml
Stock carbol fuchsin	4 ml

Filter before use.

Malachite green

Malachite green	0.8 g
Distilled water	100 ml

Method

1. Deparaffinize and rehydrate through graded alcohols to distilled water.
2. Stain in working carbol fuchsin solution, 2 min.
3. Wash well in tap water.
4. Stain in malachite green, 15–20 seconds.
5. Wash thoroughly in distilled water.
6. Repeat steps 4 and 5 until section is blue–green to the naked eye.
7. Blot sections dry, and complete drying in air.
8. Clear and mount.

Results

Helicobacter	red–magenta
Background	blue–green

Notes

The greatest problem with this method is over staining, or irregularity of staining, with Malachite green. It is valuable in demonstrating the *Legionella* bacillus in postmortem lung smears.

Toluidine blue in Sorenson's buffer for *Helicobacter*

Sections
Formalin fixed, paraffin.

Solutions
Toluidine blue in pH 6.8 phosphate buffer

Sorenson's phosphate buffer pH 6.8	50 ml
1% aqueous toluidine blue	1 ml

Method
1. Deparaffinize and rehydrate through graded alcohols to distilled water.
2. Stain in buffered toluidine blue, 20 min.
3. Wash well in distilled water.
4. Dehydrate, clear, and mount.

Results
Helicobacter	dark blue against a variably blue background

Warthin–Starry method for spirochetes
(Warthin & Starry 1920)

Sections
Formalin fixed, paraffin.

Solutions
Acetate buffer, pH 3.6

Sodium acetate	4.1 g
Acetic acid	6.25 ml
Distilled water	500 ml

1% silver nitrate in pH 3.6 acetate buffer

Developer

Dissolve 3 g of hydroquinone in 10 ml pH 3.6 buffer, and mix 1 ml of this solution and 15 ml of warmed 5% Scotch glue or gelatin; keep at 40°C. Take 3 ml of 2% silver nitrate in pH 3.6 buffer solution and keep at 55°C. Mix these two solutions immediately before use.

Method
1. Deparaffinize and rehydrate through graded alcohols to distilled water.
2. Celloidinize in 0.5% celloidin, drain, and harden in distilled water, 1 min.
3. Impregnate in preheated 55–60°C silver solution (b), 90–105 minutes.
4. Prepare and preheat developer in a water bath.
5. Treat with developer (solution c) for $3^1/_2$ minutes at 55°C. Sections should be golden-brown at this point.
6. Remove from developer and rinse in tap water for several minutes at 55–60°C, then in buffer at room temperature.
7. Tone in 0.2% gold chloride.
8. Dehydrate, clear, and mount.

Results
Spirochetes	black
Background	golden–yellow

Notes
It is wise to take a few slides through at various incubation times to insure optimum impregnation.

Modified Steiner for filamentous and non-filamentous bacteria (Steiner & Steiner 1944; modified Swisher 1987)

Sections
Formalin fixed, paraffin.

Solutions
1.0% uranyl nitrate commercially available, or

Uranyl nitrate	1 g
Distilled water	100 ml

1% silver nitrate

Silver nitrate	1 g
Distilled water	100 ml

Make fresh each time and filter with #1 or #2 filter paper before use.

0.04% silver nitrate

Silver nitrate	0.04 g
Distilled water	100 ml

Refrigerate and use for only 1 month.

2.5% gum mastic commercially available, or

Gum mastic	2.5 g
Absolute alcohol	100 ml

Allow to dissolve for 24 hours then filter until clear yellow before use. Refrigerate unused portion.

2% hydroquinone

Hydroquinone	1 g
Distilled water	25 ml

Make fresh solution for each use.

Reducing solution

Mix 10 ml of 2.5% gum mastic, 25 ml of 2.0% hydro-quinone, and 5 ml absolute alcohol. Make just prior to use and filter with #4 filter paper; add 2.5 ml of 0.04% silver nitrate. Do not filter this solution. When gum mastic is added, solution will have a milky appearance.

Method

1. Deparaffinize and rehydrate through graded alcohols to distilled water.
2. Sensitize sections in 1% aqueous uranyl nitrate at room temperature, and place in microwave oven until solution is just at boiling point, approx. 20–30 seconds; do not boil. *Alternatively*, place in preheated 1% uranyl nitrate at 60°C in a water bath for 15 min, or in microwave oven and bring to boiling point—do not boil; 2% zinc sulfate in 3.7% formalin may be substituted.
3. Rinse in distilled water at room temperature until uranyl nitrate residue is eliminated.
4. Place in 1% silver nitrate at room temperature and microwave *until* boiling point is just reached. Do not boil. Remove from oven, loosely cover jar, and allow to stand in hot silver nitrate, 6–7 min; *alternatively*, preheat silver nitrate for 20–30 min in a 60°C water bath, add slides, and allow to impregnate for $1^1/_2$ hours.
5. Rinse in three changes of distilled water.
6. Dehydrate in two changes each of 95% alcohol and absolute alcohol.
7. Treat with 2.5% gum mastic, 5 min.
8. Allow to air dry, 5 min.
9. Rinse in two changes of distilled water. Slides may stand here while reducing solution is being prepared.
10. Reduce in preheated reducing solution at 45°C in a water bath for 10–25 min, or until sections have developed satisfactorily with black micro-organisms against a light yellow background. Avoid intensely stained background.
11. Rinse in distilled water to stop reaction.
12. Dehydrate, clear, and mount.

Results *(Fig. 17.2)*

Spirochetes, cat-scratch organisms, Donovan bodies, non-filamentous bacteria of *L. pneumophila*	dark brown-black

Background	bright yellow to golden yellow

Notes

Bring all solutions to room temperature before using. All glassware making contact with silver nitrate should be chemically cleaned. Avoid the use of metal forceps in silver solutions. When doing a bacterial screen, Gram controls should be run along with diagnostic slides. As spirochetes take longer to develop, Gram controls should be used in addition to spirochete controls. When Gram controls have a yellow appearance, remove them to distilled water, and check on microscope for microorganisms. Return to silver solution if they are not ready, and repeat, realizing that spirochetes will take longer. Most solutions can be made in large quantities and kept in the refrigerator.

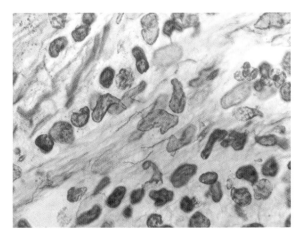

Fig. 17.2 Syphilis bacilli, *Treponema pallidum*, demonstrated here with the modified Steiner technique. The resistance to coloration is shared by *Helicobacter*, spirochetes, and *Legionella* (×100).

SOME IMPORTANT BACTERIA

Staphylococcus aureus is perhaps the most important pathogen of this group. It causes boils, wound and burn infections, and a form of cavitating pneumonia in children and adults. Septicemic states and the formation of multiple scattered abscesses sometimes occur. Staphylococci tend to form clusters (cf. streptococci). Multi-resistance to antibiotics is sometimes encountered.

Neisseria meningitidis (meningococcus) is a common cause of meningitis, and may produce a fulminating septicemia. Organisms can be seen in histological sections of meningococcal meningitis, but are difficult to see because they are usually within neutrophil cytoplasm.

Neisseria gonorrheae (gonococcus) is the cause of gonorrhea. Organisms may be seen within polymorphs in sections of cervix, endometrium, or fallopian tubes in cases of gonorrhea, but, again, are difficult to find. Members of the *Neisseria* family are generally difficult to see in histological sections, although easily detectable in smears of fresh pus or cerebrospinal fluid (CSF), characteristically in pairs. They are easier to detect using the Gram–Twort method.

Lactobacillus acidophilus (Doderlein's bacillus) is a normal inhabitant of the human vagina and is seen in cervical smears taken in the secretory phase of the cycle.

Corynebacterium vaginale is a short Gram-negative bacillus which may cause cervicitis, and is present in about 6% of women of childbearing age. It may be seen in cervical smears where it accumulates as blue-stained masses on the surface of squamous cells stained by Papanicolaou's method; these cells are known as 'clue cells'.

Helicobacter pylori is frequently seen in endoscopic biopsies. A spiral vibrio organism is heavily implicated as the organism causing many cases of chronic gastritis. It is seen as small, weakly hematoxyphilic organisms (usually in clumps) in the lumina of gastric glands, often adherent to the luminal surface of the epithelial cells. With practice, these can be identified from an H&E stain, but Warthin–Starry, Steiner, Gimenez, toluidine blue, or cresyl violet acetate methods demonstrate them more clearly. A commercial specific antiserum has recently become available for their demonstration.

Clostridium difficile causes pseudomembranous colitis, an inflammation of the large bowel. This arises following the administration of broad-spectrum antibiotics; the balance of the normal anerobic gut microflora is disturbed, allowing the organism to proliferate unchecked. *C. difficile* is difficult to stain but the 'explosive lesions' of purulent necrosis of the epithelium and lamina propria of the gut, giving rise to a 'mini volcano' effect, are a good indicator.

Listeria monocytogenes is the cause of a rare form of meningitis and may cause septicemia in humans. Focal necrosis with macrophages that contain tiny intracellular rods arranged in a 'Chinese letter' formation, and staining variably with the Gram stain, are the hallmark of this disease.

Mycobacterium tuberculosis remains a significant pathogen in developed countries where the familiar caseating granulomatous lesion and its associated 1–2-μm, blunt-ended, acid and alcohol-fast bacilli can still be seen. In Africa and other countries, this organism has developed an opportunistic relationship with AIDS, where it is a major cause of death.

Mycobacterium avium/intracellulare are representatives of a group of intracellular opportunistic mycobacteria that are frequently present in the later stages of immunosuppression, particularly that associated with AIDS. They frequently persist in spite of treatment, and are often lethal. The lesions produced are non-caseating and consist of collections of vacuolated macrophages that often contain vast numbers of organisms. On occasion, there is little evidence of a cellular reaction on an H&E-stained section, and the organism is detected only by routinely performing an acid-fast stain, such as the ZN, on all tissue from AIDS patients. This group also includes *M. kansasii*.

Mycobacterium leprae is an obligate intracellular, neurotrophic mycobacterium that attacks and destroys nerves, especially in the skin. Tissue reaction to leprosy depends on the immune status of the host; it can be minimal with a few macrophages packed with crescentic, pointed, intracytoplasmic bacilli (lepromatous leprosy), or may contain scanty organisms and show florid granulomatous response (tuberculoid leprosy). *M. leprae* is only acid-fast and can often be demonstrated with a standard Ziehl–Neelsen technique.

Legionella pneumophila was first identified in 1977 as the cause of a sporadic type of pneumonia of high mortality. The small Gram-positive coccobacillus is generally spread in aerosols from stagnant water reservoirs, usually in air-conditioning units. The bacterium may be difficult to stain except with the Dieterle and modified Steiner silver stains, and specific antiserum.

Treponema pallidum is the organism causing syphilis, and is infrequently seen in biopsy specimens as the primary lesion or 'chancre' is diagnosed clinically. The spirochete is quite obvious using dark-ground microscopy, as an 8–13-μm corkscrew-shaped microorganism that often kinks in the center. Dieterle, Warthin–Starry, or modified Steiner methods demonstrate the organism; specific antiserum is also available.

Leptospira interrogans is the organism causing leptospirosis or Weil's disease. It is a disease characterized by spirochetes, and is spread in the urine of rats and dogs, causing fever, profound jaundice, and sometimes death. Spirochetes can be seen in the acute stages of the disease where they appear in Warthin–Starry and modified Steiner techniques as tightly wound 13-µm microorganisms with curled ends resembling a shepherd's crook.

Intestinal spirochetosis appears as a massive infestation on the luminal border of the colon by spirochete *Brachyspira aalborgi* (Tomkins et al 1986). It measures 2–6 µm long, is tightly coiled, and arranged perpendicularly to the luminal surface of the gut, giving it a fuzzy hematoxyphilic coat in an H&E stain. There is no cellular response to the presence of this spirochete. It is seen well with the Warthin–Starry and the modified Steiner techniques.

Cat-scratch disease presents as a self-limiting, local, single lymphadenopathy appearing about 2 weeks after a cat scratch or bite. Histologically the node shows focal necrosis or micro-abscesses. Two Gram-negative bacteria (*Afipia felis* and *Bartonella henselae*) have been implicated. Because of the timing or maturation factor of the bacterium, it is difficult to demonstrate on paraffin sections, but the modified Steiner and the Warthin–Starry methods are valuable techniques for demonstrating this organism.

FUNGAL INFECTIONS

Fungi are widespread in nature, and humans are regularly exposed to the spores from many species, yet the most commonly encountered diseases are the superficial mycoses that affect the subcutaneous or horny layers of the skin or hair shafts, and cause conditions such as athlete's foot or ringworm. These dermatophytic fungi belong to the *Microsporum* and *Trichophyton* groups and may appear as yeasts or mycelial forms within the keratin. They are seen fairly well in the H&E stain, but are demonstrated well with the Grocott and PAS stains. As with other infections, the increase in the number of patients with diminished or compromised immune systems has increased the incidence of *systemic mycoses*, allowing opportunistic attacks by fungi, often of low virulence, but sometimes resulting in death.

When fungi grow in tissue they may display primitive asexual (imperfect) forms that appear as either spherical *yeast* or *spore* forms. Some may produce vegetative growth that appears as tubular *hyphae* that may be septate and branching; these features are important morphologically for identifying different types of fungi. A mass of interwoven hyphae is called a fungal *mycelium*. Only rarely, when the fungus reaches an open cavity, the body surface, or a luminal surface such as the bronchus, are the spore-forming fruiting bodies called *sporangia*, or *conidia*, produced.

Identification of fungi

Some fungi may elicit a range of host reactions from exudative, necrotizing, to granulomatous; other fungi produce little cellular response to indicate their presence. Fortunately, most fungi are relatively large and their cell walls are rich in polysaccharides, which can be converted by oxidation to dialdehydes and thus detected with Schiff's reagent or hexamine–silver solutions. Fungi are often weakly hematoxyphilic. Some fungi, such as sporothrix, may be surrounded by a stellate, strongly eosinophilic, refractile Splendore–Hoeppli precipitates of host immunoglobulin and degraded eosinophils.

Fluorochrome-labeled specific antibodies to many fungi are available, and are in use in mycology laboratories for the identification of fungi on fresh and paraffin sections. These antibodies have not found widespread use, however, on fixed tissue where identification still relies primarily on traditional staining methods.

An H&E stain, a Grocott methenamine (hexamine)–silver (GMS), a mounted unstained section to look for pigmentation, and a good color atlas (Chandler et al 1980) when experience fails, permit most fungal infections to be identified to levels sufficient for diagnoses. However, there is no substitute for microbiological culture.

Grocott methenamine (hexamine)–silver for fungi and *Pneumocystis* spp. organisms (Gomori 1946; Grocott 1955; Swisher & Chandler 1982)

Sections
Formalin fixed, paraffin.

Solutions

4% chromic acid *commercially available, or*

Chromic acid	4.0 g
Distilled water	100 ml

1% sodium bisulfite

Sodium bisulfite	1 g
Distilled water	100 ml

5% sodium thiosulfate

Sodium thiosulfate	5.0 g
Distilled water	100 ml

0.21% silver nitrate (stock)

Silver nitrate	2.1 g
Distilled water	1000 ml

Refrigerate for up to 3 months

(A) Methenamine–silver borate solution (stock)

Methenamine	27 g
Sodium borate decahydrate (borax)	3.8 g
Distilled water	1000 ml

Refrigerate for up to 3 months.

(B) Methenamine–silver sodium borate solution (working)

Equal parts of solutions A and B. Make fresh each time and filter before use.

0.2% light green (stock)

Light green	0.2 g
Distilled water	100 ml
Glacial acetic acid	0.2 ml

Light green (working)

Stock light green	10 ml
Distilled water	50 ml

Prepare working solution fresh before each use.

Method

1. Deparaffinize and rehydrate through graded alcohols to distilled water.
2. Oxidize in 4% aqueous chromic acid (chromium trioxide), 30 minutes.
3. Wash briefly in distilled water.
4. Dip briefly in 1% sodium bisulfite.
5. Wash well in distilled water
6. Place in preheated (56–60°C water bath) working silver solution for 15–20 minutes. Check control after 15 minutes. If section is 'paper bag brown' then rinse in distilled water and check under microscope. If it is not ready, dip again in distilled water and return to silver. Elastin should not be black. Check every 2 minutes from that point onwards. (See Note a.)
7. Rinse well in distilled water.
8. Tone in 0.1% gold chloride, 5 seconds. Rinse in distilled water.
9. Place in 5% sodium thiosulfate, 5 seconds.
10. Rinse well in running tap water.
11. Counterstain in working light green solution until a medium green (usually 5–15 seconds).
12. Dehydrate, clear, and mount.

Results

Fungi, pneumocystis, melanin	black
Hyphae and yeast-form cells of fungi	sharply delineated in black
Mucins and glycogen	taupe to dark gray
Background	pale green

Notes

a. Incubation time is variable and depends on the type and duration of fixation, and organism being demonstrated. Impregnation is controlled microscopically until fungi are dark brown. Background is colorless at this point. Over-incubation produces intense staining of elastin and fungi that may obscure fine internal detail of the hyphal septa. This detail is essential for critical identification, and is best seen on under-impregnated sections. To avoid excess glycogen impregnation in liver sections, section may be digested prior to incubation. A water bath may be used effectively to insure an even incubation temperature.
b. Borax insures an alkaline pH.
c. Sodium bisulfite removes excess chromic acid.
d. Some workers prefer a light H&E counterstain. This is especially useful when a consulting case is sent with only one slide, providing morphological detail for the pathologist.
e. Solutions A and B need to be made and stored in chemically clean glassware (20% nitric acid), as does the working solution. This includes graduates and Coplin jars. Do not use metal forceps.
f. Allow all refrigerated solutions to reach room temperature before using.

McManus' PAS method for glycogen and fungal cell walls

Fixation
10% NBF.

Sections
3–5-μm paraffin sections.

Solutions

Schiff's reagent (see p. 171), also commercially available

0.5% periodic acid solution

Periodic acid	0.5 g
Distilled water	100 ml

0.2% light green (stock)

Light green	0.2 g
Distilled water	100 ml
Glacial acetic acid	0.2 ml

This is the same stock solution used in the GMS.

Light green (working)

Stock light green	10 ml
Distilled water	50 ml

Make fresh before each use.

Method

1. Deparaffinize and hydrate slides to distilled water.
2. Oxidize in periodic acid solution for 5 minutes.
3. Rinse in distilled water.
4. Place in Schiff's reagent for 15 minutes.
5. Wash in running tap water for 10 minutes to allow pink color to develop.
6. Counterstain for a few seconds in working light green solution.
7. Dehydrate in 95% alcohol, absolute alcohol, and clear in xylene.
8. Mount in resin-based mountant.

Results

Fungal cell walls and glycogen	magenta to red
Background	pale green

Quality control/notes

A solution of 5% aqueous sodium hypochlorite reduces over-staining by Schiff's.

A SELECTION OF THE MORE IMPORTANT FUNGI AND ACTINOMYCETES

Actinomyces israelii is a colonial bacterium which can be found as a commensal in the mouth and tonsillar crypts. It can cause a chronic suppurative infection, actinomycosis, which is characterized by multiple abscesses drained by sinus tracts. Actinomycotic abscesses can be found in liver, appendix, lung, and neck. The individual organisms are Gram-positive, hematoxyphilic, non-acid-fast, branching filaments 1 micron in diameter. They become coated in 'clubs' of Splendore–Hoeppli protein when the organism is invasive. These clubs are eosinophilic, acid-fast, 1–15 μm wide, and up to 100 μm long, and stain polyclonally for immunoglobulins. This arrangement of a clump of actinomyces or fungal hyphae, which measures 30–3000 μm, surrounded by eosinophilic protein, is called a 'sulfur' granule and is an important identification marker for certain fungal groups. These granules may be macroscopically visible and their yellow color is an important diagnostic aid.

Nocardia asteroides is another actinomycete. It is filamentous and may be visible in an H&E stain, but is Grocott positive and variably acid-fast using the modified Ziehl–Neelsen for leprosy; however, it is difficult to demonstrate even with the acid-fast bacillus. Its pathology is similar to that of actinomycosis, but its organisms are generally more disseminated than those of actinomycosis.

Candida albicans is a common fungus, but with immunosuppression can become systemic. It infects the mouth as thrush, the esophagus, the vagina as vaginal moniliasis, the skin and nails, and is in heart-valve vegetations. It is seen as both ovoid budding yeast-form cells of 3–4 μm, and more commonly as slender 3–5-μm, sparsely septate, non-branching hyphae and pseudo-hyphae. While difficult to see on H&E, this organism is strongly Gram positive, and is obvious with the Grocott and PAS techniques.

Aspergillus fumigatus is a soil saprophyte and a commensal in the bronchial tree. It may infect old lung cavities (Fig. 17.3) or become systemic in immunosuppressed patients. The fungus has broad, 3–6-μm, parallel-sided, septate hyphae showing dichotomous (45°C) branching. It may be associated with Splendore–Hoeppli protein and sometimes forms fungal balls within tissue. This fungus may be seen in an H&E stain and is demonstrated well with a PAS or Grocott. When it grows exposed to air, the conidophoric fruiting body may be seen as *Aspergillus niger*, a black species that can cause infection of the ear.

Zygomycosis is an infrequently seen disease caused by a group of hyphated fungi belonging mainly to the genera *Mucor* and *Rhysopus*. They have thin-walled hyphae (infrequently septate) with non-parallel sides, ranging from 3 to 25 μm in diameter, branch irregularly, and often show empty bulbous hyphal swelling.

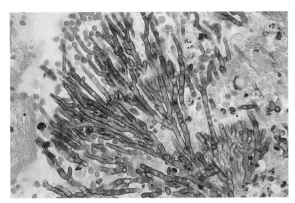

Fig. 17.3 A strong hematoxylin (Ehrlich's and eosin stain) will show the fine detail of many infectious agents. The hyphal structure identifies this as *Aspergillus* which was colonizing an old tuberculosis cavity in the lung (×100).

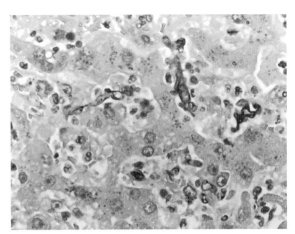

Fig. 17.5 Immunohistochemistry is being increasing applied to the demonstration of microorganisms using labeled specific antibody. This figure demonstrates *Zygomycetes*, a fast-growing fungus, with fast red chromogen (×20).

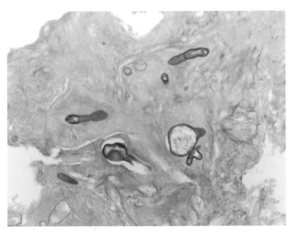

Fig. 17.4 *Rhizomucor* spp. (a cosmopolitan, filamentous fungus) is well demonstrated by this PAS stain with light green counterstain (×40).

Grocott and PAS are the staining methods of choice (Figs 17.4 and 17.5).

Cryptococcus neoformans exists solely in yeast-form cells, variable in diameter (2–20 μm) with ovoid, elliptical, and crescentic forms frequently seen. There is an extensive mucopolysaccharide coat around the yeasts that is mostly dissolved during processing, but, when present, appears as a halo around the organism and is visible with special stains such as Mayer's or Southgate's mucicarmine procedures. Yeasts may be free form or within the cytoplasm of giant cells, staining faintly with an H&E stain. The PAS and Grocott procedures demonstrate these cells well. Infection is found in the lungs and in the brain within the parenchyma or in the leptomeninges. Usually these patients are immunosuppressed.

Histoplasma capsulatum is another soil-dwelling yeast that can cause a systemic infection in humans called histoplasmosis. It is especially common along the southern border of the United States, and where there are large bird populations. The organism is usually seen within the cytoplasm of macrophages that appear stuffed with small, regular, 2–5-μm yeast-form cells that have a thin halo around them in H&E and Giemsa stains. Langhans' giant cells forming non-caseating granulomas may be present. PAS and Grocott stains demonstrate this fungus well (Fig. 17.6).

Pneumocystis carinii. There is still some debate over the taxonomy of this organism, although recent analysis of its ribosomal RNA has placed it nearer to a fungal than a protozoan classification (Edman et al 1988). It came to prominence as a pathogen following immunosuppressive therapies associated with renal transplants in the 1960s, and has become a life-threatening complication of AIDS. It most frequently causes pneumonia, where the lung alveoli are progressively filled with amphophilic, foamy plugs of parasites and cellular debris. It is found rarely in other sites such as intestines and lymph nodes. The cysts are invisible in an H&E stain, and can barely be seen in a Papanicolaou stain, as they

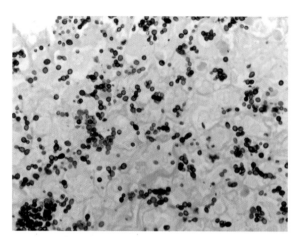

Fig. 17.6　Grocott's methenamine–silver stains a wide variety of infectious agents. Here seen with light green counterstain is the method of choice for *Histoplasma capsulatum*, a dimorphic endemic fungus (×63).

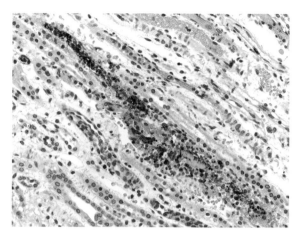

Fig. 17.7　Immunohistochemical method demonstrating Rocky Mountain spotted fever in kidney. It is caused by the bacterium *Rickettsia rickettsii*, which is carried by ticks (×20).

appear refractile when the microscope condenser is racked down. Specific antiserum is available to use; otherwise Grocott methenamine–silver is recommended.

Only electron microscopy or an H&E stain on a resin-embedded thin section will show their internal structure. The cysts are 4–6 μm in diameter and contain 5–8 dot-like intracystic bodies. The cysts rupture and collapse, liberating the trophozoites which can be seen as small hematoxyphilic dots in a good H&E and Giemsa stain; these attach to the alveolar epithelium by surface philopodia.

THE DEMONSTRATION OF RICKETTSIA

Rickettsial organisms, such as those causing Q fever, Rocky Mountain spotted fever, or typhus, rarely need to be demonstrated in tissue sections. They can sometimes be seen with a Giemsa stain, or by using the Macchiavello technique which also demonstrates some viral inclusion bodies (Fig. 17.7).

Macchiavello's stain for rickettsia and viral inclusions, modified (Culling 1974)

Sections
Formalin fixed, paraffin.

Method
1. Deparaffinize and rehydrate through graded alcohols to distilled water.
2. Stain in 0.25% basic fuchsin, 30 min.
3. Differentiate in 0.5% citric acid, 3 seconds.
4. Wash in tap water, 2 min.
5. Counterstain in 1% methylene blue, 15–30 seconds.
6. Rinse in tap water.
7. Dehydrate, clear, and mount.

Results

Rickettsia and some viral inclusions	red
Background	blue

THE DETECTION AND IDENTIFICATION OF VIRUSES

While the cytopathic effects of viruses can often be seen in a good H&E stain, and may be peculiar to a single viral group, the individual viral particles are too small to be seen with the light microscope, thus requiring the electron microscope to reveal their structure. This allows a rapid and accurate diagnosis in viral infections; an outline of the value of electron microscopy in the diagnosis of viral lesions is given in Chapter 30. Some viruses aggregate within cells to produce *viral inclusion bodies*, that may be intranuclear, intracytoplasmic, or both. These inclusion bodies may be acidophilic and usually intranuclear, or can be basophilic and cytoplasmic. Most special staining methods are modified trichromes, using contrasting acid and basic dyes to exploit these differences in charges on the inclusion body and the host cell. These methods include Mann's methyl blue–eosin stain for the Negri bodies of rabies, Machiavello's method, and more recently the elegant Lendrum's phloxine–tartrazine stain. Unfortunately, the need for optical differentiation in these methods increases the chance of technical error.

The introduction of commercially available monoclonal antibodies to viruses, which are either class- or species specific, has revolutionized the tissue detection of viruses. Hepatitis B virus is a good example of the diagnostic value of this technique where the surface antigen (HBs or Australia antigen) and the core antigen (HBc) can be specifically detected immunohistochemically, providing clinically important information about the stage of this disease. More recently, nucleic acid hybridization probes have become available and can be used to detect genomically inserted viral nucleic acid in situ, in cells and tissues that are frozen or formalin fixed. It should be remembered, however, that the detection of microorganisms using nucleic acid probes, unlike specific biotinylated antiserum, does not necessarily mean active disease.

Phloxine–tartrazine technique for viral inclusions (Lendrum 1947)

Sections
Formalin fixed, paraffin.

Solutions
Phloxine
Phloxine	0.5 g
Calcium chloride	0.5 g
Distilled water	100 ml

Tartrazine
A saturated solution of tartrazine in 2-ethoxyethanol, or cellosolve.

Method
1. Deparaffinize and rehydrate through graded alcohols to distilled water.
2. Stain nuclei in alum hematoxylin (Carazzi's or Harris's), 10 min.
3. Wash in running tap water, 5 min.
4. Stain in phloxine solution, 20 min.
5. Rinse in tap water and blot dry.

6. Controlling with the microscope, stain in tartrazine until only the viral inclusions remain strongly red, 5–10 min on average.
7. Rinse in 95% alcohol.
8. Dehydrate, clear, and mount.

Results
Viral inclusions	bright red
Red blood cells	variably orange–red
Nuclei	blue–gray
Background	yellow

Notes
All tissue is stained red with phloxine which is then differentiated by displacement with the counterstain, tartrazine. The red color is first removed from muscle, then other connective tissues. Paneth cells, Russell bodies, and keratin can be almost as dye retentive as viral inclusions, and can occasionally be a source of confusion.

Shikata's orcein method for hepatitis B surface antigen (modified Shikata et al 1974)

Sections
Formalin fixed, paraffin.

Solutions
Acid permanganate
0.25% potassium permanganate	95 ml
3% aqueous sulfuric acid	5 ml

Orcein
Orcein (synthetic)	1 g
70% alcohol	100 ml
Concentrated hydrochloric acid (gives a pH of 1–2)	1 ml

Saturated tartrazine in cellosolve (2-ethoxyethanol).

Method
1. Deparaffinize and rehydrate through graded alcohols to distilled water.
2. Treat with acid permanganate solution, 5 min.
3. Bleach until colorless with 1.5% aqueous oxalic acid, 30 seconds.
4. Wash in distilled water, 5 min, then in 70% alcohol.

5. Stain in orcein solution at room temperature, 4 hours, or in a Coplin jar of 37°C pre-heated orcein, 90 min.
6. Rinse in distilled alcohol and examine microscopically to determine desired staining intensity.
7. Rinse in cellosolve, stain in tartrazine, 2 min.
8. Rinse in cellosolve, clear, and mount.

Results

Hepatitis B-affected cells, elastic and some mucins	brown–black
Background	yellow

Notes

The success of this method largely depends on the particular batch of orcein used, and on freshly prepared solutions. This method relies on permanganate oxidizing of sulfur-containing proteins to sulfonate residues that react with orcein. Results compare well with those obtained using labeled antibodies, but the selectivity is inferior.

IMMUNOHISTOCHEMISTRY

Immunohistochemistry is now a routine and invaluable procedure in the histopathology lab for the detection of many microorganisms. There are many commercially available antibodies for viral, bacterial, and parasitic organisms. Most methods today utilize (strept)avidin–biotin technologies. These are based on the high affinity that (strept)avidin (*Streptomyces avidinii*) and avidin (chicken egg) have for biotin. Both possess four binding sites for biotin, but due to the molecular orientation of the binding sites fewer than four molecules of biotin will actually bind. The basic sequence of reagent application consists of primary antibody, biotinylated secondary antibody, followed by either the preformed (strept)avidin–biotin enzyme complex of the avidin-biotin complex (ABC) technique or by the enzyme-labeled streptavidin. Both conclude with the substrate solution. Horseradish peroxidase and alkaline phosphatases are the most commonly used enzyme labels. (Handbook of Immunohistochemical Staining Methods, 3rd edn. DAKO Corporation.)

SOME IMPORTANT VIRAL INFECTIONS

This summary is presented because of the viruses that are likely to be encountered in surgical and post-mortem histopathology and cytopathology (Table 17.3).

Viral hepatitis. To date, five hepatitis viruses have been reported, hepatitis viruses (HV) A, B, C, D, and E, that show great biological diversity, and three of which are incompletely characterized. The liver is the target organ and damage varies with the viral strain, ranging

Table 17.3 Viral infections seen in histopathology

Virus	Family	Genome	Disease
Measles	Paramyxo	SS RNA	Measles
Varicella-zoster	Herpes	DS DNA	Chickenpox, shingles
Herpes simplex	Herpes	DS DNA	Cold sores
Herpes genitalis	Herpes	DS DNA	Genital herpes
Cytomegalovirus (CMV)	Herpes	DS DNA	Cytomegalic inclusion disease
Epstein–Barr virus	Herpes	DS DNA	Glandular fever, African Burkitt's lymphoma
Human T-cell leukemia virus (HTLV-1)	Retro	SS RNA	Adult T-cell leukemia
Human immunodeficiency virus (HIV)	Retro	SS RNA	AIDS
Human papilloma virus (HPV)	Papova	DS DNA	Human wart viruses
JC virus	Papova	DS DNA	Progressive, multifocal leucoencephalopathy
Poliovirus	Picorna	SS DNA	Poliomyelitis
Molluscum virus	Pox	DS DNA	Molluscum contagiosum
Lyssavirus	Rhabdo	SS RNA	Rabies

DS = double-stranded; SS = single-stranded

from massive acute necrosis to chronic 'piecemeal necrosis' of liver cells, leading to cirrhosis. An eosinophilic 'ground glass' appearance is seen in the cytoplasm of some hepatocytes, due to dilated smooth endoplasmic reticulum that contains tubular HB surface antigen. It is this component that can be demonstrated using Shikata's orcein method, or by specific antiserum.

Herpes viruses are usually acquired subclinically during early life and enter a latent phase, to be reactivated during times of immunological stress. These viruses cause blistering or ulceration of the skin and mucous membranes, but can cause systemic diseases, including encephalitis, in immunosuppressed or malnourished individuals. The cytopathic effects of the herpes virus are well seen in Tzanck smears of blister fluid, and include the margination of chromatin along nuclear membranes, Cowdry type A ('owl's eye') inclusion bodies, and syncytial or 'grape-like' nuclei within giant cells. *Cytomegalovirus* (CMV) is sometimes seen as a systemic opportunistic infection in AIDS patients. It is seen in the endothelial cells, forming prominent intranuclear inclusions that spill into the cytoplasm where they form granular hematoxyphilic clusters. The CMV virus causes obvious cytomegaly in the cells it infects. All herpes viruses have an identical electron microscopic appearance of spherical, 120-nm, membrane-coated particles.

Papilloma viruses are a family of about 50 wart viruses that cause raised verrucous or papillomatous skin warts, or flat condylomatous genital warts. Cytologically, evidence of hyperkeratosis may be present together with koilocytosis (irregular nuclear enlargement and cytoplasmic vacuolation forming perinuclear halos). Skin verrucas are associated with HPV 1–4 strains, genital condylomas with HPV 6, 11, 16, and 18, and cervical cancer with HPV 16 and 18. These uncoated viruses measure 55 nm, are mainly intranuclear, and can be detected using electron microscopy, or immunoperoxidase and gene probes on paraffin sections.

JC virus is a papova virus that causes progressive multifocal leucoencephalopathy, a demyelinating disease, in AIDS and other immunosuppressed patients. Intranuclear hematoxyphilic inclusions may be seen within swollen oligodendrocytes.

Molluscum virus produces a contagious wart in children and young adults called molluscum contagiosum. Large eosinophilic, intracytoplasmic inclusion bodies can be seen in maturing keratinocytes, and are seen well with phloxine–tartrazine. The large 1-μm viral particles

have a typical pox virus structure: brick-shaped with a superimposed figure-of-eight nucleic acid sequence.

Rabies virus. This neurotrophic rhabdovirus forms intracytoplasmic eosinophilic inclusions best seen in the axonal hillocks of hippocampal neurons of the brain. Machiavello, phloxine–tartrazine, Mann's methyl blue–eosin, or PAS stains are recommended.

Human immunodeficiency virus (HIV) consists of at least two retrovirus strains. The virus is best seen in cultured lymphocytes and is rarely seen in tissues from AIDS patients. It produces a distinctive neuropathological lesion in AIDS encephalitis consisting of microglial nodules, or stars, containing collections of giant cells, microglia, and astrocytes. Synthetic nucleic acid probes have been prepared to HIV genomes.

Influenza virus (flu) is a contagious respiratory illness caused by influenza viruses (Fig. 17.8). It can cause mild to severe illness, and at times can lead to death. According to the Centers for Disease Control (CDC), every year in the United States, on average:

- 5–20% of the population suffers from the flu
- more than 200,000 people are hospitalized from flu complications
- about 36,000 people die from flu.

Some people, such as older people, young children, and people with certain health conditions, are at high risk for serious flu complications.

SARS (severe acute respiratory syndrome) is a viral respiratory illness caused by a coronavirus called SARS-associated coronavirus (SARS-CoV) (Fig. 17.9). SARS

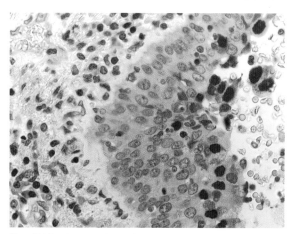

Fig. 17.8 Immunohistochemical method demonstrating Flu A (which is caused by influenza viruses) in bronchus (×40).

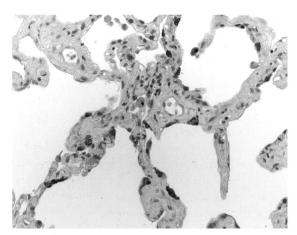

Fig. 17.9 Immunohistochemical method demonstrating the previously unrecognized SARS-associated coronavirus which is responsible for severe acute respiratory syndrome (SARS) (×20).

The CJD Surveillance Center in the USA is an invaluable source for monitoring and testing of human prion disease in the United States. The Center is supported by the CDC and by the American Association of Neuropathologists. Visit their website (http://www.cjdsurveillance.com) for details on how to submit specimens for testing; they perform these tests at no charge for laboratories in the USA. In addition, both CDC and the World Health Organization (WHO) also offer guidelines regarding the handling of suspected and known cases of prion disease. Visit http://www.cdc.gov and search for CJD for a fact sheet and other relevant information. WHO offers a manual in pdf form for downloading. It gives information about what to do should you find yourself with a suspected or known positive case in your lab: http://who.int/bloodproducts/TSE-manual2003.pdf. Remember that these types of cases should never knowingly be handled in a routine histology lab. Contact your local health department for additional guidelines.

was first reported in Asia in February 2003. Over the next few months, the illness spread to more than two dozen countries in North America, South America, Europe, and Asia before the SARS global outbreak of 2003 was contained.

PRION DISEASE

To date, more than eight transmissible neurodegenerative diseases have been described affecting the central nervous system (CNS). The diseases caused by prions include Creutzfeldt–Jakob disease (CJD) and variant CJD (vCJD), Germann–Straussler–Shienker disease, fatal familial insomnia, and kuru in humans, bovine spongiform encephalopathy (BSE, also known as 'mad cow disease'), scrapie (in goats and sheep), and chronic wasting disease (CWD) (in mule deer and elk). In addition, prions are not microbes in the usual sense because they are not alive, but the illness they cause can be transmitted from one animal to another. All usually produce a characteristic spongiform change, neuronal death, and astrocytosis in affected brains. The infectious agent is a prion, a small peptide, free of nucleic acid and part of a normal transmembrane glycoprotein which is not, strictly speaking, a virus. Antibodies have been prepared from prion protein that strongly mark accumulated abnormal protein in these diseases (Lantos 1992).

THE DEMONSTRATION OF PROTOZOA AND OTHER ORGANISMS

The identification of protozoa is most often made on morphological appearance using H&E and, particularly, Giemsa stains. The availability of antisera against organisms such as entamoeba, toxoplasma, and leishmania has made diagnosis much easier in difficult cases (Fig. 17.10).

Giemsa stain for parasites

Sections
Fixative is not critical, but B5 or Zenker's is preferred; thin (3 μm) paraffin sections. (If Zenker's is not used, post-mordant in Zenker's in a 60°C oven for 1 hour before staining.)

Solutions
Giemsa stock (commercially available) or

Giemsa stain powder	4 g
Glycerol	250 ml
Methanol	250 ml

Dissolve powder in glycerol at 60°C with regular shaking. Add methanol, shake the mixture, and allow to stand for 7 days. Filter before use.

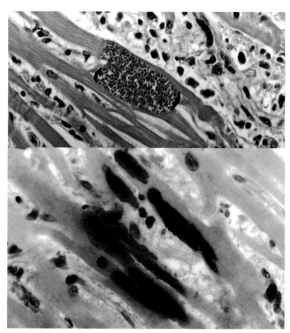

Fig. 17.10 H&E and immunohistochemical methods demonstrating the single-celled parasite *Toxoplasma gondii* in heart (×40).

Working Giemsa for parasites

Giemsa stock	4 ml
Acetate buffered distilled water, pH 6.8	96 ml

Method

1. Deparaffinize and rehydrate through graded alcohols to water.
2. Rinse in pH 6.8 buffered distilled water.
3. Stain in working Giemsa, overnight.
4. Rinse in distilled water.
5. Rinse in 0.5% aqueous acetic acid until section is pink.
6. Wash in tap water.
7. Blot until almost dry.
8. Dehydrate rapidly through alcohols, clear, and mount.

Results

Protozoa and some other microorganisms	dark blue
Background	pink–pale blue
Nuclei	blue

Protozoa

Entamoeba histolytica, the organism causing amebic colitis or dysentery, can be found in ulcers that occur in infected colon and in amebic liver abscesses. The trophozoite (adult form) measures 15–50 μm, contains a small nucleus, and has a foamy cytoplasm containing ingested red cells and white cell debris. They may be seen in granulation tissue within ulcers, or in the luminal mucus overlying normal appearing mucosa, and are PAS positive; brief counterstaining in 1% aqueous metanil yellow emphasizes the ingested red cells.

Toxoplasma gondii, a commonly encountered organism that is spread in cat litter, causes an acute lymphadenopathy which is often subclinical. Affected nodes show non-specific changes and no organisms. In AIDS and other immunosuppressed patients this protozoon causes systemic diseases, including meningoencephalitis where encysted bradyzoites and free tachyzoites can be seen in necrotic brain tissue. Cysts also occur in other tissues such as cardiac muscle, and measure up to 40 μm with tachyzoites 4–6 μm, which can be seen on H&E. A Giemsa stain can also be used, but the use of labeled specific antiserum is recommended.

Leishmania tropica is transmitted by sandfly bite and causes a chronic inflammatory disease of the skin sometimes called cutaneous leishmaniasis. The injected parasite forms (2 μm), or amastigotes, are found in large numbers within the cytoplasm of multiple swollen histiocytes that congregate in early lesions in the dermis. A related organism, *L. donovani*, causes a systemic visceral infection, kala azar, in which the organisms are seen within histiocytes in spleen, lymph nodes, liver, and bone marrow. The organisms are hematoxyphilic and can be emphasized with a Giemsa stain.

Giardia duodenalis (lamblia) is a flagellate protozoon that is ingested in cyst form from drinking water with fecal contamination; the trophozoites migrate to the duodenum where they may cause severe diarrhea and malabsorption. These organisms can easily be missed on an H&E stain, where they appear as eosinophilic, sickle-shaped flakes with indistinct nuclei resting on intestinal mucosa that may show little evidence of inflammation. When seen in a fresh Giemsa-stained duodenal aspirate, they appear kite-shaped, 11–18 μm in size, binucleate, and have faint terminal flagella.

Trichomonas vaginalis is a similar flagellate protozoon most frequently seen in a Papanicolaou stain. Inflammatory cells and mildly dysplastic squamous cells often accompany this parasite as it causes cervicitis in the female, and urethritis in both sexes.

Cryptosporidium is one of a group of protozoa (including *Isospora* and *Microsporidium*) that causes severe and relentless outbreaks of diarrhea among AIDS patients. Cryptosporidial gametes are seen on H&E stain as blue dots arranged along the mucosal surface. Mature cysts are shed into feces and are acid fast in a ZN stain of fecal smears.

WORMS

Schistosoma species cause the disease schistosomiasis or 'bilharzia'. Various manifestations of the disease differ according to the particular *Schistosoma* species involved, but granulomata containing schistosome ova are found in the liver, bowel, and bladder mucosa, and sometimes in the lungs. The ova have thick, refractile, eosinophilic walls and are easily detected in H&E-stained sections. The PAS, Grocott, and ZN techniques are positive for these ova. Where the plane of section allows, the presence of a terminal spine to the ovum indicates *S. haematobium* whereas *S. mansoni* and *japonicum* have lateral spines. Any good trichrome procedure will demonstrate worm development.

Echinococcosis. Echinococcus granulosus is a tapeworm found in dogs; humans and sheep may become intermediate hosts and develop hydatid cyst disease. These cysts form in many organs, particularly liver and lung. The walls of the daughter cysts are faintly eosinophilic, characteristically laminated, and produced by the worm, not by its host. The walls are PAS positive and Congo red positive, showing green birefringence. The scolicial hooklets survive inside old, burnt-out cysts, are of diagnostic shape, and stain brilliant yellow with picric acid.

Acknowledgments

Alan Stevens contributed this chapter for the first three editions, and he and Bob Francis updated the fourth edition. Billie Swisher contributed the chapter for the fifth edition. Our acknowledgments are due to them for their contributions. I would also like to thank Sherif Zaki, Jeannette Guarner, and Mitesh Patel for their assistance with this chapter.

REFERENCES

Brown P., Wolff A., Gajdusek D.C. (1990) A simple and effective method for inactivating virus infectivity in formalin-fixed samples from patients with Creutzfeldt–Jakob diseases. Neuropathology 40:887.

Chandler F.W., Kaplan W., Ajello, L. (1980) A colour atlas and textbook of the histopathology of mycotic diseases. London: Wolfe Medical, pp. 109–111.

Churukian C.J., Schenk, E.A. (1982) A method for demonstrating Gram-positive and Gram-negative bacteria. Journal of Histotechnology 5(3):127.

Crowder C, Taylor H. (1996) Modified Fite stain for demonstration of mycobacterium species in tissue sections. Journal of Histotechnology 19(2):133–134.

Culling C.F.A. (1974) Handbook of histopathological and histochemical techniques, 3rd edn. London: Butterworths.

Edman J.C., Kovacs J.A., Masur H. et al. (1988) Ribosomal RNA sequence shows *Pneumocystis carinii* to be a member of the fungi. Nature 334:519.

Gimenez D.F. (1964) Staining rickettsia in yolk sac cultures. Stain Technology 39:135–140.

Gomori G. (1946) A new histochemical test for glycogen and mucin. American Journal of Clinical Pathology 16:177.

Grocott R.G. (1955) A stain for fungi in tissue sections and smears. American Journal of Clinical Pathology 25:975.

Kinyoun J.J. (1915) A note on Uhlenhuth's method for sputum examination for tubercle bacilli. American Journal of Public Health 5:867–870.

Kuper S.W.A., May J.R. (1960) Detection of acid-fast organisms in tissue sections by fluorescence microscopy. Journal of Pathology and Bacteriology 79:59.

Lantos P.L. (1992) From slow virus to prion; a review of the transmissible spongiform encephalopathies. Histopathology 20:1.

Lendrum A.C. (1947) The phloxine–tartrazine method as a general histological stain for the demonstration of inclusion bodies. Journal of Pathology and Bacteriology 59:399.

McMullen L., Walker M.M., Bain L.A. et al. (1987) Histological identification of campylobacter using Gimenez technique in gastric antral mucosa. Journal of Clinical Pathology 464–465.

Ollett W.S. (1947) A method for staining both Gram positive and Gram negative bacteria in sections. Journal of Pathology and Bacteriology 59:357.

Shikata T., Uzawa T., Yoshiwara N. et al. (1974) Staining methods of Australia antigen in paraffin section—detection of cytoplasmic inclusion bodies. Japanese Journal of Experimental Medicine 44:25.

Steiner G., Steiner G. (1944) New simple silver stain for demonstration of bacteria, spirochetes, and fungi in sections of paraffin embedded tissue blocks. Journal of Laboratory and Clinical Medicine 29:868–871.

Swisher B.L. (1987) Modified Steiner procedure for microwave staining of spirochetes and nonfilamentous bacteria. Journal of Histotechnology 10:241–243.

Swisher B.L., Chandler F.W. (1982) Grocott methenamine silver method for detecting fungi: practical considerations. Laboratory Medicine 13:568–570.

Swisher B.L., Nicholson M.A. (1989) Development of staining controls for *Campylobacter pylori*. Journal of Histotechnology 12:299–301.

Tomkins D.S., Foulkes S.F., Goodwin P.G.R., West A.P. (1986) Isolation and characterization of intestinal spirochetes. Journal of Clinical Pathology 39:535.

Twort F.W. (1924) An improved neutral red, light green double stain for staining animal parasites, microorganisms and tissues. Journal of State Medicine 32:351.

von Lichtenberg F. (1991) Pathology of infectious diseases. New York: Raven Press.

Warthin A.S., Starry A.C. (1920) A more rapid and improved method of demonstrating spirochetes in tissues.

American Journal of Syphilis, Gonorrhea, and Veneral Diseases 4:97.

WEBSITE

'Man and Microbes'. Microbiology at Leicester. Available: http://www.microbiologybytes.com/iandi/1a.html

FURTHER READING

Boenisch T., ed. (2001) Immunochemical staining methods handbook, 3rd edn. Carpinteria, CA: DAKO Corporation.

Luna L., ed. (1968) Manual of histologic staining methods of the Armed Forces Institute of Pathology, 3rd edn, New York: McGraw-Hill, pp. 158–159.

Neelsen F. (1883) Ein Casuistischer Beitrag zur Lehre von Tuberkulose. Zentralblatt fur die Medizinischen Wissenschaften 21:497.

Ziehl F. (1882) Zur Farbung des Tuberkelbacillus. Deutsche Medizinische Wochenschrift 8:451.

18

Bone

Gayle M. Callis

NORMAL BONE

Two types of bone can be recognized macroscopically in the normal adult human skeleton. Cortical or compact bone is the solid, hard, and immensely strong bone that form the shafts of long bones, e.g. femur, tibia, etc., and exterior surfaces of the flat bones, e.g. ribs and skull.

Trabecular, cancellous, or spongy bone is found in the diaphysis, epiphysis, and marrow cavities of long bones, vertebrae, and centers of flat bones. It is a mesh of bone strands each about 1 mm thick and, although it looks less solid than cortical bone, this arrangement of trabeculae, particularly in the femoral head and vertebrae, forms an almost ideal weight-bearing structure.

The three major components of bone are mineral, cells, and an organic extracellular matrix, i.e. collagen fibers and ground substance. These are dynamic components for, as cells are dying and being replaced, the collagen and mineral are being eroded and reformed continually throughout healthy adult life. This process is called remodeling and consists of resorption and deposition taking place in equilibrium so that the volume and shape of bones stays more or less constant. In later life, remodeling slows down, and deposition may not keep up with resorption, causing increased bone porosity and brittleness, and, in extreme cases, the disease osteoporosis.

The main bulk of bone is approximately 70% mineral and 30% organic components by weight. Bone cells, as opposed to marrow cells, are relatively sparse.

Bone collagen

The bone collagen differs from other collagen in the body in that it becomes mineralized and is laid down in bands or lamellae roughly parallel to one another. The collagen fibers within each lamella tend to lie next each other but at an angle to the fibers in adjacent lamellae. A cement or proteoglycan ground substance outlining these fibers is seen in sections only at the reversal or cement lines. The organization of collagen lamellae is responsible for the distinctive micro-anatomical patterns of bone which are easily seen with polarized light microscopy (Fig. 18.1)

The simplest pattern occurs on the periosteal and endosteal surfaces of compact bone as circumferential lamellae, and in trabecular or non-Haversian bone where lamellae are roughly parallel to the surface. Cortical bone is composed of Haversian systems or osteons in which concentric lamellae surround channels (Volkmann's canals) containing one or more blood vessels. These tubular structures run longitudinally in the bone and are packed closely together with irregular interstices filled by the remnants of older osteons (Fig. 18.2). Cement lines outline the boundaries of osteons, and some trabecular and circumferential lamellae.

Another collagen fiber arrangement forms non-lamellar or woven bone and is found in immature bone and some pathological conditions. This collagen is not deposited in the lamellae but in thick, short, randomly oriented bundles. When viewed with polarized light, these appear as coarse fibers resembling a woven tweed fabric.

Unmineralized collagen or osteoid forms a border or seam on surfaces of newly formed bone, and after osteoid is deposited there is a lag before it becomes mineralized. Osteoid is normally around 15 μm thick, covering only a small proportion of the surfaces, but in some diseases, e.g. rickets or osteomalacia, is much thicker and widespread. On inactive surfaces osteoid is very thin, difficult

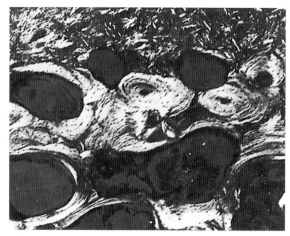

Fig. 18.1 Lamellar and non-lamellar (woven) bone of normal rib from child aged 2¹/₂ years. Celloidin section; polarized light.

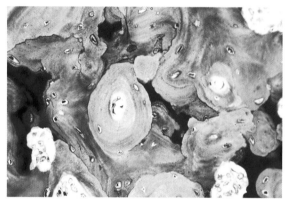

Fig. 18.2 Haversian systems (osteons, Volkmann's canals, and bone cells) in ground section of undecalcified bone in methacrylate, acid etched/surfaced stained with Sanderson's rapid bone stain. (original magnification ×40.)

to see, and is completely absent where resorption is taking place.

Bone mineral

The mineral of bone is mainly calcium and phosphate combined with hydroxyl ions to form hydroxyapatite crystals. The mineral is approximately 38% calcium and thought to be deposited as amorphous calcium phosphate in the initial mineralization phase. This transforms to hydroxyapatite by addition of hydroxyl ions to form a crystal lattice into which carbonate, citrate, and fluoride ions as well as magnesium, potassium, and strontium

can be substituted or included. Carbonate is present in large quantities but probably only in the hydration shell and on crystal surfaces.

The hydroxyapatite forms needle-like crystals about 22 nm in length, resulting in an enormous total crystal surface area. Thus, the mineral fulfils the obvious function of giving strength and rigidity while approximately 20% remains in the amorphous form to provide a readily available buffer for maintaining total body chemical equilibrium, e.g. pH, enzyme systems.

Bone cells

There are three types of bone cell other than the marrow cells belonging to the hemopoietic system.

Osteoblasts

Although the name suggests immaturity, osteoblasts are fully differentiated to carry out the primary function of bone formation by producing and laying down osteoid. They are seen on surfaces of actively forming bone as plump cells with basophilic cytoplasm and eccentric nuclei distal to the bone surface. The cytoplasm is basophilic due to ribonucleic acid, and before becoming fully differentiated frequently contains glycogen. Acid phosphatase is found in osteoblasts and the surrounding tissues, but decreases at onset of calcification. Upon completion of bone formation duties, most osteoblasts revert to a quiescent undifferentiated state and reside among the heterogeneous cell population.

Osteocytes

In one respect osteoblasts do represent immature cells for some are trapped in the osteoid matrix they lay down, and become mature osteocytes residing in tiny spaces or lacunae within the bone. Lacunae are connected to each other and to the vascular spaces by canaliculi, tiny channels into which osteocyte processes project for the purpose of passing fluids and dissolved substances necessary for cell metabolism (see Fig. 18.6 p. 347).

Osteoclasts

These are the cells responsible for bone resorption or erosion. Osteoclasts are large multinucleated giant cells whose cytoplasm contains numerous mitochondria and alkaline phosphatase. They occur in small clusters or singly on bone surfaces undergoing resorption and are often seen in the depressions (Howship's lacunae) they are actively eroding. These surfaces have an irregular outline and lack osteoid (Fig. 18.3). The direction of resorption is random, with no relationship to lamellar structure. Osteoclasts respond to altered mechanical stresses on the skeleton and to growth, and their activity contributes to remodeling. Osteoclasts respond to hormones that can either stimulate or inhibit their activity. When resorption halts, the process of bone formation resumes (osteoid, mineralization, etc.). Cement lines will occur at the junction between old and newly formed bone.

Development and growth

Bone develops in two different ways according to the site and shape of the bone. It begins early in the embryo and is not complete until approximately 15 years of age.

Intramembranous ossification

This occurs in flat bones, e.g. skull, sternum, pelvic bones. A fibrous membrane first develops at the bone formation site in which mesenchymal cells differentiate into osteoblasts that begin the bone formation process by laying down osteoid. This starts in small islets that gradually unite to become trabeculae and finally form an external layer of compact bone.

Endochondral ossification

This occurs in long bones and major parts of the skeleton. This type of bone development begins with differentiation of mesechymal cells at sites where bone will be formed, but this bone is laid down in a cartilage model that resembles the final shape of the bone. This cartilage model becomes covered with a connective tissue sheath or perichondrium and grows by both apposition and interstitially. Appositional growth or the laying down of more cartilage begins towards the exterior and is mainly responsible for increased diameter; interstitial growth is by cells dividing within the model and mainly occurs towards the extremities resulting in increased length.

In the central part of the model, cells continue to differentiate, cartilage begins to calcify, blood vessels invade, and the cartilage is broken up into strands. Ossification, by differentiation of perichondral cells into osteoblasts, begins around the exterior of the primary ossification site at the center of the model. Osteoblasts invade the strands of calcified cartilage and deposit osteoid that soon becomes calcified. This process continues and secondary ossification sites appear at each end of the model, separated from a now bony shaft by cartilage growth or epiphyseal plates capable of interstitial growth. Once bone has ossified, it can only grow by apposition. Remodeling is continuous; in some places deposition exceeds resorption, in others this is reversed and results in the characteristic shape of the bone. When bone is fully grown, the three ossification sites unite and the cartilage growth plates disappear.

BONE TECHNIQUES

Techniques for the demonstration of bone and its components are possibly more varied and difficult than for any other tissue. They include:

- for decalcified bone: frozen, paraffin, or celloidin sections, and transmission electron microscopy (EM)
- for mineralized bone: frozen, plastic for microtomed or sawn/ground sections, scanning and transmission EM.

Mineralized sections are used for microradiographic and histomorphometric studies as well as polarized and fluorescent light microscopy. The technique chosen for examination of bone is influenced by the initial clinical diagnosis, case urgency, and the extent of investigation.

Specimens arriving in the laboratory can vary in size from a needle biopsy a few millimeters long to a whole arm or leg amputation, or large specimens in need of special immediate attention.

Biopsies

For diagnosis of tumor, hemopoietic disorders, infection, etc. These are treated much like soft tissue except that a

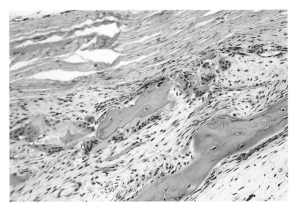

Fig. 18.3 Osteoclasts lining trabecular bone. Decalcified bovine rib, 3-μm paraffin section. Hematoxylin and eosin stain. (Original magnification ×40.)

bone biopsy usually needs decalcification in order to produce paraffin sections. Whenever possible, specimen radiography of large or multiple bone fragments helps select the sample for processing. A bone marrow biopsy is usually removed with a Jamshidi needle for diagnosis of metabolic bone disease. Metabolic bone diseases are diagnosed using trabecular bone taken from the iliac crest, an accessible bone site representative of skeletal bone as a whole. This biopsy is removed with a bone trephine (Byers & Smith 1967) to produce a 6–8 × 2-cm bone core large enough for bone histomorphometry (p. 358).

Sections are required to assess the relationship between mineralized and unmineralized bone (osteoid). Consequently, mineralized bone sections embedded in methyl methacrylate (MMA) plastic is the preferred method for metabolic bone disease work (see p. 351). It is also possible to produce adequate frozen sections from an undecalcified bone biopsy (see p. 350). The silver impregnation method of Tripp and McKay (1972) demonstrates bone and osteoid in a decalcified, paraffin-embedded bone section, but MMA-embedded bone remains the chosen method.

Amputation specimens

As a result of tumor, chronic osteomyelitis, and gangrene, large amputation specimens are often delivered to the laboratory immediately after removal. They often are not in any container and without fixative, and must be dealt with as soon as possible. The majority of the limb is usually discarded and the area or lesion with actual or suspected involvement in the disease process retained for final evaluation. Skin, excess muscle, and connective tissue should be cut away, and either excess bone sawn or a joint disarticulated above and below the lesion. The relevant portions should be immersed into a large volume of fixative to insure adequate fixation. If it is not possible to care for the specimen for several hours after receipt, it should be refrigerated at 4°C. An available mortuary area has a dual advantage for both limb storage and subsequent sample preparation on an available autopsy table.

Resection specimens

Benign or low-grade malignant tumors and arthritic femoral heads resemble large biopsy specimens and frequently have an established diagnosis and are considered less urgent.

Fixation

Unless immediate diagnosis is needed using cryomicrotomy, all bone specimens must be totally fixed before subjecting them to any decalcification and processing procedures. Complete fixation helps protect bone and surrounding soft tissue from the damaging effects of acid decalcification. Ten per cent neutral buffered formalin (NBF) is suitable for both paraffin and non-tetracycline-labeled bone in MMA, with some fixatives reserved for specialized procedures. Alcoholic formalin or 70% ethanol fixation can be used to fix tetracycline-labeled mineralized bone in MMA, but is not recommended for bone destined for acid decalcification as alcohol can slow or prevent decalcification. Fixatives containing chloroform (Carnoy's) and mercury (B-5, Zenker's, Susa) should be avoided due to extreme chemical toxicity in addition to mercury making bone radio-opaque and unsuitable for specimen radiography.

Fixation proceeds faster by reducing the size of the bone, opening the bone, and removing excess skin and soft tissue surrounding the lesion. Large specimens can be bisected or reduced in size by sawing into multiple slabs, and immersed into fixative immediately, or no longer than 48 hours after initial fixation, then cut into smaller pieces and put into fresh fixative.

Sawing

A good band saw is an essential piece of equipment in a bone histology laboratory. Inexpensive, small, light-weight hobby shop or handyman's bench band saws designed to cut through wood, plastic, rubber, and some thin metals are useful. These saws cut through cortical bone slowly with cuts no deeper than 7.5 cm and saws for cutting dry materials may need wheel modifications to prevent blade slippage when cutting wet, fatty bone. A 'Wetter' or a meat cutter's saw overcomes these problems with heavier, rigid, floor-standing construction, strong coarse blades for deeper cuts, blade-cleaning devices, and debris catchers. The meat cutter's saw can be water-cooled to prevent heat damage to bone due to high speed sawing, and is capable of full-length cuts through long bones and appendages, e.g. femur, tibia, foot.

Suitable blade specifications on small saws are 0.5-cm width and 12 to 16 teeth per inch (tpi), making finer, cleaner cuts than a larger saw blade 1.25 cm wide with 6 tpi. Blades in specifications needed are available from tool companies.

Soft tissues and dense connective tissue, e.g. tendons, should be removed before sawing or the sample will drag through the blade. The first cut is made through the midplane, then approximately 3–5 mm thick slabs are cut parallel to the first cut. A saw guide plate or wood block held against the first cut edge ensures an even slice. It is safer for workers to hold thinner bones between two wood blocks that will not ruin blades. Sawing should be at a slow even rate to match speed of blade cutting into the bone. Pushing the bone produces uneven cuts, and may jam or break a blade.

Bone slabs should be fixed for an additional 24–48 hours especially if they appear pinkish-red or partially fixed. After sawing, any bone dust or debris adhering to slab surfaces can be cleaned away using a slow stream of water and a soft brush. Care must be taken not to push debris into marrow spaces or to wash slabs excessively before the bone is totally fixed.

Fine detail specimen radiography

Radiographs of bone slabs, blocks, or fragments are useful for four main purposes:

1. To examine the nature and extent of a lesion.
2. To provide a diagram of lesion prior to block selection for processing.
3. To check progress of decalcification, i.e. decalcification endpoint test.
4. To confirm the presence of foreign materials, e.g. prosthetic devices, metal or glass fragments implanted by trauma.

Thin bone slices give sharper image radiographs than a whole specimen or clinical radiographs. The use of 'soft' X-rays (of low kV) and high-contrast X-ray film provides finer detail and clarity (Fornasier 1975). Fine grain photographic film can be used, but is slower than the X-ray film, and after development unenlarged contact prints must be made from a negative. A standard clinical X-ray machine can be used if operated at its lowest kV setting, but the long exposures needed for slow high-contrast film are less suitable for precise results.

The 'Faxitron' (Faxitron Inc, USA) cabinet X-ray system, used for both bone work and mammography, is a tabletop unit measuring 56 cm wide × 51 cm deep × 89 cm high. The energy output is 10–110 kV with 3 mA tube current. In addition to the manual exposure capability, the unit should be equipped with its automatic exposure timer with 5 second to 60 minute setting at 1-second intervals. The cabinet has adjustable shelf levels for film-to-source distances of 31–61 mm and is fully lead lined to shield the operator from X-rays. A special door interlock safety device automatically turns off the X-ray beam if the door is opened during operation.

X-ray film (Kodak X-OMAT 2, Ready Pak; Kodak Ltd.) is used for specimen radiography. Initially, a bone slab should be radiographed using the automatic exposure timer, then exposure time, kV, and mA recorded. This eliminates guesswork for a first exposure and provides the correct exposure time and kV for a repeat radiograph or for subsequent manual exposures of adjacent bone slabs of the same thickness.

An example of manual exposure requirements is as follows:

- bone slab 3–5 mm thick on polyethylene sheet (moisture barrier)
- Kodak X-OMAT 2, Ready Pak (Kodak Ltd.)
- film to source distance (FTSD), 50 cm (lowest shelf level)
- settings, 30 kV (3 mA)
- exposure time approximately 1 min.

Exposure time is dependent on specimen thickness (thicker slabs require longer exposures), film to source distance (longer distance requires more time), and type of film used. Large, whole bones, e.g. proximal end of femur with metal prosthesis, can be radiographed using X-OMAT 2, FTSD (upper shelf), longer exposure time (approx. 8 minutes), and higher kV (70 kV). Soft tissues, cartilage, and tumor are more easily seen in underexposed radiographs, useful for evaluating surrounding soft tissue involvement by a bone tumor, e.g. osteosarcoma. The X-ray film can be developed quickly in a radiology department and viewed without delay.

Selection of blocks

In urgent cases of suspected tumor or infection, an attempt should be made to select a sample with the least mineralization in order to provide the quickest possible diagnosis. These pieces can be fixed, rapidly decalcified, and processed to meet urgency requirements.

Iliac crest trephine biopsies can be bisected longitudinally: half for decalcification and paraffin techniques, and half for undecalcified bone MMA sections. However, metabolic bone disease laboratories usually prefer a whole trephine bone core for plastic embedment. The Buehler Isomet Low Speed saw (Buehler Ltd., USA) uses a thin diamond-impregnated blade with a water-cooling bath and is ideal for bisecting these biopsies. This metallurgical saw can make precise, debris-free cuts through 8-mm thick bone cores, other cortical or trabecular and MMA-embedded bone specimens. Scalpel blades, fretted wire or jewellers' saws have been used to cut trephine biopsies but with damaging results. These cutting devices can crush or fracture fine trabeculae creating 'fracture artifact', and force bone fragments into marrow spaces, spoiling the bone histology. Jamshidi needle biopsies should remain whole for paraffin and plastic methods.

If a specimen radiograph is available, a diagram or 'map' of the lesion can be made from the X-ray and a representative sample selected from the mapped area of interest for processing.

The ideal thickness of bone pieces is 3–5 mm. If bone slabs are too thick, both decalcification and processing are prolonged while overly thin bone slabs (less than 2 mm) tend to release from paraffin wax during sectioning. The dense collagen matrix tends to prevent adequate paraffin wax penetration and thin pieces are not held firmly in the softer paraffin embedding media during microtomy.

Decalcification

In order to obtain satisfactory paraffin or celloidin sections of bone, inorganic calcium must be removed from the organic collagen matrix, calcified cartilage, and surrounding tissues. This is called decalcification and is carried out by chemical agents, either with acids to form soluble calcium salts or with chelating agents that bind to calcium ions. Even after decalcification, the dense collagen of cortical bone is remarkably tough and tends to harden more after paraffin processing. Occasionally, small foci of calcifications in paraffin-embedded or frozen tissues can be sectioned without much noticeable damage to the knife or disruption of surrounding tissue. After hematoxylin staining, these foci usually appear cracked and as dark purple granular masses with lighter purple halos.

The choice of decalcifier is influenced by four interdependent factors: urgency of the case, degree of mineralization, extent of the investigation, and staining techniques required.

Any acid, however well buffered, has some damaging effects on tissue stainability. This problem increases with acidity of solutions, i.e. lower pH, and length of decalcification periods. Consequently, the rapid decalcifiers are more likely to adversely affect any subsequent staining. This is most noticeable in cell nuclei with the failure of nuclear chromatin to take up hematoxylin and other basic dyes as readily as soft tissues never exposed to acid solutions. The staining by acid dyes is also less affected, but eosin can stain tissue a deep, unpleasant, brick red without its many differential shades. These effects on H&E staining can be reduced by doing the decalcification endpoint test, post-decalcification acid removal, and adjustment of the stain procedure (see p. 341).

Decalcifying agents

As noted previously there are two major types of decalcifying agent, i.e. acids and chelating agents, although Gray (1954) lists over 50 different mixtures. Many of these mixtures were developed for special purposes with one used as a fixing and dehydrating agent. Other mixtures contain reagents, e.g. buffer salts, chromic acid, formalin, or ethanol, intended to counteract the undesirable swelling effects acids have on tissues. Many popular mixtures used today are from the original formulas developed many years ago (Evans & Krajian 1930; Kristensen 1948; Clayden 1952). For most practical purposes, today's laboratories seem to prefer simpler solutions for routine work. Provided the bone is totally fixed and treated with a decalcifier suitable for removal of the amount of mineral present, the simple mixtures work as well or better than more complex mixtures.

Acid decalcifiers

Acid decalcifiers can be divided into two groups: strong (inorganic) and weak (organic) acids. As Brain (1966) suggested, many laboratories keep an acid from each group available for either rapid diagnostic or slower, routine work.

Proprietary decalcifiers

The components in proprietary decalcifying solutions are often trade secrets. Manufacturers provide Material Safety Data Sheets (MSDS) that frequently indicate the type and concentration of acid. Their product data sheets usually indicate if a solution is rapid or slow, give decalcification instructions and warnings against prolonged use. Rapid proprietary solutions usually contain hydrochloric acid (HCl) whereas slow proprietary mixtures contain buffered formic acid or formalin/formic acid. A study (Callis & Sterchi 1998) found that dilution of a proprietary HCl solution was not deleterious for effective decalcification or staining, and this is an option if a strong mixture is considered too concentrated. Although proprietary mixtures have no obvious advantages over solutions prepared in laboratories, their usage is increasingly popular in busy laboratories because they are reliable, time and cost effective while addressing safety issues by eliminating handling and storage of concentrated acids.

Strong inorganic acids, e.g. nitric, hydrochloric

These may be used as simple aqueous solutions with recommended concentrations of 5–10%. They decalcify rapidly, cause tissue swelling, and can seriously damage tissue stainability if used longer than 24–48 hours. Old nitric acid is particularly damaging, and should be replaced with fresh stock. Strong acids, however, tend to be more damaging to tissue antigens for immunohistochemical staining, and enzymes may be totally lost.

Strong acids are used for needle and small biopsy specimens to permit rapid diagnosis within 24 hours or less. They can be used for large or heavily mineralized cortical bone specimens with decalcification progress *carefully* monitored by a decalcification endpoint test (Callis & Sterchi 1998).

Aqueous nitric acid, 5–10% *(Clayden 1952)*

Nitric acid	5–10 ml
Distilled water to	100 ml

Perenyi's fluid *(Perenyi 1882)*

10% nitric acid	40 ml
Absolute ethanol	30 ml
0.5% chromic acid	30 ml

Mix shortly before use; chromic acid must be collected for proper disposal.

Formalin–nitric acid *(use inside a fume hood)*

Formaldehyde (37–40%)	10 ml
Distilled water	80 ml
Nitric acid	10 ml

Weak, organic acids, e.g. formic, acetic, picric

Of these, formic is the only weak acid used extensively as a primary decalcifier. Acetic and picric acids cause tissue swelling and are not used alone as decalcifiers but are found as components in Carnoy's and Bouin's fixatives (pp. 69 and 70). These fixatives will act as incidental,

although weak, decalcifiers and could be used in urgent cases with only minimal calcification. Formic acid solutions can be aqueous (5–10%), buffered or combined with formalin. The formalin–10% formic acid mixture simultaneously fixes and decalcifies, and is recommended for very small bone pieces or Jamshidi needle biopsies. However, it is still advisable to have complete fixation before any acid decalcifier is used. The salts, sodium formate (Kristensen 1948) or sodium citrate (Evans & Krajian 1930), are added to formic acid solutions making 'acidic' buffers. Buffering is used to counteract the injurious effects of the acid, but this, in addition to low 4–5% formic acid concentration, results in increased time needed for complete decalcification. Formic acid is gentler and slower than HCl or nitric acids, and is suitable for most routine surgical specimens particularly when immunohistochemical staining is needed. Formic acid can still damage tissue, antigens, and enzyme histochemical staining, and should be endpoint tested. Decalcification is usually complete in 1–10 days, depending on the size, type of bone, and acid concentration. Dense cortical or large bones have been effectively decalcified with 15% aqueous formic acid and a 4% hydrochloric acid–4% formic acid mixture (Callis & Sterchi 1998).

Aqueous formic acid

90% stock formic acid	5–10 ml
Distilled water to	100 ml

Formic acid–formalin *(after Gooding & Stewart 1932)*

90% stock formic acid	5–10 ml
Formaldehyde (37–40%)	5 ml
Distilled water to	100 ml

Buffered formic acid *(Evans & Krajian 1930)*

20% aqueous sodium citrate	65 ml
90% stock formic acid	35 ml

This solution has a pH of approximately 2.3.

Chelating agents

The chelating agent used for decalcification is ethylenediaminetetracetic acid (EDTA). Although EDTA is nominally 'acid', it does not act like inorganic or organic acids but binds metallic ions, notably calcium and magnesium. EDTA will not bind to calcium below pH 3 and is faster at pH 7–7.4; even though pH 8 and above gives optimal binding, the higher pH may damage alkaline-sensitive protein linkages (Callis & Sterchi 1998). EDTA binds to ionized calcium on the outside of the apatite crystal and as this layer becomes depleted more calcium ions reform from within; the crystal becomes progressively smaller during decalcification. This is a very slow process that does not damage tissues or their stainability. When time permits, EDTA is an excellent bone decalcifier for immunohistochemical or enzyme staining, and electron microscopy. Enzymes require specific pH conditions in order to maintain activity, and EDTA solutions can be adjusted to a specific pH for enzyme staining. EDTA does inactivate alkaline phosphatase but activity can be restored by addition of magnesium chloride.

EDTA and EDTA disodium salt (10%) or EDTA tetrasodium salt (14%) are approaching saturation and can be simple aqueous or buffered solutions at neutral pH of 7–7.4, or added to formalin. EDTA tetrasodium solution is alkaline, and the pH should be adjusted to 7.4 using concentrated acetic acid. The time required totally to decalcify dense cortical bone may be 6–8 weeks or longer, although small bone spicules may be decalcified in less than a week.

Formalin–EDTA (Hillemann & Lee 1953)

EDTA, disodium salt	5.5 g
Distilled water	90 ml
Formaldehyde (37–40% stock)	10 ml

EDTA (aqueous) pH 7.0–7.4

EDTA, disodium salt	250 g
Distilled water	1750 ml

If solution is cloudy, adjust to pH 7 with approximately 25 g sodium hydroxide. Solution will clear.

Factors influencing the rate of decalcification

Several factors influence the rate of decalcification, and there are ways to speed up or slow down this process. The concentration and volume of the active reagent, including the temperature at which the reaction takes place, are important at all times. Other factors that contribute to how fast bone decalcifies are the age of patient, type of bone, size of specimen, and solution agitation. Mature cortical bone decalcifies slower than immature, developing cortical or trabecular bone. Of all the factors, the effectiveness of agitation is still being debated.

Concentration of decalcifying agent

Generally, more concentrated acid solutions decalcify bone more rapidly but are more harmful to the tissue. This is particularly true of aqueous acid solutions, as various additives, e.g. alcohol or buffers that protect tissues, may slow down the decalcification rate. Remembering that 1 N and 1 M solutions of HCl, nitric, or formic acid are equivalent, Brain (1966) found that 4 M formic acid decalcified twice as fast as a 1 M solution without harming tissue staining, and felt it was more advantageous to use the concentrated formic acid mixture. With combination fixative–acid decalcifying solutions, the decalcification rate cannot exceed the fixation rate or the acid will damage or macerate the tissue before fixation is complete. Consequently, decalcifying mixtures should be compromises that balance the desirable effects (e.g. speed) with the undesirable effects (e.g. maceration, impaired staining).

In all cases, total depletion of an acid or chelator by their reaction with calcium must be avoided. This is accomplished by using a large volume of fluid compared with the volume of tissue (20:1 is usually recommended), and by changing the fluid several times during the decalcification process. Brain, however, pointed out that if a sufficiently large volume of fluid is used (100 ml per g of tissue) it is not necessary to renew the decalcifying agent even though depletion is less apparent in a larger volume.

Ideally, acid solutions should be endpoint tested and changed daily to ensure the decalcifying agent is renewed and that tissues are not left in acids too long or overexposed to acids, i.e. 'over-decalcification.'

Temperature

Increased temperature accelerates many chemical reactions including decalcification, but it also increases the damaging effects acids have on tissue so that, at 60°C, the bone, soft tissues, and cells may become completely macerated almost as soon as they are decalcified.

The optimal temperature for acid decalcification has not been determined although Smith (1962a) suggested 25°C as the standard temperature, but in practice a room temperature (RT) range of 18–30°C is acceptable. Conversely, lower temperature decreases reaction rates and Wallington (1972) suggested that tissues not completely decalcified at the end of a working week could be left in acid at 4°C over a weekend. This practice may result in 'over-decalcification' of tissues, even with formic acid. A better recommendation is to interrupt decalcification by briefly rinsing acid off bone, immersing it in NBF, and resuming decalcification on the next working day. Microwave, sonication, and electrolytic methods produce heat, and must be carefully monitored to prevent excessive temperatures that damage tissue (Callis and Sterchi 1998).

Increased temperature also accelerates EDTA decalcification without the risk of maceration but may not be acceptable for preservation of heat-sensitive antigens, enzymes, or electron microscopy work. Brain (1966) saw no objection to decalcifying with EDTA at 60°C if the bone was well fixed.

Agitation

The effect of agitation on decalcification remains controversial even though it is generally accepted that mechanical agitation influences fluid exchange within as well as around tissues with other reagents. Therefore, it would be a logical assumption that agitation speeds up decalcification and studies were done attempting to confirm this theory. Russell (1963) used a tissue processor motor rotating at one revolution per minute and reported the decalcification period was reduced from 5 days to 1 day. Others, including Clayden (1952), Brain (1966), and Drury and Wallington (1980), repeated or performed similar experiments and failed to find any time reduction. The sonication method vigorously agitates both specimen and fluid, and one study noted cellular debris found on the floor of a container after sonication could possibly be important tissue shaken from the specimen (Callis & Sterchi 1998). Gentle fluid agitation is achieved by low speed rotation, rocking, stirring, or bubbling air into the solution. Even though findings from various studies are unresolved, agitation is a matter of preference and not harmful as long as tissue components remain intact.

Suspension

The decalcifying fluid should be able to make contact with all surfaces of a specimen and flat bone slabs should not touch each other or the bottom of a container as this is enough to prevent good fluid access between the flat surfaces. Bone samples can be separated and suspended in the fluid with a thread or placed inside cloth bags tied with thread. Some workers cleverly devise perforated plastic platforms to raise samples above a container bottom to permit fluid access to samples.

Completion of decalcification

Ideally, bone should be taken from the acid solution as soon as all calcium has been removed from the bone, and this requires frequent monitoring. It is still possible that the outer parts of a sample will be over-exposed to the acid, although these parts usually stain no differently from inner portions, which are the last to be decalcified. Tissues decalcified in acids for long time periods or in high acid concentrations are more likely to show the effects of over-decalcification, whether or not all mineral has been removed.

Consequently, it is important for a laboratory to control a decalcification procedure by using a decalcification endpoint test to know when calcium removal is complete and, if incomplete, renew the decalcifying agent. If laboratories do not perform endpoint testing, it is recommended they should do so. When using formic, HCl or nitric acids, daily testing is recommended unless near the endpoint, then test every 5 hours when possible. With EDTA, weekly tests are sufficient unless solution changes are more frequent. Minimally calcified tissues and Jamshidi needle biopsies decalcified by a strong acid may be tested only once. These may be urgent cases where shorter decalcification time is allowed, but the sample must be carefully selected and incomplete decalcification is still possible. If tissue is still slightly calcified after paraffin embedment and sectioning, surface decalcification can be done (p. 343). Problem blocks should be identified as such so that proper treatment is given should further microtomy be requested.

Decalcification endpoint test

There are several methods for testing the completion of decalcification, with two considered the most reliable. These are specimen radiography, using an X-ray unit (p. 338) and the chemical method to test acids and EDTA solutions. Another method first used to test nitric acid is a weight loss, weight gain procedure that provides relatively good, quick results with all acids and EDTA (Mahwhinney et al 1984; Sanderson et al 1995). Although still used, 'physical' tests are considered inaccurate and damaging to tissues. Probing, 'needling', slicing, bending, or squeezing tissue can create artifacts, e.g. needle tracks, disrupt soft tumor from bone, or cause false-positive microfractures of fine trabeculae, a potential misdiagnosis. The 'bubble' test is subjective and dependent on worker interpretation.

Methods for chemical testing of acid decalcifying fluids detect the presence of calcium released from bone. When no calcium is found or the result is negative, decalcification is said to be complete and may entail using one extra change of decalcifier after actual completion. EDTA can be chemically endpoint tested by acidifying the used solution; this forces EDTA to release calcium for precipitation by ammonium oxalate (Rosen 1981).

Calcium oxalate test (Clayden 1952)

This method involves the detection of calcium in acid solutions by precipitation of insoluble calcium hydroxide or calcium oxalate but is unsuitable for solutions containing over 10% acid even though these could be diluted and result in a less sensitive test.

Solutions
Ammonium hydroxide, concentrated.
Saturated aqueous ammonium oxalate.

Method
1. Take 5 ml of used decalcifying fluid, add a piece of litmus paper or use a pH meter with magnetic stirrer.
2. Add ammonium hydroxide drop by drop, shaking after each drop, until litmus indicates solution is neutral (pH 7).
3. Add 5 ml of saturated ammonium oxalate and shake well.
4. Allow solution to stand for 30 min.

Result
If a white precipitate (calcium hydroxide) forms immediately after adding the ammonium hydroxide, a large quantity of calcium is present making it unnecessary to proceed further to step 3 which would also be positive. Testing can be stopped and a change to fresh decalcifying solution made at this point. If step 2 is negative or clear after adding ammonium hydroxide, then proceed to step 3 to add ammonium oxalate. If precipitation occurs after adding the ammonium oxalate, less calcium is present. When a smaller amount of calcium is present, it takes longer to form a precipitate in the fluid, so, if the fluid remains clear after 30 minutes, it is safe to assume decalcification is complete.

'Bubble' test. Acids react with calcium carbonate in bone to produce carbon dioxide, seen as a layer of bubbles on the bone surface. The bubbles disperse with agitation or shaking but re-form, becoming smaller as less calcium carbonate is reduced. As an endpoint test, a bubble test is subjective and unreliable, but can be used as a guide to check the progress of decalcification, i.e. tiny bubbles indicate less calcium present.

Radiography. This is the most sensitive test for detecting calcium in bone or tissue calcification. The method is the same as specimen radiography (p. 358) using a FAXITRON with a manual exposure setting of approximately 1 minute, 30 kV, and Kodak X-OMAT X-ray film on the bottom shelf. It is possible to expose several specimens at the same time. The method is to rinse acid from sample, carefully place identified bones on waterproof polyethylene sheet on top of the X-ray film, expose according to directions, and leave bones in place until film is developed and examined for calcifications. Bones with irregular shapes and variable thickness can occasionally mislead workers on interpretation of results. This problem is resolved by comparing the test radiograph to the pre-decalcification specimen radiograph and correlate suspected calcified areas with specimen variations. Areas of mineralization are easily identified, with tiny calcifications best viewed using a hand-held magnifier. Metal dust particles from saw blades are radio-opaque, sharply delineated fragments that never change in size. These are unaffected by decalcification, appearing as gray specks on the bone surface and can be easily removed. Spicules of metal, metallic paint, or glass forced deep into tissue by a traumatic injury are also sharply delineated but cannot be removed without damaging tissue. Radiography only indicates the presence of deeper foreign objects and care must be taken during microtomy to not damage the knife.

Treatment following decalcification

Acids can be removed from tissues or neutralized chemically after decalcification is complete. Chemical neutralization is accomplished by immersing decalcified bone into either saturated lithium carbonate solution or 5–10% aqueous sodium bicarbonate solution for several hours. Many laboratories simply rinse the specimens with running tap water for a period of time. Culling (1974) recommended washing in two changes of 70% alcohol for 12–18 hours before continuing with dehydration in processing, a way to avoid contamination of dehydration solvents even though the dehydration process would remove the acid along with the water.

Adequate water rinsing can generally be done in 30 minutes for small samples and larger bones in 1–4 hours in order not delay processing. Samples needing immediate processing, e.g. needle biopsies, can be blotted or quickly rinsed to remove acid from surfaces before proceeding to the first dehydrating fluid. It is important to avoid contaminating the first dehydrating fluid with acids, and washing bones even for a short time is good practice particularly with large bone slabs.

Acid-decalcified tissues for cryomicrotomy must be thoroughly washed in water or stored in formal saline containing 15% sucrose, or PBS with 15–20% sucrose, at 4°C before freezing. This helps avoid any residual acid in the tissue from corroding the metal knife.

Tissues decalcified in EDTA solutions should not be placed directly into 70% alcohol as this causes residual EDTA to precipitate in the alcohol and within the tissue. The precipitate does not appear to affect tissue staining since EDTA is washed out during these procedures, but may be noticeable during microtomy or storage when a crystalline crust forms on the block surface. A water rinse after decalcification or overnight storage in formal saline, NBF, or PBS should prevent this.

Surface decalcification

Surface decalcification is needed when partially decalcified bone or unsuspected mineral deposits in soft tissue are found during paraffin sectioning. This technique is done to prevent knife damage and torn tissue sections. After finding a calcification, the exposed tissue surface in a paraffin block is placed face down in 1% HCl, 10% formic, or a proprietary acid solution for 15–60 minutes, rinsed to remove corrosive acids, and re-sectioned. The acid removes a few micrometers of calcium from the tissue surface, permitting only a few sections to be cut after careful block re-orientation in the microtome to avoid wasting this thin surface decalcified layer.

PROCESSING DECALCIFIED BONE

In today's laboratories, automated computerized processors with vacuum and pressure options have improved the efficiency and quality of tissue processing, particularly bone. Open, carousel-style processors with agitation process most bone samples well, but can present some problems with adequate paraffin infiltration of dense, cortical bone and thicker slabs. Solvents used for dehydration (ethanol, isopropanol, reagent and proprietary alcohol mixtures) and clearing (xylene, xylene substitutes) will work well for bone and soft tissue processing. Paraffin waxes developed in recent years have been improved by the addition of plastic polymers and other chemicals that allow better wax penetration and sectioning. Decalcified bone sectioning is made easier after infiltration and embedding in a harder paraffin wax. Often bone infiltrated with routine paraffin for all tissues can be embedded in harder paraffin to give firmer support

of bone during sectioning. Small bone and needle biopsies containing little cortical bone can be processed with soft tissues.

Oversized, thick bone slabs require an extended processing schedule in order to obtain adequate dehydration, clearing, and paraffin infiltration. Some laboratories specialized in orthopedic work find it advantageous to dedicate a processor to extended processing schedules for bone and not interfere with routine daily soft tissue processing. With an enclosed automatic processor, time in each dehydrating, clearing solvent, and paraffin may vary from 2–4 hours, with larger bone slabs needing the longest time. Many workers prefer simple hand processing with a vacuum desiccator for dehydration and clearing steps, and infiltration in a heated vacuum oven with three changes of paraffin, up to 8 hours per change. If a bone sample has been endpoint tested for completed decalcification, but still appears chalky, mushy, and crumbles out of the block during sectioning, then dehydration, clearing, or paraffin infiltration may be incomplete. Blocks can be melted down and re-infiltrated with paraffin for up to 8 hours to see if this improves sectioning. Another possibility is reversing processing by melting paraffin from bone and going back through two changes of xylene, two changes of 100% alcohol to remove residual water, and then reprocessing back into paraffin.

Modern embedding methods using metal molds with plastic tissue cassettes have all but eliminated the necessity to mount the paraffin-embedded tissues on wood, hard rubber blocks, or metal chucks. A labeled cassette contains the tissue throughout processing and, after embedding, the plastic back of a block fits into a microtome cassette clamp. Macro-cassette systems including larger cassettes, molds, and a special block holder are available for sledge microtomes. A large specimen is the limiting factor for embedding with cassettes, and with a little creativeness the oversized bone can be embedded in a paraffin-filled metal pan or similar container, a warm hardwood block placed directly on top of bone, with all allowed to harden in place. This results in a hard back, embedded directly in the block, that can be clamped tightly in the microtome, avoiding holding onto softer paraffin which can crack under excessive clamping pressure.

Microtomes and knives

Bone biopsies and smaller primarily cancellous bone blocks can be cut on any properly maintained microtome. Many newer microtomes are more powerful, heavier, and automated, making them capable of sectioning both paraffin and plastic bone blocks. Oversized and exceptionally hard, dense bone samples too difficult to cut on a smaller microtome are easier to section on a large sledge or heavy duty motorized sliding microtome (Polycut, Leica, USA).

There is a wide choice of good microtome blades including heavy 'c' profile steel and the popular disposable blades. The disposable knives are convenient, extremely sharp, single-use blades capable of sectioning properly decalcified and processed paraffin-embedded bones. Newer microtomes come equipped with disposable blade holders, or disposable blade holder inserts can be purchased for older model microtomes. High-profile disposable blades are slightly thicker and wider than the low-profile blades, and tend to 'chatter' or vibrate less when cutting denser bones. Heavier steel knives range in size from 16 to 18 cm for small microtomes and from 200 to 300 cm for base sledge microtomes with specially designed blades for the Polycut. Because steel knives need frequent sharpening, an automatic knife sharpener is a cost-effective, time-saving device when these knives are used routinely.

Microtomy

Small bone samples and biopsies usually section well with knife angles set for routine soft tissue microtomy. Generally, disposable blades work well at the manufacturer's recommended angle settings for their high- or low-profile blades. Slight adjustment of a knife angle can be attempted if dense cortical bone sectioning is not working with the routine soft tissue knife angle, and can be increased or decreased at a microtomist's discretion. Knives must be changed frequently, sometimes after cutting one ribbon or a few sections of cortical bone. When sectioning any bone sample, a sharp knife is necessary in order to get flat, uncompressed, wrinkle-free sections, along with patience and good microtomy skills by the operator.

Longitudinal sections of cortical bone may section better when the knife cuts 'along the grain' or the length of the bone oriented at right angles to the knife. A bone of somewhat rectangular shape can be embedded or oriented in a block holder so that a smaller corner of sample is cut first with the wider area cut last. This helps reduce knife vibration and potential gouging of bone out of paraffin. When cartilage is present, it should be located near the top of a block or angled in a way to avoid compres-

sion of the softer cartilage and paraffin into the denser bone, creating wrinkles. Generally, hard tissues cut more easily if cooled by a melting ice block to allow water penetration into the tissue surface. Extensive soaking causes visible tissue swelling away from the block face and, even though the tissue cuts more easily, the sections fall apart on the water bath. A flat ice block made with water-filled polyethylene storage bags keeps blocks dry during cooling, or paraffin bone blocks can be cooled in a $-20°C$ freezer for a short time.

An optimal thickness for bone sections is the same as that for soft tissues, 4–5 μm, and cut routinely from adequately processed blocks. Bone marrow biopsies should be cut at 2–3 μm for marrow cell identification, and sliding microtome sections may vary from approximately 6 to 10 μm.

Flattening and adhesion

Bone sections adhere to slides better when glass surfaces are coated with some type of adhesive. Many laboratories now use commercially silanized Plus Charge® (Erie Scientific, NH) or poly-L-lysine-coated slides or can coat them in the laboratory. A simple coating method is to wash slides then dip in a gelatin and potassium dichromate 'subbing' solution, air dry, and store slides in a clean dry box until needed (Drury & Wallington 1980). When sectioning numerous bone blocks, 10 ml of the chrome subbing solution can be added to a 2-liter water bath or simply add a few gelatin granules to the water as it is heating. If some sections are persistently non-adherent, a solution containing amylopectin, a starch (Steedman 1960), or a high molecular weight 225 bloom gelatin in the chrome subbing mixture may be more successful. Gelatin should be used sparingly or an excess coating is stained by hematoxylin giving an unsightly blue background under and around sections.

While floating on water, cartilage and bone sections can expand more than the paraffin or other tissue components, and small folds may form as the sections dry. When this occurs, the water bath temperature should be lowered to 10–15°C below the paraffin melting point. Flattening a section by mounting a section in excess water on the slide, then holding the slide against a hot-plate to melt the wax and evaporate the water must be used with caution. Bone sections may 'explode' apart, displacing cortical bone from trabecular bone and ruining the gross morphology. Reducing the surface tension of water by floating a section on RT 10% ethanol, picking up the section on a slide, then immediately but slowly lowering the section into a warm water bath allows a section to flatten gently. If cartilage curling is a problem, drying sections flat at 37°C overnight or longer may solve this problem. Most bone sections flatten and dry without problems or special treatment provided the tissue has been properly processed and sectioned with a sharp knife.

Celloidin and double embedding

The celloidin or nitrocellulose embedding method is useful for large decalcified bone and brain section preparations but is seldom used in routine daily work, and many laboratories have largely replaced celloidin with MMA-embedded undecalcified bone section methods. Celloidin embedding does not harden cortical bone, is pliable and more elastic, with the latter qualities helping to bind tissues with different consistencies together and prevent separation from the slide during sectioning. Some staining methods demonstrating canaliculi and cement lines are superior in celloidin-embedded bone sections compared with paraffin sections (see Fig. 18.6, p. 347). The double embedding method combining celloidin and paraffin has similar advantages and disadvantages to celloidin embedding (Stevens et al 1996), but using harder paraffin, extended processing, and newer, powerful microtomes may work just as well.

The disadvantages of celloidin are the expense and reduced availability of nitrocellulose, chemical safety issues, i.e. toxic chloroform and unstable, volatile ether and nitrocellulose, extended preparation time, sections too thick for good cellular detail, and the need for a sledge microtome with a knife suitable for sectioning celloidin. Consequently, these discouraging drawbacks tend to rule out its use for routine diagnostic and other work. A standard procedure for celloidin processing and embedding is to be found in the 2nd and 3rd editions of this text. And, when used, many workers prefer the harder, low viscosity nitrocellulose (LVN) for bone.

Staining methods for decalcified bone sections

Most routine soft tissue staining methods can be used without modification for staining decalcified bone sections. Acid decalcification, particularly when prolonged or used with the heat producing methods, e.g. microwave, sonication, or electrolytic, can adversely affect the H&E and some special stains. When the temperature during decalcification exceeds 37°C, Giemsa staining may be too pink and the Feulgen stain for DNA will be negative because of excessive protein hydrolysis. Staining is successful after EDTA treatment, but the slower decalcification rate usually rules it out in favor of faster acid methods. Hematoxylin and eosin is still the primary stain used for most final diagnoses with the aid of special stains. Immunohistochemical staining is now an important aspect in disease diagnosis, and is used frequently on decalcified bone tumors, marrow, and cartilage.

Hematoxylin and eosin (H&E)

When staining sections of properly decalcified tissue no modifications to the standard H&E techniques are required. There are several ways to counteract weak nuclear staining damaged by acids and make the hematoxylin stain darker. Freshly prepared hematoxylin, particularly mixtures that lose strength over time, e.g. Harris's, Gill II and III, often stain darker than solutions near an expiration date. The routine hematoxylin staining time can be doubled or increased up to 30 minutes, or dilute hematoxylin 1:10 in distilled water and stain for several hours to overnight. Before trying overnight staining, restoration of basophilic staining can be attempted by immersing a hydrated section in 4–5% aqueous sodium bicarbonate for 10 minutes to 2 hours, rinsing well with water, and staining with hematoxylin. The acid differentiation step after hematoxylin can either be shortened to one or two fast dips in 0.5% acid alcohol or this step can be eliminated entirely. Bluing solutions should be mild bases, e.g. Scott's tap water substitute or saturated lithium carbonate, to avoid bone section loss caused by ammonia water bluing. If poor hematoxylin staining is a persistent problem, it is recommended that the decalcification method be evaluated and appropriate changes made to avoid damage to staining. Alcoholic eosin solutions, 0.5–1%, often stain bone and surrounding tissues overly red, and staining time can be shortened from 1 minute to 30 seconds, or even 10–20 rapid dips. Another excellent counterstain for differential staining of bone components is eosin Y–phloxine B.

In general, most hematoxylin solutions work well for staining bone including mercury-free Harris's, Ehrlich's, Mayer's, Cole's (p. 124), Gill II or III, and many proprietary mixtures. Some workers prefer Ehrlich's hematoxylin (p. 122) to a more specific nuclear stain, e.g. Mayer's (Fig. 18.4) for its ability to stain articular and growth plate cartilages a deeper blue to purple in contrast to the pink collagen and other tissues. In general, a hematoxylin solution can stain decalcified bone to show cement lines in Paget's diseased bone, new bone, and rapidly formed or remodeled bone provided the hematoxylin

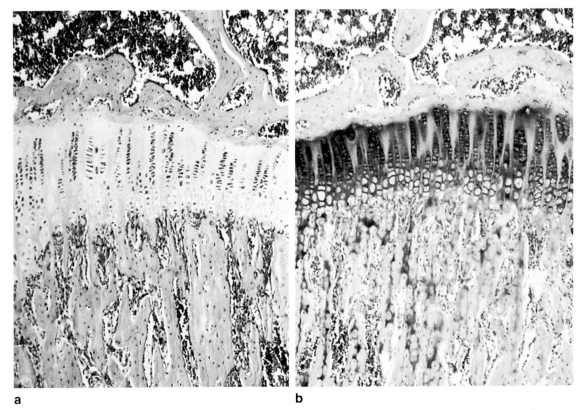

a   b

Fig. 18.4 (a) Mayer's hematoxylin and eosin. (b) Ehrlich's hematoxylin and eosin. Epiphyseal growth plate from proximal femur of an 11-week-old rat. (Original magnification ×40.)

stains darkly enough. A good H&E stain can stain all cells and bone components including osteoid as long as care is taken to adjust the staining procedure to achieve optimal results.

Collagen stains

Collagen stains can be used to demonstrate mature and finer immature fibers in certain tumors and a fracture callus. Van Gieson (VG) picro-fuchsin (p. 148) stains immature fibers a very pale orange compared to the deeper red mature fibers. A trichrome stain, i.e. Masson's, remains a standard, popular method to demonstrate collagen fibers in contrast to bone, cells, and other soft tissues. The immature collagen fibers stain distinctly but are a paler blue or green compared with darker stained mature fibers. Trichrome-stained adult or mature bone often shows areas of blue or green staining with some bright red areas that frequently have no relationship to bone structure. Osteoid is usually stained with the aniline blue or light green fiber stains.

Van Gieson demonstrates low-power microanatomy and is particularly brilliant on celloidin-embedded tissues. Polarized light microscopy may be more useful for positive identification of collagen than these stains since the finest fibers do not show distinct colors with routine light microscopy.

Cartilage and acid mucopolysaccharides

Cartilage can be stained to demonstrate mucopolysaccharides using various metachromatic staining methods or the azure method by Hughesdon (1949), recommended for its selectivity and stability.

The critical electrolyte concentration method of Scott and Dorling (1965, see p. 173) provides a more precise identification of acid mucopolysaccharides in cartilage. They used 0.05% 8GX alcian blue in pH 5.8 acetate buffer containing 0.4–0.5 M magnesium chloride to stain these strongly sulfated mucopolysaccharides blue. Another method useful for showing articular cartilage degradation of ground substances in arthritic and other diseases is safranin O-fast green (Rosenberg 1971), which stains the cartilage varying shades of red. Toluidine blue O, 0.1–1% aqueous solution, is also commonly used to stain NBF–fixed cartilage (Fig. 18.5). Workers should be aware that EDTA, as well as some fixatives and acid decalcifiers, extract proteoglycans and can result in weak cartilage staining by safranin O and possible false-negative quantitative results (Callis & Sterchi 1998).

The positive red periodic acid–Schiff (PAS; p. 171) reaction demonstrates mucopolysaccharides in new bone, calcifying cartilage, and glycogen in some early osteoblasts. PAS assists in diagnosis of some mucinous metastatic tumors and primary tumors with glycogen with a diastase digestion of glycogen to help make more precise identification of a poorly differentiated primary tumor. The PAS reaction is not affected by decalcification but prolonged treatment with strong acids should be avoided. Reticulin staining (p. 156), the silver impregnation of reticulin fibers, helps in diagnosis of bone tumors, tumor metastasis to bone, and myelofibrosis. Reticulin staining is not affected by decalcifying agents although the ammoniacal solutions can cause a section to release from the slide, necessitating the use of a stronger section adhesive.

Bone canaliculi

Osteocytes and their lacunae are large enough to be easily identified in most preparations, including H&E-stained paraffin sections of decalcified bone. Fine canaliculi radiating from lacunae are not easily seen in H&E-stained sections, but are well demonstrated with a modified Holmes' silver impregnation method on buffered, formic acid-decalcified, paraffin-embedded bone sections

(Taylor et al 1993). The latter method could be beneficial to workers without celloidin or double embedding capability even though canaliculi are often seen in thick celloidin sections heavily stained with hematoxylin.

The major problem in demonstrating canaliculi is the attempt to show spaces too fine for identification by routine staining of surrounding bone, so it is necessary to fill the spaces with a substance that appears dark against a lighter or unstained background. The simple 'air injection' method (Gatenby & Painter 1934) is done with undecalcified ground sections dried, and mounted in hot, melted Canada balsam to trap air inside the canaliculi. These look like black threads against the unstained bone and the balsam but, if sections are too thin or the balsam too fluid, the air will be displaced.

The picro-thionin method (Schmorl 1934) depends on deposition of a thionin precipitate within the lacunae and canaliculi (Fig. 18.6), although frozen or celloidin sections were recommended. Drury and Wallington

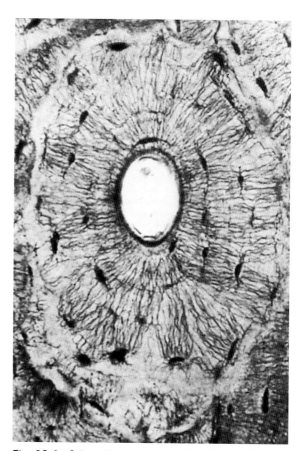

Fig. 18.6 Schmorl's picro-thionin stain showing bone canaliculi. Celloidin section of normal femoral shaft.

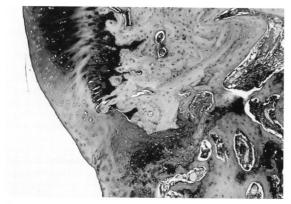

Fig. 18.5 Toluidine blue-stained articular cartilage and bone. Formic acid-decalcified rabbit femur. Paraffin section. (Original magnification ×40.)

(1980) indicated there is less channel shrinkage in these sections as compared to paraffin sections and the dye precipitate could penetrate readily. When frozen or celloidin sections are not routinely used, one of the staining methods for decalcified bone paraffin sections developed by either Taylor et al (1993) or Tornero et al (1991) could provide workers with better options to fit into routine paraffin work. Tornero's group used a microwave picro-thionin procedure and felt it gave more accurate, uniform staining of canaliculi as compared to Schmorl's method.

A later reference by Schmorl recommended aqueous 0.125% thionin and noted an alkaline solution accelerated and intensified staining by adding one or two drops of concentrated ammonia to approximately 10 ml staining solution just before use. Culling (1974) stated the pH of the thionin solution was critical, with successful staining results dependent on the amount of ammonia added, and recommended one drop of ammonia in 100 ml solution. Drury and Wallington (1980) indicated that thionin dye lots vary considerably making it necessary to adjust the ammonia content of staining solutions made from different lots in order to obtain suitable staining, and that other dyes may be used with good results, notably azure A.

Schmorl's picro-thionin method (Schmorl 1934)

Fixation
Any fixative but avoid mercuric chloride.

Decalcification
Any decalcifying solution.

Sections
Frozen or celloidin freshly cut.

Solutions
Stock solution
0.25 % aqueous thionin.

Working solution
0.125% thionin: filter 50 ml stock solution and dilute with 50 ml distilled water. Add 1 or 2 drops of concentrated ammonia immediately before use.

Saturated aqueous picric acid

Method
1. Wash sections in distilled water, 10 min.
2. Stain in thionin solution, 5–20 min or longer.
3. Wash in distilled water.
4. Immerse sections in picric acid solution, 30–60 s.
5. Wash in distilled water.
6. Differentiate in 70% alcohol until the bluish-green clouds of stain cease to form, 5–10 min or longer.
7. Dehydrate rapidly, clear in xylene, and mount in permanent mounting media.

Results

Lacunae and canaliculi	dark brown–black
Bone matrix	yellow or brownish-yellow
Cells	red

Notes
a. Agitate sections gently during steps 3–6. This is particularly important in stage 6, and change 70% alcohol frequently.
b. If bone matrix is decolorized during differentiation (step 6) restore yellow colour by returning the section to the picric acid solution for a few seconds before proceeding with dehydration.

Schmorl's modified method with 0.125% thionin solution replaced the picric acid with either phosphotungstic or phosphomolybdic acid and was preferred when staining children's bones. Culling (1974) used the modified method and recommended extended time in the alkaline thionin solution, then a few seconds' treatment in the acid, followed by fixation of the dye with dilute ammonia. This method results in blue–black canaliculi and lacunae on a sky-blue background.

Immunohistochemistry

Diagnostic immunohistochemical staining is frequently done on decalcified bone sections embedded in paraffin, e.g. bone marrow biopsies, tumors, cartilage, and uses the same staining methods and materials as for soft tissue immunohistochemistry. Care must be taken to fix bone specimens properly and decalcify with the least damaging agent in the shortest time possible in order to protect antigens from damaging effects of acids. Immunostaining is possible on 2-μm thick methyl methacrylate sections after complete removal of the plastic with warm xylene and a pressure cooker antigen retrieval method (Hand & Church 1998). Glycol methacrylate

(GMA) cannot be removed and may inhibit adequate antibody or immunoglobulin penetration to the antigenic sites.

PREPARATION OF MINERALIZED BONE

Sections demonstrating bone mineral and its relationship to the unmineralized components of bone must be prepared by methods that do not interfere with the mineral substance, i.e. undecalcified bone sections. Mineralized bone must be cut with tungsten carbide-tipped knives and need special, hard support to avoid cracked or crumbling tissue sections. Paraffin and celloidin are too soft and fail to match the hardness of bone or provide strong, solid support needed to prevent the fragmented mineralized sections.

Acrylic resins and plastics are now widely used and the preferred embedding media for undecalcified bone, and their use has revolutionized how this bone is examined. Frozen sections provide some support of cancellous bone, but the bone itself tends to look damaged and somewhat fragmented even though a diagnosis could be made from the soft tissue components.

Adhesive tape methods

Adhesive tape methods or tape transfer methods have been used to maintain the intact sections of undecalcified double-embedded bone sections during microtomy. Two methods, one for undecalcifed bone embedded in MMA (Hardt 1986) and the other for decalcified, paraffin-embedded bone (Eurell & Sterchi 1994), are used for sectioning difficult blocks. Clear adhesive packaging tape is rolled onto the trimmed block face and the cut section sticks to the tape during and after sectioning. The tape–section combination is then attached to an adhesive coated slide and either dried on a hot plate or clamped firmly between sheets of polyethylene inside a 60°C oven overnight. During the staining process, the tape releases in xylene, leaving the section 'transferred' onto the slide for subsequent staining. Plastic sections can be either transferred to a slide or stained directly on the tape. A special tape transfer system is also available for bone frozen sections.

Block impregnation for osteoid demonstration

This method is used solely for the negative demonstration of osteoid in which the calcium in mineralized bone is replaced by silver *before* decalcification and paraffin sectioning. Block impregnation techniques suffer from inherent defects of peripheral or over-impregnation near the surface with an incomplete reaction deeper in the tissues. As long as these artifacts are recognized in a finished preparation, the osteoid seams counterstained red are clearly delineated next to the blackened mineralized bone. The deeper, centrally located trabeculae are pale with only the outlines of lacunae and some blackened canaliculi. The advantage of this method is that good quality paraffin sections are easily prepared.

Silver staining of bone prior to decalcification (Tripp & Mackay 1972)

Fixation
99% ethyl alcohol.

Tissue
1–2-mm thick bone pieces.

Solutions
2% aqueous silver nitrate.

Reducer
Sodium hypophosphite	5 g
0.1 M sodium hydroxide	0.2 ml
Distilled water	100 ml

5% aqueous sodium thiosulfate (anhydrous)

Decalcifier
10% aqueous formic acid
van Gieson's picro-fuchsin (see p. 148)

Method

1. Wash in several changes of distilled water, 4 hours.
2. Place in 2% silver nitrate, 48 hours in complete darkness.
3. Rinse in three changes of distilled water, 15–20 seconds each.
4. Wash in running tap water, 4 hours.
5. Place in reducer, 48 hours.
6. Wash in running tap water, 1 hour.
7. Place in sodium thiosulfate solution, 24 hours.
8. Wash in running tap water, 1 hour.
9. Decalcify in 10% formic acid.
10. Process to paraffin wax, cut, and mount.
11. Dewax and bring sections to water.
12. Stain with van Gieson's stain, 2 min.
13. Dehydrate, clear, and mount.

Results

Edges of mineralized bone	black
Bone	brown to yellow
Osteoid	red

Notes

a. For cellular detail, an adjacent NBF-fixed, non-impregnated block should be processed.
b. Radiographic decalcification endpoint test cannot be used with the radio-opaque silver deposits.
c. Nitric and hydrochloric acid decalcifiers may attack the silver deposits.
d. NBF-fixed bone may be used provided formaldehyde is completely removed by distilled water washes before impregnation.

Frozen sections

Using a modern cryostat, patience, a slow steady cutting speed, and a tungsten carbide-tipped steel knife, frozen sections from trephine and Jamshidi needle biopsies of cortical and trabecular bone can be cut with ease and minimal section damage. A knife with a tungsten carbide edge is much harder than a steel edge and cuts calcified bone without fragmenting a section or damage to the edge. For demonstration of bone marrow cells, tumor, and calcified bone components, the hematoxylin stains cell nuclei and mineralized bone intensely blue and eosin stains osteoid and other soft tissues shades of red. Some bone with metabolic diseases, i.e. Paget's, renal osteodystrophy, and hyperparathyroidism showing advanced changes or diseased bone with moderate to severe osteomalacia, can be rapidly diagnosed on an H&E-stained frozen section. Other stains can be done on bone frozen sections including a modified Romanowsky method for patterns in bone remodeling and cartilage development (Dodds & Gowen 1994), enzyme and immunohistochemical methods. Unstained sections can be examined with polarized light to see woven and lamellar patterns in bone.

Laboratories not using MMA embedding techniques may find bone cryomicrotomy a valuable addition to their facility, and when MMA technique is available, frozen sections permit rapid diagnosis on some bone diseases. Rapid or 'snap' freezing bone samples in liquid nitrogen-cooled 2-methylbutane (isopentane) must be used carefully as some bones can shatter in the extremely cold ($-120°C$) temperature. A dry ice/isopentane bath ($-70°C$) snap freezes bone coated with 4% aqueous polyvinyl alcohol (PVA, water soluble, 124,000 MW) or embedded in optimum cutting temperature compound (OCT), gently and without shattering. Hexane can be substituted for isopentane (Dodds 1994). In brief the technique is:

1. Mount bone on cork or embed in a cryomold with OCT.
2. Snap freeze carefully in 'syrupy' (thawing) isopentane cooled by liquid nitrogen ($-120°C$) or with dry ice/isopentane ($-70°C$).
3. Place bone in cryostat at -30 to $-35°C$. Remount frozen bone onto a metal chuck with OCT to provide maximum stability during sectioning.
2. Cut section at 5–7 µm, pick up section on slide, and fix with fixative of choice. Post-fixation in 95% alcohol, 5 min, removes fat.
3. Stain in Harris, Gill II or Gill III for 1 min or longer, or desired intensity.
4. Rinse with water or a bluing reagent to 'blue' section; avoid ammonia water.
5. 1% alcoholic eosin approximately 10–30 seconds or desired intensity.
6. Dehydrate, clear, and mount in permanent mounting medium.

Notes

a. Formalin-fixed biopsies can be rinsed, immersed in 15–20% sucrose for 1–8 hours at 4°C to replace water before freezing and improve sectioning, i.e. cryoprotection.
b. Fresh frozen sections can be fixed, rinsed, then decalcified in 10% EDTA before immunostaining.
c. Enzyme staining can be done on fixed or unfixed sections.
d. A special tape transfer system (Cryojane; Instrumedics, MO) is available for cryomicrotomy of undecalcified bone and other difficult tissues, keeping sections intact and adhered to special polymer-coated slides (Schiller 1999).
e. Carazzi's or other hematoxylins can be used with staining intensity optimized for worker preference.

Plastic embedding

Mineralized bone sections are best studied when the embedding medium matches bone hardness to permit intact sections necessary to examine bone density or defects in mineralized components in relation to the bone cells, cartilage, osteoid, and other soft tissues. Synthetic resins for both EM (Epon) and light microscopy plastics (GMA, MMA) work well for these purposes. Epoxy EM resins are suitable only for ultra-thin sectioning of tiny bone pieces; their hydrophobicity causes poor stain penetration into tissues.

Methacrylates were used for specimen whole-mount displays in museums before use as support media for sections. Although Woodruff and Norris (1955) favored an *n*-butyl/ethyl methacrylate mixture, methyl methacrylate (MMA) is now the preferred plastic for undecalcified bone work. MMA mixed with polyethylene glycol (Boellaard & von Hirsch 1959) or dibutyl phthlate is softer and more elastic. Glycol methacrylate, a softer plastic than MMA, used with bone biopsies results in 'laddered' bone sections cut with glass knives. Mineralized bone specimens require extended time in dehydration, clearing, and MMA infiltration compared to decalcified bone paraffin processing.

Although some workers 'wash' the polymerization inhibitor from the monomer (Difford 1974), many now use an unwashed monomer method suitable for microtomed or sawn ground sections (D. Sterchi, private communication, 1996).

Enclosed automatic processors should not be used with toxic MMA monomers, although bone laboratories use these processors for alcohol and xylene steps but finish MMA infiltration steps with hand processing using vacuum desiccators and a vacuum source. Hand processing is commonly done for all processing steps. Approximate time per change in solvents for all processing steps depends on bone size: small, 24–30 hours; medium (3–5 mm), 48 hours or more; large, 3–7 days. A fume hood and careful chemical handling is mandatory for protection from toxic MMA fumes and other chemicals.

Procedures for MMA processing and embedding developed by Sterchi (1996) are similar to those in Chapter 29. Sterchi used two changes each of 95% and 100% ethanol; xylene or (1:1) MMA monomer/100% ethanol. MMA infiltration times are the same as processing times. Sterchi's infiltration mixtures vary from those

in Chapter 29 by using 100 ml monomer and adding to: Mixture #1, 1 g benzoyl peroxide (BPO) only; Mixture #2, 5 ml dibutyl phthlate 1 g BPO, 15 g poly methyl methacrylate powder (996,000 MW; Aldrich, MO); Mixture #3 (same as #2) but 1.5 g BPO. Embed in fresh Mixture #3, polymerize at RT or in a 37°C water bath (small bone), cure blocks for 4–6 hours at 60°C, then freeze blocks for 2 hours to remove polypropylene containers (Sanderson 1997).

Sectioning methacrylate-embedded bone

Bone embedded in MMA can be sectioned by either microtomy or sawing and grinding for thick sections (1 mm to 20 μm). Thick ground sections are necessary for microradiography (p. 357), bone containing metal or other implant material, and extremely large bones that cannot be sectioned. An ultra-miller on a large sliding microtome (Polycut E; Leica, USA) can precisely mill a perfectly flat 15–20-μm section. Ultra-milling and grinding wastes bone and must be used carefully. Thin bone sections cut more easily with a motorized microtome designed for plastic work.

Sawing

Hand sawing and grinding can be done by clamping a block in a vice, cutting a slab with a fretted wire saw, then grinding the slab to produce a section thin enough for staining and microscopic examination. Hand preparations result in thick, uneven slices with deep scratches requiring extra grinding to obtain a smooth section. This is time consuming and wastes more specimen even though adequate sections are possible with practice and careful sawing/grinding techniques.

Saws designed for cutting metallurgy samples are recommended for obtaining precise, flat, thin sections. A Micro-Grinding System (EXAKT Technologies, Oklahoma, USA) specifically developed for bone work by Donath (1988a,b) is complete with plastic embedding media, plastic slides, special saws, and a grinder/polisher. Low- or high-speed metallurgical saws (Isomet, Buehler Ltd., IL, USA) cut easily through bone blocks with or without metal implants using diamond-impregnated cut-off blades, and produce sections in need of less grinding. These machines cut wafers down to 100 μm thick and, by resetting the micrometer, precise serial sectioning is possible. These saws are water cooled to disperse heat produced by cutting while continuously cleaning the blade and block face for debris-free sections.

The blade thickness (kerf) increases with larger blade diameters and each cut with a blade wastes only as much tissue as its own thickness (kerf loss). It is advisable to use a smaller diameter blade with the thinnest kerf whenever possible. Larger blocks generally need sturdier, large-diameter blades for proper clearance through a block and no flexing of blade while cutting even though the kerf loss will be greater.

Milling cutters and precision cutting machines (Malvern Microslice, UK) can cut sections to approximately 150 μm. Sawn sections are ground and polished to produce the final thickness and remove scratches while ultra-milled sections need no further grinding or polishing. The MMA-embedded slab section is glued to white or clear plastic slides (Sanderson 1997) with cyanoacrylate glue. Glass slides are dangerous to workers due to shattering under the stresses of grinding.

Grinding and polishing

Motorized metallurgical grinder/polishers are ideal for final finishing of MMA-embedded bone wafers to a required thickness for microscopic examination and microradiography. These machines have variable speed adjustments, rotating base plates to hold self-adhesive grinding papers or polishing cloths, running water for removing debris, and even have special adapters to hold a specimen during the grinding process. Grinding papers remove scratches with progressively coarser to finer grit papers (360, 400, 600 grits), followed by polishing with an aqueous 1 μm alumina for a mirror-smooth surface. Residual fine scratches cause unsightly patterns in microradiographs and surface stained sections. A dial caliper can be used to check section thickness throughout the grinding process. Hand grinding is inexpensive, simple, and with practice will produce adequate sections but automated grinders have the advantages of speed and producing flatter sections. Unembedded cortical bone hand-ground between abrasive glass plates without support of the plastic can fracture the bone, grind away fine trabeculae, cells and soft tissues without complete removal of scratches.

Microtome sections of undecalcified bone

Automated microtomes (Leica 2165, Leica USA, or Olympus Cut 4060E, Triangle Biomedical Systems, NC) and a D profile tungsten carbide-tipped steel knife section, both MMA and GMA. Tungsten carbide knives help avoid the 'laddered' bone sections seen after cutting with glass knives. Large blocks need to be sectioned on a larger, sliding motorized microtome (Leica Polycut E or S) with special tungsten carbide knives.

Staining methyl methacrylate-embedded bone

Methacrylate bone sections can be stained in two ways depending on the type of section available. Sections, 5–10 μm thick, attached to adhesive-coated glass slides can be stained after either softening or removing the plastic. When section loss is a problem, sections can be stained by free floating in a dish or attached to adhesive tape (see p. 349). Ultra-milled or ground sections, 20–200 μm thick, glued to plastic slides, can be 'surface' stained, a unique, effective method for examination of mineralized bone and its components.

Unstained thin sections examined with polarized light demonstrate collagen patterns within the bone. There are many staining methods for MMA bone sections including methods necessary to distinguish the osteoid from the mineralized components. Microradiographic evaluation can be done on 100-μm thick sections followed by surface staining of the same section for microscopic examination and correlation of two methods. Paraffin staining methods often do not stain MMA sections well, and must be adapted for these sections by longer staining times, or plastic removal ('deplasticize') or softening with solvents ('etching') to permit stain penetration.

Stains for calcium are of prime importance and include hematoxylin, solochrome cyanin, and the von Kossa silver nitrate methods. Trichrome stains will distinguish calcified bone stained with some hematoxylin and the fiber stain from the osteoid stained with the cytoplasmic stain. Thus, a Masson's trichrome (p. 150) stains bone blue and osteoid red. A modification of this method by Goldner (1937) results in clear, brilliantly detailed staining of osteoclasts, osteoblasts, fibroblasts, and cells from marrow or tumors. Some workers feel the modified MacNeal's tertrachrome and Movat's pentrachrome methods give superior staining results for differentiating osteoid from mineralized bone (Schenk et al 1984).

Various toluidine blue methods with pH ranges of 7–9 are routinely used to specifically stain trabecular mineralization fronts, cartilage, and other bone components.

Detection of tetracycline fluorescence in bone can be done on either unstained sections or sections stained with Villanueva's mineralized bone stain (Sanderson 1997).

Surface staining methods for 20–200-µm thick polished bone MMA sections mounted on white plastic slides are helpful for examining oversized bone sections or sections containing metal implants. This staining technique provides surprisingly excellent cellular detail, and is commonly used to study the interface of the bone with a metal implant. Surface staining can be done by mildly decalcifying (acid 'etching) the exposed bone surface with 1% formic acid for 1 min to remove a few micrometers of calcium from the section to permit better dye penetration into the bone, thereby enhancing staining of bone. MMA is very hydrophobic and only certain low molecular weight dyes actually penetrate MMA for suitable staining of softer tissue components with the aid of heat or alkaline stain solutions (pH 7–9). Some methods used for surface staining include methylene blue–basic fuchsin, potassium permanganate-oxidized methylene blue (Sanderson's Rapid Bone Stain, Surgipath, USA), modified MacNeal's tetrachrome (Schenk et al 1984), and 0.75% toluidine blue in phosphate buffer, pH 7–8 (Eurell & Sterchi 1994). These methods stain calcified bone and its components distinctly, i.e. osteoid, calcification fronts, lacunae, canaliculi, osteons, osteoclasts, osteoblasts, marrow cells, collagen, and other soft tissues, various shades of dark to light blue or blue–green, and cartilage shades of deep purple to violet. Basic fuchsin, light green, and van Gieson's are used as counterstains with these methods.

Mounting after staining

Deplasticized stained sections on glass slides are mounted in the same way as paraffin sections using alcohol dehydration, xylene clearing, and mounting with a synthetic mounting medium. Free-floating sections tend to wrinkle and, while in clearing agent, can be flattened with a brush or rolled between pieces of smooth filter paper, then mounted with synthetic resin with a weight placed on top of the cover glass to keep the section flat until the medium dries. Strong clamping devices maintain flat sections briefly but cause the mounting media to retract during storage. Sections cleared with terpineol and mounted with terpene-based mounting media do not harden as well as the synthetic resins and result in an unstable mount.

Surface stained sections in MMA cannot not be dehydrated, cleared, or mounted. Methyl methacrylate is softened by alcohols, and is soluble in xylene and other mounting media solvents. Their use results in ugly cracking of plastic in and around a section. To examine surface stained sections, place a cover glass on top of the dry section and examine with the brightest light setting on the microscope. Immersion oil can be used to mount these sections, but is temporary and leaves messy oil residue on stored sections.

Hematoxylin and eosin for MMA-embedded tissue

This method is useful for diagnosis of suspected osteomalacia and distinguishes mineralized bone from osteoid, with nuclei and other soft tissues stained similarly to decalcified bone paraffin sections.

Hematoxylin and eosin (Wallington 1972)

Reagents
Cole's hematoxylin (p. 124) 1 % aqueous eosin.

Method
1. Deplasticize with xylene and hydrate sections to distilled water.
2. Stain in freshly filtered Cole's hematoxylin, 60 min with occasional agitation.
3. Wash well in alkaline tap water.
4. Stain in eosin solution, 30 min.
5. Wash in tap water.
6. Dehydrate, clear, and mount.

Results

Osteoid	pink
Calcified bone	purplish brown
Nuclei	blue

Solochrome cyanine

The solochrome cyanine stain differentiates osteoid from newly laid down bone and older bone (Fig. 18.7). The following method gives stronger sharper staining compared to 1% solochrome cyanine R in 2% acetic acid (Matrajt & Hioco 1966) but the procedures are essentially the same.

Solochrome cyanine (Hyman & Poulding 1961)

Solution

Solochrome cyanine R	1 g
Concentrated sulfuric acid	2.5 ml

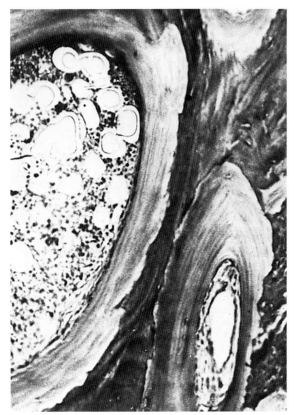

Fig. 18.7 Solochrome cyanine method showing osteoid and mineralized bone. Undecalcified section of methacrylate-embedded iliac crest biopsy from a patient with osteomalacia.

Mix well until dye incorporates into the resulting 'sludge'. Add 500 ml of 0.5% aqueous iron alum (ferric ammonium sulfate).

Mix and filter.

Method

1. Deplasticize with xylene and hydrate sections to distilled water.
2. Stain in solochrome cyanine solution, 60 min.
3. Using a microscope, differentiate in warm (30°C) alkaline tap water until mineralized areas appear blue and other areas light red. Over-differentiation causes all parts to become blue.
4. Dehydrate, clear, and mount.

Results

Mineralized bone	light blue
Calcification front	dark blue
Osteoid	light red–orange
Wide osteoid	light red–orange with pale blue and orange bands
Nuclei	blue

Staining for bone mineral

The classic von Kossa (1901) silver method is used to stain the mineral component (calcium phosphate) in bone, and is a negative stain for osteoid with the calcium component blackened by silver deposition. Osteoid is counterstained red by either the van Gieson's or safranin O (Figs 18.8 and 18.9). This can also be used as a ground section surface stain but without the acid 'etching' removal of calcium.

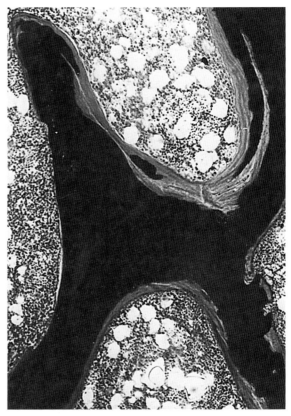

Fig. 18.8 Von Kossa's silver deposition method giving a negative demonstration of osteoid, counterstained with safranin O. Undecalcified section of methacrylate-embedded iliac crest biopsy from a patient with osteomalacia. Ground section.

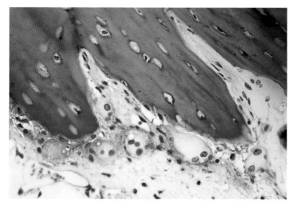

Fig. 18.9 Surface stained canine bone. Rapid bone stain counterstained with van Gieson's. Bone (red), osteocytes and giant osteoclasts (blue). Undecalcified methyl methacrylate embedded ground section. (Original magnification ×40.)

von Kossa method (modified von Kossa 1901)

Solutions

1% aqueous silver nitrate
2.5% sodium thiosulfate
1% safranin O or van Gieson's picro-fuchsin

Method

1. Deplasticize with xylene, and hydrate sections to distilled water.
2. Place in silver nitrate solution, expose to strong light for 10–60 min, and watch the mineralized bone turn dark brown to black, indicating a completed reaction.
3. Wash in three changes of distilled water.
4. Treat with sodium thiosulfate, 5 min.
5. Wash well in distilled water.
6. Counterstain as desired.
7. Dehydrate, clear, and mount.

Results

Mineralized bone   black
Osteoid   red

Notes

1. Long wavelength UV light from sunlight or a quartz halogen microscope lamp is preferable to a tungsten filament light bulb, and accelerates the reaction.
2. van Gieson's picro-fuchsin counterstaining may interfere with birefringence of osteoid

Goldner's trichrome method

This staining technique can be more valuable than the von Kossa method in investigations of metabolic diseases, e.g. Paget's, renal osteodystrophy, and hyperparathyroidism, because of excellent staining of cells. Osteoblast and osteoclast activity is easily assessed, an important factor for both diagnosis and evaluating the effects of treatment in these disorders by repeated bone biopsies. An additional advantage is that metastatic tumor cells in bone marrow are easily identified.

Solutions

Weigert's iron hematoxylin (see p. 128)

Ponceau–fuchsin–azophloxin stock solutions

Ponceau de xylidine solution

Ponceau de xylidine	0.75 g
Acid fuchsin	0.25 g
Acetic acid	1 ml
Mix, and add to distilled water	100 ml

Azophloxin solution

Azophloxin	0.5 g
Acetic acid	0.6 ml
Mix, and add to distilled water	100 ml

Final working stain solution

Ponceau–fuchsin solution	5–10 ml
Azophloxin	2 ml
0.2% acetic acid solution	88 ml

Light green solution

Light green	1 g
Acetic acid	1 ml
Mix, and add to distilled water	500 ml

Phosphomolybdic acid–orange G solution

Phosphomolybdic acid	3 g
Orange G	2 g

Dissolve in 500 ml of distilled water, and add a crystal of thymol.

Method

1. Deplasticize with xylene and hydrate sections to water.
2. Immerse sections in alkaline alcohol solution (90 ml of 80% ethanol and 10 ml of 25% ammonia), 1 hour.
3. Rinse in water, 15 min.
4. Stain in Weigert's hematoxylin, 1 hour.
5. Rinse in tap water, 10 min.

6. Rinse in distilled water, 5 min.
7. Stain in final Ponceau–fuchsin–azophloxin solution, 5 min.
8. Rinse in 1% acetic acid, 15 s.
9. Stain in phosphomolybdic acid–orange G solution, 20 min.
10. Rinse in 1% acetic acid, 15 s.
11. Stain with light green, 5 min.
12. Rinse in three changes of 1% acetic acid.
13. Rinse in distilled water, blot dry, and mount

Results

Mineralized bone	green
Osteoid	orange–red
Nuclei	blue–gray
Cartilage	purple

Demonstration of aluminum

Patients receiving hemodialysis for chronic renal failure may deposit aluminum at the mineralization sites in bone, producing an osteomalacia-like pattern. Aluminum can be demonstrated by either the aluminon or solochrome azurine methods with the latter considered the most reliable. Two newer methods eliminated staining of free-floating sections (see method below) and used sections attached to glass slides. One is a modified acidic solochrome azurine method for GMA-embedded bone sections (Huffer et al 1996), and the other is an aluminon method for the study of uremic bone fixed with NBF instead of absolute ethanol and embedded in MMA (Maloney et al 1982).

Solochrome azurine method for aluminum in bone biopsies (modified from Denton et al 1984)

Sections
Undecalcified bone embedded in MMA.

Solutions

Stock solution
1% aqueous solochrome azurine (CI 143830). Stable for long period of time.

Working solution
Adjust pH of 1% solochrome azurine stock solution to pH 5 with 25% acetic acid. This forms an important

precipitate needed for staining; do not filter this solution. Prepare working solution immediately before use and discard after use.

Method

1. Free-floating MMA sections to distilled water. Use a small Petri dish to contain all solutions for free-floating sections throughout the procedure.
2. Stain sections in working stain solution (pH 5.0) at RT for 18 h or overnight.
3. Wash gently in distilled water for 20–30 s.
4. Counterstain with 1% neutral red.
5. Wash in distilled water.
6. Blot dry and leave in drying oven overnight.
7. Mount in synthetic mounting medium.

Results

Aluminum	dark blue–purple
Nuclei and background	shades of red

Aluminon method (after Irwin 1955)

Fixation
Fix bone in absolute ethanol.

Sections
MMA, free-floating sections.

Solutions

Buffer solution

5 M ammonium chloride	60 ml
5 M ammonium acetate	60 ml
6 M HCl	10 ml

Mix, and check pH (should be approx. pH 5.2).

Working stain solution

Aurine tricarboxylic acid ('aluminon')	2 g
Buffer solution, as above	100 ml

Dissolve aluminon in few milliliters of buffer, and bring final volume to 100 ml with remaining buffer. Heat to 60°C. Filter immediately before use.

Differentiating solution

Buffer solution, as above	50 ml
1.6 M ammonium carbonate	22 ml

Check pH; should be approx. 7.2.

Method

1. Bring sections to water.
2. Stain for 5–10 min at 60°C; use freshly filtered stain, preheated to 60°C (see Notes a and b).

3. Rinse in distilled water.
4. Differentiating solution for 3–5 s.
5. Wash in distilled water.
6. Counterstain in 1% aqueous methylene blue for 1 min.
7. Rinse in distilled water.
8. Dehydrate in alcohols and mount in synthetic resin medium.

Results

Sites of aluminum	bright red
Background	blue

Notes

a. Sections embedded in MMA and other acrylics, e.g. LR White, may detach from glass slides in this 60°C solution.
b. Free-floating MMA sections often wrinkle in the 60°C solution. Multiple sections and careful handling are recommended.

Microradiography

Microradiographs are high-resolution, fine-detail contact X-rays of thinner ground sections for microscopic examination and evaluation of bone mineral density and distribution. The denser, highly mineralized areas appear almost white as fewer X-rays penetrate them, and less dense, non-mineralized areas show shades of yellowish-grey grading to black against the black background of the exposed film (Fig. 18.10).

The requirements for microradiography, even though similar to those for fine-detail specimen radiography, are even more stringent: a fairly powerful, controllable source of 'soft' X-rays (low kV), even overall section thickness, and high-resolution film or photographic plates are necessary for this procedure.

Mineralized bone sections embedded in MMA are preferred and must be perfectly flat, measure approximately 70–130 μm thick, and be free of debris and scratches. Thicker sections create blurred images and thinner sections transmit too many X-rays. Sections must be in tight, close contact with the film or plate and developed under controlled conditions for comparative work.

Microradiography has been done with X-ray crystallography units, and, although not called microradiography, even greater resolution work is accomplished with the BSEM or backscatter electron imaging scanning

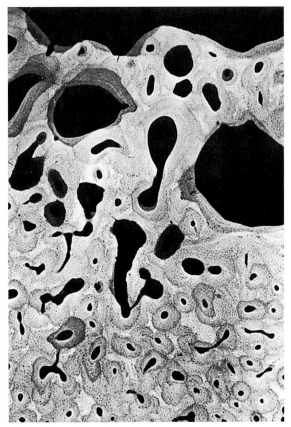

Fig. 18.10 Microradiograph of normal femoral shaft showing different densities of mineralization. The lightest areas indicate the heaviest mineral deposition.

electron microscope (Bloebaum et al 1990). The Faxitron X-ray unit produces satisfactory results, and Dunn et al (1974) described a standard procedure with this unit using 20 kV, 20-cm film to source distance (FTSD) for 75 min with 5 × 5 cm glass Kodak High Resolution Plates, Type 1A. Unfortunately, photographic plates and films suitable for microradiograpy are frequently discontinued. Workers should locate replacement film with a resolving power of 2000 lines/mm or higher and high-contrast, fine-grain emulsions, properties that help reduce long exposure times (Boivin & Baud 1984). Some workers are finding success using mammography film (Kodak MIN R 2000; Kodak, Rochester NY) at higher kV, longer FTSD, and short exposure time (L. Jenkins, personal communication, 2000). Using the example below as a guideline, workers should be able to optimize settings needed for any new film or photographic plates.

An example of microradiography using mammography film in Faxitron

(L. Jenkins, personal communication, 2000)

Bone section, approximately 100 μm thick, pressed tightly against film inside a vacuum cassette.

A Kodak MIN R 2000 mammography film.

Film to source distance (FTSD) 50 cm (lowest shelf level).

Tube, 55 kV.

Tube current, 3 mA.

Exposure time is approximately 5 s.

After exposure, the mammography film or plates must be developed exactly according to manufacturer instructions, using solutions and temperatures specified for these products, then dried. The dried film is cut to fit on a larger glass slide mounted under a larger cover glass and secured at the edges by cellophane tape. An exposed area on a photographic plate is mounted under a cover glass with Eukitt's or an equivalent medium. Examination should be made using a 10X objective on light microscope in a dark room.

Fluorescent labeling

Tetracycline antibiotics form fluorescent complexes with calcium at the sites of bone mineral deposition (Milch et al 1957, 1958) and provide an effective in vivo tracer of bone formation in these areas. The drug localizes rapidly in newly mineralized sites of bone or teeth and appears as a bright fluorescent line under UV light. Two or more doses administered to patients at known intervals provide a method for estimating the rate of bone remodeling (Frost 1983a). The measurable distances between parallel uptake lines indicate the amount of bone deposited at each time interval between doses (Fig. 18.11). In order to retain tetracycline labeling, mineralized bone is fixed in 70% ethanol or alcoholic formalin, embedded in MMA, sectioned, mounted unstained, and viewed with a UV light microscope at approximately 360–400 nm wavelength. After UV light evaluation, sections can be stained with toluidine blue for further microscopic examination.

MORPHOMETRY OF BONE

The general principles and methods of morphometry are outlined in Chapter 31 of this book; this section very

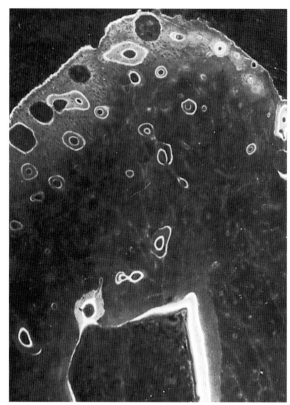

Fig. 18.11 Tetracyline-labeled rat ulna. Two doses were given at 4-week intervals and the rat euthanized after a further 7 days. Alcohol-fixed, mineralized, methacrylate-embedded section illuminated with 400 nm wavelength UV light.

briefly deals with some application of techniques to evaluate bone disorders, particularly in metabolic bone disease (MBD).

Normal bone containing trabeculae undergoes constant remodeling or resorption by the osteoclasts and formation by osteoblasts (see p. 334). In disease, remodeling can be disturbed and cause either too much or too little of one of these dynamic processes to occur in the bone.

Assessment of relative amounts of bone trabeculae, osteoid, resorption and deposition (apposition) can be made by a subjective microscopic examination of the section. This is adequate where changes are obvious, but subtle alterations may require accurate measurements to detect an abnormality. In metabolic bone disease, tetracycline is administered at specific times prior to biopsy (fluorescent labeling p. 358) to help determine the amount of active mineralization in bone (see Fig. 18.11), followed by an iliac crest biopsy (p. 335) and subsequent MMA embedment. Briefly, bone histomorphometry can be used for detection and assessment of disease severity or effects of treatments of MBD, e.g. postmenopausal osteoporosis. Recker (1990) listed eight metabolic bone diseases with tentative indications for bone biopsy although this list is anticipated to expand with acquisition of more knowledge and treatment of MBD.

Histomorphometric analysis can be done with manual, semi-automated, or automated methods. A manual method could include a standard microscope with eyepiece graticules, digitized tablets (image display), image storage, and a computer for data storage and output. Increasingly, modern automated computerized image analysis systems with a video camera, a screen with screen grid for area counting, and software designed specifically for bone work are being used to reduce time needed for measurements and calculations of final results.

A standardized, generally universal system of nomenclature, symbols, and units for bone histomorphometry was summarized by Parfitt (1988) and it is recommended that workers be familiar with and use this system. This is a terminology list of primary measurements for volume, surface, thickness, mineralization rate, formation rate, and so on. Basic measurements are confined to trabecular bone and are:

a) trabecular bone volume and surface
b) eroded (resorption) surface
c) osteoid surface
d) mineralized surface
e) osteoid thickness
f) wall thickness (of new bone layers at formation site)
g) mineral apposition rate (calcification rate) (Recker 1983).

Calculations are made from collected data (Parfitt et al 1987), and results correlated to the various diseases. Chapter 31 explains how area measurements are numerically equated with volume measurements. The derivation of some of these values is shown below:

Bone volume (%)

$$= \frac{\text{area of trabeculae}}{\text{area of trabeculae and marrow space}}$$

Osteoid volume (%)

$$= \frac{\text{area of osteoid}}{\text{area of trabeculae and marrow space}}$$

Osteoid surface (%)

$$= \frac{\text{length of trabecular surface covered by osteoid}}{\text{total length of trabecular surface}}$$

Osteoid index (%) $= \dfrac{\text{osteoid volume}}{\text{osteoid surface}}$

Resorption surface (%)

$$= \frac{\text{length of trabecular surface occupied by lacunae}}{\text{total length of trabecular surface}}$$

There are many other derived parameters used to describe bone dynamics described by Frost (1983b).

Histomorphometric values for normal males and females with relation to age, and values for the various diseases compared to age- and sex-matched normal controls are published and useful as reference guidelines (Melsen et al 1983). It is important to be aware of pitfalls in techniques for bone morphometry; these are well discussed in Recker's book (1983). An example of a problem is with serial biopsy evaluation of a severe disease, e.g. Paget's, where known variations occur from site to site and even within the same bone. It is important that each laboratory establish its own set of normal values along with careful standard operating procedures (SOP) for sample preparation, staining techniques, and microscopy used for bone morphometry. If standardized stains or magnification are not used, measurements made using different stains can result in different values for the same biopsy. A standardized magnification must be used to estimate surface values, otherwise higher values are produced with increased magnification as finer surface convolutions are resolved. Detailed discussions of bone morphometry can be found in *Bone Histomorphometry: Techniques and Interpretation* (Recker 1983); Proceedings of the International Workshop on Bone Histomorphometry (Jee & Parfitt 1980); and a useful review by Revell (1986).

TEETH

Teeth, like bone, consist largely of mineralized collagen with the bulk of a tooth a mass of dentine forming the main part of the crown and root. This mass is composed of heavily mineralized collagen bundles penetrated by dental tubules (analogous to canaliculi in bone) that pass from the odontoblasts lining the central cavity through the dentine to its exterior surface. There are no cells comparable to bone osteocytes. The dentine of the crown is covered by an enamel layer, which is an acellular substance said to be the hardest in the body. Enamel contains very little organic material and consists mainly of mineral with a few supporting collagen bundles.

The root of the tooth is covered by a cementum layer and anchored in the jawbone cavity or tooth socket by the periodontal ligament. This ligament consists of collagen fibers that are embedded in both cement and the bone surrounding the tooth cavity.

The dental pulp forms a central core within the dentine, and is lined with odontoblasts and filled with loose connective tissue containing nerves and blood vessels.

Teeth generally receive the same treatment as bone prior to sectioning. After fixation and decalcification, processing and embedment in either paraffin, celloidin, or MMA can be used to produce thin sections necessary for the study of teeth and their associated soft tissues. Celloidin embedding is useful to study a tooth or teeth in situ within the bone, although this can be done with MMA and is possible with extended paraffin procedures. Ground sections of MMA-embedded or unembedded teeth are essential for the study of mineralized components. Plastic embedment is better for maintaining soft tissue integrity that would be lost when grinding unembedded teeth. Smith (1962a,b) has discussed the advantages of cryomicrotomy of decalcified teeth and dental material for the demonstration of innervation.

Fixation

Teeth should be fixed whole in NBF. Adult teeth will require up to 4 days' fixation and for younger teeth, where the base of the pulp cavity is more open, 24 hours' fixation may be adequate.

Decalcification

Because of its high mineral concentration, enamel is almost impossible to preserve through a completed decalcification process. Brain (1966) used a long (approximately 12 weeks) decalcification procedure on a 3-mm slice of tooth in a 4 M sodium acetate–HCl buffer solution at pH 3.55. He decalcified the tooth slice until the dentine and bone were clear with an X-ray test and the enamel still opaque but soft enough for paraffin

sectioning. Plastic embedment with ground sections may be a better choice for examination of hard enamel, and teeth containing fillings or implants.

For general purposes Smith (1962a) recommended 5% trichloracetic acid as a decalcifier, although some workers prefer to decalcify teeth with EDTA or buffered formic acid solutions. Other decalcifiers can be used with choices influenced by the same factors considered with reference to bone (p. 340).

Radiography is ideal for following the progress and endpoint testing of decalcification and also reveals the presence of amalgam or metal fillings but not some implanted resin materials. Large fillings frequently become dislodged during decalcification.

Processing

Since the tooth consists mainly of very dense material, paraffin, plastic, and celloidin processing times should be extended similar to those used in bone methods.

Section cutting and adhesion

Sectioning and adhesion techniques used for bone also work for teeth (see p. 351).

Staining

Staining methods applied to decalcified or undecalcified bone and soft tissues can be used for teeth.

H&E (p. 345)	general or diagnostic work
Trichrome (p. 150)	collagen fibers in periodontal ligament
van Gieson's (p. 148)	collagen fibers in periodontal ligament
Picro-thionin (p. 348)	dental tubules
'Air injection' (p. 347)	dental tubules
Silver impregnation (p. 354)	nerve fibers in dental pulp
Sudan black (p. 194)	lipid and myelin
Microradiography (p. 357)	mineral density

REFERENCES

Bloebaum R.D., Bachus K.N., Boyce, T.M. (1990) Backscattered electron imaging: the role in calcified tissue and implant analysis. Journal of Biomaterial Applications 5:56–85.

Boellaard J.W., von Hirsch T. (1959) Die Herstellung histologischer Schnitte von nicht enkalkten Knochen mittles Einbettung, Methacrylsaureester. Mikroskopie 13:386.

Boivin G., Baud C.-A. (1984) Microradiographic methods for calcified tissues. In: Dickson G., ed. Methods of calcified tissue preparation. New York: Elsevier, Ch. 11, p. 403.

Brain E.B. (1966) The preparation of decalcified sections. Springfield, IL: C.C. Thomas, pp. 86–89.

Byers P.D., Smith R. (1967) New appliances: trephine for full-thickness iliac-crest biopsy. British Medical Journal 1:682.

Callis G.M., Sterchi D.L. (1998) Decalcification of bone: literature review and practical study of various decalcifying agents, methods and their effects on bone histology. Journal of Histotechnology 21(1):49–58.

Clayden E.C. (1952) A discussion on the preparation of bone sections by the paraffin wax method with special reference to the control of decalcification. Journal of Medical Laboratory Technology 10:103.

Culling C.F. (1974) Handbook of histopathological and histochemical techniques, 3rd edn. London: Butterworths, p. 65.

Denton J., Freemont A.J., Ball J. (1984) Detection and distribution of aluminium in bone. Journal of Clinical Pathology 37:136–142.

Difford J. (1974) A simplified method for the preparation of methyl methacrylate embedding medium for undecalcified bone. Medical Laboratory Technology 31:79–81.

Dodds R.A., Gowen M. (1994) The growing osteophyte: a model system for the study of human bone development and remodeling in situ. Journal of Histotechnology 17(1):37–45.

Donath K. (1988a) Preparation of histologic sections by a cutting–grinding technique for hard tissue and other material not suitable to be sectioned by routine methods, 2nd edn. Norderstedt: EXAKT-Kulzer Publication, pp. 1–16.

Donath K. (1988b) Die Trenn-Dünnschliff-Technik zur Herstellun hisologische Präparate von nicht schniebaren Geweben und Materialien. Der Präpauator 34:197–206. German report, translated and published by EXAKT-Kulzer Publication.

Drury R.A.B., Wallington E.A. (1980) Carelton's histological technique, 5th edn. London: Oxford University Press, pp. 199–220.

Dunn E.G., Bowes D.N., Rothert S.W., Greer R.B. III (1974) An inexpensive x-ray source for the microradiography of bone. Calcified Tissue Research 15:329.

Eurell J., Sterchi D.L. (1994) Microwaveable toluidine blue stain for surface staining of undecalcified bone sections. Journal of Histotechnology 17(4):357–359.

Evans N., Krajian A. (1930) A new method of decalcification. Archives of Pathology 10:447.

Fornasier V.L. (1975) Fine detail radiography in the examination of tissue. Human Pathology 6(5):623–631.

Frost H.M. (1983a) Choice of marking agent and labelling schedule. In: Recker R.R., ed. Bone histomorphometry: techniques and interpretation. Florida: CRC Press, pp. 37–52.

Frost H.M. (1983b) Bone histomorphometry: analysis of trabecular bone dynamics. In: Recker R.R., ed. Bone histomorphometry: techniques and interpretation. Florida: CRC Press, pp. 109–132.

Gatenby J.B., Painter T. (1934) In: The microtomist's Vade Mecum, 10th edn. London: Churchill, p. 427.

Goldner J. (1937) A modification of the Masson trichrome technique for routine laboratory purposes. American Journal of Clinical Pathology 20:237–243.

Gooding H., Stewart D. (1932) A comparative study of histological preparations of bone which have been treated with different combinations of fixatives and decalcifying fluids. Laboratory Journal 7:55.

Gray P. (1954) The microtomist's formulary and guide. London: Constable, pp. 256–260.

Hand N.M., Church R.J. (1998) Superheating using pressure cooking: its use and application in unmasking antigens embedded in methyl methacrylate. Journal of Histotechnology 21(3):233.

Hardt A.B. (1986) Modification of the tape transfer technique: reduced shattering and distortion of hard tissue sections. Journal of Histotechnology 13(3):125–126.

Hillemann H.H., Lee C.H. (1953) Organic chelating agents for decalcification of bone and teeth. Stain Technology 28:285.

Huffer W.E., Zhu J.M., Ruegg P. (1996) Modified acidic solochrome azurine stain for video image analysis of aluminum lines in bone biopsies. Journal of Histotechnology 19(2):115–119.

Hughesdon P.E. (1949) Two uses of uranyl nitrate. Journal of the Royal Microscopical Society 69:1.

Hyman J.M., Poulding R.H. (1961) Solochrome cyaniniron alum for rapid staining of frozen sections. Journal of Medical Laboratory Technology 18:107.

Irwin D.A. (1955) The demonstration of aluminum in human tissues. American Medical Association Archives of Industrial Health 12:218–220.

Jee W.S.S., Parfitt A.M., eds. (1980) Bone histomorphometry, 3rd International Workshop. Metabolic Bone Disease and Related Research 2(Suppl).

Kristensen H.K. (1948) An improved method of decalcification. Stain Technology 23:151.

Maloney N.A., Ott S.M., Alfrey A.C. et al. (1982) Histological quantification of aluminium in lilac bone from patients with renal failure. Journal of Laboratory and Clinical Medicine 99:206–216.

Matrajt H., Hioco D. (1966) Solochrome cyanine R as an indicator dye of bone morphology. Stain Technology 41:97.

Mawhinney W.H., Richardson E., Malcolm A.J. (1984) Control of rapid nitric acid decalcification. Journal of Clinical Pathology 37:1409–1415.

Melsen F., Mosekilde L., Kragstrup J. (1983) Metabolic bone diseases as evaluated by bone histomorphometry. In:

Recker R.R., ed. Bone histomorphometry: techniques and interpretation. Florida: CRC Press, pp. 265–285.

Milch R.A., Rall D.P., Tobie J.E. (1957) Bone localization of the tetracyclines. Journal of the National Cancer Institute 19:87.

Milch R.A., Rall D.P., Tobie J.E. (1958) Fluorescence of tetracycline antibiotics in bone. Journal of Bone and Joint Surgery 40A:897.

Parfitt A.M. (1988) Bone histomorphometry: standardization of nomenclature, symbols and units (summary of proposed system). Bone 99:67–69.

Parfitt A.M., Drezner M.K., Glorieux F.H. et al. (1987) Bone histomorphometry: standardization of nomenclature, symbols, and units. Journal of Bone and Mineral Research 2:595–610.

Perenyi J. (1882) Über eine neue Erhärtungsflussigkeit. Zoologischer Anzeiger 5:459.

Recker R.R. (1983) Bone histomorphometry: techniques and interpretation. Florida: CRC Press.

Recker R.R. (1990) Bone biopsy and histomorphometry in clinical practice. In: Clinical evaluation of bone and mineral disorders, primer on the metabolic diseases and disorder of mineral metabolism, 1st edn. Virginia: American Society for Bone and Mineral Research, William Byrd Press, pp. 101–104.

Revell P. (1986) Quantitative methods in bone biopsy examination. In: Pathology of bone. Heidelberg: Springer.

Rosen A.D. (1981) End-point determination in EDTA decalcification using ammonium oxalate. Stain Technology 56:48–49.

Rosenberg L. (1971) Chemical basis for the histological use of safranin O in the study of articular cartilage. Journal of Bone and Joint Surgery 53A:69–82.

Russell N.L. (1963) A rapid method for decalcification of bone for histological examination using the 'Histette'. Journal of Medical Laboratory Technology 20:299.

Sanderson C. (1997) Entering the realm of mineralized bone processing: a review of the literature and techniques. Journal of Histotechnology 20(3):259–266.

Sanderson C., Radley K., Mayton L. (1995) Ethylenediaminetetracetic acid in ammonium hydroxide for reducing decalcification time. Biotechnics and Histochemistry 70:18.

Schenk R.K., Olah A.J., Herrmann W. (1984) Preparation of calcified tissues for light microscopy. In: Dickson G., ed. Methods of calcified tissue preparation. Amsterdam: Elsevier, pp. 1–56.

Schiller B. (1999) A cost-effective system for paraffin-quality frozen sections. American Clinical Laboratory 18:8.

Schmorl G. (1934) Die Pathologisch-Histologischen Untersuchungsmethoden. Berlin: Vogel, p. 259.

Scott J.E., Dorling J. (1965) Differential staining of acid glycosaminoglycans (mucopolysaccharides) by Alcian Blue in salt solutions. Histochemie 5:221.

Smith A. (1962a) The use of frozen sections in oral histology Part I. Journal of Medical Laboratory Technology 19:26.

Smith A. (1962b) The use of frozen sections in oral histology Part II. Journal of Medical Laboratory Technology 19:89.

Steedman H.F. (1960) Section cutting in microscopy. Oxford: Blackwell.

Sterchi D.L. (1996) Kodak methylmethacrylate replacement (letter). Journal of Histotechnology 19(1):88.

Stevens A., Lowe J., Bancroft J.D. (1996) Bone. In: Bancroft J.D., Stevens A., eds. Theory and practice of histological techniques, 2nd edn. London: Churchill Livingstone, pp. 320–321.

Taylor R.L., Flechtenmacher J., Dedrick D.K. (1993) Variation of the Holmes method for histologic staining of bone canaliculi. Journal of Histotechnology 16(4):355–357.

Tornero G., Latta L.L., Godoy G. (1991) Use of microwave radiation for the histological study of bone canaliculi. Journal of Histotechnology 14(1):27–30.

Tripp E.J., Mackay E.H. (1972) Silver staining of bone prior to decalcification for quantitative determination of osteoid in sections. Stain Technology 47:129.

von Kossa J. (1901) Nachweis von Kalk. Beitrage zur pathologischen Anatomie und zur allgemeinen. Pathologie 29:163.

Wallington E.A. (1972) Histological methods for bone. London: Butterworths.

Woodruff L.A., Norris W.P. (1955) Sectioning of undecalcified bone with special reference to radiautographic applications. Stain Technology 30:174.

FURTHER READING

Chappard D., Blouin S., Libouban H., Baslé M.F., Audran M. (2005) Microcomputed tomography of hard tissues and bone biomaterials. Microscopy and Analysis 19(3): 23–25(AM).

Chevrier A., Rossomacha E., Buschmann M.D., Hoemann C.D. (2005) Optimization of histoprocessing methods to detect glycosaminoglycan, collagen Type II and collagen Type I in decalcified rabbit osteochondral sections. Journal of Histotechnology 28(3):165–175.

Dotti L.B., Paparo G.B., Clarke B.E. (1951) The use of ion exchange resin in decalcification of bone. American Journal of Clinical Pathology 21:475.

Fornasier V.L., Ho C.L. (2003) Radiological examination of calcified tissues with emphasis on bone. In: An Y.H., Martin K.L., eds. Handbook of histology methods for bone and cartilage. Totowana, NJ: Humana, pp. 531–535.

Frost H.M. (1976) Histomorphometry of trabecular bone 1. Theoretical correction of appositional rate measurements. In: Meunier P.J., ed. Bone histomorphometry, second international workshop. Toulouse: Société de la Nouvelle Imprimerie Fournie, pp. 361–370.

Mawhinney W.H., Richardson E., Malcolm A.J. (1984) Control of rapid nitric acid decalcification. Journal of Clinical Pathology 37:1409–1415.

Rittman B.R.J. (2000) Teeth and their associated tissues. Microscopy Today 00–1:18–20.

Sobel A.E., Hanok A. (1951) Rapid method for determination of ultramicro quantities of calcium and magnesium. Archives of Pathology 44:92–95.

Sudhaker Rao D. (1983) Practical approach to obtaining a bone biopsy. In: Recker R.R., ed. Bone histomorphome-try: techniques and interpretation. Florida: CRC Press, pp. 3–11.

Thomas C.B., Jenkins L., Kellen J.F., Burg J.L. (2003) End-point verification of bone demineralization for tissue engineering applications. Tissue Engineered Medical Products (TEMPs), ASTM STP 1452, Picciolo, G.L.

Villanueva A.R. (1980) Bone, Part II. Basic preparation and staining in decalcified bone. In: Sheehan D.C., Hrapchak B.B., eds. Theory and practice of histotechnology. London: C.V. Mosby, pp. 96–98.

19

Techniques in Neuropathology

Scott L. Nestor

INTRODUCTION

Classical neuropathology has relied heavily on the use of a large array of empirical staining techniques to demonstrate the specialized structures encountered within the central nervous system. Although many of the traditional staining techniques remain useful, e.g. Bielschowsky silver stain to demonstrate neuritic plaques and neurofibrillary tangles in Alzheimer's disease and the luxol fast blue stain to demonstrate myelin, great advances have been made, particularly in translational research laboratories, to identify more sensitive and specific techniques and markers to diagnose pathological material and in some instances predict clinically significant biological behavior, particularly in the area of tumor pathology. The majority of these techniques involve immunocytochemical methods utilizing antibodies directed against a specific protein marker or the even more specific in situ hybridization techniques to identify abnormal genes (see Chapter 26).

This chapter will review the cells and tissues which are encountered in a routine neuropathology practice, together with descriptions of appropriate laboratory methods for their detection. The staining of the main components of the nervous system, including tumors, is first described, and then an investigation of dementia, neurodegenerative diseases, and skeletal muscle pathology. For a detailed review of the underlying principles of silver impregnation techniques, the reader is referred to the fifth edition of this text.

STAINING OF COMPONENTS OF THE NERVOUS SYSTEM

The main geographic divisions of the central nervous system (CNS) are the brain (including cerebellum), brainstem, and spinal cord. Nerves lying outside of these areas constitute the peripheral nervous system (PNS). The major cellular structures encountered in the nervous system include:

- neurons (nerve cells)
- oligodendrocytes (CNS) or Schwann cells (PNS) (myelin production)
- astrocytes (supporting cells)
- ependymal cells (lining ventricles and spinal canal)
- microglia (monocyte–macrophage-type cells).

Neuronal cells and axons

Neurons receive and transmit electrical signals via salutatory conduction. Typically there are three elements common to most neurons:

- *cell body:* the main part of the cell containing the nucleus
- *axon:* a single elongated process carrying signals away from the cell body
- *dendrites:* one or more processes that receive inputs via connections with other nerve cells.

Morphological variations of these elements occur according to their specific neuronal function. *Motor neurons* convey signals away from the central nervous system to end-organs and muscles. *Sensory neurons* convey signals to the central nervous system from specialized receptors. *Interneurons* act as relay centers, synthesizing numerous inputs, and producing an appropriate output signal.

The cell body of a neuron contains a large nucleus with a crisp nuclear membrane, dispersed chromatin, and a prominent nucleolus. Within the cell body cytoplasm are *Nissl granules*, basophilic granules that represent rough endoplasmic reticulum (Palay & Palade

1955) and give rise to the characteristic stippled baso-philia present in many neurons. Changes in the pattern of distribution of Nissl granules occur with neuronal disease. Following neuronal damage, Nissl granules which are generally dispersed throughout the cytoplasm migrate to the cell periphery in a process termed *central chromatolysis.*

Pigments may be seen in neurons. The neuronal cyto-plasm in neurons of the substantia nigra and the locus ceruleus may contain *neuromelanin,* an insoluble dark macromolecule that is believed to be the byproduct of oxidative metabolism of catecholamine and is responsi-ble for the black or grey color identified within these neurons (Fasano et al 2006). *Lipofuscin* (lipochrome or 'aging pigment') is also frequently found in neuronal cell bodies within the pyramidal cell layer of the hippo-campus and the basal nucleus of Meynert in aged brains. These granules are yellow–brown in color and demon-strate autofluorescence and weak avidity for acid-fast stains. In contrast to neuromelanin, lipofuscin granules are not homogeneously argentophilic but stain around their edges only. Occasionally in aged brains and those with Alzheimer's disease these granules may become condensed within a small vacuole in a condition described as 'granulovacuolar degeneration'. Large amounts of lipofuscin-like pigment (see p. 207) accumu-late in the various forms of inherited lysosomal storage diseases, Batten's disease, neuronal ceroid lipofuscinoses (Bennett & Hofmann 1999).

Neurofibril is a term used to describe a complex network of fibrils seen running through the cytoplasm and processes of neurons, following silver impregnation staining. This staining pattern is due to the presence of three main cytoskeletal components: microtubules, (composed of α-tubulin, β-tubulin, microtubule-associ-ated proteins (MAPs), and tau proteins), neurofilaments (intermediate filament specific to neurons), and micro-filaments (actin) (Matus 1987). In certain degenerative diseases such as Alzheimer's disease, *neurofibrillary tangles* form in the cell body and are composed of an abnormally phosphorylated protein (tau protein) aligned into paired helical filaments (Kosik et al 1986).

Nerve cell processes are of two main types, the axons and dendrites. The *axon* (nerve fiber) is usually single and arises from a conical projection of the neuron ('axon hillock'). In a motor neuron, the axonal cell process may be up to 1 meter long, and in its course it may be ensheathed in an insulating layer of myelin (see later). The axon contains neurofibrils but no Nissl granules.

The *dendrites* are short multiple cell processes which arborize widely to make contact with other neurons at synapses. Dendritic processes may contain Nissl gran-ules, in contrast to axonal processes. The distal end of an axon terminates at either the cell body or dendrite of another neuron to form a synapse, or in a specialized nerve ending, e.g. the motor end-plate of muscle.

TECHNIQUES FOR STAINING NEURONS

The general architecture of the neuron is seen in routine hematoxylin and eosin preparations (p. 126). The hema-toxylin and van Gieson technique (p. 148) is a popular stain as it highlights vascular changes, emphasizes myelin staining, and provides crisp cellular cytology. A method for the application of the hematoxylin and van Gieson technique for nitrocellulose sections has been detailed in a previous editions of this text and is not included here.

Techniques for staining Nissl substance

Nissl stains may be used alone or combined with the luxol fast blue myelin stain, not so much to demonstrate Nissl substance but as a stain to show the cellular pattern useful for evaluating neuronal populations (Schochet & McCormick 1979). Nissl granules can be demonstrated with many basic dyes, e.g. neutral red, methylene blue, azur, pyronin, thionin, toluidine blue, and cresyl fast violet. Variation in stain, pH, and length of differen-tiation will enable some stains either to highlight Nissl substance only, or to include the nuclei of neurons and glia. The granules are distributed in the cytoplasm and dendrites of neurons; for practical class work, the anterior horn cells of the spinal cord, being both very large and rich in this substance, are ideally suited for the practice of these stains (Fig. 19.1). Einarson's (1932) gallocyanin method for nucleic acids is a progressive stain particularly useful for the demonstration of Nissl substance in paraffin sections by bulk staining. Since it is only slowly progressive after optimal staining has been reached, it is difficult to overstain (Kellett 1963).

Tissue fixed in alcohol stains particularly well, especially with thionin, but this dye does not give such good results as the toluidine blue technique (Fig. 19.1) or cresyl fast violet on formalin-fixed tissue.

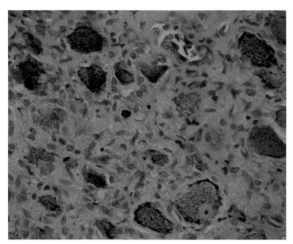

Fig. 19.1 Anterior horn cells. Notice their large size and the prominent nucleolus. Paraffin section, stained with toluidine blue. Similar results can be obtained with cresyl fast violet.

Cresyl fast violet (Nissl) stain for paraffin sections

Fixation
Alcohol, Carnoy's, or neutral formal saline.

Sections
Paraffin 7–10 μm or 25 μm (see Note b).

Preparation of stain
Cresyl fast violet	0.5 g
Distilled water	100 ml

Differentiation solution
Glacial acetic acid	250 μl
Alcohol	100 ml

Method
1. Dewax sections and bring to water.
2. Cover with filtered cresyl fast violet; stain for 10–20 min.
3. Rinse in distilled water.
4. Differentiate in 0.25% acetic alcohol until most of the stain has been removed (4–8 s).
5. Briefly pass through absolute alcohol into xylene and check microscopically.
6. Repeat steps 4 and 5 if necessary, giving less differentiation when repeating.
7. Rinse well in xylene and mount in Canada balsam or DPX.

Results
Nissl substance	purple–dark blue
Neurons	pale purple–blue
Cell nuclei	purple blue

Notes
a. If only Nissl substance is required to be demonstrated, the stain is acidified with 0.25% acetic acid.
b. Estimation of cortical neuronal density is made on 25-μm thick sections.

Immunohistochemistry of neurons

There are several immunohistochemical markers that can be used to detect neurons. Many of these methods identify markers which imply a neuroendocrine differentiation, and so include many cells of the diffuse endocrine system (amine precursor uptake and decarboxylation [APUD] cells). The main immunochemical markers can be divided into four groups:

1. Neuronal nuclear proteins. The neuron-associated Hu protein family (HuC, HuD, and HelNl) are RNA binding proteins restricted to the nucleus of neurons throughout the neuraxis. These stains give the distinct advantage of staining the nuclei of neuronal and neuroendocrine tissues and avoid the interpretative limitations of cytoplasmic and cytoskeletal stains (Gultekin et al 2000). Another nuclear protein, NeuN, is a neuron-specific DNA binding protein which also has the advantage of being a nuclear stain. NeuN becomes apparent around the time of initiation of terminal differentiation of the neuron (Mullen et al 1992).

2. Neuronal cytoskeletal proteins. The neurofilament proteins are the intermediate filaments specific to nerve cells, and antibodies to neurofilament proteins identify mature neuronal cells (Trojanowski et al 1984). There are three main types of neurofilament protein, NF70(L), NF150(M), and NF200(H), each having a different molecular weight and each capable of being modified by phosphorylation (Phry) (Nixon 1993). There are thus several possible different antibodies to neurofilament proteins, which may be directed to one of three molecular weight categories, or subject to variation because of post-translational modification by phosphorylation. These different neurofilament types show differential distribution in

different parts of the neuron, for example 200-kDa phosphorylated epitopes are restricted to the axon and are not normally seen in the perikaryal region (Schlaepfer 1987). This means that some neurofilament antibodies will not identify cell bodies of neurons, but only axons. Commercial antibodies against L, M, and H molecules with or without Phry are now available from various suppliers. A panel of at least two different antibodies, say one against Phry and non-Phry H and one against non-Phry M and H molecules, will act as a broad-spectrum test for the expression of neurofilament in the tissue. Care should therefore be exercised in the interpretation of results from antineurofilament antibody staining with due attention to what the antibody is raised against.

3. Neuron-specific cytoplasmic proteins. PGP9.5 and neuron-specific enolase (NSE) are examples of proteins which are expressed at high level in neurons and can be reliably detected by commercially available antisera. However, they are not specific for neuronal tissues and care must be taken in interpretation of positive staining (Ghobrian & Ross 1986; Van Eldik et al 1986; Wilson et al 1988). They are best used as part of a panel of antibodies defining a complete cell phenotype.

4. Proteins associated with neurosecretory granules are useful in establishing a neuroendocrine differentiation for cells by immunohistochemistry. *Chromogranin A* is a protein of the dense core matrix of neurosecretory granules, and antibodies to it can be used to identify cells containing dense core vesicles (Nolan et al 1985). *Synaptophysin* is a membrane glycoprotein seen in presynaptic neurosecretory vesicles. Antibodies to this protein immunostain at sites of synaptic junctions in normal cerebral and cerebellar cortex, and in the processes and cell perikarya of neuroblastomas (Gould et al 1986). Usually the neuronal cell body is only weakly stained (Fig. 19.2). It also stains cells in metastatic neuroendocrine tumors and is a useful marker of neuroendocrine differentiation (Wiedenmann et al 1988). *Synapsin I* and *synapsin II* are proteins associated with synaptic vesicles which can be detected by immunohistochemistry (Thiel 1993). Immunostaining for specific transmitter substances provides additional information on the anatomy and pathology of the nervous system. Antibodies to tyrosine hydroxylase, 5-hydroxytryptamine, somatostatin, substance P, vasoactive intestinal peptide, met-enkephalin, neurotensin, and serotonin

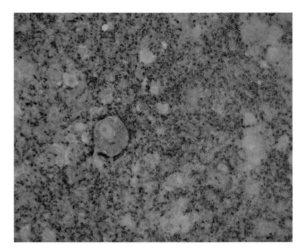

Fig. 19.2 Large neuron from area of cortical dysplasia stained with synaptophysin. Note intense staining within the neuropil and weak cytoplasmic staining.

have been identified in tumors of neuronal origin and may be applied to tissue sections to localize transmitter function (Pearson 1983; Takahashi et al 1989).

Techniques for staining axons and neuronal processes in the central nervous system

Several methods are available to demonstrate various special structures of the neuron, including axons, dendrites, terminal boutons (synaptic structures), dendritic trees, dendritic spines, degenerated axons and boutons, peripheral nerve endings, and embryonic tissue. Historically the original methods were block impregnation methods, as used by Golgi, which stain cell processes and also the cell bodies. Bielschowsky (1902) pioneered present-day methods by use of a primary 'sensitizing' silver solution which is the selectivity induction stage. A second impregnation in an ammoniacal silver solution was introduced to intensify the result, and finally reduction in formalin. Pyridine is added to some methods (Hortega) where, possibly because it is a fat solvent, it aids impregnation. Gelatin is added to reduce silver precipitation. Rinsing the section in ammoniated water prior to staining is claimed to reduce background staining. For staining axons in the peripheral nervous system, Palmgren's method uses potassium nitrate to suppress staining of reticulin. Silver techniques require attention to detail such as clean glassware and pure distilled water for a successful outcome. Stock solutions of such reagents as sodium carbonate, sodium hydroxide, and lithium carbonate should be well maintained and not more than a few months old. Demonstration of embryonic nervous tissue is best done with methods that employ the photographic principle. Examples can be found in Gallyas' 'physical development' method (1979) and Pearson and O'Neill's method (1946).

Ammoniacal silver solutions

The point at which one stops adding ammonia to dissolve precipitated silver is critical. Generally, it is best initially to add ammonia rapidly with constant shaking, and, as the end-point is approaching, add a small amount at a time with vigorous shaking to insure complete reaction before the next lot is added. It is always good to stop at a point when there are a few granules still undissolved.

Silver solutions that contain ammonia and silver nitrate only are more easily controlled. In these solutions, after the precipitate has been dissolved, a drop or two of silver nitrate can be added to absorb any excess ammonia present. If excess back titration is needed, the final solution may not have the same optimal concentration of silver ions and a 'dirtier' preparation may result. As there is a danger attending the use of ammoniacal solutions of silver (Stewart Smith 1943; Wallington 1965), they should be prepared only on the day required and discarded properly as soon as possible.

Bielschowsky's silver stain for neurofibrils, dendrites, and axons in paraffin and frozen sections, modified (Chan & Lowe 2002)

The following is a modification of Bielschowsky's method aimed at the demonstration of neurofibrils, dendrites, and axons in paraffin sections. A reproducible method requires minimal expertise. It is particularly good in showing small groups of neurons bedded in the deep nuclei of the central nervous system. To demonstrate clearly the fine and delicate neurofibrils inside neurons can be a demanding task. In order to intensify their staining without resulting in a granular preparation, a preliminary reduction step with a very dilute pyrogallol solution is introduced after the initial treatment with silver nitrate. This allows a more gradual build-up of the silver foci on the neurofibrils before the impregnation is further intensified. Da Fano's modification of Bielschowsky's ammoniacal silver solution is used, as it seems to yield a cleaner demonstration of the neuronal cell bodies, allowing the fine neurofibrils inside to be clearly seen. Often intensely stained Glees, Marsland and Erikson's, or Palmgren's preparations may show neurofibrils but their application for this particular purpose will be unreliable.

Fixation
Formal saline.

Sections
Paraffin sections, 7–10 μm. Frozen sections, 10–15 μm.

Solutions

Silver A
20% silver nitrate.

Reducer A (make fresh)
Pyrogallol	100 mg
Formalin	10 ml
80% alcohol	1200 ml

Reducer B (make fresh)
Formaldehyde	5 ml
Distilled water	95 ml

Silver B (make fresh)
To 5 ml of 20% silver nitrate add 200 μl of 40% sodium hydroxide. Add 20 ml of distilled water and shake well. Stand for a couple of minutes and discard the turbid supernatant. Repeat the washing for 5 to 6 times then add 20 ml of distilled water and 500 μl of 0.88 ammonia to dissolve the black precipitate. Shake well and add 20 μl of ammonia, a portion at a time, with vigorous shaking in between each addition until only a small amount of black granules is left. Make up to 80 ml with distilled water for use. It is essential that no excess of ammonia is added.

5% sodium thiosulfate

0.2% gold chloride

Method
1. Take sections to distilled water.
2. Cover sections with silver A for 1–2 hours in 37°C in a moist chamber. Allow 1–2 ml per section.

3. Rinse twice in distilled water and *wash in a pot* of reducer A for 3–5 min. Agitate regularly. The section should turn yellow. Because of the low concentration of pyrogallol, this solution should be changed frequently, say about once every three slides per 100 ml of the reducer.
4. Wash in three changes of distilled water, about a minute for each wash.
5. Place in silver B for 30 s. Avoid prolonged treatment as it may cause precipitation.
6. Briefly rinse in distilled water and *wash section in a pot* of reducer B for 2–5 min.
7. Wash in distilled water. Check microscopically and repeat steps 4 to 6 until the neurons are dark brown.
8. Wash in distilled water and tone in 0.2% gold chloride for 2–3 min.
9. Wash in distilled water.
10. Fix in 5% sodium thiosulfate for 5 min.
11. Wash in tap water.
12. Dehydrate, clear, and mount in DPX.

Results

Neurofibrils, dendrites, and axon	black

Notes

Before the judgment for the end-point of the impregnation is mastered, it is advisable to bring a few parallel sections through, each stained to a different intensity for comparison. Formalin-fixed frozen sections can be attached onto chrome gelatine slides for staining.

Marsland, Glees, and Erikson's method for axons in paraffin-embedded tissues
(Marsland et al 1954)

This method is popular because of its reliability. Some variants of this method use tap water to make up the reducing solution. Due to the variation in the composition of the solutes in the water supply between localities, such variants may not be successfully applied universally.

Fixation
10% formal saline.

Sections
Paraffin sections, 10–15 μm.

Solutions

Ammoniacal silver solution

Absolute alcohol	20 ml
20% silver nitrate	30 ml

Add 0.88 ammonia drop by drop until the resulting precipitate is just dissolved. Add an additional 5 drops of ammonia.

Reducing solution

Formalin	10 ml
Distilled water	100 ml

Method

1. Remove wax with xylene. Rinse in second dish of xylene.
2. Rinse in absolute alcohol.
3. Dip into 0.5–1.0% celloidin. Remove slide and allow excess celloidin to drain off. Remove celloidin from back of slide and wash in 70% alcohol for 1–5 min to harden.
4. Wash well in distilled water.
5. Place in 20% silver nitrate for 15–60 min at 37°C.
6. Wash in 10% formalin for 10–15 seconds. Sections should be pale yellow to brown.
7. Drain slides and, without washing, flood sections with ammoniacal silver solution and leave for 30 seconds.
8. Drain off silver solution and flood with 10% formalin for 1–2 min. Examine under the microscope and if necessary repeat steps 7 and 8.
9. Wash in distilled water.
10. Fix in 5% sodium thiosulfate for 1–5 min.
11. Wash, dehydrate. Remove celloidin in absolute alcohol. Clear and mount in DPX.

Results

Nerve fibers	dark brown–black
Background	light brown

Notes

Paraffin sections are celloidinized as a routine in silver methods. Some workers believe that the film of celloidin helps to trap any precipitates that may form, as it can be removed with alcohol during dehydration before mounting. This may, however, be considered an optional step. Where it does help is to increase the matrix density of the tissue, thus retaining a bit more of the silver solution after the main bulk is drained away at step 8. It also slows down the penetration of the formalin into the section. This, in a way, exaggerates the differences in reaction rate between tissue components (see text above on silver impregnation). This explains the fact that if too high a concentration of celloidin is used, which forms a thick film, the staining may be hampered as a result. Sections may be toned if desired.

If repeating steps 7 and 8 because of understaining, use 1% formalin in step 8. Alternately after step 8, further intensification can be controllably achieved by mixing 10 μl of the ammoniacal silver solution with 10 ml of 10% formalin and immediately flooding the slide. Agitate gently for 30 s to 1 min. This process can be repeated a number of times without detrimental effect on the background staining.

Techniques for staining axons in the peripheral nervous system

There are many silver impregnation methods in use that work well with the peripheral nervous system. These are modified to suppress staining of collagen and reticulin, which do not present a problem in methods destined for use in the central nervous system. Bodian's method (Mallory 1961) uses a silver proteinate (Protargol) in solution with metallic copper. The silver proteinate impregnates axons while the copper in the solution impairs uptake by connective tissue. Following development in hydroquinone, a very fine localization is achieved. Due to variability in the composition of silver proteinate, successful application of the technique relies on the selection of workable batches of Protargol by careful testing. Holmes's method (1943) uses a boric acid-buffered impregnating solution containing pyridine to achieve the correct pH for adequate staining. Immunocytochemical staining with antibodies to PGP9.5 shows fine localization to axons. Immunostaining for phosphorylated neurofilament protein of 200-kDa type shows good localization to axons. However, in biopsies that are primarily fixed in glutaldehyde, silver stains appear to give better results for routine use.

Palmgren's method for nerve fibers in paraffin-embedded material
(Palmgren 1948)

Fixation
Formal saline or Bouin's fixative.

Sections
Paraffin or double-embedded sections, 6–10 μm. Sections should be coated with nitrocellulose.

Preparation of solutions

Acid formalin

40% formaldehyde	25 ml
Distilled water	75 ml
1% nitric acid	0.2 ml

Silver solution

Silver nitrate	15 g
Potassium nitrate	10 g
Distilled water	100 ml
5% acetic acid	1 ml

Reducer

Pyrogallol	10 g
Distilled water	450 ml
Absolute ethanol	550 ml
1% nitric acid	2 ml

Allow to stand. for 24 hours before using.

Toning bath

Gold chloride	1 g
Distilled water	200 ml
Glacial acetic acid	0.2 ml

Intensifier

50% ethyl alcohol	100 ml
Aniline oil	2 drops

Fixing bath
5% sodium thiosulfate.

Method
1. Take sections to distilled water.
2. Wash sections in acid formalin for 5 min or longer.
3. Wash in three changes of distilled water for 5 min.
4. Leave in silver solution for 15 min at 20–25°C or 4–5 min at 35°C.
5. Without rinsing, drain the slide and add reducer that has been heated to 40–45°C. Rock the slide gently and add fresh reducer. Leave for 1 min. A

beaker placed on a hotplate is useful for this stage.

6. Rinse in 50% alcohol for 5–10 seconds.
7. Wash in three changes of distilled water. Examine microscopically and, if necessary, repeat from step 2, reducing the time in the silver solution and decreasing the temperature of the reducer to 30°C.
8. Tone in gold chloride until yellow–brown has faded.
9. Transfer directly into intensifier for 15 seconds or longer. Sections which contain nervous tissues *only* should be intensified after previously rinsing in 2% oxalic acid.
10. Wash in tap water.
11. Fix for a few seconds in 5% sodium thiosulfate.
12. Wash in water.
13. Dehydrate and remove nitrocellulose in absolute alcohol. Clear and mount.

Result

Nerve fibers   brown or black

Notes

a. Sections can be fixed in hypo (step 11) after stage 7 and mounted without toning.
b. The reducer keeps for several months.
c. As mentioned in the text above, at step 5 the ratio between the reducing agent and silver nitrate that was carried over greatly influences the contrast of the preparation.

Linder's method for nerves in paraffin sections of soft and mineralized tissue
(Linder 1978)

Fixation
Formal saline, formal calcium, or Bouin's fluid.

Sections
Paraffin, 6–10 µm. Mineralized tissues are decalcified with formic acid or EDTA.

Preparation of solutions

Buffer stock solution

2,4,6-Collidine	6.6 ml
Distilled water	450 ml

Adjust to pH 7.2–7.4 with 10% nitric acid, and make up to 500 ml with distilled water.

Diluted buffer

Buffer stock	8 ml
Distilled water	92 ml

Silver cyanate impregnating solution

Distilled water heated to 60°C	84 ml
1% silver nitrate	4 ml
0.38% sodium cyanate	4 ml
Buffer stock solution	8 ml

Physical developer stock solution

Sodium sulfite ($Na_2SO_3 \cdot 7H_2O$)	20 g
Sodium tetraborate ($Na_2B_4O_7 \cdot 10H_2O$)	4.75 g
Distilled water	450 ml

Heat the solution to about 50°C, and add gelatine (Belgium Gold label) 10 g.

Physical developer working solution

Physical developer stock solution	95 ml
2% hydroquinine	5 ml
1% silver nitrate	2 ml

Add the silver nitrate, stirring constantly.

Method

1. Remove paraffin, celloidinize sections and bring to distilled water.
2. Place in dilute buffer; soft tissues are left for 10–20 minutes at 60°C, decalcified tissues overnight at 40–45°C.
3. Transfer directly to silver impregnating solution; soft tissues are incubated for 10–30 min at 60°C, decalcified tissues are incubated for 90 min at 40–45°C.
4. Wash in several changes of distilled water for a total of about 3 min.
5. Transfer sections into the physical developer working solution at about 25°C. The progress of development can be monitored by washing with distilled water and examining under the microscope. When results are judged optimal, the sections are washed in distilled water, dehydrated, cleared in xylene, and mounted in Canada balsam or DPX.

Results

Myelinated and non-myelinated nerve fibers	black
Striated muscle fibers	brown

Notes

The technique can be carried out on a hotplate.

Constant stirring is essential when adding the silver nitrate in the physical developer working solution to prevent a white precipitate.

Sodium cyanate requires careful handling under safety regulations.

Techniques for staining degenerate nerve fibers

Several methods have been developed which suppress the staining of normal axons and enhance the staining of degenerate axons (Glees 1946; Nauta 1950; Nauta & Gygax 1951; Chambers et al 1956; Fink & Heimer 1967). The work of Eager is closely linked with later developments of such techniques (Eager & Barnett 1966; Eager 1970; Eager et al 1971). These methods work best when applied to tract tracing studies in experimental anatomy and the study of axonal and neuronal damage in experimental pathology as seen in the examples in Chan and Scholtz (1988) and Iizuka et al (1990).

The method given here relies on treatment of formalin-fixed frozen section material with uranyl nitrate, prior to impregnation with ammoniacal silver and subsequent reduction in an alcoholic solution. This method is of use when the presence of degenerate fibers is known, where control materials of similar nature can be used to monitor it carefully. However, because of the capriciousness of the technique it is usually unreliable as a 'search stain' for degenerate fibers. Semi-thin resin-embedded sections of tissue are much more appropriate for the detection of abnormal nerve fibers in the peripheral nervous system. In preparations of teased fibers, axonal degeneration appears as linear clusters of gray to black globules.

More recently, a method to detect degenerating axons, based on physical development applied to frozen sections of brains fixed in formalin, has been described. This involves pretreatment with alkaline hydroxylamine, washing in acetic acid, impregnation in silver nitrate in the presence of ferric ions, washing in citric acid, physical development, and washing in acetic acid (Gallyas et al 1980).

Eager's method for degenerating axons (Eager 1970)

Fixation
Formal saline.

Sections
Frozen, 30 μm.

Preparation of solutions

Ammoniacal silver solution

1.5% silver nitrate	40 ml
95% ethanol	24 ml
0.88 ammonia	4 ml
2.5% sodium hydroxide	3.6 ml

Reducer

Absolute alcohol	90 ml
Distilled water	810 ml
1% citric acid	27 ml
10% formalin	37 ml

Method

1. Place frozen sections into 2% formalin.
2. Rinse sections in distilled water.
3. Transfer sections into 2.5% uranyl nitrate for 5 min.
4. Rinse in distilled water and place in ammoniacal silver. Leave until brown, 3–15 min.
5. Transfer directly to reducer and leave until no further color change occurs, 2–5 min.
6. Rinse in distilled water.
7. Fix in 0.5% sodium thiosulfate.
8. Wash, dehydrate, clear, and mount.

Results

Degenerating fibers	brown to black
Normal fibers	pale yellow

Note
Uranyl nitrate can be replaced with 0.5% phosphomolybdic acid.

Vital staining of nerve fibers and endings with methylene blue

Renewed interest has been shown in vital staining of nerve fibers and end-plates in muscle biopsies since the work of Coers (1952). The principle of the technique, according to Ehrlich (1886), is that methylene blue injected into muscle fibers is absorbed and converted to its leuco base by reducing agents in alkaline solution; the leuco base formed is reoxidized into methylene blue by oxygenation (Fig. 19.3). For biopsies, the surgeon locates the motor point and injects the dye into the distal cut end of the muscle while it is still attached proximally. Pieces of tissue removed from the body before injection are pinned out and, using the finest needle, are injected with 10–20 ml of methylene blue. Coers and Woolf (1959) use 0.03–0.05% methylene blue (zinc free) in physiological saline, but this strength can usefully be increased for supravital staining.

Alternatives to vital staining are metal impregnation methods such as Schofield's silver impregnation technique for peripheral nerve endings (cited in Drury & Wallington 1980). Immunohistochemistry demonstration for S100 protein sometimes can show the outline of these structures by highlighting the supporting cells around them.

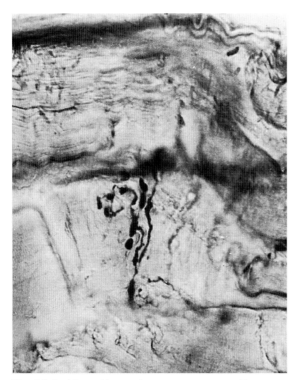

Fig. 19.3 Nerve fiber with numerous sprouts. Frozen section stained with methylene blue.

Supravital staining of nerve fibers and endings

Preparation of solutions
Methylene blue solution
Medicinal methylene blue (zinc free)	50 mg
Distilled water, pyrogen free	100 ml
Sodium chloride	0.85 g

Dissolve in the order stated.

Ammonium molybdate (stored at 4–6°C)
Ammonium molybdate	8 g
Distilled water	100 ml

Method
1. Inject methylene blue into the tissue and leave for 5–10 minutes.
2. Excise the tissue and cut longitudinally into strips no thicker than 3 mm.
3. Place tissue on Kleenex tissue soaked in saline in a Petri dish. A suitably sized funnel is inverted over the specimen and oxygen passed at the rate of 1–4 liters per minute for 1 hour. The specimen should be turned during this time in order to expose all surfaces.
4. Transfer tissue to cold ammonium molybdate and leave overnight at 4–6°C.
5. Wash in several changes of distilled water for 30 min. Squash preparations (see Note e below) or frozen sections are now made.
6. Fix tissues in 10% formalin for 24 hours.
7. Cut frozen sections at 50–100 μm.
8. Sections are dehydrated in absolute alcohol and cleared in xylene.

Results
Nerve fibers and endings   blue

Notes
a. If oxygenation is insufficient, the nerve ending will not appear stained.
b. Excessive oxygenation causes the subneural apparatus to be stained and confuses the picture.
c. Unwanted adipose tissue should be removed before oxygenation.
d. Oxygen bubbled through water helps to keep the specimen moist; otherwise drops of saline must be applied to avoid drying.
e. Squash preparations can be made in the following manner (Bone 1972).

After step 5, the tissue is dissected to obtain thin lengths of fibers. They are placed on filter paper, another filter paper placed on top, and the whole is pressed firmly on the bench. The flattened tissue is peeled off the paper and placed between two slides, which are put in a dish of absolute alcohol. The slides are kept firmly pressed together whilst in the alcohol. Eventually the slides are separated and the tissues blotted dry before returning to fresh absolute alcohol. The tissue is cleared in xylene and mounted in Canada balsam or DPX.

Golgi block impregnation techniques

The block impregnation techniques originally developed by Golgi give tremendous insight into the three-dimensional nature of the neuron and its processes. For many years these methods were of mainly historic interest, but they have recently been found of use in evaluating loss of dendritic arborization and dendritic spine density in neurons in the cerebral cortex, for example in degenerative diseases and dementia (Scheibel 1978; Garey et al 1998). Following impregnation of tissue blocks, thick sections are cut and mounted. The unexplained phenomenon which makes the method so useful is that only a few cells become impregnated, giving a clear picture of neuronal architecture uncluttered by surrounding cell processes. The morphology of individual neurons and their processes can also be investigated by intracellular injection of fluorescent dye in fixed brain slices. This technique uses micromanipulators to localize micropipettes. Dye is delivered into single cells by micro-iontophoresis (Buhl 1992). Golgi's (1873) original method was to harden fresh tissue in potassium dichromate, followed by immersion in weak silver nitrate ('slow method'). In a later modification (Golgi 1875), osmium tetroxide and potassium dichromate were used for hardening the tissues ('rapid method') before silvering. Combining the methods, Golgi fixed the tissue initially in dichromate, followed by the osmium tetroxide–dichromate mixture and then silvered it ('mixed method'). Golgi (1879) was able to obtain similar results using mercuric chloride after hardening in dichromate, but it is the method of Cox (1891) that has proved most successful.

Moliner (1957, 1958) modified the Golgi–Cox method by the addition of tungstate to the impregnating solu-tion. Fox Clement et al (1951) used formalin-fixed tissue in a zinc chromate–formic acid bath; thin slices were then cut and immersed in silver nitrate. Bertram (1958) reported the failure of some sources of zinc chromate. Tunturi (1973), using the Golgi technique, treated the tissues in formalin after the silver bath, followed by a second impregnation in silver nitrate, finally treating again with 10% formalin. With this modification, myelinated axons were also stained.

A variety of counterstaining methods have been adapted for use with this technique (Turcotte & Ramon-Moliner 1965; Smyser 1973). Inadequate tissue preservation and long postmortem delay are factors which can adversely affect staining quality and morphology (Williams et al 1978; de Rutter 1983). The technique has been adapted for plastic sections (Kirby 1978). More recently, the technique has been adapted for use with paraffin embedding, allowing combined immunohisto-chemical staining (Pugh & Rossi 1993).

Golgi–Cox method adapted for wax embedding (Pugh & Rossi 1993)

In this method, after impregnation of tissue slices in a Golgi–Cox solution, tissue is embedded in wax. After section cutting, the sections are blackened and may be counterstained. The Golgi block can be used for other purposes after sections are deimpregnated with iodine/sodium thiosulfate. In this way, routine histology can be used to complement serial sections impregnated by the Golgi–Cox method. The extent and the degree of impregnation vary through the thickness of the block and with the duration of impregnation.

Fixation
Integral in method.

Sections
None: fresh tissue slices.

Preparation of solutions
Golgi–Cox fixation/impregnation solution

a. 5% mercuric chloride ($HgCl_2$)	20 ml
b. 5% aqueous potassium dichromate ($K_2Cr_2O_7$)	20 ml
c. 5% aqueous potassium chromate ($KCrO_4$)	20 ml
d. Distilled water	40 ml

Mix a with b. Mix c with d, then add to the mixture of a and b.

Method

1. Fresh tissue slices, not thicker than 5 mm, are placed on a layer of glass wool and left in the Golgi–Cox fluid in the dark for up to 16 weeks at 20–25°C.
2. Blocks are washed overnight in 1% solution of $K_2Cr_2O_7$.
3. Blocks are processed into paraffin wax using the following schedule:

70% ethanol	2 hours
100% ethanol	4 × 2 hour changes
Chloroform	3 × 2 hour changes
Wax (56°C)	4 × 2 hour changes

4. Sections are cut between 5 and 200 μm.

Blackening

1. Dewax sections in xylene and take to water.
2. Drain and invert over a fully saturated solution of NH_3. Allow 10 min for sections up to 10 μm, 15 min for sections up to 30 μm, and 30 min for sections above 30 μm.
3. Wash in running water for 5 min.
4. Immerse in 15% Amfix to decolorize the background (approx 10 min).
5. Wash in running water for 5 min.
6. Dehydrate, clear, and mount in DPX.

Results

A proportion of neurons and their dendritic processes	black
Occasional astrocytes in subpial layer	black
Occasional astrocytes in white matter	black

Notes

a. Mercuric chloride should be pure and dissolved by boiling (HAZARDOUS).
b. Before step 6 it is possible to counterstain thinner sections with a standard H&E technique or 0.1% cresyl fast violet. Sections may also be processed for combined immunohistochemistry.
c. Blackened or unblackened sections may be de-impregnated as follows to allow conventional staining:
   1. Lugol's iodine, 5 min.
   2. Wash in running tap water, 1 min.
   3. 5% sodium thiosulfate, 5 min.
   4. Wash in running tap water, 1 min.

MYELIN

Techniques for demonstration of myelin

Myelin is the insulating layer that facilitates the rapid electrical conduction along axons in the central and peripheral nervous systems. In the central nervous system a single oligodendrocyte can support up to 50 myelin sheaths, while multiple Schwann cells are required to form the myelin sheaths required for a single axon in the peripheral nervous system. Each cell wraps up to 100 concentric layers of highly specialized plasma membrane around the axon. Chemically, myelin consists of specific proteins, lipids, and cerebrosides. There are histological techniques for the demonstration of normal myelin and also specific methods for the identification of myelin degeneration products as the result of a disease process (see also Chapter 12). Immunohistochemical methods and in situ hybridization techniques utilizing appropriate mRNA probes are now available to detect the specific proteins present in myelin sheaths. These techniques, however, are not currently utilized on a routine basis in most clinical neuropathology practices.

Historically, the classical methods for the demonstration of myelin involved a tissue chromate mordant followed by tissue processing, staining in hematoxylin, and subsequent differentiation in potassium permanganate, oxalic acid, and sodium sulfate. This method, associated with the names of Weigert, Pal, and Kultschitsky, gives brilliant staining but is time consuming in practice. Several other methods are available for formalin-fixed paraffin-processed tissue which, because of their ease of use, have largely replaced older techniques. Certain myelin stains can be combined with a Nissl stain to demonstrate myelin and neuronal localization.

Loyez' method (1910) uses a mordant in 4% iron alum followed by staining in lithium carbonate–hematoxylin and subsequent differentiation. Weil's method (1928) uses iron alum and hematoxylin simultaneously to achieve similar results. In both of these techniques sections are regressively stained and two-stage differentiation is used. Firstly 4% iron alum removes lightly bound stain into solution with free mordant, and secondly a borax–ferricyanide solution (Weigert's differentiator) acts as an oxidizing agent and removes non-specifically bound dye lake.

Luxol fast blue is a copper phthalocyanine dye which is employed in myelin staining of paraffin-processed tissue (Kluver & Barrera 1953), and can be combined with Nissl staining, periodic acid–Schiff (PAS) and hematoxylin methods (Fig. 19.4).

The solochrome cyanine stain is a simple and rapid technique for demonstration of myelin, both in the central nervous system and, particularly, in sections of peripheral nerve (see Chapter 18).

Demonstrating myelinated fibers in the peripheral nervous system requires careful microscopic control, as individual fibers are important in histological evaluation. Lipid histochemical methods for normal myelin, based on its sphingomyelin content, are discussed in Chapter 12, and the uses of combination techniques to demonstrate both normal and degenerate myelin on page 208.

Immunocytochemical staining of myelin is seen with antibodies to S100 protein (Van Eldik et al 1986), and with Leu-7, an antibody originally described as a marker for a subset of lymphocytes, but cross-reacting with myelin-associated glycoprotein (Swanson et al 1987). Other substances which identify myelin by oligodendrocyte staining include galactocerebroside (Raff et al 1978), myelin basic protein (MBP) (Sternberger et al 1977), myelin-associated glycoprotein (MAG), carbonic anhydrase C (Ghandour et al 1980), P0, P1 and P2 proteins (Mukai 1983), and αB crystallin (Iwaki et al 1989). None of these immunocytochemical methods has taken the place of conventional myelin stains; however, detection of S100 protein immunoreactivity is useful in identifying tumors derived from the cells forming myelin in peripheral nerves (Schwann cells) (Swanson et al 1987). Moreover, the demonstration of myelin basic protein can

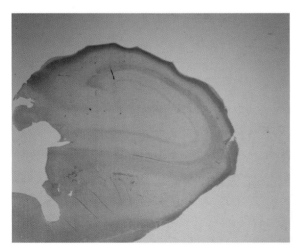

Fig. 19.4 Macrosection of a human hippocampus demonstrating geographical variation in myelin content. Luxol fast blue and hematoxylin.

be applied to less matured brain to insure that over-differentiation of the thinly and sparsely myelinated structures does not occur. Generally speaking, in frozen and glutaldehyde-fixed paraffin sections, the staining of the myelin figures is more complete as compared to formalin-fixed paraffin material.

Weil's method for myelin sheaths
(Weil 1928)

In this method, the mordant and dye are mixed in the staining solution.

Fixation
Formal saline or formal calcium.

Sections
Paraffin, 10–15 μm. Frozen, 20–30 μm. Nitrocellulose, 20–30 μm.

Frozen sections are brought through alcohols up to xylene and back again to water.

Preparation of stain

4% aqueous iron alum	50 ml

50 ml of 1% hematoxylin made from 10% alcoholic hematoxylin (5 ml) and distilled water (45 ml).

Mix together immediately before use.

Method
1. Wash sections in distilled water.
2. Place sections in stain for 10–45 min at 50–60°C.
3. Wash well in tap water.
4. Differentiate in 4% iron alum, just long enough to distinguish the gray matter or the degenerated areas.
5. Wash well in several changes of distilled water.
6. Complete the differentiation in Weigert's borax ferricyanide solution (see Appendix I).
7. Wash well in several changes of distilled water, followed by tap water.
8. Dehydrate, clear, and mount.

Results

Myelin	black
Background	yellow

Note
This is a good method for frozen sections. As with all hematoxylin stains, acid alcohol can be used to differentiate the sections.

Solochrome cyanine technique for myelin in paraffin sections (Page 1965)

Fixation
Formal saline or formal calcium.

Sections
Paraffin, 6–10 µm. Cryostat section, 10 µm.

Preparation of solution

Solochrome cyanine RS	0.2 g
Distilled water	96 ml
10% iron alum	4 ml
Concentrated sulfuric acid	0.5 ml

Method
1. Take sections to water.
2. Stain for 10–20 min at room temperature.
3. Wash in running water.
4. Differentiate in 5% iron alum until all the nuclei are unstained. Wash frequently in distilled water, and examine.
5. Wash in running tap water.
6. Counterstain if desired.
7. Dehydrate, clear, and mount.

Result
Myelin sheaths	blue

Notes
a. The staining solution keeps well.
b. Borax–ferricyanide may be used for differentiation but its action is slow.
c. Neutral red, Piero-Ponceau S, or van Gieson can be used for counterstaining.

Kluver and Barrera luxol fast blue stain for myelin with Nissl counterstain
(Kluver & Barrera 1953)

Fixation
Formalin.

Sections
Paraffin, 10–15 µm.

Preparation of solutions

Luxol fast blue

Luxol fast blue	1 g
Methanol (absolute)	1000 ml
10% acetic acid	5 ml

Mix reagents and filter. This solution may then be stored for up to 18 months before use.

Cresyl violet solution

Cresyl violet	0.5 g
Distilled water	100 ml

Filter before use.

Cresyl violet differentiator

Alcohol	100 ml
Glacial acetic acid	250 µl

Method
1. Take sections on slides to 95% alcohol (*not* water).
2. Stain in luxol fast blue solution, 2 hours at 60°C, or 37°C overnight.
3. Wash in 70% alcohol.
4. Wash in tap water.
5. Differentiate in saturated lithium carbonate solution until gray and white matter are distinguished. This may be more easily controlled by using 0.05% lithium carbonate followed by 95% alcohol instead.
6. Wash in tap water.
7. Check differentiation under the microscope. Repeat step 5 if necessary.
8. Stain in cresyl violet solution, 10–20 min.
9. Wash in tap water.
10. Differentiate in cresyl violet differentiator, 4–8 s.
11. Check differentiation under microscope (Nissl and nuclei only).
12. Dehydrate, clear in xylene, and mount.

Result
Myelin	blue–green
Cells	violet–pink

Methods for staining degenerate myelin

In the course of demyelinating diseases or following neuronal death the axon and/or associated myelin dies; this can be detected in several ways:

1. Marchi technique for early degeneration products (10–15 days after injury).
2. Neutral lipid stains for late degeneration products (5–6 weeks after injury) (see Chapter 12).

3. Loss of normal myelin staining with an established technique (Weil, Kluver & Barrera).

Myelin loss may occur with such processes as infarction, multiple selerosis, following chemotherapy with 5-fluorouracil and levamisole, and in several primary degenerative diseases of the central nervous system; hence its detection is important in neuropathological practice. In the normal state, myelin is hydrophilic due to its high content of polar phospholipids, but following degeneration it becomes hydrophobic with formation of cholesterol esters. Both normal myelin and degenerate myelin can be stained by osmium tetroxide; however, the osmiophilia of normal myelin is blocked by pretreatment with a strong oxidizing agent, and this phenomenon allows the detection of degenerate myelin by the *Marchi technique*. Following myelin loss, the degenerate products are phagocytosed by macrophages. The myelin debris may be apparent within macrophage cytoplasm and demonstrated with these techniques and occasionally with the routine myelin stains. It is occasionally useful to confirm the presence of macrophages utilizing immunohistochemical markers such as HAM-56, or CD-68 (KP-1). Assesment of the preservation of axons utilizing silver stains such as Bielschowsky is sometimes useful to differentiate pure demyelination from a more destructive lesion such as an infarct.

Stains for neutral lipids, such as oil red O, can effectively demonstrate myelin degeneration in formalin-fixed frozen sections during this period of myelin–lipid phagocytosis, and this is an effective way of looking for tract degeneration when negative myelin staining is equivocal and the use of a Marchi method is not established in the laboratory. Lipid combination methods are discussed in Chapter 12.

The Marchi method for degenerate myelin

The discovery that it is possible selectively to block osmium staining of normal myelin by treatment with potassium dichromate is the basis of the Marchi technique. There are three variants of the method using different oxidizing agents, namely potassium dichromate in Marchi, potassium chlorate in Swank–Davenport, and sodium iodate in Busch techniques. Marchi's method may be prone to artifact, the so-called 'pseudo-granulation'. Busch's method can over-oxidize and give a very pale result. The Swank–Davenport method seems to give the most reliable demonstration. Smith et al (1956) investigated the effects on the Marchi

method of the time interval between the occurrence of the lesion and death and the length of time in fixative. They showed that material stored in formalin for over 8 years can still give clear positive staining, although it depends on whether the positive material is intracellular or extracellular. After myelin degenerates, the Marchi-positive material is at first extracellular and remains so for about 10 weeks, after which time an increasing amount becomes phagocytosed and therefore intracellular. There are certain disadvantages to the Marchi technique, mainly the poor penetrating ability of osmium tetroxide (necessitating the use of a thin tissue block), the toxic nature and costliness of osmium tetroxide, and the occurrence of occasional false-positive artifacts. Smith et al (1956) described these artifacts in detail and indicated how they could be distinguished from true degeneration; the reader is advised to refer to this article. The following measures may help to reduce the incidence of artifacts.

Prevention of artifacts

1. Tissues must be handled with the minimum of stretching or bruising.
2. Tissues must not be allowed to dry.
3. Large blocks must not be thicker than 3 mm. Small blocks can be up to 5 mm thick.
4. Do not let tissues overlap in Marchi's solution. Tissues must lie flat.
5. Impregnation should be carried out in the dark.
6. Better impregnation is achieved if the tissue is turned over every day.
7. After impregnation, wash the tissues for at least 24 hours in running water.
8. Frozen sections have fewer artifacts than embedded sections. Try cutting frozen sections and if necessary embed later.

Marchi's method, Swank–Davenport modification (Swank & Davenport 1935)

Fixation
Formal saline.

Sections
Frozen.

Preparation of impregnating solution

1% osmium tetroxide	20 ml
1% potassium chlorate	60 ml

| Formaldehyde | 12 ml |
| Glacial acetic acid | 1 ml |

Osmium is highly toxic and should be used in a fume cupboard.

Method

1. Cut thin slices of tissues, 3–5 µm thick.
2. Rinse tissues for 5–10 min in 1% potassium chlorate.
3. Transfer tissues to the impregnating solution and leave for 7–12 days at room temperature, in the dark.
4. Wash in running tap water for 1–2 days.
5. Cut frozen sections at 25–90 µm. Mount in glycerine jelly, or dehydrate, clear, and mount in Canada balsam, or
6. Dehydrate and embed in paraffin wax or nitrocellulose.

Results

Degenerate myelin—*black* (Fig. 19.5). Depending on the age of the demyelination, the reaction products may vary from being ring-shaped, coarse, irregular, extracellular globules or fine intracellular granules inside macrophages.

Normal myelin   *light brown*

Notes

The times of impregnation are not critical within the limits given.

The proportioning of the chemicals is critical, the concentration of the mixture is not.

Poirer et al (1954) suggested that the impregnating solution was too strong and could be diluted to one-third of its original strength.

Sections can be counterstained in light green or, if frozen sections are used, red Sudan dyes may be used.

SUPPORT CELLS: THE NEUROGLIA

The term neuroglia refers to the supporting cells of the central nervous system and comprises four main types: ependymal cells, astrocytes, oligodendrocytes, and microglia.

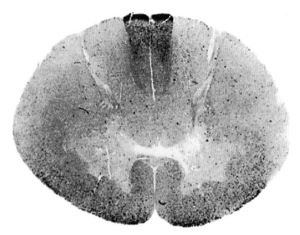

Fig. 19.5 Cervical cord showing areas of early myelin degeneration. Celloidin section, stained with the Swank–Davenport method.

Techniques for staining ependymal cells

These are ciliated epithelial cells which line the ventricles of the brain and the central canal of the spinal cord. They are well demonstrated with conventional stains (H&E). Unlike other epithelial cells, ependymal cells lack a basement membrane, but have cilial basal bodies (blepharoplasts) which may be demonstrated with phosphotungstic acid hematoxylin (PTAH) (Rubinstein 1972). By immunoperoxidase methods, ependymal cells and ependymal tumors generally express vimentin, S100, and the intermediate filament protein, glial fibrillary acidic protein (GFAP). Occasionally luminal surfaces of ependymal tumors demonstrate immunoreactivity for epithelial membrane antigen but do not express epithelial intermediate filament (cytokeratins). The demonstration of nuclear immunoreactivity with the use of the proliferation marker MIB-1 (Ki-67), which is expressed in the G1, S, G2, and M phases of the cell cycle, and the nuclear phosphoprotein p53, which is a cell cycle regulatory protein, may be useful in grading ependymal tumors, with the higher grade tumors demonstrating more cells positive for these markers (Rushing et al 1998). A relatively new technique, chromogenic in situ hybridization (CISH), has been used to demonstrate polysomy of chromosome 7 in certain histological variants of ependymal tumors (Santi et al 2005). This technique, unlike fluorescence in situ hybridization (FISH), does not require the use of a fluorescence microscope to visualize the abnormality.

Techniques for staining astrocytes

Astrocytes are multi-processed 'star shaped' cells. In normal tissue, this morphology is only seen with special stains, as with H&E sections only the nucleus is generally visible, being oval and vesicular, with small chromatin granules. There are several techniques for staining of astrocytes. With gold impregnation staining (e.g. Cajal's gold sublimate), two sorts of astrocyte can be identified: fibrous and protoplasmic. Fibrous astrocytes are mainly found in white matter and have small cell bodies with long processes containing metal-impregnated fibrils after staining. Protoplasmic astrocytes have more frequent processes that are shorter and thicker than those of fibrous astrocytes. They also lack the wealth of fibrils within processes. The tips of some astrocyte processes terminate around small vessel walls as specialized foot processes forming part of the blood–brain barrier. Specialized astrocytes, present in the cerebellar cortex and having processes arranged radially in one direction, are termed 'Bergmann astrocytes'.

Immunohistochemical demonstration of astrocytes is mainly performed by staining for *glial fibrillary acidic protein* (GFAP), one of the intermediate filament proteins. Astrocytes can also be detected with antibodies to S100 protein, αB-crystallin, and glutamine synthetase.

The identification of astrocytes is important in neuropathology as they react promptly to local tissue injury, e.g. by increase in size in response to cerebral edema, or to metabolic disturbances such as liver failure. Characteristically the astrocytes develop prominent pink cytoplasm, the nucleus is eccentric, and processes become prominent. Such cells are termed 'reactive astrocytes'. Astrocytes proliferate following damage to the central nervous system and will fill defects left by loss of specialized nervous tissue with glial fibers. This is termed astrocytic *gliosis* and its identification is important in analysis of disease processes in the CNS (Fig. 19.6).

Astrocyte stains may be performed to demonstrate normal astrocytes, and reactive or gliotic astrocytes, but are frequently used to demonstrate neoplastic astrocytes within an astrocytic tumor, i.e. astrocytoma, anaplastic astrocytoma, glioblastoma multiforme, or mixed tumors such as oligoastrocytoma, ganglioglioma, and others.

For the demonstration of normal astrocytes, Cajal's gold sublimate method gives delicate staining of processes; it may also be used for reactive astrocytes. Protoplasmic astrocytes may be stained by a silver method using physical development (Gallyas 1981).

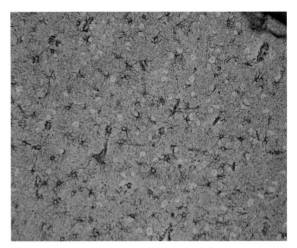

Fig. 19.6 Reactive astrocytes in white matter, stained by anti-GFAP–immunoperoxidase technique with hematoxylin nuclear counterstain. Fine GFAP-containing processes form a felt-like mat in which the stellate cell bodies are evident.

For the demonstration of gliosis, particularly in large sections, the Holzer technique or the Hortega lithium carbonate technique are both very effective, although the Holzer method uses aniline which requires careful handling. A silver method for paraffin sections has been developed which is good at detecting pathological astrocytes (Kitoh & Matsushita 1980). Unlike normal astrocytes, reactive astrocytes stain well with PTAH, but the associated staining of myelin limits its use to astrocytes in the gray matter or in areas of myelin loss.

For more sensitive and specific demonstration of astroglial differentiation in a neoplasm, the previously discussed stains are generally not considered adequate. These tumors demonstrate variable positive immunoreactivity for the intermediate filament proteins vimentin, GFAP, and some cytokeratins (AE1-AE3) (Cosgrove et al 1989). The absence of immunoreactivity for cytokeratin is often helpful to exclude metastatic carcinoma. The use of the cytokeratin CAM 5.2 (CK8–CK18) has limited cross-reactivity and is therefore a better choice for the exclusion of metastatic carcinoma. Immunoreactivity for the calcium binding protein S100 is usually demonstrated in the pattern similar to GFAP, but this marker also is positive in many other tumors, including melanoma. The demonstration of GFAP immunoreactivity is considered most useful, and is the method of choice in most laboratories to demonstrate astrocytic differentiation, but may also be expressed in ependymoma, some oligodendroglial tumors, and choroid plexus lesions (Eng & Rubinstein 1978; Velasco et al 1980; Eng & DeArmond 1983; Dogliani et al 1987). GFAP immunoreactivity is not specific for astrocytes, and positive immunostaining must be interpreted cautiously together with morphology. Immunoperoxidase demonstration of glutamine synthetase has also been used as a marker of astrocytic differentiation (Pilkington & Lantos 1982). In addition to speciation of astrocytic tumors, additional information concerning the proliferative activity as well as genetic alterations may be useful for classification and grading purposes. The MIB-1 (Ki-67) proliferation marker is often useful to help discriminate tumors of different grades, with the higher grade neoplasms demonstrating more cells within the cell cycle, but considerable overlap is demonstrated between tumor grades. Immuno-reactivity for the p53 protein and epithelial growth factor receptor (EGFR) are mutually exclusive findings that have been used to differentiate astrocytic tumors that progress from lower grade neoplasms, i.e. secondary glioblastoma, from tumors that start out as glioblastoma (primary glioblastoma) (Watanabe et al 1996). In addition to p53 and EGFR, other markers (p16, MDM2, and Bcl-2) have been demonstrated, but at least one study (Newcomb et al 1998) failed to demonstrate a survival benefit in this more detailed evaluation of these high-grade tumors.

Good results are obtainable from formalin-fixed tissues. However, improvements are possible if tissues are primarily or secondarily fixed in formal ammonium bromide for Cajal's and Hortega's methods, and in Helly's fixative for Mallory's PTAH and Holzer's crystal violet stain. Alternatively, sections of formalin-fixed tissue can be pretreated by the Globus method (1927) using ammonia and hydrobromic acid. Please refer to the fourth edition for Globus' method and Hortega's silver impregnation technique for astrocytes.

PTAH stain for astrocytes

Fixation
Formalin.

Sections
Paraffin, 5–10 μm.

Solutions
PTAH (naturally ripened)
Hematoxylin	1 g
Phosphotungstic acid	20 g
Distilled water	1000 ml

Permanganate
Potassium permanganate	1 g
Distilled water	100 ml

Oxalic acid
Oxalic acid	5 g
Distilled water	100 ml

Method
1. Take section to water.
2. Mordant sections in Zenker's for 60 min at 50°C.
3. Wash in running tap water, 15 min.
4. Place in Lugol's iodine, 15 min.
5. Decolorize in 95% alcohol for 60–90 min.
6. Wash in distilled water, three changes.
7. Oxidize in permanganate solution, 3–5 min.
8. Decolorize in oxalic acid solution, 5 min.
9. Stain in PTAH solution, 12–24 hours at room temperature.
10. Rinse rapidly with 96% alcohol.
11. Dehydrate rapidly in three changes of absolute alcohol.
12. Clear in xylene; mount.

Result
Astrocyte fibrils	blue
Nuclei	blue
Myelin	blue
Neurons	pink

Note
The mordanting in a mercuric fixative, such as Zenker's, enhances staining of glial fibrils.

Cajal's gold sublimate method for astrocytes modified for paraffin sections
(Chan & Lowe 2002)

The chemical union involved in the reaction is unknown. The presence of the mercuric chloride in the gold bath is vital for a successful impregnation. This can be shown by performing a spot test on filter that can induce the reduction of gold chloride into metallic gold. As the gold chloride solution diffused radially outwards, when it reached the right concentration, a black staining began to form. Further out, a purplish staining occurred. This resulted in two concentric rings, one purple and one black, with an unstained center. When the spot test was repeated with the addition of mercuric chloride to the solution, not only did the reduction take place much sooner but the center of the spot was also darkly stained, although to a lesser extent. Moreover, the outer ring now took on a ruby red color. Such phenomena showed the importance of the concentration of gold chloride and the role of mercury in influencing the success of the method. The latter possibly formed a complex with the gold ions so they could be readily reduced. It also altered the color of the background staining as compared to what one might get by using gold chloride on its own.

Naoumenko and Feigin (1961) modified Cajal's method for paraffin sections by post-fixing sections in formal ammonium bromide and reducing the concentration of gold chloride in the impregnation solution. However, the method is variable. In order to intensify the impregnation, various heavy metals were added to the impregnation solution and the pH was also varied. It was found that the addition of copper could accelerate and intensify the reaction while acetic acid could suppress non-specific background impregnation. Spot tests were applied, and confirmed the finding. Free-floating paraffin sections were used because better penetration of the chemicals into the tissue could be achieved.

Fixation
Formal saline.

Sections
Loose paraffin sections, 15–20 μm. Frozen, 20 μm.

Solutions

a. 5% mercuric chloride
Prepared by dissolving in distilled water with gentle heat.

b. Gold chloride solution

1% brown gold chloride	8 ml
Distilled water	40 ml

c. 5% cupric sulfate, hydrated

d. Glacial acetic acid

e. Formal ammonium bromide

Ammonium bromide	0.6 g
Formalin	14 ml
Distilled water	100 ml

Gold sublimate impregnating solution

Solution b	10 ml
Solution e	40 ml

Method

1. Dewax loose paraffin sections in xylene and bring them down to distilled water through graded alcohol.
2. Rinse sections in several changes of distilled water.
3. Place in formal ammonium bromide for 3 days. Sections should not overlap.
4. Rinse thoroughly with distilled water.
5. Place sections in the gold sublimate impregnating solution and leave at room temperature (20–22°C) in subdued light for $1^1/_2$ hours. Sections must lie flat and not overlapping; allow 10 ml of solution per section. To the impregnation bath, for every 10 ml of solution, add 120 μl of glacial acetic acid and 40 μl of solution c. Mix well and make sure that the sections remain flat and not overlapping. After 3 hours of total impregnation, at regular intervals check sections microscopically. Proceed if the astrocytes are clearly visible; otherwise return sections to the gold bath for further staining for up to 8 hours.
6. Place sections in 1% acetic acid for 30 min.
7. Rinse in distilled water.
8. Place section in 5% sodium thiosulfate for 10 min.
9. Rinse sections in distilled water, dehydrate, clear, and mount.

Results

Fibrous and protoplasmic astrocytes	dark purple to black
Background	purple

Notes
When loose sections are to be mounted, they can be picked up onto slides. Drain well and blot a couple of times with a pack of 3 to 4 sheets of blotting paper (this will prevent the section from sticking to the paper). Carefully immerse section into alcohol and blot again. Repeat this procedure with xylene.

It is advisable to bring a few sections through, each impregnated for a different length of time. One of them will give the optimal result.

A number of variants of Cajal's recipe exist. A few variants are seen in Table 19.1. The authors have applied this method to glial neoplasms. The well-differentiated components of the tumors stain well while the undifferentiated cells stain grayish.

Astrocyte staining in paraffin sections
(Kitoh & Matsushita 1980)

This method allows staining of astrocytes in formalin-fixed paraffin-embedded sections.

Fixation
Formalin-fixed paraffin-processed tissues.

Sections
Sections are cut at 5–10 μm.

Reagents
2% aqueous silver nitrate (step 7)
Ammoniacal silver solution (step 8)

Absolute alcohol	20 ml
20% silver nitrate	30 ml

Add strong ammonia drop by drop until the resulting precipitate is just dissolved. Add an additional 5 drops of ammonia.

Method
1. Post-fix in 5% mercuric chloride solution for 30 min to 1 hour at 56°C.
2. Place in 0.5% iodine in alcohol, 5 min.
3. Place in 0.5% sodium thiosulfate, 5 min.
4. Immerse in 0.25% potassium permanganate, 3 min.
5. Place in 2% oxalic acid, 2 min.
6. Mordant in 2% iron alum, 45 seconds.
7. Place in 2% silver nitrate solution for 30 min.
8. Impregnate in fresh ammoniacal silver nitrate solution for 10–15 min at 56°C.
9. Reduce in neutral buffered formalin and 2% iron alum.
10. Tone in 0.2% gold chloride.
11. Fix in 5% sodium thiosulfate.
12. Dehydrate, clear, and mount in DPX.

Result

Astrocytes	black

Nerve cells, nuclei of oligodendrocytes, and microglial cells may also be faintly stained.

Steart's modification of Holzer's method for astrocytic processes and glial fibers

This method derives from Holzer's technique (1921) and has been modified for application to paraffin sections on slides by Steart (personal communication, 1988). Use of a mordant has been claimed by some authors to be beneficial; however, this has not been found necessary, in the author's experience, with fixed tissue under a year old.

Fixation
Formalin, Helly's, or Bouin's fixatives.

Sections
Paraffin, 6–10 μm.

Preparation of solutions
Mordant

1% phosphomolybdic acid	10 ml
Absolute alcohol	40 ml

Chloroform–alcohol mixture

Chloroform	160 ml
Absolute alcohol	40 ml

Table 19.1 Variants of Cajal's recipe				
	Cajal	Davenport	Drury & Wallington	Penfield & Cone
Mercuric chloride AR	0.5 g	0.5 g	0.4 g	1.0 g
Distilled water	60 ml	50 ml	60 ml	50 ml
1% gold chloride (brown)	10 ml	10 ml	10 ml	10 ml

Crystal violet stain

Crystal violet	2 g
Absolute alcohol	20 ml
Chloroform	80 ml

Differentiating solution

Aniline oil (HAZARDOUS)	80 ml
Chloroform	120 ml
Ammonia, concentrated	10 drops

Filter before use.

Method

1. Bring sections to absolute alcohol.
2. Flood slide with mordant for 5–10 min.
3. Pour off and wash in absolute alcohol.
4. Flood slide with chloroform–alcohol mixture.
5. Drain off and quickly pour on the crystal violet stain, agitating for 30 seconds.
6. Drain slide and rapidly wash off excess stain in running tap water.
7. Pour on 10% potassium bromide solution and continue until no green discoloration remains.
8. Drain slide and blot with dry, fluff-free, filter paper. Allow to air dry.
9. Differentiate in differentiating solution until the background is nearly colorless. The time for this can be very variable and should be controlled under the microscope. In prolonged cases, tip off differentiator and add fresh.
10. Rinse well in xylene.
11. Mount in synthetic mountant.

Results

Glial fibrils	blue
Nuclei	pale blue
Background	colorless

Notes

a. The quality of the crystal violet is important in this method and there seems to be some batch-to-batch variation in stain retention and differentiation. If difficulties arise, it is advisable to change the concentration of the stain solution and repeat.
b. In some cases, particularly where formalin fixation has been prolonged, an additional stage using Anderson's mordant is helpful, as detailed below.
c. This technique should be performed in a fume cupboard due to the hazardous nature of aniline oil.

d. The addition of ammonia or acetic acid to the differentiation solution favors the staining of glial fibrils. Some variants incorporate hydrochloric acid in it, which seems to enhance the staining of the reactive astrocytes.

Anderson's neuroglia mordant

Solutions

Solution 1

Sodium sulfite (crystal)	5 g
Oxalic acid	2.5 g
Potassium iodide	5 g
Iodine	2.5 g
Distilled water	100 ml
Dissolve in the above order and then	
add glacial acetic acid	5 ml

Solution 2

5% ferric chloride

Mix equal volumes of solutions 1 and 2 immediately before use.

Method

1. Take sections to water.
2. Place sections in Anderson's mordant for 10 min.
3. Transfer to Lugol's iodine for 5 min.
4. Wash in distilled water.
5. Bleach in 5% sodium thiosulfate, 3–5 min.
6. Place sections in 0.25% potassium permanganate for 5 min.
7. Bleach in 0.25% oxalic acid for 2–5 min.
8. Wash in tap water and then in distilled water.
9. Return sections to 95% alcohol and stain by Steart's method above, from step 2.

Techniques for demonstrating oligodendrocytes

The oligodendrocytes are the cells that form myelin within the white matter of the central nervous system. A single oligodendrocyte may be responsible for the myelin of numerous nerve fibers. Oligodendrocytes are also seen in gray matter, where they are thought to act as support cells for neurons. In H&E-stained sections and Nissl-stained sections, the oligodendrocyte is identified by its small (7 μm), dense, rounded nucleus. The cytoplasm is not distinguishable from the surrounding tissues but may form an artifactual 'halo' around the nucleus after formalin fixation and paraffin processing.

The demonstration of oligodendroglial cells is usually an anatomical/histological exercise and their demonstration by metal impregnation techniques is rarely called upon for diagnostic purposes. The silver carbonate method of Penfield (see p. 387) uses frozen sections of formalin-fixed tissue and will show oligodendroglial processes in very fresh human tissue. Unfortunately, autolytic processes in autopsy material frequently lead to a poor result. Weil & Davenport's method (see below) may be applied to paraffin sections but suffers from the same problem of rapid autolysis of oligodendroglia, leading to a poor result. Oligodendroglia may be demonstrated by immunohistochemical methods using antibodies to galactocerebroside, myelin basic protein, or carbonic anhydrase C (Sternberger et al 1977; Raff et al 1978; Ghandour et al 1980). Tumors derived from oligodendrocytes generally do not react with these antibodies (Schwechheimer et al 1992). Oligodendroglial tumors may, however, demonstrate variable immunoreactivity for some of the same stains demonstrated in astrocytic tumors (GFAP, vimentin, S100, and aberrant p53 expression), but at the present time there is no adequate marker that is sufficiently sensitive and specific enough to demonstrate tumors derived from oligodendrocytes. There is a tumor marker identified in low-grade oligodendroglioma and oligoastrocytoma which, unlike many other markers, allows one to predict the response to a specific combination chemotherapy treatment with procarbazine, lomustine, and vincristine (PCV). This marker is the 1p/19q deletion which is readily demonstrated with the FISH technique (Buckner et al 2003).

Techniques for demonstrating microglia

Microglia are cells of the mononuclear phagocytic system which are residents of the central nervous system and under normal circumstances are inconspicuous. When in the reactive state in H&E sections they may appear as small, dense, rod-shaped nuclei in the neurophil. The origin of these cells has been controversial, with some claims for a neuroectodermal origin (Oehmichen 1982). However, recent work supports a derivation from monocytes which are incorporated into the CNS in development (Perry et al 1985; Cuadros & Navascues 1998). Inactive microglia are static cells in the normal CNS, with a dendritic morphology, often called 'resting' microglia. Following brain injury these inactive microglia undergo phenotypic change by expressing cell surface markers more like peripheral macrophages and become phagocytic. The numbers of phagocytic cells in the area of injury is supplemented by cells derived from blood monocytes which enter the CNS from blood vessels as part of an inflammatory process.

Functionally, the resting microglia express macrophage markers by immunohistochemistry and also weakly express surface class II major histocompatibility complex antigens (MHCII). It is probable that this cell is the antigen-presenting cell of the CNS, similar in type to Langerhans cells in skin, and interdigitating cells in lymphoid follicles (Matsumoto et al 1986; Woodroofe et al 1986; Hayes et al 1987; Lowe et al 1989a,b). The normal microglia are ATPase positive, non-specific esterase negative, acid phosphatase negative, HLA-DR positive, LCA positive, CD1 (T6)-positive and weakly CD4 (T4) positive (Lowe et al 1989a,b). Most of the phagocytic microglia seen in inflammatory states are typical monocytes derived from blood vessels, and have a primary phagocytic role. As the central nervous tissue contains abundant lipids, these phagocytic microglia assume a *foam cell* appearance with vacuoles containing lipid.

Microglial cells in the nervous system appear as rod-shaped nuclei in conventional stained sections. In silver carbonate-stained material, fixed microglia are seen to have numerous branching processes (dendritic morphology) and can be seen in normal brain. Phagocytic microglia are also well demonstrated by silver techniques. While silver impregnation methods (such as Penfield's and Weil & Davenport's methods) demonstrate cells with dendritic morphology, they are unfortunately not specific and are prone to considerable variation, depending on fixation and staining conditions. Many impregnation techniques for demonstrating microglia are derived from the studies of Ramon, Cajal, and his student Del Rio Hortega. Only a few of the techniques will be cited, but for a comprehensive treatment of the methods the reader should consult Penfield and Cone (1937) and Cox (1973).

Immunohistochemistry

Immunohistochemistry is the most reliable method for the demonstration of microglia. Microglia stain positively with antisera which detect CD68 (KP-1), a peripheral macrophage marker; EBM/11 (Dakopatts) works in frozen sections while KP-1 (Dakopatts) (Pulford et al 1989) works in formalin-fixed paraffin-processed tissues. Microglia can also be stained by antisera to class II MHC using antibodies to HLA-DR (Woodroofe et al 1986; Hayes et al 1987; Graeber et al 1994); this is low in resting cells but high in activated cells. *Leucocyte common antigen* (CD45) is faintly positive in resting microglia, hence staining is weak in normal brain. The monoclonal antibody Ki-M1P also stains microglia (Paulus et al 1992). Microglia may be demonstrated by lectin staining using *Ricinus communis* agglutin-1 or mistletoe lectin-1 (Mannoji et al 1986; Suzuki et al 1988). They may also be detected with immunohisto-chemical methods to detect ferritin, reactive microglia, and macrophages, being more strongly stained with anti-ferritin than resting cells (Kaneko et al 1989). Immunoperoxidase staining for leucocyte common antigen (LCA) is the most reliable method for the unequivocal demonstration of tumors derived from lymphoid elements in the CNS (formerly termed microg-lioma, now termed cerebral lymphoma). As with all lym-phomas, a phenotype for the tumor may be established by further immunochemical techniques.

Penfield's combined oligodendroglia and microglia method (Penfield 1928)

Fresh, well-fixed tissue is essential for the demonstra-tion of these cells and their processes. Pathological forms are more readily impregnated.

Fixation
Formalin ammonium bromide or formal saline.

Sections
Frozen sections, 15–20 μm.

Preparation of solution
Silver carbonate solution
10% silver nitrate	5 ml
5% sodium carbonate	20 ml

Ammonia is added, sufficient to dissolve the precipitate.

Distilled water up to	75 ml

Filter before use.

Method
1. Leave sections in 1% ammonia overnight to remove the formalin.
2. Transfer directly to 5% hydrobromic acid and leave for 1 hour at 37°C.
3. Wash in three changes of distilled water.
4. Place sections for 1 hour or more in 5% sodium carbonate.
5. Impregnate sections in silver carbonate solution for 3–5 min.
6. Transfer directly to 1% formalin in distilled water.
7. Wash in distilled water.
8. Tone in 0.2% gold chloride until gray.
9. Wash in water.
10. Fix in 5% sodium thiosulfate for 2–5 min.
11. Wash, dehydrate, clear, and mount in Canada balsam.

Results
Microglia and oligodendroglia	dark gray

Notes
Steps 1–3 are for formalin-fixed tissue only.

If the impregnation is prolonged, astrocytes are faintly stained.

The distinction between microglia and oligo-dendroglia is made morphologically.

Weil and Davenport's method for microglia and oligodendroglia (Scott's modification for paraffin and frozen sections)

This is a modification of Stern's (1932) method. By adding silver nitrate to ammonia, a diamino silver solution is produced, with no excess ammonia. Scott (1971), using unmounted paraffin sections, claims better results using 5% silver nitrate for making the impregnating solution.

Fixation
Formal ammonium bromide or formal saline.

Sections
Paraffin sections are cut at 15–20 μm and transferred directly into two successive baths of xylene. Place sections in absolute alcohol, then in 50% alcohol.

Wash in distilled water. Frozen sections are cut at 20–25 μm and left in 10% ammonia for 2 hours before staining.

Preparation of solution

To 2 ml of concentrated ammonia, add 5% silver nitrate, until a slight permanent turbidity is formed. The solution should be orange–brown in color.

Method

1. Wash sections well in distilled water.
2. Impregnate in silver solution for 3–4 seconds.
3. Transfer to 3% formalin in distilled water, moving them continuously. Leave for 30 seconds.
4. Wash in distilled water.
5. Fix in 5% sodium thiosulfate for 2–5 min.
6. Wash, dehydrate, clear, and mount in Canada balsam.

Results

Oligodendroglia, microglia, and astrocytes   *black*

Notes

a. Use of 10% silver nitrate with 10% formalin increases selectivity for microglia.
b. Use of 15% silver nitrate with 15% formalin increases selectivity for oligodendroglia.

HISTOLOGICAL INVESTIGATION OF DEMENTIA

With the increase in the aging population it has become apparent that neurodegenerative diseases resulting in dementia are a common contribution to morbidity in this age group. In establishing the cause of a dementia, special staining techniques are usually required for the demonstration of specific structural abnormalities. The main causes of dementia are:

- Alzheimer's disease
- vascular dementia (multi-infarct dementia)
- dementia with Lewy bodies
- frontotemporal dementias.

Of considerable public health importance is dementia caused by Creutzfeldt–Jakob disease (CJD), especially now that variant CJD (which fortunately is on the decline, but has led to the death of over 150 people) has been linked to the oral consumption of contaminated food products from cattle infected with bovine spongiform encephalopathy (BSE) (Hilton 2006). In the laboratory setting, histological examination of a brain to ascertain the cause of dementia is often a staged process, with sequential application of special stains and immunohistochemical techniques depending on initial histological findings. A scheme for the staged histological examination of brain has been published for use in specialist laboratories (Lowe 1998).

Alzheimer's disease is characterized by two main abnormalities:

1. Neurons develop intracellular filamentous inclusions termed *neurofibrillary tangles*. These may be detected with several silver stains and appear as skeins of filament around the nucleus, also extending into the axonal hillock of the cell body. They may also be detected by immunohistochemistry (see later).
2. Amyloid is deposited in the cerebral cortex, derived from a fragment of a neuronal cell membrane protein termed Alzheimer amyloid precursor protein (APP). Deposits of amyloid become surrounded radially by dilated and distorted neuronal processes to form *senile plaques*. These structures can be demonstrated with silver techniques, by amyloid staining methods, or by immunohistochemistry for the amyloid protein (termed Aβ-protein or βAPP) after formic acid pretreatment of sections.

Vascular dementia is characterized by multiple areas of cerebral infarction (Munoz 1991). In addition, many cases of mixed dementia are encountered where the changes of Alzheimer's disease are also present.

Dementia with Lewy bodies is characterized by the histological features of Alzheimer's disease with the addition of the presence of neuronal inclusions in the cerebral cortex termed *cortical Lewy bodies*. These can be detected by immunohistochemistry for the protein α-synuclein (Dickson 1999; Goedert 1999) or the protein ubiquitin (Lowe et al 1993).

Frontotemporal dementias are characterized by neuronal loss in the frontal and temporal lobes of the brain. There are several histological subgroups in this category, each characterized by the presence of distinct inclusions in neurons detected by immunohistochemistry (Cooper et al 1995; Lowe 1997).

The evolution in classification of dementia has been greatly advanced by the widespread use of immunohistochemical methods for the assessment of neurodegenerative pathology. Such methods have revealed a 'new' set of markers of disease and are now an essential part of the pathological diagnostic workup of cases. Appropriate immunochemical reagents for diagnosis include antisera to phosphorylated tau protein, α-synuclein, ubiquitin, αB crystallin, and neurofilament protein (Munoz 1999).

With the identification of protein accumulations as common characteristics of several neurodegenerative diseases it is also possible to classify diseases according to their dominant protein accumulation. Hence the proposition of a group of tauopathies, α-synucleinopathies, and ubiquitin filament disorders (Dickson 1999; Goedert 1999).

Huntington's disease as well as several other genetic degenerative diseases of the brain is characterized by the common genetic background of a CAG triplet-repeat expansion in the responsible gene. These disorders can result in accumulation of polyglutamine-containing inclusions in nuclei of nerve cells as well as in some nerve cell processes. Such inclusions can be detected by antisera to ubiquitin. Protein aggregates forming inclusions are a common factor in the pathogenesis of many common neurodegenerative disorders (Schulz & Dichgans 1999).

Stains for detection of the changes of Alzheimer's disease

The stains used to detect changes of Alzheimer's disease generally polarize into two types:

- Those that are very sensitive to amyloid detect all plaques and may detect a minority of tangles. This is true of the methenamine silver technique described below.
- Those that are very sensitive for the detection of tangles may detect the abnormal nerve processes around plaques but do not stain amyloid. This is true of the Gallyas technique described below, as well as of modifications of Palmgren's stain (Cross 1982).

Several silver-staining methods are optimized to detect both structures but do so at the expense of underestimating either plaques or tangles. This is true of the modified Bielschowsky technique, which underestimates the total amount of amyloid in sections (Lamy et al 1989). In many laboratories, specific staining of plaques and tangles is performed by immunohistochemistry using commercially available antisera. Plaques are detected

using antisera to Aβ-protein after formic acid pretreatment of sections (Dako). Tangles are detected by immunostaining for phosphorylated tau protein. Tau protein is a microtubule-binding protein which accumulates in an abnormally phosphorylated form in Alzheimer's disease (Dickson 1999).

Guidelines for the histological diagnosis of Alzheimer's disease have been published and are suitable for use in a general pathology laboratory, including descriptions of reliable special staining techniques (Mirra et al 1993; Working Group 1997). Assessment of histological changes is by comparison with standard reference pictures included in the paper.

Thioflavine S method for plaques and tangles

This method uses a fluorescent dye which binds to the amyloid and fibrillar material in the abnormal structures. Sections require viewing under a fluorescence microscope with filters for thioflavine S.

Fixation
Formalin.

Sections
Paraffin-processed or frozen.

Solution
Thioflavine S	1 g
Distilled water	100 ml

Method
1. Take sections to water.
2. Stain in thioflavine solution, 7 min.
3. Wash in 80% alcohol, three changes.
4. Dehydrate, clear, and mount in fluorescence-free mountant.
5. View using fluorescence microscopy.

Notes
a. This method is sensitive and will detect all types of plaque.
b. A control section of a known positive case is a useful addition to this method.
c. Plaques and tangles may also be demonstrated by the alkaline Congo red method, and subsequently demonstrated under polarized light microscopy. This is insensitive compared to the silver stains detailed below.

Gallyas stain for neurofibrillary tangles
(Gallyas 1971)

This method gives superb staining of tangles and nerve cell processes containing the abnormal tau protein in Alzheimer's disease. It will not detect amyloid, although plaques may show up because of their surrounding abnormal nerve cell processes (Fig. 19.7).

Fixation
Formalin-fixed tissues.

Sections
Paraffin processed sections, 8 μm thick.

Solutions

1. 5% periodic acid

2. Alkaline silver iodide solution

Sodium hydroxide	40 g
Potassium iodide	100 g
Distilled water	500 ml
1% silver nitrate	35 ml

Dissolve the sodium hydroxide in water, then add the potassium iodide and wait till dissolved. Slowly add the silver nitrate and stir vigorously until clear. Then add distilled water to give a final volume of 1000 ml.

3. 0.5% acetic acid

4. Developer working solution

Add 3 volumes of stock solution II to 10 volumes of stock solution I. Stir and add 7 volumes of stock solution III. Stir and wait to clear.

Stock solution I

Sodium carbonate (anhydrous)	50 g
Distilled water	1000 ml

Stock solution II (dissolve consecutively)

Distilled water	1000 ml
Ammonium nitrate	2 g
Silver nitrate	2 g
Tungstosilicic acid	10 g

Stock solution III (dissolve consecutively)

Distilled water	1000 ml
Ammonium nitrate	2 g
Silver nitrate	2 g
Tungstosilicic acid	10 g
Formaldehyde (conc)	7.3 ml

5. 0.1% gold chloride

6. 1% sodium thiosulfate ('hypo')

7. 0.1% nuclear fast red in 2.5% aqueous aluminum sulfate

Method

1. Take sections to distilled water.
2. Place in 5% periodic acid for 5 min.
3. Wash in distilled water for 5 min twice.
4. Place in alkaline silver iodide solution for 1 min.
5. Wash in 0.5% acetic acid for 10 min.
6. Place in developer solution (prepare immediately before use) for 5–30 min.
7. Wash in 0.5% acetic acid for 3 min.
8. Wash in distilled water for 5 min.
9. Place in 0.1% gold chloride for 5 min.
10. Rinse in distilled water.
11. Place in 1% sodium thiosulfate solution for 5 min.
12. Wash in tap water.
13. Counterstain in 0.1% nuclear fast red for 2 min.
14. Wash in tap water.
15. Dehydrate, clear, and mount in DPX.

Results

Neurofibrillary tangles and plaque neurites	black
Nuclei	red

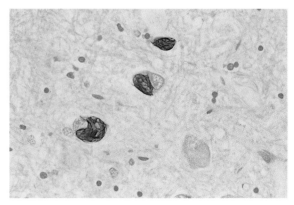

Fig. 19.7 Tangles in neurons stained by the Gallyas silver technique.

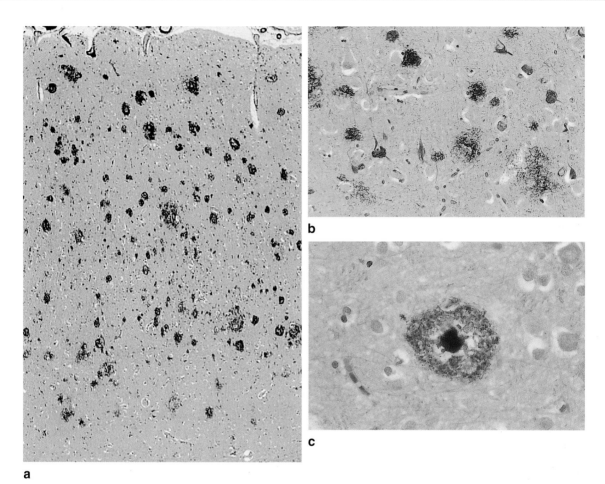

a

b

c

Fig. 19.8 Methenamine silver (Haga–Yamaguchi). (a) Low power micrograph showing senile plaques in cerebral cortex from a case of Alzheimer's disease. (b) Plaques and tangles in cortex from a case of Alzheimer's disease. (c) High power micrograph of a senile plaque showing dense core and less dense peripheral halo.

Haga methenamine silver method for senile plaques (Haga et al 1989; Yamaguchi et al 1990)

This is an excellent screening stain for the presence of amyloid plaques. While it detects a few tangles, it should not be regarded as a tangle-sensitive stain (Fig. 19.8). To diagnose Alzheimer's disease, a stain to detect tangles should also be used.

Fixation
Formalin fixed.

Sections
Paraffin 8 μm.

Solutions
Working solution
5% hexamine	500 ml
5% sodium tetraborate	25 ml
5% silver nitrate	25 ml

Add the reagents in the above order, i.e. silver nitrate last.

10% formalin in tap water

Method

1. Take sections to water.
2. Rinse in distilled water.
3. Place sections in 'working solution' for 3–4 hours at 60°C.
4. Check microscopic appearance of plaques and tangles at regular intervals until stained black.
5. Rinse in distilled water.
6. Place sections in 10% formalin in tap water for 5 min.
7. Rinse in tap water.
8. Place sections in 5% sodium thiosulfate for 5 min.
9. Rinse in tap water.
10. Dehydrate, clear, and mount in DPX.

Results

Amyloid plaques	black
Some tangles (rare)	black
Background	yellow–brown

Modified Bielschowsky stain for plaques and tangles (Yamamoto & Hirano 1986)

This stain was originally derived from Gros–Schulze's modification of the Bielschowsky method and was refined by Glenna Smith in the neuropathology laboratory at Montefiore Medical Center, New York. It gives a good compromise between sensitivity for plaques and tangles and can be used as a single stain for diagnosis of Alzheimer's disease.

Fixation
Formalin.

Sections
Paraffin sections, cut at 6–8 μm.

Solutions

Silver nitrate solution

Silver nitrate	20 g
Distilled water	100 ml

Developer

Formalin	20 ml
Distilled water	100 ml
Concentrated nitric acid	1 drop
Citric acid	0.5 g

Evaporated ammonia

Evaporate 200 ml of 28% ammonium hydroxide by leaving in an open beaker for 20 min in a fume cupboard at room temperature.

'Hypo'
1% sodium thiosulfate.

Method

1. Take sections to water.
2. Place slides in 20% silver nitrate for 20 min.
3. Place slides in distilled water while performing step 4 below.
4. To silver nitrate add evaporated ammonia, drop by drop, stirring vigorously until precipitate turns clear. Add two more drops of ammonia. Return slides to this solution for 15 min in the dark.
5. Add three drops of evaporated ammonia to a jar of distilled water. Immerse slides in this solution.
6. Add three drops of developer to the jar containing the ammonia–silver solution and stir. Allow slides to remain in this until inclusions are black with a tan background. This requires microscopic control and takes 2–5 min.
7. Wash in distilled water.
8. Wash in 'hypo' for 5 min.
9. Wash in distilled water.
10. Dehydrate, clear, and mount in DPX.

Result

Tangles	black
Plaques	black
Background	brown

Inclusion bodies in neurodegenerative disease

Several diseases of the nervous system are termed 'neurodegenerative' disease. They are generally diseases of old age and are the result of degeneration in specific neuronal groups, with the formation of intracellular inclusion bodies. The main degenerative diseases that result in inclusion bodies are Alzheimer's disease, Parkinson's disease, and motor neuron disease.

With the advent of immunohistochemical techniques, inclusion bodies can be specifically identified as an aid to diagnosis. Most of the inclusion bodies are filamentous and based on abnormalities of the cytoskeleton of neurons, detectable with antisera to the cytoskeletal protein. The protein ubiquitin is common to many inclusion bodies of diverse type, making antisera against ubiquitin particularly useful in diagnosis (Lowe et al 1988, 1989a,b, 1993). The protein α-synuclein, a normal neuronal protein mainly found in synapses, has been recognized as a component in several types of inclusion body (Dickson 1999; Goedert 1999). The main inclusion bodies in diagnostic practice are shown in Table 19.2.

Transmissible neurodegenerative diseases

Several diseases of the nervous system are termed transmissible neurodegenerative diseases. They are charac-

terized by accumulation of an abnormal protein in the brain termed *prion protein (PrP)* associated with vacuolation in affected brain areas, called spongiform change. Alternative names for this group of diseases are 'spongiform encephalopathies' or 'prion disorders' (Weihl & Roos 1999). The importance of this group of diseases for laboratory practice is that the agent responsible, believed to be a protein-only agent, can be transmitted by inoculation and is also highly resistant to normal disinfection methods. For example, formalin fixation is ineffective at inactivating the agent. Wax-embedded material is still infective by inoculation. The main disease in humans is sporadic Creutzfeldt–Jakob disease (sCJD), a rapidly progressive form of dementia. Less common are familial CJD (fCJD), iatrogenic CJD (iCJD) Gerstmann–Sträussler–Scheinker syndrome (GSS), a familial as well as transmissible form of cerebellar disease, fatal familial insomnia (FFI), fatal sporadic insomnia (FSI), and variant Creutzfeldt–Jakob disease (vCJD), a form of disease linked to bovine spongiform encephalopathy in cattle

Table 19.2 Inclusion body immunostaining		
Inclusion	**Disease**	**Immunostaining**
Neurofibrillary tangle	Alzheimer's disease	Tau protein (Fig. 19.9), ubiquitin
Lewy body (Fig. 19.10)	Parkinson's disease	α-Synuclein, ubiquitin
Cortical Lewy body (Fig. 19.11)	Dementia with Lewy bodies	α-Synuclein, ubiquitin
Motor neuron disease inclusion	Motor neuron disease	Ubiquitin (Fig. 19.12)
Glial cytoplasmic inclusion	Multiple system atrophy	α-Synuclein, ubiquitin, tau protein
Pick body	Pick's disease	Tau protein, chromogranin A, ubiquitin

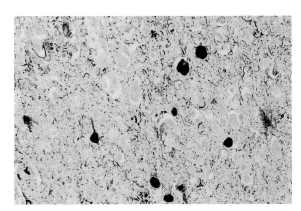

Fig. 19.9 Immunostaining for tau protein shows tangles in neurons. In the background are large numbers of positively stained neurophil threads.

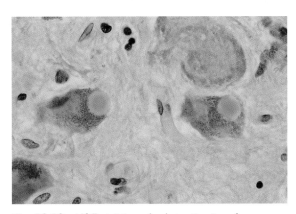

Fig. 19.10 H&E staining of substantia nigra from a patient with Parkinson's disease. The brown color is normal neuromelanin. Two neurons contain rounded inclusions with a pale 'halo' region which are Lewy bodies.

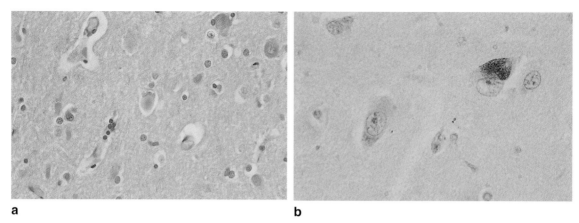

a   **b**

Fig. 19.11 (a) H&E staining of cerebral cortex showing cortical Lewy bodies, from a patient with Lewy body dementia. (b) Anti-ubiquitin immunostaining detects cortical Lewy bodies with great sensitivity.

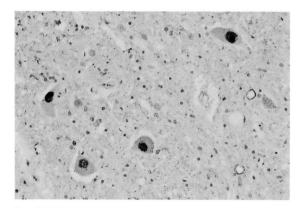

Fig. 19.12 Anti-ubiquitin immunostaining detects inclusion bodies in spinal cord motor neurons in motor neuron disease (amyotrophic lateral sclerosis).

(Collinge 1999). Prion diseases are classed as group three biological agents in the healthcare setting, without the risk of aerosol contamination. Fixed and unfixed materials must be handled according to appropriate safety protocols. Autopsies on recipients of human-derived tissues or tissue extracts should also be considered as being in a high-risk category of carrying a transmissible agent. At highest risk are patients who have received pituitary-derived hormones, and dura mater used in neurosurgical operations. Diagnosis of this type of disease is based on conventional histology and identification of the characteristic vacuolation (spongi-

form change) in the brain. Diagnosis may be assisted by immunohistochemical demonstration of accumulation of prion protein. However, complex digestion pretreatment steps are required to reveal immunoreactivity (Hayward et al 1994).

A detailed protocol for routine practice has been produced incorporating appropriate health and safety guidelines (Bell & Ironside 1993). Detailed discussion on laboratory diagnosis of vCJD has also been published (Ironside et al 2000). It is possible to render tissues practically non-infectious, i.e. greatly reducing the infectivity titer, by immersion of *small pieces of tissue* in formic acid for 1 hour, allowing safer handling in the histology laboratory (Brown et al 1990). After adequate treatment, the blocks of tissue should become almost translucent. Work surfaces and instruments may be sterilized in 2 M sodium hydroxide for 1 hour. Glassware can be cleaned in sodium hypochlorite (20,000 ppm). In cases of vCJD, prion protein, and hence an infective hazard, also resides in lymphoid tissues such as tonsil, lymph node, spleen, and bone marrow (Ironside et al 2000).

NEUROPATHOLOGY LABORATORY SPECIMEN HANDLING

The advance made in neurosciences in recent years means that histological methods are only one facet to the investigation of function and diseases of the nervous system, and are supplemented by microbiological, immunological, biochemical, and molecular genetic techniques. The histologist will, however, often be the person who is responsible for the appropriate collection and preservation of tissues.

The following are the main specimens encountered by a neuroscience histology service:

1. tumor samples from neurosurgery
2. brain biopsy from neurosurgery
3. whole brain from autopsy
4. spinal cord from autopsy
5. peripheral nerve biopsy
6. pituitary gland from neurosurgery
7. skeletal muscle biopsy.

An important aim of a neuropathology laboratory service is to facilitate the diagnosis of disease processes by preserving samples in a way that will allow appropriate investigative techniques to be performed later. This will usually be under the direction of a clinical pathologist who will choose techniques according to the diseases which are likely to be present, as judged by clinical investigations.

Brain and spinal cord biopsies

These will usually be performed for tumor, or for neuro-degenerative diseases (including infective processes). Tissue samples are usually very small and the laboratory frequently receives material fresh for rapid diagnosis or appropriate specimen processing. Ideally samples are received as soon as possible from the theater. Because of the small biopsy size, tendency to dry in transit, and the 'sticky' nature of specimens, biopsies are best placed for transport on a sterile fine polythene sheet which is wrapped over the sample by folding in two. This eliminates drying, contamination, and allows even very small (less than 1 mm) fragments to be transported safely.

In the laboratory a stereomicroscope may be used to facilitate the identification of gray matter, white matter, and abnormal tissue. For rapid diagnosis tissue may be taken for frozen section by freezing in isopentane cooled in liquid nitrogen in a suitable supporting medium for cryostat sections. Tissue from the nervous system is also amenable to diagnosis by smear preparations (see below). A small sample of biopsy material may be fixed in glutaraldehyde for electron microscopy if clinically indicated. The bulk of the sample should be fixed in an adequate volume of neutral buffered 10% formalin for conven-

tional paraffin processing. If the sample is large enough a portion may be retained in the frozen state for possible biochemical investigation.

Smear preparations of brain tissue for rapid diagnosis

A small piece (1 mm) of tissue is placed at one end of a plain glass slide. A second plain glass slide is used to crush the specimen, and then is drawn across the slide to produce a uniform smear. Unlike blood film preparation, the two slides are held flat together during smearing, maintaining a gentle and even pressure. Practice with this method and familiarity with normal smear appearances are achieved by using fresh postmortem tissue from known sites in the CNS. Alternatively the tissue may be lightly touched to a single glass slide allowing a few cells to adhere to the slide in order to minimize handling artifacts. The slides are immediately fixed in acetic alcohol. Staining is with H&E. Aqueous toluidine blue is another effective stain. The latter shows the glial fibrils well.

This technique allows rapid sampling of several areas from a biopsy. All cell types in the CNS are readily identifiable by this method (Ironside et al 2000). Certain lesions may be too tough to smear, and reliance must be placed on frozen sections.

Peripheral nerve biopsies

Nerve biopsy is a specialized procedure which should ideally be performed after consultation between the laboratory and the clinician. Nerve is tremendously prone to histological artifacts due to handling, and it is imperative that this is kept to a minimum. In modern practice the usual reason for peripheral nerve biopsy is a neuropathy of unknown origin. In these circumstances the most useful investigative techniques are high-resolution histology after glutaraldehyde fixation and resin processing, and examination of teased osmicated fibers for myelin pattern. Because most of the changes seen in nerve are subtle, paraffin sections lack the resolution required for precise diagnosis and hence special techniques are required. However, for the confirmation of inflammatory disorders, the lesion sometimes can be very focal. In this incidence, serial sections through the paraffin block plus immunohistochemistry for various types of inflammatory cells often help.

Peripheral nerve biopsies are ideally received fresh in the laboratory wrapped atraumatically in gauze lightly moistened with normal saline to prevent drying. The biopsy is usually 2–4 cm long for a typical diagnostic sural nerve sample. Using a new scalpel blade the traumatized cut ends are removed and frozen in isopentane cooled in liquid nitrogen. These may be used for frozen sections or biochemical assays. The main portion of the sample should be allowed to adhere to a piece of card for about 30 seconds and then fixed in 0.05 M phosphate-buffered glutaraldehyde to facilitate later processing into epoxy resin.

Histology of paraffin preparations of peripheral nerve, fixed in formalin, shows marked distortion and shrinkage. The preferred fixatives for paraffin sections are Heidenhain–Susa, or Bouin's (p. 70). In each case fixation should be less than 24 hours to prevent samples becoming brittle.

Following fixation in glutaraldehyde, the myelin will have hardened enough to allow the nerve to be cut into small blocks. Pieces 1 mm in size are osmicated and embedded in epoxy resin (see Chapter 29). Semi-thin (1–3 μm) sections of transversely oriented tissue are cut and stained with toluidine blue. Such tissue blocks can be used subsequently for ultrastructural studies if necessary. If Araldite resin is used, sections can be stained with multi-colored methods such as methylene blue and basic fuchsin (Huber et al 1968).

For paraffin processing, fixed material is processed and cut at 6–8 μm. It is always helpful to include a transverse and a longitudinal segment for examination. Sections are usefully stained with H&E, a trichrome stain to assess fibrosis, a myelin stain, and an axon stain. Immunoperoxidase methods may also be applied to look for macrophage infiltration using antibodies against leucocyte common antigen or macrophage-specific antigens. The examination of the pattern of myelin formation along individual axons can give information on whether there have been past episodes of myelin loss with remyelination. This is performed on teased nerve fibers. Features of segmental demyelination can only be observed in such preparations.

Preparation of teased nerve fibers
(Asbury & Johnson 1978)

Nerve fibers can be processed to glycerine or unpolymerized Araldite for teasing. The latter method produces a firmer consistency to the individual fibers

and is easier to work with. The stiffness of the fibers also relates to the amount of osmication and the concentration of the osmium used. Please refer to the former edition for the method using glycerine. Very occasionally, the demyelination may be focally affecting a few fascicles of the nerve. It will be good practice to examine the semi-thin sections first before teasing the fibers.

Tissue
Fresh nerve.

Fixation
Segment of nerve is fixed in 0.1 M phosphate buffered 3.6% glutaraldehyde, 4–16 hours.

Method
1. Wash twice in phosphate buffer, 15 min.
2. Under a stereomicroscope using two pairs of fine forceps, carefully remove the epineurium by only gripping and pulling the connective tissue. Separate the nerve into individual or small bundles of fascicles. This allows a uniform osmication, disregarding the variation in size of the specimen that one may have received.
3. Osmicate in 0.1 M phosphate-buffered 2% osmium tetroxide, 4 hours.
4. Wash twice in phosphate buffer, 15 min.
5. Briefly rinse in distilled water and process through 50, 80, and 95% alcohol for 10 min each.
6. Dehydrate in two changes of 100% alcohol, 15 min each.
7. Process through two changes of propylene oxide, 15 min each.
8. Mixed in equal parts of propylene oxide and araldite CY212 resin for 1 hour.
9. Mixed in unpolymerized Araldite CY212 resin overnight (the specimen can be kept in this resin at 4°C for up to 1 year).

To tease fibers

Place processed nerve on a glass slide under a stereomicroscope in a pool of unpolymerized Araldite. Using fine forceps and sharp needles, remove the perineurium from a fascicle. Keep dividing the nerve bundles into halves until single or small bundles of two to three fibers (black) can be careful teased out. When separating a smaller bundle from a larger one, it is helpful to hold onto the smaller one and pull the larger one slowly away. Slide the fiber across the slide in a trail of resin onto an adjacent slide. Care should be taken to insure that the fibers to be examined are aligned in parallel across the slide.

For diagnostic purposes, in order to avoid possible sampling errors, at least 100 fibers should be sampled (Dyke et al 1984). However, in severely demyelinated cases, it may sometimes prove difficult to get enough black fibers. When enough fibers are obtained, use the fine forceps to pick up a small droplet of *partially polymerized* resin. Apply a thin line of the resin along one of the aligned ends of the parallel-arranged fibers (the resin should not touch the fibers at this stage). Trim a coverslip to size. Hold the coverslip at an angle to the surface of the slide and carefully touch the line of resin with the lower edge of the coverslip. Carefully lower the coverslip until it almost touches the slide, and let go. Lay the slide on a flat surface in a 37°C oven and let the resin slowly spread longitudinally along the fibers to fill the entire gap between the slide and the coverslip. Ring the coverslip with nail varnish. Any trapped bubbles should be left undisturbed. With practice, this mounting technique will allow the well-aligned, loosely attached fibers to remain undisturbed and without overlapping on the slide. Fibers are measured for internode lengths and diameters using eyepiece graticules.

Skeletal muscle samples

Biopsy samples of skeletal muscle may be taken either using a biopsy needle or at open operation. The aim of histology is to provide an undistorted picture of muscle fiber architecture. A detailed evaluation of muscle disease relies heavily on enzyme histochemistry which necessitates the use of cryostat sections of unfixed skeletal muscle. (See Chapter 20, which describes the appropriate method for processing the skeletal muscle biopsy as well as detailed enzyme histochemistry techniques.)

Routine histochemical stains include:

H&E	morphology
Gomori trichrome	inclusion bodies, connective tissue ragged red fibers, and tubular aggregates
PAS ± diastase	glycogen
Oil red O	lipid content

ATPase pH 9.4	myosin loss and myofiber atrophy of Type 1 and 2 fibers
	pH 4.6 Type 2B myofibers
	pH 4.3 Type 2C myofibers
NADHTR (nicotinamide adenine dinucleotide [reduced] tetrazolium reductase)	internal fiber architecture: mitochondria and tubular aggregates
Alkaline phosphatase	regenerating myofibers; immune connective tissue disorders
Acid phosphatase	inflammatory cells; necrotic fibers; enhanced lysosomal enzyme activity
Non-specific esterase	inflammatory cells; necrotic myofibers; enhanced lysosomal enzyme activity
Cytochrome c oxidase (COX)	mitochondrial disorder
Succinic dehydrogenase (SDH)	mitochondrial disorder
Myoadenylate deaminase (MAD)	enzyme deficiency
Myophosphorylase	type V glycogenosis (McArdle's disease)

Dystrophy-related immunostains include:

Dystrophin 1, 2, and 3 (Fig. 19.13a,b)
Sarcoglycans (α, β, γ, and δ)
Dysferlin
Merosin
Caveolin
Calpain-3
Emerin

A small portion of muscle may be fixed for electron microscopy if clinically indicated. The sample may be fixed lightly stretched, longitudinally in a special clip, or stretched out by pinning and fixed with a few drops of buffered glutaldehyde. After a few minutes, it will be stiffened and can be put into the main bulk of fixative. Staining of motor end-plates and axons may be performed on fresh tissues (Coers 1982). A detailed description of muscle histology and biopsy handling is given by Carpenter and Karpati (2001).

Additional techniques for handling postmortem material were presented in the fifth edition.

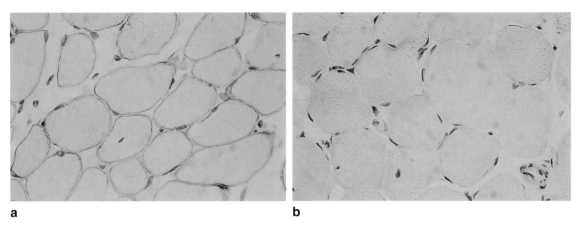

a   b

Fig. 19.13   (a) In a normal muscle dystrophin is localized beneath the cell membrane of muscle fibers. (b) In Duchenne muscular dystrophy, this staining pattern is absent.

Acknowledgments

Gordon Cox contributed this chapter for the first two editions. For editions three and four it was updated by James Lowe. For edition five it was updated by Kwok-Kee Chan and James Lowe. Our acknowledgments are due to them for their contributions.

REFERENCES

Asbury A.K., Johnson P.C. (1978) Pathology of peripheral nerve. Philadelphia: Saunders.

Bell J., Ironside J. (1993) How to tackle a possible Creutzfeldt–Jakob disease necropsy. Journal of Clinical Pathology 46:193–197.

Bennett M.J., Hofmann S.L. (1999) The neuronal ceroid-lipofuscinoses (Batten disease): a new class of lysosomal storage disease. Journal of Inherited Metabolic Disease 22:534–544.

Bertram E.G. (1958) Zine chromate solutions for impregnation of nervous tissue. Stain Technology 33:187.

Bielschowsky M. (1902) Die Silberimprägnation der Axenzylinder. Zentralblatt für Neurologie 21:579.

Bone Q. (1972) Some notes on histological methods for peripheral nerve. Journal of Medical Laboratory Technology 29:319.

Brown P., Wolff A., Gajdusek D.C. (1990) A simple and effective method for inactivating virus infectivity in formalin-fixed tissue samples from patients with Creutzfeldt–Jakob disease. Neurology 40:887–890.

Buckner J.C., Gesme D. Jr., O'Fallon J.R. et al. (2003) Phase II trial of procarbazine, lomustine, and vincristine as initial therapy for patients with low-grade oligodendroglioma or oligoastrocytoma: efficacy and associations with chromosomal abnormalities. Journal of Clinical Oncology 21(2):251–255.

Buhl E.H. (1992) Intracellular Lucifer yellow injection in fixed brain slices. In: Bolam J.P., ed. Neuroanatomy: a practical approach. London: Oxford University Press, pp. 187–212.

Cajal S., Ramon Y. (1913a) Contribucion al conocimiento de la neuraglia del cerebro humano. Travaux du Laboratoire de Récherches Biologiques de l'Université de Madrid 2:255.

Cajal S., Ramon Y. (1913b) Sobre un nuevo proceder de impregnacion de la neuroglia y sus resultados en los centios nerviosos del hombres y animales. Travaux du Laboratoire de Récherches Biologiques de l'Université de Madrid 2:219.

Carpenter S., Karpati G. (2001) Pathology of skeletal muscle, 2nd edn. New York: Oxford University Press.

Chambers W.W., Chung-Yu-Liv, Chan-Nao-Liu. (1956) A modification of the Nauta technique for staining of degenerating axons in the central nervous system. Anatomical Record 124:391–392.

Chan K.K., Lowe J. (2002) Techniques in neuropathology. In: Bancroft J.D., Gamble M., eds. Theory and practice of histological techniques, 5th edn. Edinburgh: Churchill Livingstone, pp. 371–414.

Chan K.K., Scholtz C.L. (1988) The effect of the gene for microphthalmia (*mi*) on the dorsal lateral geniculate nucleus of the cinnamon mouse. British Journal of Experimental Pathology 69:255–264.

Coers C. (1952) The vital staining of muscle biopsies with methylene blue. Journal of Neurology, Neurosurgery, and Psychiatry 15.

Coers C. (1982) Pathology of intramuscular nerves and nerve terminals. In: Mastaglia F.L., Walton J., eds. Skeletal muscle pathology. Edinburgh: Churchill Livingstone, pp. 483–507.

Coers C., Woolf A.L. (1959) The innervation of a muscle. Oxford: Blackwell.

Collinge J. (1999) Variant Creutzfeldt–Jakob disease. Lancet 354(9175):317–323.

Cooper P.N., Jackson M., Lennox G. et al. (1995) Tau, ubiquitin, and αB-crystallin immunohistochemistry define the principal causes of degenerative frontotemporal dementia. Archives of Neurology 52:1011–1015.

Cosgrove, M., Fitzgibbons, P.L., Sherrod, A. et al. (1989) Intermediate filament expression in astrocytic neoplasms. American Journal of Pathology 13(2):141–145.

Cox G. (1973) Neuroglia and microglia. In: Cook H.C., ed. Histopathology—selected topics. London: Baillière Tindall.

Cox W. (1891) Imprägnation des centralen nervensystem mit quecksilbersalzen. Archiv für Mikroskopische Anatomie 37:16–21.

Cross R.B. (1982) Demonstration of neurofibrillary tangles in paraffin sections: a quick and simple method using a modification of Palmgren's method. Journal of the Institute of Medical Laboratory Science 39:67–69.

Cuadros M.A., Navascues J. (1998) The origin and differentiation of microglial cells during development. Progress in Neurobiology 56(2):173–189.

de Rutter J.P. (1983) The influence of post mortem fixation delay on the reliability of the Golgi silver impregnation. Brain Research 266:143–147.

Dickson D.W. (1999) Tau and synuclein and their role in neuropathology. Brain Pathology 9(4):657–661.

Dogliani C., Dell'orto P., Coggi G. et al. (1987) Choroid plexus tumours: an immunocytochemical study with particular reference to the co-expression of intermediate filament proteins. American Journal of Pathology 127:519–529.

Drury R.A.B., Wallington E.A. (1980) Carleton's histological technique, 5th edn. London: Oxford University Press.

Dyke P.J., Thomas P.K., Lambert E.H., et al. (1984) Peripheral neuropathy, 2nd edn. Philadelphia, PA: W.B. Saunders.

Eager R.P. (1970) Selective staining of degenerating axons in the central nervous system by a simplified method: spinal cord projections to external cuneate and inferior olivary nuclei in the cat. Brain Research 22:137–141.

Eager R.P., Barnett R.J. (1966) Morphological and chemical studies of Nauta-stained degenerating cerebellar and hypothalamic fibres. Journal of Comparative Neurology 126:487–510.

Eager R.P., Chi C.C., Wolf G. (1971) Lateral hypothalamic projections to the hypothalamic ventromedial nucleus in the albino rat: demonstration by means of a simplified ammoniacal silver degeneration method. Brain Research 29:128–132.

Ehrlich P. (1886) Ueber die Methelenblaureaction der Lebenden Nervensubstance. Deutsche Medizinische Wochenschrift 12:49.

Einarson L. (1932) A method for progressive selective staining of Nissl and nucleus substance in nerve cells. American Journal of Pathology 8:295.

Eng L.F., DeArmond S.J. (1983) Immunocytochemistry of the glial fibrillary acidic protein. In: Zimmermann H.M., ed. Progress in neuropathology. New York: Raven Press, vol. 5, pp. 19–39.

Eng L.F., Rubinstein L.J. (1978) Contribution of immunohistochemistry to diagnostic problems of human cerebral tumours. Journal of Histochemistry and Cytochemistry 26:513–522.

Fasano M., Bergmasco B., Lopiano L. (2006) Modifications of the iron–neuromelanin system in Parkinson's disease. Journal of Neurochemistry 96(4):909–916.

Fink R.P., Heimer L. (1967) Two methods for selective silver impregnation of degenerating axons and their synaptic endings in the central nervous system. Brain Research 4:369–374.

Fox Clement A., Ubeda-Purkiss M., Ihrig K., Biagioli D. (1951) Zinc chromate modification of the Golgi technic. Stain Technology 26:109–114.

Gallyas F. (1971) Silver staining of Alzheimer neurofibrillary changes by means of physical development. Acta Morphologica Academiae Scientiarum Hungaricae 19:1–8.

Gallyas F. (1979) An improved silver stain for developing nervous tissue. Stain Technology 54:193–200.

Gallyas F. (1981) Silver staining of protoplasmic astrocytes by physical development. Acta Morphologica Academiae Scientiarum Hungaricae 29:169–176.

Gallyas F., Wolff J.R., Boettcher H., Zaborszky L. (1980) A reliable method for demonstrating axonal degeneration shortly after axotomy. Stain Technology 55:291–297.

Garey L.J., Ong W.Y., Patel T.S. et al. (1998) Reduced dendritic spine density on cerebral cortical pyramidal neurons in schizophrenia. Journal of Neurology, Neurosurgery, and Psychiatry 65(4):446–453.

Ghandour M.S., Langley P.K., Vincendon G. et al. (1980) Immunochemical and immunohistochemical study of carbonic anhydrase II in adult rat cerebellum: a marker for oligodendrocytes. Neuroscience 5:559–571.

Ghobrian M., Ross E.R. (1986) Immunocytochemistry of neuron-specific enolase: a re-evaluation. In: Zimmermann H.M., ed. Progress in neuropathology, New York: Raven Press, pp. 199–221.

Glees P. (1946) Terminal degeneration within the nervous system as studied by a new silver method. Journal of Neuropathology and Experimental Neurology 5:54.

Globus J.M. (1927) The Cajal and Hortega glia staining methods. A new step in the preparation of formaldehyde fixed material. Archives of Neurology and Psychiatry 18:263–271.

Goedert M. (1999) Filamentous nerve cell inclusions in neurodegenerative diseases: tauopathies and alpha-synucleinopathies. Philosophical Transactions of the Royal Society of London. Series B, Biological Sciences 354(1386):1101–1118.

Golgi C. (1873) Sulla struttura della sostanza grigia del cervello. Gazzetta Medica Lombarde 33:244–246.

Golgi C. (1875) Sui gliomi del cervello. Rivista Sperimentale di Freniatria Medicina Legale della Alieranjieni Mentale 1:66–78.

Golgi C. (1879) Di una nuova reazione apparentemente nera della cellule nervose cerebrali ottinuta col bicloruro di mercurio. Archive per le Scienze Mediche 3:1–7.

Gould V.E., Lee I., Wiedenmann B. et al. (1986) Synaptophysin: a novel marker for neurons, certain neuroendocrine cells, and their neoplasms. Human Pathology 17:979–983.

Graeber M.B., Bise K., Mehraein P. (1994) CR3/43, a marker for activated human microglia: application in diagnostic pathology. Neuropathology and Applied Neurobiology 20:406–408.

Gultekin S.H., Rosai J., Demopoulos A. et al. (2000) Hu immunolabeling as a marker of neural and neuroendocrine differentiation in normal and neoplastic human tissues: assessment using a recombinant anti-Hu Fab fragment. International Journal of Surgical Pathology 8(2):109–117.

Haga C., Yamaguchi H., Ikeda K., Kosaka K. (1989) PAM modified methenamine silver stain for senile plaques—comparison with β-protein immunostaining. Dementia (Japan) 3:417–422.

Hayes G.M., Woodroofe M.N., Cuzner M.L. (1987) Microglia are the major cell type expressing MHC class II in human white matter. Journal of Neurological Science 80:25–37.

Hayward P.A.R., Bell J., Ironside J.W. (1994) Prion protein immunochemistry: reliable protocols for the investigation of Creutzfeldt–Jakob disease. Neuropathology and Applied Neurobiology 20:375–383.

Hilton D.A. (2006) Pathogenesis and prevalence of variant Creutzfeldt–Jacob disease. Journal of Pathology 208(2): 134–141.

Holmes W. (1943) Silver staining of nerve axons in paraffin sections. Anatomy Record 86:157–187.

Holzer W. (1921) Uber eine neue method der Gliafases Farbung. Zentralblatt für die gesamte Neurologie und Psychiatrie 69:354–360.

Huber J.D., Parker F., Odland G.F. (1968) A basic fuchsin and alkalinized methylene blue rapid stain for epoxy-embedded tissue. Stain Technology 43:83–87.

Iizuka H., Sakatani K., Young, K. (1990) Neural damage in the rat thalamus after cortical infarcts. Stroke 21:790–794.

Ironside J.W., Head M.W., Bell J.E. et al. (2000) Laboratory diagnosis of variant Creutzfeldt–Jakob disease. Histopathology 37(1):1–9.

Iwaki T., Kume-Iwaki A., Liem R.K., Goldman J.E. (1989) αB-crystallin is expressed in non-lenticular tissues and accumulates in Alexander's disease brain. Cell 57: 71–78.

Kaneko Y., Kitamoto T., Tateishi J., Yamaguchi K. (1989) Ferritin immunohistochemistry as a marker for microglia. Acta Neuropathologica 79:129–136.

Kellett B.S. (1963) Gallocyanin–chrome alum: a routine stain for Nissl substance in paraffin sections. Journal of Medical Laboratory Technology 20:196–198.

Kirby M.L. (1978) Plastic embedding Golgi sections for light microscopy: a quick method. Stain Technology 53: 239–242.

Kitoh T., Matsushita M. (1980) A new staining method of astrocytes for paraffin section. Acta Neuropathologica 49:67–69.

Kluver H., Barrera A. (1953) A method for the combined staining of cells and fibres of the nervous system. Journal of Neuropathology and Experimental Neurology 12:400.

Kosik K.S., Joachim C.L., Selkoe D.J. (1986) Microtubule-associated protein tau is a major component of paired helical filaments in Alzheimer disease. Proc Natl Acad Sci U S A 83:4044–4048.

Lamy C., Duyckaerts C., Delere P. et al. (1989) Comparison of seven staining methods for senile plaques and neurofibrillary tangles in a prospective series of 15 elderly patients. Neuropathology and Applied Neurobiology 15:563–578.

Linder J.E. (1978) A simple and reliable method for the silver impregnation of soft or mineralised tissue. Journal of Anatomy 127:543.

Lowe J. (1997) Degenerative non-Alzheimer dementias. Brain Pathology 7:1047–1051.

Lowe J. (1998) Establishing a pathological diagnosis in degenerative dementias. Brain Pathology 8:403–406.

Lowe J., Lennox G., Jefferson D. et al. (1988) A filamentous inclusion body within anterior horn neurones in motor neurone disease defined by immunocytochemical localisation of ubiquitin. Neuroscience Letters 94:203–210.

Lowe J., Aldridge F., Lennox G. et al. (1989a) Inclusion bodies in motor cortex and brainstem of patients with motor neurone disease are detected by immunocytochemical localisation of ubiquitin. Neuroscience Letters 105:7–13.

Lowe J., Maclennan K.A., Powe D.G. et al. (1989b) Microglial cells in human brain have phenotypic characteristics related to possible function as dendritic antigen presenting cells. Journal of Pathology 159:143–149.

Lowe J., Mayer R.J., Landon M. (1993) Ubiquitin in neurodegenerative diseases. Brain Pathology 3:55–65.

Loyez M. (1910) Coloration des fibres nerveuses par la méthode à l'hematoxyline au fer après inclusion à la celloidine. Compte Rendu des Séances de la Société de Biologie 69:511.

Mallory F.B. (1961) Pathological technique. New York: Hatner.

Mannoji H., Yeger H., Becker L.E. (1986) A specific histochemical marker (lectin *Ricinus communis* agglutinin 1) for normal human microglia and application to routine histopathology. Acta Neuropathologica (Berlin) 71:341–343.

Marsland T.A., Glees P., Erikson L.B. (1954) Modification of the Glees silver impregnation for paraffin sections. Journal of Neuropathology and Experimental Neurology 13:587.

Matsumoto Y., Hara N., Tanaka R., Fujiwara M. (1986) Immunohistochemical analysis of the rat central nervous system during experimental allergic encephalomyelitis, with special reference to Ia-positive cells with dendritic morphology. Journal of Immunology 136:3668–3676.

Matus A. (1987) Putting together the neuronal cytoskeleton. TINS 10:186–188.

Mirra S.S., Hart M.N., Terry R.D. (1993) Making the diagnosis of Alzheimer's disease. A primer for practicing pathologists. Archives of Pathology and Laboratory Medicine 117:132–144.

Moliner E.R. (1957) A chlorate–formaldehyde modification of the Golgi method. Stain Technology 32:105–116.

Moliner E.R. (1958) A tungstate modification of the Golgi–Cox method. Stain Technology 33:19–29.

Mukai M. (1983) Immunohistochemical localization of S-100 protein and peripheral nerve myelin proteins (P2 protein, P1 protein) in granular cell tumors. American Journal of Pathology 112:139–146.

Mullen R.J., Buck C.R., Smith A.M. (1992) NeuN, a neuronal specific nuclear protein in vertebrates. Development 116(1):201–211.

Munoz D.G. (1991) The pathological basis of multi-infarct dementia. Alzheimer Disease Associated Disorders 5:77–90.

Munoz D.G. (1999) Stains for the differential diagnosis of degenerative dementias. Biotechnic and Histochemistry 74(6):311–312.

Naoumenko J., Feigin I. (1961) A modification for paraffin sections of the Cajal gold–sublimate stain for astrocytes. Journal of Neuropathology and Experimental Neurology 20:602–604.

Nauta W.J.H. (1950) Uber die sogenannte terminale Degeneration im Zentralnervensystem und ihre Darstellung durch Silberimprägnation Schweiz. Archives of Neurology and Psychiatry 66:353–376.

Nauta W.J.H., Gygax P.A. (1951) Silver impregnation of degenerating axon terminals in the central nervous system. (1) Technic (2) Chemical notes. Stain Technology 26:5–11.

Newcomb E.W., Cohen H., Lee S.R. et al. (1998) Survival of patients with glioblastoma multiforme is not influenced by altered expression of *p16*, *p53*, *EGFR*, *MDM2* or *Bcl-2* genes. Brain Pathology 8(4):655–667.

Nixon R. (1993) The regulation of neurofilament protein dynamics by phosphorylation: clues to neurofilament pathobiology. Brain Pathology 3:29–38.

Nolan J.A., Troganowski J.Q., Hogue-Angletti R. (1985) Neurons and neuroendocrine cells contain chromogranin: detection of the molecule in normal bovine tissues by immunochemical and immunohistochemical methods. Journal of Histochemistry and Cytochemistry 33:791–798.

Oehmichen M. (1982) Are resting and/or reactive microglia macrophages? Immunobiology 161(3–4):246–254.

Page K. (1965) A stain for myelin using solochrome cyanin. Journal of Medical Laboratory Technology 22:204.

Palay S.L., Palade G.E. (1955) The fine structure of neurons. Journal of Biophysics and Biochemical Cytology 1:69–88.

Palmgren A. (1948) A rapid method for selective silver staining of nerve fibres and nerve endings in mounted paraffin sections. Acta Zoologica 29:377–392.

Paulus W., Roggendorf W., Kirchner T. (1992) Ki-M1P as a marker for microglia and brain macrophages in routinely processed human tissues. Acta Neuropathologica (Berlin) 84:538–544.

Pearson A.A., O'Neill S.L. (1946) A silver gelatine technique for staining nervous tissue. Anatomical Record 95:3, 297.

Pearson J. (1983) Neurotransmitter immunocytochemistry in the study of human development, anatomy, and pathology. In: Zimmermann H.M., ed. Progress in neuropathology. New York: Raven Press, vol. 5, pp. 41–97.

Penfield W. (1928) A method of staining oligodendroglia and microglia. American Journal of Pathology 4:153.

Penfield W., Cone W. (1937) Neuroglia and microglia (the metallic methods). In: McClung C.E., ed. McClung's handbook of microscopical technique. New York: Paul B. Hoeber, pp. 489–521.

Perry V.H., Hume D.A., Gordon S. (1985) Immunohistochemical localisation of macrophages and microglia in the adult and developing mouse brain. Neuroscience 15:313–326.

Pilkington G.J., Lantos P.L. (1982) The use of glutamine synthetase in the diagnosis of cerebral tumours. Neuropathology and Applied Neurobiology 8:227–236.

Poirer L.J., Ayotte R.A., Gauthier C. (1954) Modification of the Marchi technic. Stain Technology 29:71–75.

Pugh B.C., Rossi M.L. (1993) A paraffin wax technique of Golgi–Cox impregnated CNS that permits the joint application of other histological and immunocytochemical techniques. Journal of Neural Transmission. Supplementum 39:97–105.

Pulford K.A.F., Rigney E.M., Micklem K.J. et al. (1989) KP1: a new monoclonal antibody that detects a monocyte/macrophage associated antigen in routinely processed tissue sections. Journal of Clinical Pathology 42:414–421.

Raff M.G., Mirsky R., Fields K.L. et al. (1978) Galactocerebroside: a specific cell surface antigen marker for oligodendrocytes in culture. Nature (London) 274:813–816.

Rubinstein L.J. (1972) Tumours of the central nervous system. Washington, DC: Armed Forces Institute of Pathology.

Rushing E.J., Brown D.F., Hladik C.L. et al. (1998) Correlation of bcl-2, p53, and MIB-1 expression with ependymoma grade and subtype. Modern Pathology 11(5): 464–470.

Santi M., Quezado M., Ronchetti R., Rushing E.J. (2005) Analysis of chromosome 7 in adult and pediatric ependymomas using chromogenic in situ hybridization. Journal of Neurooncology 72(1):25–28.

Scheibel A.B. (1978) Structural aspects of the aging brain: spine systems and the dendritic arbor. In: Katzman R., Terry R.D., Bick K.L., eds. Alzheimer's disease: senile dementia and related disorders. New York: Raven Press, Vol. 7, pp. 353–373.

Schlaepfer W.W. (1987) Neurofilaments: structure, metabolism, and implications in disease. Journal of Neuropathology and Experimental Neurology 46:117–129.

Schochet S.S., McCormick W.F. (1979) Basic neuropathology. In: Schochet S.S., McCormick W.F., eds. Essentials of neuropathology. New York: Appleton-Century-Crofts, pp. 2–6.

Schulz J.B., Dichgans J. (1999) Molecular pathogenesis of movement disorders: are protein aggregates a common link in neuronal degeneration? Current Opinion in Neurology 12(4):433–439.

Schwechheimer K., Gass P., Berlet H.H. (1992) Expression of oligodendroglia and Schwann cell markers in human nervous system tumors. An immunomorphological study and western blot analysis. Acta Neuropathologica 83(3):283–291.

Scott T. (1971) A rapid silver impregnation technique for oligodendroglia, microglia and astrocytes. Journal of Clinical Pathology 24:578.

Smith M.C., Strick S., Sharp P. (1956) The value of the Marchi method for staining tissue stored in formalin for prolonged periods. Journal of Neurology, Neurosurgery, and Psychiatry 19:62–64.

Smyser G.S. (1973) Counterstaining Golgi–Cox impregnation with luxol-fast blue as a myelin stain. Stain Technology 48:53–57.

Stern J.B. (1932) Neue Silberimprägnations Versuche zur Darstellung der Mikro- und Oligodendroglia (An Celloidin-serienschnitten anwendbare Methode). Zeitschrift für die gesamte Neurologie und Psychiatrie 138:50a.

Sternberger N., Tabira T., Kies M.W. et al. (1977) Immunocytochemical staining of basic protein in CNS myelin. Transactions of the American Society of Neurochemists 8:157.

Stewart Smith G. (1943) A danger attending the use of ammoniacal solutions of silver. Journal of Pathology and Bacteriology 55:227.

Suzuki H., Franz H., Yamamoto T. et al. (1988) Identification of the normal microglial population in human and rodent nervous tissue using lectin histochemistry. Neuropathology and Applied Neurobiology 14:221–227.

Swank R.L., Davenport H.A. (1935) Chlorate–osmic formalin method for degenerating myelin. Stain Technology 10:87–90.

Swanson P.E., Manivel J.C., Wick M.R. (1987) Immunoreactivity for Leu-7 in neurofibrosarcoma and other spindle cell tumours of soft tissue. American Journal of Pathology 126:564.

Takahashi H., Wakabayashi K., Kawai K. et al. (1989) Neuroendocrine markers in central nervous system neuronal tumors (gangliocytoma and ganglioglioma). Acta Neuropathologica 77(3):237–243.

Thiel G. (1993) Syapsin I, synapsin II and synaptophysin: marker proteins of synaptic vesicles. Brain Pathology 3:87–95.

Trojanowski J.Q., Lee V.M., Schlaepfer W.W. (1984) An immunohistochemical study of human central and peripheral nervous system tumours using monoclonal antibodies against neurofilaments and glial filaments. Human Pathology 15:248–257.

Tunturi A.R. (1973) A method for impregnating myelinated axons in adult central nervous system. Stain Technology 48:297–304.

Turcotte A., Ramon-Moliner E. (1965) Counterstaining solution for sections stained with the Golgi–Cox method. Stain Technology 40:310–311.

Van Eldik L.J., Jensen R.A., Ehrenfried B.A., Whetsell W.O. (1986) Immunohistochemical localization of S100β in human nervous system tumors by using monoclonal antibodies with specificity for the S100β polypeptide. Journal of Histochemistry and Cytochemistry 34: 977–982.

Velasco M.E., Dahl D., Roessmann V., Gambetti P. (1980) Immunohistochemical localisation of the glial fibrillary acidic protein in human glial neoplasms. Cancer 45:484–494.

Wallington E.A. (1965) The explosive properties of ammoniacal silver solutions. Journal of Medical Laboratory Techniques 22:220.

Watanabe K., Tachibana O., Sata K. et al. (1996) Over-expression of the EGF receptor and p53 mutations are mutually exclusive in the evolution of primary and secondary glioblastomas. Brain Pathology 6(3):217–223.

Weihl C.C., Roos R.P. (1999) Creutzfeldt–Jakob disease, new variant Creutzfeldt–Jakob disease, and bovine spongiform encephalopathy. Neurologic Clinics 17(4): 835–859.

Weil A. (1928) A rapid method for staining myelin sheaths. Archives of Neurology and Psychiatry 20:392.

Wiedenmann B., Kuhn C., Schwechheimer K. et al. (1988) Synaptophysin identified in metastases of neuroendocrine tumours by immunocytochemistry and immunoblotting. American Journal of Clinical Pathology 87:560–569.

Williams R.S., Ferrante R.J., Caviness V.S. (1978) The Golgi rapid method in clinical neuropathology; the morphological consequences of suboptimal fixation. Journal of Neuropathology and Experimental Neurology 37:13–33.

Wilson P.O.G., Barber P.C., Hamid Q.A. et al. (1988) The immunolocalization of protein gene product 9.5 using rabbit polyclonal and mouse monoclonal antibodies. British Journal of Experimental Pathology 69:91–104.

Woodroofe M.N., Bellamy A.S., Feldmann M. et al. (1986) Immunocytochemical characterisation of the immune reaction in the central nervous system in multiple sclerosis: possible role for microglia in lesion growth. Journal of Neurological Science 74:135–152.

Working Group (1997) Consensus recommendations for the postmortem diagnosis of Alzheimer's disease. The National Institute on Aging, and Reagan Institute Working Group on Diagnostic Criteria for the Neuropathological Assessment of Alzheimer's Disease. Neurobiology of Aging 18(4 Suppl):S1–S2.

Yamaguchi H., Haga C., Hirai S. et al. (1990) Distinctive, rapid, and easy labeling of diffuse plaques in the Alzheimer brains by a new methenamine silver stain. Acta Neuropathologica 79:569–572.

Yamamoto T., Hirano A. (1986) A comparative study of modified Bielchowsky, Bodian and thioflavin S stain on Alzheimer's neurofibrillary tangles. Neuropathology and Applied Neurobiology 12:3–9.

FURTHER READING

Cajal S., Ramón Y. (1913a) Contribución al conocimiento de la neuroglia del cerebro humano. Travaux du Laboratoire de Récherches Biologiques de l'Université de Madrid 2:255.

Cajal S., Ramon Y. (1913b) Sobre un neuvo proceder de impregnación de la neuroglia y sus resultados en los centros nerviosos del hombre y animales. Travaux du Laboratoire de Récherches Biologiques de l'Université de Madrid 2:219.

Glees P. (1943) The Marchi reaction: its use on frozen sections and its time limit. Brain 66:229–232.

Swank R.L., Davenport H.A. (1934) Marchi's staining method. Studies of some of the underlying mechanisms involved. Stain Technology 9:11.

Weigert C. (1891) Zur markscheidenfürbung. Deutsches Medizinisches Wochenschrift, 1184.

20

Enzyme Histochemistry and its Diagnostic Applications

Scott L. Nestor and John D. Bancroft

INTRODUCTION

This chapter outlines principles, describing some classical and important methods including methods of diagnostic value. Enzymes are vital components of biological systems; as the catalysts of most biochemical reactions they are essential for the metabolic processes occurring within the tissue. They may be free and soluble in the cytoplasm or body fluids (lysoenzymes) or bound to specific cell components (desmoenzymes).

To achieve a satisfactory enzymatic reaction, the presence of co-factors is required. These are often metal ions, frequently magnesium and manganese (activators), and compounds such as the nucleotides, nicotinamide adenine dinucleotide (NAD), and nicotinamide adenine dinucleotide phosphate (NADP), which are coenzymes. Enzymes are classified into groups according to their effect on substrates. For enzyme histochemistry to be applied to tissue sections, suitable preparation of the tissue is necessary. The way the tissue is handled, and the subsequent sections produced, depends upon the information required from the finished section. Surgical specimens require specialized fixation, handling, and processing. Muscle biopsies require enzyme methods to produce a definite diagnosis, most of the methods being applied to unfixed sections.

It is important to be aware of the different techniques available. As a rule there is little point in applying enzyme methods to paraffin-embedded tissue but there are a few exceptions to this statement, for instance the demonstration of chloroacetate esterase. The range of methods of preservation of the tissue and enzyme at our disposal is considerable. The first decision to be made is whether the tissue is to be fixed or frozen. Tissues frozen to $-70°C$ or below are well preserved and there is little loss of enzyme activity; the tissue can be stored for some time. Alternatively a fixative is used, with the choice governed by the subsequent method. Freezing for preservation is employed where fixation or subsequent processing will affect the results of the demonstrating method, as with the ATPase methods. Most specimens are fixed on arrival in the laboratory: formaldehyde-based fixatives are suitable for most techniques. Bancroft and Cook (1994) discuss the drawbacks of routine processing on tissue constituents.

Fixation and enzyme histochemistry

Enzymes are labile and their preservation is of the utmost importance. The mitochondria in which many of the oxidative enzymes are located are rapidly damaged when the blood supply is cut. Freezing and subsequent thawing of blocks or sections damage organelles such as lysosomes, which contain many of the hydrolytic enzymes. Hydrolytic enzymes therefore tend to show considerable diffusion if demonstrated on frozen, unfixed sections. The post-fixation of the sections does little to prevent this diffusion.

Tissues to be used for the demonstration of the majority of hydrolytic enzymes may be subjected to controlled fixation, which, whilst decreasing the amount of demonstrable enzyme within the section, does allow for a considerably sharper localization of the remaining enzyme activity. Fixation will destroy many of the oxidative enzymes; there are a few exceptions to this, and these are indicated in the relevant enzyme methods. For the demonstration of hydrolytic enzymes, histochemical techniques are usually applied to sections that have been prefixed in cold (4°C) formal calcium; this technique is discussed in detail in Chapter 4 and readers are referred to this chapter before proceeding with the methods of demonstration.

Smears

During the development of enzyme histochemistry, there have been several reports of the use of cytological smears for cytochemical identification and evaluation of cells. Such smears, whose preparation may be achieved in various ways, include blood, bone marrow, and tissue cell suspensions. Three of the most useful enzymes are non-specific esterase, acid phosphatase, and chloroacetate esterase. It is usual to fix smears before histochemical staining to preserve cell structure and enzyme localization. Various fixatives have been used, with a formalin variant being the most popular. Formalin vapor appears to be superior to either paraformaldehyde or glutaraldehyde solutions for the demonstration of non-specific esterase and acid phosphatase, but many histochemists prefer cold (4°C) formal calcium. The technique of preparing imprint smears is simple and rapid, and provides valuable diagnostic information if carried out correctly. Fresh tissue is cut and the new surface touched gently against a clean glass slide, avoiding excess pressure as this distorts cells. The slides are rapidly air-dried and stored unfixed at −70°C if staining is not immediately required. Lymph nodes are handled in a similar manner.

ENZYME TYPES

Oxidoreductases

This is a large and important group to the enzyme histochemist. These enzymes were previously known as oxidases and dehydrogenases, and are often referred to as oxidative enzymes. The following are included in this class:

Oxidases: catalyze oxidation of a substrate in the presence of oxygen

Peroxidases: catalyze oxidation of a substrate by removing hydrogen, which combines with hydrogen peroxide

Dehydrogenases: catalyze oxidation of a substrate by removal of hydrogen

Diaphorases: catalyze oxidation of NADH and NADPH by removal of hydrogen.

Other important groups

Transferases

These enzymes catalyze the transfer of the radicals of two compounds without the loss or uptake of water. There are several subgroups.

Hydrolases

Catalyze the introduction of water or its elements into specific substrate bonds, although in some instances water may be removed. These enzymes include:

- esterases
- lipases
- phosphatases
- glycosidases
- peptidases
- pyrophosphatases.

Lyases

These catalyze the removal of groups from substrates by mechanisms other than hydrolysis, this process resulting in the formation of carbon double bonds. A subclass of this group is the decarboxylases.

NOMENCLATURE

The above classification of enzymes is biochemical, and in histochemistry the situation is less precise (Bancroft & Hand 1987). The nomenclature of enzymes was originally haphazard and confusing. Different workers have used on occasion two or more names for the same enzyme, or conversely the same name has been used for two or more enzymes. In 1898, Duclaux suggested enzymes be named after the substrate upon which they acted with the added suffix 'ase'. For example, the term sucrase indicates an enzyme acting on sucrose. Later it became necessary to name not only the substrate but also the type of reaction, e.g. cholinesterase. Further definition also proved necessary to differentiate between two enzymes catalyzing similar reactions, but under different conditions, e.g. acid phosphatase and alkaline phosphatase (Bancroft & Hand 1987).

TYPES OF HISTOCHEMICAL REACTION

There are four main types of histochemical reaction available for the demonstration of enzymes:

- simultaneous capture (coupling, conversion, and chelation)
- post-incubation coupling (conversion and chelation)
- self-colored substrate (solubility change)
- intra-molecular rearrangement.

Simultaneous capture or coupling

This is the most important of the techniques available for the demonstration of enzymes. The principle applies to the long-established metal precipitation techniques of Gomori as well as to the azo dye methods. The simultaneous coupling principle, when considered in the context of azo dye methods for hydrolytic enzymes, involves the use of a suitable substrate and a diazonium salt. The 'coupler' formed by the reaction between the enzyme and the substrate is known as the primary reaction product (PRP). This PRP then combines with the diazonium salt to produce the final reaction product (FRP). This is normally seen as a visible colored deposit. The main problem with this type of method is the diffusion of the PRP that can occur. This diffusion is likely to be governed by three factors:

- rate of hydrolysis of the substrate
- diffusion coefficient of the PRP for the buffer
- rate of coupling of the PRP with the diazonium salt.

These factors can be manipulated to improve the localization of the enzyme by altering the substrate used and by modifying the diazonium salt. The type of substrate employed, choice of diazonium salt, and rate of coupling all affect the rate of hydrolysis. The substrate must be soluble in water or in the buffer medium used, allowing maximum hydrolysis by the enzyme. If the concentration of soluble substrate is too high then inhibition of the rate of hydrolysis of the substrate will occur.

The buffer medium has to be at a pH at which the enzyme will exhibit maximal activity and the substrate show reasonable solubility. Included in the incubating medium for this type of reaction is the diazonium salt required for the production of the colored final reaction product (cf. post-incubation coupling). Each diazonium salt also has an optimal pH for its most efficient rate of coupling. This means that for an acid phosphatase reac-

tion a diazonium salt is used that will couple at an acid pH level, and for an alkaline phosphatase a salt such as fast red TR, which will couple well at pH 9.4, is required.

The diazonium salts, as well as having an optimal pH range for coupling, also have a critical concentration level, for an excess of diazonium salt will cause an inhibition of the rate of formation of the final reaction product. In practice it is apparent that 1 mg per 1 ml of incubating medium gives satisfactory results.

Post-incubation coupling

In this type of method, the enzyme will hydrolyze the substrate in the manner described above to produce a primary reaction product. The PRP has to be sufficiently insoluble and remain at the site of production for the duration of the initial incubation, and for the subsequent reaction to produce the final reaction product, which is carried out in a separate solution.

The advantages of this type of method are in cases where a long first incubation stage is necessary, as most diazonium salts decompose slowly when in aqueous solution. A further advantage is that the optimal pH level for the enzyme activity can be employed in the first incubation and the different optimal pH for coupling employed in the separate second stage of the reaction. The disadvantage of this type of reaction lies in the fact that the PRP in almost all instances is soluble to some extent, with the result that some diffusion of the PRP occurs before suitable coupling to a diazonium salt can be carried out.

Self-colored substrate

This type of reaction is only occasionally used. It involves using a colored substrate that is also soluble; during the hydrolysis the enzyme removes the soluble grouping without affecting the color. The PRP produced in this instance is both insoluble and colored, and the further stage of coupling with a diazonium salt is unnecessary. Only a limited number of enzyme-sensitive solubilizing groups are known and the use of the method is therefore restricted.

Intramolecular rearrangement

This type of technique uses soluble substrates, which, after hydrolysis, undergo molecular rearrangement to give a colored insoluble reaction product.

Diazonium salts

These and the closely related tetrazolium salts react with the primary reaction product of enzymatic histochemical reactions to produce a highly colored and insoluble reaction product. The salts themselves are usually colorless, but a few are dyes, e.g. pararosanilin and fast garnet GBC. Enzymatically released naphthols or related compounds, when coupled with diazonium salts, form the chromophore azo group which is visible as a color reaction. The solubility of diazonium salts is limited, especially in the alkaline pH range.

THE USE OF CONTROLS

Controls are a necessary part of enzyme histochemistry. Substrates, diazonium salts, and other chemical solutions used will deteriorate with time, leading to the possible failure of the method; occasionally false positives may be produced. A positive control should be carried through when incubating test sections, to show that all the chemical solutions are working. Omission of the substrate from the incubating medium and the inclusion of specific enzyme inhibitors (if available) affords adequate control measures. If further controls are deemed necessary, competitive inhibitors may be added to the incubating solution. Sections may also be pre-treated by immersing them in boiling water for a few minutes, and then processing through the rest of the method, or by 'incubating' in distilled water. In each case, the absence of reaction product indicates that the positive results obtained with the authentic techniques are yielding useful information about the distribution of the enzyme. Non-specific background staining is also excluded as a possible source of error if control sections give negative results. Any activity in negative control sections must be regarded as a false result.

HYDROLYTIC ENZYMES

The phosphatases

These are enzymes that are capable of hydrolyzing organic phosphate esters. They are classified on the basis of their optimal pH levels; those that exhibit maximum activity at around pH 9.0 are termed 'alkaline phosphatases', whilst those whose peak is around pH 5.0 are called 'acid phosphatases'. Most of these enzymes are non-specific, i.e. they will catalyze the hydrolysis of a wide range of organic phosphate esters, but there are a few enzymes that will only act upon a specific substrate, an example being glucose-6-phosphatase, which is capable of dephosphorylating glucose 6-phosphate at pH 6.5. This enzyme is considered a 'specific phosphatase' although it reacts at an acid pH. The phosphatases can therefore be divided into:

- alkaline phosphatases
- acid phosphatases
- specific phosphatases.

Alkaline phosphatases

These enzymes are localized in cell membranes in the kidney and many other tissues.

Techniques for demonstration of alkaline phosphatases

The theoretical considerations of the type of method available have been discussed earlier in this chapter; the theory of the individual techniques is considered, along with the practical details.

Metal precipitation

Gomori (1939) described the original method. Gomori published further improvements in 1951 and this improved method, in a slightly modified version, is given below. The technique is a simultaneous coupling reaction in which the enzyme hydrolyzes the substrate, sodium β-glycerophosphate, to produce phosphate ions. This primary reaction product reacts with calcium ions to form calcium phosphate, and this in turn is treated with cobalt nitrate to produce a precipitate of cobalt phosphate. This reaction product cannot be seen with the light microscope and further treatment is needed with dilute ammonium sulfide to produce a visible black precipitate of cobalt sulfide. This should be seen as a granular deposit under ideal conditions. The flow chart below, modified from Bancroft (1975), summarizes the reaction.

	enzyme	
Sodium β-glycerophosphate (substrate)	———	phosphate ions (PRP) (invisible)
Phosphate ions + calcium ions	———	calcium phosphate (invisible)
Calcium phosphate + cobalt ions	———	cobalt phosphate (invisible)
Cobalt phosphate + sulfide ions	———	cobalt sulfide (insoluble visible)

Alkaline phosphatase: the Gomori calcium method (Gomori 1951, modified)

Fixation
Formal calcium at 4°C.

Sections
Pre-fixed cryostat preferred.

Preparation of incubating medium

2% sodium β-glycerophosphate	2.5 ml
2% sodium veronal	2.5 ml
2% calcium nitrate	5 ml
1% magnesium chloride	0.25 ml
Distilled water	1.25 ml

The final pH of the incubating medium should be between 9.0 and 9.4. The sodium veronal acts as the buffer vehicle and the magnesium ions as an enzyme activator.

Method
1. After suitable fixation, bring sections to water, incubate at 37°C for 25 min to 6 hours. (See Note b.)
2. Wash well in distilled water.
3. Repeat wash.
4. Treat sections with 2% cobalt nitrate, 3 min.
5. Wash well in distilled water.
6. Repeat wash.
7. Immerse sections in 1% ammonium sulfide, 2 min.
8. Wash well in distilled water.
9. Counterstain in 2% methyl green (chloroform extracted).
10. Wash well in running tap water.
11. Mount in glycerin jelly.

Results

Alkaline phosphatase activity	brownish-black
Nuclei	green

Notes
a. It is convenient to keep the stock solutions made up in batches of 20 ml.
b. The incubation time varies according to the type of preparation, cryostat sections requiring the shortest time.

Azo dye methods
These are also simultaneous coupling techniques; the original method was described by Menton et al (1944) and modified by Gomori (1951). This type of reaction involves the use of a diazonium salt. These salts, discussed earlier, provide a means of visibly locating the reaction product produced by the action of the enzyme on the substrate. Two types of substrate are employed; the first type is a simple organic phosphate (e.g. sodium α-naphthyl phosphate). The primary reaction product formed by enzymic hydrolysis of this type of substrate is moderately insoluble but some diffusion does occur.

The second type of substrate is those phosphates which contain substituted naphthol groupings (e.g. naphthol AS-BI phosphate). The primary reaction product produced by the enzymatic hydrolysis of this type of substrate is extremely insoluble and the diffusion of the PRP is minimal, hence a better localization of the final reaction product is obtained. The disadvantage of using substituted naphthols as substrates is their high cost. In their favor is the better localization of the final reaction product and the stability of solutions containing substituted naphthols.

Using simple naphthols
The hydrolysis of these substrates produces α-naphthol. This primary reaction product is coupled to a suitable diazonium salt, i.e. fast red TR.

Alkaline phosphatase: azo dye coupling method using α-naphthyl phosphate

Fixation
Formal calcium at 4°C. Formal vapor.

Sections
Pre-fixed cryostat preferred.

Preparation of incubating medium

Sodium α-naphthyl phosphate	10 mg
0.2 M Tris buffer (stock solution A) pH 10.0	10 ml
Diazonium salt (fast red TR)	10 mg

The final pH of the incubating medium should be between 9.0 and 9.4. The sodium α-naphthyl phosphate is dissolved in the buffer, the diazonium salt is added and the solution well mixed. The solution is then filtered and used immediately.

Method

1. After fixation, bring sections to water, incubate at room temperature for 10–60 min.
2. Wash in distilled water.
3. Counterstain in 2% methyl green (chloroform extracted).
4. Wash in running tap water.
5. Mount in glycerin jelly.

Results

Alkaline phosphatase activity	reddish-brown
Nuclei	green

Note

The final pH of the incubating solution is about 9.2. If paraffin sections are used, the incubating time will need to be extended.

Substituted naphthols

The principles of the reactions using these substrates are the same as those involved with the simple organic phosphates. The substituted substrates, which are prepared commercially for histochemical techniques, are complex mixtures; they are extremely insoluble in water, far more so than other substrates. They need to be dissolved in a solvent. These substrates produce a sharper localization of FRP than is seen with unsubstituted naphthols. The hydrolysis of the substrates produces an insoluble naphthol derivative which then couples with a suitable diazonium salt, i.e. fast red TR, to produce a red-colored insoluble azo dye at the site of enzyme activity.

Alkaline phosphatase: naphthol AS-BI method (substituted naphthol)

Fixation

Formal calcium at 4°C. Formal vapor.

Sections

Pre-fixed cryostat preferred.

Preparation of solutions

a. Naphthol AS-BI stock solution

Naphthol AS-BI phosphate	25 mg
N,N-dimethyl formamide	10 ml
Distilled water	10 ml
Molar sodium carbonate	2–6 drops

The reagents are added in the above order, sufficient molar sodium carbonate is added until the pH is 8.0, then add:

Distilled water	300 ml
0.2 M Tris buffer, pH 8.3	180 ml

The solution, which is faintly opalescent, is stable for many months.

b. Incubating solution

Stock naphthol AS-BI solution	10 ml
Fast red TR	10 mg

Shake well, filter, and use immediately.

Method

1. After fixation and bringing sections to water, incubate at room temperature for 5–15 min.
2. Wash in water.
3. Counterstain in 2% methyl green (chloroform extracted).
4. Wash well in running tap water.
5. Mount in glycerin jelly.

Results

Alkaline phosphatase activity	red
Nuclei	green

Notes

This is a reliable method that gives sharp localization of the enzyme. There are two points to watch in the technique. The molar sodium carbonate changes the pH rapidly and care must be taken not to make the solution too alkaline. The reaction is fast, and care must be taken not to over-incubate.

Techniques for the demonstration of acid phosphatases

The principles for these methods are identical to those discussed under the heading Alkaline phosphatases. So at this point only the rationale of the techniques given is included. The metal precipitation technique was described by Gomori (1941) and is based on his alkaline phosphatase technique. In this method sodium β-glycerophosphate is used as the substrate in a buffer medium at pH 5.0. The hydrolysis of the substrate produces phosphate ions as the primary reaction product; this is treated with lead ions to produce a precipitate of lead phosphate. The precipitate is not visible at the light microscope level, so further treatment with ammonium sulfide is necessary to produce a visible precipitate of lead sulfide at the site of enzyme activity (Fig. 20.1).

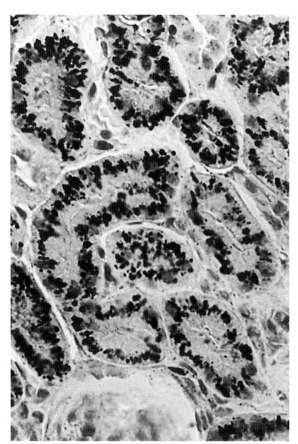

Fig. 20.1 Acid phosphatase activity in rat kidney showing localization in tubular epithelial cells. Tissue block prefixed in formal calcium; Gomori's metal chelation method. Compare this coarse granular final reaction product with that in Fig. 20.2.

the incubating medium should be approximately 5.0.

Method

1. Place sections in incubating solution at 37°C for 0.5–2 hours.
2. Wash in distilled water.
3. Immerse in 1% ammonium sulfide (fresh), 2 min.
4. Wash well in distilled water.
5. Counterstain in either 2% methyl green, or Mayer's carmalum.
6. Wash in tap water.
7. Mount in glycerin jelly.

Results

Acid phosphatase activity	black
Nuclei	green or red

Azo dye methods

As with the alkaline phosphatase methods, two types of substrate can be used, either the simple organic phosphate, e.g. sodium α-naphthyl phosphate, or the phosphates that contain substituted naphthol groupings, such as naphthol AS-BI phosphate. The advantages and disadvantages are discussed under alkaline phosphatases. In using simple naphthols the hydrolysis of the substrate by the enzyme produces α-naphthol. This primary reaction product is coupled to a suitable diazonium salt, i.e. fast garnet GBC, which gives a red insoluble azo dye final reaction product at the site of enzyme activity.

Acid phosphatase: the Gomori lead method

Fixation
Formal calcium at 4°C. Formal vapor.

Sections
Pre-fixed cryostat preferred.

Preparation of incubating solution

0.05 M acetate buffer pH 5.0	10 ml
Sodium β-glycerophosphate	32 mg
Lead nitrate	20 mg

The lead nitrate must be dissolved in the buffer before the sodium β-glycerophosphate is added. The pH of

Acid phosphatase: azo dye coupling method

Fixation
Formal calcium at 4°C. Formal vapor.

Sections
Pre-fixed cryostat preferred.

Preparation of incubating medium

Sodium α-naphthyl phosphate	10 mg
0.1 M acetate buffer, pH 5.0	10 ml
Fast garnet GBC	10 mg

The sodium α-naphthyl phosphate is dissolved in the buffer and the diazonium salt added. The solution is then filtered and used immediately.

Method

1. Incubate at 37°C for 15–60 min.
2. Wash in distilled water.
3. Counterstain in 2% methyl green (chloroform extracted).
4. Wash in running tap water.
5. Mount in glycerin jelly.

Results

Acid phosphatase activity	red
Nuclei	green

Using substituted naphthols

This method was published by Burstone (1958), when he recommended naphthol AS-BI phosphate as the substrate; the primary reaction product, produced by the enzyme hydrolyzing this substrate, is extremely insoluble. Barka (1960) recommended the use of hexazonium pararosanilin (Davis & Ornstein 1959), as the most suitable diazonium salt. The preparation of the diazonium salt is time consuming. The advantage of better localization of the final reaction product, and stability to alcohols and xylene, allowing the preparations to be dehydrated to xylene and mounted in a resinous medium, make this salt the one of choice (Fig. 20.2).

Acid phosphatase: the naphthol AS-BI phosphate method (Burnstone 1958, modified by Barka 1960)

Fixation
Formal calcium at 4°C. Formal vapor.

Sections
Pre-fixed cryostat preferred.

Preparation of solutions

a. **Substrate solution**

Naphthol AS-BI phosphate	10 mg
Dimethyl formamide	1 ml

b. **Buffer solution**

Sodium acetate (3H$_2$O)	1.94 g
Sodium barbitone	2.94 g
Distilled water	100 ml

c. **Sodium nitrite solution**

Sodium nitrite	400 mg
Distilled water	10 ml

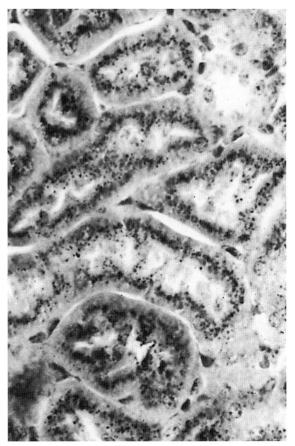

Fig. 20.2 Acid phosphatase activity in rat kidney tubules. Tissue block prefixed in formal calcium. Azo dye method using a substituted naphthol as substrate and hexazonium pararosanilin as diazonium salt.

d. **Pararosanilin HCl stock solution**

Pararosanilin hydrochloride	1 g
Distilled water	20 ml
Hydrochloric acid (conc.)	5 ml

Heat gently, cool to room temperature, and filter.

e. **Distilled water**

Preparation of incubating solution

Solution a	0.5 ml
Solution b	2.5 ml
Solution c	0.4 ml
Solution d	0.4 ml
Solution e	6 ml

For the success of this technique it is essential that equal parts of solutions c and d are mixed together and allowed to stand for 2 min before being added to the incubating medium. The final pH should be between 4.7 and 5.0; it is adjusted if necessary with 0.1 M NaOH.

Method

1. Incubate sections at 37°C for 15–60 min.
2. Wash in distilled water.
3. Counterstain in 2% methyl green (chloroform extracted).
4. Wash in running water.
5. Either mount in glycerin jelly, or dehydrate rapidly through fresh alcohols to xylene and mount in DPX.

Results

Acid phosphatase activity	red
Nuclei	green

Note

This is a reliable method giving sharp localization of the enzyme. There are three points to watch in the preparation of the incubating solution: that solution c (sodium nitrite) is fresh, the pH of the final incubating solution is correct, and the incubating solution is filtered.

Methods of demonstration of specific phosphatases

5-nucleotidase

This is a metal precipitation technique of Wachstein and Meisel (1957). Adenosine 5-phosphate is the substrate. The enzyme acts on the substrate and, in the presence of magnesium ions as an activator, produces phosphate ions. These are precipitated by lead ions also present in the incubating medium to produce lead phosphate. Ammonium sulfide is used to convert the lead phosphate to lead sulfide, which is seen as a brown precipitate at the site of enzyme activity. The method is carried out at pH 7.5 and non-specific alkaline phosphatase activity may also be demonstrated.

5-Nucleotidase: lead method
(Wachstein & Meisel 1957)

Fixation

Unfixed preferred, or formal calcium at 4°C.

Sections

Cryostat, free floating.

Preparation of incubating medium

1.25% adenosine 5-phosphate	4 ml
0.2 M Tris buffer, pH 7.2	4 ml
2% lead nitrate	0.6 ml
0.1 M magnesium sulfate	1 ml
Distilled water	0.5 ml

Method

1. Incubating medium at 37°C for 30 min to 1 hour.
2. Fix in formal saline if unfixed sections used.
3. Transfer sections with glass rod to distilled water.
4. Repeat wash in fresh distilled water.
5. 1% ammonium sulfide, 3 min.
6. Wash well in distilled water.
7. Repeat wash.
8. Mount on microscope slides and allow to dry partially in the usual way.
9. Mount in glycerin jelly.

Result

5-nucleotidase	blackish-brown deposits

Note

There is a considerable loss of enzyme activity with pre-fixed blocks, so the recommended method is to use cryostat sections of unfixed material.

Glucose-6-phosphatase

This is a metal precipitation technique. There are a number of variations of the method and the one given is by Wachstein and Meisel (1956). The enzyme will hydrolyze glucose 6-phosphate in the presence of lead ions to form a precipitate of lead phosphate. This is then converted to a precipitate of lead sulfide by treatment with dilute ammonium sulfide. Control sections for both acid and alkaline phosphatases should be employed as both may be demonstrated by this technique. Since glucose-6-phosphatase is a sensitive enzyme that is destroyed during fixation, unfixed sections should be employed and the sections post-fixed after incubation.

Glucose-6-phosphatase: lead method
(Wachstein & Meisel 1956)

Fixation
None.

Sections
Cryostat, unfixed.

Preparation of incubating medium

0.125% glucose 6-phosphate	4 ml
Tris maleate buffer pH 6.7, see Appendix 3	4 ml
2% lead nitrate	0.6 ml
Distilled water	1.4 ml

Method
1. Place fresh unfixed cryostat sections into incubating medium at 37°C for 5–20 min.
2. Wash well in distilled water, two changes, 2 min. each.
3. Immerse sections in 1% ammonium sulfide, 2 min.
4. Wash in distilled water.
5. Fix sections in 10% formaldehyde, 15–30 min.
6. Wash in distilled water.
7. Mount in glycerin jelly.

Result
Glucose-6-phosphatase activity   brownish black

Note
It is advisable to use sections 15 μm thick. Although less convenient, better results may be obtained by incubating the section free-floating.

Adenosine triphosphatase (ATPase)

The ATPase reaction is a metal precipitation technique, originally described by Wachstein et al (1960). The enzyme produces phosphate from the substrate adenosine triphosphate (ATP); in the Wachstein lead method, the released phosphate ions combine with lead ions to produce a precipitate of lead phosphate, which in turn is converted to lead sulfide by treatment with dilute ammonium sulfide. This is seen as a dark brown or black precipitate at the site of enzyme activity. Adenosine triphosphatase can also be demonstrated by a metal precipitation technique similar to the calcium–cobalt method of Gomori described in relation to alkaline phosphatase. This method is the technique of choice for skeletal muscle biopsies.

Esterases

These are enzymes which are capable of hydrolyzing carboxylic acid. There are a considerable number of enzymes capable of hydrolyzing carboxylic acids and some of these may be demonstrated histochemically. Most of the enzymes have an optimal pH between 5.0 and 9.0. Each enzyme is often capable of hydrolyzing a number of different substrates, and many different enzymes are capable of hydrolyzing the same substrates. The majority of esterase enzymes are able to hydrolyze α-naphthyl acetate as a substrate; these enzymes are called 'non-specific' esterases. This group can be subdivided by the specific action of the enzymes upon a substrate and by the effect of specific inhibitors. The majority of the specific esterases are, however, also capable of hydrolyzing a simple ester such as α-naphthyl acetate. Non-specific esterases are usually divided into three groups (Pearse 1972):

- carboxylesterases
- arylesterases
- acetylesterases.

Specific esterases are subdivided as follows:

- acetylcholinesterases
- cholinesterases
- lipases.

The classification of non-specific esterases given above is based on the most suitable substrate that the enzyme will hydrolyze. This classification is also used when the effects of organophosphate inhibitors are considered. Pearse (1972) recommends that the following terminology should be used for 'non-specific' esterases:

- A esterases (arylesterases)
- B esterases (carboxylesterases)
- C esterases (acetylesterases).

Inhibitors

To separate the different esterase enzymes the use of inhibitors is necessary. Their use allows a more accurate identification of the specific enzymes. The most useful inhibitors are the organophosphates, which include diethyl-p-nitrophenyl phosphate (E600) and diisopropyl fluorophosphate (DFP), and some aromatic mercuric compounds of which the most useful is p-chloromercuribenzoate.

Scheme for identifying non-specific esterases

To demonstrate whether esterase activity is due to either 'A', 'B', or 'C' esterases, the following technique should be employed. Sections are incubated in a 10 μM solution of E600 in buffer at pH 5.3 for 1 hour at 37°C. Following this treatment the B esterase is inhibited. Any esterase activity remaining is due to A or C esterases. These can be distinguished by incubating a section in a solution of *p*-chloromercuribenzoate (PCMB) at a concentration of 100 μM which will inhibit any A esterase but will activate C esterase (Pearse 1972).

The practical methods for non-specific esterases will also demonstrate some specific esterases, e.g. cholinesterases. The cholinesterases as a group are inhibited by eserine in a concentration of 10 μM whereas the A, B, and C esterases are unaffected.

Methods for non-specific esterase

The substrates used for the demonstration of esterases can be hydrolyzed by a number of enzymes, so suitable controls and inhibitors should be used. The method given below will also demonstrate lipases and cholinesterases.

α-Naphthyl acetate method (Gomori 1950)

This method employs a naphthyl acetate as the substrate; the enzyme releases a naphthol during the hydrolysis of the substrate. The α-naphthol is then coupled with a suitable diazonium salt to produce an insoluble azo dye at the site of enzyme activity. Gomori, who modified the original method of Nachlas and Seligman (1949), used fast blue B as the diazonium salt; this salt, however, has been largely replaced by hexazotized pararosanilin, which gives better localization of the enzyme (Davis & Ornstein 1959).

Non-specific esterase: α-naphthyl acetate method (Gomori 1950; Davis & Ornstein 1959)

Fixation
Formal calcium at 4°C. Formal vapor.

Sections
Pre-fixed cryostat preferred.

Preparation of solutions
a. Substrate solution

α-Naphthyl acetate	50 mg
Acetone	5 ml

b. Buffer solution

Disodium hydrogen phosphate (Na_2HPO_4)	2.83 g
Distilled water	100 ml

c. Sodium nitrite solution

Sodium nitrite	400 mg
Distilled water	10 ml

d. Pararosanilin HCl stock solution

Pararosanilin hydrochloride	2 g
2 M hydrochloric acid	50 ml

Heat gently, cool to room temperature, and filter.

e. Distilled water

Preparation of incubating medium

Solution a	0.25 ml
Solution b	7.25 ml
Solution c	0.4 ml
Solution d	0.4 ml
Solution e	2.5 ml

It is important that equal parts of solutions c and d are mixed together before adding to the incubation medium. Adjust pH to 7.4 if necessary with additional solution b.

Method
1. After suitable fixation, bring sections to water.
2. Incubate at 37°C for 2–20 min.
3. Wash in running water.
4. Counterstain in 2% methyl green (chloroform extracted).
5. Wash well in tap water.
6. Dehydrate rapidly through fresh alcohol to xylene, and mount in DPX.

Results

Esterase	reddish brown
Nuclei	green

Indoxyl acetate methods

As an alternative method, the indoxyl acetate technique can be used. This technique of Barnett and Seligman (1951) and Holt and Withers (1952) gives excellent localization. The enzyme hydrolyzes bromo-indoxyl acetate to produce bromo-indoxyl; this is then oxidized to an insoluble azo dye.

Non-specific esterase: indoxyl acetate method (Holt & Withers 1952)

Fixation

Formal calcium at 4°C. Formal vapor.

Sections

Pre-fixed cryostat preferred.

Preparation of incubating medium

5-Bromo-4-chloro-indoxyl acetate	1 mg
Ethanol	0.1 ml
Tris buffer (0.2 M), pH 7.2	2 ml
Potassium ferricyanide	17 mg
Potassium ferrocyanide	21 mg
Calcium chloride	11 mg
Distilled water	7.9 ml

The 5-bromo-4-chloro-indoxyl acetate is dissolved in the ethanol and the buffer is then added. The remaining chemicals are dissolved in the distilled water and the solution is mixed. It is important that the solution is freshly prepared.

Method

1. After suitable fixation, bring sections to water.
2. Incubate at 37°C for 15–60 min.
3. Rinse in tap water.
4. Counterstain in Mayer's carmalum for 5 min.
5. Rinse in tap water.
6. Mount in glycerin jelly, or
7. Dehydrate through graded alcohols to xylene.
8. Mount in DPX.

Results

Esterase activity	blue
Nuclei	red

ESTERASE DEMONSTRATION IN PARAFFIN SECTIONS

Certain esterases can be demonstrated in formalin-fixed paraffin sections, although most esterase enzymes are destroyed by fixation and tissue processing.

Methods for demonstration of the specific esterases

Lipase

The term applies to a group of enzymes which have the ability to hydrolyze long-chain esters, particularly those containing saturated fatty acids. The enzymes are found mainly in the pancreas and to a lesser degree in the adrenals and liver. There is a considerable overlap with non-specific esterase in the demonstration of lipases as they are both capable of hydrolyzing the same substrates. The lipase method relies upon the enzyme hydrolyzing the substrate Tween 60, to produce fatty acids. The fatty acids combine with calcium ions to form relatively insoluble calcium soaps, which are treated with lead ions, and finally by ammonium sulfide, to form visible dark brown to black lead sulfide deposits at the site of activity.

Lipase: Tween method (Gomori 1952)

Fixation

Formal calcium at 4°C. Acetone at 4°C.

Sections

Cryostat, paraffin.

Preparation of solutions

Solution a
Tris buffer, pH 7.2

Solution b

Tween 40, 60, or 80	5 g
Tris buffer, pH 7.2	100 ml
Thymol	1 crystal

Solution c

Calcium chloride	200 mg
Distilled water	10 ml

Solution d

Lead nitrate	1 g
Distilled water	50 ml

Preparation of incubating medium

Solution a	9 ml
Solution b	0.6 ml
Solution c	0.3 ml

Method

1. After suitable fixation, bring sections to water.
2. Incubate at 37°C for 2–8 hours. If paraffin sections, leave for 24 hours.
3. Rinse sections in three changes of distilled water.
4. Place sections in preheated lead nitrate solution (solution d) at 55°C for 10 min.

5. Rinse sections in distilled water for 2 min.
6. Wash in tap water for 10 min.
7. Place sections in 1% ammonium sulfide for 3 min.
8. Rinse in distilled water.
9. Wash in tap water.
10. Counterstain in Mayer's carmalum for 5 min.
11. Wash in tap water for 1 min.
12. Mount in glycerin jelly.

Results

Lipase activity	yellow to brown–black
Nuclei	red

Note

It is advisable to have a control section which is processed through the whole technique, except that the incubating medium lacks Tween. Paraffin sections, according to Gomori, should be fixed in acetone. Formalin-fixed frozen sections work well. Pancreas is the most suitable control tissue.

Cholinesterases

The most important of the specific esterases are the cholinesterases. Two enzymes can be demonstrated, acetyl cholinesterase (true) and cholinesterase (pseudo). Acetyl-cholinesterases, which are mainly found in the nervous system and muscle, will hydrolyze acetyl thiocholine. The pseudo-cholinesterases will hydrolyze esters of choline other than the acetyl esters more rapidly than will true cholinesterase. If differentiation between the two enzymes is required, duplicate sections and two substrates are required, acetyl and butyrylthiocholine iodide.

Acetylcholinesterase (from Filipe & Lake 1983)

Preparation of tissue

Cryostat sections of snap-frozen tissue cut at 10 μm are air-dried and fixed for 30 s in 4% formaldehyde in 0.1 M calcium acetate (formal calcium).

Frozen sections of formal calcium–gum sucrose-treated blocks of tissue.

Incubation medium

Acetylthiocholine iodide	5 mg
0.1 M acetate buffer pH 6.0	6.5 ml
0.1 M sodium citrate	0.5 ml
30 mM copper sulfate	1 ml
Distilled water	1 ml
4 mM iso-octamethyl pyrophosphoramide (iso OMPA)	0.2 ml

Add 1.0 ml 5 mmol/L potassium ferricyanide just before use.

Method

1. Rinse the fixed sections for 10 seconds in tap water.
2. Incubate at 37°C for 1 hour in the above medium.
3. Wash briefly in tap water.
4. Treat with 0.05% p-phenylene diamine dihydrochoride in 0.05 M phosphate buffer pH 6.8 for 45 min at room temperature.
5. Wash in tap water.
6. Treat with 1% osmium tetroxide for 10 min at room temperature.
7. Wash well in tap water, counterstain lightly (10 seconds) in Carrazzi hematoxylin (or Mayer's hemalum), wash, dehydrate, clear, and mount in DPX.

Results

Nerve fibers and cells containing acetylcholinesterase are stained dark brown to black.

Notes

Do not counterstain too heavily and thoroughly dehydrate, because areas with strong activity are resistant to dehydration.

Beware of areas of red blood cells (RBCs) that appear to have nerve fibers lying over. This is due to the acetylcholinesterase of the RBC membrane.

β-Glucuronidase

This enzyme is found in many tissues including proximal convoluted tubules of kidney, endometrial epithelium, and other epithelial tissues. It is not a single enzyme but is a group of enzymes, having specificity for the β-glycoside linkage of a wide range of glucuronides. It is generally regarded that the principal localization of β-glucuronidase is within lysosomes. There are numerous methods available for the demonstration of β-glucuronidases (Pearse 1972). The method given here is a simultaneous coupling method using a substituted naphthol glucuronide (naphthol AS-BI glucuronide) as a substrate; the primary reaction product is coupled with hexazotized pararosanilin.

β-Glucuronidase: naphthol AS-BI method
(Hayashi et al 1964)

Fixation
Formal calcium at 4°C. Formal vapor.

Sections
Pre-fixed cryostat preferred.

Preparation of solutions

a. *Sodium bicarbonate solution*

Sodium bicarbonate	210 mg
Distilled water	50 ml

b. *Substrate solution*

Naphthol AS-BI glucuronide	14 mg
Solution a	0.6 ml
0.1 M acetate buffer, pH 5.0	50 ml

c. *Hexazonium pararosanilin solution*

Pararosanilin HCl stock solution	0.3 ml
4% sodium nitrite (fresh)	0.3 ml

d. *Incubating solution*

Solution b	5 ml
Solution c	0.3 ml
Distilled water	5 ml

The pararosanilin is added before use, and the pH of the solution adjusted with M NaOH to 5.2. Suitable control sections are liver and kidney.

Method
1. Place sections in incubating medium at 37°C, 20–40 min.
2. Wash well in distilled water, 2 min.
3. Counterstain in 2% methyl green (chloroform washed), 4 min.
4. Wash rapidly in tap water.
5. Dehydrate through graded alcohols to xylene.
6. Mount in DPX.

Results

Glucuronidase activity	red
Nuclei	green

Notes
The pH of the incubating solution should be between 5.0 and 5.3, and the sodium nitrite should be freshly prepared.

Leucine aminopeptidase (LAP)

The method of choice is the metal chelation technique of Nachlas et al (1957a,b), which is reliable and easy to perform. The action of the enzyme on the substrate produces β-naphthylamine which is coupled to the diazonium salt, fast blue B, producing an azo dye, which is then chelated with copper ions.

Leucine aminopeptidase
(Nachlas et al 1957a,b)

Fixation
Formal calcium at 4°C.

Sections
Pre-fixed cryostat preferred.

Preparation of solutions

a. *Substrate solution*

L-Leucyl-4-methoxy β-naphthylamide	4 mg
Ethyl alcohol	0.1 ml
Distilled water	4.9 ml

b. *Sodium chloride*

Sodium chloride	425 mg
Distilled water	50 ml

c. *Copper sulfate*

Copper sulfate	798 mg
Distilled water	50 ml

d. *Potassium cyanide solution*

Potassium cyanide	65 mg
Distilled water	50 ml

e. *0.1 M acetate buffer, pH 6.5*

Incubating medium

Substrate solution a	0.5 ml
Solution e	5.0 ml
Solution b	4.0 ml
Solution d	0.5 ml
Fast blue B salt	5 mg

Method
1. Place sections in incubating medium, 15 min to 2 hours.
2. Rinse in saline, solution b, 2 min.
3. Immerse in copper sulfate, solution c, 2 min.
4. Rinse sections in saline, 2 min.
5. Counterstain in 2% methyl green, 3 min.
6. Wash in water.

7. Dehydrate through graded alcohols to xylene.
8. Mount in DPX.

Results

LAP activity	red
Nuclei	green

OXIDATIVE ENZYMES

Reactions for oxidative enzymes

These enzymes are usually demonstrated by simultaneous coupling methods, which involve the oxidation of the substrate and the consequent reduction of a tetrazolium salt, giving a relatively insoluble formazan deposit at the site of enzyme activity. The oxidation is brought about in two ways. Firstly, a number of enzymes catalyze the reaction between the substrate and atmospheric oxygen; these are termed oxidases. A second group remove hydrogen from the substrate and transfer it along a hydrogen acceptor pathway; these enzymes include the dehydrogenases.

Tetrazolium salts

For the demonstration of many oxidative enzymes, tetrazolium salts are used as a hydrogen acceptor. On reduction they will form a colored deposit. Two tetrazolium salts are in common use at the present time, monotetrazolium and ditetrazolium. The ditetrazolium salt, ditetrazolium chloride-nitro, known as NBT (Nachlas et al 1957a,b), produces a highly colored formazan deposit that is insoluble in lipid, whereas the monotetrazolium 3-(4,5-dimethyl thiazolyl-2)-2,5-diphenyl tetrazolium bromide (MTT) (Pearse 1957) produces a finely granular formazan which is soluble in lipids.

Oxidases

These enzymes oxidize substrates by catalyzing the reaction between substrate and oxygen. A number of these enzymes can be demonstrated histochemically and play an important role in diagnosis, e.g. tyrosinase (DOPA oxidase) and the peroxidases.

Reactions for oxidases

Tyrosinase

This enzyme catalyzes the oxidation of tyrosine to dihydroxyphenylalanine (DOPA) and its final oxidation to melanin pigments. The method given below can be used to demonstrate cells capable of producing melanin. Okun et al (1969, 1970) have shown, however, that the peroxidases are also capable of catalyzing the oxidation of tyrosine.

The method given below is from Okun et al (1969) and is applied to frozen sections.

Tyrosinase–DOPA reaction for frozen sections (Okun et al 1969; Pearse 1972)

Fixation and sections

Fresh frozen or formalin-fixed cryostat sections.

Preparation of solutions

Control incubating solution (A)

0.1 M phosphate buffer (pH 7.4)	10 ml

Test incubating solution (B)

L-Tyrosine	2 mg
DL-DOPA	0.2 mg
0.1 M phosphate buffer (pH 7.4)	10 ml

Control incubating solution (C)

DL-DOPA	0.2 mg
0.1 M phosphate buffer (pH 7.4)	10 ml

Control incubating solution (D)

L-Tyrosine	2 mg
DL-DOPA	0.2 mg

0.1 M phosphate buffer (pH 7.4), 10 ml, and add 1 mg sodium diethyldithiocarbamate.

Method

1. Label four serial or near serial sections, 'A, B, C, and D'.
2. Place the sections in the appropriate solutions (i.e. slide A in solution A, etc.) for 3 hours at 37°C.
3. Rinse in phosphate buffer, pH 7.4, 2 min.
4. Wash in distilled water, 2 min.
5. Dehydrate through graded alcohols to xylene and mount in DPX.

Results

Section A	Pre-formed pigment only seen
Section B	Black pigments absent from other sections in melanin synthesis
Section C	Little induced pigment
Section D	No new pigment seen

Note

Only sections B and C demonstrate enzyme activity.

Monoamine oxidase

This enzyme is involved in the breakdown of epinephrine (adrenaline) and 5-hydroxytryptamine. It is demonstrated by the oxidation of tetra nitro-blue tetrazolium (TNBT).

Monoamine oxidase: tetrazolium method
(Glenner et al 1957)

Sections
Unfixed cryostat.

Incubating solution

Tryptamine hydrochloride	25 mg
Sodium sulfate	4 mg
Tetra nitro-blue tetrazolium (TNBT)	5 mg
0.1 M phosphate buffer, pH 7.6	5 ml
Distilled water	15 ml

Method
1. Place sections in incubating medium at 37°C, 45 min.
2. Wash in running tap water, 2 min.
3. Place sections in 10% formal saline, 30 min.
4. Wash well in tap water, 2 min.
5. Mount in glycerin jelly.

Results

Monoamine oxidase activity	bluish-black

Cytochrome oxidase

Many tissues are rich in this enzyme. It is involved in the main oxidation pathway. The enzyme is also known as cytochrome A3.

Cytochrome oxidase (Seligman et al 1968)

Sections
Cryostat sections (fresh).

Incubating solution

Catalase (20 μg/ml) (4 mg in 10 ml; remove 2.5 ml and make up to 50 ml in distilled water)	1 ml
Cytochrome c (type 2)	10 mg
0.1 M phosphate buffer, pH 7.4	9 ml
3,3′-Daminobenzidine tetrahydrochloride (DAB)	5 mg

Adjust pH to 7.4 before use with 0.1 M NaOH or 0.1 M HCl as required.

Method
1. Incubate sections at room temperature for 2–3 hours.
2. Rinse in distilled water.
3. Fix in formal calcium, 15 min.
4. Counterstain in hematoxylin, 15 seconds.
5. Wash and blue.
6. Dehydrate, clear, and mount in DPX.

Results
Brown reaction product at sites of cytochrome oxidase activity.

Notes
All muscle fibers should demonstrate activity, but type 1 fibers are the most strongly positive. All fibers are negative in congenital cytochrome oxidase deficiency.

Occasional negative fibers are seen in aging, and in mitochondrial cytopathy syndromes.

DAB is carcinogenic: handle with care.

Dehydrogenases

These enzymes have the ability to remove hydrogen from a substrate and transfer it along the oxidative pathway. The released hydrogen is accepted by the coenzymes NAD or NADP, or the dehydrogenase enzyme itself can act as an acceptor, in which case no coenzyme is required. The hydrogen ions are transferred to a tetrazolium salt. The reduction of the tetrazolium salt by the hydrogen produces a formazan deposit, which can be seen at the site of enzyme activity (Fig. 20.3). Of the dehydrogenases that are capable of acting as hydrogen acceptors, the two most often demonstrated are succinate and α-glycerophosphate dehydrogenases.

Histochemical demonstration

The demonstration of dehydrogenase enzymes relies upon the reduction of tetrazolium salts by hydrogen ions. This is done by the transfer of hydrogen from the substrate to an artificial hydrogen acceptor system, the tetrazolium salts. A number of these salts are available and three are in common use: MTT, NBT, and TNBT. The following methods can employ any of the three salts. To apply a dehydrogenase method it is convenient to make a stock solution of the tetrazolium salt and of the substrate solutions (see below and Tables 20.1a and 20.1b).

Tetrazolium solution (MTT)

MTT (2 mg/ml distilled water)	2.5 ml
0.2 M Tris buffer (pH 7.4)	2.5 ml
0.5 M cobalt chloride	0.5 ml
0.05 M magnesium chloride	1 ml
Distilled water	2.5 ml

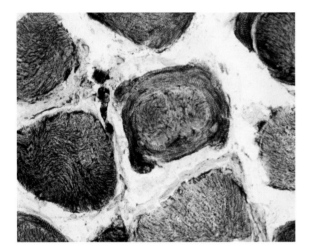

Fig. 20.3 NADH diaphorase activity in a human striated muscle biopsy. The type I fibers stain darkly due to the quantity of mitochondria. Detail of sarcoplasmic reticulum demonstrates a 'ring fiber' in the center of the image.

The pH of this solution is adjusted to 7.0 if necessary. Aliquot and store at −20°C until required.

Tetrazolium solution (NBT)

NBT 4 mg/ml distilled water	2.5 ml

(TNBT may be used in the same concentration.)

0.2 M Tris buffer (pH 7.4)	2.5 ml
0.05 M magnesium chloride	1 ml
Distilled water	3 ml

Aliquot and store at −20°C until required.

Stock substrate solutions

Employing coenzymes

These enzymes include lactate, malate, glucose 6-phosphate, isocitrate, and glutamate dehydrogenases. The substrates for these enzymes are prepared as molar solutions, as given in Table 20.1a.

Enzymes not requiring coenzymes

These are succinate and α-glycerophosphate dehydrogenases. The substrates are prepared as a 2.5 M solution of succinate and a molar solution of α-glycerophosphate, given in Table 20.1b.

Final incubating solutions

These are prepared according to Tables 20.2a and 20.2b.

Table 20.1a Substrates prepared as molar solutions

Substrate	Wt. required to make 1 M solution	Correct pH with
Sodium DL-lactate	1.25 ml in 10 ml	—
Sodium hydrogen malate	1.55 g in 10 ml	40% NaOH
Glucose 6-phosphate (disodium salt)	0.3 g in 1 ml	M HCl
DL-Isocitric acid (trisodium salt)	2.7 g in 10 ml	M HCl
L-Glutamic acid (Na salt)	1.87 g in 10 ml	M HCl

The substrate is used at neutral pH and the above solutions should be adjusted to pH 7.0–7.1 if necessary.

Table 20.1b Stock solution of the tetrazolium salt and substrate solutions

Substrate	Wt. required to make stock solution	Correct pH with
Disodium succinate (SD)	1.35 g in 10 ml	M HCl
Disodium α-glycerol phosphate (α-GDP)	3.15 g in 10 ml	M HCl

Adjust pH of substrate solutions to 7.0–7.1 if necessary.

Table 20.2a Incubating solutions

Dehydrogenase	Substrate solution, ml	Tetrazolium solution, ml	Coenzyme
Lactate (LD)	0.1	0.9	2 mg NAD
Malate (MD)	0.1	0.9	2 mg NAD
Glucose 6-phosphate (G6PD)	0.1	0.9	2 mg NADP
Isocitrate (ICD)	0.1	0.9	2 mg NAD
Succinate	0.1	0.9	Nil
*α-Glycerophosphate	0.1	0.9	Nil

*The stock tetrazolium solution should be specially prepared and saturated with menadione (vitamin K3).

Table 20.2b Stock solution of the tetrazolium salt and substrate solutions

	Substrate solution	Tetrazolium solution, ml	Distilled water, ml	Coenzyme
NAD diaphorase	Nil	0.9	0.1	2 mg NADH
NADP diaphorase	Nil	0.9	0.1	2 mg NADPH

Adjust final pH to 7.0–7.1.

Diaphorases

For the demonstration of these enzymes the stock tetrazolium solution, distilled water, and the coenzyme only are required (see Table 20.2b).

Standard dehydrogenase technique

Method

The method given below applies to all types of dehydrogenases.

Fixation

Unfixed cryostat section, 5–7 μm.

Method

1. Incubate sections in appropriate incubating solution at 37°C for 30–60 min.
2. Transfer sections to 15% formal saline, 15 min.
3. Wash in distilled water.
4. Counterstain in 2% methyl green if required.
5. Wash in distilled water.
6. Mount in glycerin jelly.
7. If NBT has been used as the tetrazolium salt, dehydrate through alcohols to xylene, and mount in DPX.

Results

Enzyme	black formazan deposit with MTT purple formazan deposit with NBT
Nuclei	green

Notes

Mayer's carmalum is a suitable counterstain with NBT. A rinse in acetone will remove soluble pink formazan when NBT is used.

DIAGNOSTIC APPLICATIONS

Enzyme histochemical techniques are not widely applied to surgical and necropsy material for diagnostic purposes, mainly because of the total or partial loss of enzyme activity that occurs when a tissue is routinely fixed and processed into paraffin. Some enzyme methods can be usefully applied to paraffin and acrylic resin-embedded sections, provided controlled fixation, dehydration, and embedding procedures are used, usually at low temperatures. Tissues prepared in this way require modifications of the enzyme histochemical methods to take account of the reduction in active enzyme in the tissues. An outline of the principles of enzyme histochemistry applied to acrylic resin sections is given in Chapter 29.

A few enzymes are still identifiable in routinely processed paraffin sections, e.g. chloroacetate esterase, and valuable information can be obtained prospectively and retrospectively by such methods. However, for the most part, cryostat sections of fresh frozen material are required for most enzyme histochemical techniques, and retrospective investigation of tissue samples received in the laboratory in fixative is not usually feasible. The current common uses of enzyme histochemistry in surgical histopathology laboratories can be summarized:

- skeletal muscle biopsy
- rapid and easy detection of ganglia and nerves in cases of suspected Hirschsprung's disease
- demonstration of specific lactase or sucrase deficiency in jejunal biopsies
- demonstration of various white blood cells
- demonstration of mast cells
- miscellaneous.

It should be appreciated that enzymes can be demonstrated by means other than histochemical techniques; for example, sites of muramidase (lysozyme) activity can be located by an immunochemical method (see Chapter 21).

Skeletal muscle biopsy

The application of enzyme histochemical methods to cryostat sections of unfixed skeletal muscle shows the presence of different fiber types, and changes in the number, size, and relative proportions of the different fibers are valuable in establishing the diagnosis. Muscle biopsy samples are of two types: open biopsy specimens, or needle biopsy samples, from a moderately affected site that has not been traumatized with electromyography needles or injections. In most instances local anesthetic is sufficient.

Open muscle biopsies

These are received in the laboratory as strips of skeletal muscle, preferably tied at each end to a piece of orange stick. The biopsy sample should be received fresh (unfixed) in the laboratory as soon as possible after surgical removal; it is transported from operating theater to laboratory wrapped in gauze soaked in normal saline, then squeezed till just damp, to minimize drying. Long delays between surgical removal and freezing can result in freezing artifact. If a long delay is inevitable (e.g.

during transport from one hospital to another), subsequent freezing artifact can be minimized by coating the biopsy specimen in glove powder. In this situation it is usually better for the tissue to be frozen at the hospital of origin and transported to the second hospital in the frozen state. On arrival, the muscle biopsy is cut into suitable block-sized pieces (say 0.5 cm in diameter and 0.5 cm thick, bulkier blocks may show freezing artifact), and oriented so that transverse sections will be cut.

Needle biopsy samples

These are taken by a Bergstrom needle and can be quickly and easily obtained under local anesthesia, after nicking the skin with a sharp scalpel blade. It is possible to obtain four or five samples of skeletal muscle from different parts of the muscle through the same small skin incision, by altering the direction of needle introduction. The biopsy samples are placed on a gauze dampened by saline and transferred to the laboratory as quickly as possible. Under dissecting microscope control, biopsies are gently manipulated and trimmed so that the fibers in each are running in the same direction, and a composite block is made of all the samples, any trimmings being placed in glutaraldehyde fixative for possible electron microscopy. The composite block is mounted upright on a cork disc in optimal cutting temperature compound (OCT) such that sectioning will produce transverse cutting of the fibers.

Whether the sample is an open biopsy or needle biopsy, it is vital that freezing be as rapid as possible, since slow freezing will produce ice crystal artifact which may hamper accurate diagnosis. As detailed in Chapter 7 there are a number of techniques available for freezing tissue blocks. For muscle biopsy work the only acceptable technique is to freeze with an agent such as isopentane, with a high rate of thermal conductivity, previously super-cooled with liquid nitrogen. The isopentane is placed in a beaker, and is frozen solid by suspending the beaker in a flask of liquid nitrogen at −160°C. After removal from the liquid nitrogen, the isopentane is placed on the bench at room temperature to thaw. When some of the solid isopentane has converted to liquid, the muscle biopsy is oriented on a cork disc in OCT compound. The cork is then frozen onto the chuck. Immediately afterwards, the block is placed in the cryostat chamber to warm to a suitable cutting temperature (−23°C). Muscle cuts well, and sections of 8–10 μm are easily obtained unless there is extensive fatty replacement (e.g. in severe muscular dystrophy) when it may be necessary to section the muscle at a cryostat temperature of −30°C.

In addition to H&E stain and others, special enzyme histochemical techniques are necessary to demonstrate some of the structural abnormalities of diagnostic importance. The following methods are used routinely.

Adenosine triphosphatase

Adenosine triphosphatase (at pH 9.4, 4.6, and 4.2) methods are used in combination to distinguish between type 1 and type 2 fibers (Fig. 20.4), and to further subdivide the type 2 fibers into 2A, 2B, and 2C subtypes (Table 20.3). This distinction is diagnostically important since some muscle diseases have characteristic patterns of loss, atrophy, or grouping of specific fiber types or subtypes. Some types of structural fiber abnormality (e.g. periodic paralysis) are also demonstrated by the ATPase methods.

NADH diaphorase

NADH diaphorase demonstrates mitochondria and the fine detail of the sarcoplasmic reticulum of the fiber. It is used to detect minor or early structural abnormality in the sarcoplasmic reticulum network of the fiber, as well as mitochondrial abnormalities, e.g. the mitochondrial myopathies. Other dehydrogenase enzymes such as succinate and lactate dehydrogenases (SDH and LDH) will also demonstrate major mitochondrial abnormalities, but are less useful for sarcoplasmic reticulum.

Phosphorylase also distinguishes between type 1 and 2 fibers but fades quickly; it is used to exclude McArdle's disease, a primary phosphorylase deficiency.

Other methods, which can be applied when there is clinical suspicion of a specific enzyme deficiency, are for cytochrome oxidase, phosphofructokinase, and aldolase.

These additional methods are occasionally applied in some laboratories: acid phosphatase (see p. 410) to identify macrophages in necrotic fibers and abnormal lysosomal activity in muscle fibers; non-specific esterase to demonstrate atrophic denervated myofibers, neuromuscular junctions, and also abnormal lysosomal enzyme activity (Fig. 20.5); alkaline phosphatase to demonstrate reactive blood vessels and connective

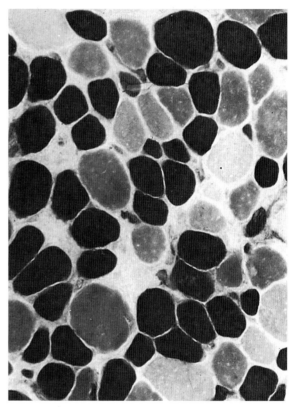

Fig. 20.4 ATPase activity in a human striated muscle biopsy. The section was pre-incubated at pH 4.2 to distinguish between type 1 fibers (dark staining) and type 2 fibers (paler staining).

Fiber type	ATPase pH 4.2	ATPase pH 4.6	ATPase pH 9.4	NADH diaphorase, SDH, and LDH	Phosphorylase
Type 1	+++	+++	+	+++	+/−
Type 2A	−	−	+++	++	+++
Type 2B	−	+++	+++	+	+++
Type 2C	+	+++	+++	++	+++

Table 20.3 Differential enzyme staining of skeletal muscle fibers (based on Dubowitz 1985)

Small regenerating fibers are usually strongly NADH positive, irrespective of fiber type. Type 2C fibers are a very small minority in normal human muscle.

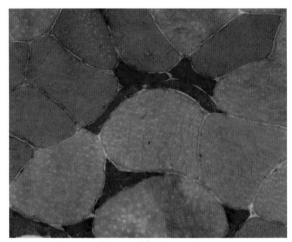

Fig. 20.5 Non-specific esterase activity in human striated muscle biopsy. Type 1 fibers stain slightly darker than type 2 fibers. Also note the small, darkly staining, angular, atrophic denervated fibers.

tissues in some inflammatory myopathies and regenerating myofibers; and cholinesterase to highlight atrophic fibers (see p. 417) and to demonstrate intramuscular nerve twigs.

Adenosine triphosphatase (ATPase)

Sections
Unfixed cryostat.

Solutions

a. 0.1 M glycine buffer

Glycine	0.75 g
NaCl	0.585 g

Make up to 100 ml with distilled water.

b. 0.1 M glycine buffer with 0.75 M CaCl$_2$

0.1 M glycine buffer (solution a)	50 ml
0.75 M CaCl$_2$ (11.03 g · CaCl$_2$ · 2H$_2$O in 100 ml distilled water)	10 ml

Mix, then add approx. 22 ml 0.1 M NaOH until pH 9.4.

c. 0.1 M solution veronal-acetate buffer pH 4.2 and pH 4.6 (see Appendix III)

d. Incubating solution

ATP	5 mg
Solution b	10 ml

Adjust to pH 9.4 with 0.1 M NaOH or 0.1 M HCl if necessary.

Method (at pH 9.4)
1. Incubate freshly cut sections in incubating solution d at 37°C.
2. Rinse well in distilled water.
3. Immerse in 2% cobalt chloride for 5 min.
4. Rinse well in tap water, then in three changes of distilled water.
5. Immerse in dilute (1:10) ammonium sulfide solution for 30 seconds (in fume cupboard).
6. Rinse well in running tap water.
7. Stain lightly in Harris's hematoxylin, blue in tap water (see Note).
8. Mount in glycerin jelly or dehydrate, clear, and mount in DPX.

Method (at pH 4.2 and 4.6)
1. Pre-incubate freshly cut sections at 4°C in appropriate 0.1 M veronal-acetate buffer (solution c above) for 10 min.
2. Rinse briefly in distilled water.
3. Proceed as from step 1 in the pH 9.4 method above.

Results
See Table 20.3.

Note
Only the pH 4.2 sections need counterstaining in hematoxylin. Sections must be well washed after the cobalt chloride and ammonium sulfide steps.

Phosphorylase (after Meijer 1968)

Sections
Unfixed cryostat.

Incubating solution *(add the reagents in the following order)*

0.1 M acetate buffer pH 5.9	100 ml
0.1 M magnesium chloride	10 ml
Glucose 1-phosphate	1 g
Glycogen (oyster/rabbit liver)	20 mg
ATP salt	50 mg
Sodium fluoride	1.8 g
Ethanol	20 ml
Polyvinyl pyrolidine	9 g

Store at −20°C.

Method

1. Incubate in solution at 37°C for 90 min.
2. Wash in 40% ethanol for 5 seconds; air dry.
3. Fix in ethanol for 3 min; air dry.
4. Wash in 1:30 Lugol's iodine for 5 min.
5. Mount in 9:1 glycerin jelly/Lugol's iodine.

Results

Phosphorylase activity   blue/black

Notes

The solution is kept in a closed Columbia jar and is frozen after each incubation. Replace when its potency is diminished.

Phosphofructokinase (PFK) and aldolase
(Abe & Shimizu 1964; Bonilla & Schotland 1970)

These two methods are carried out concurrently. The integrity of the metabolic pathway via fructose 1,6-diphosphate must be demonstrated if possible PFK deficiencies are to be investigated.

Sections
Unfixed cryostat.

Solutions

a. 0.2 M sodium cacodylate

Sodium cacodylate	4.28 g
Distilled water	100 ml

b. 0.2 M HCl

HCl	1.7 ml
Distilled water	100 ml

c. pH 7.0 cacodylate buffer

0.2 M sodium cacodylate (solution a)	25 ml
0.2 M HCl (solution b)	3.2 ml
Distilled water to	100 ml

Check pH and adjust with 0.1 M NaOH or 0.1 M HCl.

d. pH 8.6 cacodylate buffer

0.2 M sodium cacodylate (solution a)	25 ml
Distilled water to	100 ml

Check pH and adjust to pH 8.6 (see Note a).

e. Aldolase incubating solution

40 mg sodium fructose 1,6-diphosphate in 5 ml distilled H_2O	5 ml
NAD	2.5 mg
NBT (nitro-blue tetrazolium)	5 mg
Cacodylate buffer pH 8.6 (solution d)	5 ml
$MgCl_2$ (one small crystal = 2 mg)	2 mg

Mix, check pH, and adjust to 8.6 if necessary. Use immediately.

f. PFK incubating solution

80 mg fructose 6 phosphate in 1 ml distilled water	1 ml
NBT	5 mg
NAD	20 mg
ATP	10 mg
Cacodylate buffer pH 7.0 (solution c)	9 ml
$MgCl_2$ (one small crystal = 2 mg)	2 mg

Mix, check pH, and adjust to pH 7.0 with 0.1 M HCl or 0.1 M NaOH. Use immediately.

Method

1. Incubate freshly cut cryostat sections in appropriate freshly prepared incubating solutions (c and f) for 30–90 min at 37°C.
2. Rinse in distilled water.
3. Fix in formal calcium for 10–60 min.
4. Rinse in distilled water.
5. Mount in glycerin jelly.

Results

Aldolase/phosphofructokinase   purplish-blue

Negative controls may show pale staining due to 'nothing dehydrogenase' (see Note c).

Notes

a. These methods are temperamental and pH sensitive. It is vital that every solution is prepared with care. There tends to be a large swing in pH at the adjustment of the final pH of the incubating solutions, and it is often necessary to dilute the 0.1 M solutions of HCl and NaOH.

b. Pre-fixation of the freshly cut cryostat sections in 80% ethanol for 20 min at 4°C, followed by air drying for 30 min, has been recommended. In our experience this produces a fainter final reaction product.

c. It is essential to incubate adjacent test sections in 'negative control' incubation mixtures in parallel. The negative control incubation mixtures are as in solutions (e) and (f), but omitting sodium fructose 1,6-disphosphate from the aldolase mixture (i.e. use 5 ml distilled water alone), and omitting the fructose 6-phosphate from the phosphofructokinase mixture (i.e. use 1 ml of distilled water). If possible, it is good practice to use known positive control sections (fresh cryostat sections of muscle in which there is no suspicion of PFK deficiency) in the test and negative control incubations for enzymes.

Myoadenylate deaminase
(Fishbein et al 1978)

Sections
Fresh cryostat.

Solution

Adenosine 5'-monophosphate	4 mg
Distilled water	7.0 ml
Nitro-blue tetrazolium (5 mg/ml in distilled water)	2.0 ml
3 M potassium chloride	0.7 ml

Add potassium chloride slowly while stirring. Adjust pH to 6.1, then add, dropwise, 5 mg dithiothreitol dissolved in 0.3 ml distilled water just before using.

Method
1. Incubate at room temperature for 1 hour.
2. Rinse briefly in distilled water.
3. Mount in glycerin jelly.

Results
The deep blue reaction end-product is more intense in type 1 muscle fibers.

Notes
Dithiothreitol attacks electrodes. Avoid contact totally when adjusting pH of solution. For control use 4 mg inosine 5'-monophosphate instead of AMP.

Demonstration of mast cells and white cells of the myeloid series

Chloroacetate esterase techniques have recently been applied to formalin-fixed paraffin sections to assist in the identification of tissue mast cells and myeloid white cells (Leder 1964). Two methods are suitable: the fast blue RR method, which gives a vivid blue reaction product (particularly intense in mast cell cytoplasm), and the pararosanilin method which gives a pinkish-red reaction product. For high-resolution work the latter method is preferred for two reasons. The final reaction product is insoluble and the section can therefore be dehydrated, cleared, and mounted in DPX, whereas the more soluble reaction product in the fast blue RR method necessitates mounting in glycerin jelly. Furthermore, the most suitable nuclear counterstain with the pink pararosanilin method is hematoxylin, whereas the other method requires a red nuclear counterstain such as Mayer's carmalum. In the circumstances under which these methods are usually applied (e.g. identification of leukemic myeloid cells in skin or lymph node), the nuclear detail of the esterase-positive cells may be vital to the diagnosis. A crisp hematoxylin nuclear stain in a DPX-mounted section is much more informative than a carmalum nuclear stain in a glycerin jelly-mounted section, particularly at high magnification.

Chloroacetate esterase (fast blue RR) method for paraffin sections
(after Burstone 1957)

Fixation and sections
Formalin-fixed paraffin.

Incubating medium

Naphthol AS-D acetate (dissolved in 0.5 ml dimethylformamide)	5 mg
Distilled water	25 ml
0.2 M Tris buffer (pH 7.1)	25 ml
Fast blue RR salt	30 mg

Mix reagents in order given, shake well, and filter. Check that pH is below 7.1.

Method

1. Paraffin sections to water.
2. Incubate sections in freshly filtered incubating medium at room temperature, 5 min to several hours.
3. Rinse in water.
4. Counterstain nuclei in Mayer's carmalum 10–15 min.
5. Wash in water and mount in glycerin jelly.

Result

Esterase activity	shades of blue (intense in mast cells, variable in myeloid cells)
Nuclei	red

Note

The method will fail if the pH of the incubating medium rises much above pH 7.1 because of spontaneous substrate breakdown. Incubation times are variable; mast cells and mature neutrophils become strongly positive in a short time, but myeloid precursors take longer.

Chloroacetate esterase (pararosanilin) method for paraffin sections

(after Moloney et al 1960)

Sections

Formalin-fixed paraffin.

Preparation of solutions

a. Substrate solution

Naphthol AS-D chloroacetate	10 mg
Dimethylformamide	1 ml

b. Buffer solution

0.1 M Michaelis buffer pH 6.8–7.6 (see Appendix III)	30 ml

c. Pararosanilin HCl stock solution

Pararosanilin hydrochloride	2 g
2 M HCl	50 ml

Heat gently till solid dissolves, cool to room temperature, and filter.

d. Sodium nitrite solution

Sodium nitrite	400 mg
Distilled water	10 ml

e. Hexazotized pararosanilin solution

Pararosanilin HCl stock solution c	0.4 ml
Sodium nitrite, solution d, freshly prepared	0.4 ml

Mix well, allow to stand for 30 seconds, then use immediately.

Preparation of incubating medium

To 0.8 ml freshly prepared hexazotized pararosanilin (solution e), add 30 ml 0.1 M Michaelis buffer (solution b), and adjust pH to 6.3 with HCl, then immediately add the substrate (solution a). The resultant solution, which resembles pink milk, is filtered, and the clear pale pink filtrate is used as the incubating medium.

Method

1. Paraffin sections to water.
2. Incubate sections in freshly prepared filtered incubating medium, 30 min to 1 hour (see Note a).
3. Rinse in water.
4. Counterstain nuclei in Mayer's hematoxylin, 5 min.
5. Blue in Scott's tap water.
6. Rinse in water, dehydrate, clear, and mount in DPX.

Results

Mast cells and neutrophils	red
Myeloid cells	pinkish red
Nuclei	blue–black

Notes

Mast cells stain early and strongly (after 30 min) followed by mature neutrophils. Immature myeloid cells need longer incubation (1 hour).

Detection of nerves and ganglia in suspected Hirschsprung's disease

In the normal colon and rectum, there are ganglion cells in both the submucosa and the so-called myenteric plexus between the circular and longitudinal muscle of the outer bowel wall. These ganglia, and their associated nerves, are responsible for colonic motility.

In Hirschsprung's disease in children, a variable segment of the rectum and colon is devoid of ganglion cells ('aganglionic segment'). In the affected segment peristalsis is impossible and the large bowel becomes obstructed. The diagnosis may be suspected clinically and radiologically but requires histological confirmation, usually by the examination of one or more suction biopsy specimens of rectal mucosa and submucosa.

Histological examination of rectum and colon is also required during the surgical treatment of the condition when the limits of the aganglionic segment must be accurately identified so that it can be completely resected. The colon with a normal ganglion component can be anastomosed to the rectal remnant, restoring normal structural and functional continuity. Samples of rectum and colon wall, usually the muscle layers, are removed at operation to determine where the bowel becomes normally ganglionated. Therefore specimens for the identification of ganglion cells in Hirschsprung's disease are of two types: small suction biopsies, and open biopsies obtained during operation.

Small suction biopsies

These biopsies, which hopefully contain mucosa and submucosa, are removed to establish or refute the diagnosis of aganglionic Hirschsprung's disease. For these biopsies, there is no urgency and, if submucosa is present, they can be processed into paraffin, sectioned at a number of levels, and stained with H&E to identify ganglion cells in the submucosa. However, the presence of an adequate sample of submucosa in rectal suction biopsies is not always guaranteed, particularly in newborn babies, and sometimes the sample is of mucosa and muscularis mucosae only. Fortunately there are increased numbers of abnormally thick nerve twigs in the mucosal lamina propria in aganglionic Hirschsprung's disease, and this fact can be used to strongly suggest a diagnosis when the biopsy sample consists of mucosa only. For this reason it is advisable to receive the rectal sample immediately after biopsy, fresh and unfixed, on a piece of moistened filter paper in a sealed container to prevent drying out.

The biopsy sample is oriented under dissecting microscope control so that sectioning will include mucosa and any submucosa, stuck to a cork disc with a small amount of OCT, then snap-frozen at −170°C in isopentane cooled in liquid nitrogen (see p. 99) and sectioned in a cryostat. Preliminary sections are stained with H&E and the submucosa examined for the presence of ganglia. If insufficient submucosa is present, or if no ganglia are seen after examination of a number of H&E-stained levels, then two or three sections are stained by the cholinesterase method to demonstrate the fine nerve twigs in the mucosal lamina propria.

This method also demonstrates the larger nerves in the submucosa as well as any submucosal ganglion cells present. It is extremely difficult to distinguish between ganglion cells and medium-sized nerves cut transversely, so the method is not particularly useful for highlighting ganglion cells, because of lack of specificity and difficulty in interpretation.

Cholinesterase (after Karnovsky & Roots 1964)

Sections

Unfixed cryostat or cold formal calcium–gum sucrose-fixed sections.

Incubating solution

Acetyl thiocholine iodide	5 mg
0.1 M acetate buffer (pH 6.0)	6.5 ml
0.1 M sodium citrate (2.94 g/100 ml)	0.5 ml
30 mM copper sulfate (0.58 g/100 ml)	1 ml
Distilled water	1 ml
5 mM potassium ferricyanide (0.165 g in 100 ml)	1 ml

Add in order, mixing well at each stage.

Method

1. Incubate at 37°C for 15–120 min.
2. Rinse in distilled water.
3. Lightly counterstain in hematoxylin.
4. Dehydrate, clear, and mount.

Results

Cholinesterase activity	red/brown

Note

For rectal biopsies incubate for 60–90 min; muscle biopsies for 90 min. Check under microscope after 1 hour.

Open biopsies during operation

These comprise either the full thickness of the bowel wall or a wedge of the muscle component of the wall including both circular and longitudinal layers. In these circumstances there is no problem with paucity of material, but speed is essential.

The biopsy is quickly oriented such that sections will include longitudinal and circular muscle layers and the myenteric plexus, which runs between. Cryostat sections are stained with hematoxylin and eosin, and the slide searched for ganglion cells in the myenteric plexuses and any submucosal tissue included in the biopsy.

In most cases this simple technique is all that is required, but the search for ganglion cells is sometimes aided by the examination of frozen sections on which a non-specific esterase (pararosanilin method, see p. 415) has been performed. Ganglion cells are strongly positive for this enzyme; we have rarely found this necessary provided the frozen section is of good quality and the H&E staining crisp. The quality of H&E staining is improved, both in these larger biopsies and the small mucosal suction biopsies, if the frozen section is briefly post-fixed in acetic alcohol before staining.

Jejunal biopsies

Jejunal biopsies are usually taken for the investigation of malabsorption, mainly to assess whether the jejunal villi have a normal structure. In one of the most important causes of malabsorption, celiac disease, the villi become atrophic and the jejunal mucosal surface is flat. Treatment by a gluten-free diet leads to clinical improvement, and the jejunal villi develop again if the gluten-free diet is maintained. Jejunal biopsies may be taken initially to establish the presence of villous atrophy, and subsequently to monitor the improvement on treatment. Failure to improve suggests incomplete adherence to the diet, and repeat biopsy shows persisting villous atrophy rather than histological improvement.

For the assessment of jejunal mucosal biopsies in suspected celiac disease, the specimen can be examined under the dissecting microscope and the presence or absence of villi noted. Paraffin sections stained with H&E are used to assess villus height, gland hyperplasia, and intensity of inflammatory cell infiltrate in the lamina propria. Alternatively, the biopsy can be snap frozen, sectioned in a cryostat, and H&E stained for rapid diagnosis. This method has the advantage that an alkaline phosphatase method can be applied; alkaline phosphate activity resides on the enterocyte surface, and is a sensitive marker of structural and functional integrity of the mucosal absorptive cells. This is particularly useful in assessing histological recovery. Acid phosphatase demonstrates some of the inflammatory cells in the lamina propria, and also identifies lysosomal activity in villous enterocytes and glandular crypt epithelial cells. Jejunal

biopsies may be taken for the investigation of suspected primary lactase or sucrase deficiencies. Specific enzyme histochemical methods exist for both enzymes. Lactase and sucrase are localized to the luminal surfaces of the enterocytes, and in the normal jejunum there is an almost continuous line of enzyme activity on the mucosal surface, except at the tips of the villi where enzyme activity is normally sparse or absent.

Lactase (indigogenic procedure according to Lojda et al 1979)

Sections
Unfixed cryostat or cold formal calcium–gum sucrose fixed.

Incubation solution

5-Bromo-4-chloro-3-indoxyl-β-D-fucoside	5 mg
5-Bromo-4-chloro-3-indoxyl-β-D-fucopyranoside	5 mg
Dissolve in *N,N*-dimethylformamide	0.5 ml
0.1 M citric acid phosphate buffer pH 6	10 ml
a. 65% potassium ferricyanide (50 mM)	0.83 ml
b. 11% potassium ferrocyanide (50 mM)	0.83 ml

Method
1. Incubate sections in the medium at 37°C for 1 hour in a closed container to avoid evaporation.
2. Rinse in distilled water.
3. Fix in 4% formaldehyde for 5 min at room temperature.
4. Rinse in distilled water.
5. Counterstain in Mayer's carmalum for 5 min.
6. Wash, dehydrate, clear, and mount.

Results

Enzyme activity	turquoise

Note
The medium is expensive but can be used repeatedly. After incubation it can be stored in a closed vial at −20°C. The potency of the incubation solution lessens with use and therefore sections may need increasing lengths of time in the solution as it ages.

Sucrase (after Lojda et al 1979)

Sections

Unfixed cryostat, or cold formal calcium–gum sucrose fixed.

Solutions

Hexazotized pararosanilin solution

Pararosanilin HCl stock (see p. 415)	0.4 ml
Sodium nitrite solution	0.4 ml

Add pararosanilin solution dropwise to sodium nitrite until the solution is corn colored; leave to stand for 1 min.

Then add: 0.1 M citric acid/phosphate buffer pH 7.0	9.2 ml

Mix well and adjust pH to 6.5.

Incubating solution

Freshly hexazotized pararosanilin solution	10 ml
2.0 mg 6-bromo-2-naphthyl-α-D-glucoside dissolved in 0.5 ml N,N-dimethyl-formamide	0.5 ml

Filter before use.

Method

1. Incubate for 1 hour at room temperature.
2. Rinse in distilled water.
3. Immerse in 4% formaldehyde for 30 min.
4. Wash, counterstain in hematoxylin for 30 seconds to 1 min.
5. Wash, dehydrate, clear, and mount in DPX.

Results

Sucrase activity	orange/red

Note

Incubating time may be longer than 1 hour depending on the potency of the solution.

MISCELLANEOUS DIAGNOSTIC APPLICATIONS OF ENZYME HISTOCHEMISTRY

There are many isolated examples of the diagnostic use of enzyme histochemistry. Examples include the use of acid phosphatase in the identification of prostatic carcinoma, e.g. when the tumor is infiltrating the colon or bladder wall, or in bone metastases. The application of acid and alkaline phosphatase methods to cryostat sections of jejunal mucosal biopsy specimens in gluten enteropathy and the use of alkaline phosphatase methods in vascular endothelial tumors are other examples. Acid and alkaline phosphatases may also be demonstrated in osteoclasts and active osteoblasts in unfixed frozen sections of trabecular bone, although cryostat sections of bone tissue are technically difficult to obtain. Sectioning is facilitated if the trabecular bone is decalcified, but such treatment may destroy tissue enzymes. If decalcification is to be undertaken, an ethylenediaminetetra-acetic acid (EDTA) solution (10 g in 100 ml 0.1 M phosphate buffer pH 7.1) is the least damaging to enzyme activity. Decalcification is carried out at 4°C for as short a time as feasible, depending on the size of the specimen and amount of calcified bone present.

Acknowledgments

This chapter is a merging of Enzyme histochemistry and Diagnostic applications of enzyme histochemistry. John Bancroft wrote the former chapter for the previous first four editions and the latter was written by Janet Palmer and Alan Stevens for editions three and four. Edition five was written by John Bancroft. Our acknowledgments are due to them for their contributions.

REFERENCES

Abe T., Shimizu N. (1964) Histochemical method for demonstrating aldolase. Histochemie 4:209.

Bancroft J.D. (1975) Histological techniques, 2nd edn. London: Butterworths.

Bancroft J.D., Cook H.C. (1994) Manual of histological techniques and their diagnostic applications. Edinburgh: Churchill Livingstone.

Bancroft J.D., Hand N.M. (1987) Enzyme histochemistry. R.M.S. Handbook No. 14. Oxford: Oxford Science Publications.

Barka T. (1960) A simple azo dye method for histochemical demonstration of acid phosphatase. Nature 187:248.

Barnett R.J., Seligman A.M. (1951) Histochemical demonstration of esterases by production of indigo. Science 114:579.

Bonilla E., Schotland D.L. (1970) Histochemical diagnosis of muscle phosphofructokinase deficiency. Archives of Neurology 22:8–12.

Burstone M.S. (1957) Esterase activity of developing bones and teeth. Archives of Pathology 63:164.

Burstone M.S. (1958) Histochemical demonstration of acid phosphatases with naphthol AS-phosphates. Journal of the National Cancer Institute 21:523.

Davis B.J., Ornstein L. (1959) High resolution enzyme localisation with a new diazo reagent hexazonium pararosaniline. Journal of Histochemistry and Cytochemistry 7:297.

Dubowitz V. (1985) Muscle biopsy: a practical approach. London: Baillière Tindall.

Filipe M.I., Lake B.D., eds. (1983) Histochemistry in pathology. Edinburgh: Churchill Livingstone.

Fishbein W.N., Armrustmacher V.W., Griffin J.L. (1978) Myoadenylate deaminase deficiency—a new disease of muscle. Science 200:545–548.

Glenner G.G., Burtner H.J., Brown G.W. (1957) The histochemical demonstration of monoamine oxidase activity by tetrazolium salts. Journal of Histochemistry and Cytochemistry 5:591.

Gomori G. (1939) Microtechnical demonstration of phosphatase in tissue sections. Proceedings of the Society for Experimental Biology and Medicine, NY, 42:23.

Gomori G. (1941) Distribution of acid phosphatase in the tissues under normal and under pathologic conditions. Archives of Pathology 32:189.

Gomori G. (1950) An improved histochemical technique for acid phosphatase. Stain Technology 25:81.

Gomori G. (1951) Alkaline phosphatase of cell nuclei. Journal of Laboratory and Clinical Medicine 37:526.

Gomori G. (1952) Histochemistry of esterases. International Review of Cytology 1:323.

Hayashi M., Nakajima Y., Fishman W.H. (1964) The cytologic demonstration of β glucuronidase employing naphthol AS-BI glucuronide and hexazonium pararosanilin; preliminary report. Journal of Histochemistry and Cytochemistry 12:293.

Holt S.J., Withers R.F.J. (1952) Cytochemical localisation of esterases using indoxyl derivates. Nature 170:1012.

Karnovsky M.J., Roots L. (1964) A 'direct-coloring' thiocholine method for cholinesterase. Journal of Histochemistry and Cytochemistry 12:219.

Leder L.D. (1964) Uber die selektive fermentcytochemische Darstellung von neutrophilen myeloischen Zellen and Gewebsmastzellen im Paraffinschnit. Kurze wissenschaftliche Mitteilungen 42, 11:553.

Lojda Z., Gossrau R., Schiebler T.H. (1979) Enzyme histochemistry: a laboratory manual. Heidelberg: Springer.

Meijer A.E.F.H. (1968) Improved histochemical method for the demonstration of the activity of α glucan phosphorylase. Histochemie 12:244–252.

Menton M.L., Junge J., Green M.H. (1944) Coupling azo dye test for alkaline phosphatase in kidney. Journal of Histochemistry and Cytochemistry 5:420.

Moloney W.C., McPherson K., Fliegelman L. (1960) Esterase activity in leukocytes demonstrated by the use of naphthol AS-D chloro-acetate substrate. Journal of Histochemistry and Cytochemistry 8:200.

Nachlas M.M., Seligman A.M. (1949) The histochemical demonstration of esterase. Journal of the National Cancer Institute 9:415.

Nachlas M.M., Crawford D.T., Seligman A.M. (1957a) Histochemical demonstration of leucine aminopeptidase. Journal of Histochemistry and Cytochemistry 5:264.

Nachlas M.M., Tsou K.C., De Souza E. et al. (1957b) Cytochemical demonstration of succinic dehydrogenase by the use of a new p-nitrophenyl substituted ditetrazole. Journal of Histochemistry and Cytochemistry 5:420.

Okun M.R., Edelstein L., Nebaur G., Hamada G. (1969) The histochemical tyrosine-dopa reaction for tyrosinase and its use in localizing tyrosinase activity in mast cells. Journal of Investigation and Dermatology 53:39.

Okun M.R., Edelstein L.M., Or N. et al. (1970) Histochemical differentiation of peroxidase-mediated from tyrosinase-mediated melanin formation in mammalian tissues. Histochemie 23:295.

Pearse A.G.E. (1957) Intracellular localisation of dehydrogenase systems using monotetrazolium salts and metal chelation of their formazans. Journal of Histochemistry and Cytochemistry 5:515.

Pearse A.G.E. (1972) Histochemistry, theoretical and applied, 3rd edn. Edinburgh: Churchill Livingstone, vol. 2.

Seligman A.M., Karnovsky M.J., Wasserkrug H.L., Honker J.S. (1968) Non-droplet ultrastructural demonstration of cytochrome oxidase activity with a polymerising osmiophilic reagent, DAB. Journal of Cell Biology 38:1.

Wachstein M., Meisel E. (1956) On the histochemical demonstration of glucose-6-phosphate. Journal of Histochemistry and Cytochemistry 4:592.

Wachstein M., Meisel E. (1957) Histochemistry of hepatic phosphatases at a physiological pH. American Journal of Pathology 27:13.

Wachstein M., Meisel E., Niedzwiedz A. (1960) Histochemical demonstration of mitochondrial adenosine triphosphatase with the lead-absorption triphosphate technique. Journal of Histochemistry and Cytochemistry 8:387–388.

21

Immunohistochemical Techniques

Peter Jackson and David Blythe

INTRODUCTION

The recent introduction of prognostic and predictive markers in immunohistochemistry has made a tremendous impact on patient treatment and management. This has been made possible by the gradual development of immunohistochemical methodologies over the past 60 years which allow the identification of specific or highly selective cellular epitopes in formalin-fixed paraffin-processed tissues with an antibody and appropriate labeling system. The present trend in diagnostic laboratories is to try to avoid the use of frozen sections as much as possible and to perform immunohistochemical investigations on formalin-fixed paraffin-embedded tissue.

Many antibodies are now available to identify epitopes that survive the rigors of formalin fixation and paraffin embedding. In cases where morphology and clinical data alone do not allow a firm diagnosis, then immunohistochemistry is invaluable and, with the ever-increasing use of prognostic and predictive markers the pathologist is faced with a decision that could profoundly affect patient therapy and management (Fig. 21.1).

In 1941 Albert H. Coons described a revolutionary new way of visualizing tissue constituents using an antibody labeled with a fluorescent dye. Visualization of the labeled complex was achieved by the use of a fluorescence microscope. The first fluorescent dye to be attached to an antibody was fluorescein isocyanate, but fluorescein isothiocyanate soon became the label of choice because the molecule was much easier to conjugate to the antibody and more stable (Riggs et al 1958). Fluorescein compounds emit a bright apple-green fluorescence when excited at a wavelength of 490 nm. Following the early work the technique has been enor-

mously expanded and developed. New labels have been introduced, including red, yellow, and blue fluorochromes. This permits the simultaneous visualization of several labeled antibodies on a single preparation. At the present time fluorescein isothiocyanate and rhodamine are among the most popular fluorochromes. This methodology, whilst useful in some diagnostic areas, such as determining the nature of protein deposits in skin and renal diseases, and bacteria in infected material, has certain limitations. A fluorescence microscope is necessary to visualize the fluorochrome which also has a tendency to fade, but more importantly and probably the greatest disadvantage of immunofluorescence is that it is difficult to demonstrate the morphological detail of the labeled cell and the associated tissue components. The success of immunohistochemistry in some areas of pathology stimulated interest in the development of alternative antibody labeling techniques that would avoid the difficulties and limitations associated with immunofluorescence.

Many limitations were overcome with the introduction of enzymes as labels. Cells that have been labeled with an enzyme such as horseradish peroxidase, conjugated to an antibody, and visualized with an appropriate chromogen such as diaminobenzidine (DAB) (Nakane & Pierce 1966), can be counterstained with traditional nuclear stains such as hematoxylin. This permits the simultaneous evaluation of both specific immunohistochemistry and morphological detail. In 1970 Sternberger et al described the peroxidase–anti-peroxidase (PAP) technique. Engvall and Perlman in 1971 reported the use of alkaline phosphatase labeling and Cordell et al (1984) described the alkaline phosphatase–anti-alkaline phosphatase (APAAP) technique. Heggeness and Ash (1977) proposed the use of avidin–biotin

433

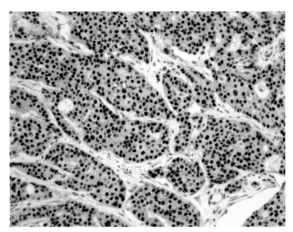

Fig. 21.1 Formalin-fixed paraffin-embedded section of breast carcinoma showing strong expression of estrogen receptor. Pressure cooker antigen retrieval for 2 minutes using Vector antigen unmasking fluid.

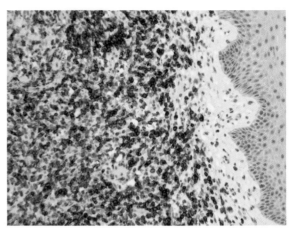

Fig. 21.2 CD5 demonstration in a formalin-fixed paraffin-embedded section from a nasal biopsy showing extra nodal T-cell lymphoma.

for immunofluorescence. This technique was modified by Guesden et al (1979) and Hsu et al (1981) who used a horseradish peroxidase label. Avidin–biotin labeling, and more recently streptavidin–biotin labeling, is one of the more popular techniques used in diagnostic laboratories; however, the labeled polymer detection systems are rapidly growing in popularity and appear certain in time to become the labeling system of choice for many laboratories.

Another significant advance was the introduction of a one-step (direct) labeling system based on the application of a primary antibody to which a labeled long-chain dextran polymer had been conjugated. These antibodies are marketed by Dakocytomation as EPOS (Extended Polymer One-step Staining) reagents. This method did not gain popularity (see UK National External Quality Assessment Scheme [NEQAS] data, Journal of Cell Pathology 1998, 1999) presumably because the level of sensitivity of some of the less avidly labeled antibodies did not live up to expectations. The technique does offer an opportunity for laboratories to provide an increasing amount of immunohistochemistry within a shorter period.

Dextran polymer technology was further enhanced when Dakocytomation introduced the EnVision⁺ detection system. Vyberg and Nielsen (1998) reported that this technology when used in an indirect technique offered comparable sensitivity to a traditional three-stage avidin–biotin technique and avoided the labeling of endogenous biotin. Since its introduction several more

labeled polymer antibody detection techniques have been introduced, notably ImmPress™ (Vector Laboratories) and the Novocastra™ Polymer Detection System (NovoLink™).

Over the last thirty years, many myths surrounding the preservation and presentation of antigens in formalin-fixed paraffin-embedded tissues have been dispelled. In the 1970s it was thought that routine paraffin processing destroyed many epitopes and that certain antigens could never be demonstrated in paraffin sections. However it was found that many antigens are not lost but are masked by the processes involved in formalin fixation and paraffin processing.

Certain epitopes, for example the proliferation antigen, Ki67 and T cell antigens CD5 (Fig. 21.2) and CD8, can only be demonstrated in formalin-fixed, paraffin wax-processed tissue after heat pre-treatment, and then only with certain monoclonal antibody clones. Antibodies such as those directed against the leukocyte common antigen (clones PD7/2B11) and the CD20 antigen (clone L26) produce enhanced staining after citrate buffer (pH 6.0) heating and, surprisingly, heat pre-treatment allows for considerably increased dilution factors. The demonstration of antigens such as cyclin D1 (with clone DCS-6), on the other hand, is better in a high pH solution (Tris–EDTA, pH 10.0). However, the use of the cyclin D1 rabbit monoclonal antibody (clone SP4) from Labvision UK precludes the use of high pH antigen retrieval solutions (Fig. 21.3).

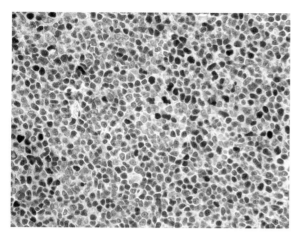

Fig. 21.3 Formalin-fixed paraffin-embedded section of lymph node, showing cyclin D1 expression in a mantle cell lymphoma. Antigen retrieval with the pressure cooker and citrate buffer pH 6.0 and Labvision rabbit monoclonal (clone SP4) primary antibody.

IMMUNOHISTOCHEMISTRY THEORY

Definitions

Immunohistochemistry

Immunohistochemistry is a technique for identifying cellular or tissue constituents (antigens) by means of antigen–antibody interactions, the site of antibody binding being identified either by direct labeling of the antibody, or by use of a secondary labeling method.

Antigens

A molecule that induces the formation of an antibody and bears one or more antibody-binding sites. These are highly specific topographical regions composed of a small number of amino acids or monosaccharide units and are known as antigenic determinant groups or epitopes.

Antibodies

Antibodies belong to the class of serum proteins known as immunoglobulins. The terms antibody and immunoglobulin are often used interchangeably. They are found in blood and tissue fluids, as well as many secretions. The basic unit of each antibody is a monomer. An antibody can be monomeric, dimeric, trimeric, tetrameric, or pentameric. The monomer is composed of two heavy and two light chains. If it is cleaved with enzymes such as papain and pepsin, two Fab (fragment binding antigen) fragments and an Fc (fragment crystallizable) fragment are produced. They are formed in the humoral immune system by plasma cells, the end cell of B-lymphocyte transformation after recognition of a foreign antigen. There are five types of antibody found in the blood of higher vertebrates: IgA, IgD, IgE, IgG, and IgM. IgG is the commonest and the most frequently used antibody for immunohistochemistry. The IgG molecule is composed of two pairs of light and heavy polypeptide chains linked by disulfide bonds to form a Y-shaped structure. The terminal regions of each arm vary in amino acid sequence and are known as 'variable domains'. This variability in amino acid provides specificity for a particular epitope and enables the antibody to bind specifically to the antigen against which it was raised.

Antibody–antigen binding

The amino acid side-chains of the variable domain of an antibody form a cavity which is geometrically and chemically complementary to a single type of antigen epitope as described by Capra and Edmundson in 1977. The analogy of a lock (antibody) and key (antigen) has been used, and the precise fit required explains the high degree of antibody–antigen specificity seen. The associated antibody and antigen are held together by a combination of hydrogen bonds, electrostatic forces, and van der Waals' forces.

Affinity

Affinity is the three-dimensional fit of the antibody to its specific antigen and is a measure of the binding strength between the antigenic epitope and its specific antibody-combining site.

Avidity

Avidity is a related property referring to the heterogeneity of the antiserum which will contain various antibodies reacting with different epitopes of the antigen molecule. A specific but multivalent antibody is less likely to be removed by the washing process than a monovalent antibody. Avidity therefore is the functional combining strength of an antibody with its antigen.

Antibody specificity

This refers to the characteristics of an antibody to bind selectively to a single epitope on an antigen.

Sensitivity

This refers to the relative amount of antigen that an immunohistochemical technique is able to detect. A technique with high sensitivity is able to detect smaller amounts of antigen than a technique with low sensitivity. If used to detect the same amount of antigen, the technique with high sensitivity would produce a larger signal than a method with low sensitivity.

Production of primary reagents

Polyclonal antibodies

Polyclonal antibodies are produced by immunizing an animal with a purified specific molecule (immunogen) bearing the antigen of interest. The animal will mount a humoral response to the immunogen and the antibodies so produced can be harvested by bleeding the animal to obtain immunoglobulin-rich serum. It is likely that the animal will produce numerous clones of plasma cells (polyclonal). Each clone will produce an antibody with a slightly different specificity to the variety of epitopes present on the immunogen. A polyclonal antiserum is therefore a mixture of antibodies to different epitopes on the immunogen. Some of these antibodies may cross-react with other molecules and will need to be removed by absorption with the appropriate antigen. The antiserum will probably contain antibodies to impurities in the immunogen. Antibodies raised against the contaminating immunogens are often of low titer and affinity, and can be diluted out to zero activity for immunolabeling. In consequence of the high possibility of a wide spectrum of antibodies being present in the host animal in response to previous antigen challenges, serum removed from the animal before injection of the immunogen is important as a negative or pre-immune control. For precise details of polyclonal antibody production see De Mey and Moeremans (1986).

Monoclonal antibodies

The development of the hybridoma technique by Kohler and Milstein in 1975 to produce monoclonal antibodies has revolutionized immunohistochemistry by increasing enormously the range, quality, and quantity of specific antisera. Detailed descriptions of the technique have been given by Gatter et al (1984) and Ritter (1986).

The method combines the ability of a plasma cell or transformed B lymphocyte to produce a specific antibody with the in vitro immortality of a neoplastic myeloma cell line; a hybrid with both properties can be produced. With the technique of cloning, this cell can be grown and multiplied in cell culture or ascitic fluid, theoretically to unlimited numbers. By careful screening, hybrids producing the antibodies of interest, without cross-reactivity to other molecules, can be chosen for cloning. The original antigen need not be pure, for hybrids reacting to unwanted antigens or epitopes can be eliminated during screening. The result is a constant, reliable supply of one pure antibody with known specificity.

This approach to the production of monoclonals has dramatically increased the number of antibodies available for immunohistochemistry and has allowed for further evolution with the ability to identify more antigens in paraffin sections. Detailed comparisons of the values and limitations of polyclonal and monoclonal antibodies have been given by Warnke et al (1983) and Gatter et al (1984).

Lectins

Lectins are plant or animal proteins that can bind to tissue carbohydrates with a high degree of specificity according to the lectin and the carbohydrate group (Brooks et al 1996). Since the carbohydrates may be characteristic of a particular tissue, lectin binding may have diagnostic significance (Damjanov 1987). They can be labeled in similar ways to antibodies, or identified by using lectin-specific antibodies as secondary reagents (Leatham 1986).

Labels

Enzyme labels

Enzymes are the most widely used labels in immunohistochemistry, and incubation with a chromogen using a standard histochemical method produces a stable, colored reaction end-product suitable for the light microscope. In addition, the variety of enzymes and chromogens available allow the user a choice of color for the reaction end-product.

Horseradish peroxidase is the most widely used enzyme, and in combination with the most favored chromogen, i.e. 3,3′-diaminobenzidene tetrahydrochloride (DAB), it yields a crisp, insoluble, stable, dark brown reaction end-product (Graham & Karnovsky 1966). Although DAB has been reported to be a potential carcinogen, the risk is now thought to be low (Weisburger et al 1978).

Horseradish peroxidase is commonly used as an antibody label for several reasons:

- Its small size does not hinder the binding of antibodies to adjacent sites.
- The enzyme is easily obtainable in a highly purified form and therefore the chance of contamination is minimized.
- It is a stable enzyme and remains unchanged during manufacture, storage, and application.
- Endogenous activity is easily quenched.
- A wide range of suitable chromogens is available. These include:

3-amino-9-ethylcarbazole, a potential carcinogen (Graham et al 1965; Kaplow 1975)	red
4-chloro-1-naphthol (Nakane 1968)	blue
Hanker–Yates reagent (Hanker et al 1977)	dark blue
α-naphthol pyronin (Taylor & Burns 1974)	red–purple

It should be noted that some of these chromogens produce reaction products which are soluble in alcohol and xylene, and therefore the sections require aqueous mounting. Whilst neutral phosphate-buffered glycerin jelly is one of the more traditional aqueous media, other commercial products are now available, which have improved preservation qualities and resolution compared with the traditional aqueous mountants. After drying in a hot oven these mountants give a hard permanent covering of the section. For long-term storage it is advisable additionally to use a coverslip and resinous mountant on top of the hardened aqueous mountant.

Endogenous peroxidase activity is present in a number of sites, particularly neutrophil polymorphs and other myeloid cells. Blocking procedures may be required, the hydrogen peroxide–methanol method (Streefkerk 1972) being the most popular.

Calf intestinal alkaline phosphatase is the most widely used alternative enzyme tracer to horseradish peroxidase, particularly since the development of the alkaline phosphatase–anti-alkaline phosphatase (APAAP) method in 1984 by Cordell et al. Fast red TR used with naphthol AS-MX phosphate sodium salt gives a bright red reaction end-product that is soluble in alcohol. New fuchsin has been reported as giving a permanent insoluble red product (Malik & Daymon 1982) when mounted in resinous mountant, but it is the experience of many workers in the field that the resistance of the reaction product to resinous mounting is inconsistent.

Endogenous alkaline phosphatase activity is usually blocked by the addition of levamisole to the substrate solution. Levamisole selectively inhibits certain types of alkaline phosphatase, but not intestinal or placental when used at a concentration of 1 mM. Twenty per cent glacial acetic acid is a better blocker of endogenous alkaline phosphatase activity as it inhibits all types of alkaline phosphatase.

Some workers use glucose oxidase as a tracer and it can be developed to give a navy blue reaction (Suffin et al 1979). This label lends itself to immunohistochemistry on animal tissue, as there is no endogenous enzyme activity in animals.

Bacterial-derived β-D-galactosidase has also been used as a tracer and can be developed using the indigogenic method to give a permanent turquoise-blue reaction end-product (Bondi et al 1982). Endogenous enzyme activity is not a problem as the endogenous mammalian enzyme has a different optimum pH from the tracer enzyme.

In recent years, commercial companies have produced a whole range of different substrate kits, especially for peroxidase and alkaline phosphatase. Many of these not only produce reaction products that are resistant to organic solvents, but also provide a range of contrasting colors for those attempting to immunostain more than one antigen in a given section.

Colloidal metal labels

When used alone colloidal gold conjugates appear pink when viewed using the light microscope. A silver precipitation reaction can be used to amplify the visibility of the gold conjugates (Holgate et al 1983a). In addition, both gold and silver-enhanced gold conjugates can be visually emphasized using polarized incident light (epi-illumination) microscopy (Ellis et al 1988) (Figs 21.4a, b).

Silver may also be used as a conjugate, and it gives a yellow color that is visible directly (Roth 1982). Other metals such as ferritin may be used, but they have not found wide usage among immunohistochemists using light microscope techniques. Colloidal gold has much wider usage with the electron microscope.

Fluorescent labels

These are discussed in detail in Chapter 24.

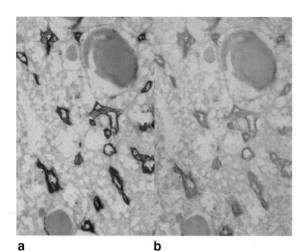

a   **b**

Fig. 21.4 (a) Endothelial cells demonstrated by the immunogold silver staining method; (b) viewed by epi-polarized illumination.

Radiolabels

The use of radioisotopes as tracers requires autoradiographic facilities, and developed from the need for quantitation in immunohistochemistry. Internally labeled antibodies are not widely available and labeling, at present, often limits the activity of the antibody. Techniques involving the use of radioisotopes as tracers have been discussed by Hunt et al (1986).

IMMUNOHISTOCHEMICAL METHODS

There are numerous immunohistochemical staining techniques that may be used to localize and demonstrate tissue antigens. The selection of a suitable technique should be based on parameters such as the type of specimen under investigation, the type of preparation under investigation, e.g. frozen sections, paraffin sections, resin sections or cytological preparations, and the degree of sensitivity required.

Traditional direct technique

The primary antibody is conjugated directly to the label. The conjugate may be either a fluorochrome (more commonly) or an enzyme (Fig. 21.5a). The labeled antibody reacts directly with the antigen in the histological or cytological preparation. The technique is quick and easy to use. However, it provides little signal amplification

and lacks the sensitivity achieved by other techniques. Its use is mainly confined to the demonstration of immunoglobulin and complement in frozen sections of skin and renal biopsies. Low levels of antigen present in certain tumors may not be demonstrated by this technique and this could be crucial to an accurate and comprehensive diagnosis.

New direct technique (Enhanced Polymer One-step Staining method)

This method was first reported by Pluzek et al in 1993, and is available under the commercial name of Enhanced Polymer One-step Staining (EPOS), from Dakocytomation. A large number of primary antibody molecules and peroxidase enzymes are attached to a dextran polymer 'backbone', hence increasing the signal amplification and providing greater sensitivity compared to the traditional direct technique. However, the technique is not widely used, probably due to the limited number of primary antibodies available.

Two-step indirect technique

A labeled secondary antibody directed against the immunoglobulin of the animal species in which the primary antibody has been raised (Fig. 21.5b) visualizes an unlabeled primary antibody. Horseradish peroxidase labeling is most commonly used, together with an appropriate chromogen substrate. The method is more sensitive than the traditional direct technique because multiple secondary antibodies may react with different antigenic sites on the primary antibody, thereby increasing the signal amplification. The techniques offers versatility in that the same labeled secondary antibody can be used with a variety of primary antibodies raised from the same animal species.

Polymer chain two-step indirect technique

This technology uses an unconjugated primary antibody, followed by a secondary antibody conjugated to an enzyme (horseradish peroxidase) labeled polymer (dextran) chain (Fig. 21.5c). This dextran chain has up to 70 molecules of enzyme and 10 molecules of antibody attached. Conjugation of both anti-mouse and anti-rabbit secondary antibodies enables the same reagent to be used for both monoclonal (rabbit and mouse) and polyclonal (rabbit) primary antibodies. The method is biotin free and therefore does not react with endogenous biotin. In addition to being quick, reliable, and easily

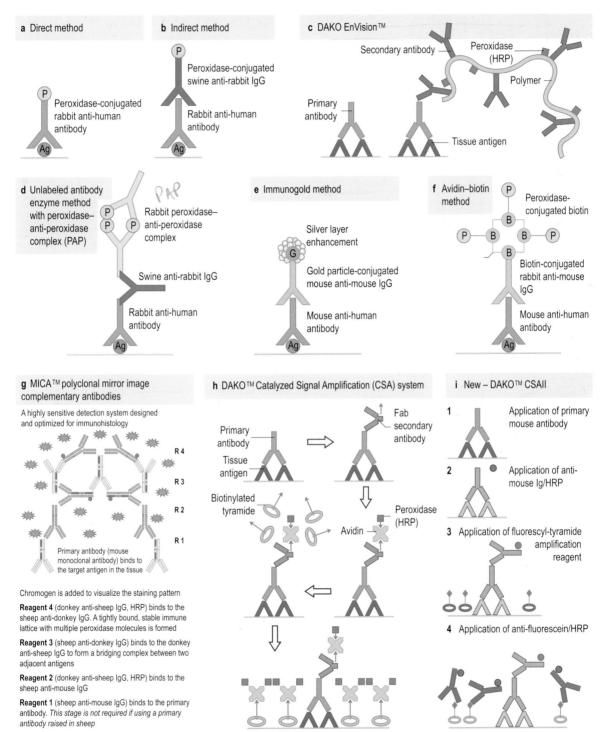

Fig. 21.5 Schematic representation of immunohistochemical techniques. HRP, horseradish peroxidase. (c), (h) and (i) used with permission from Dakocytomation™ Systems. (g) Used with permission from DAKO UK, Ltd.

reproducible, the technique offers great sensitivity. The technique is proving useful for multi-color staining on single slide preparations.

Unlabeled antibody–enzyme complex techniques (PAP and APAAP)

The original immunoenzyme bridge method using enzyme-specific antibody (Mason et al 1969; Sternberger 1969) became rapidly superseded by the improved technique using a soluble peroxidase–anti-peroxidase complex (PAP) (Sternberger et al 1970). These complexes are formed from three peroxidase molecules and two anti-peroxidase antibodies (Fig. 21.5d), and are used as a third layer in the staining method. They are bound to the unconjugated primary antibody, e.g. rabbit anti-human IgG, by a second layer of 'bridging' antibody that is usually a swine anti-rabbit applied in excess so that one of its two identical binding sites binds to the primary antibody and the other to the rabbit PAP complex.

Alkaline phosphatase antibodies raised in mouse, by the same principle, can be used to form the alkaline phosphatase–anti-alkaline phosphatase complexes (APAAP). This method, first developed by Cordell et al in 1984, lends itself to amplification by further application of the bridge and APAAP reagent. For unknown reasons, this form of amplification with the APAAP is not so successful with the PAP technique, as excessive background can sometimes be a serious drawback. These techniques have largely been replaced by streptavidin/biotin methods or polymer-based techniques.

Immunogold silver staining technique (IGSS)

The use of colloidal gold as a label for immunohistochemistry was introduced by Faulk and Taylor (1971). It can be used in both direct and indirect methods and has found wide usage in ultrastructural immunolocalization. It is not widely used in light microscope immunohistochemistry even after the advantages of silver development reported by Holgate et al (1983a). In this method the gold particles are enhanced by the addition of metallic silver layers (Fig. 21.5e) to produce a metallic silver precipitate which overlays the colloidal gold marker and which can be seen with the light microscope. The technique uses silver lactate as the ion supplier and hydroquinone as the reducing agent in a

protective colloid of gum arabic at pH 3.5. In some instances section pre-treatment with Lugol's iodine and sodium after dewaxing and rehydration may be required to improve staining intensity. The method is generally accepted to be more sensitive than the PAP technique, but suffers from the formation of fine silver deposits in the background, especially in inexperienced hands, and can be confusing when trying to identify small amounts of antigen. Modifications to the original technique have been reviewed by De Mey et al (1986).

(Strept)avidin–biotin techniques

This is a three-step technique, which has an unconjugated primary antibody as the first layer, followed by a biotinylated secondary antibody (raised against the species of the primary animal). The third layer is either a complex of enzyme-labeled biotin and streptavidin, or enzyme-labeled streptavidin (Fig. 21.5f). The enzyme can be either horseradish peroxidase or alkaline phosphatase, used with a chromogen of choice.

These methods rely on the marked affinity of the basic glycoprotein avidin (MW 67 kDa) for the small (MW 244 Da) water-soluble vitamin biotin. However, avidin has two distinct disadvantages when used in immunohistochemistry. It has a high isoelectric point of approximately 10 and is therefore positively charged at neutral pH. As a result, it may bind non-specifically to certain negatively charged structures such as cell nuclei. Avidin, being a glycoprotein, also has a tendency to react with lectins via the carbohydrate moiety, again causing non-specific staining. These problems can be overcome by the substitution of streptavidin (MW 60 kDa) for avidin. Streptavidin has now largely replaced the use of avidin in immunohistochemical detection techniques.

Streptavidin can be isolated from the bacterium *Streptomyces avidini*, and like avidin it has four high-affinity binding sites for biotin, although in practice, due to the molecular arrangement of these binding sites, fewer than four biotin molecules actually bind. Biotin (vitamin H) is easily conjugated to antibodies and enzyme markers. Up to 150 biotin molecules can be attached to one antibody molecule, often with the aid of spacer arms. By spacing the biotins, the large streptavidin has room to bind and maximize its strong affinity for biotin. The streptavidin–biotin technique can employ either enzyme label bound directly to the streptavidin (Guesden et al 1979); alternatively, the enzymes are biotinylated and the biotinylated label, forming the streptavidin–biotin complex (Hsu et al 1981), occupies 75% of the streptavidin-binding sites. Usually the latter is commercially supplied as two separate reagents, biotinylated label and streptavidin, and they are added together 30 minutes before use in order for the complex to form fully. Careful stoichiometric control ensures that some binding sites remain free to bind with the biotinylated secondary antibody. As a large number of biotins can be attached to a single antibody, then numerous labeled streptavidin molecules may be bound to it. This results in increased sensitivity compared to the previously described enzyme techniques and allows a higher dilution of the primary antibody. Tissues rich in endogenous biotin such as liver and kidney will require the use of an avidin/biotin block before applying the primary antibody.

Together with the indirect polymer-based techniques, the labeled streptavidin–biotin technique is the most widely used methodology in diagnostic immunohistochemistry.

Hapten labeling technique

Bridging techniques using haptens such as dinitrophenol and arsanilic acid have been advocated (Jasani et al 1981, 1992). In this technique, the hapten is linked to the primary antibody and a complex is built up using an anti-hapten antibody and either hapten-labeled enzyme or hapten-labeled PAP complex.

Mirror Image Complementary Antibody labeling technique (MICA)

Mangham and Isaacson reported this system in 1999. The principle of the technique involves the sequential use of mutually attractive antibodies. This is achieved by raising antibodies against each antibody's species which enables each antibody to be both antigen and antibody in respect to each other. The first antibody is directed against the tissue/cell-bound antigen. If this is a mouse anti-human, the next antibody will be sheep anti-mouse followed by peroxidase-conjugated donkey anti-sheep. Sheep anti-donkey follows this and then peroxidase-conjugated donkey anti-sheep (Fig. 21.5g). These steps attach a large number of peroxidase enzymes to the antibody–antigen below and it is said by the authors, after DAB visualization, to be over 60 times more sensitive than conventional avidin–biotin systems. While the advantages of this technique include the economy of

primary antibody and the avoidance of endogenous biotin, it is time consuming and without automation does not lend itself to routine use.

Biotinylated tyramide signal amplification

Bobrow et al first described the use of biotinylated tyramide to enhance signal amplification, in 1989. Subsequent work by Adams in 1992 and King et al in 1997 enabled the development of a highly sensitive detection system. In conjunction with heat-induced epitope retrieval techniques, the use of biotinylated tyramide amplification enabled many antigens which had previously been unreactive in formalin-fixed paraffin-embedded tissue to be demonstrated. Antibodies could be used at far greater dilutions than in conventional techniques. The biotinylated tyramide amplification reagent was first available commercially from DuPont; this was subsequently followed by the CSA (Catalyzed Signal Amplification) kit from Dakocytomation.

The technique is based around the streptavidin–biotin technique. Application of the primary antibody is followed by subsequent incubations in biotinylated secondary antibody and then either horseradish peroxidase-labeled streptavidin or streptavidin–biotin–horseradish peroxidase complex. The critical stage is the subsequent treatment with the biotinylated tyramide amplification reagent. The bound peroxidase label in the presence of hydrogen peroxide catalyses the biotinyl tyramide to form free biotin radicals. These reactive biotin molecules bind covalently to proteins adjacent to the site of the reaction. Further incubation in either horseradish peroxidase-labeled streptavidin or streptavidin–biotin–horseradish peroxidase complex results in additional enzyme being deposited at the site of the reaction (Fig. 21.5h).

The technique does have certain disadvantages; excessive background staining can be problematic, especially in tissues rich in endogenous biotin, although the use of a commercial avidin–biotin blocking kit reduces endogenous biotin demonstration. The incubation time in the biotinylated tyramide reagent is critical in preventing high background. Many users have experienced problems with consistency of results and reproducibility. Improved commercial reagents, in terms of antibodies and detection reagents, have now limited the impact and use of this technique. However, it still remains the method of choice for the demonstration of certain tissue antigens in formalin-fixed paraffin-embedded tissue and in formalin-fixed methyl methacrylate resin sections.

Biotin-free catalyzed signal amplification (CSA II)

In an attempt to reduce the problems associated with endogenous biotin in conventional tyramide signal amplification, Dakocytomation produces a biotin-free system, available commercially as Catalysed Signal Amplification system II (CSA II) for use with mouse monoclonal antibodies. Following incubation in primary antibody, a secondary anti-mouse immunoglobulin conjugated to horseradish peroxidase is bound to the primary antibody. The third layer involves peroxidase-catalyzed deposition of fluorescyl tyramide, which in turn is reacted with peroxidase conjugated anti-fluorescein, producing a greatly enhanced signal (Fig. 21.5i). This technique can be adapted easily to automated immunostaining protocols. Although a useful technique, in our hands the results fail to match the high sensitivity of conventional tyramide amplification.

Unmasking of antigen sites

A prerequisite for all routine histological and cytological investigations is to ensure preservation of tissue architecture and cell morphology by adequate and appropriate fixation (see Chapter 4). The fixative of choice will depend on the individual laboratory, the most popular choice of fixatives for routine histology are formalin based, either as a 10% solution or with the addition of different chemical constituents. Prompt fixation of thin (3 mm thickness) slices of tissue is essential to achieve consistent demonstration of tissue antigens. Delayed fixation or poor fixation may cause loss of antigenicity or diffusion of antigens into the surrounding tissue. Following fixation most material is routinely processed to paraffin wax to facilitate section cutting (Chapter 7).

The concept that antigens can be masked by the chemical processes involved in formalin fixation and paraffin processing and that some form of unmasking of these antigens is required dates far back into the history of immunohistochemistry (Brandtzaeg 1983). The majority of antigen unmasking studies have been applied to formalin-fixed material. When formalin-based fixatives are used, intermolecular and intramolecular cross-linkages are formed with certain structural proteins; these are responsible for the masking of the tissue antigens. This adverse effect has been thought to be the result of the formation of methylene bridges between reactive sites on tissue proteins (Bell et al 1987; Mason & O'Leary 1991). These reactive sites include primary amines, amide groups, thiols, alcoholic hydroxyl groups, and cyclic aromatic rings. The degree of masking of the antigenic sites depends upon the length of time in fixative, temperature, concentration of fixative, and availability of other nearby proteins able to undergo cross-linkages.

It must be remembered that tissue sections are unique to the laboratory of origin. Differences in the type and duration of fixation, together with variations in tissue processing schedules, reagents, and the manner by which sections are dried after microtomy, are important considerations. There are varying differences in the way these processes are performed by different laboratories. This lack of standardization of the basic processes of histology culminates in the production of a unique preparation. As a consequence, it is often found that one method of antigen unmasking may provide optimal results for one laboratory but not for another. Therefore, each method of antigen unmasking should be carefully evaluated using the laboratory's own material—digestion or heating times may need to be slightly modified to the times stated in the methods subsequently listed.

The Hematological Malignancy Diagnostic Service and the Histopathology Diagnostic Oncology Services at the Leeds Teaching Hospitals handle a great number of cases from outside laboratories, each showing great variation in the quality of fixation, decalcification (where applicable), and processing. In the majority of cases an accurate tumour immunophenotype can be achieved.

Many of the antigens masked during routine processing can be revealed by using one of the following techniques:

- Proteolytic enzyme digestion
- Microwave oven irradiation
- Combined microwave oven irradiation and proteolytic enzyme digestion
- Pressure cooker heating
- Decloaker heating
- Pressure cooker inside a microwave oven
- Autoclave heating
- Water bath heating
- Steamer heating.

Before pre-treatments are employed, the sections are dewaxed, rinsed in alcohol, and washed in water.

Proteolytic enzyme digestion

Pre-treating formalin-fixed routinely processed paraffin sections with proteolytic enzymes to unmask certain antigenic determinants was described by Huang et al (1976), Curran and Gregory (1977), and Mepham et al (1979). The most popular enzymes employed today are trypsin and protease, but other proteolytic enzymes such as chymotrypsin, pronase, proteinase K, and pepsin may also be used. The theory behind the unmasking properties of these proteolytic enzymes is not fully understood; it is generally accepted that the digestion breaks down formalin cross-linking and hence the antigenic sites for a number of antibodies are uncovered.

For some antigens, proteolytic digestion can be detrimental to their demonstration, occasionally producing false-positive or false-negative results. Digestion times need to be tailored to individual antibodies and to fixation time. Under-digestion results in little staining due to the antigens not being fully exposed. Over-digestion can produce false-positive staining, high background levels, and tissue damage. There can be a fine balance between under- and over-digestion when using proteolytic enzymes. Duration of enzyme digestion, enzyme concentration, use of a coenzyme, such as calcium chloride with trypsin, temperature, and pH must be optimized to produce consistent high-quality immunohistochemical staining. Different batches of enzyme may vary in quality and each new batch of enzyme should be tested prior to routine use. Enzymes produced specifically for immunohistochemical use are now widely available from commercial sources; these have been produced for use with automated immunostaining machines, are easy to use, and give good consistent results.

The use of heat-induced epitope retrieval techniques has largely replaced proteolytic digestion. However, for the demonstration of immunoglobulins and complement in formalin-fixed paraffin-embedded renal biopsies and for a number of other individual antigens proteolytic digestion is still favored by many.

Heat-mediated antigen retrieval techniques

Heat-based antigen retrieval methods have brought a great improvement in the quality and reproducibility of immunohistochemistry and have widened the use of immunohistochemistry as an important diagnostic tool in histopathology. The rationale behind the heat pretreatment methods is unclear and several different theories have been suggested. One theory is that heavy metal salts (as described by Shi et al 1991) act as a protein precipitant, forming insoluble complexes with polypeptides, and that protein-precipitating fixatives display better preservation of antigens than do cross-linking aldehyde fixatives.

Another theory is that during formalin fixation intermolecular and methylene bridges and weak Schiff bases form intramolecular cross-linkages. Theses cross-linkages alter the protein conformation of the antigen, which may prevent it from being recognized by a specific antibody. It is postulated that heat-mediated antigen retrieval removes the weaker Schiff bases but does not effect the methylene bridges, so the resulting protein conformation is intermediate between fixed and unfixed.

Another possible theory was described by Morgan et al (1997), who postulated that calcium coordination complexes formed during formalin fixation prevent antibodies from combining with epitopes on tissue-bound antigens. The underlying theory of calcium involvement is that hydroxy-methyl groups and other unreacted oxygen-rich groups (e.g. carboxyl or phosphoryl groups) can interact with calcium ions to produce large coordinate complexes which can mask epitopic sites by steric hindrance. The high temperature weakens or breaks some of the calcium coordinate bonds, but the effect is reversible on cooling, because the calcium complex remains in its original position. The presence of a competing chelating agent at the particular temperature at which the coordinate bonds are disrupted removes the calcium complexes. Evidence to support this theory comes from the chemical nature of some of the antigen retrieval reagents, such as citrate buffer and EDTA. In addition it has been shown that the inclusion of calcium ions with an unmasking reagent inhibits its effectiveness (Morgan et al 1994).

Microwave antigen retrieval

Shi et al (1991) first established the use of microwave heating for antigen retrieval. However, the use of heavy metal salts posed a significant risk to the health and safety of the users. Gerdes et al (1992) used microwave antigen retrieval with a non-toxic citrate buffer at pH 6.0 and demonstrated the Ki67 antigen, which had previously thought to be lost during formalin fixation and paraffin processing. The results were equivalent to those seen in frozen sections. Cattoretti et al (1993) established microwave oven heating as an alternative to proteolytic enzyme digestion. The method improved the demonstration of well-established antibodies such as CD45 and

CD20 and enabled the demonstration of a wide range of new antibodies, such as CD8 and P53.

Numerous antigen retrieval solutions have been described; probably the most popular are 0.01 M citrate buffer at pH 6.0 and 0.1 mM EDTA at pH 8.0. Although an expanding range of commercially available antigen buffers at both high and low pH ranges is available, some are designed to improve the staining of specific antigens.

Most domestic microwave ovens are suitable for antigen retrieval and operate at 2.45 GHz corresponding to a wavelength in vacuo of 12.2 cm (Fig. 21.6). Uneven heating and the production of hot-spots have been reported by some workers using the microwave oven. However, we have found that by using a volume of buffer between 400 and 600 ml in a suitably sized microwave-resistant plastic container, the problems of uneven heating are minimized. A batch of 25 slides in a plastic staining rack can be irradiated at one time and accurate, even antigen retrieval achieved. The actual heating time will depend on the following factors:

- Wattage of the oven. Most domestic ovens use a magnetron with an output between 750 and 1000 W. An important point to remember is that the output of the magnetron will decrease with age and frequency of use. The magnetron should be checked for efficiency annually.
- Choice of antigen retrieval buffer.
- Volume of buffer being used.
- Fixation of the tissues under investigation, in terms of fixative used and duration of fixation. This is an important factor, although not as critical as when

using proteolytic enzyme digestion. Tissue fixed for extended periods of time will require extended irradiation times. Conversely, poorly fixed tissues may require a reduction in the heating time.

- Thickness of the tissue sections, 3-μm sections require less antigen retrieval than 5-μm sections.
- Antigen to be demonstrated. Certain nuclear antigens may require increased heating times.

If extended heating times are used with a small volume of buffer, the buffer may need topping up with distilled or de-ionized water; this should be performed half-way through the total heating duration. At no stage should the sections be allowed to dry out during the antigen retrieval.

Pressure cooker antigen retrieval

Norton et al (1994) suggested the use of the pressure cooker as an alternative to the microwave oven. By using the pressure cooker, Norton et al (1994) provided evidence that the batch variation and production of hot and cold spots in the microwave oven could be overcome. Pressure cooking is said to be more uniform than other heating methods. A pressure cooker at 15 psi (103 kPa) reaches a temperature of around 120°C at full pressure. It is this increased temperature that appears to be a major advantage when unmasking certain nuclear tissue antigens such as bcl-6, P53, P21, estrogen receptor, and progesterone receptor.

The demonstration of these antigens can sometimes be weak when using microwave antigen retrieval.

It is preferable to use a stainless steel domestic pressure cooker, because aluminum pressure cookers are susceptible to corrosion from some of the antigen retrieval buffers (Fig. 21.7). The pressure cooker should have a capacity of 4–5 litres, thus allowing a large batch of slides to be treated at the same time. As with the microwave oven heat pre-treatments, the use of Superfrost Plus microscope slides or strong adhesives such as Vectabond or APES is required.

Steamer

Although quite a popular method in some parts of the world, steam heating appears to be less efficient than either microwave oven heating or pressure cooking (Pasha et al 1995). Times in excess of 40 minutes are sometimes required, but the method does have the advantage in being less damaging to tissues than the

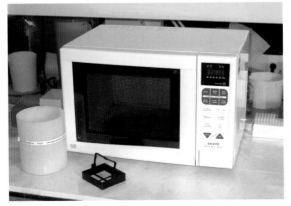

Fig. 21.6   Domestic microwave oven.

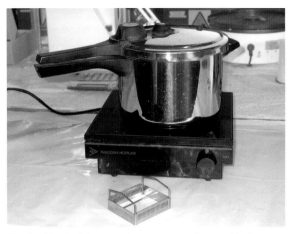

Fig. 21.7 Stainless steel pressure cooker and halogen hotplate.

other heating methods. Commercially available rice steamers are adequate for this purpose.

Water bath

Kawai et al (1994) demonstrated that a water bath set at 90°C was adequate for antigen retrieval. However, by increasing the temperature to 95–98°C antigen retrieval was improved and the incubation times could be decreased. The technique has the advantage of being gentler on the tissue sections because the temperature is set below boiling point. By using a lower temperature than other heating methods the antigen retrieval buffer does not evaporate and expensive commercial antigen retrieval solutions can be safely re-used. The method has the disadvantage in that the antigen retrieval times are increased compared to other methods. This method is recommended with the Dakocytomation Hercept test for HER2 expression.

Autoclave

This method offers an alternative form of heat-mediated antigen retrieval, producing good results for nuclear antigens such as MIB1, P21, and P53.

Advantages of heat pre-treatment

Some antigens previously thought lost in routinely processed paraffin-embedded sections are now recovered by heat pre-treatment. Many antigens are retrieved by uniform heating times, regardless of length of fixation, e.g. up to several weeks in formal saline (Singh et al 1993). The demonstration of heavy-chain immunoglob-

ulins is more reliable and reproducible than when proteolytic digestion is employed. The dilution factors of some primary antibodies ascertained with traditional methods can be increased when using heat pre-treatment.

Pitfalls of heat pre-treatment

Care should be taken not to allow the sections to dry after heating, as this destroys antigenicity. The boiling of poorly fixed material often damages nuclear detail.

Fibrous and fatty tissues tend to detach from the slide. This can sometimes be overcome by extending the drying times on Superfrost Plus microscope slides or coated slides at 56°C. Alternatively, Vectabond- or APES-coated slides can be dipped in 10% formal saline for 1–2 minutes and air dried before picking up sections. This tends to improve the adhesion, probably by adding more aldehyde groups to the slide surface.

Not all antigens are retrieved by heat pre-treatment, and the range of staining of some primary antibodies, e.g. PGP9.5, a neuroendocrine marker, is altered (Langlois et al 1994).

Combination of microwave antigen retrieval and trypsin or chymotrypsin digestion

A combination of microwave antigen retrieval followed by 30 seconds of trypsin digestion enables more reliable identification of light chain restricted plasma cells in myeloma compared with the use of trypsin alone. Furthermore, this technique has been shown to be helpful in identifying the restricted light chain in AL amyloidosis involving renal biopsies. A drastically reduced digestion time is necessary as heat pre-treatment increases the sensitivity of sections to subsequent proteolytic digestion. Time trials will need to be undertaken to ascertain the optimal pre-treatment times. Further work has shown that the reverse is also true: proteolytic digestion (by either trypsin or chymotrypsin) increases the sensitivity of the tissue sections to microwave antigen retrieval. Hence proteolytic digestion can be carried out before or after microwave heating.

Commercial antigen retrieval solutions

There are numerous commercial antigen retrieval solutions available. They can be either specialized high pH solutions (recommended by certain users for cyclin D1) or lower pH 6.0 for more general use. These solutions may be a mixture of different chemicals, such as citrate and EDTA in the Antigen Unmasking Fluid available from Vector. These offer advantages over the 'in house' retrieval solutions, in that they are ready to use, require no pH calibration, and are fully certified to comply with laboratory accreditation procedures; however they can be expensive.

Recommendation on the use of expensive commercial retrieval fluids

If cheap 'in house' fluids are employed then flushing out the hot buffer at the end of the heating cycle with cold running water is accepted practice. If, however, an expensive commercial fluid is employed, many workers now transfer the hot container with the aid of oven gloves to a sink of cold running water and allow the solution and slides to cool for 10–15 minutes. The slides are then transferred promptly to cold running water and the expensive retrieval fluid retained and re-used again and again. (See Table 21.1 for recommended retrieval methods for certain diagnostic antigens.)

Detection of low levels of antigen

Enhancement and amplification

The optimum dilution of primary antibody for diagnostic immunohistochemistry is defined as the concentration of the primary antibody which gives the optimal specific staining with the least amount of background staining. The optimal dilution will depend upon the type and duration of fixation. Serial dilutions of antibody will often give the distribution of reactivity shown in Figure 21.8.

Poor reaction in area 1 is due to steric hindrance of the labeling antibody accessing the primary antibody (the prozone effect). This is due to the primary antibody being used too concentrated.

Suboptimal reaction in area 2 is caused by inadequate presence of primary antibody, i.e. primary antibody used too diluted.

The optimum concentration of primary antibody is that measured below the apex of the peak and the use of several control sections with varying expression of antigen will aid the determination of a correct working dilution of primary antibody for that particular laboratory. Interlaboratory variations in the choice of fixative, duration of fixation, paraffin processing, section treatment, and the immunohistochemical detection system

used make this dilution of primary antibody unique to the laboratory that produced the paraffin section and accounts for the great variation in the dilution of primary antibodies used from laboratory to laboratory.

The dilutions of primary antibodies and labeling systems for diagnostic immunohistochemistry should be ascertained on material where the antigen levels are adequate but not excessive. Occasionally situations arise where some tumors shed much of their antigen, e.g. prostatic tumors often express less prostate-specific antigen than normal prostatic glands. Enhancement and amplification by modification of demonstration techniques may be required to identify low levels of antigens. This can be achieved by the following methods:

1. Increasing the concentration of the primary antibody. Usually this can be accomplished with most monoclonals without increasing the background staining significantly, as this type of antibody, especially in the form of tissue culture supernatant, does not contain any non-specific contaminants. Polyclonal antibodies can give excessive background problems and it is advisable to use a casein blocking solution as described in the Methods section and sometimes the addition of a small amount of detergent, e.g. 0.01% Tween, to the washes helps to reduce background staining. Further details on dealing with background appear later in the text.

2. Prolonging incubation with the primary antibody overnight, at 48°C or at ambient temperature, can enhance staining. Many immunohistochemists employ this methodology for their routine work because higher dilution of primary reagents is achieved, allowing costs to be reduced. Dilutions must not be excessive, otherwise low levels of antigen will not be detected, resulting in false-negative staining.

3. Increasing the concentration of bridge reagent beyond the optimal dilution, or repeated application of the bridge reagent, marginally increases the sensitivity of the avidin–biotin systems. Furthermore, in the case of the CD15 primaries, which are IgM subclass antibodies, LeBrun et al (1992) reported that an IgM link, as opposed to a broad-spectrum immunoglobulin bridge reagent, improves the rate of detecting CD15-positive Reed–Sternberg and Hodgkin cells (Fig. 21.9). Charalambous et al not only confirmed this work in 1993, but they also indicated that when microwave antigen

Table 21.1 Antibodies and pre-treatments

Antibody	Clone	Species	Supplier	Dilution	Pre-treatment
α1-Antichymotrypsin	—	Poly	Dakocytomation	1/100	Trypsin
α1-Antitrypsin	—	Poly	Dakocytomation	1/4000	Trypsin
α1-Fetoprotein	—	Poly	Dakocytomation	1/800	Trypsin
α1-Synuclein	KM51	M	Novo Castra	1/50	PC
Androgen receptor	AR441	M	Dakocytomation	1/50	PC
Alzheimer precursor protein	22C11	M	Chemicon	1/2500	PC
AUA	AUA-1	M	Skybio	1/100	Trypsin
ACTH	02A3	M	Dakocytomation	1/50	None
AE1	AE1	M	Biogenex	1/50	Trypsin
AE1 + AE3	AE1/3	M	Biogenex	1/100	Trypsin
Alk protein	ALK-1	M	Dakocytomation	1/50	PC or MWO
Amyloid P component	—	Poly	Dakocytomation	1/2000	PC or MWO
Bcl-2	124	M	Dakocytomation	1/100	PC or MW0
Bcl-6	PG-B6p	M	Dakocytomation	1/20	PC
Ber EP4	Ber EP4	M	Dakocytomation	1/200	Trypsin
BOB-1	—	Poly	Santa Cruz	1/500	PC or MW0
CA125	OV185H	M	Novo Castra	1/100	PC
Calcitonin	—	Poly	Dakocytomation	1/300	None
Caldesmon	h-CD	M	Dakocytomation	1/100	PC
Calponin	CALP	M	Dakocytomation	1/100	PC
CD1a	010	M	Immunotech	1/20	PC or MWO
CD2	271	M	Novo Castra	1/100	PC
CD3	PS1	M	Novo Castra	1/50	PC or MW0
CD4	1F6	M	Novo Castra	1/50	PC
CD5	4C7	M	Novo Castra	1/50	PC or MW0
CD7	272	M	Novo Castra	1/100	PC
CD8	C8/144B	M	Dakocytomation	1/100	PC
CD10	270	M	Novo Castra	1/20	PC
CD15	LeuM1	M	Becton Dickinson	1/20	PC or MWO
CD20	L26	M	Dakocytomation	1/200	PC or MWO
CD21	2G9	M	Novo Castra	1/50	PC
CD23	1B12	M	Novo Castra	1/50	PC
CD30	Ber-H2	M	Dakocytomation	1/50	PC
CD31	JC70	M	Dakocytomation	1/50	PC
CD34	Qbend 10	M	Dakocytomation	1/100	PC or MWO
CD43	DF-T1	M	Dakocytomation	1/50	PC or MWO
CD45	2B11 + PD7/26	M	Dakocytomation	1/200	PC or MWO
CD45RA	4KB5	M	Dakocytomation	1/50	PC or MWO
CD45RO	UCHL1	M	Dakocytomation	1/100	PC or MWO
CD56	1B6	M	Novo Castra	1/100	PC or MWO
CD63	1/C3	M	Novo Castra	1/50	None
CD68	PGM-1	M	Dakocytomation	1/200	PC or MWO
CD71	309	M	Novo Castra	1/10	PC
CD75	LN-1	M	Novo Castra	1/20	PC
CD79a	JCB117	M	Dakocytomation	1/100	PC or MWO

Table 21.1 (*continued*)

Antibody	Clone	Species	Supplier	Dilution	Pre-treatment
CD83	1H4b	M	Novo Castra	1/50	PC
CD99	12E7	M	Dakocytomation	1/50	PC
CD117	—	Poly	Dakocytomation	1/200	PC or MWO
CD138	MCA681	M	Serotec	1/200	PC or MWO
CEA	5A	M	Dakocytomation	1/600	PC or MWO
c-erb B2	—	Poly	Dakocytomation	1/800	PC
Chromogranin A	—	Poly	Dakocytomation	1/5000	PC or MWO
CK7	OV-TL 12/30	M	Dakocytomation	1/100	PC or MWO
CK14	LL002	M	Novo Castra	1/50	PC or MWO
CK20	Ks20.8	M	Dakocytomation	1/100	PC or MWO
CK8/18	5D3	M	Novo Castra	1/500	Trypsin
Cytokeratin	CAM5.2	M	Becton Dickinson	1/20	PC or MWO
Cytokeratin	MNF116	M	Dakocytomation	1/100	PC or MWO
Cytokeratin	LP34	M	Dakocytomation	1/10	MWO + Trypsin
Cyclin D1	SP4	M*	Labvision	1/20	PC
Desmin	D33	M	Dakocytomation	1/200	PC or MWO
Epithelial membrane antigen	E29	M	Dakocytomation	1/500	PC or MWO
EGFR	113	M	Novo Castra	1/100	PC
Estrogen receptor	6F11	M	Novo Castra	1/30	PC
Factor VIII	—	Poly	Dakocytomation	1/2000	PC or MWO
Fascin	5SK-2	M	Dakocytomation	1/500	PC or MWO
FSH	C10	M	Dakocytomation	1/100	Trypsin
GFAP	—	Poly	Dakocytomation	1/300	Trypsin
Growth hormone	—	Poly	Dakocytomation	1/300	None
Glucagon	—	Poly	Dakocytomation	1/1500	None
Glycophorin C	Ret 40f	M	Dakocytomation	1/200	PC or MWO
Granzyme B	Grb-7	M	Dakocytomation	1/25	PC
HLA-DR	TAL-1B5	M	Dakocytomation	1/100	PC or MWO
H.Pylori	—	Poly	Dakocytomation	1/200	PC
IgA	—	Poly	Dakocytomation	1/800	MWO
IgD	—	Poly	Dakocytomation	1/200	MWO
IgG	—	Poly	Dakocytomation	1/1000	MWO
IgM	—	Poly	Dakocytomation	1/500	MWO
Kappa	—	Poly	Dakocytomation	1/2000	MWO
Lambda	—	Poly	Dakocytomation	1/2000	MWO
LMP-1	CS1-4	M	Dakocytomation	1/100	PC
Lysozyme	—	Poly	Dakocytomation	1/1000	PC or MWO
Mast cell tryptase	AA1	M	Dakocytomation	1/1000	PC or MWO
Melanoma monoclonal	HMB45	M	Dakocytomation	1/50	PC or MWO
Mesothelial cell	HBME-1	M	Dakocytomation	1/100	None
MIB1	Ki67	M	Dakocytomation	1/200	PC or MWO
Myeloperoxidase	—	Poly	Dakocytomation	1/4000	PC or MWO
MUM-1	—	Poly†	Santa Cruz	1/500	PC
MUM-1	Mum1p	M	Dakocytomation	1/50	PC
MyoD1	5.8A	M	Dakocytomation	1/50	PC or MWO

Table 21.1 (*continued*)

Antibody	Clone	Species	Supplier	Dilution	Pre-treatment
Myogenin	F5D	M	Dakocytomation	1/50	PC or MWO
NFP	ZF11	M	Dakocytomation	1/250	PC or MWO
OCT-2	—	Poly	Santa Cruz	1/500	PC
PAX-5	24	M	Becton Dickinson	1/250	PC
Progesterone receptor	PgR636	M	Dakocytomation	1/100	PC
P21	SX118	M	Dakocytomation	1/15	PC
P53	D0-7	M	Dakocytomation	1/40	PC
PGP9.5	—	Poly	Dakocytomation	1/500	Trypsin
PLAP	—	Poly	Dakocytomation	1/100	MWO
PSAP	PASE/4LJ	M	Dakocytomation	1/1000	None
PSA	—	Poly	Dakocytomation	1/1000	None
PU-1	G148-74	M	Becton Dickinson	1/100	PC
S100	—	Poly	Dakocytomation	1/250	Trypsin
Smooth muscle actin	1A4	M	Dakocytomation	1/150	None
Synaptophysin	Sy38	M	Dakocytomation	1/100	PC
Tau	—	Poly	Dakocytomation	1/1500	None
Tdt	SEN28	M	Novo Castra	1/100	PC or MWO
TIA-1	2G9	M	Immunotech	1/100	PC
TSH	0042	M	Dakocytomation	1/100	None
TTF-1	8G7G3/1	M	Dakocytomation	1/50	PC or MWO
Thyroglobulin	—	Poly	Dakocytomation	1/5000	None
Ubiquitin	—	Poly	Dakocytomation	1/1000	PC
Vasointestinal polypeptide	—	Poly	Novo Castra	1/200	Trypsin
Vimentin	V9	M	Dakocytomation	1/500	PC or MWO
Zap-70	2F3.2	M	Upstate	1/100	PC

M = monoclonal antibody, M* = rabbit monoclonal, PC = pressure cooker with 0.01 M citrate buffer pH 6.0, MWO = microwave oven (800 W), Poly† = goat polyclonal.

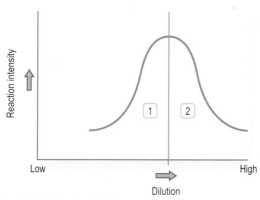

Fig. 21.8 Antibody dilution curve.

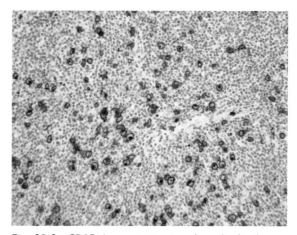

Fig. 21.9 CD15 demonstration in a formalin-fixed paraffin-embedded section of Hodgkin's disease.

recovery was used in place of trypsin, further amplification was achieved.

4. Chemical enhancement of the reaction end-product of the peroxidase–diaminobenzidine method can be achieved by the addition of imidazole (Straus 1982), heavy metals such as copper or cobalt (Hsu & Soban 1982), osmication, or treatment with gold chloride. Colloidal gold labeling can be enhanced dramatically using silver salts with the IGSS technique (Holgate et al 1983b).

5. Repeated applications of the bridge and label increase the sensitivity of the APAAP technique. Whilst the initial primary, bridge and label are incubated for 30 minutes each, the repeated applications of bridge and label require only 10 minutes each. After two such repeats enhancement is usually sufficient for most antibodies.

6. Changing the chromogen substrate used. Some chromogen substrate solutions, especially for alkaline phosphatase, give a more intense reaction product than other reagents. For example nitro-blue tetrazolium is not only more intense than fast red, but can be left on overnight to give probably the most intense reaction of all chromogens available today. The only drawback is that the blue–black reaction product does not contrast well with hematoxylin counterstaining. Improved commercial formulas of traditional substrates are superior to 'in house' formulas.

7. Techniques for elevating the sensitivity of the extended polymer labeled antibodies and other pre-diluted reagents are more restricted. The disadvantage of pre-diluted antibodies is that the dilutions selected are not necessarily suitable for the multitude of fixation and processing protocols employed. Hence weak staining can only be overcome by increasing the incubation times, elevating the temperature to 37°C, or chemical enhancement of the diaminobenzidine reaction product, or other appropriate substrate.

8. Tyramide signal amplification. Bobrow and fellow workers in 1989 described a novel signal amplification method, catalyzed reporter deposition, and its application to immunoassays. In 1992 the same group proposed that this method would be suitable for immunohistochemistry. Erber et al and King et al in 1997 quite independently published data showing that this novel signal amplification system employed with avidin–biotin systems showed greater sensitivity

than that provided by the more conventional avidin–biotin methods.

Multiple labels

The availability of several chromogens for a particular enzyme, each of which produces a different colored reaction end-product, and the variety of techniques now available, can be used in conjunction to localize in the same section. If the primary antibodies are raised in the same species and are of the same subclass, cross-reactivity between reactions must be eliminated. This can be accomplished by eluting with glycine-HCl buffer between each reaction (Nakane 1968), by build-up of the reaction components to mask the reactive sites (Sternberger & Joseph 1979; Hsu & Soban 1982) (Figs 21.10 and 21.11) or by the destruction of binding sites after each reaction with hot formalin vapor (Wang & Larsson 1985). However, it is simpler to use primary antibodies raised in different species or of different subclasses. These can then be sequentially localized by the indirect or other more elaborate techniques using non-overlapping secondary reagents and different chromogens. These techniques have been described in more detail by Mason and Sammons (1978), Gu et al (1981), Mason and Woolston (1982), Mason et al (1983), and Van Noorden et al (1986).

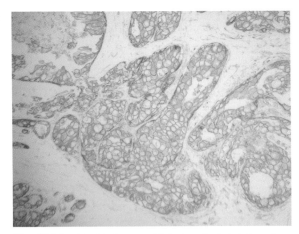

Fig. 21.10 Double immunohistochemical staining of formalin-fixed paraffin-embedded section of breast carcinoma shows HER2 membrane staining with DAB as the chromogen and smooth muscle actin stained with Vector SG chromogen.

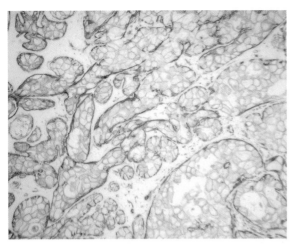

Fig. 21.11 Double immunohistochemical staining shows the smooth muscle actin demonstrated with DAB and the HER2 with Vector SG.

IMMUNOHISTOCHEMISTRY IN PRACTICE

Workload

As a result of heat antigen retrieval methods, there is a continual increase in the numbers of antibodies effective on paraffin sections. Many of these antibodies can have a direct impact on diagnosis, prognosis, or treatment. As a consequence the immunohistochemist is often overwhelmed with requests and either additional staff or automation are sought to overcome the increasing demand. If automation is selected, it does not mean that the immunohistochemist loses control of the activity. On the contrary, automation usually allows the immunohistochemist time to develop the service and improve the staining of some antigens.

Choice of technique

The choice of technique to suit the needs of particular types of work is governed by some important factors.

Frozen sections

Although the use of frozen sections for diagnostic purposes is decreasing, immunohistochemistry on frozen sections remains an important histological tool. Although frozen sections have certain inherent disadvantages compared to paraffin sections, including poor morphology, limited retrospective studies, and storage of mate-

rial, it should be considered the gold standard when evaluating and assessing new antibodies. When evaluating a new antibody the results achieved on paraffin (or resin) sections can be compared to the results achieved on frozen sections.

Poor morphology often associated with frozen sections can be improved by ensuring the frozen sections are thoroughly dried both before and after the sections are fixed in acetone. The acetone not only assists with the preservation of the antigen and related morphology, but also destroys most harmful infective agents.

Cytological preparations

The use of immunohistochemistry on cytological preparations is increasing. Acetone-fixed smears or cytospins are often preferred by the immunohistochemist as acetone allows a wide range of primary antibodies to be employed without destroying the epitopes they are attempting to identify. Many cytology laboratories still insist on fixing cytological preparations in alcohol as opposed to acetone and consequently the number of antigens demonstrable is limited, although perhaps the morphology is superior.

Formalin-fixed, routinely processed paraffin-wax sections

The aim of immunohistochemistry is to achieve reproducible and consistent demonstration of antigens with the minimum background staining whilst preserving the integrity of tissue architecture. Adequate and appropriate fixation is the cornerstone of all histological and immunohistochemical preparations. Good fixation is the delicate balance between under-fixation and over-fixation. Ideal fixation is the balance between good morphology and good antigenicity. The demonstration of many antigens depends heavily on the fixative employed and on the immunohistochemical method selected. Prompt fixation is essential to achieve consistent results. Poor fixation or delay in fixation causes loss of antigenicity or diffusion of antigens into the surrounding tissue. There is no one fixative that is ideal for the demonstration of all antigens, and certain antigens necessitate the use of frozen sections—although the modern trend is to utilize fixed paraffin sections wherever possible. Most laboratories use formulas based on formalin such as unbuffered 10% formal saline or 10% neutral buffered formalin, but some groups prefer picric acid fixation (Bouin's) or mercuric fixation (formal mercury or B5). The choice of fixation among pathologists was initially based on morphological appearance and the clarity of established staining techniques using dyes which were the mainstay of diagnostic histopathology long before the advent of immunohistochemistry. As most pathology teaching and learning is based on these traditional techniques, with all the artifacts they produce, immunohistochemistry has had to tailor itself to this type of material in order to become an effective diagnostic aid.

Blocking endogenous enzymes

If enzymes similar to those used as the antibody label are present in the tissue they may react with the substrate used to localize the tracer and give rise to problems in interpretation. Inhibiting the endogenous enzyme activity prior to staining can eliminate false-positive reactions produced in this way. Peroxidase and substances giving a pseudo-peroxidase reaction are present in some normal and neoplastic tissues, e.g. leucocytes and erythrocytes, and various methods have been described for the destruction of their activity. The most frequently used method is preincubation of the sections in absolute methanol containing hydrogen peroxide (Streefkerk 1972). Incubation in absolute methanol containing 0.5% hydrogen peroxide for 10 minutes at room temperature has been reported to produce an almost complete abolition of endogenous peroxidase activity, without affecting the immunoreactivity of antigens (Delellis et al 1979). The mechanisms of inhibition and details of other methods have been reviewed by Straus (1976).

There are many types of alkaline phosphatase within the human body, and most endogenous alkaline phosphatase activity can be blocked using a 1 mM concentration of levamisole in the final incubating medium. The alkaline phosphatase used in the labeling system is usually intestinal in nature and remains unaffected by levamisole at the recommended concentration. Using 20% acetic acid can block intestinal alkaline phosphatase. However, the acidic treatment may damage some antigens.

The other commonly used enzyme labels, glucose oxidase and bacterial β2-galactosidase, do not present a problem. The former does not have active endogenous enzyme in mammalian tissue; the latter does, but the label and chromogen react at a different pH from the mammalian enzyme.

An alternative to chemical inhibition of endogenous enzyme activity has been described by Robinson and Dawson (1975), and is similar to multiple labeling. In this method, the endogenous peroxidases are first local-ized by using one chromogen and then, following immunohistochemical staining, the enzyme tracer is localized by an alternate chromogen which yields a reaction end-product in a contrasting color. Thus, endogenous activity and specific activity can be distinguished easily by their differently colored reaction end-products. A wide range of chromogenic substrates is now commercially available (Vector Laboratories), many of which produce colored end-products that are not removed or decolorized by the dehydrating and clearing agents commonly used in immunohistochemistry.

Blocking background staining

The major causes of background staining in immunohistochemistry are hydrophobic and ionic interactions and endogenous enzyme activity. Background staining may be specific, e.g. fibrinogen in blood vessels and immunoglobulins in serum-bearing tissues, or non-specific due to the apparent affinity of certain tissue components. Non-specific uptake of antigen, particularly the high affinity of collagen and reticulin for immunoglobulins, can cause high levels of background staining.

Hydrophobic interactions are the result of the cross-linking of amino acids, both within and between adjacent protein molecules. Proteins are rendered more hydrophobic by aldehyde fixation and the extent of hydrophobic cross-linking of tissue proteins is primarily a function of fixation.

Tissues that give background staining as a result of hydrophobic interactions include collagen and other connective tissues, epithelium, and adipocytes (Kraehenbuhl & Jamieson 1974). Hydrophobic bonding can be minimized by the addition of a blocking protein, by the addition of a detergent such as Triton X (Hartman 1973), or the addition of a high salt concentration, 2.5% NaCl, to the buffer (Grabe 1980). Some workers advocate the addition of the blocking serum to the diluted primary antibody (Delellis et al 1979).

Non-specific staining is most commonly produced because the primary antibody is attracted non-immunologically to highly charged groups present on connective tissue elements. Positive staining is due not to localization of the antigen but to non-specific attachment of the primary antibody to connective tissues. Because the primary antibody is attached to connective tissue moieties the subsequent labeling antibodies will be attracted not only to primary antibodies located on the specific antigen but also to the antibody bound to the connective tissue elements.

The most effective way of minimizing non-specific staining is to add an innocuous protein solution to the section before applying the primary antibody; the added protein should saturate and neutralize the charged sites thus enabling the primary antibody to bind to the antigenic site only.

Traditionally, non-immune serum from the animal species in which the second (bridging) antibody was raised is used as a blocking serum. In practice any animal serum or protein (e.g. casein) can be used for this purpose as long as the protein used as a block cannot be recognized by any of the subsequent antibodies used in the technique.

In frozen sections and cytological preparations tissue receptors for the Fc portion of antibodies may give rise to additional problems. Fc receptors are present on several cell types such as macrophages and monocytes, and are largely destroyed by formalin fixation and paraffin processing. If necessary Fab fragments of antibodies that lack the Fc portion should be used.

Several authors have also found that enzymatic digestion reduces non-specific background staining (Huang et al 1976; Curran & Gregory 1977; Denk et al 1977).

Controls

Controls validate immunohistochemical results. It is essential that any method using immunohistochemistry principles include controls to test for the specificity of the antibodies involved. Polyclonal antibodies usually contain antibodies specific for several antigenic determinants on the antigen and, as many related molecules have components in common (e.g. gastrin and cholecystokinin), false-positive results can be obtained. Although monoclonal antibodies potentially eliminate this problem, epitope similarities are seen between some molecules and unwanted cross-reaction can occur.

The criteria for specificity have been outlined by Nairn (1976), and problems relating to specificity discussed by Petrusz et al (1976, 1977). In general, for immunochemical staining to be specific it must be shown firstly that no staining occurs in the absence of the primary antiserum, and secondly that staining is inhibited by adsorption of the primary antibody with the relevant antigen prior to its use, but not by adsorption with other related or unrelated antigens. In practice, to evaluate the results of immunohistochemical staining, the following immunological and non-immunological specificity controls can be undertaken.

Negative control. This involves either the omission of the primary antibody from the staining schedule or the replacement of the specific primary antibody by an immunoglobulin which is directed against an unrelated antigen. This immunoglobulin must be of the same class, source, and species.

Positive control. As the absence of staining in a test section does not necessarily imply that the antigen is not present, the use of a section of known positivity is always advisable. Positive elements within test sections, e.g. normal reactive lymphocytes when staining with an antibody to the leukocyte common antigen to identify a suspected lymphoma, are the best form of positive control.

Absorption control. The ideal negative control is to demonstrate that immunoreactivity is abolished by preabsorption of the specific primary antibody with the purified antigen. If staining does occur after absorption then the staining must be due to a contaminating antibody and not to the antigen–antibody interaction under investigation. This type of control is necessary in the characterization and evaluation of new antibodies. This may be regarded as the ultimate test for specificity (Fig. 21.12). It is rarely used in diagnostic work, as well-characterized antibodies are available. For reasons of economy absorption should be carried out at the highest possible dilution of the primary antibody compatible with consistent unequivocal staining as the higher the concentration of antibody, the more antigen will be required for neutralization.

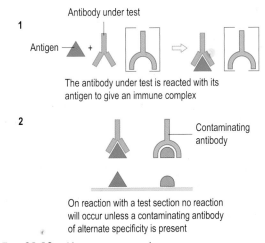

Fig. 21.12 Absorption control.

The practicalities of this type of control have been described by Van Noorden et al (1986).

An additional useful control is a blocking control in which the binding between the primary antibody and conjugated antibody in the traditional indirect method, or between the bridging antibody and the PAP in the unlabeled antibody method, is blocked. This is achieved by interposing between incubations of the two relevant antibodies incubation in unlabeled immunoglobulin of the type present in the labeled antibody.

When localizing immunoglobulin some workers consider it is advisable to include an anti-albumin 'control', as non-immunological cells in poorly fixed or post-mortem tissue are known to passively take up immuno-globulin and other serum proteins. Anti-albumin-stained sections will help to identify these false-positive cells.

Finally, it can be beneficial to check the inhibition treatment for endogenous enzymes by staining a slide histochemically after the inhibition procedure. If residual activity is present, interpretation of the immunochemically stained slides may be aided by staining an untreated slide to reveal the sites of endogenous enzyme activity.

Practical aspects of immunohistochemical staining

The practical aspects of immunohistochemical staining are simple and straightforward, as the techniques entail only sequential incubations in antibodies and labeling systems separated by washes in buffer. To obtain optimal staining and prevent the non-specific precipitation of antibody onto the sections, it is essential to insure that each antibody is used at an appropriate dilution, does not evaporate off during incubation, and is completely removed, if unbound, before the next specific antibody or reagent is added.

Dilution of immune serum/antibodies

For optimal staining to occur it is necessary to use the primary specific antibody at the correct dilution. Incorrect dilutions can give rise to false-negative results, particularly in antigen-rich tissues (Bigbee et al 1977).

When applying an untested antibody to a tissue section containing the relevant antigen, a broad dilution series should be used to insure that false-negative results do not occur. Selection of the cleanest dilution with intense signal, particularly on normal cells, is not always the optimal dilution for diagnostic material. Tumor cells can sometimes exhibit fewer antigens than the normal cells of origin. Dilutions that identify normal cells may be too dilute to demonstrate the tumor cells that originate from them. It is recommended that dilution factors are not set at the extreme end of the range and, where possible, it is useful to test out dilution factors on known neoplastic material when appropriate.

In theory, in multi-layer techniques each separate stage ought to be titrated against the other antibody stages and the optimal concentration selected for each. In practice, most commercially supplied primary antibodies and labeling systems are provided with a recommended dilution range. It is usually only the primary antibody dilution that needs to be adjusted.

Washes

To prevent the formation of antigen–antibody complexes that will precipitate onto the sections and give rise to problems with interpretation and background staining, it is necessary to remove the unbound antibody before incubation in the next layer. This is achieved by washing the sections between antibody incubations in Tris-buffered saline (TBS). This solution may be made up in bulk for convenience.

For routine work, a few brief washes, with TBS, will usually suffice. In the past some workers recommended the addition of detergent, such as BRIJ 96 (Sigma), to the washing solutions (Heyderman & Monaghan 1979). Today the most popular surfactant is Tween 20, often used in concentrations of 0.01–0.05%.

Buffer solutions and heat-mediated antigen retrieval fluids

0.5 M Tris-buffered saline

Distilled water	10 liters
Sodium chloride	85 g
TRIS (hydroxymethyl) aminomethane	60.5 g

Adjust pH to 7.6 with 50% hydrochloric acid.

Tris-buffered saline containing bovine serum albumin (BSA-TBS)

TRIS (hydroxymethyl) aminomethane	12.14 g
Sodium chloride	45 g
Bovine serum albumin	5 g
Sodium azide	6.5 g
Distilled water	5 liters

Adjust final pH to 8.2 with 1 M HCl.

Veronal acetate buffer

Sodium acetate trihydrate	0.972 g
Sodium barbitone	1.472 g
Distilled water	247.5 g
0.1 M HCl	2.5 ml

Heat-mediated antigen retrieval fluids

Citrate buffer

Citric acid (anhydrous)	21 g
Distilled water	10 liters

Adjust pH to 6.0 using 1 M HCl.

Tris–EDTA

Tris	14.4 g
EDTA	1.44 g
1 M HCl	1 ml
Tween 20	0.3 ml
Distilled water	600 ml

Add the Tris, EDTA, and acid to the distilled water and adjust pH to 10 with hydrochloric acid, then add the Tween.

Incubation methods

Manual

To prevent evaporation of antibodies, incubations must be carried out in a moist atmosphere. This is most easily obtained by placing the slides on perspex strips which run the length of a lidded staining trough, in the bottom of which is a pool of water or a layer of moist tissue paper.

It is advisable to leave a small gap between adjacent slides so that cross-contamination of antibodies cannot occur. The use of moist incubation chambers means that it is not necessary to flood the slide with antiserum and, if the area around the section is dried thoroughly with a tissue before application of the antibodies and labeling systems, just a few drops of reagent should suffice. Also the use of a wax pen around the sections assists with retaining the reagents on the sections.

Automated incubation methods

There are now many instruments available offering various levels of automation of immunohistochemical techniques. Currently there appear to be two types of

reagent delivery system. Capillary action is used by the Shandon Sequenza, Shandon Cadenza, and Ventana TechMate (supplied by Dako & Ventana in Europe), and spray delivery is used by the Dako Autostainer, LabVision Instrument, Leica HistoStainer, Ventana Nexes, and BioGenex Optimax. The latest innovation in immunostaining is the development of automated systems capable of carrying out both antigen retrieval and immunostaining, e.g. the Bond Max autostainer and the use of polymer-labeled antibodies.

Increased workloads necessitate the use of automated immunostaining. Automation ensures standardization of technique and quality of immunostaining and should give staff more time to perform other laboratory functions. Selection of a suitable autostainer should be made after consideration of factors such as capacity, flexibility, and cost per slide.

Fixation and paraffin-wax block immunohistochemistry

Many publications have discussed the merits and drawbacks of particular fixatives for immunohistochemistry on diagnostic histopathological material, with some recommending specific fixatives for certain epitopes. Most diagnostic laboratories are faced with a request for certain antigens subsequent to the routine processing and hematoxylin and eosin stage. It is therefore important to establish a fixation and processing procedure that allows for good morphology and maximizes the ability of the immunohistochemist to identify the antigens that aid diagnosis. It should also, with prior arrangement with the surgeons and theater staff, be possible to receive fresh specimens soon after surgery in order that material can be selected for routine processing and frozen storage. The latter should be snap frozen using liquid nitrogen and stored at −80°C. If required, this material can be used for preparing imprints for fluorescent in situ hybridization (FISH) techniques or as a source of RNA and DNA for molecular biology techniques or for cutting frozen sections, for the demonstration of antigens not readily demonstrated in paraffin-wax sections.

Retrospective studies are often hampered by a lack of knowledge of the duration of fixation. Banks (1979) indicated that prolonged fixation reduces immunoreactivity. Acidic fixatives such as Bouin's fluid can, over a 24-hour fixation period, reduce or destroy the immunoreactivity of some diagnostic antibodies, such as UCHL1 (CD45RO). A similar picture is seen with mercury-containing fixatives (Bilbe et al 1989, unpublished data, and Gillibrand 1991, unpublished data). Formalin fixation can have a similar effect, but tends to occur over a period of weeks rather than days. Certain antibodies such as CD20 and CD45 are less affected by fixation times. According to Singh et al (1993), microwave pretreatment enables the retrieval of antigens after formalin fixation of up to 2 years' duration. In general the use of heat-mediated antigen retrieval has enabled a greater consistency of immunohistochemical staining over a wide range of different fixatives and fixation times (Figs 21.13 and 21.14). Most individual laboratories will employ a single fixative used over a range of fixation

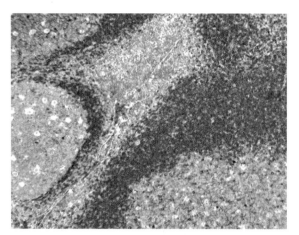

Fig. 21.13 Demonstration of IgM in a formalin-fixed paraffin-embedded section of reactive tonsil, using a labeled streptavidin–biotin immunoperoxidase technique with DAB as the chromogen.

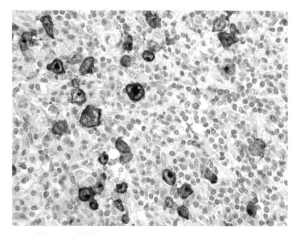

Fig. 21.14 CD30 demonstration in a formalin-fixed paraffin-embedded section of Hodgkin's disease. Note the strong staining of both membrane and Golgi apparatus.

times between 18 and 72 hours, for which a single standardized heat methodology can often be applied. For referral laboratories dealing with a wide range of material from different sources where the fixation regimes are unknown, more than one retrieval method may be necessary.

The advance in molecular technology has enabled the production of duplicate synthetic peptide sequences that survive routine processing techniques. One such peptide has been produced for the human CD3 antigen, fixed in a formalin fixative and subsequently used to raise a polyclonal antibody (Mason et al 1989). This reagent has proved to be successful in the detection of T-cells and related lymphomas in routinely processed paraffin sections. With the aid of either proteolytic digestion or heat antigen retrieval, polyclonal anti-CD3 is an excellent example of how immunohistochemistry has adapted to the prevailing conditions in histopathology.

Beyond the routine techniques there is occasion to employ other methods, usually in research or specialist laboratories. One such example is the demonstration of hormones and neuropeptides that require special fixation (Van Noorden et al 1986); for these hormones the use of freeze-dried material which is then vapor-fixed in *p*-benzoquinone or diethyl pyrocarbonate, and subsequently paraffin embedded, is recommended (Pearse & Polak 1975).

Method selection

The majority of immunohistochemists in the United Kingdom employ either a streptavidin–biotin system or a polymer chain two-step indirect method for routine work (data from the UK National External Quality Assessment Scheme for Immunocytochemistry). The peroxidase–diaminobenzidine reaction end-product, because of its resistance to processing to resinous mounting media and its long-term storage qualities, is also preferred. The storage qualities are particularly important when diagnoses are under review over prolonged periods of time.

Preparative techniques

Preparing paraffin wax sections for immunostaining

1. Cut 3–4 µm sections and place on clean electrostatically charged glass slides (we recommend Superfrost Plus slides). If using uncharged slides

an adhesive should be used. Commercial products such as APES or Vectabond are successful in assisting with section adhesion.

2. Dry the sections overnight in a 37°C incubator. Alternatively the sections may be placed on a hot-plate at 60°C for 15 minutes. Certain antigens, such as estrogen and progesterone receptors, show a reduction in staining when heated on a hot-plate and therefore this is not recommended.

3. Where possible sections should be cut fresh. Sections stored for several weeks prior to immunostaining may show reduced staining intensity. This is the case with estrogen and progesterone receptors.

4. Dewax sections in xylene and bring to absolute alcohol. Xylene substitutes such as Histoclear may be used. To ensure complete removal of wax the xylene/histoclear may be warmed to 37°C in an incubator.

5. If required, remove fixation pigments.

6. Block endogenous peroxidase activity by incubating in 0.5% hydrogen peroxide in methanol for 10 minutes. This stage may be performed after the primary antibody has been bound onto the antigenic site. It is thought by many users that the methanol/hydrogen peroxide step may slightly alter some of the more labile antigenic epitopes, leading to weak demonstration. We have certainly found this to be the case with the demonstration of CD2 and CD4 in paraffin sections.

7. Rehydrate, wash well in running water.

8. Perform the required/preferred antigen retrieval techniques as detailed below.

Antigen retrieval techniques

Proteolytic enzyme methods

The digestion media outlined below must be freshly prepared as their activity decreases with time. Digestion methods with proteolytic enzymes are usually limited to sections taken from formalin-fixed, paraffin-embedded tissues, in order to enable those antigens that are blocked by the cross-linking of the formalin fixative to be uncovered for binding to the relevant antibody. However, not all antigens are blocked and therefore do not require this treatment.

Optimal times for digestion are dependent on fixation parameters. These vary according to specimen size, temperature of fixative, duration of fixation, and the rate of penetration of the fixative. With such variables a fixed digestion time does not always achieve optimal staining. Usually a uniform time, established on controls, is used in the initial stages. Antibodies such as those for pan-cytokeratin will react to a satisfactory standard even when the digestion time is suboptimal, but others such as immunoglobulin light chains require a more precise methodology.

The following methods should be used as a guideline only; we would recommend that individual laboratories determine digestion times on their own material.

Trypsin/chymotrypsin methodology

1. Incubate sections in pre-warmed distilled water at 37°C.
2. Prepare 0.1% trypsin in 0.1% calcium chloride in distilled water (at 37°C). Adjust pH to 7.8 using 0.1 M sodium hydroxide solution.
3. Incubate the sections in the trypsin solution for 10 minutes at 37°C.
4. Wash sections in cold running tap water to prevent further digestion.
5. Proceed with the immunostaining method of choice.

N.B. A successful alternative to trypsin is chymotrypsin (Sigma C-4129) (Miller et al 1995).

Protease methodology

1. Incubate sections in pre-warmed distilled water at 37°C.
2. Prepare 0.1% protease (Sigma type XXIV, P-8038) in distilled water (at 37°C). Adjust pH to 7.8 using 1 M sodium hydroxide solution.
3. Incubate the sections in the protease solution for 6 minutes at 37°C.
4. Wash sections in cold running tap water to prevent further digestion.
5. Proceed with the immunostaining method of choice.

Using 0.05% protease may be preferred; by using a less concentrated solution the possibility of over-digesting the tissue sections is decreased. Digestion times will require increasing but are not as critical as with the 0.1% protease solution.

Pepsin methodology

1. Incubate sections in pre-warmed distilled water at 37°C.

2. Prepare 0.4% pepsin solution in 0.01 M hydrochloric acid (pH 2.0) at 37°C.
3. Incubate the sections in the pepsin solution for 15–60 minutes at 37°C.
4. Wash sections in cold running tap water to prevent further digestion.
5. Proceed with the immunostaining method of choice.

Certain antigens, e.g. basement membrane proteins, give improved staining if the digestion is performed by pepsin.

Heat-mediated antigen retrieval

There are now many heat retrieval methods employing different types of equipment and various retrieval solutions. The equipment includes: microwave oven, pressure cooker, steamer, autoclave, and water bath. Among the various solutions citrate buffer at pH 6.0, EDTA at pH 8.0, and Tris–EDTA (pH 9.9 or 10.0) are the most popular. However, commercial fluids with secret formulas are gaining popularity.

In order to prevent section damage or detachment (due to the vigorous boiling of the antigen retrieval solution) the sections should be picked up on electrostatically charged slides or on slides coated with a strong adhesive such as Vectabond (Vector Laboratories) or aminopropyltriethoxysilane (APES).

Microwave oven heating methodology
Large batch microwaving (see Fig. 21.6). Jessup reported in 1994 that it is possible to achieve relatively even exposure of antigen across the tissue section by heating 10 slides in a plastic slide rack in a deep microwavable container (e.g. Addis 9400) holding 600 ml of fluid. This method has since been developed and a maximum of 25 sections can be heated per batch. With this type of tall narrow container, the height of the fluid above the slides is such that no topping up is needed, as there is no risk of the slides drying out over a 30-minute heating cycle. A loose lid is required to reduce the volume of fluid lost, but allows the steam to escape.

1. Using a plastic staining rack, place up to 25 sections in 600 ml of 0.01 M citrate buffer, pH 6.0.
2. Irradiate on high power (800 W) for 22 minutes.
3. Carefully remove the container from the microwave oven and flood with cold water.
4. Proceed with the immunostaining method of choice.

For suboptimally fixed material we recommend reducing the volume of buffer to 400 ml and the heating time to 15 minutes.

Coplin jar method
Two or three slides are placed in a suitable buffer in a Coplin jar and covered with aerated cling-film and heated in a 800-W domestic microwave oven for 10 min (some antigens require 15 min, e.g. CD3) at full power, pausing only to top up the fluid. It is advisable to place a microwavable plastic tray under the Coplin jar in order to contain the spillage from boiling. Coplin jar methodology allows even exposure of antigens over uniform heating cycles, provided no more than three slides are heated at any one time.

This method may be preferred when using expensive commercial antigen retrieval buffers. However, we would recommend the large batch method for ease of use and consistency.

Pressure cooker antigen retrieval methodology
Use a 5-liter domestic stainless steel pressure cooker with an operating pressure of 15 psi. To bring the pressure cooker to boil use either a halogen hotplate or domestic electric hotplate (see Fig. 21.7). A maximum of three racks of 25 slides each can be pre-treated at one time.

1. Add 1.5 liters of appropriate antigen retrieval buffer into the pressure cooker and bring to the boil (without securing the lid).
2. When the antigen retrieval buffer is boiling, carefully place the slide racks into the hot solution and seal the lid.
3. Allow the pressure cooker to reach full pressure (15 psi), then incubate for 2 minutes—timing starts only when full pressure is reached.
4. Transfer the pressure cooker to a sink and run cold water over the lid until all of the pressure is released.
5. Flood the pressure cooker with cold water. Do not remove the slides until cool.
6. Proceed with the immunostaining method of choice.

Plastic pressure cookers are now available for heating in a microwave oven, but they have a lower operating pressure than the stainless steel versions and as a consequence the heating time at full pressure has to be significantly increased.

Steamer antigen retrieval methodology
This method uses a domestic rice steamer.

1. Place 1 liter of distilled water into the base of the steamer and insert a dry plate into the base.

2. Place steaming tray onto the dry tray.

3. Place the rice bowl into the steaming chamber.

4. Fill the incubation tray with 200 ml of appropriate antigen retrieval buffer and place in the chamber.

5. Place the lid onto the top of the steaming chamber.

6. Set the timer for 1 hour 15 minutes. The equilibration of the bath/rice chamber contents to 95°C is achieved after around 45 minutes.

7. Remove the lid and place the slides in the heated antigen retrieval buffer, then replace the lid.

8. Incubate sections for 30 minutes.

9. Remove the antigen retrieval buffer from the chamber and allow the sections to cool for 15 minutes.

10. Wash sections in water.

11. Proceed with the immunostaining method of choice.

Water bath antigen retrieval methodology

This method uses a conventional laboratory water bath.

1. Place the appropriate antigen retrieval buffer in a plastic Coplin jar.

2. Place the Coplin jar into the water bath and heat to 95–98°C (do not allow to boil).

3. Place slides into the pre-heated buffer and incubate for 30 minutes.

4. Remove the container from the water bath and allow to cool for 15 minutes at room temperature.

5. Wash sections in water.

6. Proceed with the immunostaining method of choice.

Autoclave antigen retrieval methodology

1. Add 250 ml of appropriate antigen retrieval buffer into the incubation chamber, place in the sections.

2. Place a lid over the incubation chamber to avoid excess evaporation.

3. Place the incubation chamber into the autoclave and close the lid.

4. Set the time for 15 minutes at 120°C.

5. Release the pressure, remove the incubation chamber, and flood with cold water.

6. Proceed with the immunostaining method of choice.

Combination of trypsin digestion and microwave antigen retrieval methodology

1. Incubate sections in pre-warmed distilled water at 37°C.

2. Prepare 0.1% trypsin in 0.1% calcium chloride in distilled water (at 37°C). Adjust pH to 7.8 using 0.1 M NaOH.

3. Incubate the sections in the trypsin solution for 30 seconds at 37°C.

4. Wash sections in cold running tap water to prevent further digestion.

5. Using a plastic staining rack, place sections in 600 ml of 0.01 M citrate buffer pH 6.0. Use a microwaveable plastic container.

6. Irradiate on high power (800 W) for 15 minutes.

7. Carefully remove the container from the microwave and flood with cold water.

8. Proceed with the immunostaining method of choice.

Examples of immunostaining protocols for routine diagnostic antigens

Testing all the clones available for a particular epitope would be too costly. Most manufacturers and suppliers provide a data sheet with each of their antibodies, which will give recommendations as to their use. If a more independent guide is sought then the *Manual of Diagnostic Antibodies for Immunohistology* by Leong et al (1999) is recommended.

The following information is based on the experiences of the University College London immunohistochemistry laboratory, the Hematological Malignancy Diagnostic Service, and the Department of Histopathology and Molecular Pathology at the Leeds Teaching Hospitals NHS Trust.

Immunohistochemistry for immunoglobulin light chains in formalin-fixed paraffin-wax sections

This is one of the most difficult of all techniques to perform. The retention of the immunoglobulin in the appropriate cells with good fixation is a prerequisite of producing good light chain demonstration. Furthermore, light chain restriction is an important criterion when identifying B-cell lymphoma, and this restriction is one of few markers of malignancy available to immunohistochemists today. Prompt fixation in either a buffered or unbuffered 10% formalin solution is essential. Lymph nodes and other dense lymphoid tissue should be sliced as soon as possible in order to facilitate the penetration of the fixative. Ideally, fixation of 18–72 hours is acceptable, but once fixation time is extended to several weeks, demonstration of light chain immunoglobulin becomes increasingly difficult.

Accuracy of staining has been verified by comparing immunohistochemical results on sections with flow cytometric analysis of fresh lymphoid tissue. Flow cytometric analysis requires fresh (not previously frozen) tissue to be perfused with an isotonic solution and any red cell contamination to be lysed with ammonium chloride. The lymphocytes are labeled with a fluorescently conjugated primary antibody, washed with an isotonic solution, and analyzed on a flow cytometer. Flow cytometric analysis is the optimum method for immunophenotyping lymphomas on fresh tissue; however, many laboratories do not have the resources to undertake this and many lymphomas present as formalin-fixed paraffin-embedded blocks.

Sections of reactive tonsil provide the ideal control material for light chain demonstration. Tonsil sections should show marked demonstration of the mantle zone and follicle center B-cells together with intense plasma cell staining (Fig. 21.15). The T-cell zone should have little staining. Background immunoglobulin, caused essentially by non-specific uptake, is seen on follicular dendritic cells, some connective tissue and epithelia.

On the test material, if there is any doubt, it is important to establish that small round B-cells are present with a series of B markers. This will usually assist with identifying B-cells at different maturation stages. Once achieved, immunoglobulin staining can be compared with the control section. If there are only a few plasma cells and little else staining then it is almost certain that the antigen retrieval has been under-achieved. Increasing the antigen retrieval times on duplicate sections will increase the reactivity, and perinuclear space and surface staining of the light chains on the B-cells will indicate optimal retrieval. In addition, intense cytoplasmic staining of immunoglobulin in plasma cells should be seen. Excessive antigen retrieval, either by heat or proteolytic digestion, will cause staining of large amounts of reticulin and could remove some of the cells and protein structures from the slide.

Reliable light chain demonstration on paraffin sections can be achieved using streptavidin–biotin methods or polymerase chain-based techniques, with diaminobenzidine as the preferred chromogen. We would recommend antigen retrieval using microwave oven heating with citrate buffer. However, results from the UK NEQAS Immunocytochemistry scheme show certain participants of the scheme achieving good results with proteolytic digestion, with combined microwave oven heating and trypsin digestion, and with the pressure cooker. The choice of antigen retrieval will depend upon the individual laboratory and their fixation and processing regimes. Polyclonal primary antibodies are recommended.

Immunohistochemistry on renal and skin biopsies

Direct immunofluorescence tests performed on skin biopsy and renal biopsy specimens to demonstrate specific patterns of immunoglobulin and complement deposition have clarified the diagnostic entities within the group of vesiculobullous diseases and glomerular nephritis. In glomerular nephritis there is usually immunoglobulin and complement deposition in relation to the glomerular basement membrane. The bullous lesions are thought to be caused by an autoimmune response producing large amounts of antibody that is deposited either on the epidermal basement membrane or intercellularly in the epidermis. The pemphigus group of diseases is characterized by antibodies, usually IgG, directed against the the intercellular substance of squamous epithelium. The pemphigoid group of bullous diseases is characterized by antibody, usually IgG, directed against the basement membrane zone (Figs 21.16 and 21.17).

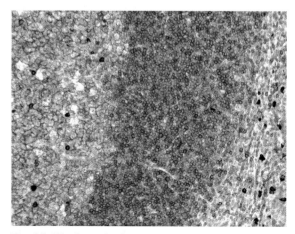

Fig. 21.15 Formalin-fixed paraffin-embedded section of reactive tonsil demonstrating kappa light chain immunoglobulins. Strong staining of plasma cells, follicular dendritic cells, and mantle zone B cells are clearly visible. Antigen rerieval using the microwave oven and citrate buffer pH 6.0.

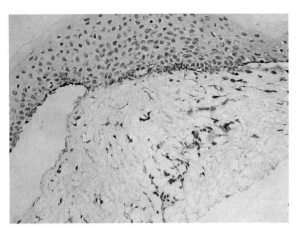

Fig. 21.16 Formalin-fixed paraffin wax-processed section of skin with a bullous pemphigoid blister, immunostained for IgG using protease digestion and an indirect technique. The bullous lesion and basement membrane clearly show IgG deposition.

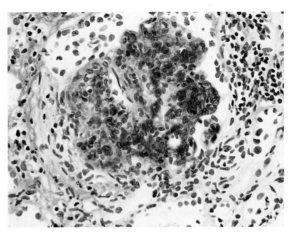

Fig. 21.18. Formalin-fixed paraffin wax-processed section of renal biopsy with IgA nephropathy, immunostained for IgA using protease digestion and labeled with an indirect immunoperoxidase staining method. IgA is clearly demonstrated.

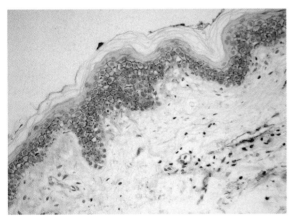

Fig. 21.17 IgG demonstration in a bullous pemphigus formalin-fixed paraffin-embedded section of skin.

McIver and Mepham reported in 1982 that immunoperoxidase was their established method for demonstrating immunocomplexes in renal biopsies. Also in the same year Turbitt et al described an immunoperoxidase method to demonstrate autoantibodies in the bullous lesions of pemphigoid and pemphigus.

Today, even with the disadvantage of having to split the biopsy for frozen and paraffin processing (and for electron microscopy for renals), the method of choice for many, certainly in the UK, is still frozen section immunofluorescence coupled with paraffin section morphology.

While the frozen fluorescence technique requires a high degree of skill, there is no doubt that the paraffin-wax method provides a difficult technical challenge. Furthermore, such is the capriciousness of this method that maintaining the standards of an established immunoperoxidase technique for these purposes requires a dedicated and highly skilled immunohistochemist. There are some important reasons why opinion is divided as to the preferred technique.

Wax-embedded paraffin sections of renal biopsies

In most cases renal disease affects the glomeruli. Hence this is an important technique especially when glomeruli are absent in the portion selected for fluorescence and electron microscopy, but are found in the paraffin-processed sample. It is essential that proteolytic digestion is employed, and an indirect peroxidase labeling system is recommended as this avoids endogenous biotin staining. In addition relatively inexpensive polyclonal antibodies can be used effectively at extremely high dilutions (Figs 21.18 and 21.19).

Protocol outline

1. Fix for 3–24 hours in a formalin fixative, e.g. 10% formal saline, 10% neutral buffered formalin.

2. Proteolytic digestion is necessary and is best achieved by using 0.1% protease type XXIV (Sigma) for 45 minutes.

3. Non-immune serum is essential, especially when polyclonal antibodies are employed.

4. Polyclonal antibodies, as described in Table 21.2, are used at high dilutions for 60 minutes followed by swine anti-rabbit peroxidase-labeled secondary antibody for 25 minutes. A high-quality DAB is employed as the chromogen (Dakocytomation DAB+).

An alternative protocol was published by Boyd SM and Ronan JE (Dakofacts Vol. 8. No. 1) using trypsin digestion with Envision reagents.

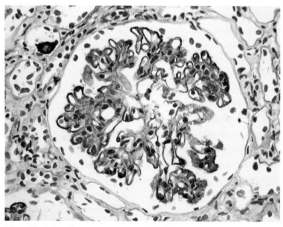

Fig. 21.19   Demonstration of IgG membranous nephropathy in a formalin-fixed paraffin-embedded renal biopsy.

Immunoperoxidase staining method for formalin-fixed paraffin wax-embedded skin biopsies

Reports suggest (W. Merchant, personal communication) that this technique can be effective on paraffin sections. However, it must be considered one of the most capricious methods employed by immunohistochemists today. Direct immunofluorescence on frozen sections is generally preferred as its relatively low level of sensitivity, compared with avidin–biotin peroxidase, reduces the labeling of non-specifically bound immunoglobulins and complement in the various tissue elements. The following immunoperoxidase protocol (Saaeda, personal communication) has, at the time of writing, proved to be successful in a number of cases, but is not always reliable.

Protocol outline

1. Fix for 3–24 hours in formalin, e.g. 10% formal saline, 10% neutral buffered formalin, and routinely process to paraffin wax.

2. Cut sections at 3–4 μm onto Superfrost Plus slides and dry overnight at 37°C.

3. Treat sections with 0.1% protease XXIV (Sigma) in Tris-buffered saline, pH 7.6, for 10 min.

4. Minimize non-specific binding by treating sections with 10% casein solution (Vector Laboratories) for 10 minutes.

5. Incubate sections in primary antibody at the dilutions shown in Table 21.3 for 30 minutes.

6. Treat sections with ChemMate EnVision (DakoCytomation) reagent for 30 minutes.

7. Visualise with DAB+ (DakoCytomation) for 5 minutes.

Table 21.2	Immunocomplexes in renal biopsies			
Antibody	**Species**	**Supplier**	**Dilution**	**Pretreatment**
IgA	Rabbit	Dakocytomation	1/20000	Protease
IgM	Rabbit	Dakocytomation	1/500	Protease
IgG	Rabbit	Dakocytomation	1/20000	Protease
C3c	Rabbit	Dakocytomation	1/800	Protease
Clq	Rabbit	Dakocytomation	1/400	Protease
Fibrinogen	Rabbit	Dakocytomation	1/30000	Protease
Kappa	Rabbit	Dakocytomation	1/20000	Protease

Table 21.3 Immunocomplexes in skin biopsies

Antibody	Species	Supplier	Dilution	Pretreatment
IgA	Rabbit	Dakocytomation	1/25,000	Protease
IgG	Rabbit	Dakocytomation	1/25,000	Protease
IgM	Rabbit	Dakocytomation	1/20,000	Protease
C1q	Rabbit	Dakocytomation	1/10,000	Protease
C3c	Rabbit	Dakocytomation	1/20,000	Protease
Fibrinogen	Rabbit	Dakocytomation	1/30,000	Protease
Lambda	Rabbit	Dakocytomation	1/20,000	Protease

8. Besides using positive controls for each particular antibody it is essential that normal skin should always be employed to monitor the background levels.

This highly sensitive method ensures good labeling of dilute primary antibody binding to the target. The background levels of normal non-specifically bound immunoglobulins and complement are subdued. This latter point is achieved because the high dilutions of primary antibody, coupled with the short incubation times and Tween TBS washes, insure weak labeling of the less concentrated non-specific uptake staining that so often causes considerable interpretation difficulties. In Fig. 21.16 the basement membrane is quite clearly positive for IgG.

Frozen section immunofluorescence

Advantages of this method are:

1. It usually involves a simple, rapid, and sensitive direct technique.
2. It is easily reproduced.
3. Histopathologists, experienced with fluorescent antibody techniques in renal and skin biopsies, find little difficulty with interpretation.

Disadvantages are:

1. The production of good-quality frozen sections from small biopsies sometimes requires a high degree of skill.
2. A fluorescence microscope is required.
3. Immunofluorescent labeling has poor storage qualities, and can often fade within days of the sections being immunostained.

4. The morphology of the tissue is not easily seen, and hence a substantial part of the biopsy is processed to paraffin wax.

Paraffin-wax section immunoperoxidase

Advantages:

1. All or a substantial part of the biopsy (except for renals where a small portion is processed for electron microscopy) is formalin fixed and paraffin processed.
2. Immunolocalization and morphology are clearly seen in the same section.
3. Peroxidase has good long-term storage qualities, especially if diaminobenzidine chromogen is employed.
4. An expensive fluorescence microscope is not required.
5. Processing, section cutting, and storage of blocks are compatible with a routine diagnostic service.

Disadvantages:

1. A more time-consuming, sensitive technique, employing proteolytic enzyme antigen retrieval, is required.
2. Proteolytic digestion must be tailored to fixation time.
3. The technique requires a high degree of skill to insure a reliable level of reproducibility.
4. To the experienced histopathologist interpretation offers little difficulty. However, for those with experience of only frozen-section immunofluorescence, paraffin-wax immunoperoxidase interpretation is more difficult.

Immunohistochemistry on frozen section and non-gynecological cytology smears

Frozen sections

1. Cut 6-μm frozen sections and place on Superfrost Plus microscope slides or adhesive-coated slides.
2. Air dry the sections at room temperature overnight (in urgent cases dry for a minimum of 1–2 hours).
3. Fix sections in absolute acetone at room temperature for 20 minutes. Allow sections to air dry. If required the sections may be stored at this stage at −20°C or lower. Prior to storage, the slides should be wrapped in foil and then placed in the freezer with a desiccant. When required, the sections should be allowed to return to room temperature before unwrapping.
4. Rehydrate in TBS, apply optimally diluted primary antibody. Antibodies should be diluted in TBS; avoid the use of commercial antibody diluents or the use of detergents such as Triton or Tween. Chromatolysis and loss of nuclear membranes on frozen sections is compounded by the action of detergents.
5. For frozen sections an endogenous peroxidase-blocking step is not included, as this can be damaging to the antigens to be demonstrated. The use of a negative control for the identification of endogenous peroxidase activity is preferable. If the endogenous peroxidase activity is excessive then an alternative enzyme tracer, such as alkaline phosphatase, should be considered.

Cytology preparations

Smears, imprints, cytospins, etc. should be air dried for 1–3 hours and then fixed or stored as outlined for frozen sections.

Immunohistochemical staining techniques

Avidin–biotin techniques

In these techniques either peroxidase or alkaline phosphatase may be used as the enzyme label.

Labeled streptavidin/streptavidin–biotin complex technique for monoclonal antibodies

1. Rinse sections in TBS, incubate in 10% casein solution for 10 minutes.
2. Drain off excess casein.
3. Incubate in optimally diluted primary antibody for 60 minutes.
4. Wash slides in TBS.
5. Incubate in optimally diluted biotinylated secondary antibody for 30 minutes.
6. Wash slides in TBS.
7. Incubate in optimally prepared labeled streptavidin or streptavidin–biotin complex for 30 minutes. When using a streptavidin–biotin complex the reagents should be mixed 30 minutes before use in order for the complex to form.
8. Wash slides in TBS.
9. Incubate in DAB substrate solution.
10. Wash in running water, counterstain in hematoxylin, dehydrate, clear, and mount.

Modifications required for rabbit primary antibody

Step 5. Replace with biotinylated swine anti-rabbit secondary. Many of the commercial streptavin–biotin kits are supplied with a multi-species secondary link which can be used for both mouse and rabbit primary antibodies.

N.B. When using a goat primary antibody an appropriate biotinylated secondary antibody raised against the goat species must be used.

Polymer techniques

Dakocytomation envision detection technique

1. Rinse sections in TBS, incubate in 10% casein solution for 10 minutes.
2. Drain off excess casein.
3. Apply optimally diluted primary monoclonal antibody for 60 minutes.
4. Wash slides in TBS.
5. Incubate with Envision polymer reagent for 30 minutes.
6. Wash slides in TBS.
7. Incubate in freshly prepared DAB solution for 10 minutes.
8. Rinse in TBS and transfer to running water.
9. Counterstain in hematoxylin, dehydrate, clear, and mount.

Novolink polymer detection technique

1. Following antigen retrieval, rinse sections in TBS.
2. Drain off excess TBS and block endogenous peroxidase activity using Peroxidase Block RE7101, for 5 minutes.
3. Wash in TBS for 5 minutes.
4. Incubate with Protein Block RE 7102 for 5 minutes.
5. Wash in TBS.
6. Apply optimally diluted primary antibody for 60 minutes.
7. Wash slides in TBS.
8. Incubate with Post Primary Block RE7111 for 30 minutes.
9. Wash slides in TBS.
10. Incubate with Novolink Polymer RE7112 for 30 minutes.
11. Wash slides in TBS.
12. Incubate in freshly prepared DAB solution for 10 minutes.
13. Rinse in TBS and transfer to running water.
14. Counterstain in hematoxylin, dehydrate, clear, and mount.

Tyramide signal amplification techniques

Tyramide signal amplification of the labeled streptavidin biotin method

1. Rinse sections in TBS, incubate in 10% casein solution for 10 minutes.
2. Drain off excess casein.
3. Incubate in optimally diluted primary antibody for 60 minutes.
4. Wash slides in TBS.
5. Incubate in optimally diluted biotinylated secondary antibody for 20 minutes.
6. Wash slides in TBS.
7. Incubate in labeled streptavidin (or streptavidin–biotin complex) for 20 minutes.
8. Wash slides in TBS.
9. Incubate slides in biotinylated tyramide reagent for 5 minutes.
10. Wash in TBS.
11. Re-incubate sections in labeled streptavidin (or streptavidin–biotin complex) for 20 minutes.

12. Wash slides in TBS.
13. Incubate in DAB substrate solution.
14. Wash in running water, counterstain in hematoxylin, dehydrate, clear, and mount.

N.B. The incubation in biotinylated tyramide should be strictly adhered to, otherwise unacceptably high levels of background staining can be encountered.

Dakocytomation CSAII detection method

1. Rinse sections in TBS, incubate in 10% casein solution for 10 minutes.
2. Drain off excess casein.
3. Incubate in optimally diluted primary antibody for 15–60 minutes.
4. Wash slides in TBS.
5. Apply anti-mouse immunoglobulins–HRP reagent for 15 minutes.
6. Wash slides in TBS.
7. Incubate in amplification reagent for 15 minutes. *N.B.* This incubation should be undertaken in the dark.
8. Wash slides in TBS.
9. Apply anti-fluorescein–HRP for 15 minutes.
10. Wash slides in TBS.
11. Incubate in DAB substrate solution.
12. Wash in running water, counterstain in hematoxylin, dehydrate, clear, and mount.

Alkaline phosphatase techniques

Alkaline phosphatase–anti-alkaline phosphatase (APAAP) for monoclonal antibodies

1. Rinse sections in TBS.
2. Drain off excess TBS and incubate in 10% casein for 10 minutes.
3. Incubate in primary antibody at optimal dilution for 30–40 minutes.
4. Wash in TBS.
5. Incubate in optimally diluted unconjugated rabbit anti-mouse bridge antibody for 30 minutes.
6. Wash in TBS.

7. Incubate in alkaline phosphatase–anti-alkaline phosphatase complex at the optimal dilution for 30 minutes.
8. Wash in TBS.
9. Incubate in substrate medium of choice, for example fast red solution.
10. Wash in running tap water.
11. Counterstain and mount as desired.

Notes

a. The reaction end-product may be enhanced by repeating steps 5–8 once or twice with a reduction of the incubation times to 10 minutes.
b. As the alkaline phosphatase label is usually intestinal, it is resistant to blocking with levamisole at the concentrations described and hence it is included in the substrate mixture. Levamisole blocks most other types of alkaline phosphatase.

Immunogold techniques

These techniques lend themselves to electron microscopy more than to the light microscope. The labeling intensity of gold alone, even using 20 nm colloidal gold, is usually not sufficiently intense to be of value for light microscopy. However, the work of Holgate et al (1983a,b) showed that silver enhancement increased the sensitivity of the method considerably. The Lugol's iodine and thiosulfate step appears to be essential for this technique to work on routinely processed paraffin sections. This method uses serum bovine serum albumin in Tris buffered saline (BSA–TBS).

Indirect immunogold technique for monoclonal antibodies

Method

1. Take sections to distilled water.
2. Treat sections with Lugol's iodine for 5 minutes, clear with 2.5% sodium thiosulfate, and then wash well in running tap water.
3. Take sections to BSA–TBS (0.1% bovine serum albumin in TBS, pH 8.2), drain and wipe off excess around section.
4. Incubate in 1/20 normal goat serum (NGS) in BSA–TBS for 10 minutes.
5. Drain, wipe off excess serum.

6. Incubate in primary antibody optimally diluted in BSA–TBS for 30–60 minutes.
7. Gently wash in TBS.
8. Incubate in gold-conjugated secondary antibody at optimal dilution in BSA–TBS for 60 minutes.
9. Repeat step 7.
10. Wash in 0.1 M phosphatase buffered saline (PBS), pH 7.6, for three 2-minute changes.
11. Post-fix with 2% glutaraldehyde in PBS for 10–15 minutes.
12. Wash well in several changes of distilled water and enhance staining with silver. (See silver enhancement procedure below.)
13. Counterstain, dehydrate, clear, and mount.

Silver enhancement

The intensity of the gold label may be enhanced by incubation of the sections in a silver solution.

Solutions

a. **Citrate buffer stock solution**

Trisodium citrate	23.5 g
Citric acid	25.5 g
Distilled water	100 ml

b. **Silver solution**

Silver lactate	110 mg
Distilled water	15 ml
Prepare fresh.	

c. **Hydroquinone solution**

Hydroquinone	950 mg
Distilled water	15 ml
Prepare fresh.	

d. **Gum acacia**

50% gum acacia solution	7 ml

e. **Silver enhancement solution**

Silver lactate solution	15 ml
Hydroquinone solution	15 ml
Molar citrate buffer	10 ml
Distilled water	60 ml
50% gum acacia solution	7 ml

Method

1. Rinse the sections in 0.2 M citrate buffer for 2 minutes.
2. Incubate the sections in freshly prepared silver enhancement solution at room temperature,

protected from the light. Development will take place in approximately 5 minutes.

3. Wash well in distilled water.
4. Wash in 2% sodium thiosulphate, 1 minute.
5. Wash well in running water.
6. Counterstain if desired.
7. Dehydrate, clear, and mount.

Visualization substrates for alkaline phosphatase methods

The methods for the visualization of alkaline phosphatase activity are based on the coupling of substituted naphthol to a suitable azo dye. The most commonly used dyes are fast red TR and hexazotized new fuchsin. Nitro-blue tetrazolium methods are also gaining popularity, as they seem to be most sensitive. The following is recommended for histological preparations.

Fast red TR solution

Naphthol-AS-MX phosphate, free acid	4.0 mg
N,N-dimethyl formamide	0.2 ml
Molar Tris–HCl buffer, pH 8.2	9.8 ml
Levamisole	2.4 mg
Fast red TR salt	10 mg

Dissolve the naphthol-AS-MX phosphate in N,N-dimethyl formamide in a glass vial and then add the Tris buffer. Add and dissolve the levamisole and fast red TR salt and immediately filter onto the sections. Incubate the sections for 10–20 minutes and, as the bright red reaction product is soluble in alcohol, mount in an aqueous medium. A blue reaction product can be obtained by using 4 mg fast blue BB instead of fast red TR salt in the above recipe. Counterstaining with hematoxylin would not be appropriate with blue salt.

Alternative fast red substrate solution recommended for cytological preparations

This solution described by Ponder and Wilkinson (1981) would appear to be more effective against endogenous alkaline phosphatase in pleural aspirates than the previous solution (Happerfield, personal communication).

Solution

Naphthol AS-BI phosphoric acid sodium salt	5.0 mg
N,N-dimethyl formamide	0.2 ml
Veronal acetate buffer, pH 9.2	9.8 ml
Levamisole	2.5 mg
Fast red TR salt	5.0 mg

This solution is prepared by dissolving the naphthol AS-BI in N,N-dimethyl formamide in a glass vial. Add the buffer, levamisole, and mix. Immediately before staining, dissolve the fast red salt in the substrate solution and filter before use.

Hexazotized new fuchsin
(Malik & Daymon 1982)

Naphthol-AS-BI phosphate	5.0 mg
N,N-dimethyl formamide	60 µl
Molar Tris–HCl buffer, pH 8.7	10 ml
Molar levamisole	10 µl
4% sodium nitrite (freshly prepared)	50 µl
5% new fuchsin in 2 M HCl	20 µl

Add the new fuchsin to the sodium nitrite, mix for 30–60 seconds and then add the Tris buffer and levamisole. Immediately before staining, add the naphthol AS-BI phosphate, dissolved in the N,N-dimethyl formamide, and filter directly onto the sections. Incubate for 20 minutes. The reaction end-product is bright red, but whilst this is considered to be resistant to dehydration, clearing in xylene, and mounting in resinous mounting media, it is not always consistent. Therefore, it is advisable to water-mount. A modified new fuchsin method proposed by Stein et al in 1985 is more complex than the first, but many users agree that the final reaction product is much more intense.

Modified new fuchsin method

Solution 1	
Molar 2-amino-2-methy-1,3-propanediol	18 ml
Molar Tris–HCl buffer, pH 9.7	50 ml
Sodium chloride	600 mg
Levamisole	28 mg
Solution 2	
Naphthol AS-BI phosphate	35 mg
N,N-dimethyl formamide	0.42 ml

Dissolve the naphthol AS-BI phosphate in *N,N*-dimethyl formamide.

Solution 3

New fuchsin (5 g in 100 ml 2 N HCl)   0.14 ml

Sodium nitrite (freshly prepared, 40 mg in 1 ml distilled water) 0.35 ml

Mix the new fuchsin with the freshly prepared sodium nitrite and incubate this mixture for 60 seconds at room temperature whilst agitating.

Mix solutions 1 and 2 and then add solution 3. Adjust the pH to 8.7 by adding HCl. Mix well, filter through ordinary filter paper directly onto slides, and incubate for 20 minutes.

Nitro blue tetrazolium method for alkaline phosphatase (McGadey 1970)

Buffer solution

0.2 M Tris–HCl, pH 9.5, containing 10 mM MgCl$_2$

Solution A

5 mg 5-bromo-4-chloro-3-indolyl phosphate (BCIP) is dissolved in 0.1 ml dimethyl formamide (DMF) and then in 1.0 ml of the above buffer.

Solution B

5 mg nitro-blue tetrazolium is dissolved in 0.1 ml DMF.

Solutions A and B are added, with continuous stirring, to 30 ml of the above buffer and filtered. Once filtered, incubate immediately for 20 minutes. The intense blue–black reaction product at the site of alkaline phosphatase activity is soluble in alcohol and xylene, hence aqueous mounting is recommended.

More detailed descriptions of these and various other methods are available in many books published on immunohistochemical methodology (Bullock & Petrusz 1982, 1983, 1985; Polak & Van Noorden 1986; Jasani & Schmid 1993; Kirkham & Hall 1995).

Double staining

The aim is to immunolabel two antigenic sites each with a distinct probe so that the site of each antigen of interest can be unequivocally determined in a single preparation. Any antigen that can be immunolabeled by light microscopy can be detected in multiple immunolabeling studies. In theory any number of antigens can be immunolabeled in one preparation provided distinct antibody labels are used to localize each antigen. Antibody labels for multiple antibody labeling should provide sufficient contrast to be easily distinguishable from each other at all magnifications. The most important considerations in the successful performance of double labeling techniques are to select two different immunohistochemical visualization systems which do not show cross-reactivity and which are preferably commercially available, and to select two different chromogens which show maximum color contrast and which allow discrimination between a mixed color at sites of co-localization and the separate colors. All types of double staining methods have to satisfy these two important demands.

Acknowledgments

Graham Robinson contributed the origins of this chapter for the second edition. In the third edition Graham Robinson, Ken Maclennan, and Ian Ellis updated it. Keith Miller revised it for the fourth and fifth editions. Our acknowledgments are due to them for their contributions.

REFERENCES

Adams J.C. (1992) Biotin amplification of horseradish peroxidase in histochemical stains. Journal of Histochemistry and Cytochemistry 40:1457–1463.

Banks P.M. (1979) Diagnostic applications of an immunoperoxidase method in hematopathology. Journal of Histochemistry and Cytochemistry 27:1192.

Bell P.B., Rundquist I., Svenson I., Collins U.P. (1987) Formaldehyde sensitivity of a GFAP epitope removed by extraction of the cytoskeleton with high salt. Journal of Histochemistry and Cytochemistry 35:1375–1380.

Bigbee J.W., Kosek J.C., Eng L.E. (1977) The effects of primary antiserum dilution on staining of 'antigen-rich' tissue with the peroxidase anti-peroxidase technique. Journal of Histochemistry and Cytochemistry 25(6):443–447.

Bobrow M.N., Harris T.D., Shaughnessy K.J., Litt G.J. (1989) Catalysed reporter deposition, a novel method of signal amplification in a variety of formats. Journal of Immunological Methods 125:279–285.

Bobrow M.N., Litt G.J., Shaughnessy K.J. et al. (1992) The use of catalyzed reporter deposition as a means of signal amplification in a variety of formats. Journal of Immunological Methods 150(1–2):145–149.

Bondi A., Chieregatti G., Eusebi V. et al. (1982) The use of β-galactosidase as a tracer in immunohistochemistry. Histochemistry 76(2):153–158.

Brandtzaeg P. (1983) Tissue preparation methods for immunocytochemistry. In: Bullock G.R., Petrusz P., eds.

Techniques in immunocytochemistry. New York, Academic Press, Vol. 1, pp. 1–75.

Brooks S.A., Leathem A.J.C., Schumacher U. (1996) Lectin histochemistry. Microscopy handbook 36. Oxford: Bios Scientific Publishers.

Bullock G.R., Petrusz P., eds. (1982) Techniques in immunocytochemistry, Vol. 1. New York: Academic Press.

Bullock G.R., Petrusz, P., eds. (1983) Techniques in immunocytochemistry, Vol. 2. New York; Academic Press.

Bullock G.R., Petrusz P., eds. (1985) Techniques in immunocytochemistry, Vol. 3. New York; Academic Press.

Capra J.D., Edmundson A.B. (1977) The antibody combining site. Scientific American 236(1):50–59.

Cattoretti G., Pileri S., Parravicini C. (1993) Antigen unmasking on formalin-fixed paraffin embedded tissue sections. Journal of Pathology 171(2):83–98.

Charalambous C., Singh N., Isaacson P.G. (1993) Immunohistochemical analysis of Hodgkin's disease using microwave heating. Journal of Clinical Pathology 46(12):1085–1088.

Coons A.H., Creech H.J., Jones R.N. (1941) Immunological properties of an antibody containing a fluorescent group. Proceedings of the Society of Experimental Biology and Medicine 47:200–202.

Cordell J.L., Falini B., Erber W. et al. (1984) Immunoenzymatic labelling of monoclonal antibodies using immune complexes of alkaline phosphatase and monoclonal anti-alkaline phosphatase (APAAP complexes). Journal of Histochemistry and Cytochemistry 32(2):219–229.

Curran R.C., Gregory J. (1977) The unmasking of antigens in paraffin sections of tissue by trypsin. Experientia 33(10):1400.

Damjanov I. (1987) Biology of disease, lectin cytochemistry and histochemistry. Laboratory Investigations 57:5–20.

Delellis R.A., Sternberger L.A., Mann R.B. et al. (1979) Immunoperoxidase techniques in diagnostic pathology. American Journal of Clinical Pathology 71(5):483.

De Mey J., Moeremans M. (1986) Raising and testing polyclonal antibodies for immunocytochemistry. In: Polack J.M., Van Noorden S., eds. Immunocytochemistry: modern methods and applications. Bristol: Wright, pp. 3–12.

De Mey J., Hacker G.W., Dewaele M., Springall D.R. (1986) Gold probes in light microscope. In: Polak J.M., Van Noorden S., eds. Immunocytochemistry: modern methods and applications, 2nd edn. Bristol: Wright, pp. 71–88.

Denk H., Syre G., Weirich E. (1977) Immunomorphologic methods in routine pathology. Application of immunofluorescence and the unlabeled antibody–enzyme (peroxidase–antiperoxidase) technique to formalin fixed paraffin embedded kidney biopsies. Beiträge zur Pathologie 160(2):187–194.

Ellis I.O., Bell J., Bancroft J.D. (1988) An investigation of optimal gold particle size for immunohistological immuno-gold and immunogold–silver staining. Journal of Histochemistry and Cytochemistry 36(1):121–122.

Engvall E., Perlman P. (1971) Enzyme-linked immunosorbent assay (ELISA). Qualitative assay of immunoglobulin G. Immunochemistry 8(9):871–874.

Erber W.N., Willis J.I., Hoffman G.J. (1997) An enhanced immunocytochemical method for staining bone marrow trephine sections. J Clin Pathol 50(5):389–393.

Faulk W.P., Taylor G.M. (1971) An immunocolloid method for the electron microscope. Immunochemistry 8(11):1081–1083.

Gatter K.C., Falini B., Mason D.Y. (1984) The use of monoclonal antibodies in histopathological diagnosis. In: Antony P.P., MacSween R.N.M., eds. Recent advances in histopathology, Vol. 12. Edinburgh: Churchill Livingstone, pp. 35–67.

Gerdes J., Becher M.H.G., Key G., Cattoretti G. (1992) Immunohistological detection of tumour growth fraction (Ki67) in formalin fixed and routinely processed tissues. Journal of Pathology 168:85–87.

Graham R.C., Karnovsky M.J. (1966) The early stages of absorption of injected horseradish peroxidase in the proximal tubules of mouse kidney: ultrastructural cytochemistry by a new technique. Journal of Histochemistry and Cytochemistry 4:291.

Graham R.C. Jr, Ladholm U., Karnovsky M.J. (1965) Cytochemical demonstration of peroxidase activity by 3-amino-9-ethylcarbazole. Journal of Histochemistry and Cytochemistry 13:150–152.

Grube D. (1980) Immunoreactivities of gastrin (G) cells II. Non-specific binding of immunoglobulins to G-cells by ionic interactions. Histochemistry 65(3):223–237.

Gu J., De Mey J., Moeremans M., Polak J.M. (1981) Sequential use of the PAP and immunogold staining methods for the light microscopical double staining of tissue antigens. Regulatory Peptides 1:365–374.

Guesden J.L., Terynck T., Avrameas S. (1979) The use of avidin–biotin interaction in immunoenzymatic techniques. Journal of Histochemistry and Cytochemistry 8:1131–1139.

Hanker J.S., Yates P.E., Metx C.B., Rustini A. (1977) A new specific, sensitive and non-carcinogenic reagent for the demonstration of horseradish peroxidase procedures. Journal of Histochemistry 9:789–792.

Hartman B.K. (1973) Immunofluorescence of dopamine B hydroxylase. Application of improved methodology to the localization of the peripheral and central noradrenergic nervous system. Journal of Histochemistry and Cytochemistry 21:312–332.

Heggeness M.H., Ash J.F. (1977) Use of the avidin–biotin complex for the localization of actin and myosin with fluorescence microscopy. Journal of Cell Biology 73:783.

Heyderman E., Monaghan P. (1979) Immunoperoxidase reactions in resin embedded sections. Investigative Cell Pathology 2:119–122.

Holgate C., Jackson P., Cowen P., Bird C. (1983a) Immuno-gold–silver staining: new method of immunostaining with enhanced sensitivity. Journal of Histochemistry and Cytochemistry 31:938–944.

Holgate C., Jackson P., Lauder I. et al. (1983b) Surface membrane staining of immunoglobulins in paraffin sections of non-Hodgkin's lymphomas using immunogold–silver staining techniques. Journal of Clinical Pathology 36:742–746.

Hsu S.M., Soban E. (1982) Colour modification of diaminobenzidine (DAB) precipitation by metalic ions and its application to double immunohistochemistry. Journal of Histochemistry and Cytochemistry 30:1079–1082.

Hsu S.M., Raine L., Fanger H. (1981) Use of avidin–biotin–peroxidase complex (ABC) in immunoperoxidase techniques: a comparison between ABC and unlabeled antibody (PAP) procedures. Journal of Histochemistry and Cytochemistry 29:577–580.

Huang S., Minassian H., More, J.D. (1976) Application of immunofluorescent staining in paraffin sections improved by trypsin digestion. Laboratory Investigation 35:383–391.

Hunt S.P., Allanson J., Mantyh P.W. (1986) Radioimmunochemistry. In: Polak J.M., Van Noorden S., eds. Immunocytochemistry. Modern methods and applications, 2nd edn. Bristol: Wright, pp. 99–114.

Jasani B., Schmid K.W. (1993) Immunocytochemistry in diagnostic pathology. Edinburgh: Churchill Livingstone.

Jasani B., Wynford-Thomas D., Williams E.D. (1981) Use of monoclonal anti-hapten antibodies for immunolocalisation of tissue antigens. Journal of Clinical Pathology 34:1000–1002.

Jasani B., Thomas N.D., Navabi H., et al. (1992) Dinitrophenol (DNP) hapten sandwich staining (DHSS) procedure. A 10 year review of its principle reagents and applications. Journal of Immunological Methods 150:193–198.

Jessup E. (1994) Antigen retrieval techniques for the demonstration immunoglobulin light chains in formalin-fixed paraffin was embedded sections. UK. NEQAS Newsletter 4:12–16.

Kaplow L.S. (1975) Substitute for benzidine in myeloperoxidase stains. American Journal of Clinical Pathology 63:451.

Kawai K., Scrizawa A., Hamana T., Tsutsumi Y. (1994) Heat induced antigen retrieval of proliferating cell nuclear antigen and p53 protein in formalin fixed paraffin embedded sections. Pathology International 44:759–764.

King G., Payne S., Walker F., Murray G.I. (1997) A highly sensitive detection method for immunohistochemistry using biotinylated tyramine. Journal of Pathology 183(2):237–241.

Kirkham N., Hall P., eds. (1995) Progress in pathology. Edinburgh: Churchill Livingstone.

Kohler G., Milstein C. (1975) Continuous cultures of fused cells producing antibody of pre-defined specificity. Nature 256:495–497.

Kraehenbuhl J.P., Jamieson J.D. (1974) Localisation of intracellular antigens by immunoelectron microscopy. International Review of Experimental Pathology 12:1–53.

Langlois N.E.I., King G., Herriot R., Thompson W.D. (1994) Non enzymatic retrieval of antigen permits staining of follicle centre cells by the rabbit polyclonal antibody to protein gene product 9.5. Journal of Pathology 173:249–253.

Leatham A. (1986) Lectin histochemistry. In: Polak J.M., Van Noorden S., eds. Immunocytochemistry: modern methods and applications, 2nd end. Bristol: Wright, pp. 167–187.

LeBrun D.P., Kamel O.W., Dorfman R.F., Warnke R.A. (1992) Enhanced staining for Leu M1 (CD15) in Hodgkin's disease using a secondary antibody specific for immunoglobulin M. American Journal of Clinical Pathology 97:135–138.

Leong A.S.-Y. Cooper K., Leong F.J.W.-M. (1999) Manual of diagnostic antibodies for immunohistology. London: Greenwich Medical Media.

Malik N.J., Daymon M.E. (1982) Improved double immunoenzymatic labelling using alkaline phosphatase and horseradish peroxidase. Journal of Clinical Pathology 35:1092–1094.

Mangham D.C., Isaacson P.G. (1999) A novel immunohistochemistry detection system using minor image complementory antibodies (MICA). Histopathology 32:129–133.

Mason D., Sammons R.E. (1978) Alkaline phosphatase and peroxidase for double immunoenzymatic labelling of cellular constituents. Journal of Clinical Pathology 31:454–462.

Mason D.Y., Woolston R.E. (1982) Double immunoenzymatic labelling. In: Bullock G.R., Petrusz P., eds. Techniques in immunocytochemistry, Vol. 1. New York: Academic Press, pp. 135–152.

Mason D.Y., Abdulaziz Z., Falini B., Stein H. (1983) Double immunoenzymatic labelling. In: Polak J., Van Noorden S., eds. Immunocytochemistry: practical applications in pathology and biology. Bristol: Wright, pp. 113–128.

Mason D.Y., Cordell J., Brown M. et al. (1989) Detection of cells in paraffin wax embedded tissue using antibodies against a peptide sequence from the CD3 antigen. Journal of Clinical Pathology 42:1194–1200.

Mason J.T., O'Leary T.J. (1991) Effects of formaldehyde fixation on protein secondary structure: a calorimetric and infrared spectroscopic investigation. Journal of Histochemistry and Cytochemistry 39(2):225–229.

Mason T.E., Pfifer R.F., Spicer S.S. et al. (1969) An immunoglobulin enzyme bridge method for localising tissue antigens. Journal of Histochemistry and Cytochemistry 17:563.

McGadey J. (1970) A tetrazolium method for non-specific alkaline phosphatases. Histochemie 23:180–184.

McIver A.G., Mepham B.L. (1982) Immunoperoxidase techniques in human renal biopsy. Histopathology 6:249–267.

Mepham B.L., Frater W., Mitchell B.S. (1979) The use of proteolytic enzymes to improve immunoglobulin staining by the P.A.P. Technique. Histochemical Journal 11:345.

Miller K., Auld J., Jessup E. et al. (1995) Antigen unmasking in formalin-fixed routinely processed paraffin wax-embedded sections by pressure cooking: a comparison with microwave oven heating and traditional methods. Advances in Anatomical Pathology 2:60–64.

Morgan J.M., Navabi H., Schmidt K.W., Jasani B. (1994) Possible role of tissue bound calcium ions in citrate-mediated high temperature antigen retrieval. Journal of Pathology 174:301–307.

Morgan J.M., Navabi H., Jasani B. (1997) Role of calcium chelation in high-temperature antigen retrieval at different pH values. Journal of Pathology 182(2):233–237.

Nairn R.C. (1976) Fluorescent protein tracing, 4th edn. Edinburgh: Churchill Livingstone.

Nakane P.K. (1968) Simultaneous localisation of multiple tissue antigens using the peroxidase-labelled antibody method: a study on pituitary glands of the rat. Journal of Histochemistry and Cytochemistry 16:557–560.

Nakane P.K., Pierce G.B. (1966) Enzyme-labeled antibodies: preparation and localisation of antigens. Journal of Histochemistry and Cytochemistry 14:929–931.

Norton A.J., Jordon S., Yeomans P. (1994) Brief high temperature heat denaturation (pressure cooking): a simple and effective method of antigen retrieval for routinely processed tissues. Journal of Pathology 173:371–379.

Pasha T., Montone K.T., Tomaszeweski J.E. (1995) Nuclear antigen retrieval utilizing steam heat (abstract). Laboratory Investigation 72:167A.

Pearse A.G.E., Polak J.M. (1975) Bifunctional reagents as vapour and liquid phase fixatives for immunochemistry. Histochemical Journal 7:179–186.

Petrusz P., Sar M., Ordonneau P., Dimeo P. (1976) Specificity in immunochemical staining. Journal of Histochemistry and Cytochemistry 24:1110.

Petrusz P., Sar M., Ordronneau P., Dimeo P. (1977) Reply to letter of Swaab et al.: 'Can specificity ever be proved in immunocytochemical staining'. Journal of Histochemistry and Cytochemistry 25:390.

Pluzek K.-J., Sweeney E., Miller K., Isaacson P.G. (1993) A major advance for immunocytochemistry: enhanced polymer one-step staining (EPOS). Journal of Pathology 169(Suppl): abstract 220.

Polak J.M., Van Noorden S., eds. (1986) Immunochemistry. Practical applications in pathology and biology, 2nd edn. Bristol: Wright.

Ponder B.A., Wilkinson M.M. (1981) Inhibition of endogenous tissue alkaline phosphatase with the use of alkaline phosphatase conjugates in immunohistochemistry. Journal of Histochemistry and Cytochemistry 29(8): 981–984.

Riggs J.L., Seiwald J.R., Burkhalter J.H. et al. (1958) Isothiocyanate compounds as fluorescent labeling agents for immune serum. American Journal of Pathology 34:1081–1097.

Ritter M.A. (1986) Raising and testing monoclonal antibodies for immunocytochemistry. In: Polak J.M., Van Noorden S., eds. Immunocytochemistry: modern methods and applications. Bristol: Wright.

Robinson G., Dawson I.M.P. (1975) Immunochemical studies of the endocrine cells of the gastrointestinal tract: 1. The use and value of peroxidase conjugated antibody techniques for the localisation of gastrin-containing cells in the human pyloric antrum. Histochemical Journal 7:321–333.

Roth J. (1982) Applications of immunocolloids in light microscopy. Preparation of protein A–silver and protein A–gold complexes and their application for the localization of single and multiple antigens in paraffin sections. Journal of Histochemistry and Cytochemistry 30: 691–696.

Shi S.R., Key M.E., Kalra K.L. (1991) Antigen retrieval in formalin-fixed paraffin-embedded tissues: an enhancement method for immunohistochemical staining based on microwave oven heating of sections. Journal of Histochemistry and Cytochemistry 39:741–748.

Singh N., Wotherspoon A.C., Miller K.D., Isaacson P.G. (1993) The effect of formalin fixation time on the immunocytochemical detection of antigen using the microwave. Journal of Pathology (Suppl): 382A.

Stein H., Gatter K., Asbahr H., Mason D.Y. (1985) Use of freeze-dried paraffin embedded sections for immunohistologic staining with monoclonal antibodies. Laboratory Investigation 52:676–683.

Sternberger L.A. (1969) Some new developments in immunocytochemistry. Mikroskopie 25:346–61.

Sternberger L.A. (1979) Immunocytochemistry, 2nd edn. New York: Wiley.

Sternberger L.A., Joseph, F.A. (1979) The unlabelled antibody method. Contrasting colour staining of paired pituitary hormones without antibody removal. Journal of Histochemistry and Cytochemistry 27:1424–1429.

Sternberger L.A., Hardy P.H., Cuculis J.J., Meyer H.G. (1970) The unlabelled antibody enzyme method of immunohistochemistry: preparation and properties of soluble antigen–antibody complex (horseradish peroxidase–antiperoxidase) and its use in identification of spirochaetes. Journal of Histochemistry and Cytochemistry 18:315.

Straus W. (1976) Use of peroxidase inhibitors for immunoperoxidase procedures. In: Feldmann G., ed. First International Symposium on Immunoenzymatic Techniques. Amsterdam, North Holland.

Straus W. (1982) Imidazole increases the sensitivity of the cytochemical reaction for peroxidase with diaminobenzidine at a neutral pH. Journal of Histochemistry and Cytochemistry 30:491–493.

Streefkerk J.G. (1972) Inhibition of erythrocyte pseudoperoxidase activity by treatment with hydrogen peroxide following methanol. Journal of Histochemistry and Cytochemistry 20:829.

Suffin S.C., Muck K.B., Young J.C. et al. (1979) Improvement of the glucose oxidase immunoenzyme technic. American Journal of Clinical Pathology 71:492–496.

Taylor C.R., Burns J. (1974) The demonstration of plasma cells and other immunoglobulin-containing cells in formalin-fixed, paraffin-embedded tissues using peroxidase-labelled antibody. Journal of Clinical Pathology 27:14–20.

Turbitt M.L., Mackie R.M., Young H., Campbell I. (1982) The use of paraffin-processed tissue and the immunoperoxidase technique in the diagnosis of bullous diseases, lupus erythematosus and vasculitis. British Journal of Dermatology 106(4):411–417.

Van Noorden S., Stuar M.C., Cheung A. et al. (1986) Localization of pituitary hormones by multiple immunoenzyme staining procedures using monoclonal and polyclonal antibodies. Journal of Histochemistry and Cytochemistry 34:287.

Vyberg M., Nielsen S. (1998) Dextran polymer conjugate two-step visualisation system for immunocytochemistry: a comparison of EnVision+ with two three-step avidin–biotin techniques. Applied Immunohistochemistry 6(1):3–10.

Wang B.L., Larsson L.I. (1985) Simultaneous development of multiple tissue antigens by indirect immunofluorescence of immunogold staining. Journal of Histochemistry 83:47–56.

Warnke R.A., Gatter K.C., Mason D.Y. (1983) Monoclonal antibodies as diagnostic reagents. Recent Advances in Clinical Immunology 3:163.

Weisburger E.K., Russfield A.B., Homburger F., et al. (1978) Testing of twenty-one environmental aromatic amines or derivatives for long-term toxicity or carcinogenicity. Journal of Environmental Pathology and Toxicity 2:325–356.

22

Immunohistochemistry Quality Control

Christa L. Hladik and Charles L. White, III

INTRODUCTION

Since the early 1980s, immunohistochemistry has gradually become established as an integral part of routine histopathology and indeed is considered by some to have transformed the discipline (Taylor et al 1996). Immunohistochemistry is now used as an aid to diagnosis in many parts of the world, from large institutions and reference centers to small district and general hospitals. Out of 200 cases reviewed by Rosai (1994), immunohistochemistry provided an 'essential' contribution to the diagnosis in 9% and a 'significant' contribution in 5% of cases. In a further 15% it helped to confirm the diagnosis reached from hematoxylin and eosin (H&E)-stained slides. Not only are immunohistochemical markers now used extensively to support diagnosis, but they are also increasingly used for prognosis or to predict the likely response to treatment, e.g. detection of estrogen and progesterone receptors and HER2/neu over-expression (Press et al 1994; Seidman et al 1996; Allred et al 1998; Pegram et al 1998; Harvey et al 1999). The extensive use of immunohistochemistry in research is evident by reference to almost any current pathology journal, where many of the papers include the use of immunohistochemical methods.

Since immunohistochemistry now plays such an integral role in diagnosis, prognosis, and research, accuracy and reliability are critical. Reproducible, high-quality results are demanded in an era of managing both time and money. Reduction of waste by repeat staining is a key goal, in addition to providing the pathologist with the highest level of quality for diagnostic purposes.

Standardization of immunohistochemical procedures has gained the attention of different organizations including the Biological Stain Commission and the US Food and Drug Administration. In the clinical laboratory today, there are many levels of quality control in immunohistochemistry applications, each monitoring a process or method that is performed by humans, machines, or both. Terms such as validation, documentation, monitoring, and troubleshooting all refer to measurements ensuring that the result is accurate and consistent.

Validating a staining process prior to implementation in the routine workload of the laboratory creates a baseline by which to compare the daily results of both chemical and technical procedures. Quality control is performed daily, within the standards set by the laboratory as well as criteria set by accrediting agencies. Standardization may not be uniform from one laboratory to another, but processes and protocols established within an individual laboratory must be followed exactly each time antibody staining is performed.

Detailed documentation throughout the process is necessary for back-tracking and troubleshooting. Documentation should include antibody dilution, control tissue, temperatures, incubation times, and the pH of solutions used. This documentation also serves as procedure validation for each step of the process to reduce human error and improve reproducibility. Automation of various steps in the process may be able to provide the laboratory scientist with helpful clues for troubleshooting when staining artifacts are observed during quality control review. For example, machine-generated error reports may be helpful to identify skipped steps and low reagent levels, both of which may contribute to commonly seen artifacts.

Both the laboratory scientist and pathologist contribute to the methods used in the laboratory. Each brings knowledge and expertise into the process. The laboratory scientist should control the processing and fixation of tissue and be knowledgeable of the chemistries used, the technology behind automation or manual staining methods, and have basic understanding of control selection and expected staining patterns. The pathologist should be responsible for tissue procurement, reviewing developmental staining, and confirming that both positive and negative tissue results are accurate, in addition to daily review of the staining quality.

Troubleshooting begins as slides are reviewed for quality and reproducible staining; this should be a daily occurrence, and is the responsibility of both the laboratory scientist and pathologist. While looking through the microscope, one should be able to differentiate artifact from true results and have the confidence that a negative result is not a result of a failed stain process. This is a skill that can be learned by gaining knowledge of the expected results for antigen binding sites, i.e. nuclear, cytoplasmic, or both. Recognition of patterns of antigen expression in either tumor or normal tissue is important, but a higher level of quality control is the ability to interpret combinations of antigen expression in the differentiation of tumor types.

If the knowledge to understand the process from beginning to end is obtained, then tracking backwards when troubleshooting is less wasteful of time and it is easier to find the point of error.

FACTORS AFFECTING STAIN QUALITY

Tissue factors

Fixation

The purpose of fixation is to preserve tissue so that it is resistant to undergoing further changes, e.g. by the action of tissue enzymes or microorganisms. The key to proper fixation is adequate time in the fixative to allow the solution to penetrate, creating uniform cellular detail throughout the tissue. The laboratory should define a standard tissue size, fixation time, and fixative for each specimen type that it processes. Fixatives must be compatible with immunohistochemical staining methods. Tissue fixation has a significant influence on immunohistochemistry as most antigens are altered during the process (Williams et al 1997).

Formalin is the most universal of fixatives and, even though it is the pathologist's choice, it can create a challenge for demonstrating certain antigens. Dabbs (2006)

characterizes formalin as 'a satisfactory fixative for both morphology and immunohistochemistry provided that a simple and effective antigen retrieval technique is available to recover those antigens that are diminished or modified'. Other fixatives, such as Bouin's, B5 (mercury), or zinc formalin influence the reproducibility of staining, each presenting a change in pH, length of required exposure, and different artifacts.

There is currently no single 'standard' fixative, and while formaldehyde-based fixatives predominate, formulations differ between laboratories and include 10% neutral buffered formalin (NBF), 10% formalin in tap water, 10% formal saline, and 10% NBF with saline (Angel et al 1989; Williams 1993; Williams et al 1997). In addition, 10% formal acetic, Bouin's fixative, Carson's fixative, B5, and Dubosq Brazil are used in some laboratories that offer an immunohistochemistry service.

Fixation time may be difficult to standardize due to the different sizes of specimens submitted to the laboratory, as the penetration of fixative into large specimens will take longer than small specimens. Prior to the advent of heat-induced antigen retrieval (HIER), laboratories usually attempted to minimize the length of fixation, as prolonged fixation resulted in irretrievable loss of many antigens, particularly membrane-associated antigens such as CD20 and Ig light chains (Miller et al 1995; Ashton-Key et al 1996). However, lack of adequate fixation, or delay in fixation, may be equally detrimental to labile antigens (Donhuijsen et al 1990; Von Wasielewski et al 1998; GEFPICS-FNCLCC 1999). Williams et al (1997) investigated the effect of tissue preparation on immunostaining to establish whether a specific preparation schedule would allow for the optimal demonstration of all antigens. Of the fixatives tested, 10% formal saline, 10% NBF (except for CD45RO), and 10% zinc formalin (except for CD3) gave the most consistent results overall and showed excellent antigen preservation. Of the fixatives previously recommended for immunohistochemistry, 10% formal acetic, B5, and Bouin's fixative all showed poor antigen preservation for the markers tested (CD20, CD45RO, CD3, vimentin, kappa Ig light chains). The period of fixation and the pH of formalin also significantly affected the immunoreactivity of some of the antigens. The use of HIER was found to reduce or eliminate most of the weak staining observed in the study.

Fixatives drive many factors for immunohistochemical staining, such as dilution, antibody incubation time, retrieval method (if applicable), type of retrieval solution, and special pretreatments (e.g. pigment removal). Depending upon the type of fixative used, protocols may require slight modifications.

Processing

Adequate tissue processing depends upon time and temperature at each step. Tissue that is adequately dehydrated using graded alcohols and infiltrated during processing will cut and adhere to slides better, especially fatty tissue such as breast. Alcoholic formalin may be used to assist with breaking down the fat, but tissue high in adipose tissue will take longer to dehydrate and penetrate on the processor. Vacuum and temperature assist with dehydration of the tissue, but high temperatures used on a processor can be detrimental to antigens that are heat sensitive. It is recommended that paraffin with a low temperature melting point be used for this reason.

Regarding paraffin processing of tissues for immunohistochemistry, in a survey of the schedules used by laboratories in the UK, Williams (1993) found nearly as many different schedules as the number of laboratories participating in the survey. Of the nine tissue processing factors investigated, only two had any significant effect on immunoreactivity. Increasing the temperature of processing from ambient to 45°C, and longer processing times for dehydration and wax infiltration, were both found to improve immunostaining. Type of processor, type and quality of reagents, time in clearing agent, use of vacuum, most of which had been suggested as possible causes of poor processing (Horikawa et al 1976; Trevisan et al 1982; Anderson 1988; Slater 1988), were found to have no effect on subsequent immunohistochemistry. Williams et al (1997) concluded that their findings, some of which were contrary to those of other studies, were explained by the variable response of different antigens to the effects of tissue preparation, and hence there was no standard universal tissue preparation schedule for the optimal demonstration of all antigens.

Microwave processing is now being introduced into some laboratories to speed the processing time and reduce turnaround time for diagnostic specimens. Microwave processing has been used successfully in conjunction with routine antibody staining. Acceptable staining was achieved when compared to tissues processed in a conventional processor (Emerson et al 2006). As with all processing, if the tissue is not completely fixed then artifacts will be introduced.

Control tissues should be processed using the same protocols established by the laboratory for everyday use. If the laboratory performs stains such as CD20 on both B5 and formalin-fixed tissue, the control employed should be processed exactly the same as the patient tissue. The laboratory may find it useful to place both formalin- and B5-fixed tissue into a control block. The combination of tissue using both types of fixative will allow for minimizing the number of control blocks that need to be maintained and will ensure that the dilution used will be adequate for tissue fixed in either fixative.

Reversal of fixation (epitope retrieval)

The quality and reproducibility of immunohistochemical staining relies upon the reversal of fixation, which allows the targeted epitope to be exposed allowing for the antigen binding site to be available. The revolution of reversing the hydrogen cross-bonds formed by formalin was introduced by Shi et al (1991). Since then, multiple mechanisms of heating buffers have allowed for the successful demonstration of antigens in tumors, including proliferation markers and oncogene expression. While there is no national or internationally recognized standard epitope retrieval protocol, internal standardization of the technique is required if the results produced by an individual laboratory are to be reliable and reproducible. Variables that require standardization in the antigen retrieval technique include the choice of heating method (e.g. pressure cooker, microwave, etc.), retrieval solution, pH, temperature, volume of the fluid, and the temperature and exposure time while heating and cooling slides. A test battery approach similar to that suggested by Shi et al (1996, 1998) can be used to establish the optimal duration and temperature for a given retrieval solution and pH.

Cattoretti et al (1993) introduced the solution most commonly used in standardized retrieval methods. They used a citrate buffer at pH 6.0, which is inexpensive, stores easily, and is readily available commercially or easily prepared in the laboratory. Equipment commonly used includes the modified pressure cooker, initially reported by Norton et al (1994). Current manufacturers have found ways to increase the safety of operating a pressure cooker and have added temperature control and quality control monitors that allow for detection of variations in temperature and pressure, which in turn can affect the quality and reproducibility of staining.

Just as the number of available antibodies has grown, so has the number of techniques used to reverse cross-linkage introduced by fixation. Many antibodies are successfully demonstrated by using a heated retrieval solution at a specific pH. These solutions range from pH 6.0 to pH 10.0, each one with a different base composition such as phosphate, Tris, or EDTA. EDTA is harsh to tissue during retrieval, and caution should be used to ensure that tissue adhesion to the slide is successful. Proper drying and complete removal of water, in addition to avoiding wrinkles or tears in the tissue, will assist with tissue adhesion to the slide.

With respect to enzymatic proteolytic 'epitope retrieval', such as trypsin digestion prior to immunostaining, the choice of enzyme usually dictates the temperature and pH of the solution, as different enzymes have different preferential pH and temperatures. For example, the optimal values for a mammalian-derived trypsin are pH 7.8 at 37°C, with 0.1% calcium chloride included as an activator (Huang et al 1976). The concentration of enzyme required is dependent on the proteolytic qualities of the product being used. A typical concentration used for many commercial trypsins employed in immunohistochemistry protocols is 0.1%. The concentration, pH, and temperature are then usually held constant, while the time of digestion is varied. The time required for optimal digestion will vary depending on the antigen under investigation, the quality (proteolytic capabilities) of the trypsin and the length of formalin fixation. For antigens that are only present in small amounts, e.g. immunoglobulin light chains on the surface of B-cells, or the epitope recognized by CD3, the time for optimal digestion may vary from case to case, depending on how long each case has been fixed in formalin.

Reagent factors

In the immunohistochemistry laboratory, there are many basic chemistry factors that contribute to a quality stain. Technical quality control requires monitoring all reagents, including kits and detection systems that are prepared by the laboratory scientist or commercial vendor. The storage conditions and expiration date of antibodies and other reagents, either prepackaged kits or raw materials, impact the reproducibility of staining results if not properly handled. Many of the barcode-driven automated immunohistochemical stainers will assist with monitoring for expired antibodies and will alert the laboratory scientist to an expired antibody or other reagent prior to staining patient tissue.

Once an antibody or reagent is validated it should be consistently prepared or used following established protocols. Documentation is needed for each staining run for each day to confirm that antibodies and reagents were used according to established guidelines. This will create a trail to back-track when troubleshooting is necessary. Documentation can be either paper or electronic (automation produced).

Buffers and diluents

The pH of reagents can influence the results of immunostaining in either a positive or negative manner. The pH of buffers used in both retrieval methods and rinsing of tissue during staining must be checked and documented prior to use, and corrected if necessary. Antibody diluents often contain components to stabilize and maintain the protein. Excessive additives such as sodium azide in the diluent may interfere with or inhibit staining.

Temperature

Storage temperature of an antibody is critical to its stability. Commercially available antibodies are accompanied by a specification sheet, which serves as a guide for proper storage in addition to many other handling instructions. Concentrated antibodies tend to have a longer shelf life than prediluted 'ready to use' antibody preparations. Concentrated antibodies can be aliquoted into cryovials, 'snap' frozen using liquid nitrogen, and stored in a −80°C freezer. This will usually allow the antibody to have a virtually indefinite shelf life. Glycerin can be added to the concentrated antibody to retard ice crystal formation that may alter an antibody.

Daily monitoring of the storage temperatures for antibodies and reagents should be documented. Alteration in both refrigerator and freezer temperatures may cause increased breakdown of reagents. Frost-free −20°C freezers should be avoided for the storage of antibodies, as this type of freezer performs freeze–thaw cycles, which will possibly alter an antibody or even destroy it.

It is important to monitor the temperature during epitope retrieval to successfully reverse formalin fixation-induced aldehyde bonds. For consistency, the temperature and cool down time should be exactly the same each time this step is performed.

Validation of antibodies

Upon receipt of an antibody in the laboratory, there are many steps that need to take place to validate its reactivity and the procedure and controls, both positive and negative, that are to be used with that antibody. Prior to starting development of an antibody it is important to be knowledgeable of its basic composition. The specification sheet that accompanies commercial antibodies should indicate: the antigen source, the host in which the antibody was raised (e.g. rabbit, mouse, or goat), the location of the antigen to which it is targeted and the recommended positive and negative control tissue sources, the protein concentration, whether applicable in formalin-fixed paraffin-embedded tissue; the classification (analyte-specific reagent, research use only, or in vitro diagnostic), and reference materials for the application of the antibody. The specification sheet also typically includes suggested staining protocols.

A new antibody should be evaluated using the vendor's recommended procedure as a baseline, and from that point variations can be introduced. If the specification sheet accompanying a commercially purchased antibody does not include a recommended protocol, then journal publications serve as useful starting points.

Knowing the basics will assist with the next step, which is choosing the type of detection complex to be used. For example, some antibodies may be found to work better with an alkaline phosphatase detection system than with a horseradish peroxidase system. It may also be important for the end-product to be of a specific color, such as the use of a red chromogen if a melanoma marker is being developed that will be used to stain tissues with intrinsic brown pigment, which may interfere with the detection of brown DAB chromogen. Also the type of retrieval solution or proteolytic enzyme will be important if tissue was formalin fixed. These factors will influence the starting point for a dilution and the level of reactivity expected.

It is recommended that a diagnostic laboratory use antibodies that are classified for 'in vitro diagnostic' (IVD) use. If an antibody is classified as an IVD, the vendor has assumed responsibility for the validation and application of the antibody. This category of antibody is not always available, so if a 'research use only' or 'analyte-specific reagent' (ASR) is used it is the responsibility of the testing laboratory to validate and document the reactivity of the antibody.

The goal for developing an antibody for use is achieving an optimal signal to noise ratio. Minimal to no background with strong labeling of the target antigen is the desired combination. Following the initial serial dilution, if the staining is too strong then a modification in the dilution may improve the staining. If a loss of foreground occurs and background remains, then addition of a blocking step, change of retrieval solution (pH), or modifying the detection system (e.g. if using an avidin–biotin system, change to polymer system) may achieve the desired result. Changing the antibody diluent may assist with increasing the antibody's reactivity while at the same time lowering background staining.

Weak initial staining may be improved with an increase of the antibody concentration. An example would be dropping from a 1 : 100 to a 1 : 50 dilution.

Negative staining may be the result of multiple factors. The first step of quality control is to repeat the initial staining to ensure that a human or mechanical error was not the cause. If still negative, increase the antibody concentration. If negative following use of a higher concentration, then modify the antibody diluent, using one of another pH or base composition. One may need to modify the retrieval solution for formalin-fixed tissues, use a more sensitive detection system including possibly an amplification system if necessary, and change control tissue (fresh cut). Most important is changing only one variable at a time, and being compulsive by documenting each step, each reagent used, and reaction time.

Antibodies are proteins and are sensitive to pH; they may be altered if exposed to a pH other than what is recommended by the manufacturer or supported by publications. It has been found that specific antibodies yield better staining intensity when either a higher or lower pH is used for the retrieval step. The opposite is also true, in that an antibody may not work as well or specifically if a proper pH is not maintained during the retrieval step.

Over-fixation of tissue may require more aggressive methods for reversing the cross-linking. In addition, some antigens may not be recovered if the tissue has been left in neutral buffered formalin for years. This is a factor that must be considered when developing an antibody if the only control or test tissue available has been stored in formalin for an extended period of time.

The final dilution for use must be confirmed on both positive and negative tissue controls prior to implementation. If a multiple tissue control block is not used for development of an antibody staining protocol, then, following the selection of the optimal concentration, an expected negative tissue should be stained with the antibody prior to implementation. False-positive staining will demonstrate whether the concentration of the antibody is too high.

Once an antibody dilution and staining method are established, each step of the process should be clearly documented and maintained in written or electronic (computer) form, in order for the laboratory scientists responsible for staining to be consistent. No staining process can be free from potential human error. The automated staining industry is making every attempt to achieve minimal human intervention, but it is imperative for the laboratory scientist to be able to reproduce what automation is doing by a manual method, to ensure their ability to troubleshoot and that they are not paralyzed if the machine malfunctions and is not available for use.

Positive and negative tissue controls

The question of how to find the appropriate control tissue is often asked. With today's computer networking, we have access to a wealth of information in addition to text books that provides data regarding expected patterns of antigen expression. Having the basic understanding of the antibody in question, including the antigen being targeted, is helpful to begin the process of choosing appropriate controls.

Steps in the selection of tissue for control purposes must be documented and the choice of both positive and negative tissues should be supported by publications. Commercial antibodies include a specification sheet that routinely lists references and, depending on the vendor, may make recommendations regarding controls. Positive controls should be used with every staining run and should be evaluated and documented for consistency of detection of the target antigen. Choosing a reliable, known, positive control tissue is necessary to achieve optimal results. It may be necessary when trying to find a positive control to stain multiple tissue types and blocks. The first step of identifying a good control is having knowledge of the tissue type, e.g. kidney, liver, etc., and, secondly, whether it is normal or tumor tissue. This information should be provided by a qualified person such as a pathologist. It is helpful if the person validating a control has access to the diagnosis for tumor controls to assist in the evaluation of expected staining patterns.

Prior to introducing a positive control into the daily staining routine, tissue should be checked for any non-specific staining using a negative reagent control (e.g. buffer in place of antibody). The fixative and processing of control tissue should be the same as the patient tissue being tested.

Tissue blocks constructed using an instrument called a tissue microarrayer that contain representative punches from multiple tissue types can serve multiple purposes. The constructed block does not have to contain a large number of punches to achieve the goal of having both positive and negative tissue controls within the same block. A basic representation of positive tumor, positive normal tissue, negative tumor, and negative normal tissue should meet the needs for developing a staining procedure (Figs 22.1 and 22.2). Multi-tissue blocks ensure that the antibody is used at the proper dilution and that the method does not introduce false-

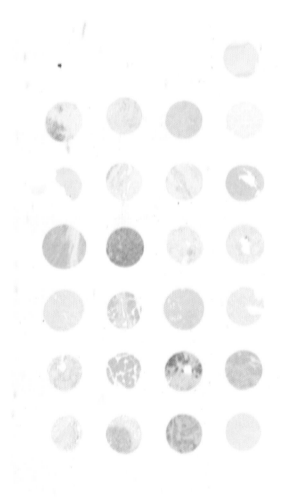

Fig. 22.1 Low-power image of a multi-tissue control stained with an antibody to polyclonal carcinoembryonic antigen (CEA). Using carefully chosen 'donor' tissues, both positive and negative tissue controls can be demonstrated on the same slide.

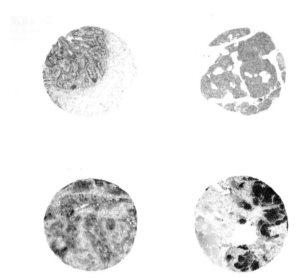

Fig. 22.2   High-power image of a multi-tissue control stained with an antibody to polyclonal CEA, demonstrating both normal tissue and tumor staining, in addition to a negative normal tissue core.

positive or -negative results. The block also serves as a day to day monitor for consistent staining. The reviewer should be familiar with the control and be able to assess whether the staining is not the same intensity or consistency as when developed.

Procedural factors

Automation has become common in the pathology laboratory today. Automation can improve the reproducibility of staining, but many laboratories still perform immunohistochemical staining manually. Manual staining procedures must be written exactly as they are to be performed. The greater the detail, the less likely human error will compromise the result. For semi-automated procedures, any step that is not automated, either pre- or post-staining, can become a factor for potential unreliable results due to human error. The challenge for the laboratory scientist is to remain on track and use tools that allow a protocol to be followed consistently. The incubation times and washing steps must not be unreasonably shortened or lengthened from the established times. A basic understanding of the reagents and how they work together will prepare a laboratory scientist to be detailed when following the procedures and will assist in obtaining reproducible quality results.

Only when there is an understanding of the relationship and chemical reactions between reagents and the effects of temperature and pH can troubleshooting of the procedure begin during the review of stained slides.

Block and slide storage conditions

Processed blocks should be kept in a cool dry place. Resealing paraffin blocks following cutting is a good practice in order for the tissue to be protected from everyday elements, such as air drying or excessive moisture. Although using fresh cut controls for each run would be ideal, it is not always feasible in a busy laboratory. In addition, repeated sectioning of a control tissue block increases the loss of usable sections, which is unavoidable with realignment of the microtome.

Precutting control slides is one way of being efficient with the laboratory scientist's time, and serial sections allow for getting the most out of a block with minimal tissue loss. Conditions for long-term storage of precut slides are important and frequently overlooked as a potential source of error in staining. Some studies have found deterioration of antigens in stored sections (Raymond & Leong 1990; Bromley et al 1994; Prioleau & Schnitt 1995). Others have found no deterioration of some markers investigated, including estrogen receptor, CD3, CD20, CD45RO, vimentin, and Ig light chains, in sections stored for up to 4 months at room temperature (Williams et al 1997; Eisen & Goldstein 1999). In general storing precut slides at room temperature is not recommended. We have found that storage of precut slides in a −20°C freezer stabilizes antigenicity for most tissue types. If a −20°C freezer is not available, precut slides can be dipped in paraffin to seal the tissue, or a button of paraffin can be created over the tissue on the slide (O'Leary 2001). The slides can then be stored at room temperature, but should be closely monitored for reactivity. These procedures require additional steps to ensure complete removal of any excess paraffin prior to staining; it can be melted away in an oven or placed on a cold plate allowing it to chip off the slide, followed by routine deparaffinization.

The temperature and duration of drying sections have been found to affect immunoreactivity for several antibodies, with drying at temperatures of greater than 60°C for greater than 4 hours being deleterious to the antigens investigated (Williams et al 1997). Henwood (2005) reported that using dry heat at a high temperature of 80°C was deleterious to the immunoreactivity of many antigens. Consequently, it is recommended that, regardless of the antigen to be demonstrated, sections should be dried overnight at 37°C or room temperature. If the sections are required more rapidly, or if greater adhesion is required prior to HIER, then drying at 60°C for no longer than 4 hours is recommended (Williams et al 1997).

Quality control documentation

When validating an antibody the documentation should include the following: antibody lot, expiration date, dilution, blocking performed (serum, avidin–biotin, and hydrogen peroxide), secondary and label (detection), and chromogen tested. The time for each step should be noted. Following evaluation of the slides for optimal signal to noise ratio, if an optimal dilution is achieved then the data will be available for creating a procedure, which can then be approved by the pathologist.

Each new batch of a detection system and chromogen should be checked and documented for the level of reactivity. The new lot should be compared to the current lot in use. A good representation of antibodies to stain would include some with enzyme digestion, some with no pretreatment, and a variety of different staining patterns (nuclear, cytoplasmic, and membrane staining). As important as positive levels of expression is a clean negative control with the new lot of detection system.

Enzyme lots should be validated prior to use, as they tend to vary from lot to lot. Additionally, if they are not shipped at the proper temperature, they may lose strength.

Antibody validation documentation should be maintained with the antibody specification sheet in either paper or electronic form.

MONITORING STAIN QUALITY

Daily slide review

All slides should be reviewed prior to sending out of the laboratory. The laboratory is responsible for providing reliable results and the burden should not rest on the receiving pathologist to troubleshoot for the laboratory. Quality control review can be performed by either a pathologist or a trained laboratory scientist. Either way, the reviewer should be able to distinguish acceptable signal to noise ratio, and demonstrate the ability of recognizing interpretable results. If a laboratory scientist is

performing the initial quality review then a pathologist should train that person in order for them to make good decisions regarding the staining patterns and intensity expected. The laboratory scientist should be able, at a minimum, to review the positive control slides for expected results.

Daily stained controls are necessary to validate the results of immunohistochemical assays. The results of staining are optimal if any interference due to non-specific staining is excluded (i.e. negative controls are not stained) and if the sensitivity of the technique is assured (i.e. positive tissue controls with low expression of the antigen in question are positive). Controls serve to monitor whether the staining protocols have been followed correctly, whether day-to-day and worker-to-worker variations have occurred, and whether the reagents continue to be in good working order (Balaton 1999).

Controls include both reagent substitution and tissue controls. Balaton (1999) recommends careful selection of sections for immunohistochemistry and the use of panels including several non-related antibodies, to avoid excessive numbers of extra slides as external controls. For example, if a colonic tumor suspected of being a carcinoma or a lymphoma is tested, test tissue containing both tumor areas and non-neoplastic areas with normal mucosa should be selected. The inclusion of external positive tissue controls is mandatory for some tests, for example those performed for infectious agents, where there is no internal positive control in the tissue under investigation. Above and beyond this, the main advantage of using external positive controls regularly is to allow for run-to-run or day-to-day comparisons of technical quality on tissue where cellular composition and its optimal staining pattern are known. External positive controls are also valuable as a baseline to test any new immunohistochemical reagents (Balaton 1999).

Ideally, antigens in positive tissue controls should be evenly distributed in the sample and, if possible, should contain the antigen of interest in low density, thereby effectively monitoring sensitivity as well as specificity of the reaction. While an external positive control should be prepared for each antibody, often the same type of tissue can be used for several antibodies. For example, a section of appendix can be used for testing antibodies to low molecular weight cytokeratins, epithelial membrane antigen, vimentin, desmin, smooth muscle actin, carcino-embryonic antigen, S-100, neuron-specific enolase, CD45, CD20, CD3, CD4, CD8, CD79a, bcl-2, Ki-67, etc.

(Balaton1999). Multi-tissue blocks allow for rapid testing of new antibodies with a limited number of slides (Rose et al 1994; Sundbland 1994).

Internal positive and negative staining controls

Many antibodies when applied to patient tissues demonstrate native tissue components that serve as internal positive controls. An example would be polyclonal CEA applied to colon, where native staining should be demonstrated in the normal crypts (Fig. 22.3). Internal controls also assist with checking that the tissue was properly fixed and processed. Vimentin has been used routinely to verify that tissue antigenicity has been retained and serves to check for antigen damage; however, vimentin is a hearty antigen, whereas others, like CD3, may not be as able to withstand harsh modifications. By using internal positive controls, each antibody can be evaluated independently.

TROUBLESHOOTING

Common reasons for artifacts include inadequately fixed and processed tissue, improperly prepared antibody dilution or reagents, and fluctuation in pH of buffers or retrieval solution during the staining process. Proteolytic enzyme exposure can exceed the established time or be inadequately removed from the tissue prior to staining. The temperature during specific steps, by which the chemical reaction is sped up or slowed down, variation in incubation times of a reagent, improper preparation of chromogen, or reagents used past an expiration date can also impact staining quality. Thickness of patient slides being different from the control, wrinkles, folds, and tears can create non-specific staining. Control tissue not properly stored can create false-negative results.

False-negative staining

False-negative staining (absence of staining of an antigen that should be present in the tissue) can occur in three different patterns. First, both the external positive control slide and the patient (test) slide may be completely negative. This is usually the easiest false-negative result to detect because the pattern of staining in the validated external positive control slide should already be known and documented. It is important, any time that both are negative, to determine the cause of the false-negative staining, to correct the problem, and to repeat the staining. The second pattern of false-negative staining occurs when the external positive control slide is negative but the patient slide shows staining in either the part of the tissue in question, or in internal positive control tissue. If known internal positive control tissue stains according to the expected pattern, it is not critical to repeat the staining process, as long as the rationale for accepting the staining result and allowing the patient slide out of the lab is documented. It is still important to determine the cause of the failure of staining in the external positive control to ensure quality in future staining runs that might employ that control. The third pattern of false-negative staining occurs when the external positive control slide stains appropriately, but the patient slide is completely negative. This can be the most difficult to detect because it may not be suspected as long as the external positive control demonstrates the expected pattern of staining. The most important clues to this third example include the lack of expected staining of internal positive control tissue, and a negative patient result that does not fit with the results of other stains that may have been performed on the same block.

Possible technical causes of false-negative staining are discussed below.

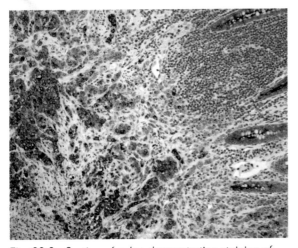

Fig. 22.3 Section of colon demonstrating staining of normal crypts for polyclonal CEA, serving as an internal positive control.

Incomplete deparaffinization

Complete removal of paraffin is necessary for an antibody to penetrate the tissue. If not adequately removed, the layer of paraffin will interfere with and even inhibit antibody binding. Xylene or xylene substitute and graded alcohol stations should be changed regularly and, if paraffin high in plastic is used, longer times in xylene with agitation will assist with complete removal. These steps are frequently overlooked as the reason for weak or false-negative staining. Deparaffinization reagents should be monitored carefully for breakdown, and setting guidelines for the number of slides run through the reagents is advised. Changing or rotating solutions every 100 slides is recommended to ensure that deterioration of these reagents does not introduce unnecessarily weak or false-negative staining.

Incorrect retrieval solution

Not all retrieval solutions work for all antibodies used in the laboratory. This is apparent from the numerous buffers available commercially and published for heat-induced epitope retrieval. If an antibody requires EDTA for optimal reaction, pretreatment of the tissue with citrate will most likely result in false-negative staining. Special pretreatments that are not 'routine' can be written on the slide to ensure that the laboratory scientist does not miss the treatment.

Inadequate heat-induced epitope retrieval temperature

For formalin-fixed tissue the use of heat-induced epitope retrieval is common practice. If the proper temperature is not reached or maintained for the defined time, adequate reversal of fixation may not be achieved. Temperature of the solution used for retrieval should be monitored and checked each time, to ensure that equipment is working properly and that the procedure is performed the same each time.

Extreme digestion using enzyme retrieval

If the tissue has been over-digested to the point at which the tissue morphology is destroyed, then antigens may no longer be available to bind antibody, resulting in a false-negative result.

Temperature

Temperature, whether too hot or cold, may have an impact on a reagent's reactivity during chemical reactions. Some automated immunohistochemical staining units use heat during various steps to speed up chemical reactions. Heat can be used successfully but also may decrease staining intensity or create a false-negative result. Antibodies are proteins and, as we learned in basic chemistry, heat can modify the structure of proteins, which may decrease the sensitivity of antibody binding during the staining process.

Antibody concentration

Both concentrated and prediluted antibodies are labeled with expiration dates. The expiration date on the bottle is determined for the recommended storage condition, usually 4°C. Antibodies stored at 4°C will decline over a period of time, and at some point will decline rapidly and produce a false-negative result.

Human error in the preparation of an antibody dilution can occur. Documentation should include the date that the antibody dilution is made in order to identify when a possible preparation error may have occurred. Pipettes used for preparing antibodies should be well maintained for accurate draws. Calibration of pipettes is recommended at least yearly.

Chromogen incompatibility

It is important to understand compatibility of chromogen and enzyme label. The standard combination is horseradish peroxidase (HRP) enzyme used with diaminobenzidine (DAB) chromogen, but other chromogens such as amino ethyl carbazole (AEC) work with HRP as well. Fast red chromogen and BCIP/NBT react only with an alkaline phosphatase enzyme. It has also been observed in our laboratory that using buffer containing detergents to blue the hematoxylin will reduce or eliminate the staining of new fuchsin-type chromogen. Reading the manufacturer's recommendations for preparation and shelf life of a prepared chromogen is important.

Positive control selection

When a positive control slide is negative and the patient slide positive, it is most likely that the incorrect control slide was used. This is probably more likely in large laboratories when several different antibodies are being run together. If the positive control has not been previously stained with the antibody in question, absence of staining could be the result of improper tissue selection; the laboratory should not use a control that has not been previously validated. Also, when serial sections are pre-cut, at some point the area of interest may have been cut through. It is useful to number the slides in the order of cutting, and to use them in numerical order, to identify at what point the positive area disappeared. As discussed previously, slide storage conditions can decrease antigenicity in the control tissue, thus causing weak or negative staining. If a control stops working, one troubleshooting step is to cut a fresh section of the same block and stain it along with a potentially negative pre-cut slide to verify that antigenicity has deteriorated in the precut stored slide.

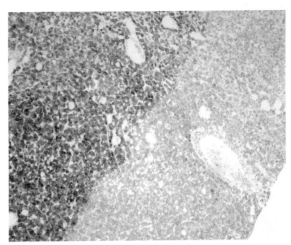

Fig. 22.4 Adenocarcinoma stained on a horizontal immunostainer with an antibody to cytokeratin 7 demonstrating incomplete coverage of the tissue section by staining reagent.

Process failure

Both human and mechanical failure may occur during the staining process. Human error usually involves missing a step, steps performed out of sequence, one of the reagents not prepared correctly, or reagent incubation time not adhered to. Shortening steps may not allow for chemical or immunological reactions to go to completion. Incorrect programming of an instrument or mislabeling of reagents or slides may also be at fault.

Instrumentation failure does occur; pumps fail, computer programs have glitches, probes get clogged, and parts just wear out. A common result is incomplete coverage of tissue with reagents; this is inherent in horizontal staining. Artifacts may appear grossly on the slide (Fig. 22.4). Equipment should be well maintained; yearly preventive maintenance is helpful to keep instruments in good working order.

False-positive staining

False-positive staining is often easier to troubleshoot than false-negative staining. If the false-positive staining is interpreted by the pathologist as real staining, the patient may be incorrectly or unnecessarily treated. When false-positive staining is observed in a patient slide only (since the staining conditions were optimized on the control), different fixation or processing of the patient tissue may be the cause. The patient negative reagent slide plays a key role in identifying such false-positive staining. In order to reduce the number of slides stained, if only one negative slide is used for a case it should be treated with the harshest of pretreatments. Harsh pretreatments include EDTA, and enzyme retrieval alone or in combination with heat-induced epitope retrieval. Reference laboratories that stain slides and blocks processed at an outside institution do not have input into the factors that cause such false-positive staining.

Poor quality of fixation

The emphasis on decreasing diagnostic turnaround times has begun to impact the quality of tissue processing. When fixation and processing times are too short, tissue may not be adequately dehydrated. The result is that the center of the tissue will be alcohol fixed during processing. If the antibody dilution and method are developed on an optimally fixed control and the patient tissue is inadequately fixed or processed, then some antibody concentrations will result in a variable immunohistochemical staining pattern that is obvious even at low power (Dabbs 2006) (Fig. 22.5).

Technical preparation

Poor technical quality of tissue sections is a common cause of false-positive staining. The results may include streaks, overall blushing across the tissue, or patches of

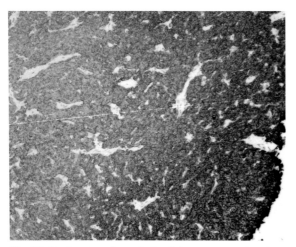

Fig. 22.5 Section of poorly fixed thymus stained with an antibody to AE1/AE3 cytokeratin cocktail demonstrating a gradient of staining from the formalin-fixed outer edge to the alcohol-fixed center.

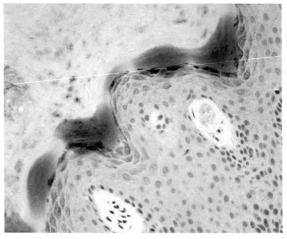

Fig. 22.6 Section of skin intended as a negative control, demonstrating trapped chromogen under the keratin layer due to tissue lifting.

positive staining. Frequently the tissue will detach more and more as the staining process progresses, creating intense artifacts.

It is logical that the final result of staining depends on good microtomy. 'The immunohistochemical stain is only as good as the section cut', as with all staining. Artifacts can be avoided if thin, wrinkle-free sections are used for immunohistochemical staining. Folds, knife lines, and holes are just a few of the examples of poor microtomy that will affect the end results. Wrinkles, tears, and folds create areas in which the reagents are not properly rinsed away and remain trapped underneath or on top of the tissue (Figs 22.6, 22.7 and 22.8). Lifting tissue will hold on to the reagents at each step, and when the colorization step is applied those areas are intensified, sometimes so much so that it is impossible to interpret the staining. All attempts should be made to create perfect tissue sections. Positively charged slides are recommended to assist with good adhesion during the exposure to heat, boiling, enzyme, and multiple washing used in the procedure. In some cases the artifact is a floater that was left from the laboratory scientist cutting the slide. Squamous cells can be identified when reviewing slides stained with cytokeratin antibodies (Fig. 22.9). Laboratory scientists should wear gloves while cutting, and clean the water bath prior to cutting immunohistochemistry slides.

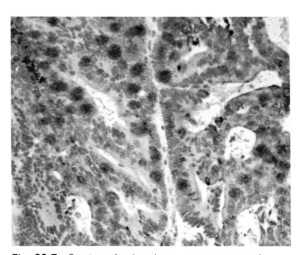

Fig. 22.7 Section of colon demonstrating trapped chromogen due to poor tissue adhesion to the slide.

Pretreatment

The pH of retrieval solutions must be monitored and be exactly the same in each use. Variation of pH in the solution will interfere with staining results. One possible effect of retrieval is non-specific staining due to the amplification of endogenous biotin in the tissue (O'Leary 2001). This is observed with avidin–biotin detection systems. Some antibodies do not require any pretreatment, and exposure to a retrieval solution or step may create non-specific nuclear staining (Fig. 22.10).

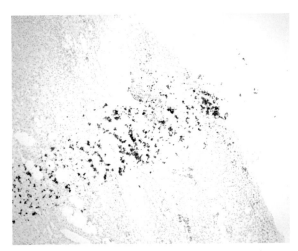

Fig. 22.8 Section of skin stained with an AE1/AE3 cytokeratin antibody cocktail demonstrating chromogen streaking across the section due to poor rinsing. Staining is present across an area expected to be negative.

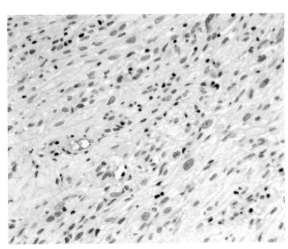

Fig. 22.10 False-positive nuclear staining demonstrated with an antibody to polyclonal myosin due to unnecessary heat-induced epitope retrieval.

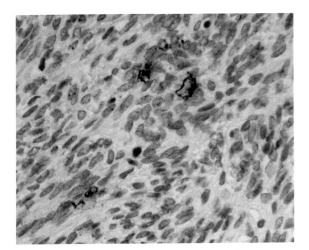

Fig. 22.9 Section of lymph node stained with an AE1/AE3 cytokeratin antibody cocktail demonstrating squamous cell contaminants resulting from the technician placing ungloved fingers into the water bath.

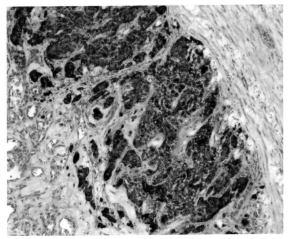

Fig. 22.11 Over-digested carcinoma stained with an AE1/AE3 cytokeratin antibody cocktail. Excessive staining creates difficulty in identifying true positive staining.

Over digestion using enzyme retrieval

There are three factors that can create non-specific staining due to over-digestion when pretreating tissue with a proteolytic enzyme. The first is prolonged time of digestion beyond what has been determined to be the optimal digestion time within the individual laboratory. The second is performing the digestion step at a warmer temperature than has been determined in the laboratory's validation process for that enzyme. Excessive heat will typically increase the rate of digestion. The third factor is inadequate rinsing following the digestion step; when the enzyme is not completely removed, it will continue to digest the tissue. All of these factors lead to over-digestion of proteins, which may then diffuse into or deposit onto the tissue, leading to diffuse, non-specific staining. A clue that over-digestion has occurred is that tissue morphology will typically be obscured (Figs 22.11 and 22.12).

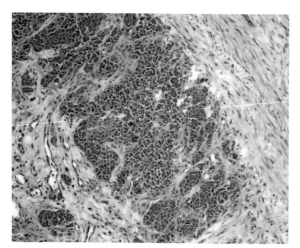

Fig. 22.12 Over-digested carcinoma (same case as in Fig. 22.11) intended as a negative reagent control slide, confirming that much of the staining observed in the patient AE1/AE3 section is non-specific staining.

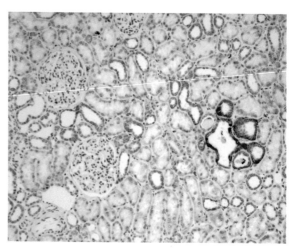

Fig. 22.14 Section of kidney intended as a negative reagent control using an avidin–biotin detection system, demonstrating non-specific biotin in some tubules.

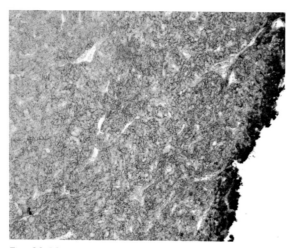

Fig. 22.13 Tissue section demonstrating edge artifact due to excessive drying.

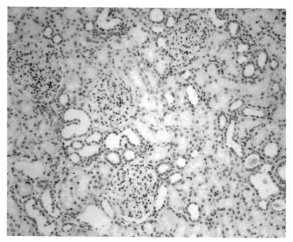

Fig. 22.15 Section of kidney (same case as in Fig. 22.14) properly blocked with avidin–biotin, demonstrating the expected absence of staining (negative reagent control).

High temperature oven exposure

Oven drying must be monitored and maintained at a constant temperature. Tissue exposed to high temperatures for long periods of time may demonstrate edge artifact (Fig. 22.13).

Intrinsic tissue biotin

Biotin is a vitamin found in high concentration in liver, kidney, and brain as well as other tissues. When using an avidin–biotin detection system, a blocking step should be added for reduction of amplification of the intrinsic tissue biotin. This is best achieved by applying unlabeled avidin and biotin. Avidin is applied first for 15 minutes, followed by rinsing with PBS; then biotin is applied for 15 minutes, followed by rinsing in PBS. Protein block or the application of the primary follows the avidin–biotin blocking step. Non-specific biotin will be easiest to identify in the negative control slide (Figs 22.14 and 22.15).

Blocking

When using horseradish peroxidase systems it is necessary to block for endogenous peroxidase commonly found in red blood cells and other tissue components (Fig. 22.16). A 3% hydrogen peroxide solution applied prior to staining will quench the peroxidase activity to eliminate non-specific staining. Staining may be observed in mast cells in a negative tissue control when inadequate quenching occurs (Fig. 22.17). Hydrogen peroxide

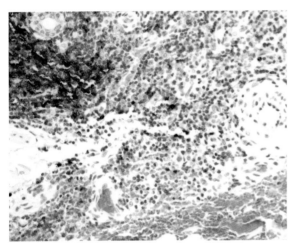

Fig. 22.16 Lymphoid tissue stained with an antibody to CD3 demonstrating non-specific staining of red blood cells (intrinsic peroxidase activity) due to inadequate quenching with hydrogen peroxide solution.

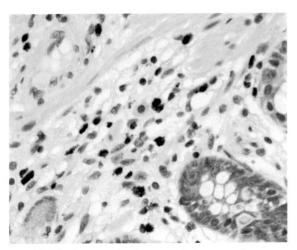

Fig. 22.17 Section of colon intended as negative reagent control demonstrating mast cell staining due to inadequate quenching of endogenous peroxidase activity within mast cells.

should be stored in dark bottles and be prepared fresh for each use.

Antibody concentration

All antibodies, whether concentrated or prediluted, should have their working dilution validated prior to implementation into the laboratory for patient care. Many times, 'prediluted' antibodies are purchased and assumed to be 'ready to use'. These antibodies should be validated by performing serial dilutions (e.g. $1:2$, $1:4$, and $1:8$) starting from the neat concentration, using both positive and negative control tissues. This will assist with choosing the proper concentration for use with the laboratory's established methods.

If non-specific staining is observed, the dilution should be taken out further until a good signal to noise ratio is achieved. Polyclonal antibodies are more sensitive than specific. Using monoclonal antibodies reduces non-specific staining, due to their specificity and affinity for one epitope.

The pH of the diluent is important to maintain the antibody in its proper structure; if the antibody deteriorates in a buffer, it can create non-specific staining and reduce the overall quality of the staining.

Detection system

Antibody to antigen binding at the molecular level is not visible to the naked eye. In order to achieve a visible reaction a complex must be built that is tagged with an enzyme to create a colored reaction product. The most commonly used chemistry is avidin/biotin or streptavidin/biotin. These systems have their challenges specifically when staining tissue types that contain intrinsic biotin, such as liver. More recently the introduction of polymer- or synthetic-based systems has allowed the elimination of biotin-induced non-specific staining, but polymer-based systems are not a cure-all for every antibody. Some polymeric complexes are large and can have difficulty reaching some epitopes, depending on their location. The utilization of polymer-based systems can shorten staining times by eliminating the need for multiple blocking steps. The increase in types of detection complexes available will allow for an improvement in the quality of staining only if the laboratory utilizes and evaluates each antibody with a variety of systems to ensure optimal results.

Species cross-reactivity

While many commercial kits are available that are ready to use, it is important for the user to understand the formulation of the kit. Kits that use 'universal' secondary reagents are directed at many primary antibody targets. This information is especially important if staining animal tissue; for example, goat anti-mouse IgG in the kit can cross-react with mouse tissue, creating a non-specific background stain. Mouse tissue typically will demonstrate blood vessel staining due to such cross-reactivity. This staining mimics endothelial cell positive staining. To avoid such non-specific staining, primary antibodies raised in a different species, and secondary reagents not directed against mouse IgG, should be used. If a primary antibody is to be used that originated in the same species being stained, special blocking steps can be introduced to minimize non-specific binding. Kits containing such blocking reagents are commercially available.

Tissue drying (wetting agents)

During the staining process tissue should remain moist and fully covered by each reagent. When the tissue dries out during a step, the edges will routinely demonstrate edge artifact. Wetting agents such as detergents may be added to the rinse buffer, in order to keep the tissue from drying out between and during the staining steps. Detergents also assist with rinsing away unbound antibodies and other reagents, keeping the staining clean. Too much of these reagents can interfere with the staining as well, so controlling the concentration in the rinsing buffer is recommended.

Chromogen

Alkaline phosphatase chromogens are sensitive to light and heat, making them susceptible to breaking down after preparation. Peroxidase chromogens can also break down, but not as quickly. When chromogen activity is depleted, it will either create a blush across the tissue or deposit debris. Chromogen precipitate and streaking can be reduced with adequate mixing, rinsing, and filtering of the chromogen prior to application (Figs 22.18 and 22.19).

An extended primary, secondary, or chromogen time may cause non-specific staining. Inadequate rinsing does not allow for proper removal of the reagents from the tissue, which may create artifacts. Clean glassware

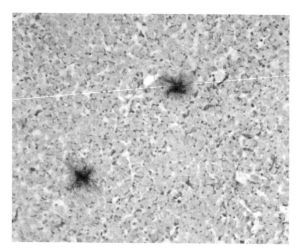

Fig. 22.18 Merkel cell tumor stained with an AE1/AE3 cytokeratin antibody cocktail using alkaline phosphatase detection with red chromogen demonstrating crystals on the surface. Crystal deposits could have been avoided by filtering the chromogen.

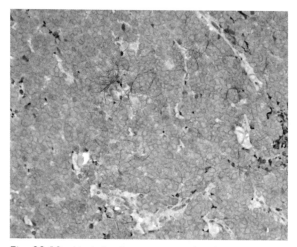

Fig. 22.19 Merkel cell tumor stained with an antibody to neuron-specific enolase using alkaline phosphatase detection with red chromogen, demonstrating 'spider web-like' precipitate across the section.

for manual staining will serve as insurance against potential artifacts.

Automation error

It has been the authors' experience that the goal of consistency is assisted by automation, but automation is not foolproof and can create unique artifacts of its own. Commonly, insufficient rinsing is observed which is amplified during the chromogen application. Horizontal staining instruments require that they be level at all times, or incomplete coverage is seen. Empty or partial draws can occur in which the probe 'thinks' it contains reagents and dispenses air bubbles onto the slide (Fig. 22.20). If reagents are not dispensed properly or do not adequately cover the tissue, staining quality is affected. Instruments that blow over the top of the tissue to mix reagents, if too close, can create a bull's eye pattern (Figs 22.21 and 22.22).

Inter-laboratory comparisons

In the desire to standardize methods a laboratory may choose to send its slides to another laboratory for comparison of staining results. Commercial programs are available for checking the quality of staining and diagnosis against other laboratories using the same stains. These programs check the proficiency of the laboratory testing personnel and pathologist. It is helpful to know

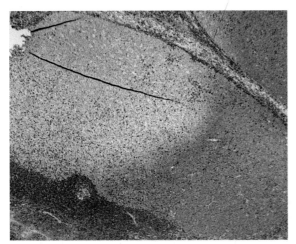

Fig. 22.20 Lymph node stained with an antibody to Bcl-2 demonstrating poor tissue coverage due to air bubbles, and non-specific staining due to poor rinsing.

Fig. 22.22 Tonsil stained with an antibody to CD3 demonstrating bull's eye artifact on the slide, visible to the naked eye, created by the stainer's blowing head being too close to the slide.

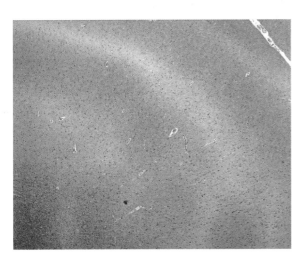

Fig. 22.21 Brain stained with an antibody to polyclonal ubiquitin using alkaline phosphatase detection with red chromogen. Bull's eye pattern created on a horizontal stainer with the blowing head too close to tissue.

how your laboratory is performing in relation to other laboratories, and it can serve as a step toward standardization of immunohistochemistry techniques.

Acknowledgments

We are grateful for the helpful editorial suggestions of Dr Jack Raisanen, and to the University of Texas Southwestern Medical Center Pathology Immunohistochemistry Laboratory for the stain preparations illustrated in this chapter. This chapter incorporates some material that was previously contributed by Anthony Rhodes and Keith D. Miller, authors of the Quality Control chapter in the fifth edition; our acknowledgment is due to them for their contributions.

REFERENCES

Allred D.C., Harvey J.M., Berardo M., Clark G.M. (1998) Prognostic and predictive factors in breast cancer by immunohistochemical analysis. Modern Pathology 11:155–168.

Anderson G. (1988) Enclosed tissue processors. IMLS Gazette 32:141–142.

Angel C.A., Heyderman E., Lauder I. (1989) Use of immunochemistry in Britain: EQA forum antibody usage questionnaire. Journal of Clinical Pathology 42:1012–1017.

Ashton-Key M., Jessup E., Isaacson P.G. (1996) Immunoglobulin light chain staining in paraffin-embedded tissue using a heat mediated epitope retrieval method. Histopathology 29:525–531.

Balaton A. (1999) Defining objectives for technical quality in immunohistochemistry. Journal of Cell Pathology 4:69–77.

Bromley C.M., Palecheck P.L., Benda J.A. (1994) Preservation of estrogen receptor in paraffin sections. Journal of Histotechnology 17:115–118.

Cattoretti G., Pileri S., Parravicini C. et al. (1993) Antigen unmasking of formalin-fixed, paraffin-embedded tissue sections. Journal of Pathology 171:83–98.

Dabbs D.J. (2006) Diagnostic immunohistochemistry, 2nd edn. New York: Churchill Livingstone.

Donhuijsen K., Schmidt U., Hirche H. et al. (1990) Changes in mitotic rate and cell cycle fractions caused by delayed fixation. Human Pathology 21:709–714.

Eisen R.N., Goldstein N. (1999) Observations on antigen preservation in unstained sections. In: Proceedings of the National Society for Histotechnology, 25th Symposium, 1–11.

Emerson L.L., Tripp S.R., Baird B.C. et al. (2006) A comparison of immunohistochemical stain quality in conventional and rapid microwave processed tissues. American Journal of Clinical Pathology 125:176–183.

GEFPICS-FNCLCC (1999) Recommendations pour l'evaluation immunohistochimique. Annals of Pathology 19: 336–343.

Harvey J.M., Clark G.M., Osbourne C.K., Allred D.C. (1999) Estrogen receptor status by immunohistochemistry is superior to the ligand binding assay for predicting response to adjuvant endocrine therapy in breast cancer. Journal of Clinical Oncology 17:1474–1481.

Henwood A.F. (2005) The effect of slide drying at 80°C on immunohistochemistry. Journal of Histotechnology 28:45–46.

Horikawa M., Chisaka N., Yokoyama S., Onoe T. (1976) Effect of stirring during fixation upon immunofluorescence. Results with distribution of albumin-producing cells in liver. Journal of Histochemistry and Cytochemistry 24:926–932.

Huang S.N., Minassian H., More J.D. (1976) Application of immunofluorescent staining on paraffin sections improved by trypsin digestion. Laboratory Investigation 35:383–390.

Miller K.D., Singh N., Wotherspoon A.C. (1995) Current trends in immunocytochemistry. Progress in Pathology 1:99–119.

Norton A.J., Jordon S., Yeomans P. (1994) Brief high temperature heat denaturation (pressure cooking): a simple and effective method of antigen retrieval for routinely processed tissues. Journal of Pathology 173:371–379.

O'Leary T.J. (2001) Standardization in immunohistochemistry. Applied Immunohistochemistry and Molecular Morphology 9:3–8.

Pegram M.D., Lipton A., Hayes D.F. et al. (1998) Phase II study of receptor-enhanced chemosensitivity using recombinant humanized anti-p185HER2/neu monoclonal antibody plus cisplatin in patients with HER2/neu-overexpressing metastatic breast cancer refractory to chemotherapy treatment. Journal of Clinical Oncology 16:2659–2671.

Press M.F., Hung G., Godolphin W., Slamon D.J. (1994) Sensitivity of HER-2/neu antibodies in archival tissue samples: potential source of error in immunohistochemical studies of oncogene expression. Cancer Research 54:2771–2777.

Prioleau J., Schnitt S.J. (1995) p53 antigen loss in stored paraffin slides. New England Journal of Medicine 332:1521–1522.

Raymond W.A., Leong A.S. (1990) Oestrogen receptor staining of paraffin-embedded breast carcinomas following short fixation in formalin: a comparison with cytosolic and frozen section receptor analyses. Journal of Pathology 160:295–303.

Rosai J. (1994) A consultant's apologia of immunohistochemistry. Applied Immunohistochemistry 2:229–230.

Rose D.S., Maddox P.H., Brown D.C. (1994) Multiblock slides: a useful technique for teaching. Journal of Clinical Pathology 47:88–89.

Seidman A.D., Beselga J., Yao T.-J. et al. (1996) HER2/neu-overexpression and clinical taxanc sensitivity: a multivariate analysis in patients with metastatic breast cancer (MBC). Proceedings, American Society of Clinical Oncology 15:104.

Shi S.-R., Key M.E., Kalra K.L. (1991) Antigen retrieval in formalin-fixed, paraffin-embedded tissues: an enhancement method for immunohistochemical staining based on microwave oven heating of tissue sections. Journal of Histochemistry and Cytochemistry 39:741–748.

Shi S.R., Cote R.J., Yang C. et al. (1996) Development of an optimal protocol for antigen retrieval: a 'test battery' approach exemplified with reference to the staining of retinoblastoma protein (pRB) in formalin-fixed paraffin sections. Journal of Pathology 179:347–352.

Shi S.R., Cote R.J., Chaiwun B. (1998) Standardization of immunohistochemistry based antigen retrieval technique for routine formalin-fixed tissue sections. Applied Immunohistochemistry 6:89–96.

Slater D.N., Cobb N. (1988) Enclosed tissue processors. IMLS Gazette 32:543–544.

Sundbland A. (1994) A simplified multitissue block. American Journal of Clinical Pathology 102:192–193.

Taylor C.R., Shi S.R., Cote R.J. (1996) Antigen retrieval for immunohistochemistry: status and need for greater standardization. Applied Immunohistochemistry 4:144–166.

Trevisan A., Gudat F., Busachi C. et al. (1982) An improved method for HBcAg demonstration in paraffin-embedded liver tissue. Liver 2:331–339.

Von Wasielewski R., Mengel M., Nolte M. (1998) Influence of fixation, antibody clones, and signal amplification on steroid receptor analysis. Breast Journal 4:33–40.

Williams J.H. (1993) Tissue processing and immunocytochemistry. UK NEQAS Immunocytochemistry News 2:2–3.

Williams J.H., Mepham B.L., Wright D.H. (1997) Tissue preparation for immunocytochemistry. Journal of Clinical Pathology 50:422–428.

23

Immunohistochemistry Applications in Pathology

Charles L. White, III

INTRODUCTION

The past three decades have witnessed the evolution of immunohistochemistry into an indispensable tool for diagnostic pathologists and for researchers who study human disease. It is widely employed in establishing diagnoses, predicting prognosis and response to therapy, and in the study of disease pathogenesis. This evolution has occurred through a series of technical advances.

The first major step in the introduction of immunohistochemistry into the routine diagnostic pathology arena was the development of methods to label antibodies with enzymes that reacted with non-fluorescent chromogenic substrates such as diaminobenzidine (DAB) (Nakane & Pierce 1966). This enabled the use of a routine visible light (rather than fluorescent) microscope for the simultaneous visualization of antigen localization and tissue morphology. The introduction of the so-called unlabelled antibody method, or peroxidase–antiperoxidase (PAP) technique (Sternberger et al 1970) provided increased sensitivity. Even greater sensitivity was subsequently obtained using avidin–biotin complexes in place of the PAP complex (Guesdon et al 1979; Hsu et al 1981). Another major advance occurred with the availability of monoclonal antibodies that could be used with paraffin-embedded tissues, thus providing a theoretically infinite supply of highly specific, well-characterized antibodies to particular antigens represented in tissues, and to infectious agents. The introduction of epitope retrieval techniques, first using enzyme digestion (Huang et al 1976) and subsequently heat pretreatment (Shi et al 1991), was another revolutionary step in using immunohistochemistry in formalin-fixed, paraffin-embedded tissues, including archival specimens that may have been in storage for decades (Shi et al 1991). Improvements in detection systems and automated technology occur continuously, ensuring that immunohistochemistry will remain an integral part of diagnostic anatomic pathology for the near future.

It is beyond the scope of this chapter to provide a comprehensive listing of all possible applications for the hundreds of immunohistochemical reagents currently available. Other excellent texts devoted entirely to that task are available (Dabbs 2006; Taylor & Cote 2006). Rather, the intent of this chapter is to provide an overview of the ways in which immunohistochemistry is commonly employed in the diagnostic pathology laboratory for the study of both neoplastic and non-neoplastic disorders, illustrated with selected disease-specific examples.

SURGICAL PATHOLOGY OF NEOPLASIA

A common problem in diagnostic pathology is the classification of neoplasms according to the type of cellular differentiation that they display. Proper classification provides important information regarding the likely clinical course and prognosis for particular disease conditions, and has a significant impact on treatment decisions by clinicians. Before the advent of immunohistochemical staining techniques that could be applied to paraffin sections, electron microscopy was widely used to identify cytoplasmic features that would indicate evidence of differentiation toward a particular tissue or cell type. Immunohistochemistry has largely replaced that application of electron microscopy.

Anaplastic tumor workup

One of the most common, and yet most basic, diagnostic applications of immunohistochemistry is in the so-called 'anaplastic tumor workup'. This involves the identification of biochemical 'signatures' of neoplastic cells that are so poorly differentiated ('anaplastic') that their light microscopic morphology alone does not closely resemble any particular mature or normal tissue type. The anaplastic tumor workup is typically applied when it is not clear by clinical, radiological, and morphological features whether a neoplasm in a given body site is primary or metastatic, or when metastases are so widespread at the time of initial diagnosis that the primary site cannot easily be determined. Such cases account for about 5% of cancer patients, ranking as the seventh most common malignancy (Ghosh et al 2005). The biochemical 'signatures' in question include the expression of particular antigens or types of antigens (e.g. epithelial, hemato-lymphoid, or melanocytic), or unique combinations of antigens.

The kinds of neoplasm that need to be considered in the 'anaplastic tumor workup' differ between children and adults. In adults, typical candidates are neoplasms composed of relatively large, pleomorphic cells with highly atypical or active-appearing nuclei (Fig. 23.1).

The differential (list of possible diagnoses) includes neoplasms of epithelial origin (carcinomas), hematopoietic origin (e.g. large cell lymphomas), melanocytic origin (melanoma), mesenchymal origin (sarcomas), and, in the central nervous system, glial origin (e.g. glioblastoma multiforme).

It is tempting to the pathologist when faced with such a case to try to make as specific a diagnosis as possible in the first round. While this may be desirable in a climate where turnaround time is a paramount consideration, it is also likely to result in significantly greater expense in that a large number of stains will be performed that are irrelevant to the eventual diagnosis. A more rational approach is to perform stains in a tiered fashion, where the first tier is designed to place a neoplasm into one of the major diagnostic categories, and the second and subsequent tiers are used to subclassify a neoplasm within the major category determined. Using this approach, a typical panel of stains that would be used in the first tier of evaluation would include:

- cytokeratin stain (positive in almost all carcinomas and only rarely in neoplasms of the other categories)
- stain for hematopoietic cells (e.g. CD45RB, or 'leucocyte common antigen')

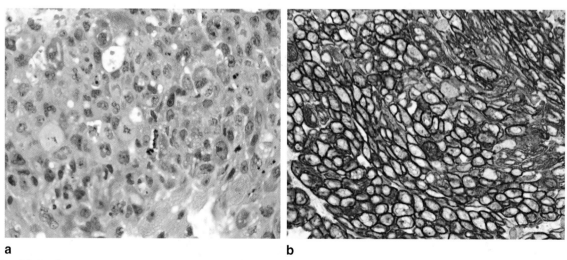

a   **b**

Fig. 23.1   Comparison of antigen expression in various anaplastic tumors of adults. A poorly differentiated carcinoma stained with H&E (a) and with an antibody to low molecular weight cytokeratin (b). Large B-cell lymphoma stained with H&E (c) and with an antibody to CD20, a B-cell marker (d). Melanoma stained with H&E (e) and with HMB45 antibody (red chromogen) demonstrating melanocytic differentiation (f). Glioblastoma multiforme stained with H&E (g) and with an antibody to glial fibrillary acidic protein (h).

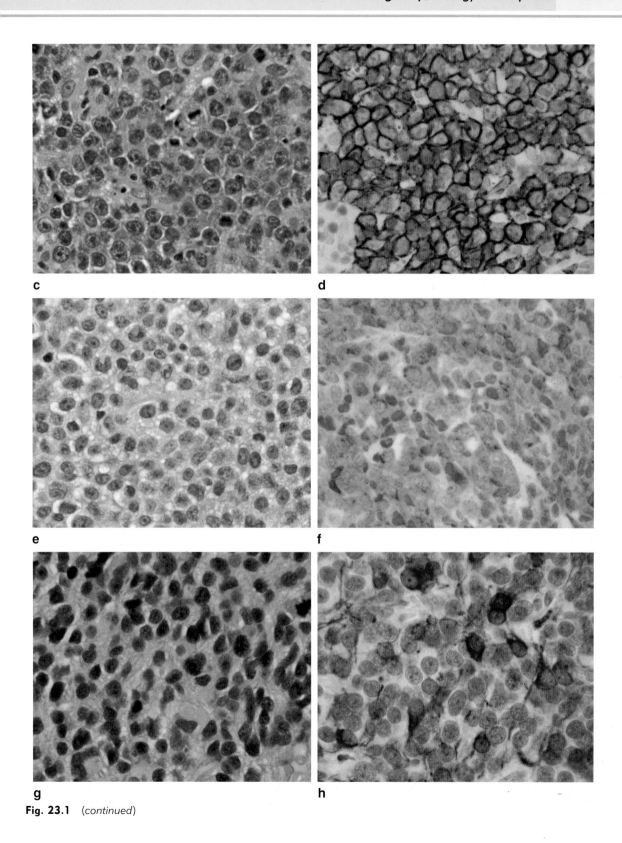

c

d

e

f

g

h

Fig. 23.1 (continued)

- stain for melanocytic differentiation (e.g. S100 protein, or more specifically, HMB45 or MART-1)
- stain for mesenchymal differentiation (e.g. vimentin)
- stain for glial differentiation (e.g. GFAP).

Some neoplasms may show immunoreactivity for more than one of the above immunohistochemical markers. For example, glial neoplasms may show staining with some cytokeratin antibodies (notoriously, AE1/AE3); some non-melanocytic neoplasms stain for HMB45; rare carcinomas and virtually all melanomas and glioblastomas stain for vimentin; some breast carcinomas stain for GFAP; and many neoplasms show S100 positivity. Thus, it is important to perform the entire panel in this first round of investigation, as well as to be familiar with the patterns of combined positivity for specific neoplastic categories.

Once the basic category of neoplasm is determined, it is often useful to analyze a more directed set of immunohistochemical markers to further characterize a neoplasm. For example, antibodies to various cytokeratins (e.g. CK7 and CK20) are often used to help differentiate among various subtypes of carcinoma, sarcomas can often be subdivided into those that show smooth muscle differentiation, endothelial differentiation, etc., and many lymphoid markers are now available for use in formalin-fixed, paraffin-embedded tissues that can be used in the subclassification of lymphomas.

'Small round cell tumors' of childhood

In children, the most common poorly differentiated neoplasms consist of small, immature-appearing cells with relatively round nuclei and scant cytoplasm—so-called 'small round blue cell tumors' (Fig. 23.2). This group typically comprises Ewing sarcoma, neuroblastoma, and other primitive neuroectodermal tumors, lymphomas, Wilms' tumor, rhabdomyosarcoma, and desmoplastic small round cell tumor. A panel of antibodies that is useful in distinguishing among these differential diagnostic possibilities, and the expected pattern of immunoreactivity, is provided in Table 23.1.

Spindle cell neoplasms

Spindle cell neoplasms are composed of thin, elongated cells typically arranged in bundles (Fig. 23.3). They may occur at virtually any site in the body, including sub-

cutaneous tissue, deep soft tissues, viscera, and central and peripheral nervous systems. Most are of mesenchymal or neuroectodermal origin. The differential diagnosis of spindle cell neoplasms includes neoplasms showing smooth muscle differentiation (leiomyomas and leiomyosarcomas), which typically show immunoreactivity for desmin, caldesmon, and smooth muscle actin; tumors of nerve sheath origin (schwannomas, neurofibromas, and malignant peripheral nerve sheath tumors), which show variable degrees of staining for S100 protein; and the more recently recognized gastrointestinal stromal tumors (GIST), which show immunoreactivity for CD117.

Neoplasia versus reactive proliferations

Many reactive proliferations result in masses ('tumors') that may clinically mimic neoplasms. More challenging to the surgical pathologist, however, is differentiating reactive processes from subtle or early manifestations of neoplasia at the microscopic level. Immunohistochemistry has been able to play an increasingly important role in this process as we learn more about the cellular and molecular mechanisms of neoplasia and are able to identify abnormalities early in the neoplastic process. These abnormalities may take the form of alterations in the normal cellular composition of a tissue, or be characterized by the expression of proteins that are not typically expressed at detectable levels in normal tissues.

A prime example of a neoplastic alteration in the normal cellular composition or structure of a tissue is the development of lymphomas. Neoplasms that arise within lymphoid tissue typically obliterate the native follicular architecture of a lymph node, in which B and T lymphocytes are localized to different regions within and around the follicles, and other antigens, such as CD21, are present on follicular dendritic cells in the centers of follicles. Reactive proliferations (Fig. 23.4), may result from localized or systemic infectious processes or other immunological challenges. These may show an alteration in the relative proportions of B and T lymphocytes and other cellular elements (e.g. histiocytes), but the underlying nodal architecture can still be demonstrated immunohistochemically. Neoplastic lymphoid proliferations, particularly non-Hodgkin lymphomas, are typically 'clonal'; i.e. composed exclusively of either B or T lymphocytes, whereas reactive proliferations typically consist of admixtures of B and T lymphocytes, even though the inciting stimulus for the reaction

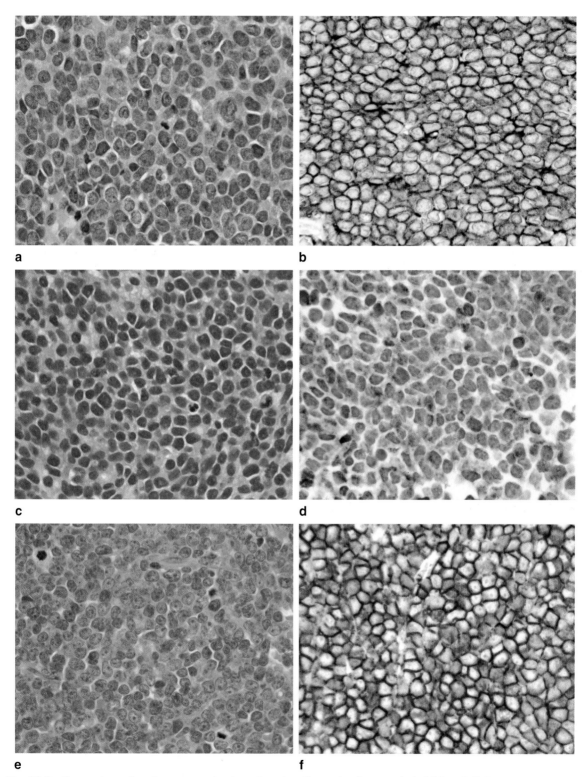

Fig. 23.2 Comparison of antigen expression in various 'small round cell tumors' of childhood. Ewing sarcoma stained with H&E (a) and with an antibody to CD99 (b). Neuroblastoma stained with H&E (c) and with an antibody to synaptophysin demonstrating neural differentiation (d). Lymphoblastic lymphoma stained with H&E (e) and with an antibody to CD79a, a marker of B-cell differentiation (f).

Table 23.1 'Small round cell tumors' of childhood: antibodies useful in distinguishing differential diagnostic possibilities, and the expected pattern of immunoreactivity

	CD99	Lymphoid markers (e.g. CD45RB)	Cytokeratin	Desmin	Neural markers (e.g. CD56, synaptophysin)	Myogenin	WT1
Ewing sarcoma/ PNET	+	–	Sometimes +	Sometimes +	+	–	–
Neuroblastoma	–	–	–	–	+	–	–
Desmoplastic small round cell tumor	+	–	+	+	+	–	+
Wilms' tumor	–		+	+ (blastema)	–	–	+
Rhabdomyosarcoma	Sometimes +	–	–	+	–	+	–
Lymphoma	+	+	–	–	–	–	–

References: Chang 2006; Ghosh et al 2005.

may favor the proliferation of one cell type over the other.

Another example of an alteration in the cellular composition of a tissue in neoplasia is the identification of subtle neoplastic proliferations in the prostate gland, where age-associated hyperplasia (enlargement of an organ due to a non-neoplastic proliferation of cells) is common. Glands containing neoplastic epithelium can be identified by the expression of α-methalacyl coenzyme A racemase (P504S, 'racemase', or AMACR) in most cells of premalignant high-grade prostatic intraepithelial neoplasia or prostatic adenocarcinoma, whereas normal cells or those of benign hyperplasia lack significant AMACR immunoreactivity (Zhou et al 2004). Similarly, antibodies to either nuclear (e.g. p63) or cytoplasmic (e.g. high molecular weight cytokeratin, CK903) antigens of basal cells associated with non-neoplastic epithelium can be used to identify areas more likely to represent normal or hyperplastic epithelium (Signoretti et al 2000; Oliai et al 2002). 'Cocktails' containing antibodies to all three of these antigens may allow increased diagnostic specificity (Fig. 23.5).

Brain neoplasia provides an excellent illustration of the abnormal expression of a protein in the earliest stages of neoplasia. Any pathologist who has had experience with primary brain neoplasms can attest to the frequent difficulty in distinguishing low-grade astrocytomas from reactive gliosis. Molecular studies of brain neoplasia have shown that mutation in the p53 tumor suppressor gene is an early event in the development of many astrocytic neoplasms (Ohgaki & Kleihues 2005) (see below for more detailed discussion of p53). Therefore, nuclear expression of p53, when present by immunohistochemical staining, can be used as evidence of true astrocytic neoplasia (Yaziji et al 1996) (Fig. 23.6).

Stains specific for particular neoplasms

Some neoplasms can be identified by the presence of specific tumor markers, such as prostate-specific antigen (PSA) in prostate, thyroglobulin in thyroid, and GCDFP-15 (gross cystic disease fluid protein) in breast. However, most neoplasms have no unique markers, and may therefore require a panel of antibodies for diagnosis. Nonetheless, in the proper context, an individual marker may allow precise identification of the primary site from which an otherwise unclassifiable neoplasm arose. An example of such a marker is thyroid transcription factor, or TTF-1, found in many neoplasms of the thyroid gland and the lung. TTF-1 can be useful in the identification of the pulmonary origin of small cell carcinomas (Fig. 23.7), which may be widely metastatic at the time of

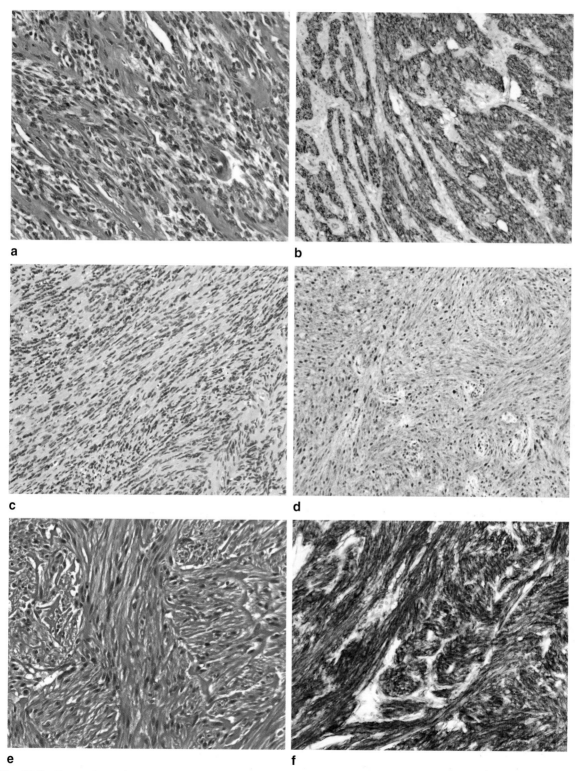

Fig. 23.3 Comparison of antigen expression in various spindle cell neoplasms. Leiomyosarcoma stained with H&E (a) and with an antibody to desmin (b). Schwannoma stained with H&E (c) and with an antibody to S100 protein (d). Gastrointestinal stromal tumor stained with H&E (e) and with an antibody to CD117 (f).

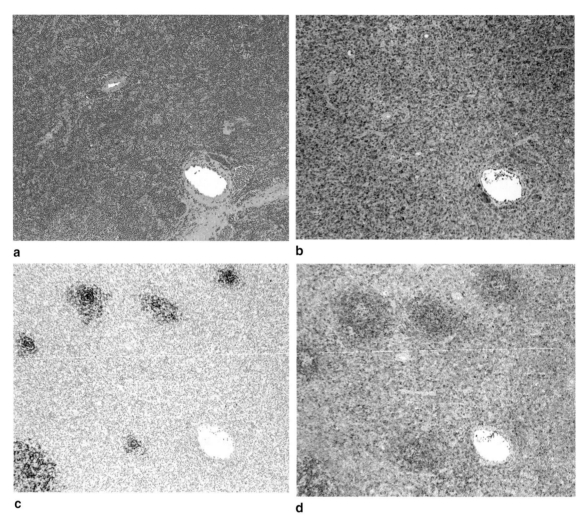

Fig. 23.4 Comparison of lymphoid hyperplasia and lymphoma in lymph nodes demonstrating alterations in proportions of normal cell types and in normal nodal architecture. Panels (a)–(d) are photomicrographs of the same field from adjacent sections of a single lymph node. In extreme lymphoid hyperplasia, nodal architecture is obscured in H&E-stained sections (a), but immunohistochemical staining may still demonstrate an admixture of CD3-immunoreactive T cells (b) and CD20-immunoreactive B cells (c); antibodies to CD20 (c) and to CD21 (a marker for follicular dendritic cells localized to germinal centers) (d) both demonstrate the presence of persistent follicular architecture. In lymphoma (e), the native architecture of the lymph node may be obliterated; in this case, there is a diffuse proliferation of CD79a-immunoreactive B cells (f) and few residual CD3-immunoreactive T cells (g).

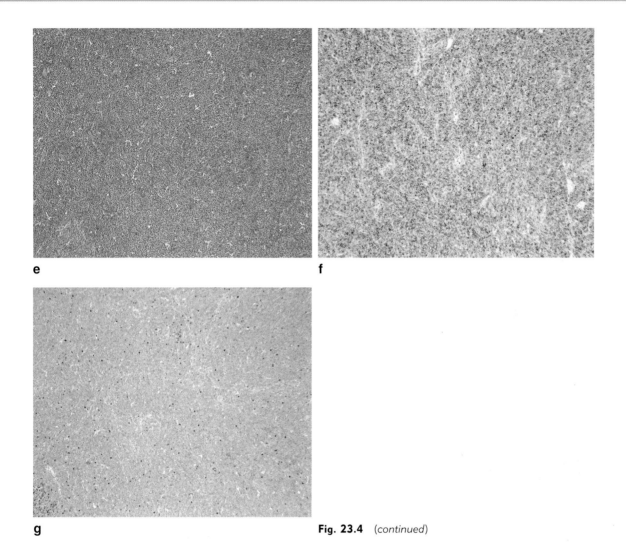

e

f

g

Fig. 23.4   (*continued*)

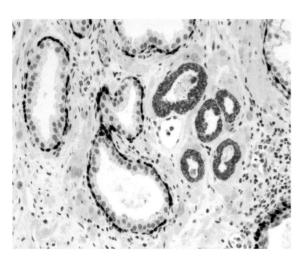

Fig. 23.5   Comparison of the morphology of neoplastic and non-neoplastic prostatic glands. A cocktail of three antibodies demonstrates p63 immunoreactivity (brown chromogen) in nuclei of the basal layer of non-neoplastic glands, high molecular weight cytokeratin immunoreactivity (brown chromogen) in the cytoplasm of the basal layer of non-neoplastic glands, and P504S immunoreactivity (red chromogen) in neoplastic glands. The antibody to P504S recognizes an enzyme known as α-methacryl-CoA racemase (AMACR), which is expressed in high amounts in neoplastic prostate epithelium. Neoplastic glands also lack the normal basal epithelial layer.

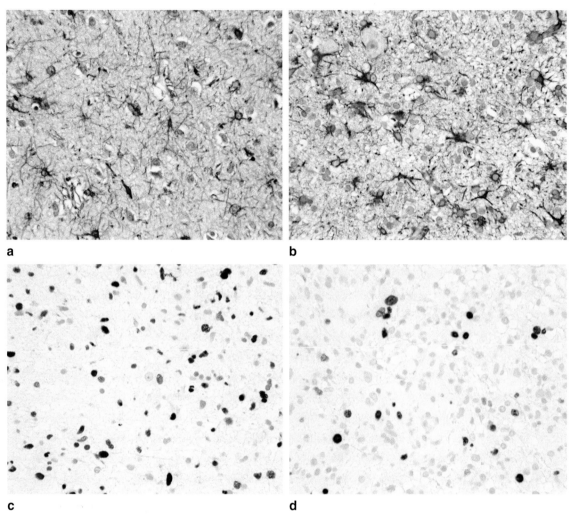

a

b

c

d

Fig. 23.6 Comparison of reactive gliosis and low-grade astrocytoma in brain tissue. In reactive gliosis, as in this example of multiple sclerosis (a), star-shaped astrocytes are prominently demonstrated by GFAP immunostaining. In low-grade astrocytomas, the same prominent GFAP immunostaining (b) may be observed; however, neoplastic astrocytes also frequently display p53 overexpression in nuclei (c), and antibodies to Ki67 antigen highlight the nuclei of proliferating cells (d). Neither p53 nor Ki67 immunoreactivity is typical of reactive gliosis.

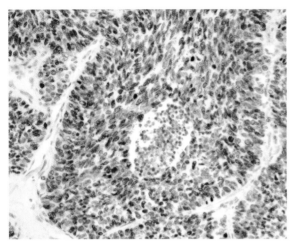

Fig. 23.7 Antibody to thyroid transcription factor (TTF-1) demonstrating nuclear immunoreactivity in this small cell carcinoma of pulmonary origin.

discovery and otherwise show little or no cytoplasmic specializations as clues to their site of origin. Such proper identification can be pivotal to determination of therapy and prognostication that is more accurate.

Unique combinations of stains for particular neoplasms

As previously noted, most neoplasms are characterized and diagnosed by the identification of patterns of immunoreactivity for several antibodies. In some instances, the staining patterns for particular antibodies may be surprising, based upon biological expectations. A prime example of such an unusual combination is renal cell carcinoma, which typically shows immunoreactivity for epithelial markers like cytokeratins, CD10 (a lymphoid marker), and vimentin (an intermediate filament protein more commonly seen in non-epithelial tissues) (Fig. 23.8). Such empirical observations may be of great utility in everyday diagnostic applications. When the pathologist is faced with an unexpected or unusual pattern of immunostaining during efforts to identify a neoplasm, a useful resource is a popular internet site known as 'ImmunoQuery' (http://www.ipox.org), which provides likely diagnoses for combinations of up to three immunostains, including statistics and references.

Stains used to predict prognosis and response to therapy

Many of the biological processes or altered proteins that can be identified by immunohistochemical techniques are related to the prognosis of a given tumor (Porter-Jordan & Lippman 1994). The mechanisms for some associations have an apparently simple basis. For example, a measure of proliferative activity can give an indication of tumor doubling time. Other associations are less clearly understood but may relate to differentiation or events occurring during tumor promotion or progression to a more anaplastic state.

Proliferation markers

The most important component of histological grade is the assessment of mitotic frequency. Objective measurements of tumor cell proliferation such as percentage of cells in mitosis and the Ki-67 labeling index have been shown to provide powerful prognostic information. Ki-67 labeling index can be assessed on paraffin sections using the MIB-1 antibody, and provides a tumor-dependent prognostic variable that can be measured (quantified) in an objective fashion.

Detection of micrometastases in lymph nodes

The presence or absence of regional lymph node metastases is the single most important prognostic indicator for most carcinomas. Often, small metastatic deposits are difficult to see by routine histological examination of serial lymph node sections. Studies have shown that the immunohistochemical detection of these micrometastases is more sensitive than routine light microscopy of H&E-stained sections. Immunohistochemical detection of micrometastases in 'sentinel lymph nodes' is especially commonly applied in cases of breast carcinoma and melanoma. The clinical and prognostic significance of identifying such micrometastases is still under investigation (Ross et al 2003; Klevesath et al 2005).

Oncogenes and growth factors

Oncogenes are normal cellular genes that become altered by mutation or by gene amplification, resulting in loss of regulation of cell growth control mechanisms.

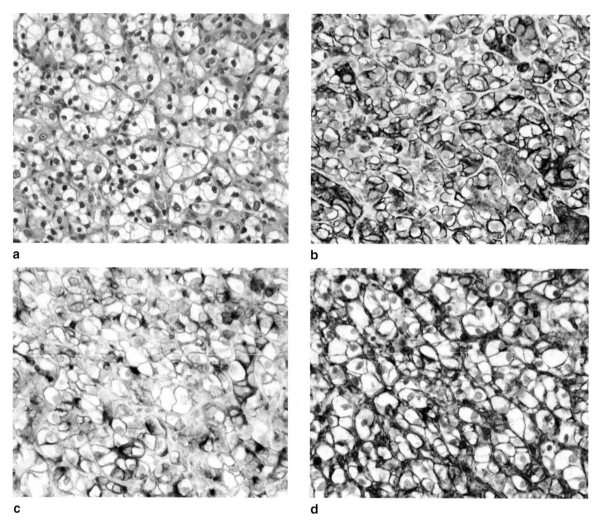

Fig. 23.8 Renal clear cell carcinoma (a) demonstrating a combination of immunoreactivity for high molecular weight cytokeratin (b), CD10 (c), and vimentin (d).

Antibodies are available against some of these oncogene products, such as HER2/neu, bcl-2, and epithelial growth factor receptor (EGFR). HER2/c-erbB-2 is a member of the type I tyrosine kinase family. HER2 protein is a transmembrane growth factor receptor that is normally expressed in a variety of epithelial cells, and overexpressed in some neoplasms, particularly human breast carcinoma, in association with amplification of the gene. Although gene amplification is associated with a poorer prognosis in breast carcinoma, studies of the humanized anti-HER2/neu monoclonal antibody trastuzumab (Herceptin™) have demonstrated a potent inhibitory activity of the antibody against tumor cell lines over-

expressing the HER2 protein. It also increases the sensitivity of experimental tumors to chemotherapy, possibly by lowering the threshold for cells to undergo apoptosis following drug exposure. Large multicenter trials have reported objective responses in a group of patients with HER2 over-expressing tumors and who had received prior combination chemotherapy (Cobleigh et al 1999), and improved response rates when combined with other chemotherapeutic agents (Slamon et al 2001). Patients suitable for this therapy require selection by demonstration of over-expression of the HER2 protein by immunohistochemistry or amplification of the gene by fluorescent in situ hybridization (FISH). A commonly used immunohistochemical method employs a kit consisting of a standardized combination of reagents (HercepTest™; DakoCytomation, Carpinteria, CA, USA) and a semi-quantitative scoring system for membrane staining intensity (Fig. 23.9). Cases with equivocal staining may be further studied for gene amplification using FISH (Dolan & Snover 2005).

Epidermal growth factor receptor (EGFR) is structurally very similar to HER2/neu. It has been detected immunohistochemically in a variety of different tissues, particularly epithelial tissues and neoplasms derived from them, and is thought to play a role in tumor progression (Mellon et al 1996). Demonstration of EGFR expression in patients with certain neoplasms, most notably colorectal carcinomas (Fig. 23.10), is used to identify patients who would be eligible for treatment with cetuximab (Erbitux™), a monoclonal antibody directed against EGFR. Unlike HercepTest™, staining intensity for EGFR is interpreted qualitatively; that is, staining results are reported simply as positive or negative.

p53 is a tumor suppresser gene located on chromosome 17p. Mutations of *p53* are the commonest molecular abnormality found in human solid tumors and are found in a high proportion of breast cancers (Elledge & Allred 1994; Ozbun & Butel 1995). The range of functions of p53 are cell type-specific and appear to be directly related to the ability of p53 to act as a specific transcriptional activator. Wild-type p53 is a negative regulator of cell growth, allowing DNA repair to occur before cell

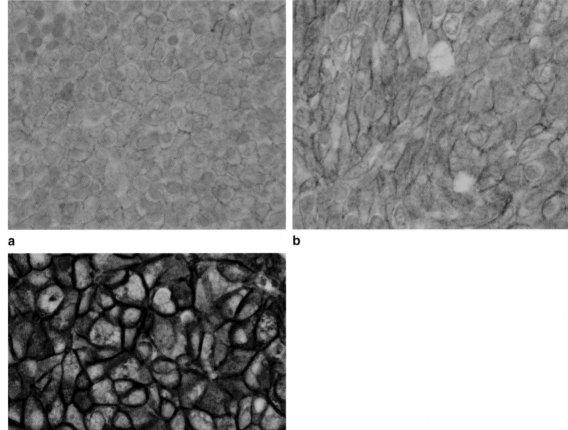

a

b

c

Fig. 23.9 Examples of different intensities of membrane staining for HER2 protein over-expression in breast carcinoma using the HercepTest™ staining system and scoring guidelines. (a) 1+ staining; (b) 2+ staining; (c) 3+ staining.

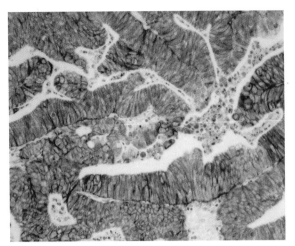

Fig. 23.10 Section of colon carcinoma demonstrating membrane staining for EGFR, used to identify patients who would be eligible for cetuximab monoclonal antibody therapy.

division, or if repair does not occur, then inducing cell death through apoptosis. p53 has been described as the guardian of the genome. Mutation of p53 is believed to result in more stable forms of the protein that form ineffective dimers around wild-type p53 and lead to a failure of growth regulation (Ozbun & Butel 1995). p53 mutation is associated with more aggressive biological phenotypes of tumors and poorer prognosis in breast cancer patients (Eeles et al 1993). Because there are so many different possible mutations in the p53 gene, it is not feasible in routine practice to screen diagnostic tissues with antibodies to specific mutated forms of the protein. Rather, antibodies raised to wild-type p53 are used. These antibodies will typically detect mutant p53 as well, and if the primary antibody is sufficiently dilute, it will selectively identify the accumulated stable mutant p53, which has a significantly longer half-life than wild-type p53 in the cell.

Predictors of therapeutic response

Some neoplasms, including carcinomas of the breast, prostate, uterus, and ovary, are often responsive to hormones, a property that has been exploited by the use of drug therapy to influence hormone levels or inhibit the effects of hormones on tumor cells. Steroid hormones bind with high specificity and affinity to intracellular receptors. These steroid receptors belong to a 'super-

family' of proteins whose function is to control the transcription of a repertoire of other cellular genes (Parker 1991). Steroid receptors such as estrogen and progesterone receptor are located in the cell nucleus. Some of the genes regulated by steroid receptors are involved in controlling cell growth and it is currently believed that these effects are the most relevant to estrogen receptor influences on the behavior and treatment of breast cancer. Approximately 30% of unselected patients with breast cancer will respond to hormone therapy such as oophorectomy (or chemical castration) or tamoxifen treatment. Immunohistochemical methods of detection of estrogen and progesterone receptors have superseded earlier ligand binding and enzyme immunochemical assays, as they require less tissue and allow formal histological assessment, thereby reducing sampling error, and they may be used on very small samples such as fine-needle aspirates. These techniques allow successful use of antibodies on tissue routinely processed in any histopathology laboratory, giving the potential for evaluation of estrogen and progesterone receptor status as part of the process of histological assessment of breast carcinoma. Most tissue fixatives can be used to preserve receptor reactivity if heat-induced epitope retrieval is used prior to staining. It is essential, however, to insure that rapid fixation occurs, and tumor specimens should be incised immediately after resection to insure rapid penetration of fixative. Use of control tissue is essential in hormone receptor assays, particularly because of the risk of false-negative classification. Positive control tissues should include not only a block of a known strongly positive tissue but also a block of tissue showing weak expression to insure that sensitivity is maintained; ideally the test block should include normal breast lobules and ducts to provide an internal control population of cells, since a proportion of these should show positive reactivity. Use of internal control cells in this fashion protects against the effects of poor fixation.

IMMUNOHISTOCHEMISTRY OF INFECTIOUS DISEASES

Immunohistochemical techniques may also be used for diagnosis of infectious processes by the identification of infectious agents in tissue sections (Fig. 23.11). In fact, in some regards, immunohistochemistry is superior to culture in that rapid results can be obtained for agents that may be difficult to grow or require long incubation.

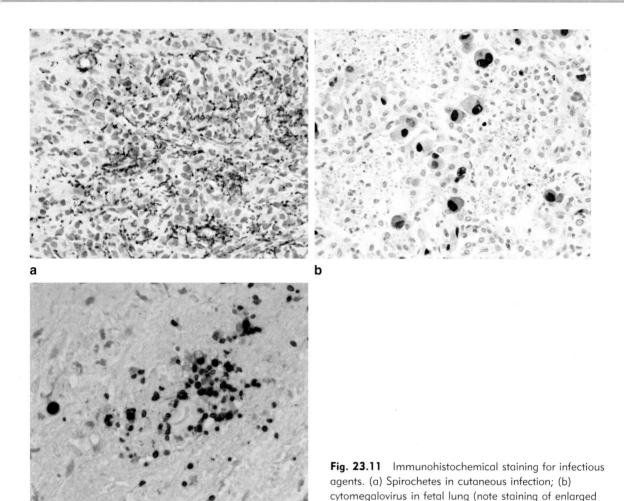

a

b

c

Fig. 23.11 Immunohistochemical staining for infectious agents. (a) Spirochetes in cutaneous infection; (b) cytomegalovirus in fetal lung (note staining of enlarged nuclei of infected cells); (c) tachyzoites of *Toxoplasma gondii* in a brain abscess.

Examples include bacteria such as *Helicobacter pylori*, *Treponema pallidum*, and some mycobateria; fungi such as *Histoplasma capsulatum* and *Coccidioides immitis*; viruses such as *Herpes simplex*, cytomegalovirus, and hepatitis B and C viruses; and parasites such as *Toxoplasma gondii* and *Pneumocystis carinii*. In addition, immunohistochemical preparations are often easier to read than conventional organism stains. As an illustration, in one study it was found that immunohistochemistry detected mycobacteria that were missed by routine acid-fast stains. Moreover, the immunohistochemical results were obtained more quickly than the culture results and were easier to read than the acid-fast stains. It was determined that immunohistochemical

methodology is more sensitive for the detection of acid-fast bacilli because the antibodies can detect fragments of mycobacteria, in contrast to the acid-fast technique, which requires that the organisms be intact (Hove et al 1998). As another example, many viruses (e.g. cytomegalovirus and *Herpes simplex* virus) may be detected by immunohistochemical studies on tissue sections or cytologic preparations before the viral cytopathic changes are recognizable to the pathologist and before the virus appears in culture.

Another important advantage of immunohistochemistry is that it can also be used to detect organisms in cytological preparations, such as fluids, sputum samples, and material obtained from fine-needle aspiration procedures. This can be very helpful in certain situations, such as the detection of pneumocystis from the sputum of an immunocompromised patient who needs rapid and precise confirmation of infection in order to begin immediate and appropriate therapy.

IMMUNOHISTOCHEMISTRY IN NON-NEOPLASTIC BRAIN DISEASES

Neurodegenerative disorders

Degenerative disorders of the nervous system include a wide range of diseases characterized by the dysfunction and death of specific, selectively vulnerable populations of nerve cells, or neurons. For most, there is no clinical test to diagnose the disorder with certainty; definitive diagnosis depends upon microscopic examination of brain tissue obtained at biopsy or, more commonly, autopsy. Immunohistochemistry allows greater specificity in diagnosis than was previously possible using standard histological stains. It has played an increasingly important role in the subclassification of neurodegenerative disorders and the development of consensus criteria for their diagnosis. The role of immunohistochemistry in the evaluation of some of the more common of these disorders is briefly discussed below.

Alzheimer's disease

Alzheimer's disease is a common neurodegenerative disorder that occurs worldwide. Advanced age is the most important risk factor for the development of Alzheimer's disease; predictably, then, its prevalence has increased steadily as the human lifespan has increased. The chief neuropathological features of Alzheimer's disease are microscopic lesions called neurofibrillary tangles and senile plaques (Fig. 23.12).

Neurofibrillary tangles are fibrillar structures present in the cytoplasm of neurons. The main constituent of neurofibrillary tangles is an abnormally phosphorylated form of tau, a microtubule-associated protein whose normal function is to stabilize the cytoskeleton of neurons (Binder et al 1985; Lang & Otvos 1992). Many antibodies are available to various tau epitopes. Neurofibrillary tangles also frequently contain ubiquitin (Mori et al 1987; Perry et al 1987; Love et al 1988; Manetto et al 1988; Bancher et al 1989), a low molecular weight

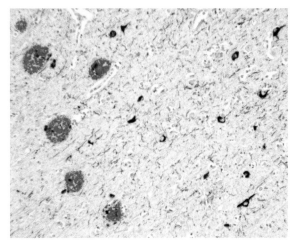

Fig. 23.12 Section of cerebral cortex in Alzheimer's disease. Simultaneous demonstration, using two monoclonal antibodies, of intraneuronal neurofibrillary tangles enriched in phosphorylated tau protein (brown chromogen), and senile plaques containing tau-rich neurites (brown chromogen) and extracellular β-amyloid (red chromogen).

protein that 'tags' damaged proteins for non-lysosomal degradation within the neuron.

Classical senile plaques are composed of two components: a peripheral crown of dystrophic (misshapen) processes of neurons, or neurites, many of which contain aggregated tau, and a central core of extracellular β-amyloid, or Aβ. β-Amyloid is a 40–43 amino acid peptide that is cleaved from a much larger, normally occurring precursor molecule called β-amyloid precursor protein (βAPP) (see below for discussion of βAPP immunostaining as a marker of reaction to acute brain injury). Either mutations in the βAPP gene, pathological cleavage of the β-amyloid peptide from βAPP, decreased clearance of β-amyloid, or a combination of these mechanisms may result in abnormal accumulations of β-amyloid in the brain and cerebral blood vessels. These deposits are easily and specifically identified by immunohistochemistry using antibodies to β-amyloid. Excessive deposits of β-amyloid in cerebral blood vessel walls may predispose elderly patients to spontaneous brain hemorrhages.

Both tangles and plaques may occur in the brains of elderly non-demented individuals, though typically in lower density and more restricted deposition than in Alzheimer's disease. The neuropathological distinction between the occurrence of neurofibrillary tangles and senile plaques of 'normal aging' and Alzheimer's disease is largely a quantitative one (Tomlinson et al 1968, 1970; Mirra et al 1991, 1993; The National Institute on Aging and Reagan Institute Working Group on Diagnostic Criteria for the Neuropathological Assessment of Alzheimer's Disease 1997). Quantitation of tangles and plaques is greatly facilitated by the use of immunohistochemical staining techniques, often in conjunction with computer-assisted image analysis.

Lewy body disorders

A spectrum of disorders is associated with the accumulation of microscopic structures called Lewy bodies. The most basic of these disorders is idiopathic (Lewy body) Parkinson's disease. Idiopathic Parkinson's disease is characterized pathologically by a selective loss of neurons from the substantia nigra, a collection of pigmented neurons in the brainstem. Many surviving neurons in the nigra may contain one or more Lewy bodies, round, eosinophilic cytoplasmic inclusions surrounded by a pale halo. Lewy bodies contain large amounts of α-synuclein (Spillantini et al 1997; Baba et al 1998; Gomez-Tortosa et al 2000), a normally occurring brain protein that may be associated with synaptic function. Mutations in the α-synuclein gene in some rare cases of familial Parkinson's disease led to the search for α-synuclein in the structural lesions of Parkinson's disease, particularly Lewy bodies. Antibodies to α-synuclein have provided a sensitive and specific tool for the detection of Parkinson's disease pathology in brain tissue.

The clinical and neuropathological features of Alzheimer's disease and idiopathic Parkinson's disease frequently coexist (Ditter & Mirra 1987; McKeith et al 1996; Brown et al 1998). One favored term for the common finding of coexistent Alzheimer's disease and idiopathic Parkinson's disease neuropathology is 'Lewy body variant of Alzheimer's disease' (Hansen et al 1990). Brain tissue in this disorder shows a similar distribution of senile plaques to that in Alzheimer's disease, but neocortical neurofibrillary tangles are usually present in smaller quantities, or may be absent altogether (Hansen et al 1993). As in idiopathic Parkinson's disease, the substantia nigra shows pigmented neuron loss and gross pallor, and there are Lewy bodies in many surviving neurons. Lewy bodies are also present in many neurons of the cerebral cortex.

In contrast to the Lewy bodies in the brainstem, cortical Lewy bodies often lack the pale halo and are therefore more difficult to identify in routine H&E-stained sections. Lewy neurites, which are abnormal neuronal processes that occur in gray matter in several locations in the Lewy body disorders, are also a prominent feature in Lewy body variant of Alzheimer's disease. α-Synuclein antibodies are useful in demonstrating neocortical Lewy bodies and Lewy neurites (Irizarry et al 1998) (Fig. 23.13).

Frontotemporal degenerations

This is a heterogeneous group of disorders that share the clinical features of prominent language and personality manifestations (McKhann et al 2001). They have a variety of pathological lesions, but most have selective neuron loss and atrophy in the frontal and temporal lobes, and ballooned neurons in the cerebral cortex. Many fall under the heading of so-called 'tauopathies', due to the primary involvement by tau pathology or mutations in the tau gene on chromosome 17 (Spillantini et al 1998). Immunohistochemistry has played a pivotal role in their identification and differentiation.

Huntington's disease

Huntington's disease is a rare genetic disorder that is inherited in an autosomal dominant pattern. The under-

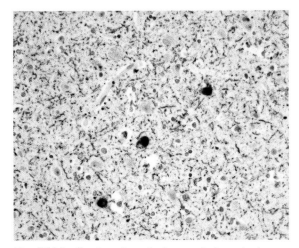

Fig. 23.13 Section of cerebral cortex in Lewy body variant of Alzheimer's disease. A monoclonal antibody to human α-synuclein demonstrates occasional Lewy bodies (larger, rounded structures) within cortical neurons, as well as a dense feltwork of fine thread-like processes of neurons, termed 'Lewy neurites'.

lying genetic abnormality is an expansion of C-A-G 'triplet repeats' in the DNA of the *huntingtin* gene on chromosome 4, which results in increased incorporation of glutamine (amino acid) residues into the huntingtin protein (Landles & Bates 2004). The resultant abnormal huntingtin protein accumulates in neurons and is detectable by immunostaining with antibodies to ubiquitin, to aggregated huntingtin, or to expanded polyglutamine tracts.

Research applications

Much current research into the cause(s) of neurodegenerative diseases is directed at identifying factors that result in the formation of paired helical filaments, the deposition of β-amyloid, cytoplasmic accumulations of α-synuclein, etc. Consequently, studies to localize and quantify the abnormal proteins that constitute the lesions of neurodegenerative disease are of central importance. Immunohistochemistry using antibodies to tau, β-amyloid, α-synuclein, ubiquitin, huntingtin, polyglutamine, and others, has become a routine tool for the sensitive detection and quantification of these abnormal proteins in both human tissues and in experimental animals that are used to model some of the features of these diseases

Brain trauma

Diffuse injury to axons in the white matter of the brain has emerged as an important consequence of head trauma, and is probably the most common neuropathological substrate in patients with persistent vegetative state. In the last few years, immunohistochemical staining for β-amyloid precursor protein (βAPP) has been validated as a method to detect axonal injury within as little as 2–3 hours of head injury (Sherriff et al 1994) (Fig. 23.14). Immunohistochemical detection of axonal injury can be useful in establishing timing of a traumatic insult (i.e. minimum survival time) in medicolegal settings. Caution is required in interpretation of staining results, however, as non-traumatic factors, such as ischemia, can also lead to the increased reactive expression of βAPP (Reichard et al 2003a, 2003b).

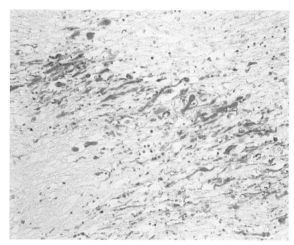

Fig. 23.14   Section of cerebral white matter. Immunohistochemical staining for β-amyloid precursor protein (βAPP) demonstrates increased expression of βAPP in an aggregate of swollen, traumatically injured axons, many of which show beaded varicosities.

IMMUNOHISTOCHEMISTRY IN MUSCLE DISEASES

General features of the muscular dystrophies

Muscular dystrophy is a clinical term that refers to a progressive loss of skeletal muscle function (weakness) due to an inherent defect in the muscle itself. The muscular dystrophies comprise a heterogeneous group of disorders with variable inheritance patterns, ages of onset, clinical distribution of muscles involved, and prognosis. Specific diagnosis of muscular dystrophy is important because of the genetic counseling implications of inherited disease, and for accurate prognostication. Routine histopathological examination of the muscle biopsy in muscular dystrophy reveals significant similarities among the disorders, including characteristic morphological changes of 'degeneration and regeneration'. Moreover, primary muscle disorders (myopathies) other than dystrophies, such as inflammatory myopathies and enzyme deficiencies, may present clinically with a similar pattern of progressive muscle weakness. In recent years, abnormalities in several muscle proteins have been identified in muscular dystrophies. Such abnormalities involve proteins located in the sarcolemma (plasma membrane), extracellular matrix, cytosol, nucleus, and other sites within muscle fibers (Vainzof & Zatz 2003). Skeletal muscle biopsy can play a pivotal role in differentiating muscular dystrophy from non-dystrophic disorders, and immunohistochemistry can assist in establishing a specific diagnosis of the dystrophies for which specific protein abnormalities (due to underlying genetic defects) are known.

Dystrophinopathies: Duchenne muscular dystrophy and Becker muscular dystrophy

The most common and severe muscular dystrophy is Duchenne muscular dystrophy, accounting for about 70% of dystrophies in males (Hoffman 1996). This disorder typically has its onset in early childhood; eventually patients become wheelchair bound, and most die by about age 20 due to respiratory insufficiency and infection. Cardiac muscle involvement is present in up to 90% of Duchenne patients (Hyser & Mendell 1988). A far less frequent form of dystrophy is Becker muscular dystrophy, which also affects males almost exclusively; Becker muscular dystrophy is also less severe than Duchenne dystrophy clinically, with onset in later childhood or adolescence, and most patients surviving into their 30s or 40s (Hyser & Mendell 1988).

Our understanding of the biology and genetics of the muscular dystrophies was revolutionized in 1987 by the discovery of the dystrophin gene (Koenig et al 1987), located on the short arm of the X chromosome, and its protein product, termed dystrophin (Hoffman et al 1987). Both Duchenne and Becker muscular dystrophies are now known to result from mutations in the dystrophin gene, and together are referred to as 'dystrophinopathies'.

The dystrophin gene is a very large gene (3 megabases of DNA), reportedly the largest gene identified to date (Anderson 2002), which is subject to a high rate of new mutations (Sadoulet-Puccio et al 1996). In general, more severe mutations result in the Duchenne phenotype, with almost complete absence of dystrophin, while less severe mutations result in the clinically less severe Becker phenotype, with dystrophin that is abnormal in size, abundance, or both (Brown 1996; Sadoulet-Puccio et al 1996). The functional defect that results from either dystrophin or sarcoglycan (see below) deficiency is

instability of the cytoskeleton of the plasma membrane of muscle fibers, rendering the sarcolemma susceptible to stress-induced fracture, and subsequent necrosis of the muscle fiber (Hoffman 1996).

Dystrophinopathies may be detected by several means, including DNA testing (e.g. to identify deletions in the dystrophin gene), immunoblot analysis of muscle tissue for dystrophin, or immunohistochemical staining of muscle biopsy tissue. With immunohistochemistry, muscle biopsies in Duchenne dystrophy show marked deficiency of dystrophin at the sarcolemma of almost all muscle fibers (Hoffman 1996). Becker dystrophy, on the other hand, may show faint dystrophin immunostaining overall, or absence of staining in only a portion of muscle fibers (Fig. 23.15).

Because the portion of the dystrophin molecule that is abnormal or deleted in Becker muscular dystrophy is variable (Comi et al 1994), multiple antibodies directed at different parts of the dystrophin molecule should be used to increase diagnostic sensitivity (Hoffman 1996). Since a positive diagnosis of disease is based upon deficient or absent membrane staining, the use of appropriate controls is important to avoid incorrect interpretation of false-negative staining. Staining of an adjacent section with an antibody to spectrin, another membrane protein, should be performed on the test specimen to exclude the possibility of non-specific membrane damage that may accompany other, non-dystrophic necrotizing myopathies or even biopsy artifact. Similarly, sections from a normal control case should be stained in the same batch as the suspected abnormal case.

Most antibodies to dystrophin are not generally applicable to paraffin sections, and must be used with frozen sections of muscle tissue; presumably, the epitopes to which they are directed do not withstand fixation or paraffin processing. The need for frozen sections of muscle for dystrophin analysis is not a significant problem, however, as most laboratories that process muscle biopsies for diagnosis of muscular dystrophy or other muscle disorders use frozen sections for enzyme histochemical analyses, which are a routine part of comprehensive muscle biopsy analysis.

We have found that, even though we perform the immunostaining on the same day that the sections are cut, in some cases antigenicity is decreased or lost through air drying of the sections prior to staining. We recently adopted the technique of immersing the

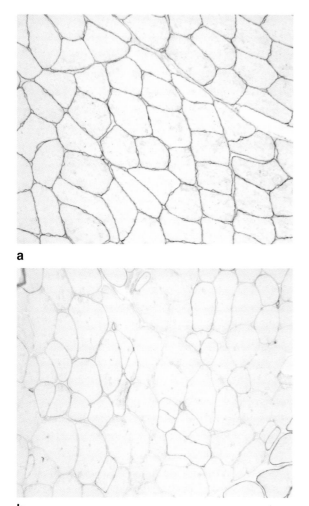

a

b

Fig. 23.15 Dystrophin expression in frozen sections of skeletal muscle using a monoclonal antibody to dystrophin. (a) Section of normal adult muscle demonstrating an even intensity of circumferential membrane staining. (b) Section of muscle from a patient with Becker muscular dystrophy, showing uneven, decreased, or absent staining for dystrophin in many muscle fibers.

mounted frozen sections in 10% horse serum in phosphate buffered saline (pH 7.4) prior to immunostaining (E.P. Hoffman, personal communication). This step preserves antigenicity and greatly enhances the quality of the immunostaining that is obtained. It is important that fresh horse serum/buffer solution be prepared from frozen aliquots of horse serum for each separate run, as storage of the horse serum at refrigerator temperatures

favors the growth of bacteria, which can then deposit on the sections in the form of bacterial colonies and interfere with staining and interpretation.

Sarcoglycanopathies

The sarcoglycans are a complex of four proteins (α-, β-, γ-, and δ-sarcoglycan) that are associated with dystrophin at the sarcolemma of skeletal and cardiac muscle (Brown 1996). Deficiency of any of the sarcoglycan proteins can result in a disorder that is similar both clinically and histopathologically to Duchenne or Becker dystrophy (Hoffman 1996). These sarcoglycanopathies, as they are called, account for about 2% of cases of muscular dystrophy (Hoffman 1996). Because the genes for the sarcoglycans are not located on the X chromosome, the sarcoglycanopathies show an autosomal recessive pattern of inheritance (1 in 4 risk factor with each pregnancy when both parents are carriers, affecting both male and female children) (Brown 1996).

Absence of any of the sarcoglycans results in the absence of all of the other proteins in the complex. Therefore, immunostaining for any one of them may be sufficient for evaluation of the entire sarcoglycan complex in a case of suspected sarcoglycanopathy (Brown 1996). Since dystrophinopathies may show a secondary reduction in sarcoglycan immunostaining, the diagnosis of a primary sarcoglycanopathy can be made only after documentation of normal dystrophin staining (Hoffman 1996).

Merosin deficiency

Congenital muscular dystrophy is a rare disorder, usually inherited in an autosomal recessive manner. About 30% of cases show a deficiency in the protein merosin (also known as α2-laminin), which is a normal component of the basal lamina of skeletal muscle (Hoffman 1996). The underlying defect is a mutation in the α2-laminin gene on chromosome 6 (Hillaire et al 1994; Helbling-Leclerc et al 1995; Brown 1996).

Acknowledgments

I am indebted to Ms Christa Hladik, Ms Ping Shang, and the University of Texas Southwestern Medical Center Pathology Immunohistochemistry Laboratory for the stain preparations illustrated in this chapter, and to Drs Charles Timmons and Amanda Rivera-Begeman and

Mr Chan Foong for their assistance in identifying illustrative cases. This chapter incorporates some material that was previously contributed by authors of chapters in the fifth edition: Ian Ellis ('Immunocytochemistry in Breast Pathology'), and Nancy J. Barr, Nancy C. Wu, and Clive R. Taylor ('Immunohistochemistry and Diagnostic Pathology'); my acknowledgment is due to them for their contributions.

REFERENCES

Anderson L.V.B. (2002) Dystrophinopathies. In: Karpati G., ed. Structural and molecular basis of skeletal muscle diseases. Basel: ISN Neuropath Press, pp. 6–23.

Baba M., Nakajo S., Tu P.H. et al. (1998) Aggregation of alpha-synuclein in Lewy bodies of sporadic Parkinson's disease and dementia with Lewy bodies. American Journal of Pathology 152:879–884.

Bancher C., Brunner C., Lassmann H. et al. (1989) Tau and ubiquitin immunoreactivity at different stages of formation of Alzheimer neurofibrillary tangles. Progress in Clinical and Biological Research 317:837–848.

Binder L.I., Frankfurter A., Rebhun L.I. (1985) The distribution of tau in the mammalian central nervous system. Journal of Cell Biology 101:1371–1378.

Brown D.F., Dababo M.A., Bigio E.H. et al. (1998) Neuropathologic evidence that the Lewy body variant of Alzheimer disease represents coexistence of Alzheimer disease and idiopathic Parkinson disease. Journal of Neuropathology and Experimental Neurology 57:39–46.

Brown R.H.J. (1996) Dystrophin-associated proteins and the muscular dystrophies: a glossary. Brain Pathology 6:19–24.

Chang F. (2006) Desmoplastic small round cell tumors: cytologic, histologic, and immunohistochemical features. Archives of Pathology and Laboratory Medicine 130: 728–732.

Cobleigh M.A., Vogel C.L., Tripathy D. et al. (1999) Multinational study of the efficacy and safety of humanized anti-HER2 monoclonal antibody in women who have HER2-overexpressing metastatic breast cancer that has progressed after chemotherapy for metastatic disease. Journal of Clinical Oncology 17:2639–2648.

Comi G.P., Prelle A., Bresolin N. et al. (1994) Clinical variability in Becker muscular dystrophy. Genetic, biochemical and immunohistochemical correlates. Brain 117(Pt 1):1–14.

Dabbs D.J. (2006) Diagnostic immunohistochemistry, 2nd edn. New York: Churchill Livingstone.

Ditter S.M., Mirra S.S. (1987) Neuropathologic and clinical features of Parkinson's disease in Alzheimer's disease patients. Neurology 37:754–760.

Dolan M., Snover D. (2005) Comparison of immunohistochemical and fluorescence in situ hybridization assessment of HER-2 status in routine practice. American Journal of Clinical Pathology 123:766–770.

Eeles R.A., Bartkova J., Lane D.P., Bartek J. (1993) The role of TP53 in breast cancer development. Cancer Survival 18:57–75.

Elledge R.M., Allred D.C. (1994) The p53 tumor suppressor gene in breast cancer. Breast Cancer Research and Treatment 32:39–47.

Ghosh L., Dahut W., Kakar S. et al. (2005) Management of patients with metastatic cancer of unknown primary. Current Problems in Surgery 42:12–66.

Gomez-Tortosa E., Newell K., Irizarry M.C. et al. (2000) α-Synuclein immunoreactivity in dementia with Lewy bodies: morphological staging and comparison with ubiquitin immunostaining. Acta Neuropathologica 99:352–357.

Guesdon J.L., Ternynck T., Avrameas S. (1979) The use of avidin–biotin interaction in immunoenzymatic techniques. Journal of Histochemistry and Cytochemistry 27:1131–1139.

Hansen L., Salmon D., Galasko D. et al. (1990) The Lewy body variant of Alzheimer's disease: a clinical and pathologic entity. Neurology 40:1–8.

Hansen L.A., Masliah E., Galasko D., Terry R.D. (1993) Plaque-only Alzheimer disease is usually the Lewy body variant, and vice versa. Journal of Neuropathology and Experimental Neurology 52:648–654.

Helbling-Leclerc A., Zhang X., Topaloglu H. et al. (1995) Mutations in the laminin alpha 2-chain gene (LAMA2) cause merosin-deficient congenital muscular dystrophy. Nature Genetics 11:216–218.

Hillaire D., Leclerc A., Faure S. et al. (1994) Localization of merosin-negative congenital muscular dystrophy to chromosome 6q2 by homozygosity mapping. Human Molecular Genetics 3:1657–1661.

Hoffman E.P. (1996) Clinical and histopathological features of abnormalities of the dystrophin-based membrane cytoskeleton. Brain Pathology 6:49–61.

Hoffman E.P., Brown R.H., Jr., Kunkel L.M. (1987) Dystrophin: the protein product of the Duchenne muscular dystrophy locus. Cell 51:919–928.

Hove M.G.M., Smith M.B., Hightower B., Pencil S.D. (1998) Detection of mycobacteria with use of immunohistochemistry in granulomatous lesions staining negative with routine acid-fast stains. Applied Immunohistochemistry 6:169–172.

Hsu S.M., Raine L., Fanger H. (1981) Use of avidin–biotin–peroxidase complex (ABC) in immunoperoxidase techniques: a comparison between ABC and unlabeled antibody (PAP) procedures. Journal of Histochemistry and Cytochemistry 29:577–580.

Huang S.N., Minassian H., More J.D. (1976) Application of immunofluorescent staining on paraffin sections improved by trypsin digestion. Laboratory Investigation 35:383–390.

Hyser C.L., Mendell J.R. (1988) Recent advances in Duchenne and Becker muscular dystrophy. Neurologic Clinics 6:429–453.

Irizarry M.C., Growdon W., Gomez-Isla T. et al. (1998) Nigral and cortical Lewy bodies and dystrophic nigral neurites in Parkinson's disease and cortical Lewy body disease contain alpha-synuclein immunoreactivity. Journal of Neuropathology and Experimental Neurology 57:334–337.

Klevesath M.B., Bobrow L.G., Pinder S.E., Purushotham A.D. (2005) The value of immunohistochemistry in sentinel lymph node histopathology in breast cancer. British Journal of Cancer 92:2201–2205.

Koenig M., Hoffman E.P., Bertelson C.J. et al. (1987) Complete cloning of the Duchenne muscular dystrophy (DMD) cDNA and preliminary genomic organization of the DMD gene in normal and affected individuals. Cell 50: 509–517.

Landles C., Bates G.P. (2004) Huntingtin and the molecular pathogenesis of Huntington's disease. Fourth in molecular medicine review series. EMBO Reports 5:958–963.

Lang E., Otvos L., Jr. (1992) A serine–proline change in the Alzheimer's disease-associated epitope Tau 2 results in altered secondary structure, but phosphorylation overcomes the conformational gap. Biochemical and Biophysical Research Communications 188:162–169.

Love S., Saitoh T., Quijada S. et al. (1988) Alz-50, ubiquitin and tau immunoreactivity of neurofibrillary tangles, Pick bodies and Lewy bodies. Journal of Neuropathology and Experimental Neurology 47:393–405.

Manetto V., Perry G., Tabaton M. et al. (1988) Ubiquitin is associated with abnormal cytoplasmic filaments characteristic of neurodegenerative diseases. Proceedings of the National Academy of Sciences of the United States of America 85:4501–4505.

McKeith I.G., Galasko D., Kosaka K. et al. (1996) Consensus guidelines for the clinical and pathologic diagnosis of dementia with Lewy bodies (DLB): report of the consortium on DLB international workshop. Neurology 47: 1113–1124.

McKhann G.M., Albert M.S., Grossman M. et al. (2001) Clinical and pathological diagnosis of frontotemporal dementia: report of the Work Group on Frontotemporal Dementia and Pick's Disease. Archives of Neurology 58:1803–1809.

Mellon J.K., Cook S., Chambers P., Neal D.E. (1996) Transforming growth factor alpha and epidermal growth factor levels in bladder cancer and their relationship to epidermal growth factor receptor. British Journal of Cancer 73:654–658.

Mirra S.S., Heyman A., McKeel D. et al. (1991) The Consortium to Establish a Registry for Alzheimer's Disease (CERAD). Part II: standardization of the neuropathologic assessment of Alzheimer's disease. Neurology 41: 479–486.

Mirra S.S., Hart M.N., Terry R.D. (1993) Making the diagnosis of Alzheimer's disease: a primer for practicing pathologists. Archives of Pathology and Laboratory Medicine 117:132–144.

Mori H., Kondo J., Ihara Y. (1987) Ubiquitin is a component of paired helical filaments in Alzheimer's disease. Science 235:1641–1644.

Nakane P.K., Pierce G.B. (1966) Enzyme-labeled antibodies: preparation and localisation of antigens. Journal of Histochemistry and Cytochemistry 14:929–931.

Ohgaki H., Kleihues P. (2005) Epidemiology and etiology of gliomas. Acta Neuropathologica 109:93–108.

Oliai B.R., Kahane H., Epstein J.I. (2002) Can basal cells be seen in adenocarcinoma of the prostate? An immunohistochemical study using high molecular weight cytokeratin (clone 34betaE12) antibody. American Journal of Surgical Pathology 26:1151–1160.

Ozbun M.A., Butel J.S. (1995) Tumor suppressor p53 mutations and breast cancer: a critical analysis. Advances in Cancer Research 66:71–141.

Parker M.G. (1991) Nuclear hormone receptors. London: Academic Press.

Perry G., Friedman R., Shaw G., Chau V. (1987) Ubiquitin is detected in neurofibrillary tangles and senile plaque neurites of Alzheimer disease brains. Proceedings of the National Academy of Sciences of the United States of America 86:3033–3036.

Porter-Jordan K., Lippman M.E. (1994) Overview of the biologic markers of breast cancer. Hematology/Oncology Clinics of North America 8:73–100.

Reichard R.R., White C.L., III, Hladik C.L., Dolinak D. (2003a) Beta-amyloid precursor protein staining in nonhomicidal pediatric medicolegal autopsies. Journal of Neuropathology and Experimental Neurology 62: 237–247.

Reichard R.R., White C.L., III, Hladik C.L., Dolinak D. (2003b) Beta-amyloid precursor protein staining of non-accidental central nervous system injury in pediatric autopsies. Journal of Neurotrauma 20:347–355.

Ross G.L., Shoaib T., Scott J. et al. (2003) The impact of immunohistochemistry on sentinel node biopsy for primary cutaneous malignant melanoma. British Journal Plastic Surgery 56:153–155.

Sadoulet-Puccio H.M., Kunkel L.M. (1996) Dystrophin and its isoforms. Brain Pathology 6:25–35.

Sherriff F.E., Bridges L.R., Sivaloganathan S. (1994) Early detection of axonal injury after human head trauma using immunocytochemistry for beta-amyloid precursor protein. Acta Neuropathologica 87:55–62.

Shi S.-R., Key M.E., Kalra K.L. (1991) Antigen retrieval in formalin-fixed, paraffin-embedded tissues: an enhancement method for immunohistochemical staining based on microwave oven heating of tissue sections. Journal of Histochemistry and Cytochemistry 39: 741–748.

Signoretti S., Waltregny D., Dilks J. et al. (2000) p63 is a prostate basal cell marker and is required for prostate development. American Journal of Pathology 157: 1769–1775.

Slamon D.J., Leyland-Jones B., Shak S. et al. (2001) Use of chemotherapy plus a monoclonal antibody against HER2 for metastatic breast cancer that overexpresses HER2. New England Journal of Medicine 344:783–792.

Spillantini M.G., Schmidt M.L., Lee V.M. et al. (1997) Alpha-synuclein in Lewy bodies. Nature 388:839–840.

Spillantini M.G., Bird T.D., Ghetti B. (1998) Frontotemporal dementia and Parkinsonism linked to chromosome 17: a new group of tauopathies. Brain Pathology 8:387–402.

Sternberger L.A., Hardy P.H., Jr., Cuculis J.J., Meyer H.G. (1970) The unlabeled antibody enzyme method of immunohistochemistry: preparation and properties of soluble antigen–antibody complex (horseradish peroxidase–antihorseradish peroxidase) and its use in identification of spirochetes. Journal of Histochemistry and Cytochemistry 18:315–333.

Taylor C.R., Cote R.J. (2006) Immunomicroscopy: a diagnostic tool for the surgical pathologist, 3rd edn. Philadelphia: Elsevier.

The National Institute on Aging and Reagan Institute Working Group on Diagnostic Criteria for the Neuropathological Assessment of Alzheimer's Disease (1997) Consensus recommendations for the postmortem diagnosis of Alzheimer's disease. Neurobiology of Aging 18:S1–S2.

Tomlinson B.E., Blessed G., Roth M. (1968) Observations on the brains of non-demented old people. Journal of the Neurological Sciences 7:331–356.

Tomlinson B.E., Blessed G., Roth M. (1970) Observations on the brains of demented old people. Journal of the Neurological Sciences 11:205–242.

Vainzof M., Zatz M. (2003) Protein defects in neuromuscular diseases. Brazilian Journal of Medical Biological Research 36:543–555.

Yaziji H., Massarani-Wafai R., Gujrati M. et al. (1996) Role of p53 immunohistochemistry in differentiating reactive gliosis from malignant astrocytic lesions. American Journal of Surgical Pathology 20:1086–1090.

Zhou M., Aydin H., Kanane H., Epstein J.I. (2004) How often does alpha-methylacyl-CoA-racemase contribute to resolving an atypical diagnosis on prostate needle biopsy beyond that provided by basal cell markers? American Journal of Surgical Pathology 28:239–243.

24

Immunofluorescent Techniques

Christa L. Hladik and Charles L. White, III

INTRODUCTION

Immunofluorescent techniques have been used for over 65 years to localize antigenically distinct molecules in tissue sections for microscopic study. This is achieved by the use of specific antibody to detect antigenic differences at the molecular level. The combination of antibody with its specific antigen does not lead to a visible change, and therefore a readily identifiable label must be irreversibly bound to the antibody so that its localization can be recognized. In immunofluorescence, this label takes the form of a fluorochrome, for example fluorescein or rhodamine, which has the property of absorbing radiation in the form of ultraviolet or visible light. This absorbed radiation causes the molecule to attain an 'excited state' leading to electron redistribution and the emission of radiation of a different wavelength. The emitted light is almost invariably of a longer wavelength and within the visible spectrum. In addition, the total emitted energy is less than that originally applied in the form of 'excitation energy'. This leads to important practical considerations in selecting suitable light sources and filters to obtain optimal results.

Since the original work of Coons, Creech and Jones (1941), immunofluorescent techniques have been extensively developed and widely applied. The method introduced by Coons et al is known as the *direct technique*, where the antibody (against pneumococci) was conjugated directly with the fluorochrome (β-anthracene) and used to detect pneumococcal antigen in the slide preparation when examined using ultraviolet light microscopy. The introduction of the sandwich or *indirect technique* by Weller and Coons (1954) was a major advance. The method cited in the original paper involved the interaction between the antigen (herpes zoster virus

monolayer) and patient serum containing antibody to this virus. After a washing step, an antibody to human immunoglobulin conjugated to a fluorochrome was applied. Fluorescence indicated a reaction between the virus preparation and antibody to the herpes zoster virus present in the patient's serum.

Immunofluorescent methods have the potential to define antigen–antibody interactions at the subcellular level, such as the detection of antibodies against mitochondria, microsomes, and smooth muscle fibers, as well as identifying small cell-surface structures such as receptors on lymphocytes. The advantage of tissue immunofluorescence methods over other common immunological methods, such as enzyme-linked immunosorbent assay (ELISA), is the ability to identify the site of antigen–antibody reactions in tissue.

Success in immunofluorescent staining techniques is dependent upon many factors, including:

- Preservation of substrate antigens and quality of sections
- Affinity and specificity of antibodies and conjugates
- Detection method used
- Proper selection of microscope and photographic equipment
- Quality control of staining procedures.

PRESERVATION OF SUBSTRATE ANTIGENS

Tissue antigens demonstrable by immunofluorescent techniques include viruses, protozoa, bacteria, enzymes, hormones, plasma proteins, cells, and cell constituents. For successful demonstration the antigen must remain sufficiently insoluble in situ but not so denatured that it will no longer react with specific antibody. A variety of

517

methods are available to preserve different antigens. For example, the use of air-dried, unfixed cryostat sections of skin or renal biopsies will allow the demonstration of chemically sensitive or otherwise labile antigens present in the tissue. In practice, unfixed cryostat sections or cell preparations are generally used whenever possible, unless the antigen under investigation is known to be soluble, in which case suitable fixation such as cold 10% neutral buffered formalin can be utilized. Ethanol and acetone are alternatives, but tissue morphology is suboptimal with these methods.

For the best quality, frozen tissue sections should be cut fresh from unfixed tissue that was properly frozen. Slow freezing can cause ice crystal formation which distorts tissue morphology and antigen binding sites, and should be avoided. There are several good methods for freezing small pieces of tissue. Quick freezing using OCT in the cryostat is a commonly used technique for skin and kidney biopsies. For muscle tissue, the method producing the fewest freezing artifacts employs isopentane cooled in liquid nitrogen. Frozen sections, preferably 4 μm thick, are produced using a cryostat and mounted on clean, positively charged slides, followed by air drying. Sections should be stained within 1–2 hours to ensure antigen preservation. Optimal cryostat temperatures for sectioning may vary depending upon the tissue type. A technical challenge associated with staining unfixed frozen sections by this technique is that they do not adhere well to the slide, occasionally floating free or partially washing off of the slide. It is a recommendation of the authors to use commercially prepared, positively charged slides to ensure tissue adhesion during the staining process; these slides will also be clean and almost free of any non-specific background staining. For storage of frozen tissue blocks, tissue should be placed in an airtight plastic bag and then in an ultra-low temperature freezer (−70°C or lower). Tissue can also be stored in a vapor-phase liquid nitrogen system. Air-dried sections on glass slides can be stored at −20°C in an air-tight container with desiccant. The hardiness of a given antigen will dictate whether slides can be successfully stored at −20°C for an extended time.

Preparation of frozen sections of kidney

Tissue preparation

Unfixed tissue to be frozen within a brief period can be placed on saline-saturated gauze and transported to the laboratory in a sealed plastic container on ice. Tissue that will not be frozen for several hours is best preserved using a transport medium such as Zeus (Zeus Scientific) or Michel medium. A pH of 7.0 to 7.2 is important to maintain during transport to reduce variable staining or other tissue artifacts. Extensive time in medium can increase autofluorescence (Carson 1997).

Method

1. If transported in Zeus or Michel medium, remove tissue from medium and rinse using phosphate buffered saline containing 10% sucrose or Zeus wash solution, three times for 10 minutes each.
2. Remove the tissue and gently roll it across a piece of paper towel to remove excess buffer. This will reduce ice crystal artifact.
3. Place the biopsy in the bottom of a plastic mold that has been pre-chilled in the cryostat, and cover with OCT.
4. Allow OCT to solidify and pop the frozen button out of the mold.
5. Place additional OCT on a chuck, using it to adhere the frozen button to the chuck.
6. Begin sectioning; cut and number slides so that when glomeruli are identified at particular levels by H&E, immunofluorescent staining can be performed on subsequent serially numbered sections that contain glomeruli.
7. The first and last sections from the series of sections used are stained with H&E.

PRIMARY ANTIBODIES AND CONJUGATES

In practice, most of the reagents used in immunofluorescent staining procedures are available commercially. However, it is useful to be familiar with the methods of production and characterization of these reagents in order to compare similar offerings from different vendors, and for troubleshooting procedures.

Antigen requirements

A preparation of highly purified antigen is the best starting material for the production of antisera. An immune response to a foreign antigen is finite and therefore the objective is to direct this response towards a limited number of antigenic determinants. With this approach, fewer purification steps are required to remove 'cross-reacting' or unwanted antibodies in the antiserum. The species of animal chosen to produce potent antisera can be relatively unimportant for some antigens but critical for others. For example, many species have been used to produce antibodies reactive against whole human IgG, including rabbits, horses, goats, chickens, and guinea pigs, but in order to produce specific antibody against the human IgG$_2$ subclass, greater selectivity is required, e.g. sheep or monkey.

Potency and specificity of antibody

Precipitating antibodies of relatively high titer are required for conjugation with fluorochromes. Such antibodies are easily detected in simple immunodiffusion tests, using antigen dilutions (e.g. Ouchterlony double diffusion). The specificity of an antiserum must also be determined prior to conjugation and this can be achieved, for example, by simple gel diffusion, immunoelectrophoresis or passive hemagglutination. A technique to highlight the presence of unwanted 'contaminating' antibodies must be selected. For example, in testing an antiserum as a specific anti-IgG reagent by immunoelectrophoresis, it would be essential to show that only a single precipitin line resulted when this antiserum was tested against whole human serum, but also it would be necessary to show that this reaction was indeed due to IgG alone. It is also vital to insure that antibodies to all subclasses of immunoglobulin are present in such antisera. Incomplete or inconclusive results in some assays may be traced to poor representation of subclass antibodies.

Preparation of antibody-rich serum for conjugation

Serum proteins have differing capacities to combine (i.e. conjugate) with fluorochromes; in particular, immunoglobulins have less affinity for fluorescein than do other more 'negatively charged' proteins, e.g. albumin and β-globulins. These latter molecules when conjugated also have a propensity to combine via electrostatic forces with tissue components, leading to high levels of nonspecific staining. Therefore purified immunoglobulins, essentially free from other serum proteins, are the best starting material for conjugation. Conjugates may be prepared from:

1. immunoglobulin-rich fractions of serum, prepared by salting-out procedures
2. chromatographically prepared fractions, usually on diethyl aminoethane (DEAE) ion exchange columns, consisting mainly of IgG
3. pure IgG fractions obtained by immunoabsorption on affinity chromatography columns
4. F(Ab)$_2$ fractions of IgG obtained by proteolytic cleavage of purified IgG (from 3 above).

These four methods are progressive in terms of the purity of the antibody preparation, and each can be used with success in different situations. For most routine applications, reagents prepared using methods 1 or 2 for purification are adequate, particularly when they can be used in high dilution. Reagents prepared using method 3 are useful where background staining is a problem. Conjugates made from F(Ab)$_2$ fragments are used when the binding of the conjugated antibody to Fc receptors is to be avoided. They may also be useful in double-staining techniques where cross-reactions between antibodies produced in different species are a problem.

Conjugation of proteins with fluorochromes

The spectral characteristics of commonly used fluorochromes are summarized in Table 24.1. Fluorescein is still the most widely used fluorochrome, having a wide absorption spectrum over the ultraviolet and blue light range with a characteristic apple-green emission. One distinct advantage of fluorescein is that the apple-green emission is rarely seen as 'autofluorescence' in mammalian tissue, which is often blue in color. Rhodamine conjugates that absorb maximally in green light, exhibiting an orange–red emission, are commonly used in two-color techniques. Two other fluorochromes that are being increasingly used are Texas red and phycoerythrin (PE). Texas red is similar in its absorption and emission characteristics to rhodamine, while PE has a maximal absorption spectrum in the blue range with a red color emission. This is a useful property, best exploited in fluorescence-activated cell sorter systems, since it allows two different emission colors to be measured simultaneously. The potential for PE and fluorescein combinations in more conventional fluorescent microscopy has not been fully exploited, mainly because of the slightly different excitation light requirements for the different fluorochromes.

Table 24.1 Spectral characteristics of commonly used fluorochromes

Fluorochrome	Absorption maximum (nm)	Emission maximum (nm)	Observed color
Fluorescein (FITC)	494	518	green
Rhodamine (TRITC)	550	580	red
Texas Red™	595	615	red
R-Phycoerythrin (PE)	565	575	orange/red

Reference: Allan 2000

The reactions employed in conjugating fluorochromes with immunoglobulin molecules are complex and vary according to the form in which the fluorochromes are presented. The isothiocyanates of fluorescein (commonly abbreviated FITC) or rhodamine (tetramethyl rhodamine isothiocyanate, or TRITC) that are commonly used can be linked covalently with different chemical groups on proteins. These include free terminal amino and carboxyl groups as well as free amino groups on lysine side-chains and free carboxyl groups in aspartic and glutamic acid residues. The reactions occur at alkaline pH, and the degree of conjugation is both time- and temperature-dependent.

Over- and under-conjugation have adverse effects on the final product. Over-conjugation yields reagents that produce high background staining, often with poor reactivity related to the interference with antigen combining sites on the conjugated antibody molecule, whereas under-conjugation results in low-level fluorescence.

Removal of free dye and assessment of degree of conjugation

This essential step is often overlooked, even in some commercial preparations, and must be carried out to remove unreacted dye that would otherwise cause non-specific staining. Dialysis against large volumes of 0.15 M NaCl at 4°C is the simplest procedure, although this may take several days. The absence of fluorescence in the dialyzing fluid is noted, preferably using a UV lamp. Alternatively the free dye can be removed by gel filtration using chromatography. A simple technique for testing commercial preparations for free dye is described by Johnson and Holborow (1986).

Performance testing of conjugates

In assessing the *sensitivity* of the reagent, the objective is to define the highest dilution of the conjugate that will detect weak reactions in the system. Such tests are therefore concerned with measuring the titer and affinity of the antibody, as well as the degree of conjugation. Tests for *specificity* are designed to determine whether the conjugate will detect the relevant antigen, and to demonstrate that other irrelevant antigens are not interfering at the dilution at which the conjugate is to be used.

Sensitivity testing

Conjugates can be used in both direct and indirect techniques. In practice, the optimal dilution of an individual conjugate is usually higher in indirect systems compared to direct systems, due to the amplification effect of the additional antibody layer. Therefore, differing methods will be required to assess the suitability of an anti-immunoglobulin conjugate in both indirect and direct techniques.

To test a conjugate for its ability to detect human immunoglobulins of IgA, IgG, and IgM classes in individual sera (via the indirect immunofluorescent technique), a 'checkerboard titration' is used. A series of dilutions of conjugate is tested against serial dilutions of a suitable serum, e.g. serum containing antinuclear antibody (ANA), using an appropriate antigen such as rat liver sections. Positive and negative results are scored (−, +/−, +, ++, +++, etc.), as well as reactions that show non-specific staining, i.e. background fluorescence unrelated to ANA reaction. The end-point titer is the highest conjugate dilution that still identifies the target antigen.

If the conjugate assessed by checkerboard titration for indirect techniques is also to be used in direct techniques the following procedures could be followed.

1. Assess the conjugate at 2-fold higher concentration. The higher concentrations required reflect the less sensitive nature of direct techniques.
2. Test the conjugate dilutions against suitable antigen substrates, such as skin and renal tissue sections from selected patients shown to contain class-specific Ig deposits, for example IgA nephropathy, skin sections from patients with dermatitis herpetiformis (IgA-specific), and pemphigoid and pemphigus (usually IgG-specific), as well as skin/renal material from systemic lupus erythematosus (SLE) patients (IgG, IgA, and IgM). A bank of well-characterized tissues can be invaluable material in this context, enabling laboratories to perform sensitivity and specificity tests to a high standard.

Specificity testing

The object of specificity testing should be to show that a suitably diluted conjugate will not cross-react with similar but distinct antigens. An anti-IgG (heavy chain-specific) conjugate, for example, should not recognize other classes of immunoglobulins, e.g. IgA, IgM, or light chains. As stated previously, the specificity of conjugates used should be proven and not assumed. Testing for specificity for use in direct procedures also requires that biopsy material is used as substrate antigen.

STAINING AND INCUBATION PROCEDURES

In the *direct* method, tissue is reacted directly with a fluorochrome-conjugated antibody specific for the material sought within the tissue. In routine practice, the direct technique is the one most often used for the examination of biopsy material from patients, e.g. kidney, skin, gut, and lymphoid tissue.

In the *indirect* method, the tissue section is initially reacted with an unlabeled specific antibody and then, in a second stage, a fluorochrome-conjugated antibody that specifically reacts with the antibody used in the first

stage is applied. This technique gives greater sensitivity when used for the detection of antigens within the sectioned tissue, but an important further advantage is that such a technique can be used for detecting the presence of antibodies within certain sera that may react with tissue components. Thus, normal tissue can be used as a substrate to detect, for instance, antinuclear antibody in patients' sera; the localization of bound anti-nuclear antibody is then determined by the use of a fluorescent conjugated anti-immunoglobulin antibody in a second stage. If a direct technique were used to determine the presence of such antibody then each individual serum would have to be conjugated with fluorescein. The indirect technique permits the use of many different sera with only a single conjugated reagent being used in a second stage.

Direct immunofluorescence staining technique

Slide preparation

Unfixed cryostat sections, air dried, 4 microns thick

Method

1. Circle the location of the tissue on the back of the slide using a permanent pen; this will assist with identifying the tissue following staining.
2. Place air-dried slides in Tris buffer pH 7.6 for 5 minutes.
3. Tap off and quickly remove excess buffer.
4. Place FITC-labeled antibody or negative serum at its previously validated concentration on to the tissue section for 30 minutes.
5. Rinse with Tris buffer to remove excess antibody.
6. Rinse with deionized water.
7. Coverslip using an aqueous mounting medium.
8. Seal the edge of the cover glass with clear fingernail polish or permanent mounting medium.
9. Place slides in a slide tray.
10. Store the slides in a cool dark place until review.

Technical note: Tissue should not be placed on the edge of the slide; proper placement is vital to ensure complete coverage of the tissue during staining.

Indirect immunofluorescence staining technique

Slide preparation

Unfixed cryostat section, air dried, 4 microns.

Method

1. Circle the location of the tissue on the back of the slide using a permanent pen; this will assist with identifying the tissue following staining.
2. Place air-dried slides in Tris buffer pH 7.6 for 5 minutes.
3. Tap off and quickly remove excess buffer.
4. Apply unlabeled antibody at its previously validated concentration on the tissue section for 30 minutes.
5. Rinse using Tris buffer pH 7.6 for 5 minutes.
6. Tap off and quickly remove excess buffer.
7. Apply Avidin D for 15 minutes.
8. Rinse using Tris buffer pH 7.6 for 5 minutes.
9. Tap off and quickly remove excess buffer.
10. Apply d-biotin to tissue for 15 minutes.
11. Rinse using Tris buffer pH 7.6 for 5 minutes.
12. Tap off and quickly remove excess buffer.
13. Apply biotinylated horse anti-mouse antibody for 25 minutes.
14. Rinse using Tris buffer pH 7.6 for 5 minutes.
15. Tap off and quickly remove excess buffer.
16. Apply fluorescein–streptavidin for 15 minutes.
17. Rinse using Tris buffer pH 7.6 for 5 minutes.
18. Rinse using deionized water for 5 minutes.
19. Coverslip using an aqueous mounting medium.
20. Seal the edge of the cover glass with clear fingernail polish or permanent mounting medium.
21. Place slides in a slide tray.
22. Store the slides in a cool dark place until review.

Technical note: Tissue should not be placed on the edge of the slide; proper placement is vital to ensure complete coverage of the tissue during staining.

MICROSCOPY

In principle, the aim of all fluorescent microscopy is to apply as much excitation energy as possible to the fluorochrome, ideally at the point of maximum absorption. This means that the potential to see the fluorescent process is maximized and the amount of emitted light is at its greatest.

The choice of light source and of excitation and secondary filters is of major importance to achieve maximum performance, and careful adjustment of condenser(s) and mirror is necessary to achieve the best results. Reference standards are available, comprising slides with wells containing standard polystyrene beads (about 10 μm) with different levels of brightness of fluorescence. This was the subject of an investigation by Rostami et al (1992). Such reference slides enable more accurate adjustment of the microscope for maximal fluorescence.

Light sources

Most fluorescent microscopes now employ mercury vapor or xenon light sources. These units can be expensive due to the requirement of an external power supply. Light output is reduced over time due to blackening of the quartz envelope. An automatic 'hour counter' is a useful asset and is usually fitted as standard.

Filters

The requirements for excitation (primary) and barrier (secondary) filters are complementary. The aim is to adapt the transmission ranges of the excitation and barrier filters to the shape of the absorption and emission curves of the fluorochromes as closely as possible. Colored glass filters have been replaced in most modern microscopes with broad or narrow band interference filters. The latter can be accurately tailored to meet the special requirements of fluorochromes, and unlike glass filters have high transmission with near vertical cut-off. In practice, broad-band excitation filters are most commonly used, where energy over a relatively wide spectrum is employed (e.g. 390–490 nm for FITC). Such filters give a high throughput of excitation energy and are particularly useful where the level of fluorescence is likely to be low. However, the contrast level of such filters can sometimes be poor, in which case narrow-band filters (450–490 nm) are of value, albeit the total excitation energy available is of a lower order. Barrier (secondary) filters are selected to absorb out excess excitation light, and allow transmission of the emitted light.

In practice this means selection of filters with a steep cut-off point, just above the emission level. An orange filter (cut-off 510 nm) is particularly suitable for FITC conjugates. The marriage of suitable excitation and barrier filters is now part of the standard equipment of modern fluorescent microscopy, and a wide and varied range is available. Manufacturers produce 'filter blocks' comprising combinations of excitation and barrier filters, along with suitable dichroic mirrors. A combination of three blocks—(1) for UV light excitation (FITC); (2) for broad-band blue light excitation (FITC); and (3) for green light excitation (TRITC)—is the most useful in routine laboratory applications.

Transmitted versus incident light illumination

Most modern fluorescent microscopes rely on incident light (epi-illumination). Compared to transmitted light, the path of the excitation light with epifluorescence is through fewer glass surfaces; hence, less light is lost due to internal absorption. Secondly, since the lens used also acts as a condenser, the area viewed equals the area illuminated. In these systems, lenses of high numerical aperture (NA) are a distinct advantage; for example, a lens with an NA of 0.9 will give twice the fluorescence intensity of a lens of similar magnification with an NA of 0.65. Increased brightness in epi-illumination systems is achieved by increasing *lens* rather than *eyepiece* magnification; an increase in eyepiece magnification will *reduce* the apparent brightness. In practice a combination of a 50× (NA 1.0) lens plus a 6.3× ocular will give a brighter image than the use of a 25× (NA 0.65) plus a 10× ocular, as well as giving a higher total magnification, i.e. 315 instead of 250. A major advantage is found in studies at the cellular level where lenses of high magnification, with correspondingly high NA, are required.

Dichroic mirrors are an essential part of incident light fluorescence. These mirrors have a dual purpose, allowing firstly *reflection* of the primary excitation light onto the prepared slides to produce fluorescence and secondly *transmission* of the emitted light through the oculars. Mirrors with different reflecting/transmission properties are compounded for use with different fluorochromes, and composite filter blocks of excitation and barrier filters, plus a dichroic mirror, make this type of illumination system particularly valuable for two-color fluorescence, since simple rapid change-over devices can be used on the microscope.

PHOTOGRAPHY

Immunofluorescent stain preparations fade with time, so stained slides do not provide a permanent record of staining results. Therefore, photo documentation of staining results when preparations are still fresh is necessary. Good photographs of preparations showing even low level of fluorescence (e.g. three or four lymphocytes showing membrane fluorescence only) can be achieved if the following points are observed:

- There should be unequivocal staining against a background that shows good contrast.
- A darkened work area is preferable, in which case the photographer should allow his or her eyes to become dark-adapted prior to viewing and photographing stained sections.
- The microscope and camera must be firmly mounted and vibration-free. Particular attention should be paid here in view of the long exposure times, compared with brightfield photomicrography (for example, vibration from a centrifuge in an adjacent room, or other mechanical equipment such as air conditioning, can lead to poorly focused images).
- The use of 'anti-fade' reagents in the mounting medium shortens exposure time significantly and is especially useful when UV or blue light is used, e.g. for FITC preparations, or when the preparation has a low fluorescence level. Mounting media containing an anti-fade reagent are available commercially.
- Camera systems that allow 100% available light to be used for photography are preferable to those using beam splitters for simultaneous observation/photography. In addition, cameras using short light paths are preferred.

QUALITY CONTROL

Quality control throughout the staining process is necessary for results to be consistent. The quality of staining should be monitored regularly and documented. Many tissues, such as kidney and muscle, may contain normal tissue elements that express the targeted antigen, thus serving as an internal positive control. Skin and heart do not typically contain the antigens that are usually targeted by immunofluorescent staining, so an external positive control must be stained along with the patient sample. A negative patient slide that omits the primary antibody should be stained with any patient tissue, to aid in the identification of false-positive staining. Possible causes and cures of false-positive staining are as follows.

Direct techniques

- False-positive staining may be observed due to inadequate rinsing following the application of the fluorochrome-conjugated primary antibody.
- Further dilution of the concentration of the fluorochrome-conjugated antibody may also reduce false-positive staining.

Indirect techniques

- False-positive staining may be observed due to inadequate rinsing following any step in the staining process.
- False-positive staining may result from inadequate blocking of intrinsic tissue biotin when using a biotinylated secondary antibody. Blocking with avidin and biotin is recommended.
- False-positive staining may result from incubation times that are too long in any given reagent, especially a fluorescein–streptavidin label.

With either direct or indirect techniques, the temperature should be controlled and excessive heat should be avoided.

IMMUNOFLUORESCENT TECHNIQUES IN DIAGNOSTIC HISTOPATHOLOGY

Many tissue immunofluorescence techniques, such as immunophenotype of lymphoid tissue and detection of infectious agents (especially viruses), have been supplanted by the use of flow cytometry and tissue immunoperoxidase staining. However, immunofluorescence is still widely used for diagnosis in evaluation of renal glomerular disease and certain skin diseases.

Renal diseases

Immunofluorescent methods, applied to frozen sections of renal tissue obtained by percutaneous needle biopsy, are of value in the diagnosis of glomerular disease. They enable the detection and localization of immunoglobulins, complement components, and fibrin within glomerular basement membrane, mesangium, and vessel walls.

Different glomerular diseases show different, sometimes specific, patterns of distribution. Some of these patterns are illustrated in Figures 24.1–24.4, and are discussed in detail in Jennette et al (1998). Most of these investigations employ the direct method, using FITC-labeled primary antibodies. However, some pathological reactions, such as the detection of C4d in renal or heart transplant biopsies in patients with suspected transplant rejection (Collins et al 1999), are better demonstrated using the indirect method (Fig. 24.5).

Skin diseases

Certain skin diseases have characteristic patterns of deposition of immunoglobulins, usually in upper dermis

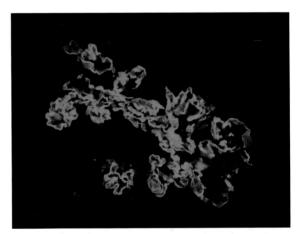

Fig. 24.1 Renal biopsy demonstrating glomerular basement membrane staining pattern, as seen in Goodpasture's syndrome.

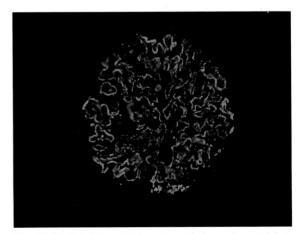

Fig. 24.2 Renal biopsy demonstrating membranous staining pattern with antibody to C3.

or at the dermoepidermal junction. This investigation is particularly useful in the diagnosis of bullous disorders of the skin, and in systemic lupus erythematosus and vasculitides. Some of the more common examples are summarized in Table 24.2 and are discussed in more detail in Farmer and Hood (2000).

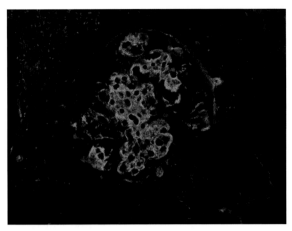

Fig. 24.3 Renal biopsy in lupus demonstrating glomerular staining for C1q.

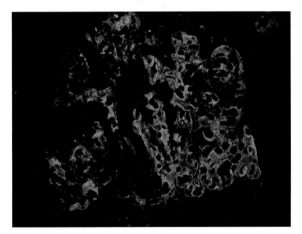

Fig. 24.4 Renal biopsy in lupus demonstrating glomerular staining for IgG.

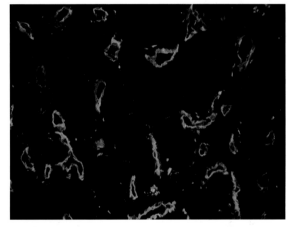

Fig. 24.5 Renal biopsy from a patient with kidney transplant rejection demonstrating staining of peritubular capillaries for C4d.

Table 24.2 Immunofluorescent patterns in selected skin diseases		
Skin disease	**Substances present**	**Location of deposits**
Pemphigus	IgG, C3	Intercellular epidermis
Pemphigoid	C3, IgG	Basement membrane zone (linear pattern)
Bullous systemic lupus erythematosus	IgG, C3 (±IgM, IgA) (granular)	Basement membrane zone
Dermatitis herpetiformis	IgA and C3 (granular)	Dermal papillae of perilesional skin (granular pattern)

Source: Farmer & Hood (2000).

Acknowledgments

We are indebted to Dr Joseph Zhou of the University of Texas Southwestern Medical Center Department of Pathology for providing the photographs of immuno-fluorescently stained renal biopsy specimens. Denis Marriott and Dr Gordon Reeves contributed this chapter for the first two editions. Denis Marriott and Stuart Carlton updated the chapter for the third edition and Stuart Carlton contributed the chapter for the fourth and fifth editions. Our acknowledgments are due to them for their contributions.

REFERENCES

Allan V.J. (2000) Protein localization by fluorescence microscopy. Oxford: Oxford University Press.

Carson F.L. (1997) Histotechnology: a self-instructional text, 2nd edn. Chicago: ASCP Press.

Collins A.B., Schneeberger E.E., Pascual M.A. et al. (1999) Complement activation in acute humoral renal allograft rejection: diagnostic significance of C4d deposits in peri-tubular capillaries. Journal of the American Society of Nephrology 10:2208–2214.

Coons A.H., Creech H.J., Jones R.N. (1941) Immunological properties of an antibody containing a fluorescent group. Proceedings of the Society for Experimental Biology and Medicine 47:200–202.

Farmer E.R., Hood A.F. (2000) Pathology of the skin, 2nd edn. New York: McGraw-Hill.

Jennette J.C., Olson J.L., Schwartz M.M., Silva F.G. (1998) Heptinstall's pathology of the kidney, 5th edn. Philadelphia: Lippincott-Raven.

Johnson G.D., Holborow E.J. (1986) Preparation and use of fluorochrome conjugates. In: Weir D.M., Herzenberg L.A., eds. Immunochemistry. Handbook of experimental immunology. Oxford: Blackwell, pp. 28.1–28.21.

Rostami R., Beutner E.H., Kumar V. (1992) Quantitative studies of immunofluorescent staining. VII. Quantitative reference standard slide for standardization of fluorescence microscopes. International Archives of Allergy and Immunology 98:200–204.

Weller T.H., Coons A.H. (1954) Fluorescent antibody studies with agents of varicella and herpes zoster propagated in vitro. Proceedings of the Society for Experimental Biology and Medicine 86:789–794.

25

Tissue Microarray

Wanda Grace-Jones

HISTORY

Tissue microarrays have been developed as a method to evaluate numerous samples of tissue in a short period. Battifora (1986) first introduced the concept of putting together multiple pieces of tissue in a single block called a sausage block. Kononen et al (1998) used this mechanism for examining several histological sections at one time by arraying them in a paraffin block. Today's tissue microarrays use multiple tissues in a single paraffin block using a precise size and shape to prepare the recipient block (Fig. 25.1). Histological techniques have an important role in the development of molecular biology.

PURPOSE

Tissue microarray has become a powerful tool which can be used in many aspects of research including cancer research. It has applications in clinical pathology and serves as quality control for new antibodies.

ADVANTAGES OF THE TECHNIQUE

This technology enables researchers and pathologists to study and evaluate diseases at an early stage. A hundred or more tissue samples are placed in one block. Many sections can be cut from the array block depending on the experience of the technologist and size of the cores. Hundreds of tissue cores are placed on a single slide for the pathologist to review.

The technique is used for a wide range of staining procedures: immunohistochemistry, in situ hybridization, fluorescent in situ hybridization, special stain control samples, and quality control sections for H&E stains. Only a small amount of reagent is used to analyze one slide, so it is cost effective in reagents used for immunohistochemistry and in situ hybridization techniques.

TMAs (tissue microarrays) have been widely used in immunohistochemistry for several years for quality control and quality assurance. They demonstrate the antibody thresholds on a single slide, which is used to optimize where the high and low signal intensities are seen.

FIXATION AND PROCESSING OF TISSUES AND CONTROLS

Fixation and processing is the most important part of the tissue preparation for histology. The most popular fixative is 10% neutral buffered formalin (NBF). It penetrates rapidly, does not over-harden tissue, and permits the use of a large variety of staining techniques. The fixative volume needs to be at least 15 to 20 times greater than the size of the tissue (see Chapter 4). Some antigens are not well demonstrated when using NBF (see Chapter 21). Pretreatment methods such as proteolytic enzyme digestion or retrieval can be performed. Extensive studies of fixation and processing have been done at our institution over the past 4 years on both large and small specimens. The following method works best in our laboratory (Table 25.1).

TISSUE MICROARRAYS CAN BE DIVIDED INTO FOUR GROUPS

Prevalence TMAs—are assembled from tumor samples of one or several types without attached clinical and pathological information. These TMAs are used to determine

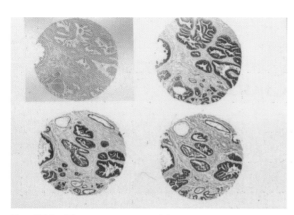

Fig. 25.1 Tissue microarray slide.

Table 25.1		
Station	Reagents	Time
1	10% NBF	2 hours
2	10% NBF	2 hours
3	70% alcohol	30 min
4	80% alcohol	30 min
5	95% alcohol	30 min
6	95% alcohol	30 min
7	100% alcohol	45 min
8	100% alcohol	45 min
9	Xylene	1 hour
10	Xylene	1 hour
11	Paraffin	1 hour
12	Paraffin	1 hour

the prevalence of a given alteration in the areas of interest in a tumor.

Progression TMAs—contain samples of different stages of one tumor type. They are used to discover associations between tumor genotype and phenotype. For example, an ideal breast cancer progression TMA would contain samples of normal breast from patients with and without breast cancer history, several different non-neoplastic breast diseases, ductal and lobular carcinoma in situ, invasive cancers of all stages, grades, and histological subtypes as well as metastases and recurrences after initially successful treatment.

Prognosis TMAs—contain samples from tumors available with clinical follow-up data. They represent a fast and reliable platform for the evaluation of clinical importance of new detected disease-related genes. Vali-

dation studies using prognosis TMAs readily reproduced all established associations between molecular findings and clinical outcome. Significant examples of these associations are found between estrogen or progesterone expression of HER-2 alterations and survival in breast cancer patients, between vimentin expression and prognosis in kidney cancer, and between Ki-67 labeling index and prognosis in urinary bladder cancer, soft tissue sarcoma, and Hurthle cell carcinoma.

Experimental TMAs—are constructed from tissues like cell lines. Cell line TMAs are optimally suited for screening purposes, e.g. tumor samples from TMA archives are also used in experimental TMAs.

DESIGNING THE GRID

Depending upon the purpose of the array, the design varies and the pathologist and technologist must determine the guidelines. In our laboratory, once the grid sheet is completed and has been reviewed and signed off, the array process can be started. The purpose for constructing the array is to assemble a simple series of 50 or more patients into one or several blocks. It is important to plan in advance how many samples will be arrayed and create a map or grid sheet which will be easy to follow (Fig. 25.2). A large number of samples (high density) can be arrayed in a 37 × 24 × 5 mm block. If you are working with a smaller number of samples (low density), use a 24 × 24 × 5 mm block.

Normal tissue controls and control cell lines are placed in columns between the tumors and normal tissue asymmetrically at one end of the block; be careful not to lose the orientation of the block. It is helpful to place a notch at the end of your cassette block to help with this. Archived blocks are used as a source of control tissue without destructive sampling. Making the tissue arrays is a project that involves many steps. Selecting the slides, collecting the blocks, and designing the grid consumes the time, rather than the array process. Setting up this process can take several weeks to a month before the array process actually will begin. Standardize the construction by making it easy to follow.

NEEDLE SIZES

0.6, 1.0, 1.5 or 2.0 mm needles can be used. 1.0 or 1.5 mm needles are recommended for general use. 0.6

TISSUE MICROARRAY GRID/MAP FORM

Cassette (place notch at this end of cassette)

1	2	3	4	5	6	7	8	9	10
A									
B									
C									
D									
E									
F									
G									
H									
I									
J									
K									
L									

Investigator's name: ______________________________

Date received: ______________________________

Fixation type: ______________________________

Tissue type: Human/Rodent/Cell lines

Tech initials: ______________________________

Date completed: ______________________________

In our laboratory, we have found that color coding the grid sheet and TMA slide can make it easier for the pathologist and investigator to review the slide

A
B
C
D
E
F
G
H

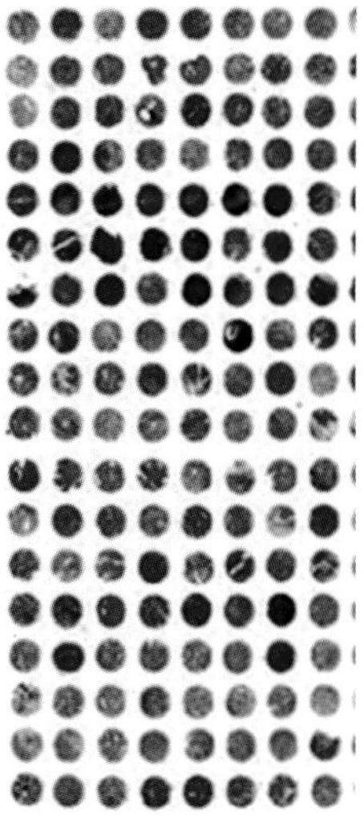

Fig. 25.2 Tissue microarray grid/map form.

needles can be used if you are coring 200 or more blocks. The use of 2.0 mm needles is not recommended by this author since damage can occur to the donor blocks.

DATABASE FOR TISSUE MICROARRAY ANALYSIS (Shaknovich et al 2003)

The first step in construction of a TMA is the selection of cases from a database and creation of a template or spreadsheet that identifies the position of each case and controls in the TMA block. During viewing and photographing of the slide, refer to core cases by position. Each case in the database is identified by the unique positions of each core on the template.

To acquire the image, each core in the TMA is identified based on the row and column position on the slide. One image per core is taken and saved as a compressed file, then named as the position identifier. Each image acquisition takes less than 1 minute, including field selection, manual focusing, and identification. It is sensible to save a set of images for each stain in a folder with a name that you can identify.

The next step is linking the images with the database, and the last is data entry. Several images from different stains can be viewed on the screen, scored, and the data entered manually into additional cells, adjacent to the image cell in the spreadsheet. This method allows examination of multiple cores and multiple stains of the same case with ease, allowing flexibility that is impossible at the microscope as it requires changing slides, stains, light sources, and identifying the correct core. Investigators can check scoring, and images can be printed and shared over the network. The collections of these images are used as an educational tool.

PREPARATION OF THE DONOR BLOCK

A pathologist reviews the file slides and blocks to determine which blocks will be arrayed. The area of interest to be sampled is marked by circling with a pilot pen or permanent fine-point marker. Some pathologists prefer to mark the blocks rather than the slides. Once the slides are reviewed and marked, the block is matched to the glass slide. Circle the area of interest on the block to match the marked slide. It is important that the block is marked in the same area of interest as the marked slide (Figs 25.3 and 25.4). Donor blocks must be at least

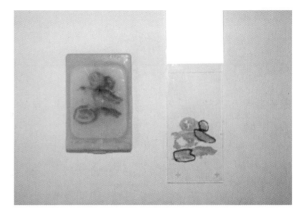

Fig. 25.3 Shows an H&E slide and the paraffin block area are matched.

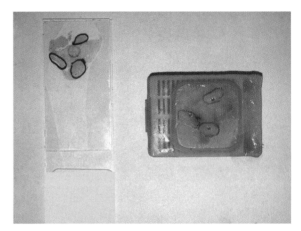

Fig. 25.4 The slide is reviewed and the area(s) of interest for the TMAs are circled.

1 mm thick to be suitable for constructing the arrays. An area site marked that is not 1 mm thick requires two cores from the same site and they are stacked on top of each other.

When marking the slides and blocks we use the following colors as indicators (Fig. 25.5):

- Red—cancer
- Green—normal
- Black—pre-invasive.

It is important to keep the blocks and slides together; a filing system of archival blocks is used for controls and a system of case studies for arraying. A sectioned H&E slide is filed behind the block.

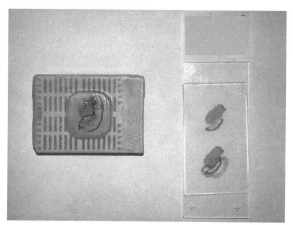

Fig. 25.5 Specific areas of interest can be identified with different colored markings; cancer areas are marked red, normal tissue green, and invasive areas black.

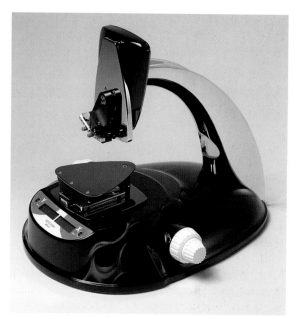

Fig. 25.7 Manual tissue arrayer MTAII, manufactured by Beecher Instruments, Inc.

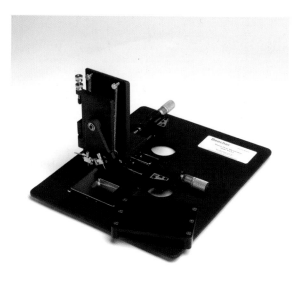

Fig. 25.6 Manual tissue arrayer MTAI, manufactured by Beecher Instruments, Inc.

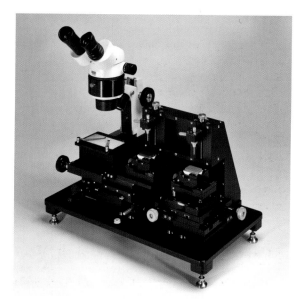

Fig. 25.8 Manual tissue arrayer MTAIII with microscope, manufactured by Beecher Instruments, Inc.

ARRAYERS

There are several different arrayers on the market today (Figs 25.6 to 25.9).

The automated arrayer is easy to use and includes a specimen tracking software system. The instrument marks, edits, and saves punch coordinates using an on-screen display and software tools. It pre-marks the punch areas. The video merge unit displays pre-marked slide images side by side to the donor block image. Some 120 to 180 cores can be punched per hour. The automated arrayer is ideal for a laboratory with a high volume of TMAs.

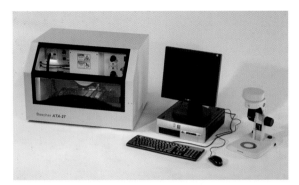

Fig. 25.9 Automated tissue arrayer ATA27, manu-factured by Beecher Instruments, Inc.

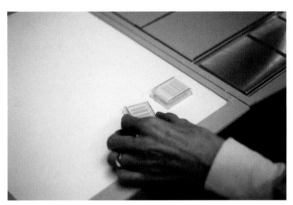

Fig. 25.10 Preparation of the recipient block. A blank block is embedded with paraffin, preferably using soft paraffin such as Paraplast X-tra.

Using a manual arrayer you have to rely on your map or grid sheet. Visual selection while punching depends on the technologist, who uses a hand-held magnifying glass or magnifying lamp attached to the counter or a base to hold the magnifying lamp in place. The pathologist marks all areas of interest on the slide and the technologist makes the movements.

Cores punched per hour depend on the experience of the worker. The average number of cores punched per hour using the manual arrayer is between 30 and 70. To prepare microarray blocks for special stain controls, or QC controls for H&E staining, an inexpensive pen extractor would be suitable.

No matter which arrayer you decide to use you need to have a quiet environment where you will not be distracted and to become familiar with the equipment by constructing a practice array block. The number of specimens per array depends on the size of the punches and the desired array density. Using a 0.6 mm needle you can construct tissue arrays with 400 or more cores per block. Using a 1.0 mm needle, you can construct about 200 cores per block. Using a 2.0 mm punch allows you to construct 50 to 100 cores per block. We prefer using the 1.0 mm needle, allowing us to get a desirable core and leaving little distortion to the donor block.

PREPARATION OF THE RECIPIENT AND DONOR ARRAY BLOCK

A blank paraffin block is prepared and used as the recipient for the tissue samples. It is best to use a soft paraffin

Table 25.2 Typical core spacing and number of cores using various needle sizes

Needle size	Spacing between samples	Array format	# Cores
0.6 mm	0.2 mm	20 × 20 cores	400
1.0 mm	0.3 mm	16 × 13 cores	208
1.5 mm	0.4 mm	11 × 9 cores	99

and to make sure there are no holes in the paraffin block caused by air bubbles (Fig. 25.10). Typical core spacing and number of cores using various needle sizes are shown in Table 25.2.

To ensure the alignment of the punches, first move the recipient punch into position and make a mark in the paraffin. Then do the same for the donor punch. Move the needles to the position of the first punch with the X or Y micrometer adjustment controls. The position of the punches over the block can be made by gently pushing down on them until a mark is made in the paraffin. Continue to make adjustments with the micrometer knobs until the desired position is attained, then zero the micrometers.

The empty recipient block is placed in the holder and the attachment screws are tightened to keep the block from slipping. Place the recipient block notched edge to the left of the block holder. Making a hole in the first position begins the array process. The smaller needle is used to create the hole. First the depth stop is adjusted and its nut is tightened to stop the needle at the correct

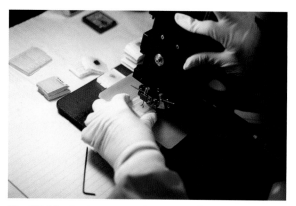

Fig. 25.11   In the preparation stage of making the TMA at the arrayer the bridge is placed over the recipient block.

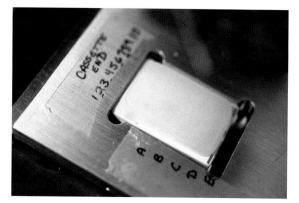

Fig. 25.12   The donor tissue has been placed in the appropriate location in the recipient block.

depth. The needle is pushed downwards by hand; the depth stop limits this motion and the handle in the needle is used to rotate the needle. The downward pushing pressure is relieved and springs will pull the needle upwards. The stylet is used to empty the needle. Do not remove the stylets from the needles during the array process. The donor block bridge is placed over the recipient block and the turret is moved to switch the larger needle into a vertical sampling position (Fig. 25.11). The donor block is moved under the sampling needle. The larger needle is used to retrieve the sample. The H&E slide is moved out of the way and the needle is pushed downwards to retrieve the sample. The depth stop does not block the needle motion from the donor block. Care must be taken to prevent the needle from entering too deep. Depending on the tissue type and the purpose of the study it is best to have three punches of the same site. This way the tissue sample is well represented in evaluation of prognostic markers. Use of a four block indexer allows four replicate blocks to be made at the same time. Cut down the length of the donor core if it is too tall to fit in the recipient punch; this can be done by ejecting the core with the stylus and placing it on a clean flat surface. Use a clean razor blade to cut the core to the desired length; the core is then placed into the recipient block using a pair of forceps (Fig. 25.12).

SMOOTHING AND SECTIONING

The array block must be smooth and level before sectioning. There are two methods in use in our laboratory.

Method 1

Place a clean microscope slide on top of the array block and warm in a 35–37°C oven checking at intervals of 3 minutes. Do not leave the block in the oven or the paraffin will melt causing loss of tissue orientation. Move the slide in a gentle circular motion and press. You will notice circles on the slide. Place the slide and block in the refrigerator or freezer. Once cooled, the slide will separate from the array block.

Method 2

Heat a clean microscope slide to around 70–80°C and touch it to the array block surface. The surface of the block will begin to melt. Move the slide in a circular motion and place the slide and block in the refrigerator or freezer.

MICROTOMY

Set the temperature in your water bath at 37°C. Gently face off the array block on a dedicated microtome. Cut sections at 4–5 microns. Always use positively charged slides for the microarray sections. A hundred or more sections, depending on the skill of the technologist, can be cut from the array block. Place the sections on the slide in the same orientation. Stain one slide for H&E; unstained slides are placed in a box and stored at −20°C. Sections can be cut a day or two before they are stained. To avoid contamination place in a slide box and store.

Sectioned TMA blocks should be dipped in paraffin to avoid loss of antigens.

Excessive soaking or freezing can cause the tissue to swell and keep the array block from ribboning well. The ability to study archival tissue specimens is important. To collect samples, cores can be placed into Eppendorf tubes and labeled.

DISTORTION OF THE TISSUE BLOCK

In most cases the tissue block can be cored several times with minimal distortion. When you section the cored block it is still possible in most cases to make a diagnosis.

TROUBLESHOOTING AND TIPS

- Core does not come out of the punch easily—punch tip is bent or distorted. Change the punch.
- Tissue core was pushed too deep—remove the sample with the small punch and place a new sample in the same position.
- Insufficient spacing of cores—can cause minor cracks or stress on the core when sectioning.
- Thinning of TMA cores in block—this is a result of repeated sectioning of the same block where cores are uneven in block.
- Loss of tissue on water bath—due to folds, wrinkles, and mishandling of ribbon.
- Re-facing block—when sections are cut to accommodate slides for stains requested. If the block is filed and then pulled for cutting of extra slides, the block is repositioned and re-faced. This is why it is important to use a dedicated microtome.
- Re-facing angle—shortens the life of the tissue microarray block which is called thinning. Make sure the cassette is completely flat on top of the mold.

DEFINITIONS

Dedicated microtome: a microtome used only for TMAs.
Donor block: a tissue paraffin block that contains tissue of the desired type to be placed into the tissue microarray recipient block.
High density: large number of samples arrayed in a $37 \times 24 \times 5$ mm block.

Histological section: a flat ribbon of paraffin and embedded tissue cut from a paraffin block on a microtome. The thickness of the section can vary, but a typical thickness is 4 microns.
In situ hybridization: an assay for nucleic acids on site fixed tissue sections by the use of heat to first denature and then to reanneal with specific DNA or RNA probes.
Low density: small number of samples arrayed in a $24 \times 24 \times 5$ mm block.
QA: quality assurance.
Recipient block: the blank paraffin block into which the tissue cores are inserted to form the tissue microarray.
Scoring: quantitative comparison of normal versus diseased tissue samples.
Standardization: to compare with or conform an assay of unknowns to established standards.
Tissue Microarray: a recipient paraffin block consisting of tissue specimen cores.
TMA technology: a technology where hundreds of tissue cores are arranged in a single glass slide for analysis by immunostaining, in situ hybridization, or fluorescent in situ hybridization.
Tissue paraffin block: a sample of tissue that has been fixed in formalin, processed to remove water, then infused with molten paraffin, which hardens in and around the tissue in the base mold. The paraffin is cut on a microtome to produce thin histological sections which are placed on glass slides. These donor blocks can be selected for TMA studies.
Tissue spot: the tissue sample present on a section of a tissue microarray that corresponds to the tissue core.

MAINTENANCE OF THE ARRAYER

During the array process, it is useful to clean any residual paraffin from the punches, sampling block, and block holders. Wipe clean with a 5×5-cm gauze sponge. Do not soak any parts in xylene. X-Y or Z rails should be oiled once every few months.

Punches need to be replaced periodically: they are made of a thin tube and can bend. The tip of the punch may become dulled after several hundred punches. The replacement punch is correctly positioned when the groove in the punch hub is firmly placed against the metal rod in the v-block. Make sure it does not wobble.

Alignment of the replacement punches should be checked prior to beginning an array. Clean work area at the end of each day.

Acknowledgment

The author acknowledges the information gained from the NSH workshop no. 89 in 2003, 'Tissue microarrays: principles and practice', given by Helen Fedor and Angelo DeMarzo MD, PhD.

REFERENCES

Battifora H. (1986) The multitumor (sausage) tissue block: novel method for immunohistochemical antibody testing. Laboratory Investigation 55:244–248.

Kononen J., Bubendorf L., Kallioniemi A. et al. (1998) Tissue microarrays for high-throughput molecular profiling of tumor specimens. Nature Medicine 4:844–847.

Shaknovich R., Celestine A.,Yang L., Cattoretti G. (2003) Novel relational database for tissue microarray analysis. Archives of Pathology and Laboratory Medicine 127(4): 492–494.

FURTHER READING

Brady J. The Science Advisory Board: Tissue microarrays: bringing histology up to speed. Online. Available: http://www.scienceboard.net/community/perspectives.63.html

Enghardt M.H., Aghassi N.B., Bond C.J., Elston D.M. (1995) A simplified multitissue control block. Journal of Histotechnology 18:51–55.

Flores G. (2005) Tissue microarrays go coreless. Scientist 19:38–39.

Jensen T.A., Hammond M.E. (2001) The tissue microarray—a technical guide for histologists. Journal of Histotechnology 24:283–287.

26

Molecular Pathology—In Situ Hybridization

Diane L. Sterchi

INTRODUCTION

In molecular pathology the emphasis is on assessing gene expression, morphology, and using gene expression analysis to validate large numbers of targets.

Molecular pathology techniques have been used in the clinical laboratory to aid in the diagnosis and monitoring of treatment regimens of many infectious diseases such as HIV, hepatitis B, and tuberculosis (Netterwald 2006). These tests are usually performed on serological or other body fluids such as sputum and seminal fluid. Currently the most well known and most advertised molecular testing is for human papillomavirus (HPV).

Clinical and especially research laboratories may use additional molecular pathology techniques, such as blotting methods that are used to study extracted ribonucleic acid (RNA) and deoxyribonucleic acid (DNA). Blotting methods consist of extracting DNA and/or RNA from homogenized tissues and then analyzing these nucleic acids using dot, Southern and northern blotting filter hybridization methods (Sambrook et al 1989). Blotting techniques such as these are powerful tools for the qualitative analysis of extracted nucleic acid from fresh or frozen cells and frozen tissues.

The polymerase chain reaction (PCR) is included in molecular pathology methods. PCR is a common method of creating copies of specific fragments of DNA. PCR rapidly amplifies a single DNA molecule into many billions of molecules. In one application of the technology, small samples of DNA, such as those found in a strand of hair at a crime scene, can produce sufficient copies to carry out forensic tests. PCR may also be used in addition

to in situ hybridization (ISH) to study a specific genome of a tissue (Innis et al 1990).

All of this leads to the role the histology laboratory plays in molecular pathology. In the histology laboratory the main method used in molecular pathology is in situ hybridization. John et al (1969) and Gall and Pardue (1969) described the technique of in situ hybridization almost simultaneously.

In situ hybridization is a method of localizing and detecting specific mRNA sequences in preserved tissue sections or cell preparations by hybridizing the complementary strand of a nucleotide probe to the sequence of interest.

In situ hybridization consists of denaturing (breaking apart) DNA/RNA strands using heat. A probe (a labeled complementary single strand) is incorporated with the DNA/RNA strands of interest. The strands will anneal (nucleotides bonding back together) with their homologous partners when cooled (Fig. 26.1). Some will anneal with the original complementary strands, but some will also anneal or hybridize with the probe. As probes increase in length, they become more specific. The chances of a probe finding a homologous sequence other than the target sequence decreases as the number of nucleotides in the probe increases. Optimal probe size for in situ hybridization is small fragments of about 200–300 nucleotides. However, probes may be as small as 20–40 base pairs (bp) or as large as 1000 bp.

The detection of specific nucleic acid sequences—RNA, viral DNA or chromosomal DNA—in cells, tissues or whole organisms by in situ hybridization has numerous applications in biology, clinical and anatomical pathology, and research.

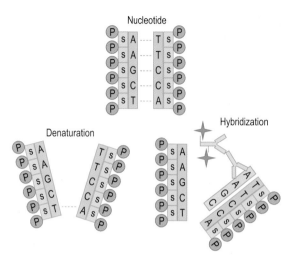

Nucleotide

Denaturation

Hybridization

Fig. 26.1 The genetic information for humans is encoded in billions of nucleotides, the building blocks of the DNA code, arranged in a double helix molecule. Nucleotides consist of a base, a sugar (S), and a phosphate (P). The DNA code is written in an alphabet that uses four letters to represent each of the bases. (A) = adenine, (T) = thymine, (C) = cytosine, (G) = guanine. These bases will form pairs. (A) will only pair with (T). (G) will only pair with (C). Therefore, double-stranded DNA consists of two strands of homologous nucleotides. The *genetic code* in DNA is in triplets such as ATG. The base sequence of that triplet in the partner strand is therefore TAC.

ISH methods may employ radiolabeled probes that are visualized on a photographic film or photographic emulsion. However, most of these probes do not work well on routinely fixed, processed tissues, require the use of frozen sections, and take around 20–50 days' exposure before seeing results. The development of non-radiolabeled probes that perform well on routine surgical and autopsy specimens has extended the field of anatomic pathology.

Detection of mRNA is particularly useful if the protein product is quickly degraded or rapidly transported out of the target cell.

In ISH detection, immunohistochemistry (IHC)-like methods may be incorporated to detect the labeled (biotin, digoxygenin (DIG)) probe. So the question arises, why not just do IHC? It is well-established, reliable, and less time consuming than ISH. IHC has been employed in the clinical and research arenas for several decades and has become a routine procedure in the histology

laboratory. IHC has provided diagnostic procedures and a close look at the proteins within and on the cell membranes. So why do ISH? The advantages of ISH over IHC are:

1. high degree of specificity.
2. DNA and mRNA are not as sensitive to formalin fixatives.
3. probe–target hybrid is stronger than antibody–antigen complex.
4. provides an alternative means of detection when reliable antibodies are not available.
5. provides a diagnosis at the molecular level.

It is important to understand the 'how and why' of the different stages in the ISH process in order for the testing to result in a functional outcome. This chapter focuses on the 'how and why' of ISH and general procedures on tissue sections.

APPLICATIONS

There are many modifications to ISH methods that relate to the application needs. Although the demonstration of DNA and RNA sequences by in situ hybridization is a valuable research tool, according to Warford and Lauder (1991) and Mitchell et al (1992), it is also used diagnostically in:

- detection of abnormal genes
- identification of viral infection
- tumor phenotyping.

In situ hybridization alone can provide cytological information on the location and alteration of genomic sequences in chromosomes. Traditionally the technique has been applied to metaphase chromosome spreads (Davis et al 1984; Lux et al 1990), but it has been shown to be applicable to interphase nuclei (Hopman et al 1988; Poddighe et al 1992). Routine paraffin wax preparations of tissues can be used and 'interphase cyto-genetics', as the method is termed, can provide direct information on chromosomal abnormalities in unselected tumor cell populations. Chromogenic in situ hybridization (CISH) is a method 'that enables the detection of gene expression in the nucleus using a conventional histochemical reaction' (White 2005); it is used for the detection of abnormal genes and to identify a gene therapy treatment direction. CISH can be used as

In situ

In the normal location. An 'in situ' tumor is one that is confined to its site of origin and has not invaded neighboring tissue or gone elsewhere in the body.

In situ hybridization

A technique that identifies and quantifies nucleic acid sequences within cells.

Integration

The combining of a foreign segment of DNA with cellular DNA sequences, causing the expression and replication of foreign DNA.

Intron

A segment of a gene situated between exons that is removed before translation of messenger RNA and does not function in coding for protein synthesis.

In vitro transcription

Using a DNA template to synthesize a RNA sequence in the presence of RNA polymerase and nucleotide triphosphates.

Kilobase

A measure of length of nucleic acids. One kilobase (kb) equals 1000 nucleotides of single-stranded nucleic acid. (kbp) refers to kilobase pairs of double-stranded DNA.

Melting temperature

The temperature at which the hydrogen bonds between complementary nucleotides will break, causing the dissociation of double-stranded nucleic acid. It is dependent on the G+C content of the DNA.

mRNA

Messenger RNA carries the message of the DNA to the cytoplasm of the cell where protein is made. Single-stranded RNA synthesized from a DNA template during transcription binds to ribosomes and directs protein synthesis.

Missense mutation

A single base substitution in DNA that changes a codon for one amino acid into a codon for a different amino acid.

Mutation

A change in the sequence of nucleotides in DNA.

Nick translation

Incorporating a labeled deoxyribonucleotide triphosphate into DNA.

Nonsense codon

A codon that does not code for an amino acid, but is a signal to terminate protein synthesis.

Northern blot

A cellulose or nylon membrane to which RNA molecules have been attached by capillary action. The transferred RNA is hybridized to single-stranded DNA probes. Northern blot technique is often used to measure expression (transcription) of a gene for which a specific cDNA is available for use as a probe. A gel-based laboratory procedure that locates mRNA sequences on a gel that are complementary to a piece of DNA used as a probe.

Nucleotide

The unit of DNA or RNA that consists of a phosphate group, a sugar, and a base.

Oligonucleotide

A short piece of nucleic acid that can be used as a hybridization probe.

Oncogene

A gene whose activity is associated with the conversion of normal cells to cancer cells.

Operator

The segment of DNA to which the repressor binds; it controls the expression of adjacent genes.

Operon

The sequence of bases in DNA that contain one or more structural genes together with the operator controlling their expression.

Phage

A virus that infects a bacterium. Phages are often used to produce recombinant DNA molecules.

Plasmid

A piece of DNA that can replicate independently of the chromosome or be incorporated into it. A plasmid is inherited, but not required for the host cell's growth or reproduction. Plasmids can be used to produce recombinant DNA.

Probe

A single-stranded piece of labeled DNA or RNA that will bind to a complementary sequence (target).

Promotor

The region of DNA, at the start of a gene, that the RNA polymerase binds to before beginning transcription.

Random priming
A method for labeling double-stranded DNA to produce a probe.

Recombinant DNA
The production of a single piece of DNA from two different sources.

Replication
The process by which an exact copy of parental DNA or RNA is made with the parental molecule serving as a template.

Restriction endonuclease
An endonuclease that is specific for a particular nucleotide sequence.

Reverse transcriptase
An enzyme that will synthesize a complementary sequence of DNA from a RNA template.

RNA
Ribonucleic acid. A nucleic acid that plays an important role in protein synthesis and other cell activities.

RNA polymerase
An enzyme that catalyzes the synthesis of RNA from a DNA template, using nucleotide triphosphates as substrates.

RNases
Ubiquitous RNA degrading enzymes.

rRNA
Ribosomal RNA is a component of ribosomes and functions as a non-specific site for making polypeptides.

Sense strand
The DNA strand that RNA polymerase copies to produce mRNA, rRNA, or tRNA.

Southern blot
The analysis of DNA sequences. It identifies and quantifies the DNA sequences using a specific hybridization protein.

Stringency
Conditions employed in hybridization reactions used to control the specificity of probe binding. The highest stringency conditions ensure the probe will bind only to completely complementary sequences. Lower stringency conditions will allow binding to sequences with some mismatching.

Template
A strand of DNA or RNA that specifies the base sequence of a newly synthesized complementary strand of DNA or RNA.

Transcription
The process by which a DNA sequence is copied into a complementary RNA sequence.

tRNA
Transfer RNA is a short-chain type of RNA present in cells that transfers specific amino acids in the formation of proteins.

Translation
The process by which the genetic message carried by the mRNA directs the synthesis of polypeptides; protein synthesis.

REAGENT PREPARATION

Listed here are formulas and methods on how to prepare the reagents for most ISH methods. The majority of these reagents can be purchased pre-mixed or in a kit for easy mixing. Keep in mind that different reagents may be suggested with some ISH methods, as you will see further in this chapter. The reagents listed here are for use in a universal no-frills or special equipment ISH procedure. Purchasing the reagents pre-mixed or in kits is convenient and safer to use, and provides some comfort that they are mixed according to manufacturer's specification and guaranteed by the vendor. This may cut down the possibility of human error. Some laboratories have limited budgets and find that pre-mixed reagents and kits are not an option. They can be expensive and expire before all of the reagents are used. To aid those laboratories in getting started, a reagent preparation list follows.

Diethylpyrocarbonate (DEPC) treated water

Diethylpyrocarbonate	1 ml
Distilled water	1000 ml

Stir while bringing to a boil for 10 min (in fume hood). Autoclave to expel DEPC.

2% aminoalkylsilane (positively charged slides)

Aminoalkylsilane (AAS)* stored at 4°C	5 ml
Dry acetone	250 ml

Dip clean slides in 2% AAS for 1 min. Rinse in three changes of deionized water.

Note

These slides may be purchased pre-coated. Make sure they are RNA/DNA free.

Proteinase K

Proteinase K	100 mg
Buffer #1	5 ml

Aliquot and freeze below −20°C.

Hyaluronidase

Hyaluronidase	20 mg
Buffer #1	20 ml

0.1 M triethanolamine (make fresh)

Triethanolamine	0.1 ml
DEPC water	100 ml
Acetic anhydride	0.25 ml*

*Add just prior to use. Stir for 5 minutes, then add an additional 0.25 ml, and stir for another 5 min.

1 M Tris (stock)

Trizma base	60.55 g
DEPC water	500 ml
Adjust pH to 8.0 with conc. HCl	20 ml*

*Autoclave.

1 M magnesium chloride (stock)

Magnesium chloride	20.34 g
DEPC water	100 ml*

*Autoclave.

5 M sodium chloride (stock)

Sodium chloride	29.22 g
DEPC water	100 ml*

*Autoclave.

Maleic acid buffer

Maleic acid	100 mM
Sodium chloride	150 mM

Mix 1:10 with water and adjust pH to 7.5, or add Tween 20 (0.3% v/v) for a washing buffer.

Buffer #1: Tris buffered saline, pH 7.5

1 M Tris (stock)	10 ml
5 M sodium chloride (stock)	3.3 ml
1 M magnesium chloride (stock)	0.2 ml
Deionized water	86.7 ml

Adjust pH to 7.5 with HCl.

Buffer #2: Tris buffered saline, pH 9.5

1 M Tris (stock)	10 ml
5 M sodium chloride (stock)	2 ml
1 M magnesium chloride (stock)	5 ml
Deionized water	83 ml

Adjust pH to 9.5 with sodium hydroxide (NaOH).

20× Saline sodium citrate (SSC) buffer

Sodium chloride	348 g
Sodium citrate	167.4 g
DEPC water	1600 ml

Adjust to pH 7.4 with dilute acetic acid, stirring vigorously. Autoclave.

2× SSC

20× SSC	10 ml
DEPC water	100 ml

1× SSC

20× SSC	5 ml
DEPC water	95 ml

Denhart's solution

Ficoll	100 mg*
Polyvinylpyrrolidone	100 mg*
Bovine serum albumin	100 mg
DEPC water	500 ml

*May cause increase in background.

Prehybridization solution

Deionized formamide	5 ml*[1]
20× SSC	2 ml
Denhart's solution	0.10 ml*[2]
50% dextran sulfate	2 ml
Salmon sperm DNA (10 mg/ml)	0.30 ml*[3]
Yeast tRNA (10 mg/ml)	25 ml*[4]

[1] purified = less non-specific staining
[2] reduces non-specific probe binding
[3] denature by boiling for 10 min
[4] blocks non-specific staining

Hybridization solution

Prehybridization solution	1 ml
Labeled probe (500 ng/25 μl)	10 ml

Detection method reagents: pick one

1. Streptavidin–alkaline phosphatase	0.01 ml
Buffer #1	5 ml
2. Anti-digoxygenin	0.01 ml
Buffer #1	2.50 ml

3. Horseradish peroxidase (HRP)   0.01 ml
   Buffer #1   5 ml

Colorimetric detection reagents: pick one

1. *BCIP–NBT*
   5-bromo-4-chloro-3-indolyl
   phosphate (BCIP)   0.5 mg/ml
   nitro-blue tetrazolium salt (NBT)   0.3 mg/ml
2. *AEC*
   3-amino-9-ethylcarbazole (AEC)   0.08 g
   acetone   10 ml
   0.05 M acetate buffer   200 ml
   hydrogen peroxide (30%)   0.10 ml
3. *DAB*
   Diaminobenzidine (DAB)   22 mg
   Tris buffer   50 ml
   Hydrogen peroxide (30%)   0.2 ml

PROBES AND THEIR CHOICE

Probe choice is based on the type of sequence you are trying to detect. The technologist needs to optimize the conditions he or she uses as much as possible. The strength of the bonds between the probe and the target plays an important role. The strength decreases in the order RNA–RNA to DNA–DNA. Various hybridization conditions such as concentration of formamide, salt concentration, hybridization temperature, and pH influence this stability.

A probe is a labeled bit of DNA or RNA used to find its complementary sequence or locate a particular clone. The choice of probes will depend on availability, sensitivity, and resolution required. The sensitivity of the probe will depend on the degree of substitution and the size of the labeled fragments. Degree of substitution refers to the original nucleotide substituted by the labeled analogues. The sensitivity of detection correlates with the amount of label substituted. In general, probes with 25–32% substitution yield the highest sensitivity. There are several different types of probe. Each has unique characteristics that must be considered for each application.

Probe type and means of synthesis

There are essentially four types of probe that can be used in performing in situ hybridization.

Oligonucleotide probes are usually 20–50 bases in length. They are produced synthetically by an automated chemical synthesis employing a specific DNA nucleotide sequence (of your choice). These probes are resistant to RNases and are small which allows for easy penetration into the cells or tissue of interest. However, the small size has it disadvantage in that it covers fewer targets. The label should be positioned at the 3′ or the 5′ end. To increase sensitivity one can use a mixture of oligonucleotides that are complementary to different regions of the target molecule. Oligonucleotide protocols can be standardized for many different probes regardless of the target genes being measured. Another advantage of oligonucleotide probes is that they are single stranded, therefore excluding the possibility of renaturation.

Single-stranded DNA probes are a much larger size range ($\approx$200–500 bp) than oligonucleotide probes. Single-stranded DNA probes can be prepared by a primer extension on single-stranded templates by RT-PCR of RNA, or by an amplified primer extension of a PCR-generated fragment in the presence of a single antisense primer, or by the chemical synthesis of oligonucleotides. PCR-based methods are much easier and probes can be synthesized from small amounts of starting material. Moreover, PCR allows great flexibility in the choice of probe sequences by the use of appropriate primers.

Double-stranded DNA probes can be prepared by nick-translation, random primer, or PCR in the presence of a labeled nucleotide, and denatured prior to hybridization in order for one strand to hybridize with the mRNA of interest. They can also be produced by the inclusion of the sequence of interest in bacteria, which is replicated, lysed, and then the DNA is extracted and purified. The sequence of interest is removed with restriction enzymes. Random priming and PCR give the highest specific activities. These probes are less sensitive than single-stranded probes, since the two strands have a tendency to rehybridize to each other, thus reducing the concentration of probe available for hybridization to the target. Nevertheless, the sensitivity obtained with double-stranded probes is sufficient for many purposes, although they are not widely used today.

RNA probes (cRNA probes or riboprobes) are thermostable and are resistant to digestion by RNases. These probes are single stranded and are the most widely used probes with ISH. RNA probes are generated by in vitro transcription from a linearized template using a promoter for RNA polymerase that must be available on the vector DNA containing the template (SP6, T7, or T3). RNA polymerase is used to synthesize RNA complementary to the DNA substrate. Most commonly, the probe sequence is cloned into a plasmid vector so that it is flanked by two different RNA polymerase initiation sites enabling either sense-strand (control) or antisense (probe) RNA to be synthesized. The plasmid is linearized with a restriction enzyme so that plasmid sequences are not transcribed, since these may cause high backgrounds.

When comparing double-stranded to single-stranded probes, single-stranded probes provide a few advantages over double-stranded probes such as:

- The probe does not self-anneal in solution so the probe is not exhausted.
- Large probe chains are not formed in solution, thus probe penetration is not affected.

If high sensitivity is required, single-stranded probes should be used (Table 26.1).

PROBE PREPARATION AND LABELING

To visualize where the probe has bound within your tissue section or within your cells, you must attach a detectable label to your probe before hybridization. Two major choices must be made for the preparation of a probe.

- What type of nucleic acid is to be used (DNA or RNA, single or double stranded)?
- What type of label is to be incorporated into the probe?

A vital consideration is the length of the probe, and the means by which this is controlled depends on the type and the method of synthesis. There are two methods of probe labeling. They are:

- Direct: The reporter molecules (enzyme, radioisotope or fluorescent marker) are directly attached to the DNA or RNA.
- Indirect: A hapten (biotin, digoxygenin, or fluorescein) is attached to the probe and detected by a labeled binding protein (typically an antibody).

Methods for incorporation of labels into DNA are nick translation and random primer methods.

Oligonucleotide probe labeling

- 5'-end labeling:
  The 5' end of DNA or RNA undergoes direct phosphorylation of the free 5'-terminal OH groups. The free 5'-OH substrates can be labeled using T4 polynucleotide kinase. This method is usually used for radiolabeling. Non-radiolabels use a covalent linker.
- 3'-end labeling:
  Terminal dexoxynucleotidyl transferase (TdT) is used to add a labeled residue to the 3' end of a synthetic oligonucleotide that is approximately 14–100 nucleotides in length. These probes provide excellent specificity but only moderate sensitivity. See oligonucleotide 3'-end labeling procedure in this chapter (see Procedure 26.1).
- 3' tailing:
  A tail containing labeled nucleotides is added to the free 3' end of double- or single-stranded DNA using TdT. These probes are more sensitive than the 3'-end labeled but can produce more non-specific background. Oligonucleotide tailing kits are commercially available.

It should be noted that the use of commercially available labeling kits can greatly assist in making methods simpler to undertake while providing results of an assured standard.

Purification of labeled probes

Sephadex G-50 column

Sephadex matrix traps unincorporated labeled probes. The labeled probes are excluded from the pores of the matrix and spun through the column. The labeled probes are collected in the eluent. Other brand name spin columns are commercially available.

Sephadex G-50 chromatography

Purifies probes, but fractions of the eluent have to be collected and tested for the presence of label. There are smaller sized columns available than the ones described above that fit into ordinary microcentrifuges.

Selective precipitation

This can be used to remove interferences from a mixture. A chemical reagent is added to the solution, and it selectively reacts with the interference to form a precipitate. The precipitate can then be physically separated from

Table 26.1   Probe types

Probe	Labeling	Advantages	Disadvantages
dsDNA	Random primers	Easy to use Subcloning unnecessary Choice of labeling methods High specific activity Possibility of signal amplification (networking) Readily available	Re-annealing during hybridization (decreased probe availability) Probe denaturation required, increasing probe length and decreasing tissue penetration Hybrids less stable than RNA probes
ssDNA	Primer extension	No probe denaturation needed No re-annealing during hybridization (single strand) More sensitive Stable	Technically complex Subcloning required Hybrids less stable than RNA probes Template binding
ssRNA	DNA polymerase transcription	High specific activity No probe denaturation needed No re-annealing Unhybridized probe enzymatically destroyed, sparing hybrid	Subcloning needed Less tissue penetration RNase labile May have higher levels of non-specific binding to tissue components, thus increasing the chance of higher background and lower penetration of the probe into the tissue
Oligo	5′ end 3′ end 3′ tailing	No cloning or molecular biology expertise required Stable Good tissue penetration (small size) Constructed according to recipe from amino acid data No self-hybridization Limited labeling methods Short oligonucleotide sequences can be directly manufactured Can use multiple probes, no competition between probes	Limited labeling methods Lower specific activity, so less sensitive Dependent on published sequences Less stable hybrids

the mixture by filtration or centrifugation. Under this premise, unincorporated labeled nucleotides can be eliminated by ethanol precipitation in the presence of a DNA carrier. Mononucleotides remain in the supernatant. Labeled and/or purified probes can be concentrated by ethanol precipitation and can be stored at −20°C. Do **not** purify biotinylated probes by phenol/chloroform extraction, as this will destroy the biotin.

Spin columns provide a simple way of purifying nucleic acid sequences from labeling reagents. This is achieved by centrifuging the labeling solution through a column of packed G-50 Sephadex, Sephacryl S-400, or Probe Quant G-50, in which the labeling reagents are retained but the larger nucleic acid sequences are excluded and, therefore, are recovered in the eluent.

METHOD

Preparation of columns

1. Plug the barrel of a 1.0 ml disposable syringe with sterile siliconized glass wool (GE) or polyallomer wool. Fill the syringe with a slurry of 5 g Sephadex G-50 (Roche 1273973), Sephacryl S-400 (GE 17-0609-10), or Probe Quant G-50 (GE 27-5335-01), pre-swollen (this may take a couple of hours) in 100 ml of 1× Tris buffer, pH 8.0.
2. Let the Tris buffer drain out, fill the syringe again with Sephadex slurry. Continue addition of Sephadex until the syringe is filled with gel when the Tris buffer has drained out.
3. Insert the syringe into a polypropylene 10 ml centrifuge tube. Centrifuge at 3000× g for 5 min in a bench centrifuge. Do not be alarmed at the appearance of the column. Continue to add Sephadex until the packed column volume after centrifugation is 0.9 ml.
4. Add 100–200 µl of 1× Tris buffer, pH 8.0, to the top of the column and re-centrifuge. Do this three times. Collect the last eluent in an uncapped 1.5 µl Eppendorf tube and measure its volume, which should be 100 µl. If significantly different, add another 100 µl of Tris buffer and centrifuge again.

Use the column immediately or cap with laboratory film (parafilm) and leave at 4°C until required.

Note

If the columns are not used immediately, it will be necessary to repeat step 4 before adding the labeling solution for purification.

Spin columns can also be prepared following the same method, but using a 2 ml disposable syringe, when the purification of a scaled-up labeling reaction is required.

Use of columns

1. Place a 1.5 ml sterile Eppendorf tube uncapped under the column. Add the probe solution to the top of the column and centrifuge at 3000× g for 5 min.
2. Measure volume, cap Eppendorf, and transfer to −20°C for storage.

Estimating the labeling efficiency and testing the probe

It is always good practice to estimate the yield of labeled nucleic acids. This confirms a successful labeling reaction before performing the staining.

Before using a labeled probe, it is useful to prepare and demonstrate test strips to gauge the degree of label incorporation. This may be done by using the normal detection procedure for the ISH method on dots of labeled nucleic acid sequence and a labeled control applied at matching descending concentrations to a positively charged nylon membrane. Some technicians will prepare several test strips from one labeled sequence to compare the sensitivity of different detection systems. The nylon membrane is subjected to an immunological detection which can be either a colorimetric or chemiluminescent method depending on which protocol is used. Direct comparison of the signal intensities of sample and control allows estimation of labeling yield. Kits for this technique are commercially available where the labeled control is already on a test strip. A much quicker method to estimate the yield of your labeled nucleic acids is to use a bioanalyzer that can give you quantitative results in as little as 30 minutes.

Described below is a method for estimating labeling efficiency of the nucleic acid using a dilution series followed by a spot test.

PREPARATION OF THE DILUTION SERIES

1. Dilute the labeling probe using dilution buffer to a starting concentration of 2.5 pmol/µl.
2. Make a dilution series in Eppendorf tubes of purified probe to give nucleic acid concentrations of 300 pg/µl, 100 pg/µl, 30 pg/µl, 10 pg/µl, 3 pg/µl, and one tube containing diluent only. Ensure that all tube volumes are equal. Repeat the same dilution series with your control or used pre-labeled (with control) test strips.
3. Apply 1 µl drops from each tube onto the nylon membrane (Roche). The control dilutions should be lined up with the test sample dilution concentration. For an example of placing spots, see Fig. 26.2.
4. Label the position of each application with a pencil on the side of the strip (not on the strip).

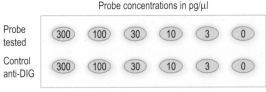

Probe concentrations in pg/µl

Fig. 26.2

5. Fix the nucleic acid to the membrane by either baking the membrane for 30 min at 120°C or using a UV light.
6. Wash the membrane briefly in washing buffer.
7. Immerse in blocking solution for 10 min.
8. Incubate with reagents used in ISH detection technique.

Note

Dilute reagents in blocking solution and use this solution for washing.

9. Detect enzyme using the same solutions and procedure as for ISH method.
10. Rinse in double distilled water and blot dry.

COMMERCIALLY MADE PROBES

Custom designed, pre-made cloned DNA and oligonucleotide sequences and labeling kits are commercially available and their use can greatly assist in making methods simpler to undertake while providing results of an assured standard. Depending on the type of laboratory you have and how many ISH requests you receive, premixed reagents and pre-labeled probes can be cost effective. The kits, reagents, or ordering the labeled probes can cut down on precious technologist time, and for the novice technologist they come with instructions. However, this does not mean that the theory behind ISH can be ignored. The technologist must understand ISH to order labeled probes and the ISH kits.

Probe concentration

For DNA probes the concentration of the probe will be ~0.5–2 µg/ml. Oligonucleotide probes can be used with or without acetylation. Probes without acetylation pretreatment of the sample will have a concentration of ~50–200 ng/ml and may provide more intense results

with minimal background. For probes with acetylation pre-treatment, a higher concentration of oligonucleotide probe may be used without incurring non-specific background staining.

Length of probe

As mentioned previously in choosing a probe, one must consider the length of the probe. Longer probes give weaker signals and they penetrate less effectively into the cross-linked (fixed) tissue. The extent of weaker signals and penetration depends also on the nature of the tissue, the choice of fixative, and whether a pretreatment has been carried out.

The length of probe can be controlled in either the synthesis reaction or the subsequent partial cleavage. In nick-translated probes the DNA length is determined by the amount of DNase in the reaction, while in random priming the length is determined by concentration of the primer. Long RNA probes may show poor tissue penetration; while chemical shortening (hydrolysis) enhances tissue penetration, it also increases the likelihood of non-selective binding to other non-targeted gene sequences.

Once a probe is prepared, the size should be checked. If the probe is too small, it may yield low signals with high background. It is necessary to know if a reduction of probe size (length) improves both the signal for the tissue and the preparation method used.

DETECTION

The choice of detection system will be principally determined by the probe label used and secondly by the ISH procedure type. One must consider the sensitivity and resolution required.

Colorimetric detection substrate systems include horseradish peroxidase with either 3-amino-9-ethylcarbazole (AEC) or 3,3'-diaminobenzidine tetrahydrochloride (DAB) substrates. AEC forms a reddish brown product which is alcohol soluble, therefore aqueous mounting media are required. Methyl green/blue has been the most often used counterstain in earlier publications but is losing popularity. DAB forms a brownish product that is compatible with solvent-based mounting solutions, and is good for permanence. Alkaline phosphatase systems can use BCIP/NBT (5-bromo-4-chloro-3-indolyl phosphate/nitro-blue tetrazolium) or fast red. BCIP/NBT forms a purple/blue alcohol-insoluble stain. Eosin is a compatible counterstain if a nuclear target is expected, or nuclear fast red if the target is cytoplasmic. Fast red forms an intense red product which is alcohol soluble and an aqueous mounting media is required. Methyl green or blue is compatible if a nuclear target is expected, or light hematoxylin if the target is cytoplasmic.

Detection methods can be direct or indirect. Incorporation of a stable hapten to a probe is the cornerstone of non-radiographic detection. Hybridized probes can be detected by enzymatic reactions that produce a colored precipitate at the site of hybridization. The most commonly used enzymes for this application are alkaline phosphatase (AP) and horseradish peroxidase (HRPO). Although these enzymes can be conjugated directly to nucleic acid probes, such enzyme-coupled probes are often inappropriate for in situ hybridization to tissue preparations because probe penetration is hampered by the presence of the conjugated enzyme. Therefore, indirect methods are preferred (Knoll & Lichter 1995).

Biotin, fluorochromes (fluorescein), and digoxygenin (DIG) are the most common labels used. Probes that are labeled with these reporter molecules are usually detected by an AP or HRPO conjugate to avidin (for biotin) or antibodies (for DIG). Fluorescein and DIG have an advantage over biotin in that they produce lower levels of background signals in tissues that contain high amounts of endogenous biotin.

Direct detection of a fluorescent label is often employed for the demonstration of multiple chromosome targets (Nederlof et al 1989), but when single target sequences are to be identified indirect methods may be used.

To reduce non-specific staining (particularly of collagen) by indirect detection reagents it is advisable to pre-incubate preparations in a Tris (Triton-X-100 or Tween) buffer solution containing bovine serum albumin. It may also prove beneficial to use this solution as the diluent for the primary detection reagent. However, at this step it is more important to use a Fab fragment of an antibody as this may reduce background staining.

Indirect detection procedures offer increased sensitivity. The selection of the enzyme and substrate (De Jong et al 1985) should be included in weighing the benefits of different detection systems. A substrate system that employs conjugated antibodies such as anti-DIG or anti-FITC that are conjugated with AP together with the application of a colorimetric BCIP/NBT that can be cycled to produce an insoluble blue/black precipitate over a period of 24 hours is recommended. Another substrate system one could use for a more intense fluorescent signal is a fluorescent 2-hydroxy-3-naphthoic acid-2'-phenylanilide phosphate (HNPP) with fast red TR.

The main advantages of this procedure are low levels of non-specific staining, simplicity, and the use of an enzyme substrate system that can produce an insoluble blue/black precipitate.

Many commercially available probes for ISH are labeled with biotin. When used in combination with streptavidin detection systems, high sensitivity can be achieved. A disadvantage of that combination is having a widespread endogenous tissue distribution. Substantial quantities of endogenous biotin are, for example, present in the liver and kidney (Wood & Warnke 1981), and other tissues, such as pituitary, submandibular gland, thyroid, and parathyroid. Furthermore, proliferating cells may often produce enough biotin to make the discrimination between true and false-positive results difficult. However, methods of blocking endogenous biotin have greatly improved and work well to prevent false positives.

Digoxygenin (Herrington et al 1989) in combination with a Fab fragment–enzyme conjugate detection system currently provides results of equal or superior sensitivity to biotin, with extremely low non-specific background staining. Another label that may be used in conjunction with a single-step detection method is fluorescein. Using this label it is possible to undertake rapid ISH methods in which target sequences of moderate to high copy number can be demonstrated in a working day.

SAMPLE PREPARATION

Fixation

Fixation is an initial step in specimen preparation or can be an intermediate step in a protocol, as in methods using cryostat sections. The duration, type, and temperature of fixation may also differ according to preparation. Together these factors will have an effect, not only on the preservation of the tissue, but also on the retention of nucleic acid and the resistance of DNA and RNA to nuclease digestion. The choice of fixative will have an influence on the conservation of nucleic acids and their availability for hybridization. Specimens that are immersion-fixed prior to paraffin embedding appear to be unaffected by 'normal' contamination levels of nucleases, thus indicating that only the hybridization solutions need to be scrupulously free of the enzymes.

The functional groups involved in base pairing are protected in the double helix structure of duplex DNA. RNA is fairly unreactive to cross-linking agents.

Methanol/acetic acid fixation is recommended for metaphase chromosome spreads. Cryostat sections may be fixed with 4% formaldehyde (~30 minutes), Bouin's fixative, or paraformaldehyde vapor fixation. This fixation also helps to secure the tissue to the slide.

Proteins surround DNA and RNA target sequences and the extensive cross-linking of these proteins may mask the target nucleic acid. Therefore, permeabilization procedures may be required.

After the tissue is removed from the patient or animal, it must be fixed to prevent autolysis, inhibit bacterial/fungal growth, and make it resistant to damage from subsequent processing. There are two main groups of fixatives based on their reaction with soluble proteins. They are coagulant and non-coagulant fixatives. Coagulant fixatives are ethanol and mercuric chloride, and are not the preferred fixative for use with ISH since ethanol dehydrates, coagulates, and precipitates cellular proteins, nucleic acids, and carbohydrates. Covalent bonding does not occur with ethanol fixatives and the tissue components, so mRNA is not anchored within the tissue and is likely to be lost during post-fixation processing procedures. For ISH, non-coagulant, cross-linking aldehydes (formaldehyde, paraformaldehyde, and glutaraldehyde) are recommended.

Tissues fixed for ISH should retain mRNA within the tissue but not raise background. Both background and signal are generally higher on perfused-fixed paraffin tissue sections than on frozen sections. The signal to noise (S/N) ratio on perfused-fixed tissue sections is better.

Most commonly, tissue specimens are routinely fixed in 10% buffered formalin, processed overnight in an automatic tissue processor, and embedded in paraffin. Fixation time of 8–12 hours is optimal. Keep in mind that the longer the fixation, the more rigorous the enzyme digestion is required to optimize the signal. Alcohol-fixed tissues should be post-fixed with an aldehyde fixative to prevent the diffusion of mRNA (if you are looking at RNA).

Slide/section preparation

Sections are cut—4–6 μm on an alcohol-cleaned microtome using positively charged or hand-coated slides. Sections are drained well and then air-dried at room temperature. After deparaffinization, place slides in an alcohol-cleaned staining container of DEPC water. The staining container is then placed in the heated water bath at 23–37°C and held until the start of ISH. Gloves must be worn to prevent contamination, and all utensils, such as brushes and forceps, are cleaned with alcohol and kept within the cleaned area designated for ISH.

Proteolytic digestion

The use of formaldehyde-based fixatives prior to paraffin embedding of specimens will mask nucleic acid sequences. Digestion is a important step when performing ISH. Digestion improves probe penetration by increasing cell permeability with minimal tissue degradation. Although the nucleic acid is not directly affected by proteolytic digestion, it is important to control this step carefully as under-digestion will result in insufficient exposure of the nucleic acid while over-digestion can sufficiently weaken the protein structure surrounding the sequence to bring about its loss into subsequent solutions. mRNA sequences tend to be loosely associated with proteins while DNA targets are intimately associated with histone and other nuclear proteins. Due to these differences, the concentration of proteolytic enzyme required to unmask mRNA will be less than that necessary to expose DNA.

The selection of the proteolytic enzyme is important. This should be of molecular biology grade to ensure the absence of nuclease activity. Proteinase K and pepsin are two enzymes commonly used for digestion. The use of proteinase K has an advantage over other proteolytic enzymes because during incubation it digests any nucleases that might be present. However, higher concentrations of the enzyme may be required depending on the tissue fixation time (Fig. 26.3).

Nuclease digestion is used as a negative control. Treatment of same tissue/patient tissue sections with RNase A will demonstrate that ISH signals are due to RNA hybridization.

Proteoglycan digestion is required for bone and cartilage. Kidney and brain may also need proteoglycan digestion if the signal is weak. Post-fixation in 4% paraformaldehyde is necessary after digestion to prevent tissue loss. In addition, post-fixation after digestion (for all digestions) prevents leaching and will inhibit RNase activity.

When in situ hybridization methods are used to demonstrate mRNA sequences, non-specific attachment of digoxygenin and fluorescein-labeled oligonucleotides to epithelial tissues can create non-specific results. To minimize this interaction, preparations can be acetylated after proteolytic digestion and before post-fixation. Acetylation decreases non-specific binding of the probe to the tissue. Positive charges on the tissue are neutralized by reducing electrostatic binding of the probe.

Prehybridization is intended to reduce non-specific binding. Sites in the tissue become saturated with the components of the prehybridization solution preventing non-specific binding. The purpose of the prehybridization solution is to equilibrate the specimen with the hybridization solution prior to the addition of the probe, and to allow anionic macromolecules to block sites of potential non-specific probe interaction. The prehybridization solution contains all the ingredients of the hybridization mixture except the probe. Non-complementary sequences such as bovine serum albumin (BSA at 1 mg/ml), Denhardt solution (Ficoll, BSA, and polyvinylpyrrolidone all at 0.02%), and tRNA are used to reduce non-specific binding. Most data indicate that blocking is required, but a separate prehybridization step may not be necessary. In some cases, adequate blocking may be accomplished during the hybridization step. Electrostatic binding of probes to the tissue and slides can be neutralized by treatment in TEA buffer containing 0.1 M triethanolamine.

Hybridization

Hybridization is the cooling after denaturization, in the presence of a complementary probe, that results in hydrogen bonding of the two strands of nucleic acids. The probe must form stable hydrogen bonds with the target with minimal hybridization with non-target sequences. The probe and target sequences must be single stranded. Simultaneously heating the probe and target to high temperatures may increase the consistency and sensitivity of detection. This can only be met if care is taken to precisely control this step of the in situ hybridization procedure. Control is achieved through balancing the various components of the hybridization solution and hybridizing at an optimal temperature for the correct length of time.

If a DNA probe is employed or a DNA target demonstrated, then it is essential that these are rendered single stranded. This is achieved by using dry heat with the hybridization solution placed over the specimen, which is then covered with a coverslip, plastic sheet, or cap. The denaturation will differ according to the percentage of guanine–cytosine base pairs within the target sequence

of interest. When there is a high percentage of guanine–cytosine base pairs, the third hydrogen bond associated with the base pair will occur at a higher melting temperature (TM) than in the sequences in which adenosine and thymidine pairing predominates. Overheating, i.e. above 100°C, at this stage may compromise specimen preservation.

At the molecular level, hybridization involves an initial nucleation reaction between a few bases, followed by hydrogen bonding of the remaining sequences. The control of temperature during hybridization is crucial as variations will influence the specificity (stringency) of annealing. RNA and DNA hybrids are formed optimally at about 25°C below their TM. When lower temperatures are used, some partial homologous annealing may occur. Although this situation should be avoided, it can be usefully employed to screen for sequences with partial homology, e.g. human papillomavirus subtypes. By incorporating formamide, a helix-destabilizing reagent, annealing may be maintained using lower temperatures, e.g. 37°C, at which tissue preservation is not affected.

Stringency can also be altered by adjusting the availability of monovalent cations in the hybridization solution. These cations are usually supplied by sodium chloride and their action is to regulate the degree of natural electrostatic repulsion between the probe and target sequences. When used at high concentration their effect is to produce conditions of low stringency, while at low concentrations only sequences with complete homology can hybridize.

Anionic macromolecules are often included in the hybridization solution to reduce non-specific interactions of the probe. Sonicated and denatured salmon sperm DNA can shield non-homologous nucleic acid sequences from the probe and reduce the opportunity for cellular electrostatic interactions. Dextran sulfate will also reduce the possibility of cellular electrostatic interactions and locally concentrate the probe, enhancing the rate of hybridization. Particular attention should be taken to ensure that hybridization solutions are prepared using reagents free from nuclease contamination.

The rate of annealing will be influenced by time and temperature as well as by the composition of the hybridization solution as discussed above. Due to steric constraints, in situ hybridization proceeds at a slower rate than in blotting methods. However, high probe concentrations can be used to compensate for this factor. Hybridization times of 1–2 hours for biotinylated and

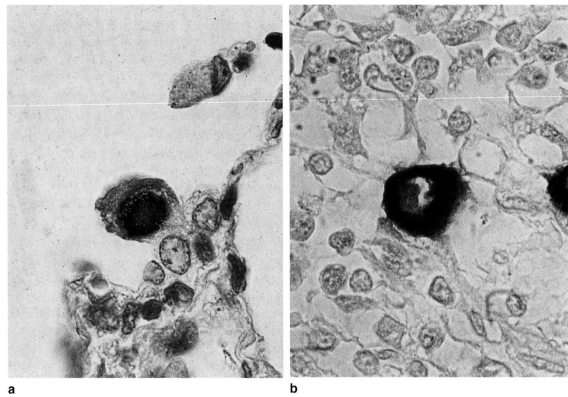

a   b

Fig. 26.3 Example photographs of ISH. Human cytomegalovirus (HCMV) demonstrated by in situ hybridization in paraffin wax sections. (a) HCMV DNA in infected lung, proteinase K pretreatment 50 μg/ml for 1 hour at 37°C. (b) HCMV early gene RNA transcript in AIDS infected bowel, proteinase K pretreatment at 15 μg/ml for 30 min at 37°C.

fluorescein-labeled probes are often effective but with digoxygenin-labeled probes, overnight hybridization may be required to provide high sensitivity.

Post-hybridization washes are used to adjust the stringency of hybridization. The sections must be rinsed with solutions that contain high concentrations of salt to remove the unbound probe. Subsequent washing with solutions containing decreasing salt concentrations and increasing temperature reduces mismatching of base pairs. Longer probes and those with higher G+C content are more stable and increases in temperature and formamide concentration are the destabilizing factors. By reducing the concentration of formamide in the hybridization solution, but maintaining a constant temperature, annealing conditions will become less stringent, thereby increasing the sensitivity of mRNA detection when using fluorescein-labeled oligonucleotide probes.

Controls

It is essential to include controls to verify ISH results. A positive and no-hybridization control should always be included when undertaking an ISH procedure. The positive control should contain the target sequence being demonstrated and be prepared the same as the test samples. It should receive the same solutions and go through the same procedural steps as the test samples. This will provide a gauge for the overall performance of the technique. If the same positive control is used from run to run, it will help validate the ISH staining reproducibility.

Other controls may be incorporated to test the validity of your results. The number and type of controls to be incorporated into the technique is determined at the discretion of the laboratory's personnel and standard operating procedures. As mentioned under the digestion section earlier in this chapter, nuclease digestion can be used as a negative control.

Equipment and reagent preparation

DNA and RNA can be degraded by nuclease activity. Indeed, the use of high concentrations of DNase and RNase are useful in confirming the nucleic acid type specificity of hybridization. However, at much lower concentrations, nucleases present on the skin may contaminate solutions used in hybridization methods sufficiently to degrade the quality of naked DNA and RNA. For this reason, in addition to the wearing of gloves, elaborate precautions are often taken to ensure the absence of nucleases from solutions used in hybridization techniques.

TREATMENT OF SOLUTIONS AND GLASSWARE TO DESTROY NUCLEASE ACTIVITY

DNase is destroyed by autoclaving. RNase is resistant to heat inactivation and therefore other procedures should be used as described below.

Preparation of DEPC-treated water

Add diethylpyrocarbonate (DEPC) (Sigma D5758) to pure water to a final concentration of 0.1%. This should be done in a fume hood. Shake well to dissolve and allow it to stand overnight. Autoclave the solution and container the following day.

Preparation of DEPC-treated solutions

Prepare solutions, then add DEPC to 0.1%. Shake and leave overnight, then autoclave.

Note

Adding full-strength DEPC directly to a buffer may alter the buffering properties. Solutions that require a buffer of that type should be made up in RNase-free glassware using pre-mixed autoclaved DEPC-treated water.

Preparation of glassware

Treat glassware at 200°C overnight or, if delicate:

1. Wash in a mild/low suds soap or RNase Away solution.

2. Rinse in double distilled nuclease-free water until detergent is removed.
2. Soak in 3% aqueous hydrogen peroxide, 10 min.
3. Rinse in DEPC-treated water.
4. Dry and protect from dust.

Most laboratories purchase DEPC-treated water and use sterile plastic disposable containers in place of the glassware. The information is in this chapter is for those laboratories that prefer to prepare their own DEPC water and use glass bottles for buffer storage.

UNIVERSAL ISH METHOD (NO FRILLS OR SPECIALIZED EQUIPMENT)

Day 1

1. Deparaffinize slides completely. Three changes of xylene and/or substitute for 4–8 min each.

Note

Incomplete deparaffinization may cause a weak reaction.

2. Dehydrate through two changes 100% EtOH, 1 change 95% EtOH for 3 min each. Rinse in DEPC-treated water or use slides already in warmed DEPC-treated water. Rinse in warmed (23–37°C) Tris/saline buffer #1, pH 7.5, and drain.
3. De-proteinize sections in freshly prepared proteinase K solution at 23–37°C, in a moist chamber for 15 min.
4. Rinse in Tris/saline buffer #1 at room temperature for 5 min. If necessary, digest proteoglycans and/or acetylation before going to next step.
5. Dehydrate slides through one change of 95% EtOH and two changes 100% EtOH for 2 min each. Air-dry for 5 min. **This step is omitted if prehybridizing (next step).**
6. Apply the prehybridization solution by putting 1–2 drops (60–100 μl) on the sections. Incubate in a moist chamber at room temperature for 1 hour. Blot off *all* excess prehybridization solution before adding the probe.
7. Apply hybridization fluid (probe) and cover with a heat-resistant film (microwave wrap, coverslips, or chambers). The probe is tailed with either biotin–dUTP or digoxygenin–dUTP.
8. Initiate hybridization by denaturing slides for 5–10 min at 92–100°C (try not to exceed 100°C).

Use a preheated 'metal' tray to set slides on for optimal denaturization. Cool slides to 37–42°C and incubate in humidity chamber for 18–24 hours. Agitation may enhance reaction. Since this method is not using a commercial kit, the staining continues on day 2.

Day 2

9. Rinse slides twice in 2×SSC and twice in 1×SSC for 5 min each at 37°C.
10. Apply a 5% blocking solution at 37°C for 10 min.
11. Rinse in buffer #1 for 2 min, followed by a 10-min rinse in buffer #2.
12. Add 1–2 drops of detection reagent to each slide (streptavidin–AP or anti-digoxygenin–AP). Incubate in humidity chamber for 20–30 min at 37°C. During the incubation period, prepare the substrate and warm to 37°C.
13. Rinse slides in three changes of buffer #3 for 5 min each.
14. Incubate in substrate for 30–60 min at 37°C.
15. Stop reaction by washing in buffer at 37°C for 2 min. Rinse in two changes of distilled water (DW) for 2 min each.
16. Rinse in two changes of DW for 2 min each.
17. Counterstain; this is dependent on the chromogen selected. For BCIP/NBT use nuclear fast red, eosin, or methyl green. For DAB use hematoxylin or methyl green. Go on to step 18 if using BCIP/NBT or DAB. For AEC use methyl green and coverslip out of distilled water using an aqueous mounting medium. Do not go through alcohols or clearing.
18. Dehydrate in increasing concentrations of alcohol.
19. Clear using xylene and coverslip in permanent mounting resin (Doran & Sterchi 2000).

TROUBLESHOOTING

Tissue sections fall off

- adhesive absent/insufficient poly-L-lysine or amino-alkylsilane (AS) on slide
- insufficient adhesion time/temperature
- over-digestion (too long/too concentrated)
- overzealous coverslip removal (use pliable wrap, AS slips, or well covers)
- denaturation too long or temperature too high (93–98°C is ideal)
- excessive slide agitation.

Weak staining (tissue preparation)

- slides incompletely deparaffinized (add an additional xylene/substitute step to insure that all the paraffin has been removed)
- slides not dehydrated or drained prior to addition of probe (water in tissue will dilute probe)
- over-fixation (increase digestion time)
- insufficient digestion (increase time, concentration, or type of digesting reagent).

Weak staining (hybridization/detection)

- probe insufficiently biotinylated
- probe concentration too dilute (hybridize longer)
- probe or target DNA insufficiently denatured (increase time of denaturation, check the temperature of the hot start)
- incomplete hybridization (prehybridize, increase hybridization time, lower temperature if too high, or check stringency)
- buffer wrong pH (should be alkaline, pH 9.5)
- reagents too cold (warm reagents to 23°C).

High background

- skipped blocking step
- probe too concentrated
- slides dried out during incubations
- washes omitted or shortened
- detergent wash buffer not used after label incubation
- incubated substrate too long.

'Negative' positive control

- wrong probe
- reagents bad (improper storage)
- digestion absent (enzymes are unstable)
- denaturation absent (increase temperature)
- omitted step in protocol
- mixed detection reagents improperly.

Inconsistent staining (stringency conditions)

Stringency conditions are conditions that if a related but non-homologous probe binds to the target:

- non-homologous sequences hybridize/some mismatch (low stringency—high salt concentration, low temperature, low formamide concentration)
- complete binding only if homologous (high stringency—low salt concentration, high temperature, high formamide concentration).

RT-PISH

In situ hybridization–polymerase chain reaction overview

PCR is used to detect minute quantities of DNA or RNA in tissue sections or intact cells and to visualize, by light microscopy, the individual cells expressing or carrying specific genes. It is also used to detect low copy numbers of nucleic acid sequences in viral infections, gene mutations, gene alterations, chromosomal translocations, gene therapy, and low-level gene expression.

Conventional in situ PCR is a means to amplify small amounts of DNA or RNA down to a single copy of a gene, to an exponential accumulation of the same sequences consisting of millions or billions of identical copies for detection, sequencing, cloning or diagnosis.

There are several ways in which one can perform PISH methods. There is the direct in situ PCR, indirect in situ PCR, and reverse transcription–PCR. In all methods, tissues should be fixed to preserve both the DNA and the RNA. Tissues are cut slightly thicker for the RT-PISH method described here. Thicker sections are thought to contain more target. Tissue pre-treated with proteinase K is necessary.

Primers are usually 18–28 nucleotides long and it is important to design a pair of primers that has little or no homology to any other sequences in the tissue, to each other or within themselves. For animal tissue, it is better to select the sequence that several (but similar) species can use as the primers for PISH.

Controls are important in each step of the procedure. This is to ensure there are no false positives or negatives. Validation of the amplification is the most important reason for the controls but confirmation of the subsequent hybridization/detection is also important.

Examples of controls would be:

- omission of the primers, using unrelated primers
- have good positive and negative tissues
- destroy the target before subjecting it to PISH

- use a known cell line
- verify results with conventional PCR.

See PISH Procedure 26.2

Procedure 26.1

Oligonucleotide 3'-end labeling with DIG-ddUTP

Terminal transferase is used to add a single modified dideoxyuridine triphosphote (DIG-ddUTP, biotin-ddUTP, or fluorescein-ddUTP) to the 3' ends of an oligonucleotide. In this method, DIG-ddUTP will be used. The method described here has been modified from the Boehringer Mannheim procedure. Now the method is described from Roche Applied Science Laboratory. The reagents in this procedure may be purchased in a kit (Roche).

Contents of labeling reagents: The amounts to prepare listed here are the amounts supplied in the kit. The kit will accommodate 25 labeling reactions. If you require other amounts, just adjust your volume calculations for less or more.

1. *Reaction buffer pH 6.6 (this is a 5×concentrated solution)*
    1 M potassium cacodylate
    0.125 M Tris-HCl
    1.25 mg/ml bovine serum albumin
    Prepare 50–100 µl

2. *CoCl₂ solution*
    25 mM cobalt chloride
    Prepare 50–100 µl

3. *DIG-ddUTP solution*
    1mM digoxygenin-11-ddUTP in double distilled water
    Prepare 25 µl

4a. *Terminal transferase 1 (newer method)*
    25 µl terminal transferase, in the following:

    60 mM potassium phosphate (pH 7.2 at 4°C)
    150 mM potassium chloride
    1 mM 2-mercaptoethanol
    0.5% Triton X-100
    50% glycerol
    Prepare a solution with a concentration of 400 units/µl

4b. *Terminal transferase 2 (older method)*
    1 µl (50 units) terminal transferase, in the following:

200 mM potassium cacodylate

200 mM potassium chloride

1 mM EDTA

0.2 mg/ml bovine serum albumin

50% glycerol

Add enough double-distilled water to make a final volume of 20 µl.

5. *0.2 M EDTA (pH 8.0) made in double distilled water.*

Procedure

1. Dissolve 100 pmol of the purified oligonucleotide in 10 µl of sterile double distilled water.
2. Add the following to a sterile microcentrifuge tube on ice:

   4 µl of 5× concentrated reaction buffer

   4 µl of 25 mM cobalt chloride (CoCl$_2$)

   1 µl DIG-ddUTP solution. For this labeling we will use DIG-ddUTP.

   1 µl of terminal transferase (400 units/µl)
3. Mix and centrifuge briefly.
4. Incubate at 37°C for 15 min, then place on ice.
5. Stop the reaction by adding 2 µl of 0.2 M EDTA (pH 8.0)

Procedure 26.2

Direct PCR amplification protocol

1. Fix the tissue with a cross-linking fixative.
2. Cut sections at 5–7 µm on an alcohol-cleaned microtome and knife.
3. Place 2–3 sections on positively charged coated slides (spaced evenly apart). Dry overnight flat on a slide warmer, 50–55°C, and then an additional 30 min before deparaffinization.
4. Deparaffinize in three changes of xylene for 3–5 min each. Dehydrate in two changes 100% ethanol for 5 min. Air dry.
5. Digest for 30–90 min. Do not let slides dry out. A humidity chamber is helpful for this step*.

   *Quick test for sufficient digestion is: Place slide under a microscope; using a 40× objective look at one cell. When you can count 20 dots in nucleus, digestion is complete.
6. After digestion, rinse slides in double distilled water for 1 min.
7. Dehydrate slides in two changes of 100% ethanol for 2 min each. Air dry for 5 min.

Note

Depending on the type of thermocycler used, the slides are treated differently. For example, some thermocyclers have coverwells that seal and snap tight over the individual tissue section. Other thermocyclers just have a heat block to sit the slides on. To accommodate the individual thermocycler, you may need to circle the tissue with a hydrophobic pen.

8. Cover tissue with PCR mixture and cover with glass coverslip, autoclave wrap or coverwell (use what is recommended by manufacturer of thermocycler).
9. Line the slide girdle of the thermocycler with aluminum foil to prevent leakage from the slides and equipment contamination. For this procedure a Perkin-Elmer thermocycler was used, which was the recommendation of the manufacturer.
10. Place the slides in the aluminum foil trough. Cover each slide with 2 ml of mineral oil.
11. Heat thermal block to 80°C and place on hold for 10 min while setting the thermocycler program. The amplification program used is 15 cycles of 1 min at 96°C, 1 min at 59°C, and 1 min at 72°C.

Note

Amplification program settings will vary.

12. Remove slides from thermocycler and gently remove coverslips, etc. Rinse slides in two changes of xylene for 3 min each to remove mineral oil. Dehydrate and remove xylene with two changes of 100% ethanol for 3 min each. Air dry.
13. Wash slides three times for 5 min each in buffer #1.
14. Place slides in 150 mM NaCl with 0.2% BSA at 50°C for 10 min (this solution should be prewarmed).
15. Drain NaCl from slides and cover with 100 µl alkaline phosphatase-conjugated anti-digoxygenin (1:50 dilution in 0.1 M Tris pH 7.5 with 0.1 M NaCl) for 30 min at 37°C in a humidity chamber.
16. Rinse slides in 0.1 M Tris pH 9.5 with 0.1 M NaCl for 1 min.
17. Incubate slides in NBT/BCIP solution (10 µl of NBT/BCIP in 2.0 ml Tris pH 9.5 with 0.1 M NaCl) for 5–15 min. Check the proper end-point under the microscope.

18. Wash slides in distilled water for 2 min. Counterstain with nuclear fast red for 5 min. Rinse in distilled water for 1 min, dehydrate, clear, and mount.

Reagent list for the RT-PISH procedure 26.2

Digestion reagents

1. Pepsin or trypsin at 2 mg/ml (mild digestion)

Note

Stock solution is 20 mg pepsin + 9.5 ml sterile water + 0.5 ml 2 N HCl.

2. Protease K (harsh)

Dilute 1.0 ml proteinase K at 1 mg/ml in 150 ml of PBS.

Use at 55°C.

3. Buffer #1

4. 20× SSC

5. 2× SSC

6. Formamide SSC

Formamide	50 ml
2× SSC	50 ml

7. PCR mixture

00.25 μM primers
10 μM dATP
10 μM dCTP
10 μM GTP
3.5 μM dTTP

TROUBLESHOOTING DIGESTION

If there is no or a weak signal, you need to increase digestion by 10 minutes.

Suggested digestion times are indicated in Table 26.2.

Table 26.2 Suggested digestion times adjusted to fixation time

Fixation time (hours)	Enzyme	Digestion time (minutes)
4	Pepsin or trypsin	10
15	Pepsin or trypsin	90
24	Pepsin or trypsin	120

Acknowledgments

The author would like to acknowledge Tony Warford and Lamar Jones for writing the first two versions of this chapter. Some of their writing remains in this chapter. Special thanks go to Maureen Doran for her technical sharing, to Dr Bruce Gitter for his scientific review, and to Eli Lilly and Company for the support and time to write this chapter.

REFERENCES

Davis M., Malcolm S., Rabbitts T.H. (1984) Chromosome translocation can occur on either side of the c-myc oncogene in Burkitt lymphoma cells. Nature 308:286–288.

De Jong A.S.H., Van Kessel-Van Vark M., Raap A.K. (1985) Sensitivity of various visualization methods for peroxidase and alkaline phosphatase activity in immunoenzyme histochemistry. Histochemical Journal 17: 1119–1130.

Doran M., Sterchi D.L. (2000) Let's do in situ (workshop no. 67). Milwaukee, WI: National Society for Histotechnology.

Gall J.G., Pardue M.L. (1969) Formation and detection of RNA–DNA hybrid molecules in cytological preparations. Proceedings of the National Academy of Sciences USA 63:378–383.

Goldsmith C.S., Tatti K.M., Ksiazek T.G. et al. (2004) Ultrastructural characterization of SARS coronavirus. Emerging Infectious Diseases 10(2):320–326.

Haugland R.P., Spence M.T.Z., eds (2005) The handbook: a guide to fluorescent probes and labeling technologies, 10th edn. Paisley: Invitrogen.

Herrington C.S., Burns J., Graham A.K. et al. (1989) Interphase cytogenetics using biotin and digoxigenin labeled probes II: Simultaneous differential detection of human and papilloma virus nucleic acids in individual nuclei. Journal of Clinical Pathology 41:601–606.

Innis M.A., Gelfand D.H., Sminsky J.J. et al., eds (1990) PCR protocols: a guide to methods and applications. New York: Academic Press.

Janneke C., Alers P-J.K., Kees J. et al. (1999) Effect of bone decalcification procedures on DNA in situ hybridization and comparative genomic hybridization: EDTA is highly preferable to a routinely used acid decalcifier. Journal of Histochemistry and Cytochemistry 47(5):703–709.

John H.A., Birnstiel M.L., Jones K.W. (1969) RNA–DNA hybrids at the cytological level. Nature 223:582–587.

Hopman A.H., Ramaekers F.C., Raap A.K., et al. (1988) In situ hybridization as a tool to study numerical chromosome aberrations in solid bladder tumors. Histochemistry 89:307–316.

Kendall C.H., Roberts P.A., Pringle J.H. et al. (1991) The expression of parathyroid hormone messenger RNA in normal and abnormal parathyroid tissue. Journal of Pathology 165:111–118.

Knoll J.H.M., Lichter P. (1995) Current protocols in molecular biology. In situ hybridization and detection using nonisotopic probes. New York: Wiley.

Lux S.E., Tse W.T., Menninger J.C. et al. (1990) Hereditary spherocytosis associated with deletion of human erythrocyte ankyrin gene on chromosome 8. Nature 345:736–739.

Madrid M.A., Lo R.W. (2004) Chromogenic in situ hybridization (CISH): a novel alternative in screening archival breat cancer tissue samples for HER-2/neu. Breast Cancer Research 6(5):R593–R600.

Mitchell B.S., Dhami D., Schumacher U. (1992) In situ hybridization: a review of methodologies and applications in the biomedical sciences. Medical Laboratory Sciences 49:107–118.

Nederlof P.M., Robinson D., Abuknesha R. et al. (1989) Three-color fluorescence in situ hybridization for the simultaneous detection of multiple nucleic acid sequences. Cytometry 10:20–27.

Netterwald J. (2006) Molecular testing? Emerging technologies show promise for helping to prevent spread of the epidemic disease. Advance for Medical Laboratory Professionals April:17–18.

Poddighe P.J., Ramaekers F.C.S., Hopman A.H.N. (1992) Interphase cytogenetics of tumors. Journal of Pathology 166:215–224.

Pringle J.H., Ruprai A.K., Primrose L. et al. (1990) In situ hybridization of immunoglobulin light chain mRNA in paraffin sections using biotinylated or hapten-labeled oligonucleotide probes. Journal of Pathology 162:197–207.

Pringle J.H., Barker S. et al. (1992) Demonstration of Epstein-Barr virus in tissue sections by in situ hybridization for viral RNA. Journal of Pathology 167(Suppl):133A.

Pringle J.H., Baker J. Colloby P.S. et al. (1993) The detection of cell proliferation in normal and malignant formalin-fixed paraffin-embedded tissue sections using in situ hybridization for histone mRNA. Journal of Pathology 169 (Suppl):144A.

Ruprai A.K., Pringle J.H., Angel C.A. et al. (1991) Localization of immunoglobulin light chain mRNA expression in Hodgkin's disease by in situ hybridization. Journal of Pathology 164:37–40.

Sambrook J., Fritsch E.F., Maniatis T. (1989) Molecular cloning—a laboratory manual, 2nd edn. Cold Spring Harbor: Cold Spring Harbor Laboratory Press.

Van den Berg F., Schipper M., Jiwa M. et al. (1989) Implausibility of an aetiological association between cytomegalovirus and Kaposi's sarcoma shown by four techniques. Journal of Clinical Pathology 42:128–131.

Wakamatsu N., King D.J., Seal B.S. et al. (2005) Detection of Newcastle disease virus RNA by reverse transcription polymerase chain reaction using formalin-fixed, paraffin-embedded tissue and comparison with immunohistochemistry and in situ hybridization. [abstract] American Association of Veterinary Laboratory Diagnosticians 48:166.

Warford A., Lauder I. (1991) In situ hybridization in perspective. Journal of Clinical Pathology 44:177–181.

White J. (2005) An introduction to chromogenic in situ hybridization. Journal of Histotechnology 28:229–234.

Wood G.S., Warnke R. (1981) Suppression of endogenous avidin binding activity in tissues and its relevance to biotin–avidin detection systems. Journal of Histochemistry and Cytochemistry 29:1196–1204.

Xiao Y., Sato S., Oguchi T. et al. (2001) High sensitivity of PCR in situ hybridization for the detection of human papillomavirus infection in uterine cervical neoplasias. Gynecologic Oncology 82(2):350–354.

Yan S.J., Blomme E.A.G. (2003) In situ zymography: a molecular pathology technique to localize endogenous protease activity in tissue sections. Veterinary Pathology 40:227–236.

FURTHER READING

Darby I.A., ed. (2000) In situ hybridization protocols, 2nd edn. Totowa, NJ: Humana Press.

Wilkinson D.G., ed. (1999) In situ hybridization: a practical approach, 2nd edn. New York: Oxford University Press.

27

Genetic Testing: Utilization of Fluorescent In Situ Hybridization (FISH)

Caroline Astbury

INTRODUCTION

Genetic testing can be defined as the analysis of human DNA, RNA, chromosomes, proteins, or metabolites, performed in order to detect inherited or disease-related genotypes, mutations, phenotypes, or karyotypes for clinical purposes (Kroese et al 2004). The scope of genetic testing is vast, incorporating many disciplines and sub-disciplines, including diagnostic testing (both cytogenetic and molecular), clinical research, biochemical genetics, pharmacogenetics, and forensic science. Additionally, there is a broad selection of methods and techniques available to undertake genetic testing; the backbone of the clinical molecular diagnostic laboratory is the polymerase chain reaction (PCR) and its many modifications. In the clinical cytogenetic laboratory, chromosome analysis is the gold standard. The advent of fluorescent in situ hybridization (FISH) or molecular cytogenetics, as it is also known, has enabled a huge advance in the diagnostic and prognostic capability of the clinical cytogenetic laboratory.

In situ hybridization, utilizing radiolabeled probes, had been used by laboratories for a number of years. However, the long exposure periods associated with autoradiography were impractical for clinical applications. The development of biotin-labeled DNA probes in the mid-1980s allowed fluorescent detection of the centromeric or alpha-satellite sequences of chromosomes (Pinkel et al 1986). The major advantage was thus the quick and easy detection of fluorescent DNA probe sequences that allowed for a high sensitivity assay, with utility in the clinical context.

METHODOLOGY

The basic steps in a FISH procedure include the fixation of the DNA, as either metaphase chromosomes or interphase nuclei, on a slide; the DNA is then denatured in situ, so that it becomes single stranded. This target DNA is then hybridized to specific DNA probe sequences, which are labeled with fluorochromes to allow for their detection. The labeled probe is added in excess, so probe binding to target DNA occurs. Fluorescence microscopy then allows for visualization of the probe on the target material; analysis of the probe signals includes observation of gain of signals, loss of signals, positioning of signals, or fusion of signals.

PROBES

The majority of probes used in the clinical cytogenetic laboratory are commercially made in the United States and sold as analyte-specific reagents (ASRs). Commercially available FISH probes tend to fall into three categories:

1. Repetitive sequences (such as the centromeres or alpha-satellite regions of chromosomes).
2. Whole chromosome sequences (including the short arm, centromere, and long arm of the chromosome).
3. Unique sequences (ranging in size from 1 kb to >1 Mb of DNA).

With the availability of data from the Human Genome Project (www.genome.ucsc.edu), virtually any sequence of DNA may be used as a FISH probe for the study of specific regions of the chromosome. Several laboratories utilize the Human Genome Project to create 'homebrew' probes, such as bacterial artificial chromosomes. These probes are essentially research based and are not subject to the same regulations as commercially available probes.

LABELING

Commercially available probes are generally directly labeled, such that the fluorochrome is directly attached to the probe nucleotides. This technique involves no other detection of the probe before analysis. Probes may also be indirectly labeled, via incorporation of a hapten (such as biotin or digoxygenin) into the DNA via nick translation or PCR. The probes are then detected using a fluorescently labeled antibody (such as strepavidin and anti-digoxygenin). Currently, directly labeled probes may be labeled in green (such as SpectrumGreen™ or fluorescein), red (SpectrumOrange™ or Texas Red), blue (SpectrumAqua™), or gold (SpectrumGold™). The ability of a fused green and red FISH signal to be seen as yellow under a fluorescent microscope is helpful in several hematological FISH studies, as detailed below.

TISSUE TYPES

FISH can be applied to a variety of clinical specimens, providing there is DNA in the sample. Cultured cells, such as amniocytes, chorionic villi cells, lymphocytes, cells from bone marrow aspirates, or cells from solid tumors, will yield metaphase spreads. Metaphase spreads are used routinely in the clinical cytogenetic laboratory and are stained with a selection of special stains to allow interpretation of chromosomal regions and rearrangements; these spreads may also be used for FISH analysis. Analysis of FISH on metaphase spreads allows the exact position of the target signals to be determined and whether they are in their normal location or not. One major advantage of FISH is that it does not require either cultured cells or metaphase spreads, and can therefore be applied to interphase or non-dividing cells, including uncultured amniocytes (used for prenatal diagnosis), peripheral blood smears (used in rapid newborn blood

analysis), or bone marrow aspirate smears. In addition, FISH may be performed on paraffin block sections, disaggregated cells from paraffin blocks, touch preparations from lymph nodes or solid tumors. FISH may, therefore, be used when metaphase chromosomes are unavailable, such as from archival material or when using samples of poor quality.

CLINICAL APPLICATIONS

In the clinical cytogenetic laboratory, FISH is used for both constitutional and acquired chromosomal analyses. Microscopy and standard banding techniques allow for the detection of rearrangements of approximately 3 Mb or greater. FISH is a necessary adjunct in delineating rearrangements, such as subtle deletions or duplications, that would not be defined by standard banding techniques. In addition, FISH may help to identify marker (generally supernumerary and of unknown origin) chromosomes, which is particularly important in the prenatal setting.

CONSTITUTIONAL ABNORMALITIES

Microdeletion syndromes

Microdeletion or contiguous gene syndromes are caused by a small deletion of genetic material which results in the loss of several genes from one chromosomal region. Generally, these deletions are <2 Mb in size. There are several, clinically recognized, microdeletion syndromes (Table 27.1). Commercially available FISH probes are used to provide a definitive diagnosis for a clinically determined disorder (Fig. 27.1).

Subtelomeric rearrangements

The subtelomeric regions of chromosomes are located immediately proximal to the terminal telomeric repeated DNA sequences found at the end of each chromosome. The subtelomeric regions are unique sequence and highly gene rich. FISH probes (Fig. 27.2) consisting of unique sequence DNA have been designed for the subtelomeric regions of every chromosome except for: (1) the acrocentric short arms (chromosomes 13, 14, 15, 21, and 22); (2) the short arms of the X and Y chromosome, which share sequence homology;

Table 27.1   Common microdeletion or contiguous gene syndromes

Syndrome	Chromosomal region	FISH probe to relevant gene(s)
Angelman	15q11.2-15q13	SNRPN, D15S10
Miller–Dieker	17p13.3	LIS1
Prader–Willi	15q11.2-15q13	SNRPN
Smith-Magenis	17p11.2	SHMT1, TOP3, FLI1, LLGL1
Velocardiofacial/DiGeorge	22q11.2	TUPLE1
Williams	7q11.2	ELN

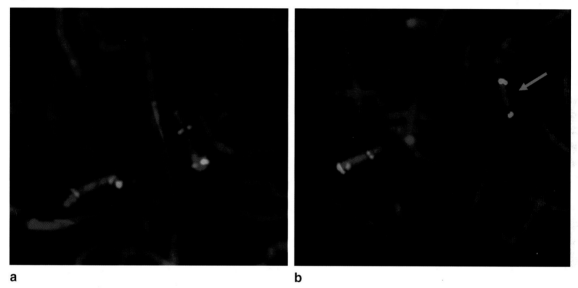

a   b

Fig. 27.1   Fluorescent in situ hybridization (FISH) images of the SNRPN probe set used in the diagnosis of Prader–Willi and Angelman syndromes, with SNRPN at 15q11.2 and PML at 15q22 labeled in SpectrumOrange™, and D15Z1 at 15p11.2 labeled in SpectrumGreen™. The D15Z1 and the PML probes are used as internal controls in this probe set. (a) A partial metaphase spread from a peripheral blood specimen. This is the normal signal pattern, with two green signals and four red signals, indicating there is no deletion of any of these probes. (b) A partial metaphase spread from a peripheral blood specimen, showing a deletion of one SNRPN locus at 15q11.2 (red arrow), indicating that this patient has the clinical diagnosis of either Prader–Willi syndrome or Angelman syndrome.

and (3) the long arms of the X and Y chromosome, which also share sequence homology (Knight et al 1997).

Cryptic rearrangements involving the subtelomeric regions have been proposed as a cause of idiopathic mental retardation, particularly in cases with prenatal onset of growth delay and a positive family history of mental retardation (de Vries et al 2001). Patients with moderate to severe mental retardation have a higher frequency of subtelomeric rearrangements, as do patients

with dysmorphic features and mental retardation (Jalal et al 2003).

Prenatal studies

One of the major advantages of FISH is the ability to rapidly detect numerical abnormalities (aneuploidy) in uncultured cells. The turnaround time is generally estimated at 24 to 48 hours. In high-risk pregnancies including those associated with advanced maternal age

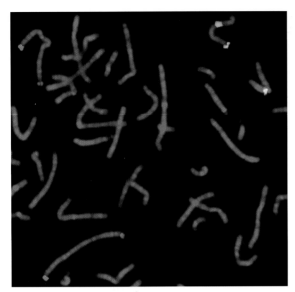

Fig. 27.2 Representative FISH image of one of the probe sets from the ToTelVysion™ (Vysis, Downers Grove, IL, CA) Multi-Color Probe mixture on a partial metaphase spread from a peripheral blood specimen. The two chromosomes 2 are labeled with SpectrumGreen™ on their short arms and with SpectrumOrange™ on their long arms. The long arms of the X chromosome and the Y chromosome are labeled with both SpectrumGreen™ and SpectrumOrange™, resulting in a fused yellow signal. In addition, there is a Spectrum Aqua™ signal on the centromere of the X chromosome. This is the normal signal pattern for this probe set.

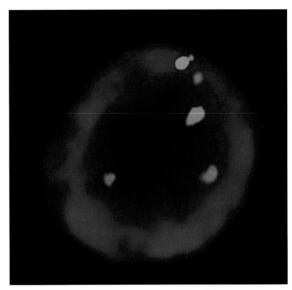

Fig. 27.3 Representative FISH image of the Aneu-Vysion™ (Vysis, Downers Grove, IL, CA) probe set with probes for chromosome 13 (labeled in SpectrumGreen™) and chromosome 21 (SpectrumOrange™) on an interphase cell from an uncultured amniocyte sample. Three red signals are seen for chromosome 21, indicating that this fetus has Down's syndrome.

(older than 35 years), abnormal ultrasound findings, or abnormal maternal screening results, FISH is used as an adjunct to standard cytogenetic analysis to provide aneuploidy screening for chromosomes 13, 18, 21, and the X and Y chromosomes. Aneuploidy of these chromosomes accounts for the most common abnormalities detected prenatally (Fig. 27.3). FISH technology on prenatal (generally amniocyte) samples has been found to be effective, sensitive, and specific (Tepperberg et al 2001).

Acquired abnormalities

FISH probes have been developed for the majority of recurrent chromosomal aberrations found in hematological malignancies (Table 27.2). One of the commercial suppliers of hematological FISH probes is Vysis, an Abbott Laboratories Company (Downers Grove, IL, USA). Their hematological FISH probes are currently divided into four types:

1. Dual color/single fusion probes.
2. Extra signal probes.
3. Dual color/break apart probes.
4. Dual color/dual fusion probes (Fig. 27.4).

With the dual color, single fusion probes, the DNA probe hybridization targets are located on one side of each of the two genetic breakpoints in the specific translocation (for example, chromosomes 9 and 22 in the case of the Philadelphia chromosome associated with chronic myelogenous leukemia). The extra signal, or ES, probes are designed to reduce the frequency of normal cells with an abnormal FISH signal pattern due to random co-localization of probe signals in the nucleus. In this type of probe set, one larger probe (labeled in one color) spans one breakpoint in the specific translocation, while the other probe (labeled in another color) flanks the breakpoint of the other gene involved in the translocation.

Table 27.2 Commercially available FISH probes for hematological diseases

Chromosomal aberration	Gene(s)	Associated disease[a]
t(8;14)(q24;q32)	MYC/IgH	ALL, NHL, MM
t(8;21)(q22;q22)	ETO/AML1	AML
Trisomy 8	8cen[b]	AML, CML
t(9;22)(q34;q11.2)	ABL/BCR	CML, ALL, AML
t(11;14)(q13;q32)	CCND1/IgH	NHL, MM
del(11)(q22.3)	ATM	CLL
11q23 rearrangements	MLL	ALL, AML
t(12;21)(p13;q22)	TEL/AML1	ALL
Trisomy 12	12cen[b]	CLL
del(13)(q14.3)	D13S319	CLL, NHL, MM
t(14;18)(q32;q21)	IgH/BCL2	NHL
14q32 rearrangements	IgH	NHL, MM
t(15;17)(q22;q21.1)	PML/RARA	APL
inv(16)(p13q22) or t(16;16)(p13;q22)	CBFβ	AML
del(17)(p13.1)	TP53	CLL, MM, NHL

[a] Abbreviations: ALL = acute lymphocytic leukemia; AML = acute myelogenous leukemia; APL = acute promyelogenous leukemia; CLL = chronic lymphocytic leukemia; CML = chronic myelogenous leukemia; MM = multiple myeloma; NHL = non-Hodgkin's lymphoma.
[b] Cen = centromere of chromosome (and, therefore, not a gene).

Dual color, break apart probes are used when a specific gene may have several different chromosomal partners, for example the *MLL* gene, rearrangements of which are seen in a small percentage of acute myelogenous leukemia and in acute lymphocytic leukemia. These probes are designed in two colors, one on either side of the breakpoint in a specific gene; when the gene is disrupted due to a translocation, the probe is seen as two separate colors (red and green), rather than as one fused signal pattern (yellow). The fourth probe set, the dual color/dual fusion probes, is designed to reduce the number of normal nuclei showing an abnormal signal pattern due to random co-localization; large probes (in different colors) span both breakpoints involved in the rearrangement. In a truly abnormal cell, two fusion signals are generally seen, representing the specific chromosomal translocation, as well as a red and a green signal, representing the normal and uninvolved chromosomes.

Solid tumors

Solid tumors are often difficult to grow in culture, and metaphase spreads can be hard to obtain. FISH is useful in detecting specific rearrangements in interphase cells

of solid tumors that have diagnostic and prognostic implications. Some soft tissue masses, such as Ewing's sarcoma or synovial sarcoma, may be difficult to diagnose by morphology alone. Most Ewing's sarcomas (Taylor et al 1993) contain translocations between the *EWS* gene (on chromosome 22) and various other chromosomal partners, the most common of which juxtaposes the *EWS* gene with the *FL1* gene (on chromosome 11). A break apart, dual color FISH probe has been designed which is telomeric and centromeric to the *EWS* gene. In a normal cell, two yellow or fused signals are seen, while in an abnormal cell, one yellow, one red, and one green signal are seen, representing the disruption and translocation of the *EWS* gene. A break apart FISH probe has also been designed to detect the translocation between the X chromosome and chromosome 18 seen in more than 90% of synovial sarcomas (Fig. 27.5). Such translocations bring the *SYT* gene on chromosome 18 into contact with either the *SSX1* or *SSX2* gene on the X chromosome (Geurts van Kessel et al 1997). Chromosomal rearrangements involving the *CHOP* gene on chromosome 12 are common in myxoid/round cell liposarcomas (Aman et al 1992). This FISH probe, also a break apart probe, will detect a translocation involving

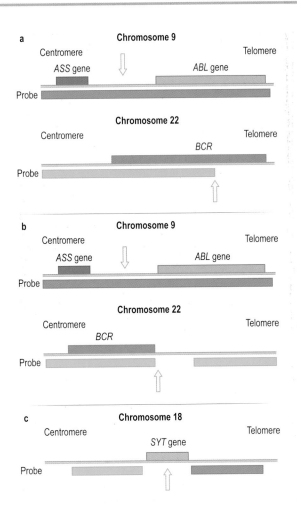

Fig. 27.4 (a) Diagram illustrating the design of a dual color, extra signal probe set. This probe set is used to identify the Philadelphia chromosome, which results from the translocation between chromosomes 9 (labeled with SpectrumOrange™) and 22 (SpectrumGreen™) in chronic myelogenous leukemia (CML) and some cases of acute lymphocytic leukemia (ALL). The arrows indicate the breakpoints on the chromosomes. The extra signal is due to the presence of the *ASS* gene, also labeled in SpectrumOrange™, which remains on the derivative chromosome 9, following the translocation. (b) Diagram illustrating the design of the dual color, dual fusion signal probe set. This probe set is also used to identify the translocation between chromosomes 9 and 22 seen in CML and some cases of ALL. The arrows indicate the breakpoints on the chromosomes. The two fusion signals arise due to the fusion of part of the red signal on chromosome 9 with part of the green signal on chromosome 22, and vice versa. (c) Diagram illustrating the design of a dual color, break apart probe. This probe is used to identify translocations involving the *SYT* gene on chromosome 18 seen a majority of synovial sarcomas. The probe is labeled in both SpectrumGreen™ and SpectrumOrange™, forming a yellow or fused signal in a normal cell; a translocation in an abnormal cell will disrupt this fused yellow signal, creating a separate red and green signal. (Diagrams adapted from Vysis product information with permission from Abbott Molecular Inc).

the *CHOP* gene, but not the specific chromosomal translocation partner. The *PAX3* and *FKHR* genes form an abnormal fusion gene in alveolar rhabdomyosarcoma. Again, a FISH probe detects the translocation between chromosomes 2 and 13 which is a significant finding in this form of tumor (Biegel et al 1995). Amplifications of the *MYCN* oncogene on chromosome 2 are seen in childhood neuroblastoma (Taylor et al 2000). This FISH probe is designed to detect extra copies of the gene.

Breast cancer

Breast cancer is the leading cause of death among Caucasian and African American women. A great deal of money and research has been targeted toward the improvement of early detection and effective therapies. This area of genetic testing has arisen because of the advances made in the field of pharmacogenomics, in which therapeutic drug development is dependent upon genetic variations in an individual. One of the major advantages of FISH is the ability to study paraffin-embedded tissue, permitting the analysis of both fresh and archival samples. This has been extremely helpful in the analysis of breast cancer tissue specimens. The *HER2* gene on chromosome 17 has been shown to be overexpressed or amplified in approximately 25% of breast cancers (Kallioniemi et al 1992). Amplification of the *HER2* gene and/or overexpression of its protein product is associated with poor prognosis, an increased risk for recurrence, and a shortened survival time (Press et al 1997). There are two types of test commonly used to determine *HER2* status: 1) immunohistochemistry, which measures the level of expression of the gene; and 2) FISH, which measures the number of copies of the

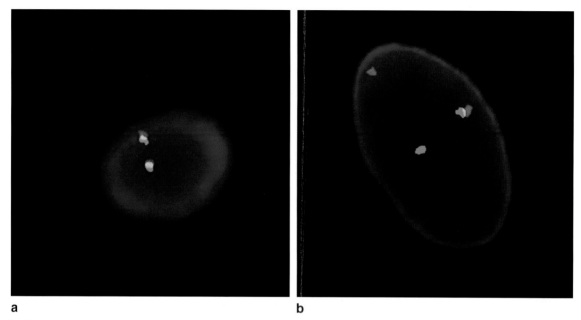

a   b

Fig. 27.5   Representative FISH images of the *SYT* dual color, break apart probe on interphase cells from a bone marrow sample. The *SYT* gene is located on chromosome 18 and translocations involving this region are seen in the majority of synovial sarcoma patients. (a) Two yellow or fused signals (both SpectrumOrange™ and SpectrumGreen™ present) are seen, which is the normal signal pattern. (b) One fused yellow signal is seen, representing the normal chromosome 18, as well as a separate red and green signal, indicating that a translocation has occurred. The *SYT* gene is translocated to the X chromosome and forms an abnormal fusion protein with either the *SSX1* or *SSX2* gene. This analysis was performed in an interphase cell and, therefore, the specific translocation partner of the *SYT* gene cannot be determined.

gene. Assessment of *HER2* status (Pegram & Slamon, 2000) is useful for determining chemotherapy responsiveness and selection for targeted monoclonal antibody therapy (Herceptin® (Trastuzumab), Genentech, Inc, South San Francisco, CA). FISH (for example, the PathVysion™ DNA probe kit from Vysis) has been approved by the United States Food and Drug Administration (FDA) as the most sensitive and specific methodology for *HER2* detection. The highest Herceptin® response is seen in FISH-positive breast cancer patients; therefore, knowledge of the status of *HER2* amplification is vital to treatment strategies for some breast cancer patients.

The PathVysion™ FISH procedure for the detection of *HER2* amplification will be described in detail later on. In brief, 4-μm sections of paraffin-embedded breast cancer tumor samples are prepared, the tumor areas are scored by a pathologist, and a FISH analysis with the *HER2* gene in combination with the alpha-satellite probe for the centromere of chromosome 17 is performed. The number of *HER2* and chromosome 17 signals is scored, the ratio of the two is determined, and a ratio of greater than 2.2 is taken to indicate amplification of the *HER2* gene (Fig. 27.6). These results are then interpreted in conjunction with clinical and pathological findings to determine the best treatment option for patients with stage II, node-positive breast cancer.

Bladder cancer recurrence screening

Bladder cancers are among the most frequent of adult cancers. Chromosomal aberrations, such as aneuploidy for chromosomes 3, 7, 9, and 17, have been found to be associated with histological progression in bladder cancer (Nemoto et al 1995). A FISH assay has been developed by Vysis, the UroVysion™ assay, which consists of a panel of probes for the centromeric regions of chromosomes 3, 7, and 17, as well as a probe for a region on the short arm of chromosome 9 (9p21). The UroVysion™ assay is designed to detect a gain of chromosomes 3, 7, and 17, and/or homozygous loss of chromosome 9p21. Both findings have been associated with recurrence of bladder cancer (Fig. 27.7).

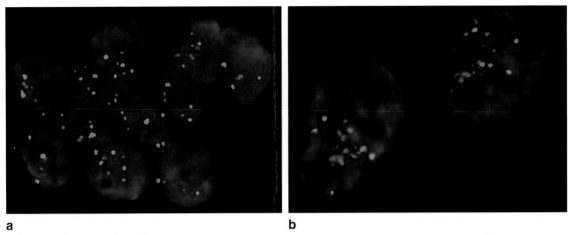

Fig. 27.6   Representative FISH images of the PathVysion™ (Vysis, Downers Grove, IL, CA) probe set with probes for the centromere of chromosome 17 (labeled in SpectrumGreen™) and the *HER2* probe (labeled in SpectrumOrange™) on a paraffin-embedded sample of two patients with breast cancer. (a) The signal ratio of the two probes was determined to be 1.13 in this sample and, therefore, no amplification of the *HER2* gene was seen. (b) The signal ratio of the two probes was determined to be 5.48 in this sample and, therefore, amplification of the *HER2* gene was determined to have occurred.

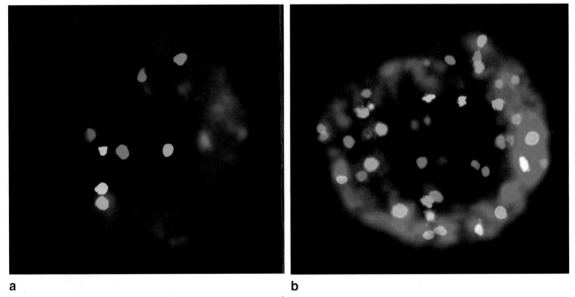

Fig. 27.7   Representative FISH images of the UroVysion™ (Vysis, Downers Grove, IL, CA) probe set with probes for the centromeres of chromosome 3 (labeled in SpectrumRed™), chromosome 7 (SpectrumGreen™), and chromosome 17 (SpectrumAqua™). The chromosome 9p21 probe is labeled in SpectrumGold™. (a) Two signals with each of the probes can be seen in this cell from a urine sample of a patient previously diagnosed with bladder cancer; this is the normal signal pattern. (b) This FISH image is from an abnormal cell found in a urine sample of a patient previously diagnosed with bladder cancer. The extra copies of chromosomes 3, 7, and 17 indicate aneuploidy of these chromosomes and perhaps a recurrence of the bladder cancer.

General FISH procedure

Sample requirements

1. Fixed metaphase or interphase chromosomes on a microscope slide or coverslip are required. Do not bake the slides (as is performed for slides that will be G-banded for routine chromosome analysis). Aging of slides is essential to obtaining good FISH signals, as it hardens the DNA, removes water, and may increase signal intensity. If slides are made and used in a FISH analysis the same day, then artificial aging must be performed, by placing slides for a minimum of 2 hours in a 37°C oven. Alternatively, if the slides have been stored at room temperature for less than 3 weeks, then the slides may be aged in 2× SSC at 73°C for 2 minutes or at 37°C for 60 minutes (followed by dehydration in an ethanol series).
2. For analysis with metaphase FISH probes, at least 15 metaphases per 22 × 22 mm area are required for a complete analysis.

Solutions

20× SSC

sodium chloride	175.32 g
sodium citrate	88.20 g
ddH$_2$O	800 ml

pH to 7.0 with 1N HCl. Bring to 1 liter with ddH$_2$O. Store at room temperature. Expiration: 6 months.

2× SSC

20× SSC	50 ml
ddH$_2$O	450 ml

Store at room temperature. Expiration: 6 months.

Ethanol series

	70%	80%	95%	100%
Ethanol (ml)	350	400	475	500
ddH$_2$O (ml)	150	100	25	0

Store at −20°C.

Denaturation solution (70% formamide/2× SSC)

Formamide	35 ml
20× SSC	5 ml
ddH$_2$O	10 ml

Bring pH to 7.0 with 1 N HCl. Store at 4°C. Expiration: 1 week.

Post-wash solution (2× SSC/0.1% Nonidet P-40 (NP-40))

20× SSC	50 ml
ddH$_2$O	450 ml
NP-40	500 µl

Bring pH to 7.0 ± 0.2 with 1 N NaOH. Mix well. Store at room temperature. Discard used solution at the end of each day. Expiration: 6 months.

Post-wash solution (0.4× SSC/0.3% NP-40)

20× SSC	20 ml
ddH$_2$O	977 ml
NP-40	3 ml

Bring pH to 7.5 ± 0.2 with 1 N NaOH. Mix well. Store at room temperature. Discard used solution at the end of each day. Expiration: 6 months.

DNA counterstain

Propidium iodide and DAPI (4′,6-diamidino-2-phenylindole) are fluorescent dyes used to counterstain DNA. Propidium iodide dyes the chromosomes red/orange, while DAPI stains chromosomes blue. Different concentrations of DAPI are available. Vysis provide both DAPI I and DAPI II. DAPI I is recommended when a more intense counterstain is required. It provides a more distinct banding pattern. DAPI II provides a weaker counterstain, which is useful when viewing smaller probes (unique sequences and centromeric regions).

FISH SET-UP

This FISH set-up procedure is the basic procedure for use with either commercially available probes or home brew probes. The denaturation times and temperatures may need to be adjusted depending on the specific probe used (whole chromosome paint versus centromere-specific probes, for example) and the tissue type (peripheral blood specimen slide versus amniocyte coverslip). Different commercially available probes are provided either pre-denatured and in solution with the appropriate hybridization buffer or require to be prepared with the appropriate hybridization buffer and distilled water (step 5) before denaturation. The two alternatives to denaturation of the slides/coverslips and probes are listed in step 7 (denaturation solution) and step 12 (all-in-one co-denaturation and hybridization system). The stringency of the post-wash solutions is important to remove non-specifically bound probe. The stringency of the post-wash solutions may be altered by changing the salt concentration, the temperature, or the time in each solution. Some specimen types require pretreatment before denaturation, which removes cytoplasmic proteins of the cell membrane, allowing greater accessibility of the DNA. Pretreatment is generally performed using fresh pepsin in an acid solution.

Day one

1. Place denaturation solution in water bath at 73°C (if following step 7).
2. Examine slide or coverslip to determine optimal target area.
3. Treat slide(s) in 2× SSC at 37°C for at least 30 minutes.
4. Dehydrate the slide(s) in a cold ethanol series (70%, 85%, then 100%) for 2 minutes each.
5. Allow slides to dry. Store slide(s) in covered slide box until ready to denature.
5. Pre-warm probe to room temperature for about 5 minutes. If probe does not need to be denatured, aliquot 10 µl for each 22 × 22 mm target area; if probe needs to be denatured, aliquot 7 µl hybridization buffer, 2 µl ddH₂0, and 1 µl probe into a microcentrifuge tube. Keep probe in darkness as much as possible. Return probe to freezer as soon as possible.
6. Vortex probe briefly and centrifuge for 2–3 seconds.
7. Denature the slide(s) for exactly 2 minutes in the pre-warmed denaturant at 73°C.

Note

A maximum of three slides should be denatured at one time to maintain the correct denaturation temperature.

8. Dehydrate the slide(s) in a cold ethanol series (70%, 80%, then 100%) for 2 minutes each.
9. Wipe the back of the slide(s) and place on a 37°C slide warmer to dry completely. Leave slide(s) on slide warmer until ready to apply probe mixture.
10. Denature aliquoted probe mix for 5 minutes in a 73°C water bath. Vortex probe briefly and centrifuge for 2–3 seconds.
11. Apply 10 µl probe mix to target area and cover with a 22 × 22 mm glass coverslip. Seal with rubber cement.

12. If *not* denaturing probes and slides separately, probes and slides can be co-denatured on, for example, the HYBrite™ Denaturation and Hybridization system 110/120 V from Vysis (# 30-144010) for 2 minutes at 73°C.

Note

Denaturation temperatures and times may vary depending on tissue type and type of probe.

13. Following either form of denaturation: incubate slide(s) at 37°C overnight in a humidified chamber (place moist sponge or paper towels in an airtight, opaque container).

Note

Slide(s) may be left in the Hybrite™ instrument for hybridization at 37°C for 4–16 hours. A minimum of 4 hours of hybridization is recommended for any probe.

Day two

14. Warm glass Coplin of 0.4× SSC/0.3% NP-40 to 73 ± 1°C. Do not wash more than three slides at a time, to ensure the correct wash temperature is maintained.
15. Remove coverslip and rubber cement from hybridized slide(s). Keep slides covered as much as possible and away from the light.
16. Wash slide(s) in 0.4× SSC/0.3% NP-40 at 72°C for 2 minutes. Agitate slide(s) for 1–3 seconds.
17. Wash slide(s) in 2× SSC/0.1% NP-40 at room temperature for 1 minute. Agitate slide(s) for 1–3 seconds.
18. Allow the slide(s) to dry while protected from the light.
19. Apply 20 µl of DAPI I or DAPI II to slide(s) and cover with appropriately sized glass coverslip.

Note

DAPI is a carcinogen.

Notes

For batching FISH samples, or running a FISH procedure with many steps and solution changes, automated FISH processing may be advantageous. One such pre-programmed automated system is supplied by Vysis, the VP 2000™ Processor 100V (# 30-144100), which may be used for a variety of functions, such as deparaffinization and pretreatment of FISH samples, histology/

cytology staining, special stains of chromosomes, and routine slide washing.

SPECIFIC FISH PROCEDURE: *HER2* FISH (PATHVYSION™)

Sample requirements

Formalin-fixed, paraffin-embedded breast cancer tissue specimens should be cut into approximately 4-µm sections. Slides are then floated in a protein-free water bath at 40°C. Each section is mounted on the positive side of an organosilane-coated slide in order to minimize the loss of tissue during processing. The slides are air dried. A hematoxylin and eosin (H&E) slide, scored by a pathologist, should accompany each specimen, with the areas of tumor to be scored clearly delineated.

Control slides (one negative and one positive slide) must be run at the same time as the clinical, patient slides in each specimen processing run, to ensure accuracy of signal analysis and to monitor assay performance. If the FISH assay on the control slides does not work, then the patient analysis cannot be reported. In addition, control slides must be run with each new lot of the PathVysion™ probe kit.

A more detailed reference of the procedure may be obtained from the PathVysionTM *HER-2* DNA Probe Kit product data sheet (Vysis).

Solutions needed for the VP 2000™ processor
70%, 85%, 95% ethanol

Post-hybridization wash buffer. *Note*: only one wash buffer used in this procedure.

2× SSC/0.3% NP-40

Protease I reagent
25 mg pepsin/lyophilized per 50 ml 0.01 N HCl. Make fresh.

(Also available from Vysis (#30-801260 and #30-8012550)).

Pretreatment reagent (1 M sodium thiocyanate)
Keep covered at ambient temperature. Expiration: 6 months.

0.2 N HCl
Keep covered at ambient temperature. Expiration: 6 months.

10% buffered formalin

Pathvysion™ *HER-2* DNA probe kit (Vysis #36-161060)

DAPI I

Day one
Bake slide(s) overnight at 56°C (hot plate or oven).

Day two
Slide pretreatment (as run on the VP 2000™ Processor)

1. Deparaffinization in Hemo-De (non-toxic solvent similar to xylene) for 5 minutes at ambient temperature.
2. Repeat twice.
3. 95% ethanol for 1 minute at ambient temperature.
4. Repeat.
5. 0.2 N HCl for 20 minutes at ambient temperature.
6. Rinse in water for 3 minutes at ambient temperature.
7. Pretreatment reagent for 30 minutes at 80°C.
8. Rinse in water for 3 minutes at ambient temperature.
9. Protease treatment for 10 minutes at 37°C.
10. Rinse in water for 3 minutes at ambient temperature.
11. Fixation in 10% buffered formalin for 10 minutes at ambient temperature.
12. Rinse in water for 3 minutes at ambient temperature.
13. Dehydrate for 1 minute each in ethanol series— 70%, 85%, then 95% ethanol.
14. Air dry on drying station for 3 minutes at 25°C.
15. Proceed to FISH procedure.

Notes
1. Before each run on the VP 2000™ Processor, each basin should be filled with 470 ml of the appropriate reagent. After approximately 15 runs, all solutions should be discarded and the basins refilled with fresh reagents.
2. The fixative step (11) helps to reduce tissue loss during denaturation.

FISH procedure

See general FISH procedure described previously. It is recommended that denaturation solution (step 7) is used to denature the slide(s). Denature slide(s) at 72 ± 1°C for 5 minutes.

Day three

1. Wash slide(s) in 2× SSC/0.3% NP-40 at 73 ± 1°C for 2 minutes.
2. Air dry slides in the dark.
3. Apply 20 µl DAPI I counterstain and cover with a glass coverslip.

Signal analysis

Using a 40× objective, scan several areas of tumor cells within the area corresponding to the H&E area, as designated by the pathologist. Select an area of good nuclei distribution. Using a 100× objective, begin analysis in the upper left quadrant of the selected area and, scanning from left to right, count the number of signals within the nuclear boundary of each evaluable interphase cell. Do not score nuclei with no signals or signals of only one color.

1. Thirty interphase cells are analyzed by one technologist and the results are confirmed by a second technologist. *Note*: A minimum of 20 interphase cells must be analyzed.
2. Results are recorded as the number of signals for the *HER2* probe and the number of signals for the CEP (chromosome enumeration probe) 17 probe (the centromere of chromosome 17).
3. The ratio of the average copy number of *HER2* to CEP 17 signals is calculated.
4. If the ratio of *HER2* to CEP 17 signals is borderline (between 1.8 and 2.2), then a second technologist will count an additional 30 interphase cells and a new ratio is calculated.
5. A schematic drawing of the section of the tissue analyzed should be made to indicate the area analyzed by each technologist.

Interpretation of results

1. The ratio of the average copy number of *HER2* to CEP 17 signals is calculated. If the number is less than 1.8, then the results are reported as not amplified.
2. If the ratio is >2.2, the results are reported as amplified.

3. If the ratio is between 1.8 and 2.2 the results are reported as equivocal.

Troubleshooting

One of the most common problems encountered with paraffin-embedded FISH analysis is under- or over-digestion of the tissue sample. If the tissue looks under-digested (too much cytoplasm, weak or no signals), then the incubation time in the pretreatment solution should be increased to 15–60 minutes. Over-digested tissue appears faded, with a loss of cell borders. A repeat sample must be run, with a decrease in the pretreatment time to 15–25 minutes and a decrease in the protease solution to 5–7 minutes. In addition, the denaturation time and temperature may be adjusted to increase the accessibility of the sample DNA to the probe. Formalin fixation, tissue size, and sample quality may all also affect the FISH results.

GENERAL SCORING ANALYSIS CRITERIA FOR FISH

The scoring analysis criteria described here are based on the minimum requirements of the College of American Pathologists (CAP) guidelines, as well as recommendations by the American College of Medical Genetics (ACMG).

Metaphase scoring criteria

General information

1. Only complete metaphases (i.e. with 46 chromosomes) should be scored. An exception may be made when the number of complete metaphases is low and all the chromosomes of interest are present in one field of view.
2. Analysis of 10 metaphase cells on all clinical samples is required for a complete study. If necessary, additional metaphase cells may be analyzed.
3. Record coordinates and results of at least two representative metaphase spreads analyzed on analysis sheet. At least two images should be captured if the analysis is abnormal; at least one image should be captured if the analysis is normal.
4. In cases suspected of mosaicism (more than one cell line present), additional metaphase cells should be counted.

Interphase scoring criteria

General information

1. At least 200 individual interphase cells should be analyzed. Only cells that are in a monolayer with discrete borders are countable. Cells that are overlapping or on top of each other are not countable. Not all cells are analyzable and may be skipped.
2. Signals should be discrete (not diffuse). Signals should be counted as two signals if they are greater than one signal-width apart. Signals that are closer than one signal-width apart should be counted as one signal.
3. A signal should be counted as yellow (fusion of orange and green) if they are on top of each other. A green signal and an orange signal with discrete borders are considered separate and, therefore, not a fusion (yellow) signal.

TROUBLESHOOTING FISH

There are various problems that may be encountered when setting up a FISH experiment, ranging from overdenaturation of the DNA, to weak or no FISH signals. Table 27.3 highlights some of the more common problems and their solutions; however, the list is by no means exhaustive. Commercially available probes are supplied with package inserts which generally cover a wide array of possible problems with FISH set-up and analysis.

VALIDATION OF FISH ANALYSIS IN THE CLINICAL CYTOGENETIC LABORATORY

The majority of probes and materials used for clinical FISH studies are considered to be analyte-specific reagents (ASRs) that are exempt from the FDA (probes that are FDA-approved include PathVysion™ and UroVysion™). Therefore, these probes must be independently validated by each clinical laboratory. The College of American Pathologists (CAP) and the Standards and Guidelines for Clinical Genetics Laboratories issued by the ACMG state that each probe must be validated for sensitivity (the expected signal pattern is observed) and specificity (the probe is localized to the correct chromosome and chromosomal region). If the probe is to be used on interphase cells, a reportable reference range for that probe must be established. Reportable reference ranges are generally established from a database of cytogenetically characterized cases, so that the percentage of cells exhibiting an 'abnormal' signal pattern by random

Table 27.3 Troubleshooting FISH

Problem	Possible cause	Possible solution
Slide background	Inadequate post-hybridization wash	Ensure correct wash solution and temperature Re-wash slide
	Inadequate cleaning of glass slides	Clean slides in ethanol and wipe dry with lint-free paper
Weak or no signal	Specimen inadequately denatured	Ensure correct denaturation solution and temperature. Increase denaturation time
	Specimen slides not aged	Age slides for 24 hours at ambient temperature before use
	Probe not added	Allow probe to thaw completely before use Vortex probe. Pipette slowly
	Probe inadequately denatured	Ensure correct temperature of water bath
	Counterstain is too bright	Remove coverslip. Re-wash in 2× SSC/0.1% NP-40 at ambient temperature. Dehydrate slides; reapply counterstain
Distorted chromosome morphology	Specimen over-denatured	Ensure correct denaturation solution and temperature. Repeat on new specimen with reduced time of denaturation

chance can be determined; thus, a normal cut-off for each probe can be established. Biannual or continual evaluation of the performance characteristics of each probe in clinical use is also required by the CAP.

FISH nomenclature

The 2005 International System for Human Cytogenetic Nomenclature (Editors: Shaffer and Tommerup) addresses FISH nomenclature (Chapter 13). The appropriate FISH nomenclature should accompany each FISH report on a patient, indicating whether the FISH test was performed on metaphase (ish) or interphase (nuc ish) cells, the chromosomal location, the probe name, and the number of signals observed. For example, a result indicating a deletion of the *SNRPN* gene (see Fig. 27.1) is written as: ish del(15)(q11.2q11.2)(SNPRN−), indicating that one chromosome 15 did not have the *SNRPN* signal, confirming a diagnosis of Angelman or Prader–Willi syndrome. A normal *HER2* result would be written: nuc ish (D17Z1,HER2) × 2[X], with [X] representing the number of interphase cells analyzed; in addition, the result indicates that two signals for both the centromere of chromosome 17 and the *HER2* gene were seen, and no amplification of the *HER2* gene was observed. An abnormal *HER2* result, indicating amplification of the *HER2* gene, may be written as: nuc ish (D17Z1 × 2),(HER2 × 8)[30].

Summary

Advances in genetic testing seem to occur on an almost daily basis. This chapter describes only one specialized area of genetic testing. As new FISH probes and molecular cytogenetic techniques, such as microarrays, become available and more widely used in the clinical cytogenetics laboratory, as well as the use of automation for both FISH set-up and analysis, the advances in genetic testing will continue to evolve.

REFERENCES

Aman P., Ron D., Mandahl N. et al. (1992) Rearrangement of the transcription factor gene CHOP in myxoid liposarcomas with t(12;16)(q13;p11). Genes, Chromosomes and Cancer 5(4):278–285.

Biegel J.A., Nycum L.M., Valentine V. et al. (1995) Detection of the t(2;13)(q35;q14) and *PAX3–FKHR* fusion in alveolar rhabdomyosarcoma by fluorescence in situ hybridization. Genes, Chromosomes and Cancer 12(3):186–192.

de Vries B.B., White S.M., Knight S.J. et al. (2002) Clinical studies on submicroscopic subtelomeric rearrangements: a checklist. Journal of Medical Genetics 38:145–150.

Geurts van Kessel A., dos Santos N.R., Simons A. et al. (1997) Molecular cytogenetics of bone and soft tissue tumors. Cancer Genetics and Cytogenetics 95(1):67–73.

Jalal S.M., Harwood A.R., Sekhon G.S. et al. (2003) Utility of subtelomeric fluorescent DNA probes for detection of chromosome anomalies in 425 patients. Genetics in Medicine 5(1):28–34.

Kallioniemi O.P., Kallioniemi A., Kurisu W. et al. (1992) *ERBB2* amplification in breast cancer analyzed by fluorescence in situ hybridization. Proceedings of the National Academy of Sciences USA 89(12):5321–5325.

Knight S.J., Horsley S.W., Regan R. et al. (1997) Development and clinical application of an innovative fluorescence in situ hybridization technique which detects submicroscopic rearrangements involving telomeres. European Journal of Human Genetics 5(1):1–8.

Kroese M., Zimmern R.L., Sanderson S. (2004) Genetic tests and their evaluation: can we answer the key questions? Genetics in Medicine 6(6):475–480.

Nemoto R., Nakamura I., Uchida K., Harada M. (1995) Numerical chromosome aberrations in bladder cancer detected by in situ hybridization. British Journal of Urology 75(4):470–476.

Pegram M., Slamon D. (2000) Biological rationale for *HER2/neu* (c-erbB2) as a target for monoclonal antibody therapy. Seminars in Oncology 27(5):13–19.

Pinkel D., Gray J.W., Trask B. et al. (1986) Cytogenetic analysis by in situ hybridization with fluorescently labeled nucleic acid probes. Cold Spring Harbor Symposia on Quantitative Biology 51(1):151–157.

Press M.F., Bernstein L., Thomas P.A. et al. (1997) *HER2/neu* gene amplification characterized by fluorescence in situ hybridization: poor prognosis in node-negative breast carcinomas. Journal of Clinical Oncology 15(8):2894–2904.

Taylor C., Patel K., Jones T. et al. (1993) Diagnosis of Ewing's sarcoma and peripheral neuroectodermal tumour based on the detection of t(11;22) using fluorescence in situ hybridisation. British Journal of Cancer 67(1):128–133.

Taylor C.P., Bown N.P., McGuckin A.G. et al. (2000) Fluorescence in situ hybridization techniques for the rapid detection of genetic prognostic factors in neuroblastoma. United Kingdom Children's Cancer Study Group. British Journal of Cancer 83(1):40–49.

Tepperberg J., Pettenati M.J., Rao P.N. et al. (2001) Prenatal diagnosis using interphase fluorescence in situ hybridization (FISH): 2-year multi-center retrospective study and review of the literature. Prenatal Diagnosis 21(4):293–301.

WEBSITES

American College of Medical Genetics. Standard and Guidelines for Clinical Genetic Laboratories. Online. Available: http://www.acmg.net

College of American Pathologists Laboratory Accreditation Checklists. Online. Available: http://www.cap.org/apps/docs/laboratoryaccreditation/checklists/checklistftp.html

UCSC Genome Bioinformatics. Online. Available: http://www.genome.ucsc.edu

FURTHER READING

Shaffer L.G., Tommerup N., eds. (2005) An international system for human cytogenetic nomenclature. Basel: S. Karger, ISCN.

28

Laser Microdissection

Diane L. Sterchi

INTRODUCTION

Laser microdissection is a powerful tool that can be used rapidly and reliably to procure pure single or multiple cells from specific microscopic region/regions of a tissue section for use in a variety of molecular analytical techniques. Through laser microdissection, cell acquisition is performed in a manner that preserves cell and tissue morphology while maintaining DNA, RNA, and protein integrity.

Cells may be acquired from frozen, paraffin, or plastic embedded tissue sections, blood smears, and cell cultures (living or fixed). The tissue sections may be unstained or stained using a modified hematoxylin and eosin (H&E). Other staining methods may include immunohistochemical (IHC) along with fluorochromes or chromagens, or in some cases a fluorescent in situ hybridization (FISH) technique depending on the type of subsequent testing to be performed.

The terms laser microdissection, laser capture microdissection, and laser-manipulated microdissection with laser pressure catapulting, to name a few, pertain to the instrumentation that is used for acquiring cells, each having its own unique method of cell acquisition. In some of the systems the laser moves instead of the stage. In others the tissue section/cells are attached to membranes for cutting and ablation techniques. The unique feature of all of these methods is how the excised cells are transported from the slide or culture dish to the collection vessel. Listed below are some examples of how the excised cells may be transported:

- Cells are acquired by passing the laser to the glass slide or membrane-coated slide, cutting the membrane (foil), and causing the sample to fall into a collection tube.

- The excised cells are catapulted by a photonic cloud into a microcentrifuge tube cap.
- Cells are attached to a cap lined with a thermoplastic film that forms a protrusion when hit by the laser pulse. The protrusion closes the gap between the tissue and the film. Lifting the cap will remove the target cells and keep them attached to the cap. The cap is then placed on a microcentrifuge tube for processing. The cap method can be used in conjunction with cutting cells from a tissue section and then attaching them to a cap.
- Cells or tissue fragments are propelled using an electrostatic force toward a film, and the film is pushed inside a microcentrifuge tube for collection.
- Live cells in a sterile culture dish or slide are covered with a light absorbing film. The laser cuts around the cells of interest under the film and, when the film is removed, the cells stay in the culture dish and the unwanted cells come off with the film. This method is called cell ablation. It removes the unwanted cells from the culture and the remaining cells can be washed and re-cultured.

Regardless of the system used, all systems provide a way to inspect the accession process by viewing the cells or tissue removed and the area from which they were excised.

After cell acquisition by laser microdissection, cells may then be subjected to a variety of procedures for genetic analysis, pathology studies, forensics, reproduction, and botany.

APPLICATIONS

- *Genetics:* The concept of tumor heterogeneity is important to distinguish unique properties between cell types within a tumor biopsy (Chu et al 2000). Comparative studies between normal, premalignant, and malignant cells from the same individual may provide evidence of genetic changes and may serve to predict tumor biology and therapy response. Once certain tumor characteristics are determined, the tumors may be identified with specific markers which would make it possible to classify them rapidly (Walch et al 2000).

- *Neuroscience:* The isolation of single neurons, plaque, or glial cells for genetic analysis to investigate neurodegenerative diseases such as Alzheimer's disease, Parkinson's disease, and multiple sclerosis (Luo et al 1999: Segal et al 2005).
- *Protein analyses:* Obtaining pure samples for analysis of the protein complement and to identify qualitative or quantitative differences in proteins between normal and diseased cells (Banks et al 1999: Palmer-Toy et al 2000).
- *Microarrays:* Comparing gene expression between like cells of different sizes. Providing pure cells for high-throughput cDNA microarrays in the study of normal, malignant, and metastatic cells from the same individual to trace genetic alterations during the development of neoplasia (Luzzi et al 2003).
- *Forensics:* Removing and isolating specific epithelial cells or sperm to aid in the prosecution of a sexual assault case.

- *Cell genetics:* Selecting single chromosomes or chromosome arms/bands to produce specific paint probes for reverse chromosome painting (Schermelleh et al 1999).
- *Cell ultrastructure and components:* Selecting specific cells for ultrastructural morphology, chemical, and mineral analysis using electron microscopy (Grant & Jerome 2002; Bobryshev 2005) or cell component separation using flow cytometry.

Laser microdissection has its advantages and disadvantages. An important advantage is the ability to procure a pure cell sample for molecular analysis. This means that the data from the pure cell are more specific than the data acquired when using homogenized tissue samples containing heterogeneous cells (Curran et al 2000). Other advantages are that there is minimal sample loss along with an opportunity to use a variety of staining and preparation procedures on the specimens.

Some disadvantages of laser microdissection might be the slightly diminished resolution during the visualization of the uncoverslipped sample. However, most equipment manufacturers have resolved this problem (Fig. 28.1). Another disadvantage may be that laser microdissection isolates only small amounts of material which may limit those analyses that require amplification techniques or necessitate the collection of many samples.

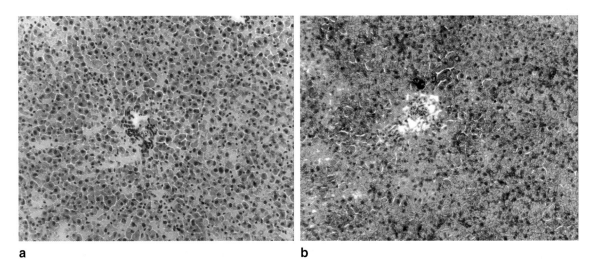

a   **b**

Fig. 28.1 An 8 μm frozen section of liver. (a) is an example of how a coverslipped frozen tissue section appears under the microscope. (b) illustrates a frozen tissue section without a coverslip and how it appears through the laser microdissection microscope. Note the resolution differences.

SAMPLE PREPARATION

The method of preparation for the tissue sections must be considered with regard to which molecular analyses are feasible and will provide reliable and meaningful results. Histology slide preparation must be performed in a fashion that does not destroy, deplete, or manipulate the cells to be studied. Sections are minimally stained to allow cell identification under the microscope. There are two major issues affecting sample collection for molecular profiling. One is reproducibility and the second is quality. In most cases molecular profiling requires frozen or fresh tissue along with as pure as possible sample to insure quality. Developed and validated protocols should be in place for reproducibility.

There are several questions that one needs to answer prior to collection of any specimen for laser microdissection. They are as follows:

- What is the tissue and specific cell population chosen for acquisition? Each tissue type may require modifications to the procedure to allow complete microdissection.
- What are the cells of interest? Cell type is important in adjusting the preparation procedure to insure proper fixation, dehydration, and identification.
- What is the size of the cells and how many are needed? Cell size and type are important in adjusting the parameters of the laser equipment for optimal cell acquisition. Also, the number of cells will determine the method of procurement and is important to the subsequent molecular analysis method.
- What needs to be isolated from the cells? Is it RNA, DNA, proteins, or specific whole cells for ultrastructural examination with transmission electron microscopy or flow cytometry?
- What is the best method of tissue collection and sample preparation? In the best case scenario, the specimen should be collected fresh and as rapidly as possible. Choosing the best preparation method depends on the answer to 'what needs to be isolated from the cells?'
- What stains are compatible with the subsequent testing and aid in the identification of the cells of interest? Before staining any laser microdissection sample, it is important to determine how that stain will interfere with the subsequent molecular analysis.

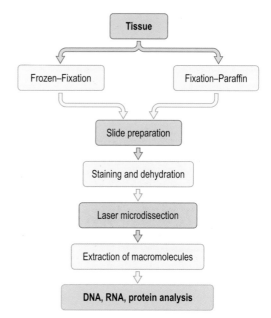

Fig. 28.2 A schematic of the basic process of sample preparation for laser microdissection.

Above is a schematic overview of the steps performed in tissue processing for laser microdissection (Fig. 28.2).

FIXATION

The effect of aldehyde-based (cross-linking) fixatives, ethanol, and acetone-based (precipitative) fixatives on RNA extraction and amplification from laser microdissected tissue is an issue (Ahram et al 2003). Ethanol-based fixatives consistently produce more polymerase chain reaction (PCR) amplification product than cross-linking fixatives (Goldsworthy et al 1999). It is also important to keep the time in any fixative to a minimum to avoid compromising the sample. Often there is no control over how long the tissue is in a fixative such as archived wet tissues and paraffin blocks (Specht et al 2000). When preparing tissue for fixation the tissue should be trimmed to around 3–5 mm^2 if possible while retaining the area of choice after removal, and either fix or freeze it immediately.

GENERAL PRECAUTIONS TO TAKE WHEN PREPARING LASER MICRODISSECTION SAMPLES

The collection and sample preparation area should be thoroughly cleaned and isolated, if possible in a 'low-traffic' area of the laboratory. Always wear gloves throughout specimen preparation and handling to prevent contamination from RNases found on human hands. Clean all dissecting instruments and laboratory bench-tops by wiping them down with a commercially available RNase decontamination cleaner or RNase-free alcohol. Change gloves after touching skin (e.g. nose, face), door-knobs, and common surfaces. Clean instruments and change gloves between each specimen collected. Keep specimens in separate containers in order to avoid cross-contamination. When preparing buffers and solutions for laser microdissection, it is essential to use RNase-free diethylpyrocarbonate (DEPC) or sterile water.

Slide preparation

Tissue sections may be mounted on plain (non-charged) membrane or foil slides. The membrane or foil slides offer support to the cells during transfer after microdissection. When using plain slides, make sure they are clean and handled only with gloved hands. It is better to open a fresh box of slides or they may be washed with a mild soap then rinsed thoroughly with de-ionized water. After rinsing they can be placed in an RNA-free cleaning solution and then rinsed with RNA-free water, making sure that the RNA-free cleaning solution is completely rinsed off the slides before they are used. Membrane slides do not need decontamination but should be kept away from excess handling and in a closed container when not in use.

Paraffin preparation

Paraffin processing may not be the optimal procedure for laser microdissection. Most often the tissues of interest for molecular research are formalin fixed and paraffin embedded (FFPE). FFPE is less damaging when extracting DNA and some proteins but it does have a profound effect on the quality and quantity of RNA isolation due to the cross-linking of the macromolecules. Most laser microdissector manufacturers have protocols on extracting RNA from FFPE.

Specimens trimmed to 3–5 mm² should be processed as soon as possible using an automatic tissue processor on a short cycle. The following settings are recommended to use with an automatic tissue processor. If the processor has vacuum available, the vacuum setting should be on the 'ON' position.

1. Rinse tissues in water briefly after fixation.
2. 70% ethyl alcohol 10–15 min 38°C
3. 80% ethyl alcohol 10–15 min 38°C
4. 95% ethyl alcohol 10–15 min 38°C
5. 95% ethyl alcohol 10–15 min 38°C
6. 100% ethyl alcohol 10–15 min 38°C
7. 100% ethyl alcohol 10–15 min 38°C
8. 100% xylene or xylene substitute 10–15 min 38°C
9. 100% xylene 10–15 min 38°C
10. Low temperature paraffin 15–20 min 52–55°C
11. Low temperature paraffin 15–20 min 52–55°C
12. Embed immediately.

Note

It is important to *not* expose the tissue to excessive (time and temperature) heating.

Microwave paraffin processing

Microwave processing may be used in place of a conventional tissue processor. It is faster, eliminates the use of xylene in the processing protocol, and produces better results with protein analysis. Specimens should be trimmed to a thickness of 2–3 mm prior to fixation (if done in the microwave) or after fixation before microwave processing. Process the tissues as soon as possible on the shortest time schedule without compromising complete processing of the tissue. The time and temperature is not listed. Most laboratories using microwave technology have established time and temperature protocols (Willis & Minshew 2002). The following is a recommendation for the solutions and the sequence to be used:

1. Fix tissues in microwave (optional).
2. 100% ethyl alcohol.
3. 100% ethyl alcohol (this second ethyl alcohol may be omitted if tissue is very small).
4. Absolute isopropyl alcohol.
5. Absolute isopropyl alcohol.

6. Paraffin.
7. Paraffin.
8. Embed immediately.

Microtomy (paraffin)

Section thickness (paraffin or frozen) depends on the size of the cells for microdissection. Section thickness ranges from 4 to 10 μm. Experience has demonstrated that larger cells require thicker sections to be cut, thus more laser power is needed. Wear gloves at all times when possible. Wearing gloves during paraffin microtomy may be difficult due to the sections sticking to the gloves via static cling. If gloves cannot be worn during sectioning, do not touch the tissue in the section when transferring to the water bath. Do not touch surrounding unclean areas with gloves and then touch tissue block, knife, or microtome. Change gloves after each animal and tissue handling. Clean microtome, knife holder, knife, and flotation bath with 100% ethyl alcohol or RNase decontamination cleaner (for RNA analysis) prior to use. Fill *clean* flotation baths with fresh clean distilled water or DEPC water and heat to preset temperature. Do not add adhesives.

Place paraffin block into the block holder on the microtome. Wipe the face of the block with 70% ethyl alcohol-dampened gauze prior to facing to remove debris. Let dry and proceed to face block. Microtome sections at 4–10 μm thick. Drain slides standing upright on a clean paper towel or an upright slide rack. Place slides into a staining rack that has been cleaned with 100% ethyl alcohol or RNase decontamination cleaner prior to use. Dry slides in a 45–65°C oven for 30–45 minutes (the least amount of time is better). If RNA extraction following paraffin microtomy is to be performed, dry slides at room temperature for 1 hour or more. Do not dry them in the oven.

Paraffin blocks should be sealed before archiving. Slides may be stored for up to 2 weeks in a cool dry place or a dessicator prior to staining and laser microdissection.

Frozen preparation

For optimal recovery of DNA, RNA, and proteins, using frozen tissue for laser microdissection is best. In general, frozen tissue yields a higher quality of amplification product than paraffin-embedded tissue.

Place snap-frozen tissue into a properly labeled vial. Keep individual tissues in separate containers in order to avoid cross-contamination. It is very important to keep tissues frozen (−70°C to −80°C) until ready to section.

After snap freezing, the tissues may be stored in a −80°C freezer for up to 6 months and will retain RNA quality. It is recommended, however, to freeze several small blocks containing the cells of interest to avoid freeze/thawing artifacts and loss of RNA quality that may occur when cutting a block more than once.

There are several ways to freeze tissues for laser microdissection. Determine the method to use by the way the specimen is received into the laboratory (frozen or in fixative) and by the procedure the laboratory is more comfortable using. Always test the different methods before deciding and applying one. Follow the general precautions and slide preparation methods before freezing the tissue (RNase-free blades, instruments, wear gloves, and clean work area).

Snap-frozen

This method is used when a time delay occurs between collection and sectioning the tissue for laser microdissection until well after collection. After freezing the tissue in liquid nitrogen, place tissue *immediately* into storage (−70 to −80°C freezer) without embedding. A brief process is listed below.

1. Remove tissue from animal.
2. Quickly trim tissue as small as possible.
3. Immerse tissue directly into liquid nitrogen.
4. Place frozen specimen into an airtight storage container and store.

Snap-frozen then embedded for cryosectioning

This method may be used with snap-frozen tissues (with liquid nitrogen) that were stored in the freezer.

1. Fill the embedding mold half full with cryo-embedding medium.
2. Remove tissue from the freezer and allow the surface of the tissue to melt a little. This takes about 1 or 2 minutes.
3. Place tissue into the embedding medium and press flat to the bottom of the mold with cutting face down.
4. Quickly fill the remainder of the embedding mold with cryo-embedding medium.
5. Immerse mold/tissue/embedding medium into a beaker of hexane or isopentane sitting in dry ice.

Note that isopentane can be poured directly over dry ice to make a slurry to freeze the tissue. Either method is acceptable for laser microdissection.

Embedding and freezing

This method may be used with fresh tissues that are to be cryosectioned immediately after freezing/embedding.

1. Fill the embedding mold half full with a cryo-embedding medium.
2. Place tissue into the embedding medium and press flat to the bottom of the mold with cutting face down.
3. Fill the remainder of the embedding mold with cryo-embedding medium.
4. Immerse mold/tissue/embedding medium into liquid nitrogen or in a beaker of hexane or isopentane sitting on dry ice.

The above freezing methods work well for most tissues, including very delicate tissues such as pancreas and spleen.

Freezing method for whole rodent brains

When freezing whole rodent brains, a 3–30% sucrose solution is normally used to prevent ice crystals from forming. For microdissection, omit the recommended sucrose solution. The sucrose solution may prevent complete freezing of the tissue and the tissue may retain moisture during cryosectioning, thus degrading the RNA.

Freeze whole rodent brains by placing the brain into ice-cold phosphate buffered saline (PBS) immediately after removal. Blot off the excess PBS and set the brain on a piece of aluminum foil overlying dry ice. Allow the brain to freeze completely. This may take 10–15 minutes. Wrap the frozen brain into the aluminum foil and place it into a sealed container. Place container and tissue into a −80°C freezer until the cryosectioning is performed.

Cryosectioning

1. Wipe down the cryostat (microtome, knife holder, knife, side panels, etc.) with 100% alcohol before using.
2. Remove one piece of snap-frozen unembedded tissue from freezer and place it into cryostat.

3. Allow the tissue to come up to the cryostat temperature.
4. Place a small amount of cryo-embedding medium on a tissue chuck.
5. Allow cryo-embedding medium to harden.
6. Add a few more drops of embedding medium and, while the embedding medium is still wet, position tissue onto the chuck with cutting area side up.
7. Allow the embedding medium between the tissue and base to harden.
8. Apply layers of embedding medium until tissue is surrounded by embedding medium and is firmly attached to the chuck. Do not touch the tissue with the tip of embedding medium applicator.
9. Trim the embedding medium into a pyramid or rectangular shape, leaving an edge free of tissue.
10. Attach chuck to microtome and face block.
11. Wipe the knife (carefully) and brush the debris off the face of the block and surrounding area.
12. Move the knife to a clean spot.
13. Cut 4–10 µm thick sections for glass slides, 3–5 µm thick for membrane-coated slides. Use a clean anti-roll plate if available.
14. Place the sections onto a clean glass slide or a membrane-coated slide.
15. Keep the slides frozen after cryosectioning by placing them in a clean slide rack inside a clean staining dish that is surrounded by dry ice, or by placing them into a −70 to −80°C freezer immediately.

If tissues were *embedded* and stored at −80°C or colder, follow the steps below:

1. Remove the frozen tissue from the freezer and place into the cryostat.
2. Allow the tissue/block to come up to the cryostat temperature.
3. Place a small amount of cryo-embedding medium on a tissue chuck and allow it to harden.
4. Add additional cryo-embedding medium to hardened embedding medium in a large enough area to cover the bottom of the frozen tissue block.
5. Position the tissue/block onto the liquid cryo-embedding medium and onto the chuck with the cutting side face up.
6. Allow the cryo-embedding medium to harden to attach tissue/block to chuck.

The inside of the cryostat, blade holder, and blade should be cleaned with 100% alcohol after each tissue. Gloves should be changed before cryosectioning the next tissue, and the knife should be moved to a different cutting area or changed.

Slides should be stained immediately after cryosectioning, and laser microdissection should be performed immediately after staining. When this is not possible, slides may be stored at various stages of the process.

Fresh-cut slides may be stored in a −70 to −80°C freezer until stained. Slides are placed in a moisture and airtight container. Storage time should be kept to less than 3 months. Once slides are removed from the freezer, stain them using the desired staining method.

Stained slides may be stored in a −70 to −80°C freezer until laser microdissection. Slides must be placed in a moisture and airtight container. Storage time should be kept to less than 1 month. Perform dehydration through graded alcohols and xylene on the stained slides just prior to laser microdissection.

STAINING

General considerations for staining tissue sections for laser microdissection are as follows.

- Keep staining time to a minimum
- Avoid excessive washings and rinsing
- Keep the color intensity of the stain as light as possible, just dark enough to recognize the cells of choice
- Use all fresh chemicals
- Stain each animal/patient separately if possible
- Change staining solutions after each animal/patient.

Paraffin hematoxylin and eosin (H&E) staining method

Slides are deparaffinized using xylene. Xylene substitutes are not ideal to use on slides for laser microdissection. Xylene substitutes leave an oily residue that sometimes interferes with the attachment of the cells to the thermoplastic film used with one of the laser microdissection instruments. The following H&E staining method is recommended. When looking at protein characterization, keep the hematoxylin staining time to a minimum and omit the eosin.

1. Xylene × 3   5–8 min (for plain glass slides)
   Xylene × 2   2–3 min (for membrane/foil slides)
2. 100% ethanol ×2   1–3 min each
3. 95% ethanol   1–15 dips
4. 70% ethanol   1–15 dips
5. Rinse slides briefly in RNase-free water
6. Hematoxylin   30–45 seconds.

Use a progressive hematoxylin to avoid the differentiation and bluing steps.

7. Rinse slides in warm RNase-free water to blue the hematoxylin.
8. Eosin   3–5 quick dips
9. 95% ethanol   1–8 dips
10. 100% ethanol × 2   1–3 min each
11. 100% xylene × 2   1–3 min each.

After the staining procedure is completed, allow slides to dry in a cool dust-free area by placing into a slide box or a desiccator with a moisture-absorbing material, recalling that moisture encourages RNase activity.

Frozen H&E staining method

1. Remove slides from the freezer or dry ice.
2. Allow slides to defrost slightly at room temperature for 30–100 seconds.
3. Wipe off all excess moisture around tissue sections and back of slide.
4. Fix tissue sections with either 70% ethyl alcohol, cold acetone, or alcohol/acetone mix if tissues were not fixed prior to freezing for 10–20 seconds. If tissue sections were fixed prior to freezing, skip this step.
5. Rinse slides briefly in RNase-free water.
6. Hematoxylin   10–15 dips.
7. Rinse slides in warm RNase-free water to blue the hematoxylin.
8. Eosin   3–5 quick dips
9. 95% ethanol   1–8 dips
10. 100% ethanol × 2   1–3 minutes each
11. 100% xylene × 2   1–3 minutes each.

After the staining procedure, allow slides to dry in a cool dust-free area by placing into a slide box or a desiccator with a moisture-absorbing material.

Immunohistochemical (IHC) staining

General rules

- When performing immunohistochemical staining procedures to identify specific cells for laser microdissection, it is important to use IHC methods that are short and direct (Fend et al 1999). Charged slides or slides with a light poly-L-lysine coating can be used to minimize section loss. To reduce the amount of moisture introduced into the tissue section that may increase RNA degradation, design a staining procedure to include minimal rinse and incubation times. For example, using biotinylated primary antibodies usually decreases the staining time. In addition, using a direct immunofluorescence staining protocol instead of a chromogen detection system (e.g. DAB) may be preferred because the cells are easier to identify using fluorescence during microdissection and the staining methods are usually very short.

CELL CULTURE PREPARATION

Cells may be grown on membrane, chamber, coated slides, culture bottles, or plates. Deciding on which processing method to use is governed by how the cells were produced or grown and whether the cells must remain alive if they can be fixed. Live cell application protocols are available from the instrument manufacturer and it is advisable to follow their recommendations. Some examples are listed below.

Culture slides (chamber, membrane)

- Cells are seeded and grown on a glass chamber slide or a membrane-prepared slide.
- Carefully aspirate the medium off the cells.
- Fix slides with either methanol or 70% ethanol for 2–5 minutes. If using chamber slides that contain more than one chamber, make sure each chamber has been fixed.
- Remove chamber walls once the cells are fixed.
- Stain as appropriate and perform laser microdissection.

Cultured cells (bottle, plate, flask)

- Cells are removed from culture plate, bottle, or flask by trypsinization and/or scraping.
- Place the detached cells into a small sterile centrifuge tube.
- Pipette a fixative (aldehyde or alcohol type) inside centrifuge tube containing cells; vortex gently and then centrifuge into a cell pellet. Agar may be added to hold cells together just before centrifugation. Do

not use fixatives if the cell pellet is to be frozen and sectioned for laser microdissection. Follow the freezing and cryosectioning protocol in this chapter.
- Fixed cell pellets are placed into a labeled cassette, processed on the biopsy short cycle, and paraffin embedded. Follow the paraffin processing protocol in this chapter.
- Blocks are sectioned and stained.

BLOOD SMEAR/CYTOSPIN PREPARATION

A cytospin preparation usually requires a predetermined number of suspended cells (e.g. 50,000 cells per 100 μl) in order to get a nice thin preparation of the cells and to guarantee that the number of cells is sufficient. Cleaned glass slides are used in the instrument and are loaded on to the cytospin equipment according to the manufacturer's instructions. Once the cytospin slide(s) preparation is complete, remove the slide(s) and drain excess liquid off (do not allow slide to dry). Fix cells immediately by immersing the slide(s) into 95% ethanol for 7–10 minutes. Transfer slide(s) to 70% ethanol for 30–60 seconds. Rinse slides in DEPC water or buffer of choice for 30–40 seconds before staining. Stain the slide(s) and perform the dehydration steps prior to laser microdissection.

TESTING RNA QUALITY PRIOR TO LASER MICRODISSECTION

RNA quality is vital for many applications following cell acquisition. In fact, it may be necessary to test the RNA quality within the tissue sample prior to laser microdissection. A typical method consists of scraping the tissue section(s) from an unstained, dehydrated slide into a 500 μl microcentrifuge tube and performing agarose gel electrophoreses on the extracted RNA sample (this may be very time consuming and requires a large amount of tissue or cells). Alternatively, the quality of the extracted RNA may be assessed on a microchip bioanalyser (this is quicker and requires less tissue).

Several manufacturers recommend this pre-testing of the RNA quality of the sample prior to staining or laser microdissection. Moreover, it is advisable to compare the RNA quality of a stained slide tissue scraping with the unstained slide to determine if the staining method chosen compromises the RNA quality. Thus, degraded or contaminated RNA preparations can be easily identified before time-consuming protocols, such as cDNA synthesis, are initiated.

REFERENCES

Ahram M., Flaig M.J., Gillespie J.W. et al. (2003) Evaluation of ethanol-fixed, paraffin-embedded tissues for proteomic applications. Proteomics 4:413–421.

Banks R.E., Dunn M.J., Forbes M.A. et al. (1999) The potential use of laser capture microdissection to selectively obtain distinct populations of cells for proteomic analysis. Electrophoresis 20:689–700.

Bobryshev Y.V. (2005) Intracellular localization of oxidized low-density lipoproteins in atherosclerotic plaque cells revealed by electron microscopy combined with laser capture microdissection. Journal of Histochemistry and Cytochemistry 53(6):793–797.

Chu S.S., Kunitake S.T., Travis J.C. (2000) Laser capture microdissection: applications in cancer research. Biomedical Products 25(4):58–62.

Curran S., McKay J.A., McLeod H.L. et al. (2000) Laser capture microscopy. Molecular Pathology. 53(2):64–68.

Fend F., Emmert-Buck M.R., Chuaqui R. et al. (1999) Immuno-LCM: laser capture microdissection of immuno-stained frozen sections for mRNA analysis. American Journal of Pathology 154:61–66.

Goldsworthy S.M., Stockton P.S., Trempus C.S. et al. (1999) Effects of fixation on RNA extraction and amplification from laser capture microdissected tissue. Molecular Carcinogenesis 25(2):86–91.

Grant K., Jerome W.G. (2002) Laser capture microdissection as an aid to ultrastructural analysis. Microscopy and Microanalysis 8:170–175.

Luo L., Salunga R.C., Guo H. et al. (1999) Gene expression profiles of laser-captured adjacent neuronal subtypes. Nature Medicine 5:117–122.

Luzzi V., Mahadevappa M., Raja R. et al. (2003) Accurate and reproducible gene expression profiles from laser capture microdissection, transcript amplification, and high density oligonucleotide microarray analysis. Journal of Molecular Diagnostics 5(1):9–14.

Palmer-Toy D.E., Sarracino D.A., Sgroi D. et al. (2000) Direct acquisition of matrix-assisted laser desorption/ionization time-of-flight mass spectra from laser capture microdissected tissues. Clinical Chemistry 46(9):1513–1516.

Schermelleh L., Thalhammer S., Heckl W. et al. (1999) Laser microdissection and laser pressure catapulting for the generation of chromosome-specific paint probes. Biotechniques 27:362–367.

Segal J.P., Stallings N.R., Lee C.E. et al. (2005) Use of laser-capture microdissection for the identification of marker genes for the ventromedial hypothalamic nucleus. Journal of Neuroscience 25(16):4181–4188.

Specht K., Richter T., Muller U. et al. (2000) Quantitative gene expression analysis in microdissected archival formalin-fixed and paraffin-embedded tumor tissue. American Journal of Pathology 158(2):419–429.

Walch A., Komminoth P., Hutzler P. et al. (2000) Microdissection of tissue sections: application to the molecular genetic characterization of premalignant lesions. Pathobiology 68:9–17.

Willis D., Minshew J. (2002) Microwave technology in the histology laboratory. HistoLogic 35(1):1–5.

FURTHER READING

Burgemeister R., Gangnus R., Haar B. et al. (2003) High quality RNA retrieved from samples obtained by using LMPC (laser microdissection and pressure catapulting) technology. Journal of Histochemistry and Cytochemistry 199(6):431–436.

De Souza A.I., McGregor E., Dunn M.J. et al. (2004) Preparation of human heart for laser microdissection and proteomics. Proteomics 4:578–586.

Emmert-Buck M., Strausberg R.L. Krizman D.B. et al. (2000) Molecular profiling of clinical tissue specimens: feasibility and applications. American Journal of Pathology 156(4):1109–1115.

Gillespie J.W., Ahram M., Best C.J. et al. (2001) The role of tissue microdissection in cancer research. Cancer Journal 7(1):32–39.

Heel K., Dawkins H. (2001) Laser microdissection and optical tweezers in research. Today's Life Science 13(2):42–48.

Lahr G. (2000) RT-PCR from archival single cells is a suitable method to analyze specific gene expression. Laboratory Investigation 80(9):1477–1479.

Lehmann U., Bock O., Gloeckner S. et al. (2000) Quantitative molecular analysis of laser-microdissected paraffin-embedded human tissue. Pathobiology 68:202–208.

Nagasawa Y., Takenaka M., Matsuoka Y. et al. (2000) Quantitation of mRNA expression in glomeruli using laser-manipulated microdissection and laser pressure catapulting. Kidney International 57:717–723.

Ren Z.P., Saellstroem J., Sundstroem C. et al. (2000) Recovering DNA and optimizing PCR conditions from microdissected formalin-fixed and paraffin embedded materials. Pathobiology 68:215–217.

Specht K., Richter T., Muller U. et al. (2000) Quantitative gene expression analysis in microdissected archival tissue by real-time RT-PCR. Journal of Molecular Medicine 78(7):B27.

Witliff J.L., Kunitake S.T., Chu S.S. et al. (2000) Applications of laser capture microdissection in genomics and proteomics. Journal of Clinical Ligand Assay 23(1):66–73.

29

Plastic Embedding for Light Microscopy

Neil M. Hand

INTRODUCTION

Paraffin wax is a suitable embedding medium for most tissues, combining adequacy of tissue support with ease of sectioning on a standard microtome. Section thicknesses of 4–6 μm are satisfactory for most diagnostic purposes, although with skill and experience thinner sections may be produced. However, there are three main areas where paraffin wax is an unsuitable embedding medium for light microscopy studies. Firstly it may not offer sufficient support; secondly it does not permit thin sections to be cut (these two factors are interrelated); and thirdly substances such as enzymes are destroyed. In these circumstances, the use of plastic instead of paraffin wax may provide superior histological preparations. The main applications of the use of plastic embedding are outlined below.

ULTRASTRUCTURAL STUDIES

In the early development of electron microscopy extremely hard ester waxes were used, but with limited success. They are totally unsuitable for ultrastructural studies, as they do not offer sufficient support for ultra-thin sections (approximately 30–80 nm) to be cut and because they are unable to withstand the high-energy electron beam that passes through the section within the electron microscope (see Chapter 30). The introduction instead of plastic/resin embedding media provided improved results and stimulated the development of electron microscopy. Nunn (1970) and Glauert (1987) discussed the properties of embedding media suitable for ultrastructural studies. This chapter will focus mainly on the use of plastic techniques for light microscopy

(LM), as details of those for electron microscopy (EM) demand different protocols and are described in Chapter 30.

HARD TISSUES AND IMPLANTS

In extremely hard tissues such as undecalcified bone, especially where the sample is large and/or when dense cortical bone is present, the difference in hardness between the tissue and the medium in which it is embedded may be so great that sectioning is exceptionally difficult, resulting in only poor-quality fragmented sections being obtained. The use therefore of a harder embedding medium such as a plastic can enable superior sections to be cut. This may be achieved either in the form of a section using a motorized microtome, or as a slice which is then ground down to the required thickness. The latter (known as a ground section) requires specialized equipment and procedures that are different from those used for conventional microtomy. Ground sections are useful if inorganic material such as an implant is present or the tissue is tooth, as these are virtually impossible to section by traditional means. These applications are discussed more fully in Chapter 18.

HIGH-RESOLUTION LIGHT MICROSCOPY

It has long been appreciated that where an accurate diagnosis and prognosis may depend on the detection of some subtle histological or cytological change, sections thinner than the usual 4–6 μm greatly facilitate accurate examination. The two best-known examples are for renal biopsy and interpretation of hematopoietic tissue, where the reduction of paraffin section thickness to about 2 μm has led to easier and more accurate diagnosis through the detection of minor histological abnormalities that are obscured in thicker sections. Experience has proved that even thinner sections combined with high-quality optics will provide a more accurate diagnosis by light microscopy of minor glomerular abnormalities in the renal biopsy. Unfortunately, even with the greatest skill and experience, it is extremely difficult to produce good-quality sections thinner than about 3 μm using a standard paraffin wax embedding technique, so the possibilities for high-resolution light microscopy are limited. In addition, the artifacts produced in wax sections often limit potential morphological improvements, so the advantages gained are less obvious than if a plastic is employed as the embedding medium.

Pathologists experienced in the use of electron microscopy have long been well aware of the increased amount of cytological detail detectable in 0.5–1 μm plastic-embedded tissue sections produced prior to ultra-thin sectioning for ultrastructural studies. It was the realization of the diagnostic value of high-resolution light microscopy in identifying certain nuclear and cytoplasmic characteristics, which are usually obscured in thicker sections, that led to an interest in plastic embedding for specific uses in diagnostic histopathology. In practice, tissue sections other than those from a renal biopsy are frequently cut at 2–3 μm (referred to as semithin sections), to combine satisfactory resolution with sufficient staining intensity and contrast. As applications and histological procedures have developed, there have been additional uses of plastic embedding for high-resolution light microscopy. Some of these will be discussed in this chapter.

PLASTIC EMBEDDING MEDIA

Plastics are classified according to their chemical composition into epoxy, polyester, or acrylic. The change in the physical state of an embedding medium from liquid to solid is called polymerization and is brought about by joining molecules together to produce a complex macromolecule made up of repeating units. The macromolecule, termed polymer (derived from the Greek word *poly* meaning 'many' and *mer* meaning 'part'), is synthesized from simple molecules called monomers ('single part'). Several ingredients are required to produce a plastic

suitable as an embedding medium for biological material and subsequent histological examination. Some of these ingredients can present potential health and safety problems, and it is important that all chemicals used in the formulation of plastics are handled and disposed of in accordance with local and legal requirements.

Epoxy plastics

Various epoxy plastics have found their widest application as embedding media for ultrastructural studies, because the polymerized plastic is sufficiently hard to permit sections as thin as 30–40 nm to be cut and is stable in an electron beam. Embedding schedules for the different epoxy resins used in electron microscopy are given in Chapter 30, and only a brief outline of their properties and uses is given here. Epoxy plastics derive their name from the active group through which they polymerize (Fig. 29.1). Epoxide or oxirane groups can be attached to an almost infinite number of chemical structures in single or multifunctional conformations. Three types of epoxy plastic are used in microscopy: those based on either bisphenol A (Araldite), glycerol (Epon), or cyclohexene dioxide (Spurr). The names in parentheses are those in common usage by microscopists and do not convey any structural property.

Epoxy embedding plastics are a carefully balanced mixture of epoxy plastic, catalyst, and accelerator, each component having a direct influence on the physical and mechanical properties of the cured plastic. The catalyst system used is of the anhydride/amine type and causes curing of the resin by the formation of ester cross-links. The anhydride catalyst can be either a long-chain aliphatic anhydride, e.g. dodecenyl succinic anhydride (DDSA), or an aromatic fused ring anhydride, e.g. methyl nadic anhydride (MNA). The long-chain anhydrides act as internal plasticizers which make blocks more flexible and generally tough, whereas MNA is a rigid molecule that results in stiffening and hardening of cured blocks. Both catalysts increase the hydrophobicity of the plastic, but this property can be reduced by oxidizing the alkyl chains and aromatic rings with peroxides.

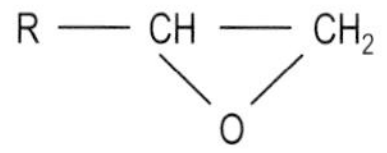

Fig. 29.1   The active epoxide group in all epoxy plastics.

The amines used as accelerators are either mono- or poly-functional. Because amines form adducts with epoxide groups, the use of poly-functional amines, e.g. dimethylamino methyl phenol (DMP 30), can result in the formation of three-dimensional structures, which are slow to diffuse and hence slow to infiltrate tissue. Thus the mono-functional amines, ethanolamine and benzyl dimethyl amine (BDMA), are more conducive to faster infiltration times. The only other common additive in epoxy plastic mixtures is dibutyl phthalate (DBP), which is present as an external plasticizer to soften the blocks, especially in 'Araldite' formulations.

The rate at which each epoxy plastic infiltrates the tissue depends on the density of the tissue and the size of the diffusing molecules. Infiltration by Araldite is slow, partly because of the formation of amine adducts, but also because the epoxy plastic itself is a large molecule. The glycerol-based epoxy plastics (Epon) have a lower viscosity but are often sold as mixtures of isomers, and care should be exercised in choosing the most suitable fraction of isomers. Cyclohexene dioxide-based plastics (Spurr) can be obtained pure and infiltrate fastest, having a low viscosity (7 centipoise at 25°C). Infiltration at higher temperatures is faster, although agglomerates can form and negate any increase in the diffusion coefficient.

The physical properties of epoxy plastics are affected considerably by their rate of polymerization. In industry, the same formulations as used in microscopy are cured at temperatures in excess of 150°C for up to several days, whereas tissue blocks at 60°C are considerably under-cured. Rapid curing for 1 hour at 120°C produces large numbers of cross-links, but hard brittle blocks; 18 hours at 60°C results in tougher blocks that are more suitable for sectioning and subsequent microscopy. Care is needed to provide a section with the right level of cross-linking to allow staining later. Sodium methoxide can be used to reduce the cross-link density of the cured plastic by trans-esterifying the ester cross-links. This allows the plastic to expand more in solvents and improves access to the tissue for stains and antibodies.

Stability in an electron beam arises from two main factors. Both aromatic and unsaturated groups can stabilize the radicals formed by electron impact, either within the aromatic ring or along an unsaturated aliphatic chain, thus preventing chain fission and depolymerization. Further stability is induced by cross-links that minimize the effects of any depolymerization that occurs by preventing creep.

Epoxy plastics have some disadvantages: they are hydrophobic and subsequent oxidation by peroxide to correct this may produce tissue damage. Both epoxide groups and anhydrides can react under mild conditions with proteins, which may reduce the antigenicity of embedded tissue. More importantly this may cause sensitization of workers who absorb them by skin contact or inhalation. The components of many epoxy plastics are toxic, and one, vinylcyclohexane dioxide (VCD), is known to be carcinogenic. Hence gloves should always be worn when handling these plastics, and adequate facilities must be provided for the removal of toxic vapors and the disposal of toxic waste (Causton 1981).

Cutting and staining epoxy sections for light microscopy

Ultra-thin section cutting and staining for electron microscopy are discussed in detail in Chapter 30. It is not possible to obtain satisfactory sections of thickness 0.5–1 μm on a standard microtome using a steel knife, so semi-thin sections are produced using a glass or diamond knife, and cut on a motorized microtome. Using specialized strips of glass and equipment, two types of glass knives can be prepared; either the more common triangular shape Latta–Hartmann knife or the Ralph knife, which has a longer cutting edge.

To an observer experienced in its interpretation, there is little doubt that for high-resolution light microscopy, toluidine blue is the most useful and informative stain applied to tissue sections embedded in an epoxy plastic. If the stain is heated and used at high alkaline pH (Chapter 30), it easily penetrates the plastic and stains various tissue components a blue color of differing shades and intensities, with no appreciable staining of the embedding medium. The staining intensity of tissue components by toluidine blue largely reflects its electron density, and the ultrastructural appearances on subsequent electron microscopy can be partly predicted by the appearances at light microscopy level. For those who prefer polychromatic stains, various formulations, e.g. Paragon, can be used which resemble H&E staining. Many staining techniques can be applied after the surface resin has been 'etched' using alcoholic sodium hydroxide (Janes 1979), but the results are not always reliable. Another type of pre-treatment consists of oxidizing osmium-fixed tissue without etching (Bourne & St John 1978) so that aqueous solutions can be stained more consistently.

A few reports have described the application of immunohistochemistry to epoxy sections for light microscopy studies following treatment with sodium ethoxide/methoxide (Giddings et al 1982; McCluggage et al 1995; Krenacs et al 2005), but this practice is seldom used routinely. In general, for the majority of occasions when high-resolution light microscopy is required, it is preferable to use acrylic plastic sections because of their easier handling and quality of staining achieved.

Polyester plastics

These plastics were originally introduced for electron microscopy in the mid-1950s, but were soon superseded by the superior epoxides for ultrastructural purposes. Nowadays they are seldom used for microscopy, although a few studies have reported embedding undecalcified bone for light microscopy studies (Mawhinney & Ellis 1983).

Acrylic plastics

The acrylic plastics used for microscopy are esters of acrylic acid (CH_2=$CH \cdot COOH$) or more commonly methacrylic acid (CH=$C(CH_3) \cdot COOH$), and are often referred to as acrylates and methacrylates respectively. They are used extensively for LM, but some have been formulated so that EM can be performed, either in addition or exclusively. Numerous mixes can be devised to produce plastics that provide a wide range of properties, with a consequence that there is a diverse range of potential uses. Butyl, methyl, and glycol methacrylate (the latter is chemically the monomer 2-hydroxy ethyl methacrylate or HEMA) were all introduced for electron microscopy, but are now rarely used (unless as a component of a mix) because the plastic disrupts in the electron beam. However, greater success has been achieved in the production and staining of semi-thin sections for high-resolution light microscopy.

Conventional acrylics are cured by complex free-radical chain reactions; that is, the intermediate chemicals formed have an incomplete number of electrons. The monomer is exposed to a source of radicals, usually produced from the breakdown of a catalyst such as benzoyl peroxide. This decomposes to produce phenyl (benzoyl-peroxy) radicals that transfer to the double bond of the acrylic monomer, and which then itself breaks to become a radical in turn. This now acts as an active site, attracting and joining another monomer by repeating the process of opening the carbon–carbon double bond and forming a covalent link. In this way a polymer is formed by joining monomeric units together to produce a long aliphatic chain. Finally, to complete the polymer, a phenyl radical instead of another monomer molecule attaches to the active site to block and terminate further reactions. Both oxygen and acetone prevent attachment of radicals and therefore should be avoided during the curing process.

Radicals can be produced spontaneously by light or heat, and consequently acrylic plastics and their monomers should be stored in dark bottles in a cool place. Acrylics contain a few parts per million of hydroquinone to prevent premature polymerization, and for most applications this can remain when preparing the embedding mixes. Benzoyl peroxide is the most common source of radicals since it breaks down at 50–60°C, but the addition of a tertiary aromatic amine, e.g. N-N, dimethyl-aniline or dimethyl p-toluidine, can cause the peroxide to break down into radicals at 0°C, so that the plastic can be cured at low or room temperature. Dry benzoyl peroxide is explosive and is supplied damped with water, or as a paste mixed with dibutyl phthalate, or as plasticized particles. In some mixes, the water is required to be removed and care must be taken to dry aliquots away from direct sunlight or heat. Azobisisobutyronitrile is another catalyst that has been used, but by far the most popular is benzoyl peroxide. Light-sensitive photocatalysts such as benzil and benzoin (various types) are used for polymerization of acrylics at sub-zero temperature using short wavelength light.

In addition to the monomer and catalyst, several other ingredients are often necessary in acrylic plastics. An amine will stimulate polymerization to proceed at a faster rate, and consequently these chemicals are termed either activators or more commonly accelerators. Other activators include sulfinic acid and some barbiturates. To improve sectioning qualities of acrylic blocks, softeners or plasticizers are often added to the mix. Examples are 2-butoxyethanol, 2-isopropoxyethanol, polyethylene glycol 200/400 and dibutyl phthalate. Some acrylic mixes require a small amount of a cross-linker to stabilize the matrix of the plastic against physical damage caused by either the electron beam (Lowicryl plastics) or staining solutions (Technovit 8100). An example of a cross-linking agent is the difunctional ethylene glycol dimethacrylate, which provides flexible hydrophilic cross-links.

Poly (2-hydroxy ethyl methacrylate) 'glycol methacrylate' (GMA) has proved to be a popular embedding medium for light microscopy since it is extremely hydrophilic, allowing many tinctorial staining methods to be applied, yet tough enough when dehydrated to section well on most microtomes. Various mixes have been reported, with a result that some may be either prepared from the ingredients or purchased as a commercial kit, but many are based on the recipe published by Ruddell (1967). Although the mixes all contain the monomer HEMA, the proportion and variety of this and other ingredients may be different, leading to dissimilar characteristics between various kits. The monomer can be contaminated with methacrylic acid, which may result in some background staining, but this can be reduced by purchasing low-acid HEMA or a high-quality proprietary kit such as JB4 (Polysciences, USA), Technovit 7100, or Technovit 8100 (Kulzer, Germany). Currently these are all available from TABB, UK. Various plastic embedding kits have been marketed under different names (especially the Technovit range), which has caused confusion (Hand 1995a), but recently there appear to be attempts to standardize their description. Butyl methacrylate is now rarely used for any histological purpose unless as an ingredient in an acrylic mix, e.g. Unicryl, (British BioCell International, UK) since it has proved unreliable and produces considerable tissue artifact during polymerization.

There are also available aromatic polyhydroxy dimethacrylate resins (LR White & LR Gold from London Resin, UK), which can be used both for light and electron microscopy since they combine hydrophilicity with electron beam stability. LR White may be polymerized by the addition of dimethyl *p*-toluidine, whereas LR Gold is cured by the addition of benzil and exposure to a quartz halogen lamp specifically for sub-zero temperature embedding. Other acrylic plastics cured at low temperature include Lowicryl HM20, HM23 (hydrophobic) and K4M, K11M (hydrophilic), and Unicryl (formerly called Bioacryl). The Lowicryls, developed in Germany (available from Polysciences, USA; TABB, UK), may be cured by the addition of a benzoin photocatalyst exposed to ultraviolet light. Though in some cases these plastics can be employed for light microscopy studies, they are really intended and are more suitable for electron microscopy.

In recent years there has been increasing interest in the renewed use of mixes based on methyl methacrylate (MMA). Although MMA continues to be widely used because of its hardness as the ideal embedding medium for undecalcified bone, other hard tissues, and tissues with stent implants (see Chapter 18), its use as the monomer in mixes specifically devised for tinctorial and immunohistochemical staining on semi-thin sections for high-resolution light microscopy has stimulated considerable attention. The author has developed various mixes and procedures suitable for these purposes that are described later in this chapter, although the proprietary Technovit 9100 is also based on MMA. Unlike epoxides, the viscosity of acrylics is low and hence short infiltration times are possible, although the size and nature of tissue, together with the processing and embedding temperature, will affect the times required.

APPLICATIONS OF ACRYLIC SECTIONS

The development of acrylic plastic embedding media has usually been stimulated by a requirement for a specific application. Most applications are for light microscopy, but as understanding of the formulation of acrylics has increased, so too have various plastics been introduced which may also be useful for some electron microscopy studies. Some of these plastics, such as the Lowicryls, have been developed mainly for electron microscopy alone (Carlemalm et al 1982; Acetarin et al 1986), whereas LR White and Unicryl (Scala et al 1992) can be used for either purpose. However, for various technical reasons, not all dual-purpose plastics are practical for routine high-resolution light microscopy studies.

Hydrophilic plastics such as GMA and LR White allow tissue to be stained without removal of the embedding medium, and have therefore become popular for routine use. Many 'simple' staining techniques may be applied, but some may require modification or present special difficulties to those used on paraffin sections. All acrylic hydrophilic media are insoluble, and consequently all staining occurs with the plastic in situ. This can cause problems in two ways, either because the medium itself becomes stained, which may affect the final appearance, or because the matrix acts as a physical barrier to particular molecules. The most obvious example where the latter occurs is the difficulty that large molecules have in penetrating the plastic matrix during immunohistochemical staining. The alternative use of hydrophobic MMA without the addition of cross-linking agents as an embedding medium permits the plastic to be dissolved, and for certain techniques this is an extremely useful property. However, hydrophobic plastics such as Lowicryl HM20 and HM23 that contain cross-linking agents are insoluble.

Acrylic plastics may be polymerized in different ways by using a chemical accelerator, heat, or light. The optimum method depends on several factors including the study required and the practicality of the method chosen. Polymerization can also be induced at low temperature, and with some Lowicryl plastics, processing and embedding can be accomplished at temperatures down to −70°C. K4M is the most popular, and is said at −35°C to enhance ultrastructural preservation and immunohistochemical staining.

Tinctorial staining

Acrylics have become popular for high-resolution light microscopy mainly because of the ease with which sections can be stained. Excellent staining may be achieved on tissue embedded in any of the various GMA mixes/kits and other acrylics such as LR White, even though the plastic cannot be removed. Numerous (but not all) routine histological staining methods may be applied, including H&E, PAS, van Gieson, alcian blue, Perls', elastic methods, Giemsa, and silver techniques for reticulin. Modifications from the standard methods for paraffin sections may be necessary and, because London Resins (Histocryl, LR White, and LR Gold) are all softened by alcohol with the possibility of section loss from the slide, alcoholic staining solutions such as those used in elastic methods should be avoided. Consequently, even hematoxylin staining on London Resins should be progressive to avoid differentiation with acid alcohol, whereas regressive staining on GMA is (with care) possible. The plastic embedding medium (especially GMA) may also become stained, but in some techniques this can be reduced by various washing procedures.

An alternative approach is to use MMA where the plastic can easily be removed prior to staining, using similar procedures and solutions but with slightly extended times to those used routinely for dewaxing paraffin sections. It is beyond the scope of this chapter to describe in detail numerous staining methods on different acrylics, but best results are achieved using either a method previously published or one that is recommended by other histologists. It should be noted that tinctorial staining of tissue embedded in MMA is possible (where no cross-linker has been added) without removing the plastic, and this is often useful for sections of undecalci-

fied bone MMA prepared as described in Chapter 18. However, this type of procedure is unsuitable for semi-thin sections described in this chapter for high-resolution LM.

Enzyme histochemistry

The ability to process, embed, and polymerize some acrylic plastics at low temperature enables several enzymes to be preserved and demonstrated in tissue sections. Many enzymes are destroyed by routine fixation and processing, but under controlled conditions several (mainly hydrolytic) enzymes may be localized, including those illustrated in Figures 29.2 and 29.3. Fixation, processing, and polymerization are all usually carried out at 4°C, and sections are dried on to a coverglass or slide at room temperature overnight (rather than at 60°C) prior to performing enzyme histochemical staining.

A variety of aldehyde fixatives have been advocated, but in the author's experience 10% formal calcium as recommended by Dawson (1972) has proved successful. Enhanced staining can be further achieved if the tissue is subsequently washed at 4°C in 3% buffered sucrose solution. Hand (1988) has also shown that enzyme

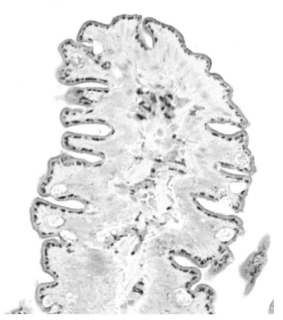

Fig. 29.2 Section of jejunum fixed in formal calcium and embedded in glycol methacrylate (JB4) showing hydrolytic acid phosphatase activity in the macrophages (lamina propria) and lysozymes in the villi using hexazonium pararosanilin. Original magnification ×325.

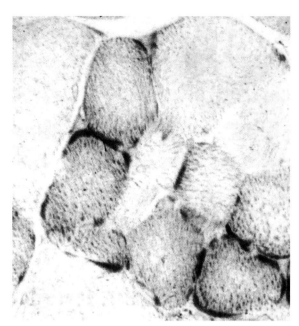

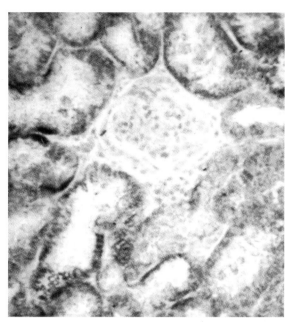

Fig. 29.3 Section of transversely cut muscle fixed in formal calcium and embedded in glycol methacrylate (JB4) showing oxidative NADH diaphorase staining in mitochondria using methyl-thiazolyldiphenyl tetrazolium (MTT). Original magnification ×325.

Fig. 29.4 Section of unfixed kidney embedded in LR Gold which has been photo-polymerized showing succinate dehydrogenase activity in mitochondria using tetra-nitro blue tetrazolium (TNBT). Original magnification ×200.

activity may also be affected during processing, infiltration, embedding, and polymerization, and therefore to achieve best results the effects of these stages on a particular enzyme should first be ascertained. Polymerization is normally carried out at 4°C using a chemical accelerator, but for methods utilizing sub-zero temperatures either an excess of catalyst or a photocatalyst has been employed.

The use of GMA for enzyme histochemical studies is preferred, as this acrylic is probably the easiest to handle and produces the best results. Various enzyme histochemical investigations have been described using several different techniques on plastic-embedded tissue including the identification of cell types (Beckstead 1983), cephaloridine nephrotoxicity in rats (Bennett 1982), and assessment of malabsorption on jejunum (Hand 1987).

A further development described by Thompson and Germain (1983) employed processing fresh (unfixed) tissue stabilized with polyvinyl pyrollidine (MW 44,000) at −25°C and embedding in LR Gold. Polymerization was induced by irradiating the plastic containing the photo-catalyst benzil with blue light from a quartz halogen lamp. This specialized procedure offers the potential to

demonstrate enzymes, including those that are sensitive to fixation, but in reality the only additional enzyme demonstrated to those that survive mild fixation has been the oxidative enzyme succinate dehydrogenase (Fig. 29.4). Other enzymes that have been demonstrated in fixed tissue include acid phosphatase, adenosine triphosphatase (membrane), alkaline phosphatase, chloroacetate esterase, dipeptidyl (amino) peptidase IV, lactase, lactate dehydrogenase, leucine aminopeptidase, β-galactosidase, glucose-6-phosphate, phosphate dehydrogenase, β-glucuronidase, γ-glutamyl transpeptidase, NADH, α-naphthyl acetate, non-specific esterase, 5'-nucleotidase, peroxidase, and sucrase.

Following successful staining, care must be taken to ensure that enzyme diffusion and loss do not occur during the washing and mounting procedures.

Immunohistochemistry

During the past 30 years, numerous reports have been published describing the application of immunohistochemistry to acrylic-embedded tissue sections, with even a GMA kit developed specifically for this use (ImmunoBed from Polysciences Inc., USA). However,

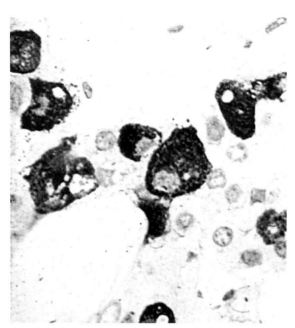

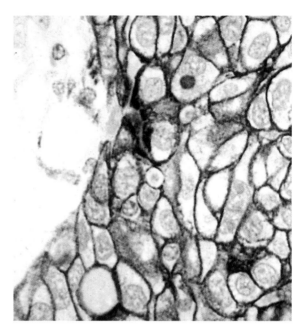

Fig. 29.5 Section of formalin-fixed pituitary embedded in methyl methacrylate showing localization of adreno-corticotrophin hormone (ACTH) with immunoperoxidase staining. Chromogen 3,3′-diaminobenzidine tetrahydrochloride (DAB). Original magnification ×500.

Fig. 29.6 Section of formalin-fixed ovarian tumor embedded in methyl methacrylate showing immunoperoxidase staining of cytokeratin 7 following pretreatment using microwave antigen retrieval. Chromogen DAB. Original magnification ×500. (Reproduced, with permission, from Hand N.M., Blythe D., Jackson P. (1996) Antigen unmasking using microwave heating on formalin fixed tissue embedded in methyl methacrylate. Journal of Cellular Pathology 1:31–37. © Greenwich Medical Media Ltd, London).

immunohistochemical staining still remains a controversial topic because the results have been mainly idiosyncratic and disappointing, leading many laboratories to abandon this type of investigation for diagnostic purposes. Further confusion has been compounded by the wide variety of plastics and techniques advocated, but a major cause of unreliable immunostaining is that many of the acrylics are insoluble in their polymerized form. Although it would be too simplistic an explanation to imply that all the problems are due to the insolubility of the polymer involved, there is no doubt that the presence of the embedding medium can present formidable difficulties (Gerrits 1988).

Many papers based on the classic publications of Beckstead (1985) and Casey et al (1988) have tried to create mild conditions by fixing, processing, and then polymerizing the plastic at low temperature in an attempt to protect sensitive antigens, and produce a 'looser' matrix that would be more conducive to allowing large immunological reagents to penetrate through to antigen sites. Unfortunately, this is not always easy to control, and further cross-linking can continue after 'polymerization' to produce super-polymerization that will inhibit access of reagents to the antigens. In addition, it has long been recognized that tissue antigens may be chemically altered by the reagents in the plastic embedding medium (Takamiya et al 1980).

A variety of complex and sophisticated staining protocols using 3,3′-diaminobenzidine tetrahydrochloride (DAB) as the chromogen have also been suggested. One particular procedure recommended by Newman et al (1983) for LR White used an enhancement technique, where DAB was intensified using a gold–sulfide–silver method to detect immunohistochemical reactivity.

Though immunohistochemistry is possible on all acrylic plastics, the non-routine procedures required, coupled with frequently poor results, do not encourage this type of histological examination for light microscopy. Against this background, an alternative concept employing a plastic based on MMA was developed (Hand et al 1989; Hand & Morrell 1990). Tissue can be fixed in formalin under routine conditions and then processed and embedded at room temperature. The plastic is polymerized using a chemical accelerator, e.g. *N,N*-dimethylaniline, although other amines have been suc-

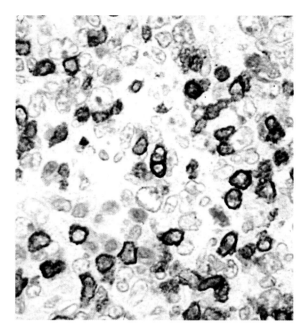

Fig. 29.7 Section of formalin-fixed lymph node embedded in methyl methacrylate showing immunoperoxidase staining of T lymphocytes with anti-CD3 following pretreatment with trypsin digestion and subsequent heat-induced antigen retrieval using a pressure cooker. Chromogen DAB. Original magnification × 500. (Reproduced, with permission, from Hand N.M. (1999) Plastic embedding for light microscopy. A guide for the histotechnologist. *Tech Sample*. Histotechnology No. HT-6. 29-35. © American Society of Clinical Pathologists.)

cessfully used. The embedding procedure is similar to that used for GMA blocks using an open molding tray system inside a glass dessicator. The main difference from other acrylics is that the polymerized plastic is soluble, and therefore can be removed prior to staining, which is particularly advantageous for immunohistochemical staining. Routine tinctorial staining is obviously possible, although the procedure is probably not suitable for the localization of many enzymes. To date, over 100 antibodies have been successfully demonstrated with excellent results including those illustrated in Figs 29.5–29.7. Further details are discussed later in this chapter relating to immunohistochemical staining on MMA sections.

IN SITU HYBRIDIZATION

Only a few methods have been described for in situ hybridization on various plastic sections using either iso-topic or non-isotopic techniques. Studies by Church et al (1997, 1998) and Doverty (2005, 2007), both using non-isotopic methods on MMA sections, have demonstrated *Sox* gene mRNA in chick tissue, and kappa and lambda mRNA in bone marrow trephines respectively.

ACRYLIC PLASTIC PROCESSING SCHEDULES

Processing and embedding schedule for glycol methacrylate using ingredients (Ruddell 1967)

Solution a

2-hydroxyethyl (glycol) methacrylate	80 ml
2-butoxyethanol	16 ml
Dried benzoyl peroxide	0.27 g

Solution b

Polyethylene glycol 400	15 parts
N,N-dimethylaniline	1 part

Fixation

Fix tissues in formalin, e.g. formal saline, neutral buffered formalin, or buffered paraformaldehyde.

Processing and embedding

1. If necessary, rinse tissue in an appropriate buffer for 15 minutes.
2. Dehydrate through 70%, 90%, and 100% ethanol. For an average block of 10 × 5 × 2 mm, use two 15-minutes changes in each solution.
3. Infiltrate in two changes of solution a, each for 1 hour.
4. Embed in the following mixture:

Solution a	42 parts
Solution b	1 part

5. Polymerize at room temperature, standing the mold in cold water to dissipate heat generated by the exothermic reaction. Polymerization should be complete in 2–4 hours.

Notes

a. Specimens should only be processed under a fume hood with extraction.
b. Processing is best achieved if the specimens are agitated continuously on a roller mixer.
c. Small aliquots of benzoyl peroxide should be dried carefully away from direct heat and sunlight as it is potentially explosive. It must be completely dis-

solved in the infiltrating solution and this may take up to 30 minutes.

d. Several block molding systems are commercially available, but the open polypropylene molding tray system enables the tissue to be attached directly onto a block stub (Polysciences Inc., USA). To achieve good polymerization, the mold should be placed inside a glass dessicator and oxygen excluded by filling the chamber with oxygen-free nitrogen. The chamber is then sealed.

e. The acrylic plastic mixes are best prepared in the quantity required, preferably using a large capped glass vial. It is advisable to measure the quantities by volume.

f. Any waste solutions containing plastic components must be handled and discarded in accordance with local and legal requirements.

Standard processing and embedding schedule for JB4 embedding medium

JB4 embedding medium is supplied as a kit, comprising two stock solutions (A and B) and separate plasticized benzoyl peroxide (C). Solution A is the infiltrating/embedding medium and solution B is the accelerator.

Fixation
Any, preferably formalin or paraformaldehyde.

Processing and embedding
1. If necessary, rinse tissue in an appropriate buffer for 15 minutes.
2. Dehydrate through 70%, 90%, and 100% ethanol as described for the previous GMA schedule.
3. Infiltrate tissue in two changes of freshly prepared catalyzed solution A (prepared by mixing 1.25 g of benzoyl peroxide plasticized (C) in 100 ml of solution A or the equivalent, until the solid is completely dissolved). Most tissues require at least 3 hours' infiltration depending on the nature and size of the tissue. Hard dense tissues such as bone are best infiltrated overnight at 4°C.
4. Embed in fresh embedding medium (add 1 ml of solution B to 25 ml of freshly catalyzed solution A or the equivalent) at room temperature in a mold. The time needed for full polymerization varies with the temperature, atmospheric oxygen, etc., but at

room temperature (22°C) it may take 1–2 hours. For enzyme histochemical investigations, better results will be obtained using pre-chilled solutions throughout, with processing and embedding at 4°C. In these circumstances, polymerization may take 6–12 hours.

Notes
See Notes a, b, c, d, e, and f from previous GMA schedule. Tissues may be taken directly into several changes of freshly catalyzed solution A from buffer, omitting the alcohols, but it may be necessary to extend the time of this partial dehydration with at least three changes. This procedure may produce better results with some enzyme methods, and lipids are also better retained.

Modified processing and embedding schedule for JB4 embedding medium

This particular schedule is especially useful for hematological bone marrow trephines to provide a firmer support medium.

Fixation
Fix tissues in formalin, e.g. formal saline, neutral buffered formalin, or buffered paraformaldehyde.

Processing and embedding
1. If necessary, rinse tissue in an appropriate buffer for 15 minutes.
2. Dehydrate through 70%, 90%, and 100% ethanol using two changes in each solution of 30 minutes.
3. Infiltrate tissue in two changes of freshly prepared catalyzed solution A (prepared by mixing 120 mg of benzoyl peroxide plasticized in 9 ml of solution A and 1 ml of methyl methacrylate monomer until the solid is completely dissolved) for 1 hour, followed by infiltration overnight at room temperature.
4. Embed in pre-chilled embedding medium (10 ml of catalyzed solution A and 450 µl of JB4 solution B) at room temperature in a mold. The time needed for full polymerization varies with the temperature, atmospheric oxygen, etc., but at room temperature (22°C) may be 1–2 hours.

Notes
See Notes a, b, c, d, e, and f from previous GMA schedule.

Processing and embedding schedule for methyl methacrylate

This schedule can be used for routine tinctorial and immunohistochemical staining, although other schedules and mixtures have been published. Care should be taken when handling MMA as it has a pungent odor and is flammable.

Infiltration solution

Methyl methacrylate monomer (unwashed)   15 ml
Dibutyl phthalate   5 ml
Dried benzoyl peroxide   1 g

Fixation

Fix tissues in formalin, e.g. 10% formalin, 10% formal saline, or 10% formal calcium, 24–48 hours.

Processing and embedding

1. Dehydrate through 50%, 70%, and 90% ethanol. For an average block of 10 × 5 × 2 mm, use 1-hour changes in each solution.
2. Complete dehydration through two changes of 100% ethanol, each for 1 hour.
3. Infiltrate in two changes of infiltration solution, each for 1 hour.
4. Infiltrate in a further change of infiltration solution overnight.
5. Embed in 10-ml aliquots of infiltration solution to which 125 µl of N,N-dimethylaniline is added. Polymerization will occur in 3–4 hours. Blythe (personal communication, 2006) recommends 250 µl of N,N-dimethylaniline for bone marrow trephines, where polymerization is achieved in 1.5–2 hours.

Notes

a. Aliquots of benzoyl peroxide should be dried carefully away from direct heat and sunlight as it is potentially explosive. It is important that no water is present before dissolving the catalyst (2 minutes) in the infiltrating solution.
b. Also see Notes a, b, d, e, and f from previous GMA schedule.

Standard processing and embedding schedule for LR White

LR White is usually supplied as a pre-mixed solution that includes catalyst in three grades (hard, medium, and soft) to match as closely as possible the hardness of the tissue being processed. (To avoid spontaneous polymerization in hot climates, it is possible to purchase the monomer and catalyst separately.) A dropper bottle containing accelerator is also supplied.

Fixation

Fix tissues in formalin or paraformaldehyde.

Processing and embedding

1. If necessary, rinse tissue in an appropriate buffer for 15 minutes.
2. Dehydrate through 70%, 90%, and 100% ethanol, using two changes of each solution for 15 minutes for a block of 12 × 10 × 3 mm.
3. Infiltrate with LR White, three changes of 60 minutes each or leave overnight, depending on nature and size of tissue block. Hard tissues such as bone and teeth benefit from vacuum infiltration during the last change of resin.
4. Polymerize using 'heat' or 'cold' (accelerator) curing. To 'heat' cure, place the molds in an incubator between 55°C and 60°C for 20–24 hours. For 'cold' curing add 1 drop of accelerator per 10 ml of resin; polymerization should occur in 15–20 minutes.

Notes

a. When 'heat' curing it is important to limit the contact of oxygen with the resin while polymerization occurs. The most convenient way of achieving this is to use gelatin capsules for small pieces of tissue, or the commercial block stub and molding tray systems for larger pieces. Alternatively a nitrogenous environment can be utilized.
b. Processing is best achieved if the specimens are agitated continuously on a roller mixer.
c. Small aliquots of benzoyl peroxide should be dried carefully, away from direct heat and sunlight as it is potentially explosive. It must be completely dissolved in the infiltrating solution and this may take up to 30 minutes.
d. Polymerization time and temperature are fundamental to the physical character of the final block. Increased temperature or time will produce highly cross-linked blocks that are brittle and may be difficult to stain.

Cutting acrylic plastic sections

Semi-thin sections of GMA, MMA, and LR White of thickness 2–3 μm may be cut with a steel knife on a standard microtome, but better quality semi-thin sections will be obtained using a glass knife on a motorized microtome. Either the triangular Latta–Hartmann or longer-edged Ralph knife is suitable, but the choice depends mainly on the mold/block size. For most routine purposes, 2–3-μm sections are satisfactory and these can be picked up using a fine pair of forceps. GMA sections will flatten immediately on contact with water at room temperature, and if a water bath is used the sections may be picked up on slides similar to paraffin sections. Using the MMA mix described, the water bath will require to be heated at 65–70°C for these sections to flatten. LR White sections are floated out on 70% alcohol or 30–40% acetone on a hot-plate at 60°C. It is advisable that all acrylic sections are picked up on grease-free slides that have been coated with an adhesive such as (2%) APES, and allowed to drain before drying on a hot-plate at 60°C for at least 30 minutes. Many histotechnologists have commented that MMA sections, especially when used for undecalcified bone marrow trephines, become detached from the slide. Whilst this is true with many MMA formulations, if the recipe described in the series of articles by Hand and in the processing schedule on page 5 is used, then this is less likely. The use of Superfrost Plus slides (without adhesive) for bone samples has proved satisfactory (D. Blythe, personal communication 2006).

Staining acrylic plastic sections

As previously described, GMA and LR White sections are stained with the plastic matrix present. LR White is softened by alcohol, so after completion of staining it is recommended that sections are blotted and dried on a hot-plate at 60°C for a few minutes before being dipped in xylene and mounted. MMA sections require the plastic embedding medium to be removed prior to staining, and this may be easily achieved by immersing the slides in xylene for 10–20 minutes at 37°C. Numerous H&E protocols can be used, but the following has proved satisfactory for GMA and LR White. For MMA sections, 30 minutes in hematoxylin and 5 minutes in 1% buffered eosin staining is preferred, but sections should be washed rapidly in water and ethanol as eosin is quickly removed.

Hematoxylin and eosin method

1. Harris's or Gill's alum hematoxylin for 10–20 minutes.
2. Wash in tap water.
3. If necessary differentiate in 1% acid alcohol for 2–3 seconds.
4. Blue in tap water.
5. Wash in water for 15 minutes.
6. Stain in filtered 1% aqueous eosin in 1% calcium chloride for 3 minutes.
7. Wash in tap water for 30 seconds.
8. Blot dry.
9. Rinse in ethanol for 20 seconds.
10. Rinse in xylene.
11. Mount in DPX.

Note
Omit steps 3 and 9 for LR White.

Immunohistochemical staining on MMA sections

Sections can be stained with a protocol and procedure that follows closely that which is used for paraffin sections, using a routine immunoperoxidase technique such as the sensitive avidin–biotin type technique that is commonly employed in many laboratories. Polymer-based immunohistochemical procedures have also been successfully employed. DAB can be used as the chromogen and intensification is not required for visualization. Incubations are carried out at room temperature and essentially the reagents and times of the various stages are as usual, although optimal staining of some antigens may require changes in pre-treatment and/or dilution of the antibody. In addition to the application of a wide range of polyclonal and monoclonal antibodies, rabbit monoclonal antibodies have also recently been successful (Doverty 2005, personal communication). To avoid poor or erroneous results, it is important during staining that sections are not allowed to dry out, which occurs faster than for paraffin sections.

As with paraffin sections, one of the most problematic aspects of immunostaining is the use of pre-treatment. Enzyme digestion with trypsin has been used for some antigens, but the introduction of heat-mediated procedures, using either a microwave oven (Hand et al 1996) or a pressure cooker (Hand & Church 1998) with sodium citrate solution has helped significantly to improve and standardize staining. However, some details of the precise procedure may differ from those for paraffin sections, and for some antigens a combination of pre-treatments may be required to achieve best results. Heat-mediated pre-treatment also retrieves antigenicity better in archival material (Hand et al 1996). For greater detail, the reader is advised to refer to a number of articles (Hand 1995b; Blythe et al 1997; Hand & Church 1997).

In recent years an amplification procedure based on tyramide has been introduced to immunohistochemistry, resulting in a highly sensitive intensification technique. Although the procedure was originally intended for paraffin sections and is useful when certain antibodies produce only a weak signal using a conventional technique, it has also been successfully applied to MMA-embedded tissue (Jackson et al 1996).

The protocols and techniques previously outlined can produce excellent immunohistochemical staining and have been used routinely, especially on undecalcified hematological bone marrow trephines (Blythe et al 1997).

Processing and embedding schedule for Lowicryl K4M (Al-Nawab & Davies 1989)

The following schedule has been used on a renal needle biopsy where 2-μm and 90-nm sections were then cut for LM and EM studies respectively.

Fixation
4% paraformaldehyde for 2 hours at room temperature.

Dehydration
1. 50% methanol at −20°C for 30 minutes.
2. 80% methanol at −20°C for 60 minutes.
3. 90% methanol at −20°C for 60 minutes.

Infiltration
4. 1 part methanol and 1 part Lowicryl K4M at −20°C for 30 minutes.
5. 1 part methanol and 2 parts Lowicryl K4M at −20°C for 60 minutes.
6. 100% Lowicryl K4M at −20°C for 60 minutes.
7. 100% Lowicryl K4M at −20°C overnight.

Polymerization
Embed the tissue in fresh Lowicryl K4M in gelatin capsules and photo-polymerize at 35°C overnight using indirect (diffuse) ultraviolet irradiation from a Philips TLAD 15 W/05 fluorescent lamp (wavelength peak at 360 nm). The capsules are suspended in ethanol baths with their lower poles immersed in alcohol to dissipate any heat build-up during the polymerization process, and then removed and irradiated at room temperature for a further 1–2 days to improve sectioning properties.

FUTURE OF ACRYLIC PLASTIC EMBEDDING

As histological diagnosis becomes ever more demanding with increasing use of sophisticated techniques, so too has the technology of plastic embedding procedures been advanced. New embedding media are being developed, and recently there has been a realization that the flexibility of acrylics can often provide the most suitable embedding medium for a range of investigations. Many applications are for high-resolution LM, but some may be used for EM. Studies such as those reported by Bowdler et al (1989) and Al-Nawab and Davies (1989) have combined both LM and EM on the same biopsy using LR White and Lowicryl K4M respectively, hence demonstrating direct comparisons between immunohistochemical techniques at light microscopy with those at the electron microscopy level.

Special acrylic plastics have been formulated for low-temperature processing and embedding of tissue, especially for EM, as temperatures above 50°C are known to promote denaturation of proteins, causing loss of enzyme activity and reduction in antigenicity. Three low-temperature embedding procedures have been used with Lowicryl plastics: freeze substitution, freeze drying, and progressive lowering temperature (PLT). Processing machines are now available that can shorten as well as standardize processing times, and reduce occasions when tissue is required to be handled.

In recent years a wide range of procedures applied to plastic sections have been described for high-resolution light microscopy. This chapter has focused mainly on the applications for semi-thin acrylic sections, because this is where most developments have occurred. How future plastic embedding media and techniques impact on routine histological practice remains to be seen, although it is probable that specialized procedures will still be required.

Acknowledgments

Alan Stevens contributed the text for this chapter for the second edition of the text. He and Jocelyn Germain updated the text for editions three and four. Our acknowledgments are due to them for their contributions.

REFERENCES

Acetarin J-D., Carlemalm E., Villiger W. (1986) Developments of new Lowicryl resins for embedding biological specimens at even lower temperatures. Journal of Microscopy 143:81–88.

Al-Nawab M.D., Davies D.R. (1989) Light and electron microscopic demonstration of extracellular immunoglobulin deposition in renal tissue. Journal of Clinical Pathology 42:1104–1108.

Beckstead J.H. (1983) The evaluation of lymph nodes, using plastic sections and enzyme histochemistry. American Journal of Clinical Pathology 80:131–139.

Beckstead J.H. (1985) Optimal antigen localization in human tissues using aldehyde-fixed plastic-embedded sections. Journal of Histochemistry and Cytochemistry 33:954–958.

Bennett R. (1982) The use of histochemical techniques on 1 micron methacrylate sections of kidney in the study of cephaloridine nephrotoxicity. In: Bach P.H., Bonner F.W., Bridges J.W., Locks E.A., eds. Nephrotoxicity: assessment and pathogenesis. Chichester: John Wiley.

Blythe D., Hand N.M., Jackson P. et al. (1997) The use of methyl methacrylate resin for embedding bone marrow trephine biopsies. Journal of Clinical Pathology 50:45–49.

Bourne C.A.J., St John D.J.B. (1978) Application of histochemical and histological stains to epoxy sections: pretreatment with potassium permanganate and oxalic acid. Medical Laboratory Sciences 35:397–398.

Bowdler A.L., Griffiths D.F.R., Newman G.R. (1989) The morphological and immunocytochemical analysis of renal biopsies by light and electron microscopy using a single processing method. Histochemical Journal 21:393–402.

Carlemalm E., Garavito R.M., Villiger W. (1982) Resin development for electron microscopy and an analysis of embedding at low temperature. Journal of Microscopy 126:123–143.

Casey T.T., Cousar J.B., Collins R.D. (1988) A simplified plastic embedding and immunologic technique for immunophenotypic analysis of human haematopoietic and lymphoid tissues. American Journal of Pathology 131:183–189.

Causton B.E. (1981) Resins: toxicity, hazards and safe handling. Proceedings of the Royal Microscopical Society 16(4):265–271.

Church, R.J., Hand, N.M., Rex, M., Scotting, P.J. (1997) Non-isotopic in situ hybridization to detect chick *Sox* gene mRNA in plastic-embedded tissue. Histochemical Journal 29:625–629.

Church R.J., Hand N.M., Rex M., Scotting P.J. (1998) Double labelling using non-isotopic in situ hybridisation and immunohistochemistry on plastic embedded tissue. Journal of Cellular Pathology 3:11–16.

Dawson I.M.P. (1972) Fixation: What should the pathologist do? Histochemical Journal 4:381–385.

Doverty L. (2005) Cyclin D1 expression in multiple myeloma: positive or negative prognostic factor? Abstract no. 91 of papers presented to the Institute of Biomedical Science Congress 2005.

Doverty L. (2007) Immunohistochemistry and in-situ hybridisation on bone marrow trephine biopsy (electronic letter). Online. Available: http://jcp.bmj.com/cgi/eletters/59/9/903.

Gerrits P.O. (1988) Immunohistochemistry on glycol methacrylate tissue: possibilities and limitations. Journal of Histotechnology 11:243–246.

Giddings J., Griffin R.C., MacIver A.G. (1982) Demonstration of immunoproteins in araldite-embedded tissues. Journal of Clinical Pathology 35:111–114.

Glauert A.M. (1987) Fixation, dehydration and embedding of biological specimens. Amsterdam: Elsevier North-Holland.

Hand N.M. (1987) Enzyme histochemistry on jejunal tissue embedded in resin. Journal of Pathology 40:346–347.

Hand N.M. (1988) Enzyme histochemical demonstration of lactase and sucrase activity in resin sections: the influence of fixation and processing. Medical Laboratory Sciences 45:125–130.

Hand N.M. (1995a) The naming and types of acrylic resins. UK NEQAS Newsletter 6:15 (letter).

Hand N.M. (1995b) Diagnostic immunocytochemistry on resin-embedded tissue. UK NEQAS Newsletter 6:13–16.

Hand N.M., Blythe D., Jackson P. (1996) Antigen unmasking using microwave heating on formalin fixed tissue embedded in methylmethacrylate. Journal of Cellular Pathology 1:31–37.

Hand N.M., Church R.J. (1997) Immunocytochemical demonstration of hormones in pancreatic and pituitary tissue embedded in methyl methacrylate. Journal of Histotechnology 20:35–38.

Hand N.M., Church R.J. (1998) Superheating using pressure cooking: its use and application in unmasking antigens embedded in methyl methacrylate. Journal of Histotechnology 21:231–236.

Hand N.M., Morrell K.J. (1990) Immunocytochemistry on plastic sections for light microscopy. Proceedings of the Royal Microsopical Society 25(2):111.

Hand N.M., Morrell K.J., MacLennan K.A. (1989) Immunohistochemistry on resin embedded tissue for light microscopy: a novel post-embedding procedure. Proceedings of the Royal Microsopical Society 24(1):A54–A55.

Hand N.M., Blythe D., Jackson P. (1996) Antigen unmasking using microwave heating on formalin fixed tissue embedded in methyl methacrylate. Journal of Cellular Pathology 1:31–37.

Hand N.M. (1999) Plastic embedding for light microscopy. A guide for this histotechnologist. Tech Sample. Histotechnology No HT-6. 29–35. American Society of Clinical Pathologists.

Jackson P., Blythe D., Quirke P. (1996) Amplification of immunocytochemical reactions by the catalytic deposition of biotin on tissue sections. Journal of Pathology 179(Suppl):23A.

Janes R.B. (1979) A review of three resin processing techniques applicable to light microscopy. Medical Laboratory Sciences 36:249–267.

Krenacs T., Bagdi E., Stelkovics E. et al. (2005) How we process trephine biopsy specimens: epoxy resin embedded bone marrow biopsies. Journal of Clinical Pathology 58:897–903.

Mawhinney W.H.B., Ellis H.A. (1983) A technique for plastic embedding of mineralised bone. Journal of Clinical Pathology 36:1197–1199.

McCluggage W.G., Roddy S., Whiteside C. et al. (1995) Immunohistochemical staining of plastic embedded bone marrow trephine biopsy specimens after microwave heating. Journal of Clinical Pathology 48:840–844.

Newman G.R., Jasani B., Williams E.D. (1983) The visualisation of trace amounts of diaminobenzidine (DAB) polymer by a novel gold–sulphide–silver method. Journal of Microscopy 132(2):RP1–RP2.

Nunn R.E. (1970) Electron microscopy: preparation of biological specimens. London: Butterworths.

Ruddell C.L. (1967) Embedding media for 1–2 micron sectioning. 2-hydoxyethyl methacrylate combined with 2-butoxethanol. Stain Technology 42:253–255.

Scala C., Cenacchi G., Ferrari C. et al. (1992) A new acrylic resin formulation: a useful tool for histological, ultrastructural, and immunocytochemical investigations. Journal of Histochemistry and Cytochemistry 40:1799–1804.

Takamiya H., Batsford S., Vogt A. (1980) An approach to post-embedding staining of protein (immunoglobulin) antigen embedded in plastic. Journal of Histochemistry and Cytochemistry 28:1041–1049.

Thompson G., Germain J.P. (1983) Histochemistry and immunocytochemistry of fixation labile moieties in resin embedded tissue. Journal of Pathology 142:(2)A6.

30

Electron Microscopy

Anthony E. Woods and John W. Stirling

The fundamental advantage of transmission electron microscopy (TEM) over conventional light microscopy (LM) is the vast improvement in resolution it offers. With this greater resolving power, the transmission electron microscope is able to reveal the substructure or *ultrastructure* of individual cells. The physical basis for this benefit lies in the formula:

$$R = \frac{0.61\lambda}{NA}$$

Where: R, the resolution, represents the capacity of the optical system to produce separate images of objects close together; λ is the wavelength of the incident illumination, and NA is the numerical aperture of the lens.

Critically, for any given lens, resolution is directly related to the wavelength of the source radiation. For example, the limit of resolution of a conventional microscope using glass lenses and white light is around 200 nm whereas a fluorescence microscope operating with shorter wavelength ultraviolet light is capable of resolving objects around 100 nm apart.

By comparison, using electromagnetic lenses and a beam of electrons accelerated to a potential of 100 kV, an electron microscope is theoretically capable of resolving approximately 0.001 nm. Although flaws in lens design restrict this potential, contemporary transmission electron microscopes are capable of resolving structures of 0.2 nm or less.

TISSUE PREPARATION FOR TRANSMISSION ELECTRON MICROSCOPY

The basic preparation methods for routine TEM are given in this chapter. More detailed discussions of these, plus alternative and specialized procedures, can be found elsewhere (Glauert 1972; Robards & Wilson 1993; Allen & Lawrence 1994; Glauert & Lewis 1998; Hayat 2000). A flow chart summarizing the steps required for preparing the basic range of diagnostic TEM specimens is given in Figure 30.1.

The fundamental principle underlying TEM is that electrons pass through the section to give an image of the specimen. However, the electron beam is only capable of penetrating around 100 nm, so, to obtain a high-quality image and optimize the resolution of the instrument, it is necessary to section the tissue to a thickness of around 80 nm.

Sectioning at this level requires tissues to be embedded in extremely rigid material; clearly the wax embedding media used in light microscopy are not suitable. In routine TEM synthetic embedding resins are used that are capable of withstanding the vacuum in the electron microscope column and the heat generated as the electrons pass through the section. Although hydrophilic media are available, in most circumstances hydrophobic epoxy resins are preferred.

SPECIMEN HANDLING

In order to preserve the ultrastructure of the cell it is crucial that samples are fixed as soon as possible after biopsy. The most sensitive indicators of postmortem change are mitochondria and endoplasmic reticulum, both of which may show signs of swelling (a reflection of osmotic imbalance) only a few minutes after the cells are separated from a blood supply.

The standard approach is to immerse the specimen in fixative (pre-cooled to 4°C) immediately after collection. Once in fixative the specimen is cut into smaller samples

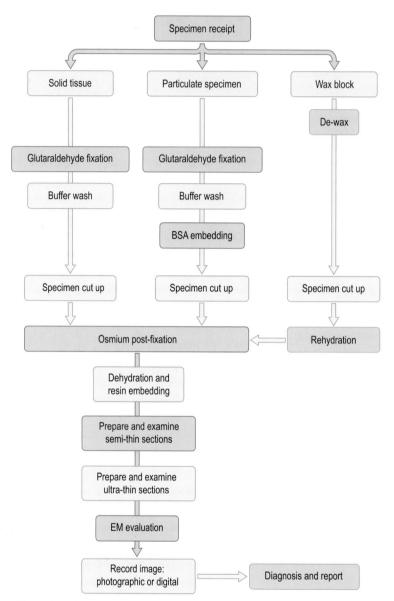

Fig. 30.1 Flow chart illustrating the major steps in the preparation of specimens for diagnosis by electron microscopy.

using a scalpel or razor blade. The final specimen size is usually of the order of 1 mm^3, although the risk of sampling error increases as the size of the sample decreases. In general, the volume of fixative should be at least ten times the volume of the tissue. It is also vital to insure that the tissue remains completely submerged in the fixative— small pieces may adhere to the inside of the lid of the biopsy container and these will be poorly fixed

even if they have been exposed to fixative vapor. Gently agitating the vial on a mechanical rotator will overcome this problem and facilitate fixation.

The importance of using small samples cannot be over-emphasized. The use of cold fixative assists in minimizing postmortem changes but fixation may be hindered as a result. In addition, the penetration rate of most TEM fixatives is quite slow, increasing the risk of artifact formation. Both of these problems are reduced with small samples. If a delay in fixation is unavoidable the specimen should be chilled, but not frozen, preferably in normal saline.

FIXATION

The fixatives used in TEM generally comprise a fixing agent in buffer (to maintain pH) and, if necessary, with various additives to control osmolarity and ionic composition. Other factors that affect fixation include fixative concentration and temperature, and the duration of fixation. The standard protocol involves primary fixation with an aldehyde (usually glutaraldehyde) to stabilize proteins, followed by secondary fixation in osmium tetroxide to retain lipids (Hayat 1981).

Fixative concentration

Glutaraldehyde is effective at a concentration of between 1.5% and 4%, with 2.5% the simplest to prepare from the 25% stock solutions available commercially. Osmium tetroxide is usually used at a concentration of 1% or 2%.

Temperature

Many practitioners prefer to place tissues in cold primary fixative solution but this is not essential. Fixation at room temperature improves the penetration rate (particularly of aldehyde fixatives) and reduces the time required for fixation but it also increases the risk of autolytic change. Osmium tetroxide is generally used at room temperature.

Duration of fixation

The time required for optimal fixation depends on a range of factors including the type of tissue, the size of the sample, and the type of fixative and buffer system used. In most circumstances, immersion of 0.5–1.0 mm^3 blocks of tissue in 2.5% glutaraldehyde fixative for 2–6 hours is sufficient. Secondary fixation in 1% osmium tetroxide for 60–90 minutes is usually effective; much longer times are required if osmium tetroxide is the primary fixative. The use of microwave irradiation can accelerate fixation times in aldehyde fixative to as little as 5–10 seconds (Leong 1994), after which the sample may be stored in buffer or processed immediately.

Buffers

Fixatives are normally buffered within the range of pH 7.2–7.6 (Robinson & Gray 1996). Ideally the osmolarity and ionic composition of the buffer should mimic that of the tissue being fixed. In general practice this is not a major requirement but, if necessary, 300–330 mOsm, the osmolarity equivalent to that of blood plasma or slightly hypertonic, is suitable for most circumstances. Non-ionic molecules such as glucose, sucrose, or dextran are used to adjust tonicity, as these will not influence the ionic constitution of the buffer. The addition of various salts, particularly calcium and magnesium, is thought to improve tissue preservation, possibly by stabilizing membranes (Hayat 1981). This is unlikely to have a major effect in routine diagnostic applications.

Phosphate buffers

Phosphate buffers (Gomori 1955) have the disadvantage of being good growth media for molds and other microorganisms. Additionally, most metal ions form insoluble phosphates, which restricts the use of this buffer (the phosphates of sodium, potassium, and ammonium are soluble). Nevertheless, phosphate buffers are the buffer of choice as they are non-toxic and work well with most tissues.

Phosphate buffer (0.1M, pH 7.4)

Stock reagents

Solution A

Disodium hydrogen orthophosphate (Na_2HPO_4 anhydrous)	14.2 g
Distilled water	1000 ml

Solution B

Sodium dihydrogen phosphate ($NaH_2PO_4 \cdot 2H_2O$)	51.6 g
Distilled water	1000 ml

Method

Mix 40.5 ml of solution A with 9.5 ml of solution B. The pH should be checked and adjusted if necessary using 0.1 M hydrochloric acid or 0.1 M sodium hydroxide.

Alternative buffers

Other buffers that have been recommended for use in TEM include cacodylate (Plumel 1948; Sabatini et al 1963), HEPES (N-2-hydroxyethylpiperazine-N'-2-ethanesulfonic acid), MOPS (3-N-morpholino propanesulfonic acid) and PIPES (piperazine-N,N'-bis(2) ethanesulfonic acid) (Good et al 1966; Good & Izawa 1972; Massie et al 1972; Salema & Brandão 1973; Ferguson et al 1980).

ALDEHYDE FIXATIVES

Glutaraldehyde

Although glutaraldehyde is the most widely used primary fixative in TEM, its fixation reactions are not well understood. The most important reaction of glutaraldehyde, that of stabilizing proteins, is thought to occur via a cross-linking mechanism involving amino groups of lysine and other amino acids through the formation of pyridine intermediaries. Lipids and most phospholipids (those that do not contain free amino groups) are not fixed and will be extracted during subsequent processing without secondary fixation (Hayat 2000).

Glutaraldehyde fixative (2.5%, buffered)

Stock reagents

25% glutaraldehyde stock solution	10 ml
0.1 M phosphate buffer, pH 7.4	90 ml

Method
Combine glutaraldehyde and phosphate buffer in proportions indicated.

Formaldehyde

Commercially supplied formaldehyde solutions (i.e. formalin) normally contain some level of formic acid and considerable quantities of methanol. As such it is a poor cytological fixative and should not be used for TEM. By contrast, formaldehyde that has been freshly prepared from paraformaldehyde powder is adequate for TEM as it lacks impurities and has the advantage of a faster penetration rate compared with glutaraldehyde. Paraformaldehyde is often recommended in electron immunohistochemistry as epitopes are less likely to be significantly altered during fixation and, if required, antigen unmasking is more effective.

Aldehyde combinations

The use of an aldehyde mixture has been proposed as a way of offsetting the disadvantages of glutaraldehyde (a slow penetration rate) and formaldehyde (less stable fixation) when applied individually (Karnovsky 1965).

Paraformaldehyde (2%)—glutaraldehyde (2.5%) fixative (buffered) (Karnovsky 1965; based on Glauert 1972)

Stock reagents

0.2 M buffer, pH 7.4 (phosphate, cacodylate)	50 ml
Paraformaldehyde	2 g
25% aqueous glutaraldehyde	10 ml
Distilled/deionized water	to 100 ml

Method
1. Completely dissolve paraformaldehyde in buffer using heat and with continuous stirring. It may be necessary to add a few drops of 1.0 M sodium hydroxide to clarify the solution.
2. Cool the solution rapidly under running water.
3. Add aqueous glutaraldehyde. Check the pH of the mixture and adjust if necessary to pH 7.4.
4. Add distilled water to make 100 ml.

Note
Adding 0.2 ml of 1.0 M calcium chloride is thought to have a membrane stabilizing effect, but may precipitate if phosphate buffer is used.

OSMIUM TETROXIDE

The use of osmium tetroxide fixation to preserve lipids is fundamental to electron microscopy (Palade 1952; Millonig & Marinozzi 1968). While primary fixation in osmium tetroxide is effective, its extremely slow penetration rate can give rise to autolytic changes. For this reason osmium tetroxide is almost always used as a secondary fixative after primary fixation in aldehyde. The penetration rate of osmium tetroxide is also higher in stabilized tissue, such that immersion for 60–90 minutes is usually sufficient for most specimens.

Osmium tetroxide is usually supplied in crystalline form sealed in glass ampoules. Extreme care should be exercised when preparing this material, and gloves and eye protection should always be worn. It is particularly important only to handle osmium tetroxide in a fumehood, as the vapor will also fix tissue.

Specimens fixed in aldehyde solutions should be washed thoroughly in buffer before immersion in osmium tetroxide to prevent interaction between the fixatives, which can lead to precipitation of reduced osmium. Osmium tetroxide can be prepared as an aqueous solution, although it can also be made in the same buffer used to prepare the primary fixative. Osmium tetroxide should be avoided if electron immunogold labeling studies are to be performed as it has the potential significantly to alter protein structure, rendering antigenic determinants unreactive.

Osmium tetroxide fixative (2% aqueous)

Stock reagent

Osmium tetroxide	1 g
Distilled/deionized water	50 ml

Method

1. Clean then score the glass ampoule with a diamond pencil and place in a dark-glass storage bottle.
2. Break the ampoule with a glass rod and add water. It may take 24 hours or longer for the osmium tetroxide to dissolve completely.
3. Prepared solutions may be stored for short periods at room temperature in the dark in a well-sealed bottle (double wrap the bottle in aluminum foil); for long periods store at 4°C. All osmium solutions should be stored inside a second closed container to prevent the leakage of osmium fumes. Osmium solutions in water should last for approximately 1 year; solutions in buffer may last only a few days before they deteriorate.
4. For a 1% working solution combine 1 : 1 with water or buffer.

Note

Osmium is readily reduced by dust and light. Only glassware that has been acid cleaned and thoroughly rinsed in distilled water should be used. Prepared solutions should be monitored during storage and discarded if a reddish color develops.

Wash buffer and staining

Rinsing the tissue in buffer after post-fixation, although not crucial, removes surplus fixative and provides an opportunity for tissue storage if necessary. An optional step at this point is to immerse tissues after post-fixation in 2% aqueous uranyl acetate. This en bloc staining procedure adds to the contrast of the final sections and improves preservation. It should be noted though that uranyl acetate can extract glycogen.

DEHYDRATION

The most common embedding compounds used in TEM are epoxy resins. These are totally immiscible with water, thus requiring specimens to be dehydrated.

Dehydration is performed by passing the specimen through increasing concentrations of an organic solvent. It is necessary to use a graded series to prevent the damage that would occur with extreme changes in solvent concentration but it is also important to keep the dehydration times as brief as possible to minimize the risk of extracting cellular constituents. The most frequently used dehydrants are acetone and ethanol. Acetone should be avoided if en bloc staining with uranyl acetate has been performed to prevent precipitation of uranium salts. Ethanol overcomes this difficulty but requires the use of propylene oxide (1,2-epoxypropane) as a transition solvent to facilitate resin infiltration. Residual dehydrant can result in soft or patchy blocks.

Commercially available 'absolute' ethanol normally contains a small percentage of water. This will severely restrict infiltration and polymerization of the resin and it is necessary to complete dehydration in anhydrous ethanol (which can be obtained commercially or prepared by using an appropriate molecular sieve). Propylene oxide is highly volatile, flammable, and may form explosive peroxides; it should be stored at room temperature in a flammable solvents facility.

EMBEDDING

The standard practice following dehydration and, if required, treatment with a transitional solvent, is to infiltrate the tissue sample with liquid resin. This usually requires gradual introduction of the resin, beginning with a 50:50 mix of transition solvent (propylene oxide) and resin followed by a 25:75 transition solvent/resin mix, then, finally, pure resin. An hour in each of the preliminary infiltration steps is usually adequate, although it is preferable to leave samples in pure resin for 24 hours. Gentle agitation using a low-speed angled rotator during these steps is recommended, as failure to completely infiltrate the tissue will cause major sectioning difficulties.

Once infiltrated, tissue samples are placed in an appropriate mold which is filled with resin and allowed to polymerize using heat. A paper strip bearing the tissue identification code written in pencil or laser-printed is included. Various shaped and sized molds are available. Capsules made from polyethylene are recommended as they are unreactive with resin, as are flat embedding molds made of silicone rubber. Polymerized blocks can be easily removed from the latter by bending the mold, which can then be re-used. Polyethylene capsules can be cut away from the block using a razor or scalpel blade, or the block can be extruded from the capsule using large forceps or pliers.

EPOXY RESINS

Epoxy resins have been the embedding medium of choice in TEM since their introduction in the mid 1950s (Glauert et al 1956). These resins contain a characteristic chemical group in which an oxygen and two carbon atoms bond to form a three-membered ring ('epoxide'). Cross-linking between these groups creates a three-dimensional polymer of great mechanical strength. The polymerization process generates little shrinkage (usually less than 2%) and, once complete, is permanent. As well as their properties of uniform polymerization and low shrinkage, epoxy resins also preserve tissue ultrastructure, are stable in the electron beam, section easily, and are ready available.

Epoxy resins usually comprise four ingredients: the monomeric resin, a hardener, an accelerator, and a plasticizer. Although manufacturers provide advice on the appropriate proportions, the hardness and flexibility of blocks and polymerization times can be manipulated by varying the amount of the individual components. It is the proportion of each component that is important; hence resins can be prepared by volume or weight. The simplest approach is to weigh the components into a disposable paper or plastic cup as unused resin can be

polymerized and discarded in the container. Thorough mixing of the components is essential. When prepared, the resin is best delivered through a non-reactive plastic syringe or pipette.

Examples of widely used epoxy resin composites include Araldite (Glauert & Glauert 1958), Epon (Luft 1961), and Spurr's resin (Spurr 1969). Although the original product names Araldite and Epon refer to epoxy resins developed by the CIBA Chemical Company and Shell Chemical Company respectively, these terms are now in general use. Araldite polymers are preferred as these react with a higher degree of cross-linking and are the most stable.

Occupational exposure to epoxy resins is a common cause of allergic contact dermatitis (Kanerva et al 1989; Jolanki et al 1990). These agents are also probable carcinogens, primary irritants, and systemically toxic (Causton 1981). Spurr's resin in particular is highly toxic and should be handled with great care (Ringo et al 1982).

ACRYLIC RESINS

Acrylic resins (methacrylates) derive from methacrylic acid [CH_2=$C\cdot(CH_3)COOH$] and acrylic acid [CH_2=$CH\cdot COOH$] and were the original synthetic media developed for use in TEM. Acrylic resins can rapidly infiltrate fixed dehydrated tissues at room temperature. However, marked variable shrinkage of tissue components was common due to unreliable polymerization and acrylic resins are relatively unstable in the electron beam. Currently available acrylics are now polymerized using a cross-linking process, hence overcoming earlier disadvantages. Acrylic monomers are of low viscosity, and both hydrophilic and hydrophobic forms are obtainable. Acrylic resins react by free radical polymerization, which can be initiated using light, heat, or a chemical accelerator (catalyst) at room temperature.

The main commercial acrylic resins are LR White and LR Gold and the Lowicryl series (K4M, K11M, HM20, and HM23). Each of these can be used for low-temperature dehydration and embedding to reduce the heat damage from exothermic polymerization and extraction by solvents and resin components (Acetarin et al 1986; Newman & Hobot 1987, 1993). These characteristics make several forms of acrylic resin ideally suited to electron immunogold labeling (Stirling 1994) and enzyme cytochemical studies.

TISSUE PROCESSING SCHEDULES

Manual tissue processing is best performed by keeping the tissue sample in the same vial throughout, and using a fine pipette to change solutions. Attaching a paper label, which is doubly secured with a length of clear adhesive tape, identifies the vial. It is advantageous to agitate tissue specimens throughout the processing cycle to enhance reagent permeation. Automated processors are available, but tend to be limited to high-throughput laboratories. A protocol for routine processing of solid tissue samples is given in Table 30.1.

PROCEDURES FOR OTHER TISSUE SAMPLES

Cultured cells

Cell cultures may be fixed in situ then separated from the substrate, centrifuged into a pellet and treated as a solid tissue. Alternatively, cells can be harvested into a centrifuge tube, pelleted lightly, resuspended in fixative, and again pelleted by gentle centrifugation. After fixation the tube is inverted to dislodge the pellet, which is then cut into cubes for further processing. Finally cell cultures can be fixed and processed while attached to the substratum, after which inverted embedding capsules are pressed onto the cell layer. Once polymerized, blocks can be separated by force or after being cooled in liquid nitrogen (see 'Pop-off' technique, below).

Cell suspensions or particulate matter

Cell suspensions (such as fine-needle biopsy aspirates, bone marrow specimens, or cytology samples) or particulate materials (including fluid aspirates, tissue fragments or products, and specimens for the assessment of ciliary structures) are best embedded in a protein support medium before processing. Blood plasma, agar, or bovine serum albumen (BSA) can be used. The addition of tannic acid (Hayat 1993) during the preparation of

Table 30.1 Standard processing schedule for solid tissue cut into 1mm³ blocks (each step is performed at room temperature unless stated otherwise)		
Primary fixation	2.5% glutaraldehyde in 0.1M phosphate buffer	2–24 hours (room temperature or 4°C)
Wash	0.1 M phosphate buffer	2 × 10 minutes on rotator
Post-fixation	1% aqueous osmium tetroxide	60–90 minutes
Wash	Distilled water	2 × 10 minutes
En bloc staining (optional)	2% aqueous uranyl acetate	20 minutes
Dehydration	70% ethanol	10 minutes on rotator*
	90% ethanol	10 minutes on rotator
	95% ethanol	10 minutes on rotator
	100% ethanol	15 minutes on rotator
	Dry absolute ethanol	2 × 20 minutes on rotator
Transition solvent (clearing)	1,2-epoxypropane	2 × 15 minutes on rotator
Infiltration	50 : 50, clearant : resin#	1 hour
	25 : 75, clearant : resin	1 hour
	Resin only	1–24 hours (with vacuum to remove bubbles)
Embedding	Fresh resin in embedding capsules	12–24 hours at 60–70°C

* Tissues may be stored at this stage.
\# As batches may vary, resin should be prepared in accordance with manufacturer's instructions.

ciliary specimens gives improved visualization of axonemal components (Sturgess & Turner 1984; Glauert & Lewis 1998). The tannic acid is thought to act as a fixative and also a mordant, facilitating the binding of heavy metal stains (Hayat 2000). Double en bloc staining with uranyl acetate and lead aspartate may also improve the visibility of dynein arms (Rippstein et al 1987).

Preparing particulate specimens

Stock reagents
15% aqueous bovine serum albumen (BSA)
0.1% tannic acid (low molecular weight) in buffer, pH 7.4 (phosphate)

Method
1. Centrifuge the material in buffer in a plastic centrifuge tube to form a loose pellet.
2. Discard supernatant and resuspend the material in glutaraldehyde fixative at room temperature for a minimum of 1 hour.
3. Centrifuge the material and carefully discard the supernatant.
4. Wash the specimen by resuspending it in buffer for 10–15 minutes.
5. Centrifuge the material to form a loose pellet.
6. Discard supernatant and introduce 0.5 ml of 15% aqueous BSA. Resuspend the specimen and allow it to infiltrate for a minimum of 1 hour.
7. Centrifuge the material and discard most of the supernatant, leaving sufficient to cover the pellet to a depth of approximately 1 mm.
8. Introduce an equal volume of glutaraldehyde fixative to form a layer above the BSA. Allow material to solidify for 2–24 hours.
9. Remove the material (this is most easily achieved by cutting away the plastic centrifuge tube) and divide into small portions.
10. Wash in four changes of buffer, each for 5 minutes.
11. Post-fix in 1% aqueous osmium tetroxide and process as normal.

For ciliary biopsies only
10. Wash in four changes of buffer, each for 5 minutes.
10a. Incubate for 15 minutes in buffered tannic acid solution.
10b. Wash in four changes of buffer, each for 5 minutes.
11. Post-fix in 1% aqueous osmium tetroxide and process as normal.

Material embedded in paraffin/cell smears

Occasionally it becomes necessary to examine the ultrastructure of a cell smear or specimen originally embedded in paraffin and intended for light microscopy. As the preservation quality may vary, considerable care must be exercised in the electron microscopic interpretation of such material. Nevertheless it is often possible to obtain information sufficient for diagnostic purposes.

Reprocessing paraffin-embedded material

Method
1. Remove the area of interest from the block, taking care not to damage the tissue.
2. Dewax the specimen by passing through several changes of xylene. The time required depends on the size of the sample but should be at least 1 hour. A minimum of three changes is recommended.
3. Rehydrate the material in a graded ethanol series.
4. Wash in water, post-fix in osmium tetroxide, and process as routine specimen (see above).

'Pop-off' technique for slide-mounted sections (after Bretschneider et al 1981)

Method
1. Remove the coverslip by soaking the slide in xylene. (This may take some time. An alternative is to firstly cool slides to −20°C for up to 1 hour, then carefully pry off coverslip with a blade.)

If additional fixation is required
2. Rehydrate the tissue in a graded ethanol series.
3. Wash in buffer and fix the tissue in glutaraldehyde fixative for 15–20 minutes.
4. Wash in buffer and post-fix in 1% osmium tetroxide for 20–30 minutes.

5. Wash in buffer or distilled water, then cover with 2% uranyl acetate for 15 minutes.
6. Dehydrate the tissue by passing the slide through 70%, 90%, 95%, 100%, and super-dry ethanol for 5 minutes at each stage.
7. Dip the slide into propylene oxide for 5 minutes. The tissue should not be allowed to dry.
8. Cover the tissue with a 2:1 mixture of propylene oxide and epoxy resin for 5–15 minutes. The tissue should not be allowed to dry.
9. Cover the tissue with a 1:2 mixture of propylene oxide and epoxy resin for 5–15 minutes. The tissue should not be allowed to dry.
10. Cover the tissue with neat epoxy resin for 5–15 minutes.
11. Drain off surplus resin mixture. Invert a freshly filled (to overflowing) embedding capsule over the section and press onto the slide.
12. Incubate the slide and capsule at 60°C for 24 hours for polymerization to occur.
13. Remove the slide and, while still warm, separate the capsule and the newly embedded tissue from the glass slide.

If additional fixation is not required

2. Dip the slide in equal parts of propylene oxide and xylene, then into propylene oxide for 5–10 minutes. The tissue should not be allowed to dry.
3. Cover the tissue with a 2:1 mixture of propylene oxide and epoxy resin for 5–15 minutes. The tissue should not be allowed to dry.
4. Cover the tissue with a 1:2 mixture of propylene oxide and epoxy resin for 5–15 minutes. The tissue should not be allowed to dry.
5. Cover the tissue with neat epoxy resin for 5–15 minutes.
6. Drain off surplus resin mixture. Invert a freshly filled (to overflowing) embedding capsule over the section and press onto the slide.
7. Incubate the slide and capsule at 60°C for 24 hours for polymerization to occur.
8. Remove the slide and, while still warm, separate the capsule and the newly embedded tissue from the glass slide.

Note

Sections (or cell cultures) are easier to prepare using the 'pop-off' method if mounted (or grown) directly on Thermanox coverslips.

ULTRAMICROTOMY

Glass knives

Knives are prepared from commercially available plate glass strips which are manufactured to a high degree of quality and dimensional precision. Before use the strips should be washed thoroughly with detergent, then rinsed in distilled water and alcohol, and dried using lint-free paper. Most knife-makers will allow knives of different cutting edge angles to be produced. Higher angle knives (up to 55°) are best suited to cutting hard materials, while softer blocks respond better to shallower (35°) angle knives. Glass squares and knives should be prepared just before use to avoid contamination and stored in dust-free, lidded boxes.

Knives should always be inspected before use. If the knife edge is correctly formed, when it is observed face-on it should be straight and even but with a small glass spur on the top right-hand end (Fig. 30.2). The edge need not be horizontal, but those that are obviously convex or concave should be discarded. The knife should also display a conchoidal fracture mark that curves across and down from the top left-hand edge of the knife until it meets, and runs parallel to, the right-hand edge of the glass. Each of these characteristics is visible macroscopically. When placed in the ultramicrotome and viewed under the microscope the cutting edge will

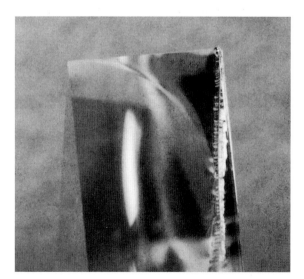

Fig. 30.2 Glass knife prepared from 6.4 mm thick glass strip. Note the straight cutting edge and conchoidal fracture mark.

appear as a bright line against a dark background. The left third of the cutting edge should appear as a smooth line and is the zone recommended for thin sectioning. The middle third is quite frequently also adequate but can show minute imperfections, and is best reserved for trimming blocks prior to sectioning and for cutting semi-thin sections.

In ultramicrotomy thin sections are floated out for collection as they are cut. This requires a small trough to be attached directly to the knife. Pre-formed plastic or metal troughs that can be fitted to the back of the knife are commercially available. These must be sealed with molten dental wax or nail varnish after attachment but they are expedient and simple to use. An alternative approach is to prepare a trough using self-adhesive PVC insulating tape. The lower edge of the trough so formed is then sealed with molten dental wax (Fig. 30.3).

Diamond knives

A well-maintained diamond knife is capable of cutting any type of resin block and most biological and many non-biological materials. Knives are priced according to the length of the actual cutting edge. Manufacturers supply diamond knives already mounted in a metal block (incorporating a section-collecting trough) designed to fit directly into the knife holder of the ultramicrotome. Diamond knives are brittle but durable and will continue to cut for quite some time provided they are kept clean and treated carefully. The cutting edge can be cleaned by carefully running a polystyrene cleaning strip (available commercially) along (never across) the edge. A diamond knife must be used only to cut ultrathin sections and should never be used 'dry' without a trough fluid.

Trough fluids

The simplest and most suitable fluid routinely used in section-collecting troughs is distilled or deionized water; 10–15% solutions of ethanol or acetone can also be used (not with a diamond knife). It is important to insure the correct level of fluid is added. If the level is too high the fluid will be drawn over the cutting edge and down the back of the knife, thereby preventing proper sectioning; if the level is too low sections will accumulate on the cutting edge and will not float out.

Block trimming

Once polymerized, blocks must be cleared of excess resin to expose the tissue for sectioning. At the completion of this process the trimmed area should resemble a flat-topped pyramid with a square or trapezium-shaped face (Fig. 30.4).

Trimming the block can be achieved manually or by using the ultramicrotome. At its simplest, manual trimming can be performed by mounting the block in a suitable holder under a dissecting microscope and removing the surplus resin with a single-edged razor blade. Although this method is quite speedy, considerable care is required to insure the ultimate cutting surface is as level as possible to facilitate sectioning. Alternatively, the block is positioned in the ultramicrotome and mechanically trimmed using a glass knife.

Semi-thin sections

Semi-thin (or 'survey') sections allow samples to be screened for specific features and to select areas for thin sectioning. Semi-thin sections should only be cut on a glass knife, never on a diamond knife.

Commonly, semi-thin sections are cut at between 0.5 and 1.0 μm from trimmed or partly trimmed blocks using the ultramicrotome and a glass knife. Sections can be cut dry (using a slow cutting speed) and picked up with forceps or directly into the flotation bath attached to the knife. Sections are transferred to a drop of water on a glass microscope slide and dried on a hot-plate at 70–80°C. Semi-thin sections can be examined using phase contrast or be stained and viewed by bright-field

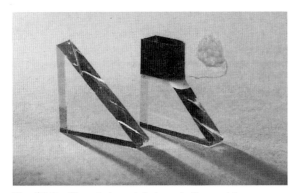

Fig. 30.3 Glass knives: left, bare knife used for trimming and semi-thin sectioning; right, knife used for ultrathin sectioning with trough [prepared from plastic (PVC) tape] fitted.

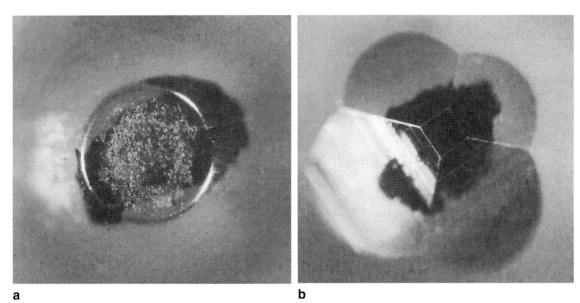

a   b

Fig. 30.4 Araldite blocks: (a) untrimmed, (b) trimmed of excess resin.

microscopy. Various cationic dyes including methylene blue, azure B (Richardson et al 1960), and crystal violet can be used for this purpose, although the most common is toluidine blue. All are applied at high alkaline pH and with heat to facilitate penetration of the resin.

Toluidine blue stain for semi-thin sections

Stock reagents

Sodium tetraborate (borax)	1 g
Toluidine blue	1 g
Distilled water	100 ml

Dissolve the borax in the distilled water and then add the toluidine blue. After filtering, the final solution can be stored at room temperature.

Method

1. Cover sections with staining solution and heat on a hot-plate at 70–80°C.
2. Allow to stain adequately (the time is not crucial— up to 60 seconds is usually sufficient), then wash thoroughly in running water. Allow section to dry.
3. Sections can be viewed dry or mounted in DPX or epoxy resin.

Note

Borax raises the pH of the final stain to around pH 11.

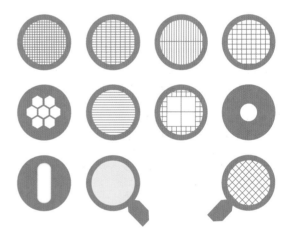

Fig. 30.5 Some examples of specimen grids (from top left): mesh (200 size); slotted (200 size); parallel with divider (200 size); mesh (50 size); hexagonal (7 size); parallel (75 size); freeze fracture; single hole; slotted; tabbed mesh (400 size); tabbed mesh (75 size).

Collection of sections

Ultrathin sections are mounted onto specimen grids for viewing. Grids measure 3.05 mm in diameter and are made of conductive material, commonly copper, nickel, or gold although silver, palladium, molybdenum, aluminum, titanium, stainless steel, nylon–carbon, and combination varieties are available. A large range of patterns and mesh sizes are available (Fig. 30.5) with 200 square mesh being commonly used although slotted, parallel bar, and hexagonal patterns are also standard. As electrons cannot pass through the metal grid bars, the choice of grid becomes a compromise between support for the sections (better with grids of smaller mesh size) and the relative proportion of exposed section (better with grids of larger mesh size). The latter provides a large area of section for viewing but with less stability.

Support films

The use of support films is generally unnecessary with contemporary, routine embedding media that have been properly prepared. If, however, larger viewing areas are required, it may be necessary to use support films to provide greater section stability.

Electron-transparent plastic films prepared from collodion, Formvar, or Butvar are commonly used. There are many methods for applying plastic films, with one of the simpler being illustrated in Figure 30.6. The major problem with using plastic films is that the conductive properties of the grid become compromised. Reinstating the thermal and electrical properties is usually achieved by adding a 5–10 nm layer of carbon in a sputter coater or vacuum-evaporating unit.

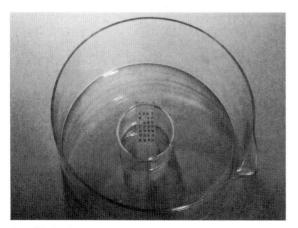

Fig. 30.6 Apparatus for application of plastic support films. The water level is raised over the level of the wire mesh, on which grids are then placed. Approximately 0.2 ml of liquid plastic film is dropped onto the water surface over the submerged grids and the solvent allowed to evaporate. The water is then drawn off, allowing the film of plastic to settle onto the grids.

Ultra-thin sectioning

The basic principles of ultramicrotomy are similar regardless of the ultramicrotome used (Reid 1975; Dykstra 1992). Difficulties with sectioning usually relate to tissue that is poorly fixed or inadequately infiltrated, an imperfectly polymerized block, or a dull knife (Table 30.2).

Specific instructions on operating particular ultramicrotomes are normally provided by the instrument manufacturer. A key element in ultramicrotomy is to insure the sections are cut at a thickness that allows optimal resolution and specimen contrast. The most effective estimate of section thickness is given by viewing the interference color reflected from the section as it is cut—this color is the result of interactions between light waves reflected from the upper and lower surfaces of the section and is directly related to section thickness (Table 30.3).

Silver to straw-colored sections (around 80 nm) are recommended. Thinner sections will give improved resolution but may not provide sufficient contrast for adequate on-screen viewing. Although it is possible to collect and examine individual sections, ribbons are easier to manage and, as the sections are in series, usually offer additional morphological information.

To collect sections, immerse the grid in the flotation fluid, then position the ribbon over the grid. If the grid is then angled slightly the ribbon of sections will fall across the diameter of the grid as it is lifted from the fluid. It is important to remove any remaining fluid by gently touching the back of the grid against lint-free absorbent paper to insure the sections become affixed. A pair of fine-point forceps should always be used to grasp the grid—this requires great care to avoid damaging the grid either before or after collecting the sections. After collecting the sections, grids should be placed on filter paper in a lidded container, such as a Petri dish, and allowed to dry completely before staining. As they are extremely fragile it is strongly recommended that grids be kept in suitable storage boxes. These not only afford protection but also provide a means of identifying individual grids.

STAINING

The purpose of staining sections in TEM is to increase the capacity of selected structural elements to scatter electrons and thus give the specimen contrast. This is achieved by introducing heavy metal atoms which

Table 30.2 Causes and remedies for common sectioning faults

Fault	Effect	Potential cause	Remedy
Scoring	Scratches, tears in section running perpendicular to cutting edge	Knife edge damaged or dirty Hard material in block	Use a new section of knife Replace knife Use diamond knife
Sections contaminated	Artifacts, dirt on section	Dirt on knife edge Dirty trough fluid Trough dirty Block face dirty	Replace knife Replace trough fluid Replace with new knife and trough Trim and re-face block
Chatter	Periodic variations in the part or all of the section running parallel to the cutting edge	Vibrations in knife, block or block holder on ultramicrotome Dull knife Block soft or unevenly polymerized Cutting speed too fast Clearance angle too great	Tighten components Replace knife Re-incubate block (60–70°C) for up to 24 hours Modify processing schedule and/or resin formulation Reduce cutting speed Reduce clearance angle
Compression	Specimen distortion with compression in the direction parallel to the cutting edge and extension in the direction perpendicular aspect	Block soft Sections too thin Cutting speed too fast Cutting edge angle too high	Re-incubate block (60–70°C) for up to 24 hours Modify processing schedule and/or resin formulation Increase section thickness Reduce cutting speed Prepare knife with shallower cutting edge angle
Section wrinkling or folding	Electron-dense bands with straight sides but of variable width	Block soft or unevenly polymerized Dull knife Block face too large Knife angle too shallow Section collection technique poor Picking up single sections	Re-incubate block (60–70°C) for up to 24 hours Modify processing schedule and/or resin formulation Replace knife Trim to a smaller block face Increase knife angle Improve technique Use ribbons

Table 30.2 (continued)

Fault	Effect	Potential cause	Remedy
Alternating thick and thin sections	Only some sections useful	Block face too large	Trim to a smaller block face
		Incorrect knife angle	Adjust knife angle
		Cutting speed too fast	Reduce cutting speed
		Dull knife	Replace knife
		Block soft or unevenly polymerized	Re-incubate block (60–70°C) for up to 24 hours
		Vibration in ultramicrotome	Modify processing schedule and/or resin formulation
		Air movement over sections during cutting	Tighten components Eliminate air drafts
Failure to cut sections as ribbon	Single sections	Upper and lower block edges not parallel	Re-trim block face
		Upper and lower block edges not straight	Re-trim block face
		Fluid level in trough too high or too low	Adjust fluid level
		Cutting speed too slow	Increase cutting speed
Skipping (sections cut on alternate strokes)	Single sections	Dull knife	Replace knife
		Clearance angle too high	Reduce clearance angle
		Knife angle too high	Reduce knife angle

Table 30.3 Relation between section thickness and interference color

Color	Section thickness (nm)
Gray	<60
Silver	60–90
Gold	90–150
Purple	150–190
Blue	190–240

deposit on the tissue components. It should be noted that image contrast can also be manipulated by changing the size of the objective lens aperture. Thus, image contrast is a function of the interactions between accelerating voltage, size of objective lens aperture, thickness of the section, and the staining used. Tissues are stained at several points during preparation (Glauert & Lewis 1998; Hayat 2000):

1. During secondary fixation (as osmium is deposited in membranes).
2. When uranyl acetate is used during the post-fixation wash.
3. By staining the sections with lead and uranium salts (en section staining).

The standard method for staining sections is to float the grids, section side down, on drops of staining solution for the required time. Alternatively, grids may be completely immersed in the solution. The procedure is carried out on a clean surface (such as a Petri dish) to minimize contamination. Normally sections are stained in uranyl acetate followed by lead citrate (Reynolds 1963). After each staining step the grid is washed under a gentle stream of distilled water or by dipping in distilled water. Finally, the grids are dried using clean lint-free filter paper. If the level of contrast achieved is not sufficient, a double lead staining method can be used (Daddow 1983).

Uranyl salts

Uranyl acetate is the uranium salt normally used in TEM although uranyl nitrate and magnesium uranyl acetate are also effective. The uranyl ions combine in large quantities with phosphate groups in nucleic acids as well as phosphate and carboxyl groups on the cell surface (Hayat 2000). Aqueous solutions of between 2% and 5%, applied en section, will give satisfactory contrast but more intense staining can be achieved in less time by using a saturated ethanolic (or methanolic) solution (~7%). Uranyl acetate is radioactive and highly toxic; its effects are cumulative and appropriate precautions should be followed.

Uranyl acetate (2% aqueous)

Stock reagents

Uranyl acetate	2 g
Distilled water	100 ml

Combine reagents in proportions indicated. Filter, divide into suitable aliquots, and store at 4°C in the dark. Centrifuge before use.

Method

1. Place droplets of the staining solution on a clean surface (as in a Petri dish).
2. Place grid section side down on the droplets for up to 10 minutes.
3. Rinse grids in three changes of distilled water.

Lead salts

Lead stains increase the contrast of a range of tissue components. Lead stains must be prepared and used carefully as lead ions have the potential to react with atmospheric carbon dioxide forming a fine precipitate of lead carbonate. The deposit appears as an electron-dense contaminant on sections and cannot be removed easily. The preparation method of Reynolds, which is in common use, addresses this problem by chelating and thus shielding the lead ion from exposure to the carbon dioxide (Reynolds 1963).

Reynolds' lead citrate stain
(Reynolds 1963)

Stock reagents

Lead nitrate	2.66 g
Trisodium citrate	3.52 g
1 M sodium hydroxide (freshly prepared)	16 ml
Distilled water (freshly prepared, carbonate-free)	84 ml

Mix the reagents in an alkaline-cleaned stoppered flask with approximately 60 ml of the water, inverting continuously for 1 minute. Allow to stand for 30 minutes with occasional mixing. Add sodium hydroxide and mix until the solution becomes clear. Make up to 100 ml with remaining water. Divide into suitable aliquots and store at 4°C. Centrifuge before use.

Method

1. Place droplets of the staining solution in a Petri dish containing a few pellets of sodium hydroxide (for preferential absorption of carbon dioxide).
2. Place grid section side down on the droplets for up to 10 minutes.
3. Rinse grids in three changes of distilled water.

DIAGNOSTIC APPLICATIONS

Here we describe only the essential features of selected diseases in which TEM plays a major diagnostic role. For in-depth analyses there are a large number of specialist texts that contain a wealth of information on the interpretation of ultrastructural morphology. For example, the ultrastructural pathology of the cell has been covered comprehensively by Ghadially (1997), renal disease by Jennette et al (1998) and Tisher and Brenner (1994), and non-neoplastic diseases by Papadimitriou et al (1992b). The ultrastructure of neoplastic diseases has been described in several texts; those by Henderson et al (1986), Erlandson (1994), and Ghadially (1985) are recommended.

RENAL DISEASE

The basic diagnostic features of the major renal diseases are outlined in Tables 30.4–30.8 and see Figures 30.7–30.20.

The location and morphology of immune complex deposits

Immune complex deposits are seen as accumulations of electron-dense, finely granular material in,

Table 30.4 Renal diseases with fine granular deposits: the ultrastructural features of post-infectious glomerulonephritis (GN), systemic lupus erythematosus, membranous GN, and IgA nephropathy

	Diagnostic ultrastructural features			
	Post-infectious GN	Systemic lupus erythematosus	Membranous GN	IgA nephropathy
Capillary wall GBM morphology: contour, width, texture	–	Normal to irregular and thickened depending on the extent and location of membrane deposits	Stage I: minimal irregular thickening Stage II: marked thickening with membrane spikes (argyrophilic by LM) Stage III: thickened membrane surrounding deposits Stage IV and V: much thickened with irregular patchy lucent areas common in stage V (Stages II–V, see Fig. 30.9)	Focal irregular thinning ('etching')
GBM deposit: type, location	Prominent subepithelial dome-shaped deposits (humps) are characteristic (Fig. 30.7): number of humps correlates approximately to intensity of inflammation. Intramembranous and subendothelial deposits may also be present	Deposits increase in extent and location with severity of inflammation. GBM deposits (subepithelial, intramembranous, and subendothelial) (Fig. 30.8) indicate severe or global inflammation. In well-established disease, deposits may be found throughout the glomerulus. SLE can mimic other diseases because of the variety of damage caused	Stage I: subepithelial deposits Stage II: subepithelial deposits with membrane spikes Stage III: intramembranous deposits Stage IV: some deposits resorbed leaving lucent areas Stage V: many deposits resorbed leaving poorly defined lucent and rarefied areas	Subendothelial deposits variable but present in some cases. Subepithelial and intramembranous deposits rare

Table 30.4 *(continued)*

	Post-infectious GN	Systemic lupus erythematosus	Membranous GN	IgA nephropathy
		Diagnostic ultrastructural features		
Capillary wall				
Visceral epithelium	Foot processes usually effaced over humps so that their outer surface is covered by epithelial cell cytoplasm	Cells may contain tubuloreticular inclusions	Foot process obliteration	Focal foot process obliteration
Endothelium, subendothelial plane	–	Tubuloreticular inclusions common in endothelial cells (see Fig. 30.20). (Note that tubuloreticular inclusions may be found in small numbers in other renal diseases)	–	–
Mesangium				
Matrix	Areas of matrix separated by cellular swelling, proliferation, and infiltration	Diffuse expansion	–	Increased
Deposits	Peripheral humps with deposits common within matrix	Minor inflammation has exclusively mesangial deposits only	Deposits absent in primary GN; may be present in secondary membranous GN	Present, sometimes nodular (Fig. 30.10)
Cells	Proliferation (endocapillary) with infiltration by inflammatory cells including macrophages and polymorphs	Diffuse but irregular proliferation with segmental inflammation	No increase	Variable mesangial cell proliferation

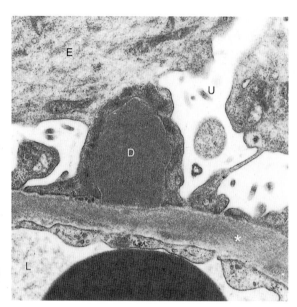

Fig. 30.7 Post-infectious GN. Typical subepithelial dome-shaped deposit (hump) (D). GBM (*), epithelial cell cytoplasm (E), urinary space (U), capillary lumen (L) with part of a red blood cell also visible. Magnification ×10,700.

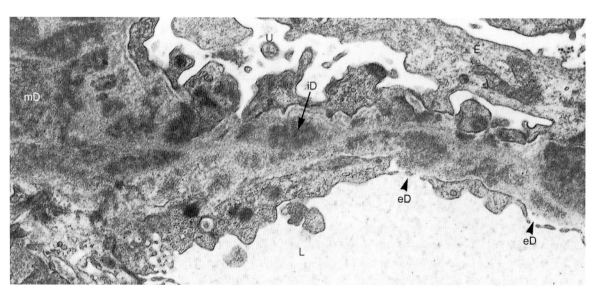

Fig. 30.8 Systemic lupus erythematosus. Subendothelial (eD) and intramembranous (iD) deposits are seen in the GBM; mesangial deposits (mD) are also present. Epithelial cell cytoplasm (E), urinary space (U), capillary lumen (L). Magnification ×15,200.

or adjacent to, the glomerular basement membrane (GBM) and mesangial matrix (Figs 30.7–30.12). Rarely, deposits may be fibrillar (Figs 30.13 and 30.14). The principal forms of deposit are (Stirling et al 1999):

- *Subepithelial (epimembranous):* raised dome-shaped deposits that protrude from the outer surface of the GBM (between the GBM and the visceral epithelial cell foot processes). Large well-formed deposits, typical of post-infectious glomerulonephritis (GN),

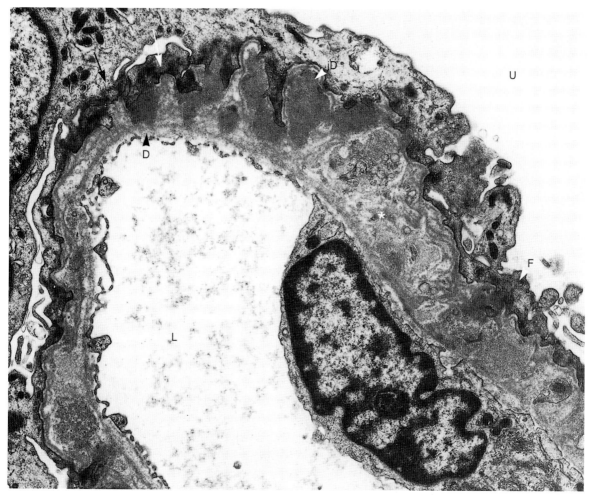

Fig. 30.9 Membranous GN stages II–V. Stage II: subepithelial deposit (D) with membrane spikes (arrows) on both sides. Stage III: intramembranous deposit (iD). Stage IV–V: thickened and disrupted GBM with patches of partially resorbed deposit and lucent areas (*). Epithelial cell foot processes are extensively effaced (F). Urinary space (U), capillary lumen (L). Magnification ×11,500.

are termed 'humps' (see Fig. 30.7). Smaller deposits are typical of membranous GN (see Fig. 30.9). In membranous GN the deposits may eventually encroach into the GBM, provoking a GBM reaction. In this case the GBM may become thickened, with 'spikes' of new membrane forming adjacent to the deposits (see Fig. 30.9). Such deposits may eventually be completely surrounded by the GBM. Finally, where deposits have been absorbed, only electron-lucent areas surrounded by thickened GBM may remain (see Fig. 30.9).

- *Intramembranous:* nodular or linear deposits that are completely incorporated into the GBM. Such deposits are typical in dense deposit disease (see Fig. 30.12).

- *Subendothelial:* linear or plaque-like deposits situated between the inner (luminal) aspect of the GBM and the endothelium (see Fig. 30.8). Subendothelial deposits may be massive and visible by LM. The latter are seen typically in systemic lupus erythematosus (SLE) as nodular hyaline 'thrombi' or 'wire-loop' capillary wall thickening (LM terms).

- *Mesangial:* deposits that lie completely within the mesangial matrix. Mesangial deposits may be massive and are seen typically in IgA disease (see Fig. 30.10).

Table 30.5   Renal diseases with fine granular deposits: the ultrastructural features of mesangiocapillary GN types I and II

	Diagnostic ultrastructural features	
	Mesangiocapillary GN Type I (with subendothelial deposits)	**Mesangiocapillary GN Type II (dense deposit disease)**
Capillary wall		
GBM morphology: contour, width, texture	Double contouring ('tram tracking' by LM) due to mesangial interposition in well-developed disease (Fig. 30.11)	Interposition in some cases
GBM deposit: type, location	Deposits mainly in interposition zone (Fig. 30.11)	Linear dense deposit, typically discontinuous (Fig. 30.12)
Visceral epithelium	Variable foot process obliteration	–
Endothelium, subendothelial plane	Interposition of mesangial cells, with deposits and new GBM-like material (Fig. 30.11)	Mesangial interposition
Mesangium		
Matrix	Greatly increased	Increased
Deposits	Present	Present, dense and finely granular
Cells	Endocapillary proliferation	Endocapillary proliferation

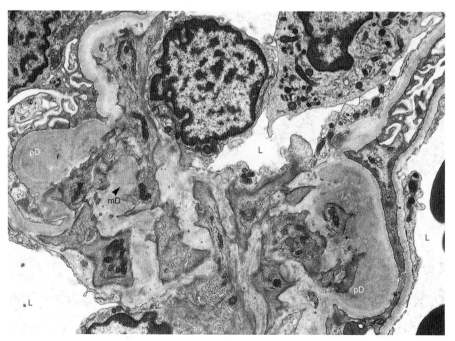

Fig. 30.10   IgA nephropathy. Areas of mesangial (mD) and nodular paramesangial (pD) deposit are seen within the mesangium. Capillary lumens (L). Magnification ×9400.

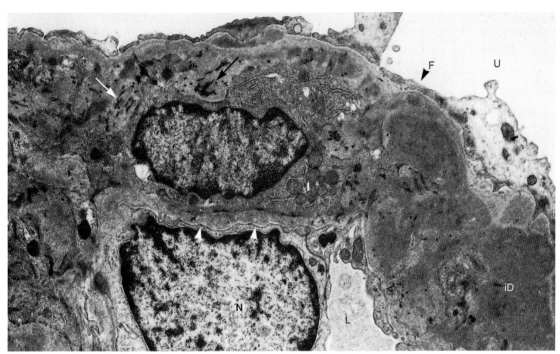

Fig. 30.11   Mesangiocapillary GN type I. The capillary wall is considerably thickened due to mesangial cell interposition (I) and the formation of new basement membrane-like material (arrow heads) giving rise to the appearance of double contouring, as seen by LM. Collagen fibers (arrows) and large areas of intramembranous deposit (iD) can also be seen in the capillary wall. Epithelial cell foot processes are extensively effaced (F). Urinary space (U), capillary lumen (L), endothelial cell nucleus (N). Magnification ×9800.

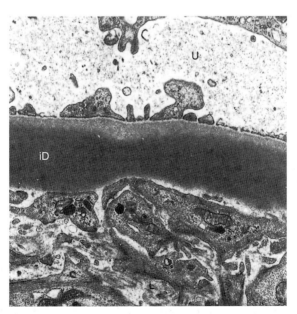

Fig. 30.12   Mesangiocapillary GN type II (dense deposit disease). A continuous linear zone of dense intramembranous deposit (iD) is seen along the length of the GBM. Cells of indeterminate type are seen in the capillary lumen (L). Urinary space (U). Magnification ×9800.

Table 30.6 Renal diseases with fibrillar deposits: the ultrastructural features of renal amyloid and immunotactoid glomerulopathy (fibrillary glomerulonephritis)

	Diagnostic ultrastructural features	
	Amyloid	Immunotactoid glomerulopathy (fibrillary glomerulonephritis)*
Capillary wall		
GBM morphology: contour, width, texture	Thickened and irregular due to deposition of amyloid fibrils	Diffuse thickening frequent
GBM deposit: type, location	Deposits Congo red positive by LM Typical amyloid deposits: extracellular fine non-branching fibrils ~7–10 nm in diameter; variable in location Fibrils tangled and irregular; not organized (Fig. 30.13)	Deposits Congo red negative by LM Extracellular non-branching fibrils or tubules ~9 to >50 nm in diameter, mostly randomly arranged but sometimes packed into parallel arrays (Fig. 30.14) (Schwartz 1998) Fibrils variable in location: subendothelial, subepithelial, and intramembranous
Visceral epithelium	Often widespread foot process obliteration	Diffuse foot process effacement may be present
Endothelium, subendothelial plane	—	—
Mesangium		
Matrix	Amyloid deposits	Expansion may be present
Deposits	Amyloid fibrils Fibrils tangled and irregular; not organized (Fig. 30.13)	Mesangial deposits present in most cases. Fibrillar/tubular, mostly randomly arranged; 9–50 nm (or greater) in diameter
Cells	—	Mild hypercellularity associated with deposits

*****Note**: some authors use ʻfibrillary glomerulonephritis' for disease where the fibril diameter averages ~20 nm, reserving 'immunotactoid glomerulopathy' for cases in which the fibrils are tubular with a diameter of ~30–50 nm; others use the terms synonymously (Alpers 1992; Verani 1993; Jennette et al 1994; Rostagno et al 1996; Strom et al 1996; Schwartz 1998).
Furthermore, some authors restrict a diagnosis of immunotactoid glomerulopathy to situations in which no underlying systemic disease has been identified (Schwartz 1998).

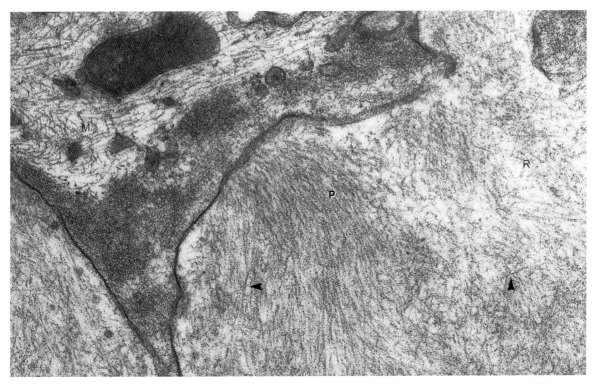

Fig. 30.13 Amyloid. Typical fine, non-branching, extracellular amyloid fibrils in the glomerular mesangium. The fibrils seen in this micrograph are arranged randomly (R) and in parallel (P). Individual fibrils (arrow heads) are 8–10 nm in diameter. Mesangial cell cytoplasm (M). Magnification ×59,300.

- *Paramesangial:* deposits within the peripheral mesangial matrix, particularly the junction of the mesangium and the GBM (see Fig. 30.10).

Variations in the thickness and/or texture of the GBM

The normal GBM has a mean thickness of approximately 390 nm (reported by Coleman et al (1986) as: mean 394 mm with a range of 356–432 nm) (Fig. 30.15).

The principal changes in the thickness and/ or texture of the GBM are (Stirling et al 1999):

- *Thickness:* the GBM may be thickened, thinned, or irregular (Figs 30.16–30.19).
- *Texture:* the GBM may be laminated, fragmented, or split. Electron-lucent zones may represent areas of resorbed deposits (see Fig. 30.9).

- *Surface structure:* the GBM may appear 'etched' (frayed or uneven).
- *Inclusions:* electron-dense granules and debris, microparticles, fibrils, fingerprint-like whorls, small vesicles and virus-like particles, fibrillar collagen and fibrin, all of doubtful or unknown diagnostic significance. Amyloid may also be found occasionally within the GBM (see Fig. 30.13).
- *Folds and wrinkles:* folds and concertina-like wrinkling may result from ischemic collapse. Eventually, folds may consolidate as a thickened and laminated area of GBM.
- *Double contouring (interposition):* the GBM appears duplicated due to the interposition of mesangial cells and matrix between the GBM and the endothelium in the capillary loop (sometimes called 'tram-tracking' when seen by LM) (see Fig. 30.11).

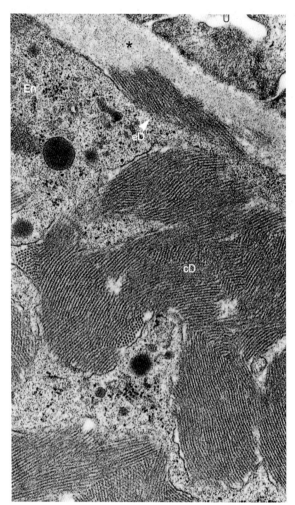

Fig. 30.14   Immunotactoid glomerulopathy (fibrillary GN). Fibrillar deposits are seen in the subendothelial zone (eD) and within the capillary lumen (cD). Individual fibrils are ~20 nm in diameter. GBM (*), endothelial cell cytoplasm (En), urinary space (U). Magnification ×29,800.

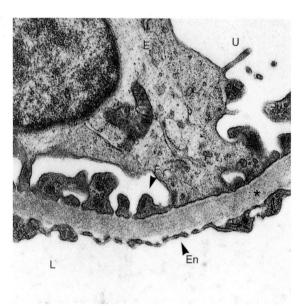

Fig. 30.15   Normal GBM. A length of normal GBM (*) with a mean width of ~390 nm. Compare this membrane with Figures 30.16–30.19, which illustrate various types of abnormal GBM at the same magnification. Urinary space (U), epithelial cell (E) and foot processes (F), fenestrated endothelium (En), capillary lumen (L). Magnification ×16,500.

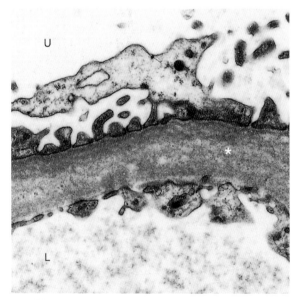

Fig. 30.16   Diabetes. In diabetes the GBM (*) typically shows uniform thickening. In this case the GBM is moderately thickened with a mean width of ~919 nm. Urinary space (U), capillary lumen (L). Magnification ×16,500.

Table 30.7 Renal diseases with or without changes in GBM thickness: the ultrastructural features of diabetic glomerulosclerosis, minimal change disease, and nephrotic focal/segmental glomerulosclerosis

	Diagnostic ultrastructural features		
	Diabetic glomerulosclerosis	Minimal change disease	Nephrotic focal/segmental glomerulosclerosis
Capillary wall			
GBM morphology: contour, width, texture	Uniform increase in GBM thickness Thickening may be considerable with GBM greater than 1000 nm in width (Fig. 30.16)	Variable thinning (Coleman & Stirling 1991) Thinning minor but GBM may be less than ~ 300 nm in width (Fig. 30.17)	Segmental sclerosis; secondary ischemic change (GBM folding and consolidation)
GBM deposit: type, location	—	—	—
Visceral epithelium	Variable foot process obliteration	Diffuse foot process obliteration is the main feature (Fig. 30.17) Microvillous transformation	Diffuse foot process obliteration. (Segmental sclerosis and foot process obliteration are essential for the diagnosis)
Endothelium, subendothelial plane	—	—	—
Mesangium			
Matrix	Increased, sometimes into nodular aggregates	—	Segmental sclerosis in some cases, especially juxtamedullary glomeruli
Deposits	—	—	—
Cells	—	—	Proliferation in some cases

- *Subendothelial widening:* the space between the endothelium and the GBM may become widened with an accumulation of flocculent material or, more rarely, cellular elements from the blood (as in hemolytic uremic syndrome).
- *Gaps:* rarely, small discontinuities are seen in the GBM. Such gaps are of unknown diagnostic significance. Although it has been speculated that GBM discontinuities are responsible for hematuria, few are seen, even in cases of macroscopic hematuria.

Morphological and numerical changes in the cellular components of the glomerulus

Changes of diagnostic significance may also occur in the cellular elements of the glomerulus. The most significant include (Stirling et al 1999):

- *Capillary endothelium:* cytoplasmic tubuloreticular inclusions may be found in the endothelial cytoplasm and are most common in SLE (Fig. 30.20).

Table 30.8 Familial renal diseases with changes in GBM thickness or texture: the ultrastructural features of benign essential hematuria and Alport's disease

	Diagnostic ultrastructural features	
	Benign essential hematuria	Alport's syndrome
Capillary wall		
GBM morphology: contour, width, texture	Variable thinning is the main feature. Thinning may be considerable with GBM less than 150 nm in width (Fig. 30.18)	Alternating areas of thinning and thickening with lamellation (basket-weave pattern) Variability in width of GBM may be extreme (reported by Stirling et al. 1999 as 127–886 nm) (Fig. 30.19) Thickness calculations may be misleading with overall GBM mean near normal value
GBM deposit: type, location	—	—
Visceral epithelium	May show focal foot process obliteration	May show focal foot process obliteration
Endothelium, subendothelial plane	—	—
Mesangium		
Matrix	—	—
Deposits	—	—
Cells	—	—

- *Visceral epithelium:* the epithelial cell foot processes may be effaced to form a continuous (or semi-continuous) layer of cytoplasm (see Fig. 30.17).
- *Mesangial cells:* mesangial cells may increase in number; the matrix may also be increased.

MALIGNANT TUMORS

Mesothelioma

Mesothelioma is morphologically diverse, with three major types generally recognized: epithelial, mixed (bimorphic, biphasic), and sarcomatoid (Henderson et al 1992). Unusual variants and subtypes also occur and mesothelioma may mimic other tumor types (Henderson et al 1992, 1997).

TEM is recommended (Comin et al 1997) when:

- the sample is small (cytological specimens, including cell block preparations)
- the histological appearances are atypical
- the immunohistochemical findings are atypical.

For an unequivocal diagnosis of mesothelioma, mesothelial hyperplasia and metastatic tumor mimicking mesothelioma, especially adenocarcinoma, must be excluded (Henderson 1982; Oury et al 1998).

Ultrastructural features that help to distinguish between epithelial mesothelioma and adenocarcinoma include:

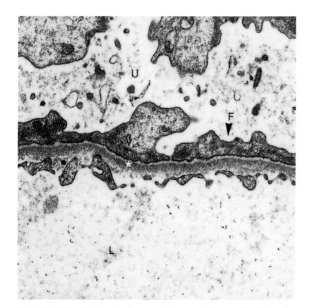

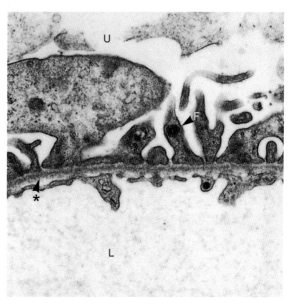

Fig. 30.17 Minimal change disease. The epithelial cell foot processes (F) are completely effaced. The GBM (*) is slightly thinned with a mean width of ~226 nm. Urinary space (U), capillary lumen (L). Magnification ×16,500.

Fig. 30.18 Benign essential hematuria. The GBM (*) is extremely thin, with a mean width of ~183 nm. The foot processes (F) are generally intact but show minor areas of effacement ('smudging'). Urinary space (U), capillary lumen (L). Magnification ×16,500.

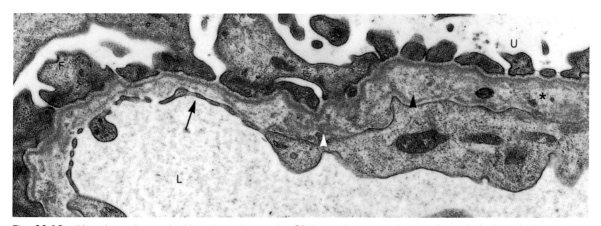

Fig. 30.19 Alport's syndrome. In Alport's syndrome the GBM may be extremely irregular with thickened, thinned, and lamellated areas. In this example the membrane is 260–900 nm in width. The thickened section of the GBM (*) is lamellated (arrow heads). Foot processes are 'smudged' (F). Thinned area (arrow), urinary space (U), capillary lumen (L). Magnification ×16,500.

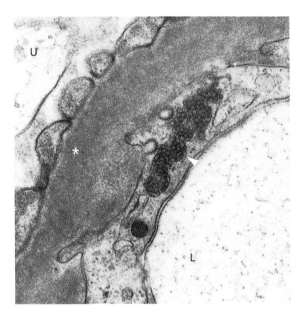

Fig. 30.20 Systemic lupus erythematosus. Tubulo-reticular inclusion (arrow head) in the cytoplasm of an endothelial cell. GBM (*), urinary space (U), capillary lumen (L). Magnification ×31,000.

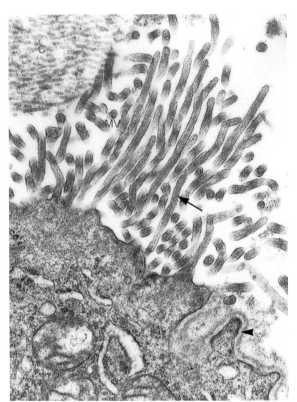

Fig. 30.21 Mesothelioma. The microvilli (MV) on the tumor cell shown here project through a discontinuous basal lamina (arrow head) and are in contact with stromal collagen fibrils (C). In mesothelioma the microvilli are much longer than those of adenocarcinoma and have an LDR greater than 11.9. The microvillus marked (arrow) is ~1900 nm long and 86 nm wide (LDR = 22). Magnification ×22,200.

- *Microvilli:* mesothelial cells have longer microvilli than those of adenocarcinoma (Fig. 30.21) (Coleman et al 1989; Henderson et al 1992) with a mean length to diameter ratio (LDR) of 11.9 (standard deviation 5.87, range 4.8–21.3) (Warhol et al 1982) versus a mean LDR of 5.28 (standard deviation 2.3, range 2.3–10).
- *Contact between stromal collagen fibrils and microvilli:* in mesothelioma, microvilli may be found interdigitating, or in contact, with stromal collagen fibrils (Fig. 30.21) (Carstens 1992). This feature is also found occasionally in adenocarcinoma and is regarded as predictive of mesothelioma rather than an absolute discriminator (Carstens 1992).
- *Cytoplasmic filaments:* intermediate filaments are common in mesothelioma. Filaments are often aggregated into tonofilaments and are characteristically seen near the nucleus (Fig. 30.22) (Henderson et al 1992).
- *Mucin granules:* for a diagnosis of mesothelioma, mucin granules must be absent.

Langerhans' histiocytosis (histiocytosis X)

In Langerhans' histiocytosis the tumor cells are similar in structure to the Langerhans' histiocyte, which is identified at the ultrastructural level by the presence of Langerhans' cell granules (Birbeck bodies or X bodies) (Fig. 30.23). Birbeck bodies are not specific for Langerhans' histiocytosis and may also be found in other disorders (Henderson et al 1986; Erlandson 1994).

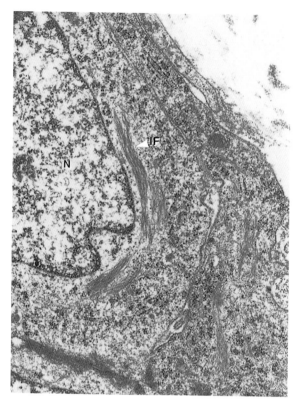

Fig. 30.22 Mesothelioma. Cytoplasmic intermediate filaments (arrow head) are common in mesothelioma, especially near the nucleus (N). Magnification ×21,500.

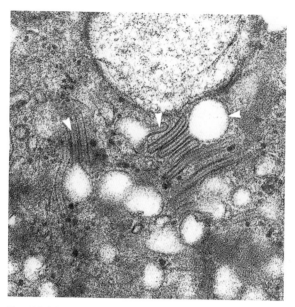

Fig. 30.23 Langerhans' cell granules (Birbeck bodies). Langerhans' cell granules (arrow heads) are typical of the Langerhans' histiocyte and the tumor cells of Langerhans' histiocytosis. The granules comprise a short rod-like structure with a clear vesicle at one end. Magnification ×54,700.

Primitive neuroectodermal (neuroepithelial) tumor (PNET) and Ewing's tumor

PNET and Ewing's sarcoma are now known to be the same tumor with variable differentiation (Grier 1997). Both tumors are defined by a translocation between the *EWS* gene on chromosome 22 with one of three ETS-like genes, especially the *FLI1* gene, on chromosome 11 (Grier 1997).

Typically, PNETs consist of cells 10–17 μm in size with little intervening stroma. The principal characteristic feature is the presence of variable numbers of cytoplasmic processes which may be elongate (sometimes sinuous and branching) or short and blunt. Within these processes, microtubules and filaments are found in small numbers. Neurosecretory granules vary in number and appearance; some are lysosomal in appearance, others are similar to typical dense-core neurosecretory gran-

ules (Henderson et al 1989). In comparison, the cells of Ewing's tumor are completely undifferentiated (Henderson et al 1989).

NON-NEOPLASTIC DISEASES

Skeletal muscle

A wide range of ultrastructural changes are seen in skeletal muscle in primary muscle diseases, as secondary events in neurological diseases and in some systemic diseases. Because it is contractile, skeletal muscle is prone to sampling artifacts and must be biopsied and processed carefully; practical guidelines are given by Pearl and Ghatak (1995) and Schochet and Lampert (1978). Only a small number of the ultrastructural changes that may be found are specific and diagnostically significant (Papadimitriou et al 1992a; Stirling et al 1999); the principal features are summarized in Table 30.9.

Table 30.9 Skeletal muscle—summary of major ultrastructural abnormalities (Schochet & Lampert 1978; Papadimitriou et al 1992a; Stirling et al 1999)

Structural element	Alteration and disease state
Satellite cells	Rare in normal muscle. Frequent in regenerating and denervated muscle. Increased in polymyositis, Duchenne muscular dystrophy, congenital myotonic dystrophy, Werdnig–Hoffman disease, and Kugelberg–Welander syndrome. May display evidence of activation and myogenic differentiation. May be confused with invading inflammatory cells.
Nuclei	Large internal nuclei in recently regenerated myofibers. Contours convoluted in atrophy and nemaline myopathy. Abundant internal nuclei found in various myopathies. Internal nuclei especially numerous, and arranged in chains, in myotonic dystrophy. Chains of internal nuclei a distinctive feature of centronuclear (myotubular) myopathy. A variety of vacuoles, inclusions, and pseudoinclusions present in a wide range of diseases. Nemaline bodies found in a few cases of polymyositis and some cases of late-onset rod diseases. Filamentous intranuclear inclusions resembling myxovirus in polymyositis and chronic distal myopathy. Fibrillar inclusions present in inclusion body myositis and polymyositis. Annulate lamellae present in a range of diseases.
Myofibrils	Hypercontracted myofibrils non-specific and often artifactual. Aberrant bundles of normal fibrils spiraling, or encircling, the long axis of myofibers are frequent in myotonic dystrophy. This feature is also observed in other diseases. Sarcomeres with disorganized myofibrils are non-specific but common in congenital myopathies (multicore and minicore diseases). Extensive disorganization of central region of type 1 myofibers is the major lesion in 'target' and 'core-targetoid' fibers. Target fibers occur in denervation, re-innervation, polymyositis, and familial periodic paralysis. Core-targetoid lesions present in denervating and myopathic conditions and in the aged. Peripheral subsarcolemmal aggregates of disorganized myofibrils and sarcoplasm are found in a variety of disorders but are characteristic of myotonic dystrophy.
Z-discs	Z-disc abnormalities are common in many disease states. Streaming of Z-disc material, Z-disc duplication, and zig-zag irregularities are the most common lesions. Characteristic rod-shaped electron-dense bodies (nemaline bodies), 6–7 μm long and similar in appearance to Z-discs, are common in nemaline myopathy. These bodies contain actin and α-actinin and are also found sporadically in other diseases. Widespread loss of Z-disc material noted in a variety of diseases. Discrete osmiophilic cytoplasmic bodies, thought to be related to Z-discs, noted in a wide range of diseased myofibers.

Table 30.9 *(continued)*

Structural element	Alteration and disease state
Mitochondria	Swelling, with deposition of osmiophilic material or formation of myelin figures, common and non-specific. Swelling may result from sub-optimal fixation. Changes in numbers common and non-specific. Re-orientation of intermyofibrillar mitochondria (in relation to myofiber) occurs in a range of diseases. Structural abnormalities common (some associated with biochemical deficiencies) and present in a wide range of diseases, including the 'mitochondrial myopathies' and 'mitochondrial encephalomyopathies'. Electron-dense granules and crystalline inclusions present in a wide range of diseases.
Transverse tubular system	Abnormalities in triads common in injured and atrophic fibers. Dilation is a common artifact but may also be present in a variety of diseases. Coalescence of T-system tubules to give a honeycomb pattern may be present in a wide range of diseases.
Sarcoplasmic reticulum	Dilation of cisternae prominent in periodic paralyses and some other diseases. Elongated tubular aggregates (probably derived from sarcoplasmic reticulum) reported in the periodic paralyses and other diseases. Cylindrical structures in a spiral pattern, and with a core of glycogen, observed in a variety of diseases.
Inclusions and deposits	Filamentous bodies; concentric laminated bodies; zebra-striped bodies; fingerprint bodies; reducing bodies; spheroidal bodies; and paracrystalline arrays present in the sarcoplasm in a range of diseases. Excessive lipid accumulation present in a wide range of diseases. Glycogen abundant in fetal muscle and regenerating myofibers. Glycogen moderately increased in a range of diseases; massively increased in various glycogenoses. Autophagic vacuoles and lipopigments present in degenerative diseases and in almost any myopathic state.

Epidermolysis bullosa—mechanobullous dermatoses

Epidermolysis bullosa (EB) is a heterogeneous group of rare, inherited or acquired diseases in which the skin blisters easily under normal levels of mechanical stress. Based on the level of blister formation within the dermal–epidermal junction, EB has traditionally been classified into three major groups: simplex, junctional, and dystrophic (Anton-Lamprecht 1992; Mellerio 1999; Pulkkinen & Uitto 1999). A fourth category, the hemidesmosomal group, has recently been recognized. In this group, blister formation is at the basal cell/lamina lucida interface at the level of the hemidesmosomes (Pulkkinen & Uitto 1999).

TEM allows the precise level of blister formation to be determined, in combination with a morphological assessment of the basement membrane components (Table 30.10) (Anton-Lamprecht 1992; Jaunzems & Woods 1997; Jaunzems et al 1997). For best results a fresh blister should be biopsied (Marinkovich 1999).

Cerebral autosomal dominant arteriopathy with subcortical infarcts and leucoencephalopathy (CADASIL)

CADASIL is a familial form of early-onset vascular dementia associated with mutations to chromosome 19 (*Notch3* gene) (Ruchoux & Maurage 1997; Kalimo et al

Table 30.10 Basic ultrastructural features of the major groups of congenital epidermolysis bullosa (EB)

EB main category	Plane of cleavage and ultrastructural features
Simplex (epidermolytic EB)	• Split above basal lamina through the cytoplasm of the basal keratinocytes causing intra-epidermal blister formation • Degenerative cytolytic changes in basal keratinocytes • Tonofilaments are clumped in EB herpetiformis (Dowling–Meara) variant
Hemidesmosomal	• Split at basal keratinocyte/lamina lucida interface at the level of the hemidesmosomes • Hemidesmosomes rudimentary
Junctional (atrophicans)	• Split at level of lamina lucida causing junctional blister formation • Hemidesmosomes abnormal and reduced in size or number
Dystrophic (dermolytic or scarring EB)	• Split below the lamina densa causing dermolytic blister formation • Anchoring fibers absent, or few, or rudimentary • Collagen degradation present in some variants

1999). In affected vessels, basophilic, periodic acid–Schiff positive deposits accumulate between the smooth muscle cells of the vessel walls (Kalimo et al 1999).

At the ultrastructural level the deposit is seen typically as extracellular electron-dense granular material that is often in contact with the vascular smooth muscle cells and sited in a small indentation (Fig. 30.24) (Bergmann et al 1996; Ruchoux & Maurage 1998). As the deposits can be patchy in distribution, multiple blocks may need to be examined.

Amyloid

Amyloid deposition is associated with a wide range of disorders and can be either hereditary or acquired. Amyloid deposits may also be focal, localized, or systemic (Gillmore et al 1997). By TEM amyloid is seen as randomly arranged extracellular non-branching fibrils. Individual fibrils are of indeterminate length and approximately 7–10 nm in diameter (see Fig. 30.13) (Harvey & Anton-Lamprecht 1992; Gillmore et al 1997).

Cornea

TEM is useful for identifying corneal deposits and inclusions, particularly amyloid and immunoglobulin deposits in diseases such as paraproteinemic crystalloidal

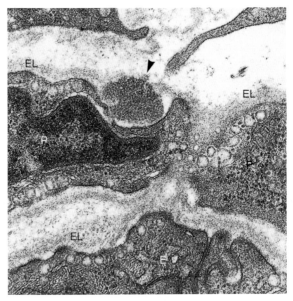

Fig. 30.24 CADASIL. In affected vessels electron-dense material (arrow head) is seen in close proximity to the pericytes or perivascular smooth muscle cells. The material is often sited (as seen here) in an indentation in the cell wall. Pericytes (P), external lamina (EL), capillary endothelial cell (E). Magnification ×38,900.

keratopathy (PCK). In PCK immunoglobulin deposits may be seen in the corneal stroma either as organized or randomly arranged extracellular tubules (Fig. 30.25) (Stirling & Graff 1995; Stirling et al 1997) or as intracellular crytalloids with a fine fibrillar substructure (Fig. 30.26) (Henderson et al 1993).

Cilia

Cilia are small motile structures approximately 5–10 μm long and 0.5 μm in diameter. Within the ciliary shaft there is a core of microtubules (the axoneme) composed of nine outer pairs of microtubules and one inner (central) pair, an arrangement referred to as the '9+2' configuration (Fig. 30.27) (Sturgess & Turner 1984; Young & Heath 2000).

A wide range of primary and secondary structural defects may be found in cilia; secondary defects, such as disorganized microtubules, can be ignored (Sturgess & Turner 1984; Carson et al 1994). Primary defects are caused by genetic abnormalities that result in immotile cilia syndrome (primary ciliary dyskinesia—PCD) (Meeks & Bush 2000). In PCD, the ciliary defects are permanent and all cilia in the body are affected (Corrin & Dewar 1992; Mierau et al 1992). The principal defects are (Sturgess & Turner 1984; Corrin & Dewar 1992; Mierau et al 1992; Carson et al 1994):

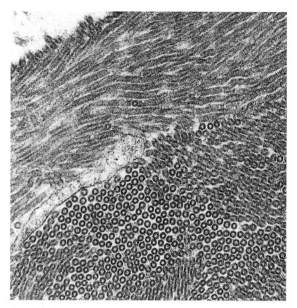

Fig. 30.25 Paraproteinemic crystalloidal keratopathy. Extracellular tubular crystalloids are found throughout the corneal stroma in this case. Tubules are thick-walled and of indeterminate length. Overall tubule diameter is 40–45 nm. The crystalloids label for κ light chains in immunogold labeling studies (Henderson et al 1993). Magnification ×38,750.

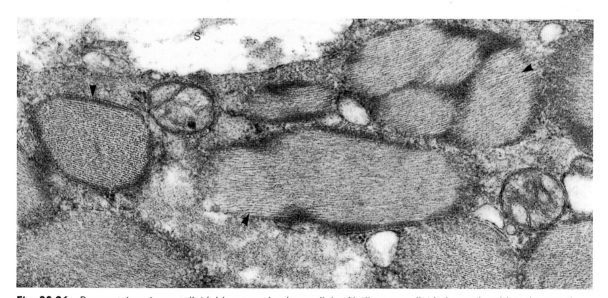

Fig. 30.26 Paraproteinemic crystalloidal keratopathy. Intracellular fibrillary crystalloids (arrow heads) in the cytoplasm of a corneal keratinocyte. Filaments are approximately 8–10 nm in diameter. The crystalloids labeled for κ light chains in immunogold labeling studies (Henderson et al 1993). Extracellular stroma (S). Magnification ×38,800.

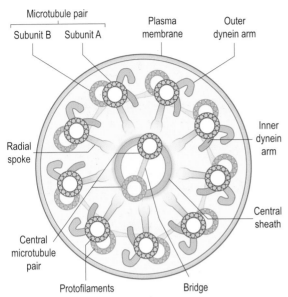

Fig. 30.27 Normal cilium. Schematic cross-section through the middle of a normal ciliary shaft to show the structure of the axoneme. The axoneme is formed from an outer ring of nine microtubule pairs with one central pair (the 9+2 configuration). The outer microtubule pairs are formed from two subunits (A and B); each subunit is formed from a ring of protofilaments. Projecting from each complete microtubule in the outer microtubule pairs (subunit A) is a pair of inner and outer dynein arms. A variety of structures (the radial spokes, bridge, and sheath) appear to link the tubule pairs together.

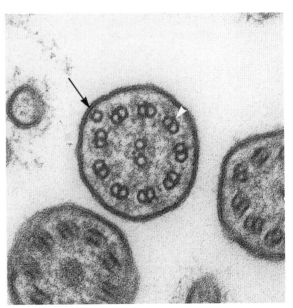

Fig. 30.28 Primary ciliary dyskinesia: dynein arm defect. The outer microtubule pairs (arrow head) lack dynein arms. A single extra displaced microtubule is also present (arrow). Magnification ×135,200.

- Dynein arms absent or short (most cases) (Fig. 30.28)
- Ciliary spokes absent
- Outer microtubular pairs absent, displaced, or discontinuous
- Central microtubular pair with one or both microtubules absent.

Observations should be made in the middle of the ciliary shaft, and approximately 50 cilia are recommended as a minimum number for examination. In routinely processed specimens the inner arms are often indistinct. However, this is undoubtedly a processing artifact and such cilia are presumed to be normal. Finally, it should be noted that not all genetic defects may result in abnormal ciliary morphology (Santamaria et al 1999).

Microsporidia

The microsporidia are a group of obligate intracellular parasites belonging to the phylum Microspora (Weber et al 1994; Curry 1998; Wasson & Peper 2000). Unclassified organisms are called by the collective name 'microsporidium' but this is not a true genus. A number of species have been identified in humans, with *Enterocytozoon bieneusi* the most common (Figs 30.29 and 30.30, and Table 30.11).

TEM plays an important role in the identification of microsporidia and is regarded by some as the gold standard for diagnosis (Curry 2000). The organisms can be examined using fecal material or tissue biopsies with standard fixation and processing protocols (Weber et al 1994).

The major ultrastructural features used for typing microsporidia (Garcia & Bruckner 1993; Bryan 1994; Weber et al 1994; Curry 1998) are as follows:

- the size and morphology of the various developmental stages

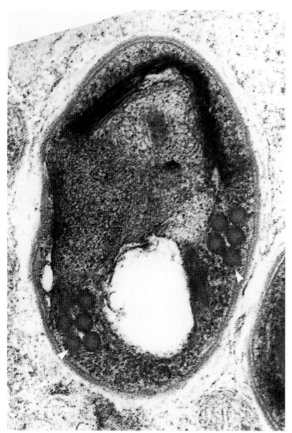

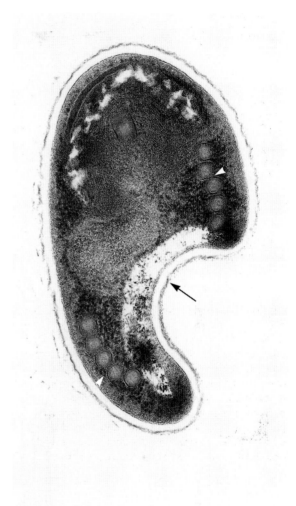

Fig. 30.29 *Enterocytozoon bieneusi.* Maturing spore showing the coils of the polar tube. In *E. bieneusi* the polar tube has a range of 4–7 coils which, in cross-section, are seen arranged in two rows on either side of the spore. The spore shown has 5–6 coils on either side (arrow heads). Electron micrograph courtesy of Dr Alan Curry. Magnification ×72,000.

Fig. 30.30 *Encephalitozoon hellem.* Spore of *E. hellem* showing the polar tube with five coils arranged in a single row on each side of the spore (arrow heads). The indentation (arrow) is an artifact caused by the collapse of the posterior vacuole. Electron micrograph courtesy of Dr Alan Curry. Magnification ×72,000.

- the configuration of the nuclei in spores and developmental stages
- the host–parasite interface
- the number of coils in the tubular extrusion apparatus in spores (Figs 30.29 and 30.30).

Table 30.11   Microsporidia found in humans

Species	Citation
Encephalitozoon hellem (Fig. 30.30)	Didier et al 1991a, 1991b
Encephalitozoon cuniculi	Pakes et al 1975; Canning et al 1986
Encephalitozoon (Septata) intestinalis	Cali et al 1993; Hartskeerl et al 1995
Pleistophora ronneafiei	Cali & Takvorian 2003
Pleistophora spp.	Canning et al 1986; Weber et al 1994
Trachipleistophora hominis	Hollister et al 1996
Trachipleistophora anthropophthera	Vavra et al 1998
Enterocytozoon bieneusi (Fig. 30.29)	Desportes et al 1985; Curry 2000
Nosema ocularum	Cali et al 1991
Vittaforma corneae (Nosema corneum)	Silveira & Canning 1995
Vittaforma sp.	Sulaiman et al 2003
*Anncaliia vesicularum**	Cali et al 1998
Anncaliia connor (Nosema connori)*	Sprague 1974; Cali et al 1998
Anncaliia algarae (Nosema algarae)*	Visvesvara et al 1999
Microsporidium ceylonensis	Ashton & Wirasinha 1973; Canning et al 1998
Microsporidium africanum	Pinnolis et al 1981

* *Anncaliia* replaces the genus *Brachiola* (Franzen et al 2006).

Acknowledgments

We thank Richard Davey (SouthPath, Flinders Medical Centre) for his assistance in preparing the illustrations for this chapter.

Graham Robinson contributed the text for this chapter for the first and second editions. Stan Terras updated the second edition, and Graham Robinson and Trevor Gray the third and fourth editions. Alan Stevens contributed to editions two, three, and four. Our acknowledgments are due to them for their contributions.

REFERENCES

Acetarin J-D., Carlemalm E., Villiger W. (1986) Developments of new Lowicryl® resins for embedding biological specimens at even lower temperatures. Journal of Microscopy 143:81–88.

Allen D.E., Lawrence F.A. (1994–1996) Tissue preparation for transmission electron microscopy. In: Woods A.E., Ellis R.C., eds. Laboratory histopathology: a complete reference. Edinburgh: Churchill Livingstone.

Alpers C.E. (1992) Immunotactoid (microtubular) glomerulopathy: an entity distinct from fibrillary glomerulonephritis? American Journal of Kidney Disease 2:185–191.

Anton-Lamprecht I. (1992) The skin. In: Papadimitriou J.M., Henderson D.W., Spagnolo D.V., eds. Diagnostic ultrastructure of non-neoplastic diseases. Edinburgh: Churchill Livingstone, pp. 459–550.

Ashton N., Wirasinha P.A. (1973) Encephalitozoonosis (Nosematosis) of the cornea. British Journal of Ophthalmology 57:669–674.

Bergmann M., Ebke M., Yuan Y. et al. (1996) Cerebral autosomal dominant arteriopathy with subcortical infarcts and leukoencephalopathy (CADASIL): a morphological study of a German family. Acta Neuropathologica (Berlin) 92:341–350.

Bretschneider A., Burns W., Morrison A. (1981) 'Pop-off' technic. The ultrastructure of paraffin-embedded sections. American Journal of Clinical Pathology 76:450–453.

Bryan R.T. (1994) Microsporidia. In: Mandell G.L. Bennett J.E., Dolin R., eds. Principles and practice of infectious diseases, 4th edn. New York: Churchill Livingstone, Part III, pp. 2513–2524.

Cali A., Takvorian P.M. (2003) Ultrastructure and development of *Pleistophora ronneafiei* n. sp., a microsporidium (*Protista*) in the skeletal muscle of an immune-compromised individual. Journal of Eukaryotic Microbiology 50(2):77–85.

Cali A., Meisler D., Lowder C.Y. et al. (1991) Corneal microsporidioses: characterisation and identification. Journal of Eucaryotic Microbiology 38:215S–217S.

Cali A., Kotler D.P., Orenstein J.M. (1993) *Septata intestinalis* n.g., n.sp., an intestinal microsporidian associated with chronic diarrhea and dissemination in AIDS patients. Journal of Protozoologyy 40:101–112.

Cali A., Takvorian P.M., Lewin S. et al. (1998) *Brachiola vesicularum*, n.g., n. sp., a new microsporium associated with AIDS and myositis. Journal of Eucaryotic Microbiology 45:240–251.

Canning E.U., Lom J., Dykova I. (1986) The microsporidia of vertebrates. New York: Academic Press.

Canning E.U., Curry A., Vavra J., Bonshek R.E. (1998) Some ultrastructural data on *Microsporidium ceylonensis*, a cause of corneal microsporidiosis. Parasite 5(3): 247–254.

Carson J.L., Collier A.M., Fernald G.W., Hu S.S. (1994) Microtubular discontinuities as acquired ciliary defects in airway epithelium of patients with chronic respiratory diseases. Ultrastructural Pathology 18:327–332.

Carstens P.H.B. (1992) Contact between abluminal microvilli and collagen fibrils in metastatic adenocarcinoma and mesothelioma. Journal of Pathology 166:179–182.

Causton B.E. (1981) Resins: toxicity, hazards and safe handling. Proceedings of the Royal Microscopy Society 16:265–269.

Coleman M., Stirling J.W. (1991) Glomerular basement thinning is acquired in minimal change disease. American Journal of Nephrology 11:437–438.

Coleman M., Haynes W.D.G., Dimopoulos P. et al. (1986) Glomerular basement membrane abnormalities associated with apparently idiopathic hematuria: ultrastructural morphometric analysis. Human Pathology 17:1022–1030.

Coleman M., Henderson D.W., Mukherjee T.M. (1989) The ultrastructural pathology of malignant pleural mesothelioma. Pathology Annual 24(1):303–353.

Comin C.E., de Klerk N.H., Henderson D.W. (1997) Malignant mesothelioma: current conundrums over risk estimates and whither electron microscopy for diagnosis? Ultrastructural Pathology 21:315–320.

Corrin B., Dewar A. (1992) Respiratory diseases. In: Papadimitriou J.M., Henderson D.W., Spagnolo D.V., eds. Diagnostic ultrastructure of non-neoplastic diseases. Edinburgh: Churchill Livingstone, pp. 264–286.

Curry A. (1998) Microsporidians. In: Cox F., Kreier J., Wakelin D., eds. Topley and Wilson's microbiology and microbial infections, 9th edn. London: Arnold, Vol. 5, pp. 411–430.

Curry A. (2000) Electron microscopy as a tool for identifying new pathogens. Journal of Infection 40:107–115.

Daddow L.Y.M. (1983) A double lead stain method for enhancing contrast of ultrathin sections in electron microscopy: a modified multiple staining technique. Journal of Microscopy 129:147–153.

Desportes I., Le Charpentier Y., Galian A. et al. (1985) Occurrence of a new microsporidian: *Enterozoon bieneusi* n.g., n.sp., in the enterocytes of a human patient with AIDS. Journal of Protozoology 32:250–254.

Didier E.S., Didier P.J., Friedberg D.N. et al. (1991a) Isolation and characterisation of a new human microsporidian, *Encephalitozoon hellem* (n.sp.), from three AIDS patients with keratoconjunctivitis. Journal of Infectious Diseases 163:617–621.

Didier P.J., Didier E.S., Orenstein J.M., Shadduck J.A. (1991b) Fine structure of a new human microsporidian, *Encephalitozoon hellem*, in culture. Journal of Protozoology 38:502–507.

Dykstra M.J. (1992) Biological electron microscopy: theory, techniques and troubleshooting. New York: Plenum Press.

Erlandson R.A. (1994) Diagnostic transmission electron microscopy of tumors. New York: Raven Press.

Ferguson W.J., Braunschweiger K.I., Braunschweiger W.R. et al. (1980) Hydrogen ion buffers for biological research. Analytical Biochemistry 104:300–310.

Franzen C., Nassonova E.S., Schölmerich J., Issi I.V. (2006) Transfer of the members of the genus *Brachiola* (Microsporidia) to the genus *Anncaliia* based on ultrastructural and molecular data. Journal of Eukaryotic Microbiology 53:26–35.

Garcia L.S., Bruckner D.A. (1993) Diagnostic medical microbiology, 2nd edn. Washington, DC: American Society for Microbiology.

Ghadially F.N. (1985) Diagnostic electron microscopy of tumours, 2nd edn. London: Butterworths.

Ghadially F.N. (1997) Ultrastructural pathology of the cell and matrix, 4th edn. Vols 1–2. Boston: Butterworth-Heinemann.

Gillmore J.D., Hawkins P.N., Pepys M.B. (1997) Amyloidosis: a review of recent diagnostic and therapeutic developments. British Journal of Haematology 99: 245–256.

Glauert A.M. (1972–1998) Practical methods in electron microscopy, Vols 1–17. Amsterdam: North Holland.

Glauert A.M., Glauert R.H. (1958) Araldite as an embedding medium for electron microscopy. Journal of Biophysical and Biochemical Cytology 4:191–194.

Glauert A.M., Lewis P.R. (1998) Biological specimen preparation for transmission electron microscopy. Practical methods in electron microscopy, Vol. 17. London: Portland Press.

Glauert A.M., Rogers G.E., Glauert R.H. (1956) A new embedding medium for electron microscopy. Nature 178:803.

Gomori G. (1955) Preparation of buffers for use in enzyme studies. Methods in Enzymology 1:138–146.

Good N.E., Izawa S. (1972) Hydrogen ion buffers. Methods in Enzymology 24:53–68.

Good N.E., Winget G.D., Winter W. et al. (1966) Hydrogen ions for biological research. Biochemistry 5:467–477.

Grier H.E. (1997) The Ewing family of tumors. Ewing's sarcoma and primitive neuroectodermal tumors. Pediatric Clinics of North America 44(4):991–1004.

Hartskeerl R.A., Van Gool T., Schuitema A.R. et al. (1995) Genetic and immunological characterisation of the microsporidian *Septata intestinalis* Cali, Kotler and Orenstein 1993: reclassification to *Encephalitozoon intestinalis*. Parasitology 110:277–285.

Harvey J.M., Anton-Lamprecht I. (1992) Stromal aberrations. In: Papadimitriou J.M., Henderson D.W., Spagnolo D.V., eds. Diagnostic ultrastructure of non-neoplastic diseases. Edinburgh: Churchill Livingstone, pp. 84–109.

Hayat M.A. (1981) Fixation for electron microscopy. New York: Academic Press.

Hayat M.A. (1993) Stains and cytochemical methods. New York: Plenum Press.

Hayat M.A. (2000) Principles and techniques of electron microscopy: biological applications, 4th edn. Cambridge: Cambridge University Press.

Henderson D.W. (1982) Asbestos-related pleuropulmonary diseases: asbestosis, mesothelioma and lung cancer. Pathology 14:239–243.

Henderson D.W., Papadimitriou J.M., Coleman M. (1986) Ultrastructural appearances of tumours. diagnosis and classification of human neoplasia by electron microscopy, 2nd edn. Edinburgh: Churchill Livingstone.

Henderson D.W., Leppard P.J., Brennan J.S. et al. (1989) Primitive neuroepithelial tumours of soft tissues and bone: further ultrastructural and immunocytochemical clarification of 'Ewing's sarcoma', including freeze-fracture analysis. Journal of Submicroscopic Cytology and Pathology 21(1):35–57.

Henderson D.W., Shilkin K.B., Whitaker D. et al. (1992) The pathology of malignant mesothelioma, including immunohistology and ultrastructure. In: Henderson D. W., Shilkin K.B., Langlois S. et al., eds. Malignant mesothelioma. New York: Hemisphere, pp. 69–139.

Henderson D.W., Stirling J.W., Lipsett J. et al. (1993) Paraproteinemic crystalloidal keratopathy: an ultrastructural study of two cases, including immunoelectron microscopy. Ultrastructural Pathology 17:643–668.

Henderson D.W., Comin C.E., Hammar S.P. et al. (1997) Malignant mesothelioma of the pleura: current surgical pathology. In: Corrin B., ed. Pathology of lung tumours. New York: Churchill Livingstone, pp. 241–280.

Hollister W.S., Canning E.U., Weidner E. et al. (1996) Development and ultrastructure of *Trachipleistophora hominis* n.g., n.sp. after in vitro isolation from an AIDS patient and inoculation into athymic mice. Parasitology 112(1):143–154.

Jaunzems A.E., Woods A.E. (1997) Ultrastructural differentiation of epidermolysis bullosa subtypes and porphyria cutanea tarda. Pathology, Research and Practice 193:207–217.

Jaunzems A.E., Woods A.E., Staples A. (1997) Electron microscopy and morphometry enhances differentiation of epidermolysis bullosa subtypes with normal values for 24 parameters in skin. Archives of Dermatological Research 289(11):631–639.

Jennette J.C., Iskandar S.S., Falk R.J. (1994) Fibrillary glomerulonephritis. In: Tisher C.C., Brenner B.M., eds. Renal pathology with clinical and functional correlations, 2nd edn. Philadelphia: Lippincott.

Jennette J.C., Olson J.L., Schwartz M.M., Silva F.G., eds. (1998) Heptinstall's pathology of the kidney, 5th edn. Philadelphia: Lippincott-Raven, Vols 1–2.

Jolanki R., Kanerva L., Estlander T. et al. (1990) Occupational dermatoses from epoxy resin compounds. Contact Dermatitis 23:172–183.

Kalimo H., Viitanen M., Amberla K. et al. (1999) CADASIL: hereditary disease of arteries causing brain infarcts and dementia. Neuropathology and Applied Neurobiology 25(4):257–265.

Kanerva L., Estlander T., Jolanki R. (1989) Allergic contact dermatitis from dental composite resins due to aromatic epoxy acrylates and aliphatic acrylates. Contact Dermatitis 20:201–211.

Karnovsky M.J. (1965) A formaldehyde–glutaraldehyde fixative of high osmolarity for use in electron microscopy. Journal of Cell Biology 27:137A.

Leong A.S.-Y. (1994) Fixation and fixatives. In: Woods A. E., Ellis R.C., eds. Laboratory histopathology: a complete reference. Edinburgh: Churchill Livingstone.

Luft J.H. (1961) Improvements in epoxy resin embedding methods. Journal of Biophysical and Biochemical Cytology 9:409–414.

Marinkovich M.P. (1999) Update on inherited bullous dermatoses. Dermatologic Clinics 17(3):473–485.

Massie H.R., Samis H.V., Baird M.B. (1972) The effects of the buffer HEPES on the division potential of WI-38 cells. In Vitro 7:191–197.

Meeks M., Bush A. (2000) Primary ciliary dyskinesia (PCD). Pediatric Pulmonology 29(4):307–316.

Mellerio J.E. (1999) Molecular pathology of the cutaneous basement membrane zone. Clinical and Experimental Dermatology 24:25–32.

Mierau G.W., Agostini R., Beals T.F. et al. (1992) The role of electron microscopy in evaluating ciliary dysfunction: Report of a workshop. Ultrastructural Pathology 16:245–254.

Millonig G., Marinozzi V. (1968) Fixation and embedding in electron microscopy. In: Barer R., Cosslett V.E., eds. Advances in optical and electron microscopy. New York: Academic Press, Vol. 2, p. 251.

Newman G.R., Hobot J.A. (1987) Modern acrylics for post-embedding immunostaining techniques. Journal of Histochemistry and Cytochemistry 35:971–981.

Newman G.R., Hobot J.A. (1993) Resin microscopy and on-section immunocytochemistry. Berlin: Springer.

Oury T.D., Hammar S.P., Roggli V.L. (1998) Ultrastructural features of diffuse malignant mesotheliomas. Human Pathology 29(12):1382–1392.

Pakes S.P., Shadduck J.A., Cali A. (1975) Fine structure of *Encephalitozoon cuniculi* from rabbits, mice and hamsters. Journal of Protozoology 22:481–488.

Palade G.E. (1952) A study of fixation for electron microscopy. Journal of Experimental Medicine 95:285–298.

Papadimitriou J.M., Henderson D.W., Spagnolo D.V. (1992a) Skeletal muscle. In: Papadimitriou J.M., Henderson D.W., Spagnolo D.V., eds. Diagnostic ultrastructure of non-neoplastic diseases. Edinburgh: Churchill Livingstone, pp. 594–614.

Papadimitriou J.M., Henderson D.W., Spagnolo D.V., eds. (1992b) Diagnostic ultrastructure of non-neoplastic diseases. Edinburgh: Churchill Livingstone.

Pearl G.S., Ghatak N.R. (1995) Muscle biopsy. Archives of Pathology and Laboratory Medicine 119:303–306.

Pinnolis M., Egbert P.R., Font R.L., Winter F.C. (1981) Nosematosis of the cornea. Archives of Ophthalmology 99:1044–1047.

Plumel M. (1948) Sodium cacodylate buffer solutions. Bulletin de la Société de Chimie Biologique 30:129–130.

Pulkkinen L., Uitto J. (1999) Mutation analysis and molecular genetics of epidermolysis bullosa. Matrix Biology 18:29–42.

Reid N. (1975) Ultramicrotomy. In: Glauert A.M., ed. Practical methods in electron microscopy, Vol. 3 Part 2. Amsterdam: North Holland.

Reynolds E.S. (1963) The use of lead citrate at high pH as an electron opaque stain based on metal chelation. Journal of Cell Biology 17:208–212.

Richardson K.C., Jarett L., Finke E.H. (1960) Embedding in epoxy resins for ultrathin sectioning in EM. Stain Technology 35:313–316.

Ringo D.L., Brennan E.F., Costa-Robles E.H. (1982) Epoxy resins are mutagenic: implications for electron micro-scopists. Journal of Ultrastructural Research 80:280–287.

Rippstein P., Cavell S., Boivin M., Dardick I. (1987) Low magnification transmission electron microscopy in diagnostic pathology. Ultrastructural Pathology 11:723–729.

Robards A.W., Wilson A.J. (1993) Procedures in electron microscopy. New York: Wiley.

Robinson G., Gray T. (1996) Electron microscopy 2: practical procedures. In: Bancroft J.D., Stevens A., eds. Theory and practice of histological techniques, 4th edn. Edinburgh: Churchill Livingstone.

Rostagno A., Vidal R., Kumar A. et al. (1996) Fibrillary glomerulonephritis related to serum fibrillar immunoglobulin–fibronectin complexes. American Journal of Kidney Disease 28:676–684.

Ruchoux M.M., Maurage C.A. (1997) CADASIL: cerebral autosomal dominant arteriopathy with subcortical infarcts and leukoencephalopathy. Journal of Neuropathology and Experimental Neurology 56(9):947–964.

Ruchoux M.M., Maurage C.A. (1998) Endothelial changes in muscle and skin biopsies in patients with CADASIL. Neuropathology and Applied Neurobiology 24(1):60–65.

Sabatini D.D., Bensch K., Barrnett R.J. (1963) Cytochemistry and electron microscopy: the preservation of cellular ultrastructure and enzymic activity by aldehyde fixation. Journal of Cell Biology 17:19–25.

Salema R., Brandão I. (1973) The use of PIPES buffer in the fixation of plant cells for electron microscopy. Journal of Submicroscopic Cytology 5:79–96.

Santamaria F., de Santi M.M., Grillo G. et al. (1999) Ciliary motility at light microscopy: a screening technique for ciliary defects. Acta Paediatrica 88(8):853–857.

Schochet S.S., Lampert P.W. (1978) Diagnostic electron microscopy of skeletal muscle. In: Trump B.F., Jones R.T., eds. Diagnostic electron microscopy. New York: John Wiley, Vol. 1, pp. 209–251.

Schwartz M.M. (1998) Glomerular diseases with organised deposits. In: Jennette J.C., Olson J.L., Schwartz M.M., Silva F.G., eds. Heptinstall's pathology of the kidney, 5th edn. Philadelphia: Lippincott-Raven, Vol. 1, pp. 369–388.

Silveira H., Canning E.U. (1995) *Vittaforma corneae* n.comb. for the human microsporidium *Nosema corneum*, Shadduck, Meccoli, Davis & Font, 1990 based on its ultrastructure in the liver of experimentally infected athymic mice. Journal of Eukaryotic Microbiology 42:158–165.

Sprague V. (1974) *Nosema connori* n.sp., microsporidian parasite of man. Transactions of the American Microscopy Society 93:400–403.

Spurr A. (1969) A low viscosity epoxy resin embedding medium for electron microscopy. Journal of Ultrastructural Research 26:31–43.

Stirling J.W. (1994) Immunogold labelling: resin sections. In: Woods A.E., Ellis R.C., eds. Laboratory histopathology: a complete reference. Edinburgh: Churchill Livingstone.

Stirling J.W., Graff P.S. (1995) Antigen unmasking for electron microscopy. Journal of Histochemistry and Cytochemistry 43:115–123.

Stirling J.W., Henderson D.W., Rozenbilds M.A.M. et al. (1997) Crystalloidal paraprotein deposits in the cornea: an ultrastructural study of two new cases with tubular crystalloids that contain IgG κ light chains and IgG γ heavy chains. Ultrastructural Pathology 21:337–344.

Stirling J.W., Coleman M., Thomas A., Woods A.E. (1999) Role of transmission electron microscopy in tissue diagnosis: diseases of the kidney, skeletal muscle and myocardium. Journal of Cellular Pathology 4(4):223–243.

Strom E.H., Hurwitz N., Mayr A.C. et al. (1996) Immunotactoid-like glomerulopathy with massive fibrillary deposits in liver and bone marrow in monoclonal gammopathy. American Journal of Nephrology 16:523–528.

Sturgess J.M., Turner J.A.P. (1984) Ultrastructural pathology of cilia in the immotile cilia syndrome. Perspectives in Paediatric Pathology 8:133–161.

Sulaiman I.M., Matos O., Lobo M.L., Xiao L. (2003) Identification of a new microsporidian parasite related to *Vittaforma corneae* in HIV-positive and HIV-negative patients from Portugal. Journal of Eukaryotic Microbiology 50(Suppl):586–590.

Tisher C.C., Brenner B.M. (1994) Renal pathology with clinical and functional correlations, 2nd edn. Philadelphia: Lippincott.

Vavra J., Yachnis A.T., Shadduck J.A., Orenstein J.M. (1998) Microsporidia of the genus *Trachipleistophora*—causative agents of human microsporidiosis—description of *Trachipleistophora anthropophthera* n.sp. (Protozoa, Microsporidia). Journal of Eucaryotic Microbiology 45:273–283.

Verani R.R. (1993) Fibrillary glomerulopathy. Kidney 2:63–66.

Visvesvara G.S., Bellosis M., Moura H. et al. (1999) Isolation of *Nosema algerae* from the cornea of an immunocompetent patient. Journal of Eukaryotic Microbiology 46(5):10S.

Warhol M.J., Hickey W.F., Corson J.M. (1982) Malignant mesothelioma. Ultrastructural distinction from adenocarcinoma. American Journal of Surgical Pathology 6(4):307–314.

Wasson, K., Peper, R.L. (2000) Mammalian microsporidiosis. Veterinary Pathology 37(2):113–128.

Weber R., Bryan R.T., Schwartz D.A., Owen R.L. (1994) Human microsporidial infections. Clinical Microbiology Reviews 7(4):426–461.

Young B., Heath J.W. (2000) Wheater's functional histology. A text and colour atlas, 4th edn. Edinburgh: Churchill Livingstone.

31

Quantitative Data from Microscopic Specimens

Alton D. Floyd

INTRODUCTION

The practice of histology and histopathology has traditionally relied upon the *subjective* interpretation of microscopic preparations by a highly trained individual. The accuracy with which such interpretations can be made is the foundation of histology and of histopathology. That said, it is important to note that these interpretations are based on *pattern recognition*, that is, overall arrangements of elements within the specimen, a task for which the human visual system is well suited. The human visual system is not well suited for quantitative functions, such as assessment of linear measurements, areas, or density of stain. The human eye is a remarkable sensor, but one that is highly adaptable. It is able to alter its sensitivity depending on the brightness of the object being viewed. The eye is also a non-linear sensor, with a response to brightness that more closely approaches a logarithmic response. These two characteristics preclude accurate assessment of the density of specimens viewed through a microscope.

Human observers do not accurately estimate physical distances and areas of specimens. The eye is reasonably good at comparisons, and most microscopists will 'estimate' sizes based on some internal specimen object, such as the diameter of red blood cells. Even with such comparisons, length and size estimates made by microscopists are neither accurate nor highly repeatable. It is the purpose of image quantitation to eliminate observer-to-observer variation, and produce evaluations that are accurate and repeatable.

In recognition of the problem of accurately describing physical measurements in microscopic specimens, manufacturers of microscopes have included various calibration devices. For spatial measurements within the object, an eyepiece (ocular) reticule is used. These reticules typically consist of either a single line, or a crossed line (like the '+' symbol) that are marked off in even increments. Reticules are also available that are in the form of a grid. For a reticule to be useful for measurement, it must be calibrated for each magnification at which it is used. This is done by use of a stage micrometer, which is a microscope slide with an accurate scale etched or photographically applied to the slide. Typically, these stage micrometers have divisions of 0.1 and 0.01 millimeters. After calibrating the reticule with a stage micrometer, the reticule can be used directly to measure linear dimensions of microscopic objects.

Microscopes also are calibrated in the 'Z' axis, which is the axis that controls stage (or nosepiece) movement. This calibration is found around the focus control knob, and is generally calibrated in microns. The 'Z' axis calibration can be used to estimate the thickness of a microscopic specimen, assuming that one can accurately determine the 'top' and 'bottom' of the focal plane through the object of interest. Accuracy can be improved by using a high numerical aperture, shallow depth of field objective, since this assists in finding the top and bottom focal plane of the object. Modern usage of 'Z' axis movement is more commonly associated with collection of a series of images at various focal planes (an image stack) that can be used subsequently to construct three-dimensional representations of the specimen.

Morphometry is the general term used to describe the measurement of size parameters of a specimen. Size is here defined as length, height, and area of an object of interest. These basic measurements can be combined to provide additional measurements, such as perimeter, smoothness, centers, etc. For some of these additional measurement parameters, it is important to understand the specific mathematical formula (algorithm) used, as there may be more than one definition of a particular parameter, and two different implementations of what appears (by algorithm name) to be an identical measurement may not be the same.

TRADITIONAL APPROACHES

The history of development of the microscope is filled with clever devices designed to assist in performing morphometry of specimens. One such device is the camera lucida, which is an optical system that projects an image of the specimen onto a surface adjacent to the microscope. This projected image can be used to draw the specimen, or to measure portions of the image. Accurate measurements within these projected images require calibration of the projection, in a manner identical to that used to calibrate reticules.

Photographic approaches have eliminated the use of the camera lucida in many laboratories, as convenient cameras have become universally available for microscopes. As with projections, a photographic system must be calibrated, using a stage micrometer. In addition to the calibration of the photographic negative, the enlarging process must also be calibrated for accurate measurements. For both camera lucida drawings and photographs, areas are generally determined using a device called a planimeter. This is a mechanical device that is used manually to trace the outline of objects of interest. Using a set of 'x' and 'y' calibrated wheels, the total area of the object is determined. For the planimeter data to be accurate, a standard area at the magnification of the specimen must be determined, and this then becomes a calibration factor used to interpret the planimeter data.

Stereology is a technique developed for analysis of metals and minerals, where generally the properties being measured relate to number, size, and distribution of some particle in the sample. Being based in geometry and probability theory, and using statistical mathematics, stereology makes specific assumptions about the object being analyzed. A general discussion of the theoretical basis of stereology can be found in DeHoff and Rhines (1968), and in Underwood (1970). Stereological techniques have been applied to many biological images,

both light and electron microscopical. General principles and applications can be found in Weibel (1979, 1980, 1990), in Elias and Hyde (1983), and in Elias et al (1978). Although there is a long history of use of stereology in histology and histopathology, the use of this technique makes assumptions about the specimen that may not be applicable. Since the foundation of stereology is statistical, the general nature of the distribution of whatever is being measured should be describable using some statistic. This condition may be met under specific conditions, such as examining the distribution of chromatin 'clumps' within a cell nucleus, where the only object being examined is a single nucleus. For highly ordered structures, such as gland elements within an organ, the organization of the structure implies that there is no statistical distribution. Stereology can make estimates of some parameters of specimens, such as area of a total image occupied by some particular component. Note that this is an estimate. Use of stereology to derive measures of the three-dimensional structure of cell and tissue specimens may provide misleading information, since the probabilities used in the mathematics assume that the entire volume of the specimen is accurately reflected in the portion measured. Due to the polarization of cell organelles, and the arrangement of tissues and organs, this is generally not the case.

While one cannot disagree that stereology has provided many useful insights into microscopic specimens, modern techniques of measurement can provide real measures of the specimen without any assumptions of the distribution pattern. The development of newer forms of microscopy (confocal) has extended this direct measurement capability to the third dimension. With the speed of modern image analysis systems, there is little justification for performing an estimate of a cell or tissue parameter when the actual parameter can be accurately measured, often in less time than is required for the stereological approach. An in-depth review of stereology can be found in the fourth edition of this book.

Electronic light microscopy

Electronic measurements of light transmitted through microscopic specimens has a long history, and roughly parallels the development of photometers, spectrophotometers, and light-detecting devices. Until recently (1980s), these devices simply detected light, and did not produce images. To use these early devices to produce images, the portion of the specimen visible to the light detector had to be restricted, and the specimen or image moved across this restricted area to generate an actual image. Many mechanisms were developed to acquire images using such techniques (Wied 1966; Wied & Bahr 1970). These mechanisms tended to be expensive, since they required high precision, and were also slow, as the image had to be acquired a small area at a time, and then 'put together' or reconstructed into a recognizable image. The majority of literature relating to quantitative light microscopy which utilized electronic measurement of light therefore was actually related to photometric and spectrophotometric studies, rather than analysis of images as currently defined.

Microscope photometry

A detailed theoretical account of microscope photometry can be found in Piller (1977). The hardware systems for obtaining data described in Piller have been superseded by modern devices, but the theoretical foundations are sound. The fundamental requirement for photometry is described by the Beer–Lambert law:

$$A = t \cdot c \cdot \varepsilon$$

where A is the absorbance, t is the path length of the absorbing material, c is the concentration of the absorbing material, and ε is the absorptivity.

In practical terms, for microscopic images, the path length (t) is approximately a constant, and for a given material being measured (usually a dye bound to the specimen) the absorptivity (ε) is also a constant. Therefore, the absorbance of the specimen is directly proportional to the concentration of the absorbing material.

Absorbance is defined as:

$$A = \text{Log} \, 1/T$$

where T is the transmittance. Transmittance is defined as the fraction of light that is transmitted through the specimen (Light through specimen/Light through blank).

A requirement of the Beer–Lambert law is that material being measured be homogeneous (there are a few other restrictions, regarding maximum absorptivities, but these are not ordinarily met in transmitted light microscopy). The requirement of homogeneity is a significant one, as we routinely examine specimens with a microscope to observe structure, and this by definition is non-homogeneous.

The measurement of non-homogeneous materials using photometry gives rise to distributional error. While one can illustrate these errors nicely with mathematical equations, microscopists can grasp the concept intuitively with a simple, classical example. Suppose you have a chamber filled with water, such as an aquarium, and you shine light through the aquarium and measure the light traversing the chamber. Now, place a capped bottle of ink in the water of the aquarium. Depending on the size of the bottle, you may note a small effect on the amount of light that passes through the chamber. If you now uncap the ink bottle, and let the ink diffuse through the aquarium contents, the amount of light that passes through the chamber will be significantly reduced. When you think about this example, note that the amount of ink in the aquarium is identical in the two cases, capped and uncapped bottle. The difference is the *distribution* of the ink. For this reason, the error that results from photometry of non-homogeneous materials is referred to as *distributional error* and can be shown to induce error as large as 50% with certain distributions.

Recognition of distributional error was the reason quantitative microscopes employed various devices to permit restricting the area of the specimen seen by the detector to a small area. This strategy was successful because of the optics of the microscope itself. A given lens resolution is defined as the ability to separate two points (point resolution). If a lens cannot separate two points, then they look like a single object. If a light detector sees an area of the specimen that is smaller than the point resolution of the microscope lens combination in use, then, by definition, that area is homogeneous, since the lens cannot see any structure in that area. For microscope lenses of 40× magnification and above, general 'area examined' sizes for photometry range from 0.25 to 0.5 micron diameter spots. Such spot sizes generally avoid significant distributional error. When such spots are generated by mechanical 'stops' or pinholes in the optical path of the microscope, they may introduce other, significant, sources of error, such as edge diffraction. These sources of error, as well as many others such as glare within the optical system, are discussed in detail in Piller (1977). The above discussion applies to absorbing images only, that is, microscope images obtained with transmitted light microscopy. Fluorescence emission microscopy and particle reflectance (autoradiography) are based on different physical principles, and require different optics and sensor configurations.

Image acquisition

As mentioned earlier, images can be acquired with systems that examine specimens a small spot at a time. Using mechanical systems such as scanning stages or Nipkow discs, an image similar to that seen through the microscope can be acquired. With a scanning stage device, the time required to acquire such an image may range into hours. In all mechanical scanning systems, the precision and repeatability required for high-quality images translate to slow, expensive, and difficult-to-use systems.

The development of television cameras provided hope for acquiring images through microscopes. Early television cameras were vacuum tube devices, and were not suitable for quantitative microscope image use. Images collected with these devices were of low resolution, and suffered from a variety of geometric and photometric distortions related to the electronics used to operate the scanning circuits of the tube, and to read out the resulting image signals.

During the decade of the 1980s, a variety of solid-state sensors were developed for television (video) purposes. One technology in particular, the CCD (Charge Coupled Device) camera, matured into a significantly useful device for microscopic imaging work. CCD cameras continue to evolve, and are the technology of choice for most photometric and imaging microscopic studies. Recently, a new technology has emerged in solid-state cameras: CMOS or Complementary Metal Oxide Semiconductor cameras. These devices promise rapid image acquisition, low cost, and the potential for some image manipulation within the camera detector itself. At this time, CMOS cameras still lag behind CCD cameras in suitability for microscope photometry, but this may change in the near future. Solid-state cameras have a number of characteristics that make them ideal for microscope imaging. The detecting element itself consists of individual sensors (pixels) that are arranged in a square or rectangular array. The physical size of individual sensors or pixels in the array is in the order of a few microns, with values of 6 to 10 micron square pixels being common (there are solid-state cameras available with rectangular pixels, but these are not suitable for quantitative image use). The technique used to manufacture solid-state detectors is similar to that used to produce electronic chips such as are used in microcomputers. Therefore sensor chips can be manufactured that may have one million or more individual sensors

(pixels) and each will have similar characteristics, such as response to light (gain and linearity). Most solid-state detectors have a reasonably linear response over a wide range of light intensities, and this implies that each pixel within the sensor is also linear. Within limits, each pixel in the sensor array also generates a similar signal to a given light input (identical gain per pixel).

Because the camera detector consists of many individual but essentially identical detectors (the pixels), each individual pixel can be considered to be a photometric detector. To use a solid-state camera detector for photometry, the image that the individual detectors (pixels) see must meet the requirements of the Beer–Lambert law, i.e. they must see a homogeneous portion of the specimen. By calibrating the microscope lens system used, and deriving the area of the specimen in square microns seen by each pixel of the solid-state camera chip, an appropriate magnification can be selected which permits accurate photometry. For modern cameras with an array size of 1024×1024 pixels, a microscope objective lens of $20\times$ magnification will achieve approximately 0.50 microns per pixel, and a $40\times$ objective will be in the range of 0.25 microns per pixel. Both of these values are close to the resolving power of the respective lenses, and therefore meet the homogeneity requirement of the Beer–Lambert law. As yet, cameras with high enough pixel density to perform photometry at lower magnifications are not commonly available, and those that do exist are both expensive and slow. With the rapid advancements in camera technology, this is expected to change in the near future.

Solid-state cameras, whether CCD or CMOS, are available in either monochrome or color versions. Color cameras may use two different techniques to generate a color image. In one approach, there are three separate detector arrays, each with a color filter in front of the array. A prism or mirror system is used to split the image coming from the microscope into three separate but identical images, so each detector sees the same image. The color filters are red, green, and blue, since a red image, a green image, and a blue image can be combined to create a full color image. This type of camera is called a three-chip color camera. The second approach to color cameras uses a single detector chip, and places a pattern of color dots over the individual pixels. Again, these color dots are red, blue, and green. The most common pattern for these dots is the Bayer pattern (Fig. 31.1). Note that in the Bayer pattern there are actually four dots per 'repeat', since for each red and each blue dot

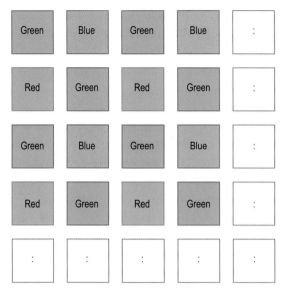

Fig. 31.1 The Bayer pattern of color filters applied to individual pixels of single-chip color cameras. Note that this effectively reduces the color resolution of the chip to one fourth that of the true number of pixels.

there are two green dots. This type of camera is called a single-chip color camera.

Because the three-chip camera has three individual detectors, and also a beam-splitting system to divide the image, these cameras are more expensive than a single-chip camera. Essentially, a three-chip camera is three separate cameras in one. The advantage of the three-chip camera is that every pixel is 'real', that is, it is generating a true signal. The disadvantage is that there may be differences in sensitivity of a 'red' pixel and a 'green' pixel that are seeing the exact same spot of an image. Use of a three-chip camera for photometry where various colors are examined requires careful calibration and correction of any variation in output between the separate detector chips.

The single-chip camera can produce excellent color images, but must be used carefully for quantitative work, and is unsuitable for photometry. The single-chip camera is unsuitable for photometry because only one pixel out of four (two in the case of green) is actually seeing the specimen at the point of maximum absorption. The other pixels in the Bayer pattern are being approximated, by assigning their 'red' value to the same value as the one real 'red' pixel in the pattern. In addition to the approximation of true signal for a given color, the Bayer pattern results in a real loss of resolution at the sensor level.

Since only one of every four pixels (for red and blue) actually sees a red or blue portion of the specimen, the true resolution of the single-chip camera is one-fourth the total number of pixels in the array. In practical terms this means that if a single pixel sees an area of the specimen that is 0.5 microns square, the true resolution of the Bayer pattern single-chip camera is 2.0 microns per pixel, for color detection. The camera does have true pixel number spatial resolution, but in colored specimens this may be reduced by the distribution of color within the specimen.

The three-chip color camera is essentially three monochrome cameras, with each camera having a different colored filter in front of the camera detector. Software is then used to combine the three separate images into a full-color image. This suggests that it is possible to use a monochrome camera to capture full-color images. A number of cameras provide a mechanism for doing this. Within the camera itself there is either an electronic filter, or a filter wheel carrying glass filters. To capture an image, three sequential images are taken, each through a different colored filter. These images are then combined to produce the full-color image. It is possible also to do this using a simple monochrome camera. One would place a red filter in the light path of the microscope, and capture a 'red' image. The same thing would then be done for 'blue' and for 'green'. The result would be three separate images of the same specimen, in different colors, and when these three-color planes are combined using software, the result is a full-color image.

Cameras used for imaging are also described in terms of signal resolution per individual pixel. This signal resolution is commonly described as *bit depth* or *gray levels* (for monochrome cameras). The signal resolution is a specification that describes the number of divisions of the signal between zero (no signal) and maximum signal. A common value is 256 levels, and these divisions are often also described as gray levels. They are based on the digital progression by powers of two, and therefore a 256-level signal corresponds to 8 bits of resolution (2 to the eighth power). Many modern cameras provide 10- or 12-bit signal resolutions. With a 12-bit camera, 4096 gray levels can be obtained. As the signal resolution increases, the susceptibility of the signal to perturbation increases. In particular, sources of electronic noise, such as internally generated heat within the detector itself, may become a problem. With high bit depth cameras, it is common to find cooling systems which lower the detector temperature, and thereby reduce electronic noise. Such cooling systems also translate to higher prices for cameras so equipped and, if the cooling system contains a fan, may introduce vibration to the microscope.

It is important to note the differences between cameras used to capture images through the microscope, and the same image viewed with the human eye. The human eye is a remarkable detector of light and of color. However, it is a non-linear, highly adaptive sensor. In addition, the resolution of the eye detector (retina) varies across the surface of the retina, being highest in the fovea. Under ideal conditions, most individuals with excellent eyesight can distinguish between 30 and 35 brightness levels (gray levels). This is a far cry from the 256 or higher number of levels seen by a digital camera. Therefore, a solid-state camera can always detect intensity variations that would be invisible to the human observer. This translates to the ability to detect finer detail within an image than can be resolved by a human observer.

The human eye adapts to light intensity, so the 30 or 35 gray levels that are detected vary depending on the intensity of the light, and the immediately preceding light exposure of the eye. This is one of the reasons why individuals must 'dark adapt' prior to doing fluorescence microscopy. The same phenomenon occurs in brightfield microscopy, but is seldom recognized. If an individual is asked to assess the density or 'darkness' of a stain, the assessment will vary depending on whether the individual has been in a dim environment or a bright environment just prior to performing the assessment.

Color capture is another area in which a camera differs from the human eye. While there is much that is still unknown as to the way in which the eye–brain combination processes color, the camera provides a fixed model. The construction of the camera itself is based on the RGB (red, blue, green) model of color. There are many other models of color, and those that incorporate intensity and saturation information appear more intuitive to human users of image systems. One common model that employs such a system is the HSI (hue, saturation, intensity) model. Software programs are available that permit images to be converted from one type of color space model to another, and often such conversions are useful when one works with full-color images.

Photographic color film is balanced for the type of light used to illuminate the scene. The type of light is specified by a 'color temperature' number. Film sold for routine color photography is generally balanced for correct color in 'sunlight', which is specified as a color temperature of 5,000° kelvin. Specialty films intended for microphotography may be balanced for 'tungsten' illumination, with a color temperature of 3,200° kelvin. Because of the narrow limits of intensity for which the film is balanced, photomicrography requires the microscope illuminator to be set to a specified level (generally bright) prior to taking a photograph. The 'color temperature' of a light source is actually a measure of the intensity of the various components of the light source, in the red, green, and blue regions of the spectrum. Photographic film records all of these components simultaneously, and there is little opportunity to 'correct' values, other than limited adjustment during processing. With a solid-state camera and capture software, the situation is different. Each of the image components (red, blue, and green) is available as an individual image. They are combined to produce the final image. Since the individual components (color planes) are available, it is possible to 'color correct' the image. This is generally done in the capture software, or the camera itself. The result is that 'white' is a true white (defined as a particular level of R, G, and B), regardless of the 'color temperature' of the microscope illuminator. This eliminates the requirement for presetting the brightness of the microscope prior to taking a picture with a solid-state camera. However, it does mean that each time the microscope is adjusted, in either magnification or illumination intensity, the user may have again to calibrate the 'white balance' of the system. Note that these same software techniques can be used to correct or modify any color image that can be converted into electronic form.

Solid-state cameras used on microscopes are generally coupled to the microscope in a manner to optimize the area of the visible field (to a user looking through the eyepieces of the microscope) that is captured. As is true of photographic cameras, the solid-state camera captures a rectangular (or in a few cases, square) portion of the circular image displayed in the microscope. The camera sensor pixels are, as previously described, quite uniform in response to light intensity. The nature of microscope lens systems, even in those that have been carefully aligned, is a higher intensity along the optical axis (center of the image) than in the periphery of the field. For an adaptive sensor such as the eye, and one with a limited number of intensity step discriminations, the field of view of a carefully aligned microscope appears to be quite uniform. That this is not the case is amply illustrated in many lectures that display photomicrographs, where a common flaw is dark corners. In the case of solid-state cameras, the increased intensity level sensitivity, as compared to the eye, accentuates this problem. Since all solid-state cameras use some type of software, either within the capture system or on the capturing computer to control the camera, this software frequently contains some type of 'field flattening' or 'background subtraction' mechanism to correct this variation in intensity from center to edge of the image. Additional details of requirements for acquiring images through microscopes using electronic cameras can be found in Shotton (1993).

IMAGE ANALYSIS

Overview

Image analysis is a broad term that may be defined quite differently by those working in diverse fields. Originally, image analysis was used to describe the extraction of numerical information from pictures. Since the process of placing pictures into a form that could be analyzed digitally was cumbersome, and the computers used to analyze such pictures were slow, image analysis was performed 'off line' and quite often at sites far removed from where the image was originally recorded. As software techniques for image analysis improved, and computers became faster and more affordable, image analysis became more widely used, in many fields and disciplines. Image analysis encompasses many areas: machine vision, graphic arts, pattern matching, photometry, optical character recognition, surveillance, security, and scores of others. While many of the same techniques are used in each of these areas (at the software level), we will restrict the remainder of this discussion to use of image analytic techniques to extract numerical data from microscopic preparations. The emphasis will be on transmitted light preparations, although in many cases identical approaches are used for fluorescence preparations.

The minimal requirement for image analysis of microscope preparations is a microscope equipped with a camera that can capture and transmit images to a computer equipped with suitable image analytic tools. The camera requirements have been discussed above. Computers suitable for image analysis range from RISC-based workstations to personal computers, either IBM PCs (or clones) or Apple PCs. A variety of sophisticated image analytic tools (programs) are available for each of these platforms. In addition to commercial offerings, there are a number of freeware or shareware programs available for personal computers. Among the best known of these is the program originally designed for the Apple computers, named NIH Image. There are now versions of this program available for the IBM (Windows) computers as well. A recent addition to the list of available image analytic programs is ImageJ, written by the original author of NIH Image. This program is also freely available, and, because it is written in the JAVA language, can run on any computer which supports JAVA (http://rsb.info.nih.gov/ij/.)

All image analysis programs must provide mechanisms to display images, read images from a source (camera or storage), and ultimately save the image and any derived data to storage. In modern computers, these functions are part of a GUI (graphical user interface) that permits the user actually to see the image and the various alterations to it during and after various image analytic or manipulation steps.

As camera resolutions increase, they often exceed the display capability of many computer displays. As an example, consider a common camera resolution available today, 1024×1310. The actual image from such a camera is larger than the common display resolution of many computers, which may be 800×600. Another common display resolution is 1024×756. In both cases, the larger image is displayed completely on the monitor. This is accomplished within the display program, by simply reducing the image to fit within the monitor resolution. Therefore the displayed image may not accurately represent the 'real' image that has been captured and is available for analysis. Some capture/display programs provide tools to permit the user to display the image at actual resolution, even though only a portion of the image is seen on the screen. Such programs allow the user to scroll over the image in order to see the entire image. Note also that many output devices, such as printers, actually reduce the size of the image, and therefore lose resolution as compared to the original image. This display resolution, which may be different from the actual image resolution, is one reason why high-resolution images may not appear as 'sharp' when viewed on a display device.

It is important to realize that an image, to the computer, is simply an array of values of the individual pixels. For 8-bit monochrome images, this would be a sequence of numbers, with values for each ranging between 0 and 255. Image file storage formats specify the number of pixels per row, and the total number of rows. This information is part of the 'header' information in the file storage, and is required for proper display and analysis of the images. The user ordinarily does not have to worry about this information, since it is taken care of transparently by the image software. Because the computer software considers the image to be an array of X by Y dimension, any pixel in the image can be individually addressed if its location is known within the array. In the case of color images, the actual image is stored as a sequence of colored pixels, i.e., red, blue, and green. To extract the 'green' image, one would read every third pixel from the file. Note that there are a variety of formats for image file storage, and the programmer should be sure to verify the 'bit order' in use prior to attempting to extract specific information.

IMAGE ANALYSIS PROCESSES

Point processes

Most forms of image analysis of microscope images start with a category of operations classically defined as *point processes*. These process are relatively simple, yet are basic to most image operations. A point process acts on an individual pixel within the image, and may modify the value of that pixel depending on the previous value. A common use of a point process is to change the value of each pixel to some other value, depending on the original value. Such an operation may make use of a LUT (look-up table). A common use for such an operation is in a pseudo-color operation, where a gray scale image is divided into a number of 'levels', i.e., all pixel values between 0 and 20 might be colored 'red', all values between 21 and 50 might be colored 'blue', etc. Since the human eye recognizes color variations much more easily than density variations, such a point operation might well make interpretation of a gray scale image easier.

Point processes are used to change the overall intensity of an image. Suppose an image is captured, and the background appears too dark. By adding a constant to every pixel, the result is an image that looks brighter. (Note: This depends on the scale being used for display of images. In this case, it is assumed that '0' is black, and '255' is white. There are systems in which this is reversed.) Often, in the process of color balancing the individual color planes of a color image, it is a point process that is used to set the 'clear' or 'background'

pixels to 'white'. Point processes can also be used to convert an image to a negative of the original image. In this process, each pixel is mapped to the value it would have if the scale of black to white values were inverted (black = 255, rather than 0). This is quite useful if the image is analyzed with a system different from the one used for capture. It is also a useful function for many intermediate image manipulations, particularly where images may be combined with one another.

Image contrast stretching is another example of a point process. In a contrast stretch (image equalization), the range of gray levels in the image is expanded. In many specimens, the actual image values cover a relatively narrow range of the total available gray values. As an example, in a nuclear preparation stained for DNA with the Feulgen procedure, the total gray levels represented by the stained nuclei occupy only about 30% of the total available levels. By contrast stretching these gray levels to cover the entire range of available values (256 levels), additional details can often be seen and/or measured in such contrast-stretched images.

By far the most common point process in image analysis is image thresholding. This is used to *segment* an image into areas that have some particular interest, such as a particular staining pattern. The action of a threshold is simple. The user selects a particular gray level (generally with some type of interactive tool in the graphical user interface). The point process then sets all pixels with a value lower than this threshold value to '0', and all values above this threshold value to '1'. In other words, the image is converted to a binary image. While this simple threshold is sufficient for some purposes, such as determining the total area in the image that is above some level (generally, the area of the image that is 'stained' by whatever is being analyzed), the simple binary image is more generally used to combine with the original image to produce some type of 'mask'. A common implementation is to combine the binary image with the original image in such a way that all '0' or background pixels are left '0', while all '1' pixels are left with their original image value. Such an operation leaves the desired portions of the image visible, with the remainder eliminated from the image. A second threshold step is often performed, thresholding from the opposite direction. After this step, a group of objects of 'medium' gray level could be separated or *segmented* from both lighter and darker objects. Another common implementation of threshold point operations is to combine the two threshold operations with a pseudo-color or LUT operation, and simply place a transparent colored mask over the desired objects, leaving the entire original image visible.

Area processes

Area processes use groups of pixels either to derive information from the image or to alter the image in some specific manner. In general, area processes involve a small portion of the image, in a two-dimensional matrix. The matrix is generally made up of an odd number of 'row' pixels and an odd number of 'column' pixels (a convolution kernel). It is the pixel in the center of this matrix that may be altered after performing the area process. Many

of the area processes are often referred to as *convolutions*. Convolutions commonly are based on matrix sizes of 3, 5, 7, or sometimes larger dimensions. In the area process, a convolution matrix is defined. The convolution matrix is placed over the image, and each pixel over which the convolution mask lies is multiplied by the number contained within the convolution mask. All of these multiplied pixel values are then summed, and the sum is used to replace the central pixel. The mask is then moved one pixel further along, and the process repeated (Fig. 31.2). Note that, in practice, the 'changed' pixel is used to construct a new image, since the process of convolution would fail if the image being analyzed were being altered during analysis. In other words, the convolution does not

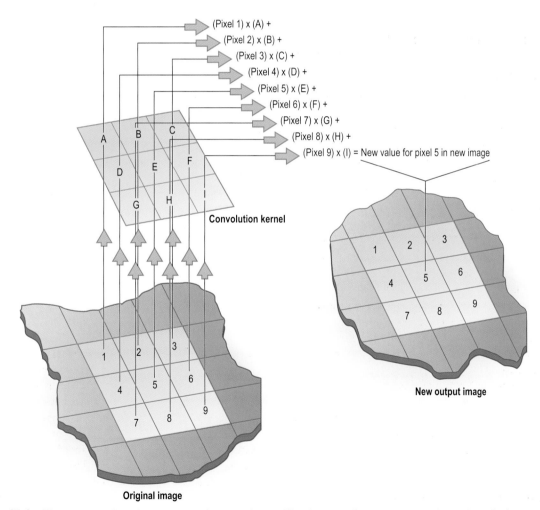

(Pixel 1) x (A) +
(Pixel 2) x (B) +
(Pixel 3) x (C) +
(Pixel 4) x (D) +
(Pixel 5) x (E) +
(Pixel 6) x (F) +
(Pixel 7) x (G) +
(Pixel 8) x (H) +
(Pixel 9) x (I) = New value for pixel 5 in new image

Convolution kernel

New output image

Original image

Fig. 31.2 The manner of implementation of a convolution. The diagram illustrates a convolution kernel of nine elements.

change the 'original' image, but creates a new, modified image based on the original (Fig. 31.3).

Area processes in general are often called spatial filtering operations, since they yield information about the rate of change of intensities within the image. In fact, it is these rates of change that are exploited by many common convolution filters. Typical area processes are those used for spatial filtering such as high-pass and low-pass filters. A low-pass filtered image will reduce the contrast of an image. Such an operation is often useful to remove unwanted noise spikes within an image. A high-pass filtered image increases contrast within the image, and is often used to improve the ability to detect edges or other structures within the image.

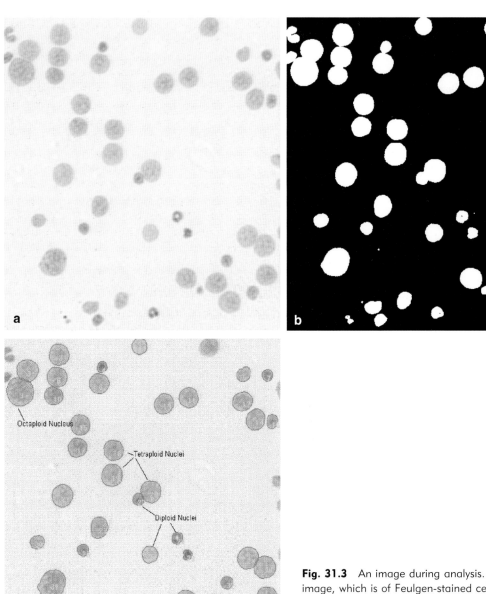

Fig. 31.3 An image during analysis. (a) is the original image, which is of Feulgen-stained cell nuclei. (b) is the image after a threshold operation that converts the image to a binary image. (c) is the final image, after isolating objects (nuclei) and separating touching nuclei. Annotations have also been added to this image.

An important type of spatial filtering is edge detection. A variety of convolution matrices are available to perform it. Often, some type of edge detection is used to perform segmentation within an image, particularly if the area to be segmented is close in gray value to other structures within the image, and thresholding is difficult.

While area processes are extremely important in image analysis, they are computationally intensive processes. As an example, a point process need only look at each pixel in an image one time. An area process, in the simplest case, must look at each pixel times the size of the convolution matrix. For a convolution matrix of 3×3, and an image of 1 million pixels, 9 million operations would have to be performed. For matrices of 7×7, 49 million operations would be required. In actuality, the number of operations required is somewhat greater than the figures given here, as impressive as they are. Because of the amount of computer processing required, image analysis requires fast computers, with large amounts of memory. Also, high-resolution, full-color images require a considerable amount of space for storage. A full-color image of 1024×1310 pixels will require almost 4 million bytes of storage (4 MB). While there are various methods of making images smaller (image compression), most of these forms of compression are 'lossy', that is, they discard image information, and this information cannot be retrieved from the stored image. Certain image storage formats allow a type of compression that is based on sequences of image data where all the pixels are the same (like large areas of background). This form of compression is called run length encoding, and does not discard any image information. However, for a typical image of a microscope specimen, where there are few or no 'constant value' areas, run length encoding may actually result in a larger image storage size than the original image. As a practical matter, any image intended for future analysis should not be stored in a compressed format, particularly in view of the low cost of large-capacity storage devices.

Frame processes

Both point processes and area processes treat the image as a series of pixels, and address each pixel in a specific manner. Frame processes, in contrast, operate on the entire image. Often frame processes use simple boolean (logic) operations to add, subtract, multiply, divide, or otherwise combine two images to produce a new third 'result' image. A common use of a frame operation is to correct a microscope image for uneven illumination. By collecting and 'temporarily' saving an image of the 'background' (when no specimen is present), the background image can then be subtracted from the specimen image. This will effectively remove any debris or other image-degrading elements that are inherent in the microscope and illuminator. A similar operation is commonly used in security systems, where a 'scene' image is collected at intervals. By subtracting the 'next' image from the previous image, any change in the 'scene' will be immediately recognized. A common biological application for a frame process would be to detect movement in a cell culture being observed at intervals. By tracking these changes over time, a 'trail' can be mapped and applied over the image to follow the movement of cells over time. Frame processes are common in many of the operators employed in image analysis systems, particularly with respect to boolean operations. They are frequently used in the display portions of image analysis systems, where they can be used to combine the results of various area processes or thresholding operations with the original image, in order to evaluate the effectiveness of a particular operation.

Geometric processes

Geometric processes are quite different from the processes discussed previously, since they are mainly used to reconstruct or correct images. Geometric processes actually move pixels within the image, and can therefore be used to correct defects such as geometric distortion. Geometric processes are used to rotate images, change scale, translate images, and produce mirror images. It is geometric processes that are used to interpolate images from 'real' size to a size that can be displayed on the monitor in use. Geometric distortion would include such image defects as a microscopic section that was attached to the slide in a manner that distorted normal morphology. In such a case, a geometric process could 'transform' the image to straighten or otherwise return it to the shape believed to be correct. Geometric processes are used to make the specimen 'look better', and to prepare the image for display or output to a print device. Until recently, geometric processes were not used extensively in microscope imaging, other than for display and printing. However, with the advent of microscope systems that can collect multiple images from various focal planes of the specimen (confocal microscopes), geometric processes have become much more widely used. These processes can be used to align 'stacks' of images which are used to reconstruct three-dimensional models of specimens.

Geometric processes can also be used to create mosaic images. A mosaic image is an image that is created from several smaller images. Using a motor-driven stage (scanning stage), an image system can travel over a slide, each time moving the exact width of the previous image, and collecting another image. Each collected image can then be 'added' to the previous one to create a large, mosaic image. With appropriate software, the area where these small images join can be a perfect, seamless match. Creation of such mosaic images requires an automatic focusing mechanism, to insure that each image collected is properly focused. While it has been suggested that such mosaic images can be retained in place of the original specimen, the resolution required to prevent loss of data (with current cameras) would mean the minimum objective magnification used to create the mosaic would be 20× and preferably 40–60×, and for large specimens this would create exceptionally large image files. Some 'virtual slide' microscopes produce image sizes that are hundreds of megabytes in size.

IMAGE ANALYSIS SOFTWARE

Many commercial image software packages are available, for both the PC and Mac personal computers. All of these offerings include the variety of image analysis processes described above, although there is little standardization of terminology for specific types of process. The user should work with each algorithm of interest, and verify that it is doing the desired function, as the implementation of common algorithms does differ from one software program to another. In general, these software systems are organized as a way to display an image. The image may be either captured from a camera, or retrieved from storage. Once the image is available, the user can select, through menus or tool bars, a variety of image manipulation tools. When the tool is applied to the image, the results can be seen immediately. Most systems also provide a mechanism to back up or undo, in case the result was not satisfactory. Such an image system is an ideal learning tool, and a user should expect to spend some time becoming familiar with any new image analysis system.

In addition to commercial software packages, there are a number of 'freeware' or 'shareware' image analysis packages available. One of the best known of these is NIH Image, written for the Mac platform, and freely available worldwide. There is also a version of this software for the PC platform. Recently, the original author of NIH Image produced a new image software package, ImageJ. This software is written in the Java language, and offers the advantage of running on any computer. ImageJ is available at no cost, and is constantly being upgraded and expanded.

Most vendors of commercial image analysis software packages provide support through user groups, and these groups are a rich source of assistance with image analysis problems. There are also a number of generic image analysis groups that maintain discussions via the internet, and these groups can provide assistance with specific image analysis problems. The internet is also a rich source of images, and a number of histology and pathology image archives are available. Note that currently most of these images are available as JPEG images. The JPEG format is a file storage format used for many internet images, and is a compressed image format (with compression based on a discrete cosine transform). Such compression is a 'lossy' format, which means that image data are lost during compression and cannot be retrieved. This is a critical issue for some types of image analysis, but is not necessarily a problem for simply viewing the image. The newer form of JPEG image is JPEG 2000. This compression uses a wavelet transform, and produces somewhat better visual results. However, it is still a 'lossy' compression format, and therefore not suitable for many types of image analysis.

SPECIMEN ANALYSIS

The goal of most image analysis of microscope images is the generation of numerical data that describe some aspect of the specimen. If the specimen is stained for some specific constituent, and the mechanism with which the stain interacts with the constituent is known, then it may be possible to use photometric techniques to produce numbers corresponding to the actual amount of the constituent present in the specimen, or in selected portions of the specimen. Generally, there will be more than one area of interest within the specimen. In the case of a specimen stained for cell nuclei, one could expect several hundred nuclei in a single image. In such a case, the first step of analysis would be to segment the objects of interest (nuclei) from the remainder of the specimen. If only the nuclei are stained, this can most likely be accomplished with a simple thresholding operation. After the nuclei are located by segmentation, it may be found that some nuclei touch each other. In such a case, additional image operations (specific area processes) may be required to separate these touching objects (see Fig. 31.3). In some cases it may be more expedient to use interactive tools, and simply draw a line between the touching objects, to effect a separation.

The above description illustrates an interesting point regarding image analysis. In many cases a particular operation may be performed in a totally automated manner, or the same result may be obtained with manual use of a particular tool. The decision of which approach to use depends on the complexity of the specimen being analyzed, the speed of the hardware and software being used, and the validity of the result. While it is difficult to deny the capability of modern image analysis programs, it is sometimes more time-advantageous simply to perform some manual intervention, thereby saving hours of analysis time. Once objects have been segmented, data can be collected from each. Common measures available include properties such as integrated optical density (absorbance), size (area), length of perimeter, shape, and a variety of other measures of the variation of intensity of pixels within the object. Many image analysis programs provide interactive tools to permit direct measurement of portions of the image. These tools commonly permit simply drawing a line on the displayed image, and having the length of this line displayed in the calibration units of the system (usually microns). Collected data can be saved, analyzed statistically, and displayed in graphs. Many programs permit direct export of data in formats compatible with common analysis tools, such as spreadsheets.

In the case of color images, analysis generally proceeds by selecting a particular color plane, which provides maximal contrast for the object(s) of interest. As an example, consider a specimen stained with an immunostain specific for some feature of cell nuclei. A common example would be a proliferation marker such as Ki-67 (MIB-1). Such a stain ordinarily results in a specimen with some number of positive nuclei, and many that are not stained. These nuclei that do not stain with the specific immunostain are then counterstained with a contrasting color. The object of the analysis of such specimens is to determine the percentage of nuclei within the specimen that are proliferating. To derive this result, we need to determine the total number of nuclei in the specimen, and then the number that stain positively.

After capturing the color image, we select the color plane that has maximal contrast for the positively stained nuclei. For a specimen that has been stained with the chromogen diaminobenzidine (DAB), the positive nuclei will be a brown color. These nuclei will have high contrast in the green or blue color plane, and if the counterstained nuclei are blue, then the blue color plane will see these counterstained nuclei as low contrast. By using a simple threshold operation, the positive nuclei can be segmented from the remainder of the specimen. From this segmented binary image alone, we can derive the total area in the specimen of positive nuclei. By switching to the red color plane, we will see high contrast in the counterstained nuclei. Unfortunately, we will also see that the DAB stain appears in the red color plane and at a density close to that of the blue counterstained nuclei. Since we already know where the DAB-positive nuclei are, from our first analysis, we can simply use a frame process to subtract the positive nuclei from the counterstain image. The result is an image that contains the counterstained nuclei, and 'holes' where the DAB-stained nuclei were. We can then threshold on the counterstained nuclei to derive an area of nuclei that did not stain with the specific proliferation stain. With these two numbers, we can add to obtain the total area of nuclei, and then divide this total into the area of positive stain and thereby obtain the desired measure, the percentage of positive staining for the specimen.

In the above example, a number of manipulations of the image were performed. In fact, most image analysis programs provide a variety of tools which can be used to significantly alter an image. This raises the issue of how much manipulation of an image is permissible in the collection of image data. The answer depends on the purpose of the analysis. When the object of the analysis is to measure some spatial property of the specimen, such as size or shape, then a variety of image tools can be employed to enhance the ability to segment the objects of interest from the remainder of the specimen. The caveat here is that the image manipulations should not alter the property being measured. In the case of photometric measurements, all image enhancement operations must be avoided. Image enhancement operations in this case include any operation that would result in the alteration of any pixel value included in the final measurement result.

It is often assumed, and frequently stated, that image analysis can be used to determine the amount of a particular material present in a specimen (a photometric measurement), assuming a stain that identifies the material of interest. This is in many ways a simplistic statement. A number of specific requirements must be met for this to hold true. First, the stain must have a defined stochiometric relationship with the material of interest. The entirety of the object containing the material must be present in the specimen. In other words, if the material of interest is confined to cell nuclei, then the specimen must contain intact nuclei. In practical terms, this means that one must provide specimens with intact nuclei. Therefore the preparation must be either a touch preparation or a cytological preparation, rather than a section. The use of sections complicates photometric measurements. In general, no intact objects (at light microscope resolution) will be present in the section. Essentially all cells, and most cellular constituents, such as nuclei, will be cut. Therefore there is no way accurately to measure their total content, since part of the content is missing. Another complicating factor is that in the architecture of many tissues every section contains fragments of overlapping cells. With most fixation and staining protocols, cell boundaries are not delineated. One simply cannot tell how much of the thickness through which light is being transmitted is due to the cell on the 'top' of the section or to the one on the 'bottom'.

A sectioned preparation can be used to measure the general concentration per unit volume of a specimen. Assuming an appropriate stain, one can define an area of known size, and sample multiple areas of the specimen with this known area (it is actually a volume, assuming constant section thickness). For this strategy to succeed, one must insure that the areas measured do not contain other, non-stained structures such as a fragment of the cell nucleus, if the material being measured is cytoplasmic in location. Although this approach is producing numerical results, it should not be assumed that the results are precise. Such analyses are more properly described as semi-quantitative and, although more accurate and reproducible than subjective visual evaluation of microscope preparations, are not truly quantitative.

Image analysis can be used to provide numerical assessment of many details of microscope specimens. An example is the thickness of an epithelial layer, or the depth of penetration of an epithelial tumor into underlying tissues. Such assessments are simple measurements of distance, but have the advantage of permitting a per-manent record to be made of the actual placement of the fiduciary mark used to perform the measurement.

Image analysis can also be used to perform repetitive measurements where many objects must be measured, or where the measurement must be restricted to a particular orientation. An example would be the measurement of the thickness of the myelin sheath around nerve fibers. For areas of cross-sectioned nerve, most myelinated nerve fibers will be cut at a slight angle, rather than a true cross-section. By measuring the long and short axes of the resulting ellipse, the myelin measurement can then be restricted to the short axis of the ellipse, insuring a true measure of the actual myelin thickness.

When many measurements must be performed on a specimen, most image analysis software permits the creation of 'scripts' or 'macros'. These are simply sequences of image analysis steps, which can be applied automatically or can be manually invoked for each object of interest. A significant advantage of defined scripts is that they insure that a particular type of measurement is performed in an identical manner each time it is performed. Scripts also insure that data are collected in precisely the same manner regardless of who performs the analysis. The general examples described here are but a brief introduction to the ways in which an image can be analyzed. Many properties of an image can be documented; with appropriate specimen-preparative methods, the subjective analyses that have been the foundation of histology and cytology may ultimately yield to precise, invariant descriptions of specific features of the cells and tissues in the majority of these microscopy specimens. While many of the tools to provide the framework for such assessments are now available, the actual data on which such descriptions might be based have yet to be collected.

In addition to actual image data, the interpretation and display of data is also an evolving science. As additional parameters are defined for a particular specimen type, one is faced with a significant increase in the number of variables. The complexity of multi-parametric data analysis is beyond the scope of this chapter, but continues to be an area of active research and progress.

SPECIMEN PREPARATION FOR IMAGE ANALYSIS

The science of cell and tissue preparation is well developed, as evidenced by the contents of this text. The techniques that have been developed and perfected over the course of many years have been designed for the subjective evaluations performed by a skilled microscopist. Stains have been developed that optimize the ability of the human eye to discriminate morphology and colors. Unfortunately, cameras used for image analysis do not mimic the human eye (see section on cameras). This means that common staining protocols will not yield optimal results for image analysis. The most common staining protocol for routine pathology is the hematoxylin and eosin (H&E) stain. Interpretation of this stain is straightforward for those trained in microscopic diagnosis. However, this stain is quite difficult to use in image analysis. If we consider the use of a monochrome camera, where all color is converted to shades of gray, the problem becomes apparent. H&E-stained specimens, when viewed as gray scale objects (like a black and white photograph), lack the sharpness and clarity that a human observer would detect when viewing the object in full color through the microscope. Light microscope images depend on absorption of light by the dyes used to stain the specimen. While the eye can readily detect the differences between the blue–purple of hematoxylin and the red of eosin, in a gray scale image there is little distinction between these two colors. The basis for this lack of differentiation is that the absorption curves of hematoxylin and eosin overlap over a considerable portion of the visible spectrum (Fig. 31.4). This overlap of absorption results in slowly varying shades of gray, rather than abrupt transitions between the blue–purple of hematoxylin and the red of eosin. This problem is not new to image analysis; it has plagued photomicrography for many years. In the case of black and white photography, one can improve the appearance of H&E-stained speci-

mens by simply substituting some other acid dye for eosin that does not have as great an absorption curve overlap with hematoxylin. Dyes that work well for this are Orange G or Naphthol Yellow S.

The H&E example illustrates the difference between optimum specimen preparation for visual observation versus preparation for image analysis. Recall that the purpose of staining is to permit the observer to detect detail within the cell or tissue specimen. Since the digital cameras used for image analysis respond differently than the eye, specimens intended for image analysis require modifications of traditional staining methods. In the case of specimens intended for analysis with monochrome (black and white) cameras, the staining protocol must be optimized to permit the *camera* to detect different portions of the specimen. Since essentially all image analysis tasks begin with methods to segregate some portions of the image from other portions, the staining methods should not use dye combinations that produce any absorption overlaps. It is also desirable that the density of the various stained components should be significantly different, so the resulting 'gray levels' are distinct. Remember, in monochrome, color disappears, as far as the camera is concerned. One should always carefully select the specimen preparation method based on the type of analysis to be performed. Careful choice of preparative (staining) method can significantly enhance the speed and accuracy of image analysis of the specimen.

As a common task in image analysis is to determine the size or area of a particular component of the specimen, in many cases the imaging task can be simplified by using single dyes, rather than combinations of dyes. If the dye is specific for a particular component of the specimen, accurate detection is simplified. Many

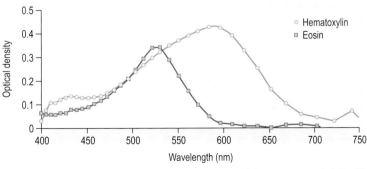

Fig. 31.4 The absorbance curves of hematoxylin and eosin, measured from a stained slide. Note the high degree of overlap of the two curves.

histochemical stains meet this criterion, and are excellent choices for image analysis, if a method is available that specifically detects the cell or tissue component of interest. When it is desired to provide some contrast to the specific stain in order to see the 'non-stained' portions of the specimens, a counterstain may be used. The choice of an appropriate counterstain should include consideration of the spectral overlap and general density of the counterstain. In most cases, the counterstain should be lightly applied, simply to provide contrast. While discussing choices of stains for image analysis, it should be mentioned that for monochrome analysis one can often effectively improve the distinction between components within the specimen by varying the color of the illumination light in the microscope. This is simply done by adding colored filters to the light path. When the desired components are stained with a blue dye, using a red filter will greatly improve the ability to detect the stained components. For objects that are stained red to magenta, a green filter will be found quite useful. Often when the specimen is stained with a method that utilizes a combination of dyes, a filter can be found that will enhance the ability to segment the monochrome image to select the component of interest.

As has been mentioned in the discussion of photometry through the microscope, accurate measurement of the concentration of a material in a stained specimen requires:

a. a stoichiometric relationship between the dye and the component of interest
b. an absorbing dye
c. an intact object, rather than a sectioned object (unless the measurement simply determines concentration per unit volume).

While many staining protocols utilize dyes that are true absorbing chromophores, there are a number of common dyes that are not true absorbing materials. Diaminobenzidine (DAB), which is commonly used as a substrate for peroxidase in immunochemical stains, is a dye that is not a true absorbing dye. DAB staining results in the deposition of a particulate in the specimen, and the concentration of this particulate gives the appearance (when observed visually) of an absorbing stain. However, when observed in reflected or incident illumination, it will be seen that DAB is a true particulate, and an effective scatterer of light. As the concentration of DAB particulate increases (darker stain), the number of particles increases and the amount of light that is scattered increases. As the DAB density increases, the scattered light may not be captured by the objective of the microscope, and the observed (as measured with an image analysis system) density of stain may become nonlinear. Light scattering is also influenced by the particle size of the DAB, and this particle size is not necessarily the same for DAB obtained from various sources. Therefore DAB is not a stain that should be employed when *concentrations* of a cell or tissue component are desired. Other chromogens for peroxidase in immunostains are true absorbing dyes, and are a more appropriate choice. DAB is useful, however, if the analytical result is simply to measure the areas stained within the specimen.

An important aspect of staining methodologies for quantitative analysis is standardization. Recall that the camera is much more sensitive than the eye. Variations in a particular preparative protocol that might not be detectable to a human observer, who may recognize 30 density levels, may become a significant source of error when these specimens are measured with an image analysis system which identifies 256 levels (8 bit) or 4096 levels (12 bit). In fact, for many types of analysis, every step of the process must be rigidly controlled, beginning with specimen collection and fixation. If the component of interest degrades with time, then the amount of time prior to fixation must be controlled. The length of time in fixative must be precisely defined also, since length of exposure to most fixatives may alter the binding of the final stain to the specimen. If the specimen displays any 'edge effect', that is, increased or decreased staining at the periphery of the specimen as compared to the center, measurements must always be taken at a specified distance from the periphery. While on the subject of fixation, it should be mentioned that common fixatives may give different results with particular staining protocols. For a quantitative study, it is imperative that all specimens included in the study be fixed in the same fixative.

Staining protocols that are routine for visual examination may prove problematic for quantitative work. Again, this relates to the increased sensitivity of image detection systems, as compared to the eye. As the length of time a specimen is exposed to a particular staining step decreases, the percentage of error that can be introduced by the physical time required to insert or remove the slides from the staining solution may become a significant source of error. In other words, if the total time in a particular staining step is only 1 minute, a variation of 10 seconds amounts to almost a 20% variation in staining time. To reduce the potential error introduced by short staining times, staining methods should be modified by decreasing stain concentrations, and then increasing staining times. As a general guide, any staining time that is shorter than 10 minutes should be extended to between 30 minutes and an hour, by reducing stain concentration. This strategy effectively controls errors introduced by the time required to physically introduce or remove specimens from staining solutions. For stains that require differentiation, often this is done with a series of dips, with differentiation controlled by an experienced technician. This type of differentiation should be optimized by changing the concentration of the differentiation solution in order to extend the differentiation steps to a defined time, preferably long enough to eliminate the effect of short times. In addition to times in actual staining solutions, stain results may also be influenced by various dehydration sequences. Standardization of every step of a stain protocol including deparaffinization, hydration, staining, differentiation, dehydration, clearing, and coverslipping will greatly improve variability of specimens analyzed with image analysis systems.

Quantitation of immunostains is commonly reported in publications. While immunostained specimens do lend themselves to morphometric measurements, photometric techniques can be used only when the chromogen employed is a true absorbing dye, and therefore diaminobenzidine is not suitable for photometric studies. Standardization of immunostaining is particularly challenging, since most staining protocols involve at least two stages of amplification, and these amplification steps are not controlled to any significant degree. To standardize an immunostaining protocol for photometric analysis, one would have to provide standards that could be used to control the various amplification steps in the staining procedure. Although such standards can be constructed, they are not commercially available, and it is rare to see any use of such controls in published works.

It has been mentioned that, for studies that purport to measure the total amount of a material present, the intact object containing that material must be present in the slide. For many cellular materials, this means that whole cells, such as from tissue cultures, be used. Another strategy is simply to disaggregate tissues and select intact cells for analysis. Sectioned material may be employed for many image analysis tasks, but generally is not suitable for measuring the total amount of material present in a given cell or tissue component. One possible exception to this is the measurement of cell nuclei constituents. However, to measure nuclei, the operator must be certain to include intact nuclei in the section, that is, nuclei which have not been sectioned on either their top or bottom surface. The difficulty with this is that, in most fixed and sectioned material, the average size of cell nuclei is approximately 7 microns in diameter. Since general practice in many laboratories is to section at under 5 microns in thickness, then all nuclei in the specimen will be sectioned. One possible way to address this is to cut thicker sections, and, while this will yield some nuclei that are intact, there is the additional problem of overlap of nuclei from top to bottom of the section.

Morphometry, or the measurement of size and arrangement of cell or tissue constituents, can be done in sections. Such studies must also be carefully controlled, since there will always be a range of 'profiles' of a given object shape in the section. As an example, imagine a perfectly round sphere in a section. If the measurement being done is the total area of the sphere, then one would obtain different values as the section passes through the sphere. The result would be a series of measurements, with only one approaching the true diameter of the sphere. Any measure taken in sections must account for this spread of values which results from the sectioning of spheroidal objects. Obviously, some objects may have shapes other than spheroids, and this particular geometry must be taken into account when establishing a measurement approach.

There are other, subtle sources of error when measuring microscopic preparations. The biological structure should be understood, and the effects of various preparative methods on that structure must be accounted for. In tissues which have oriented, linear structures, one should consider differential shrinkage. In many cases, shrinkage will be more severe at right angles to linear morphology, particularly when that linear morphology is fibrous in nature. A classic example of differential shrinkage occurs in skeletal muscle, where fiber diameter shrinks more than fiber length (and fiber length is generally difficult to measure, due to length). The act of sectioning may also induce morphological change, with compression of the section affecting the actual morphology of the specimen. When such compression artifacts are suspected, standards may be included with the specimen to assess the degree of compression. One type of standard that can be used is spherical latex particles, which may be sectioned along with the specimen. One can also use internal standards, and employ elements of the tissue structure that have known shapes to assess the degree of change introduced by the preparative process. Geometry can also provide information on the angle at which tissue elements have been sectioned. Tubular or rod-like elements within a tissue appear perfectly round when sectioned at right angles to the long axis, but appear as ellipses when sectioned at an angle. In such cases, where the diameter of the object is of interest, the minor (shorter) axis of the ellipse will provide the best estimate of the true size of the object.

'Standards' or control objects should always be included in quantitative image analysis studies. Many techniques have been developed to construct artificial standard objects, but in many cases a standard biological object can be used. For many studies of nuclear DNA content, populations of cells that contain known amounts of DNA have been used. Common cell types that have been employed in the past are sperm, and the nucleated red blood cells of various amphibian, fish, and bird species. For other cellular constituents, a common control object is a defined cell line from tissue culture. Within limits, these types of cell can be accurately characterized, and, because of the conditions under which they are grown, can be harvested in such a manner as to provide a reasonably constant control object. It must be appreciated that these control objects are biological in nature, and therefore may vary over time. Any analytical procedure using such a biological control should monitor the control itself for any potential change over time.

MULTISPECTRAL IMAGING

An emerging technique for image analysis is multispectral imaging. This technique acquires images at many specific wavelengths of light. As an example, one might collect 10 to 30 images over the wavelength range of 400 nm (blue) to 600 nm (red). Each of the selected wavelengths is narrow band, and the approach is similar to that used in chemical spectroscopy. The result is an image stack, made up of images at discrete wavelengths. When the absorbance curves for each compound (stain) within a specimen are known, the multispectral image stack can be used to accurately determine the exact location of each stain within the image. This approach is particularly powerful when the specimen contains areas of mixed stains, and the eye cannot separate the individual stains. An example would be a combination immunohistochemical stain, where one primary antibody is stained with a brown chromogen and the second with a red chromogen. The eye cannot easily separate these two colors, particularly if one is present in small amounts. Using multispectral imaging, one can generate separate images with each individual stain. By then 're-coloring', or pseudo-coloring these individual images in some highly contrasting colors, the two images can be recombined into a single, easily evaluated image. Because of the way in which color is produced in display systems, one can also employ a 'trick' and, in the case of two colors, use the pseudo-colors of 'red' and 'green'. When these two pseudo-colored images are then combined for display, any areas that contain both 'red' and 'green' color will appear in yellow. This is obviously quite useful to subjectively evaluate double-stained specimens for label co-localization. Using image logic operations, one can also generate a third image that displays only co-localized staining.

Multispectral imaging requires specific hardware to collect the 'image stack' at specific wavelengths, as well as software to permit extraction of the individual spectral information in the images. There is a variety of devices available to collect multispectral images, ranging from cameras with filter wheels in front of a monochrome sensor, cameras with electronically switchable filters, to systems using switching light sources capable of generating narrow-band light. As the hardware and software for multispectral imaging is rapidly evolving, a search of current literature should be done by those interested in employing this technique.

Acknowledgments

John Anderson contributed the origins of this chapter for the second edition. He and James Lowe updated the third edition and Trevor Gray contributed the chapter for the fourth edition. Our acknowledgments are due to them for their contributions. Data from Figure 31.4 were kindly supplied by Dr George McNamara.

REFERENCES

DeHoff R.T., Rhines F.N. (1968) Quantitative microscopy. New York: McGraw-Hill.
Elias H., Hyde D.M. (1983) A guide to practical stereology. Basel: Karger.

Elias H., Pauly J.E., Burns E.R. (1978) Histology and human microanatomy. New York: John Wiley, Appendix II.

Piller H. (1977) Microscope photometry. Berlin: Springer.

Shotton D. (1993) Electronic light microscopy. New York: Wiley-Liss.

Underwood E.E. (1970) Quantitative stereology. Reading, MA: Addison-Wesley.

Weibel E.R. (1979) Stereological methods: practical methods for biological morphometry. New York: Academic Press, Vol. 1.

Weibel E.R. (1980) Stereological methods: theoretical foundations. New York: Academic Press, Vol. 2.

Weibel E.R. (1990) Morphometry: stereological theory and practical methods. In: Gil J., ed. Models of lung disease: microscopy and structural methods. New York: Marcel Dekker, pp. 199–247.

Wied G.L. (1966) Introduction to quantitative cytochemistry. New York: Academic Press.

Wied G.L., Bahr G.F. (1970) Introduction to quantitative cytochemistry: II. New York: Academic Press.

FURTHER READING

Baak J.P.A. (1991) Quantitative pathology in cancer diagnosis and prognosis. Berlin: Springer.

Baxes G.A. (1994) Digital image processing. New York: John Wiley.

Castleman K.R. (1995) Digital image processing. Englewood Cliffs, NJ: Prentice Hall.

Crane R. (1997) A simplified approach to image processing. Upper Saddle River, NJ: Prentice Hall.

Gu J. (1997) Analytical morphology: theory, applications and protocols. Boston: Eaton.

Jahne B. (1997) Digital image processing, 4th edn. Berlin: Springer.

Jahne B. (1997) Image processing for scientific applications. Boca Raton: CRC Press.

Klette R., Zamperoni P. (1996) Handbook of image processing operators. New York: John Wiley.

Marchevsky A.M., Bartels P.H. (1994) Image analysis: a primer for pathologists. New York: Raven Press.

Parker J.R. (1997) Algorithms for image processing and computer vision. New York: John Wiley.

Rosenfeld A., Kak A.C. (1982) Digital picture processing. New York: Academic Press, Vols 1 and 2.

Russ J.C. (1995) The image processing handbook. Boca Raton: CRC Press.

Watkins C., Sadun A., Marenka S. (1993) Modern image processing: warping, morphing and classical techniques. New York: Academic Press.

Weeks A.R. (1996) Fundamentals of electronic image processing. New York: SPIE Press/IEEE Press.

Wootton R., Springall D.R., Polak J.M. (1995) Image analysis in histology. Cambridge: Cambridge University Press.

32

Ergonomics

Janet I. Minshew

INTRODUCTION

There have been many changes over recent years that have directly impacted on ergonomics in histology laboratories. The per-person workload has increased dramatically, requiring workers to perform tasks for longer periods, work faster, and take fewer breaks. Working environments are more stressful because of regulatory agency compliance issues, short turn-around times, maintaining high quality, and eliminating errors. Advancing technology has increased the use of computers for data entry and created the need to squeeze new instrumentation into already crowded work areas. To make matters worse, the average age of laboratory workers has increased, which influences characteristics such as height, quality of vision, physical strength, and tolerance levels. The one thing that has not changed in many facilities is the design of the workspace. Many older workstations were not designed with the forethought and flexibility to accommodate multiple users or today's equipment.

The combination of the physical motions associated with both histology laboratory work and a normal active lifestyle is contributing to the reports of work-related musculoskeletal disorders. These include carpal tunnel syndrome, tendonitis, and tenosynovitis. Other problems such as chronic pain, numbness, and headaches are often unreported as occupationally related injuries.

Laboratory workers should be aware of the hazards that can adversely affect their well-being and must work together with employers to develop an ergonomic program that includes determining ergonomic risk factors, finding solutions to problems, and promoting the acceptance and incorporation of positive changes in the work environment. A carefully thought out, well-executed program can result in the reduction of human suffering and the expense of workplace injuries or illnesses.

ERGONOMICS

Ergonomics is a body of knowledge about human abilities, limitations, and other characteristics that are relevant to design. It is based on one simple principle: make the task and the environment fit the person performing the work without exceeding the person's abilities or ignoring his or her limitations.

The study of ergonomics

The following principles are used by ergonomists to evaluate workplaces and design tools, machines, tasks, and environments for safe, comfortable, and effective human use. In the histology laboratory, ergonomic considerations include, but are not limited to, work habits, posture, preference for right or left handedness, arrangement and use of instrumentation and tools, countertop heights, seating, lighting, noise levels, temperatures, and vibration.

Anthropometrics

Anthropometrics—anthro (human) metric (measurements)—is the scientific study of human body dimensions, shapes, weights, and strengths. Studying the workforce provides information for the design of workstations that are adaptable, comfortable, and safe for workers. It also shows that gender, ethnic differences, and certain physical disabilities produce variations in bone structure, weight distribution, limb length, and body contours. These variations make it difficult for workers to share workstations and experience the same comfort level when performing similar tasks.

BIOMECHANICS

Biomechanics (life-machine) applies the principles of mechanics and physics to measure the forces in human movement, establish tolerances, maximize performance, and protect the safety and health of an individual. Biomechanical risk factors include exposures to excessive force, awkward posture, repetitive movement, and vibration. These risk factors are further characterized by their frequency, repetition, duty cycle, and duration of exposure. Biomechanical considerations are particularly useful in histology since almost every task is repetitive and many tasks require force and are performed in awkward positions. Risk factor information is important when selecting equipment and tools, and justifying the need for automation.

Situational analysis

Situational analysis explores the psychological, social, and physical task environment. Psychological and social factors include how work is organized and carried out (e.g. total time per shift, extended hours, pacing, and length of uninterrupted periods of work). This analysis also encompasses the quality of training, physical conditioning, and cognitive or emotional stresses, such as job demands, security, and satisfaction of the worker. Stressed, exhausted, or unhappy workers make more mistakes and incur more accidents and injuries.

Preventive measures

Preventive measures include determining and implementing motions and activities that can substitute for damaging ones. Aggravating factors may not be evident to the worker, but they usually involve either working in extreme joint positions at angles that amplify biomechanical forces or using highly repetitive movements without allowing time for rest and healing.

Biomechanical risk factors

Force

Force is defined as the amount of muscular effort required to perform a task. Usually, the degree of risk increases with the amount of force and is proportionate to the combination of all the risk factors involved. An example of this is gripping, which is a combination of a force with a posture. The risk of injury is influenced by the size of the hand and object, and the amount of exertion used during manipulation of the object. For example, a pinch grip (thumb and fingers) requires a much greater muscle exertion than a power grip (palm of hand) and has a much greater likelihood of causing injury.

It is possible that a worker can be unaware of the force necessary to accomplish a task, especially if the task is performed routinely. Some typical examples in histology are opening specimen containers and cassettes or pipetting. Using high amounts of force have been associated with musculoskeletal disorders at the forearm/wrist/hand, shoulder/neck, and lower back. Where muscular force must be exerted, the largest appropriate muscle groups available should apply the force.

Repetition

Repetitive tasks in the histology laboratory include computer data entry, manual cassette and slide labeling, embedding, microtomy, cryomicrotomy, staining, and coverslipping. These tasks require the same muscles, tendons, and joints to perform the same motions repeatedly. Performing repetitive motions for very short work cycles (30 seconds or less) for more than 50% of the workday is considered extremely high risk. Overuse can cause tight muscles, inflammation of surrounding tissues, and nerve compression or 'entrapment'.

Awkward working postures

Posture determines which muscle groups are used during physical activity. To accomplish a task, workers will often assume postures that are awkward, uncomfortable, or unbalanced. Awkward postures seen most often in histology labs are repeated or prolonged reaching, bending, twisting, grasping objects, or sitting for long periods. To avoid injury, periodically rotate tasks and alternate sitting with standing and walking. To relax muscles and renew circulation, short rest breaks (15 seconds to a few minutes) should be taken every 20 to 30 minutes. Although this may seem excessive, it actually increases productivity because the body can maintain a constant pace and not tire and slow down, as it will with sustained activity.

It is especially important to work in neutral (natural) postures which are near the midpoint of the full range of motion, where the muscles surrounding a joint are equally balanced and relaxed. The more a joint deviates from the neutral position, the greater the risk of injury.

Positions associated with injury

Wrist

Injury to the wrists results from repeatedly bending up and down (flexion/extension), and bending inward or outward (ulnar/radial deviation). To achieve a neutral position, the wrists must be straight but the palms may face either inward, toward the body, or down.

Shoulder/arms

Shoulder injuries are typically caused by holding the upper arms out to the side or above shoulder level (abduction/flexion). Injury can also result from working with slumped shoulders or having the elbows winged out away from the body.

Neck (cervical spine)

The neck supports the head and will tire rapidly when the head is tilted backwards or the neck is held forward or bent to the side (as when holding a telephone receiver on the shoulder).

Lower back

The lower back is easily injured by excessive bending and twisting at the waist, especially when lifting or with sudden movements. Whether sitting or standing, maintaining the natural 'S-curve' of the spine will help protect the lower back.

Vibration

There are two different forms of vibration that can cause injury: whole body vibration and hand–arm vibration. Hand-arm vibration is infrequent yet possible with the use of motorized hand-held tools that are used in some laboratories.

MUSCULOSKELETAL DISORDERS (MSDs)

Musculoskeletal disorders (MSDs) are sometimes confused with ergonomics; however, MSDs are actually the problem and ergonomics is a solution. They are not new and were reported as early as 1713.

MSDs occur in many forms in many different areas of the body and involve damage to the spinal discs, carti-

lage, tendons, tendon sheaths, muscles, joints, blood vessels, and nerves. They are not typically the result of a single acute event, although they can be. MSDs are usually a more gradual or chronic development, stemming from biomechanical risk factors such as prolonged repetitive, forceful, or awkward movements.

None of the common MSDs is uniquely caused by work activities. The body cannot distinguish between work and non-work movements and treats them all as cumulative. Non-work activities that can trigger MSDs include things like recreational sports (golf, tennis), hobbies (sewing, gardening), driving, and even the position of the hands while sleeping. MSDs have also been associated with vitamin B6 deficiency, thyroid conditions, obesity, diabetes, rheumatoid arthritis, previous trauma, and predispositions that are either genetically determined or a physiological response to a stressor. Women develop MSDs three times more often than men, possibly because of hormonal changes from contraceptives, pregnancy, or menopause.

The costs of MSDs directly and indirectly increase the cost of doing business. Direct costs include medical expenses and increases in worker's compensation premiums. Indirect costs, which are much higher, include employee absenteeism, turnover, and retraining. Costs can be reduced if a worker's symptoms are addressed quickly, when they are treatable. If ignored, treatment takes longer, is more expensive, and the disorder may eventually become irreversible.

Types of MSD

Some MSDs that are seen in histology laboratory workers are briefly described below.

Disorders associated with muscles

The physiological demands on a worker are either static or dynamic in nature. Static work occurs when a worker stays in a stationary position for an extended period, and dynamic work involves considerable movement. To relate this to histology, a worker who is embedding will sit for long periods with elbows bent and arms held away from the body (static) but the wrists and fingers are constantly moving (dynamic).

During prolonged static work, muscles stay contracted and the body cannot supply stressed tissues in the musculoskeletal system with enough oxygen and metabolites, nor effectively remove waste products. When performing dynamic work, muscles demand more oxygen and metabolites, but, as long as the maximum load is kept at a reasonable level, the body responds by increasing the heart rate and breathing so nutrients and waste products effectively move to and from the muscles. If the body cannot meet the muscles' demands, localized physical fatigue occurs, which manifests as tired and sore muscles. Shifting positions, finding support for tired limbs, changing movements, taking short breaks, or switching to a different activity for a while can relieve fatigue.

Normally, a worker should not be required to exert the muscles by more than 50% of their maximum level. The worker's physical endurance level usually determines the length of time they can safely spend working. No two workers are the same and each worker may experience changes in endurance for a variety of reasons.

Disorders associated with tendons

Ganglion cysts

Ganglion cysts occur on the tendon, tendon sheath, or synovial lining of the joint. They are a sign of wear and tear that is associated with repetitive wrist motion.

Tendonitis

Tendons are particularly subject to repetitive motions, awkward postures, trauma, inflammatory diseases, and the wear and tear of aging as they lose elasticity. In histology, tendon injuries occur most often during computer data entry, manual embedding, coverslipping, and possibly microtomy.

Tenosynovitis

Tenosynovitis refers to inflammation of tendon sheaths.

DeQuervain's disease occurs in the sheath surrounding the tendons that pass from the wrist to the thumb. It causes pain when the thumb is moved or during a twisting motion and is caused by repeatedly using a pinch grip (forceps), performing forceful motions with the thumb (opening cassettes), rheumatoid arthritis, or scar tissue.

Trigger finger (flexor tenosynovitis) can occur if an inflamed tendon is caught in the tendon sheath and locked into a bent position. Frequent grasping of objects (manual staining) is a leading cause.

Shoulder tendonitis

Tendon disorders of the shoulder are seen among workers performing highly repetitive movements requiring a significant use of force (manual microtomy), workers who use poor posture (shoulders slumped forward), or doing jobs requiring awkward postures relating to arm elevation or working with the arms 'winged' out away from the body (manual embedding).

Forearm and elbow tendinitis

The most common form of forearm tendonitis seen in histology workers is found in the elbow and can be traced to movements of the forearm muscles. Specific movements associated with this disorder are simultaneous rotation of the forearm and bending of the wrist (microtomy), and stressful gripping of an object combined with inward or outward movement of the forearm (manual staining or embedding).

Disorders associated with nerves

Carpal tunnel syndrome (CTS)

Excessive up and down wrist and finger movement (computer data entry and manual coverslipping) can contribute to irritation of the median nerve, which passes through the carpal tunnel and conducts impulses from the brain down the arm to the thumb, forefinger, middle finger, and half of the ring finger. Compression of the nerve causes numbness, tingling, and soreness that can lead to severe pain.

Ulnar nerve disorders

The ulnar nerve supplies feeling to half of the ring finger, the little finger, small muscles in the palm, and the muscle that pulls the thumb toward the palm. Prolonged pressure from leaning on the elbows, working with the elbows bent at right angles for long periods of time or constant bending and straightening of the wrist and fingers can lead to irritation. Prolonged pressure on the base of the palm may also cause damage to part of the ulnar nerve. Ulnar nerve damage is sometimes attributed to manual microtomy, and is exacerbated by rocking the hand wheel.

Disorders associated with nerves and blood vessels

Thoracic outlet syndrome (TOS)

TOS makes overhead activities particularly difficult. Poor posture and obesity are aggravating factors. TOS can result from injury, disease, or a congenital abnormality, such as an extra first rib. Working with outstretched arms (manual microtomy and staining) should be minimized and alternated with rest periods.

ERGONOMIC STUDIES OF HISTOLOGY PROFESSIONALS

USA, 1995

A group from the University of Michigan published the results of an ergonomic survey in the first of a three-part series of articles published in the *Journal of Histotechnology*. Carpal tunnel syndrome (CTS) was used as the model for potential work-related musculoskeletal disorders (MSDs) and the authors suspected manual microtomy to be a major contributor to the symptoms.

Results

Of the 1000 questionnaires that were randomly distributed to histology professionals, 253 were completed and returned. The responses indicated that 157 technologists complained of pain. Some 22 respondents reported a clinical diagnosis of CTS, 36 had a clinical diagnosis of MSDs other than CTS, 27 were under the care of a physician with no specific diagnosis, and 63 experienced pain but had not sought medical attention.

The data indicated that manual microtomy and coverslipping were associated with pain but there was no direct association with microtomy in clinically proven CTS and only a possible correlation with reports of other physician-diagnosed MSDs. For technologists reporting clinically diagnosed CTS, coverslipping and computer data entry were statistically significant. Embedding and computer data entry were significant among respondents with other clinically diagnosed MSDs.

Conclusion

Computer data entry contributed to clinically proven CTS and other clinically diagnosed MSDs. Manual coverslipping was clinically significant in cases of CTS and embedding was recognized as a contributor to clinically diagnosed MSDs other than CTS. Microtomy was associated with pain, especially by individuals using poor posture and non-ergonomic techniques. The third article in the three-part series described the results of a comprehensive comparison between manual and motorized microtomy and provided information regarding the ergonomic and results-oriented benefits of motorization.

Australia, 2002

Questionnaires were sent to 170 randomly selected members of the Histotechnology Group of New South Wales, Australia, to determine the nature and extent of MSDs among microtome users. It contained questions related to demographics, current and previous work history, specific task-related information, and MSD issues and their perceived associations with tasks or incidents either related or unrelated to work.

Results

One hundred completed questionnaires were returned from 60 females and 40 males. One or more musculoskeletal symptoms were reported by 63% of participants. More females (71.1%) complained of MSDs than males (50%); however, more females cut blocks and embedded cassettes than males, who tended to hold more management positions. Females also reported experiencing multiple symptoms, with 57% having up to four symptoms, and 15% having five or more. This compared to 37% and 12.5% respectively for males. Nearly 50% of females complained of neck and right shoulder symptoms, followed by symptoms in the lower back (38%), left shoulder (31.7%), and wrist (30%). There was a significant difference in shoulder symptoms between females and males: right—female 46.7% vs. male 17.5%: left—female 31.7% vs. male 5%.

Associations were made between the areas of the body affected by MSDs and the amount of time spent doing specific tasks and/or the volume of work performed. The results were:

- Blocks cut per day—lower back, hands and fingers
- Hours per day spent doing microtomy—left shoulder
- Years doing microtomy—elbow
- Number of cassettes embedded per day—left shoulder
- Number of blocks cut per session—wrist.

Conclusion

The authors felt that many routine job functions in histology were related to MSDs and they could be reduced by better job or workstation design, reduction in time spent performing microtomy, and proper task allocation and training.

ERGONOMICS PROGRAMS

Many business and industry leaders have recognized that minimizing injuries prevents human suffering and saves money, so they have been proactive in instituting ergonomics programs. They have found that instituting changes brought about by these programs increased productivity, protected workers from accidents and injuries, and has created compatibility between the work environment, worker, and task. Successful ergonomics programs protect all employees, and enable those with work restrictions, such as elderly, disabled, or pregnant workers, to perform tasks and work for longer periods. Assistance with developing an ergonomics plan is readily available via governmental and private publications and internet resources.

DESIGN CONSIDERATIONS

Human vs. machine

The proper balance of work between people and machines is sometimes difficult to determine. Automation is desirable because it reduces the physical stresses imposed on workers, but having too much automation takes away the unique value of human interaction and decision making that is based on visual interpretation and cognitive experience. Automation should be considered to replace manual tasks that require standardization (processing, and routine, special, and immuno staining) and those that contribute to MSDs (slide and cassette labeling, microtomy, and coverslipping).

Workstation design

Good workstation design is essential in creating a healthy, comfortable, and task-efficient laboratory. Workstations should follow the workflow and be planned to accommodate equipment, ancillary equipment, tools, and supplies. Consideration must also be given to the number of people who will use the space, their physical characteristics, whether they will sit, stand, or use a combination of positions, and if they need some type of aid to be able to see and reach all of the necessary components. Air quality, temperature, and humidity must be regulated and drafts must be avoided. Lighting must be task appropriate, not necessarily standard overhead lighting, and noise must be minimal.

Ideally, laboratory workstations are versatile, modular, and flexible so that they can be altered to accommodate new tasks, equipment or people. The work surface should be height adjustable, and seating should be individualized and task appropriate. Unfortunately, good workstation design is rare in histology laboratories.

Work surfaces

Generally, tasks (not the work surface itself) should be performed at elbow height whether sitting or standing, but that will vary depending upon the type of work. Working at slightly higher than elbow height is practical in a seated position for light, precision work; working at standing height is best for work that is spread out over several areas or difficult to reach or see well. Heavy work that requires upper body strength should be lower than elbow height.

There is an obvious relationship between the height of the work area and the length of the reach. Height-adjustable work surfaces are valuable for tabletop equipment that is too tall to fit under cabinetry or for workers to reach comfortably. If height adjustment is not an option, the position of the operator can be changed as long as it does not create other ergonomic or safety issues. Other alternatives include tilted work surfaces, platforms or risers for either the work or a standing worker, or, for a sitting worker, adjusting the type of seating and supplying a footrest can be beneficial. The standard fixed sitting work surface height is between 28″ and 30″ (71–76 cm) high, and is appropriate for people 5′ 8″ to 5′ 10″ (173–178 cm) in height.

Large work surfaces create long reaches and, occasionally, wasted space. Creating a cutout in a work surface is a good way to get workers closer to their work and reduce reaches, visual effort, and awkward postures.

Work surface edges should be smooth, rounded, and possibly padded if workers perform tasks while resting their fingers, palms, wrists, forearms, elbows, or knees on them. These areas of the body are more susceptible to injury because the nerves, tendons, and blood vessels are close to the skin and underlying bones.

Working positions

Workers should use different muscle groups and vary their posture (sitting, standing, walking) every hour to prevent static postures.

Sitting

Sitting is work for the human spine and musculoskeletal system, and proper seating is an extremely important ergonomic consideration. The introduction of computers into the workplace revolutionized chair design and, since that time, advances have been made. Unfortunately, along with these came multiple theories on what constitutes an ergonomic chair. Most experts will agree that the chair must first properly fit and stabilize the worker, then fit the task, and then allow posture change and a variety of movements. It must also fit into the work area configuration and provide the worker proximity to the work and a good line of vision.

There are obvious factors that are essential when selecting a chair, such as height and support, but there is a myriad of other considerations that are equally important. As an example, people with large hips need higher lumbar support and a wider seat area while people with long legs need a deeper seat. Since there is no 'perfect' chair and no workforce of 'average' sized people, selecting the correct chair is not easy; therefore, it should be individualized and done with the aid of a professional. Ergonomic chairs are more expensive than traditional chairs, but they are a worthwhile investment that can prevent MSDs and their associated costs.

Use a sitting position when:

- Working for an extended time in a fixed position
- Working with hands less than 6″ above counter height
- Writing or doing precise work
- Stability or equilibrium is required.

Sit/stand

Sit/stand seating is just what the name implies. It allows a worker with lower back or hip problems to take the weight off the back and legs by using a chair to support a standing or semi-standing position.

Use a sit/stand position when:

- Getting up and down from a sitting position is hard on the body
- Repeatedly reaching with an extended arm
- Performing tasks that require prolonged static effort.

Standing

Standing is great relief from the fatigue caused by sitting. If standing for long periods is required, a worker should stand on an anti-fatigue mat with one foot propped up and change positions often.

Use a standing position when:

- Mobility is required
- Knee clearance is unavailable
- Reaching (high, low, or extended)
- Exerting downward forces
- Lifting more than 10 pounds.

Footrests

A footrest can be used while standing or sitting. When standing, a worker should alternate feet to relieve stress on the lower back. For seated postures, a footrest should be used if the worker's feet do not touch the floor when their chair is adjusted to work comfortably at a workstation. A footrest should not be used if the worker gets up and down often or scoots the chair from one position to another when performing a task. The footrest should be adjustable in height, have the ability to tilt, and have tread that prevents slipping. If a footrest is too high it will position the hips and spine at an undesirable angle.

Reach zones or comfort zones (horizontal and vertical)

Everything should have a place and anything that is frequently used should be within a comfortable reach zone. Proper work placement reduces MSDs and increases operator efficiency. The area directly in front of the operator (zone 1) is where the majority of work should take place because the worker can maintain a neutral posture and have the greatest strength, dexterity, and visual acuity. Zones 1 and 2 are within a comfortable field of vision, which is approximately within 25″ (64 cm) from the eyes (Figs 32.1 and 32.2).

Zone 1 Objects are easily reached by pivoting at the elbows (forearm swing space). It is for fine detailed work, requires the least amount of body movement, and contains objects that are most commonly used.
Zone 2 Requires arm extension and holds objects that are used less often and do not require fine attention.
Zone 3 Requires full arm and trunk movement and holds objects that are infrequently used.
Horizontal zone 4 Requires full body movement. The worker must rise from a seated position or, if standing, take a step or turn.

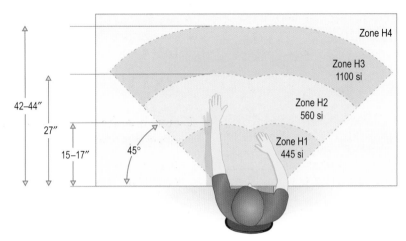

Fig. 32.1 Horizontal (H) reach zones. s.i, square inches (Lee & Nelson, Ergonomics in Lean Manufacturing. Reproduced from website with permission from Strategos, Inc.).

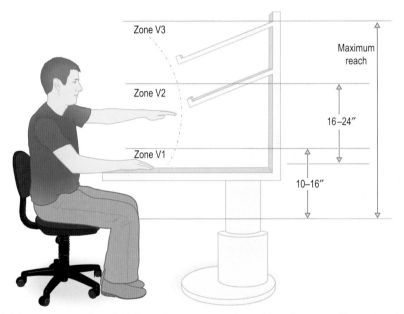

Fig. 32.2 Vertical (V) reach zones (Lee & Nelson, Ergonomics in Lean Manufacturing. Reproduced from website with permission from Strategos, Inc.).

PREVENTION

Prevention

No single mode of prevention exists; however, common sense and ergonomic controls help to minimize risk factors.

- Have the work environment and individual working habits evaluated by a person with a working knowledge of ergonomic principles. (Ergonomist, risk management consultant, or insurance agency.)
- Change as many environmental conditions as possible.
- Invest in ergonomic furniture (chairs and footrests), equipment and tools.
- Position work and frequently used objects directly in front of you.
- Automate any task requiring motions that are MSD risk factors.

- Change hazardous work habits (even if it is the way you were originally taught).
- Use the largest joints and muscles to accomplish a job.
- Be aware of your posture. Keep joints in a neutral position.
- Avoid static postures by alternating positions often.
- Exercise and stretch to strengthen the fingers, hands, wrists, forearms, shoulders, and neck before beginning repetitive, static, or prolonged activities.
- Take mini-breaks every 20–30 minutes when using static postures.
- Listen to your body. If performing a task causes discomfort, evaluate the setup and your body mechanics, and look for an alternative method.
- Recognize symptoms and *report them early*.
- Do not use splints or supports unless a physician or therapist recommends them.
- Determine if there is an underlying medical condition that may increase susceptibility to MSDs.
- Slide, push, or pull objects instead of lifting. If you must lift, use both hands.
- Carry objects close to the body at waist level.

SUGGESTIONS FOR SPECIFIC TASKS

Computer operation

- Maintain good posture with joints in a relaxed, neutral position.
- Keep the keyboard at elbow height or tilted downward.
- Use a gentle touch on the keys.
- Do not hold your thumb or little finger in the air.
- Place the mouse by the keyboard. Be aware that the burden is on one hand and finger.
- Position the top of the monitor at eye level.
- Wear glasses that allow you to keep your head upright or bent slightly forward.
- Do not cradle the phone on your shoulder while working.
- Eliminate sources of reflections and glare on the monitor screen.

Cassette and slide labeling

- Rest wrists on a padded surface when writing.
- Take rest breaks and vary tasks.

- Avoid excessive reaching.
- Use ergonomic writing utensils with large, padded grips.
- Do not use excessive force.
- Automate if possible.

Changing the solutions on the processor

- Use proper bending and lifting techniques.
- Carry containers using a power grip (whole or both hands).
- Use a stool with safe footing to reach above chest height.
- Consider acquiring a processor that assists with the transfer of fluids.

Embedding

See Figure 32.3.

- Maintain good sitting posture.
- Do not lean your arms on sharp or hard surfaces.
- Keep as many items as possible within your reach area.
- Keep joints in a neutral position. Take mini-breaks and exercise wrists and fingers.
- Alternate the motion used to open cassette lids.
- Get up periodically and walk around.
- Use ergonomic forceps.

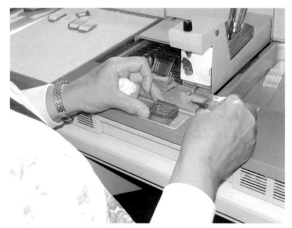

Fig. 32.3 Embedding with forceps held by pinch grip.

Manual microtomy

- Maintain good sitting posture.
- Use a well-adjusted, ergonomic chair and a footrest, if necessary.
- Do keep joints in a relaxed, neutral position.
- *Do not rock the handwheel* (wrist flexion and extension). See Figures 32.4 and 32.5.
- Use a cut-out workstation or an L-shaped extension to reach the water bath without bending at the waist and reaching over.
- Take mini-breaks often. Do exercises and practice self-massage.
- Automate as soon as possible.

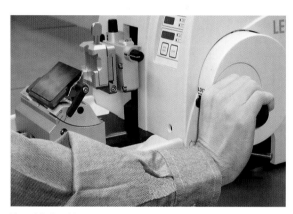

Fig. 32.4   Microtomy—wrist extension position.

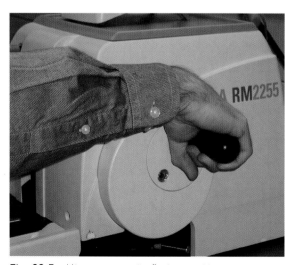

Fig. 32.5   Microtomy—wrist flexion position.

Manual staining

- Maintain good standing posture.
- Prop one foot up or stand with one foot forward, and alternate often.
- Keep work as close to the body as possible.
- Use caution when bending, lifting, and reaching.
- Avoid repeatedly dipping slides (wrist flexion and extension).
- Avoid forceps. Use slide holders and racks.
- Avoid using excessive force to squeeze bottles.
- Automate as soon as possible.

Manual coverslipping

- Automate as soon as possible; or
- Maintain correct posture with head upright and joints in a neutral position.
- Keep work at elbow height and within a close reach.
- Do not lean arms on sharp or hard surfaces.
- Alternate duties.
- Take multiple mini-breaks and do stretching exercises.
- Use ergonomic forceps.

Pipetting

- Maintain correct posture. Work at a cut-out bench if possible.
- Keep work at elbow height and as close as possible.
- Use low-profile tubes, solution containers, and waste receptacles.
- Keep wrists in a neutral position.
- Do not twist or rotate at the waist.
- Use electronic, light-touch pipettes designed for multiple finger use.
- Hold the pipetter with a relaxed grip. Alternate hands, if possible.
- Take short breaks every 20 to 30 minutes.

Cryotomy

- Keep hands as warm as possible to maintain feeling and sensitivity.
- Maintain good posture. Do not lean into the chamber.
- If standing, work with one foot propped up and alternate regularly.

- Keep ancillary items as close as possible (possibly on a cart).
- Use skills detailed under 'Manual microtomy'.

Microscopy

- Avoid static postures. Get up and move around periodically. Alternate tasks.
- Work with the head bent slightly down instead of back.
- Use a well-adjusted, ergonomic chair and sit close to the microscope.
- Use armrests with a soft, smooth surface.
- Use a microscope with ergonomically positioned controls.
- Use adjustable eyepieces or mount the microscope at a 30° angle.
- Request extenders for the microscope body if the eyepieces are still not high enough.
- Work in a place away from drafts and noise.

CONCLUSION

Work-related musculoskeletal disorders and their associated high costs are a major cause for concern in any workplace. To reduce potential occupational injuries, a safe working environment must be created, and all workers must understand, accept, and use the principles of ergonomics.

Employers should provide professional assessment of the working environment, movements associated with routine tasks, and individual work habits of employees. They should insure that job stress is minimized by encouraging task rotation, rest breaks, and employee fitness, moderating the work pace, and reducing biomechanical risks by providing automated instruments. The work environment must allow workers to feel free to offer suggestions and make reports of potential injury without repercussion.

Employees need to study the principles of proper body mechanics and insure that the movements they are using are not harmful. A simple way to do this is by watching the performance of tasks in a mirror. They must accept recommendations for safe work methods, be willing to replace bad habits with safer movements, and agree to use new methodologies and instrumentation. The worker must report MSD symptoms as soon as they are noticed and make helpful suggestions to eliminate the source.

Achieving an ergonomic environment in the histology laboratory makes it a more pleasant place to work, insure that productivity remains high and, at the same time, protects the workforce from the newest workplace hazard–*the way in which they work.*

Appendices

Updated from the previous edition by

William E. Grizzle, Jerry L. Fredenburgh and Russell B. Myers

Appendix 1   Measurement Units

SI Units (Système International d'Unités) are used throughout this text.

STRUCTURE OF SI UNITS

The SI consists of units of three types: base units, derived units, and supplementary units.

It also includes a series of prefixes by means of which decimal multiples and submultiples of units can be formed.

BASE UNITS

Seven units have been selected to serve as the basis of the system.

The four units relevant to the topics included in this book are given in Table Appendix 1.1.

DERIVED UNITS

If a base unit is multiplied by itself or by combining two or more base units, a group of units known as SI derived units are produced. Table Appendix 1.2 gives some examples.

LENGTH

The basic unit of length is the meter/metre (m) and all other units of length are expressed as multiples or sub-multiples of the metre.

VOLUME

The unit of volume is the cubic meter (m^3) but the liter (litre) 1 liter = 1000 cm^3 = 10^{-3} m^3 is allowed. Squared

Table Appendix 1.2   SI derived units

Quantity	Name of derived unit	Symbol for unit
Area	Square meter	m^2
Volume	Cubic meter	m^3
Substance concentration	Moles per cubic meter	mol/m^3

Table Appendix 1.1   SI base units

Quantity	Name of unit	Symbol for unit
Length	Meter (metre)	m
Mass	Kilogram	kg
Amount of substance	Mole	mol
Time	Second	s

Table Appendix 1.3   Non-SI units to be retained for general use

Quantity	Unit	Symbol for unit	Value in SI units
Time	Minute	min	60 s
	Hour	h	3,600 s
	Day	d	86,400 s
Volume	Liter (litre)	l	1 dm^3 = 10^{-3} m^3
Mass	Tonne	t	1,000 kg

Table Appendix 1.4	Length	
Unit	Abbreviation	Size
Meter	m	
Millimeter	mm	10^{-3} m
Micrometer	μm	10^{-6} m
Nanometer	nm	10^{-9} m
Picometer	pm	10^{-12} m

Table Appendix 1.5	Conversion of °C to °F
°C	°F
−80	−112
−70	−94
−40	−40
−20	−4
−17.7	0
−10	14
0 (water freezes)	32
10	50
20	68
30	86
40 (hot day)	104
50	122
60	140
70	158
80	176
90	194
100 (water boils)	212

and cubed are expressed as numerical powers and not by abbreviations. The volume in the histology and scientific laboratories is specified either as liters or more frequently as milliliters (ml).

TEMPERATURE CONVERSION

Several temperature scales are used, the most common of which are the Fahrenheit scale (°F) and the Celsius scale (°C). To convert from Celsius to Fahrenheit you multiply the Celsius temperature by 9/5 and add 32. Thus the temperature of boiling, 100°C, converts to (9/5) (100°C) + 32 = 180 + 32 = 212°F. Similarly, the freezing point of water is 0°C or 9/5 (0°) + 32 = 32°F. To convert from Fahrenheit you first subtract (32°F) and then multiply by 5/9. Thus the 212°F boiling point converts to (212 − 32) × 5/9 = 180 (5/9) = 100°C. Table Appendix 1.5 provides some simple conversions.

MASS

The basic unit is the kilogram (kg) and the working unit is the gram (g). The multiples and submultiples are of the gram as shown in Table Appendix 1.6.

Table Appendix 1.6	Mass	
Unit	Abbreviation	Size
Milligram	mg	10^{-3} g
Microgram	μg	10^{-6} g
Nanogram	ng	10^{-9} g
Picogram	pg	10^{-12} g

REFERENCES

Missel D.L. (1979) Proceedings of the Royal Microscopical Society 14:385.

World Health Organisation (1977) The SI for the health professions. Geneva: WHO.

Appendix II   Preparation of Solutions

INTRODUCTION

Most solutions in histology are made using water as a solvent. The agent dissolved in water to make an aqueous solution is the solute. Solutions typically are made as volume to volume and weight to volume. Consider the example of concentrated formaldehyde which is about a 37–43% solution of formaldehyde in water. This represents the maximum solubility of the molecule, CH_3CH_2O (solute), in water (the solvent) and the resulting solution is a 37–43% w/v (weight to volume) solution.

VOLUME TO VOLUME SOLUTION

Making 10% formalin from a concentrated solution of formaldehyde (37% w/v) is an example of preparing a volume to volume solution. We add one part of concentrated formaldehyde to nine parts of water and this yields a 10% solution of formalin that is actually about a 4% solution of formaldehyde. Ten per cent formalin is buffered to make 10% neutral buffered formalin—the most commonly used fixative in the USA and Europe.

For accuracy in preparing a solution, do not measure small volumes unless volume-calibrated pipettes are available. Remember the accuracy of a dilute solution is based more upon the accuracy of the measurement of the solute than of the measurement of the solvent; thus, if 1.1 ml of solute is added instead of 1 ml, the error is 10% in the concentration of a 1% solution. However, if 1 ml of solute is added to 99.1 ml instead of 99 ml of solvent, the error is of the order of 1%.

A stock solution is used to prevent having to measure small amounts of the solute, and also sometimes for molecular stability. If you have a 1% stock solution, a 0.1% solution is prepared by adding 10 ml of 1% solution to 90 ml of water, and a 0.01% solution is prepared by adding 1 ml of 1% stock solution to 99 ml of water.

In the preparation of solutions, use at least reagent grade chemicals and in general distilled or deionized water. Note the state of hydration specified on the chemical container (chemicals should not be used that are not in their original containers). The state of hydration must be considered in the molecular weight of the chemical.

In preparing various solutions, the equation, volume of solution 1 × concentration 1 = volume of solution 2 × concentration 2 ($V_1C_1 = V_2C_2$) is very useful in modifying one solution in terms of an original solution. Examples of its use are as follows:

Using 100 ml of a solution of 1% sodium hydroxide, prepare a 0.5% solution of sodium hydroxide:

$$100 \text{ ml} \times 1\% = X \text{ ml} \times 0.5\%$$
$$X \text{ ml} = 200 \text{ ml}.$$

You therefore need to add 100 ml of water to the 100 ml original solution to go from 100 ml of 1% to 200 ml of 0.5% sodium hydroxide.

Using 50 ml of 5% potassium permanganate prepare a 2% solution of potassium permanganate:

$$50 \text{ ml} \times 5\% = X \text{ ml} \times 2\%$$
$$X \text{ ml} = 125 \text{ ml}.$$

Table Appendix 2.1   Volume to volume solutions: preparation of 100 ml of a solution

% Aqueous solution	ml of solute	ml of water
1%	1 ml	99 ml
5%	5 ml	95 ml
10%	10 ml	90 ml
50%	50 ml	50 ml

For a 1-liter solution, multiply the solute and water by 10.

You therefore need to add 75 ml of water to the 50 ml original solution to go from 50 ml of 5% to 125 ml of 2% potassium permanganate.

WEIGHT TO VOLUME SOLUTIONS

Weight to volume solutions are typically used when a weight of a solute, typically a solid, is dissolved in an aqueous or other solvent. In such a preparation, one can consider the weight of 100 ml of water to be 100 grams. To make a 1% solution of potassium permanganate, add 1 gram of potassium permanganate to 99 ml of water and make the final solution up to 100 ml. This usually requires a 100-ml volumetric flask. In histology, such accuracy is seldom required and a good approximation is to dissolve the solute in 100 ml of the solvent. Just like volume to volume solutions, do not try to measure small quantities of the solute (less than 1 gram). If a dilute solution is to be made, dilute a more concentrated solution as shown below for solutions of 0.1% or less. Be careful to note the state of hydration of the chemical being used. The weight of the complexed water must be calculated and removed from the chemical weight.

To avoid measuring less than 1 g, change the preparation from weight to volume to a volume to volume solution as shown in Table Appendix 2.1.

Examples

Prepare a 0.0025% solution of sodium chloride. (Note for a % weight : volume solution you do not need the molecular weight of NaCl). Start by preparing a 2.5% solution or 2.5 g of salt in 100 ml of water. Add 1 ml of this 2.5% solution to 1000 ml of water. This would provide a 0.0025% solution without weighing or measuring small quantities.

Table Appendix 2.2   Preparation of weight to volume solutions

% Weight	Solute	Solvent
1	1 g	100 ml
2.5	2.5 g	100 ml
5	5 g	100 ml
7.5	7.5 g	100 ml
10	10 g	100 ml
0.1	10 ml of 1%	90 ml
0.01	1 ml of 1%	99 ml
0.001	1 ml of 0.1%	99 ml

Again the equation $V_1C_1 = V_2C_2$ is very useful.

How many milliliters of water do you add to 100 ml of 20% sodium chloride to obtain a 7.5% solution?

$$100 \text{ ml} \times 20\% = X \text{ ml} \times 7.5\%$$

$$X \text{ ml} = 2000/7.5 = 267 \text{ ml}$$

Thus you need to add 167 ml of water to the 100 ml of 20% solution to produce 267 ml of a 7.5% solution.

MOLAR SOLUTIONS

These are based upon the molecular weight of the solute. The molecular weight is stated on the label of the container of the chemical or it can be looked up in the Merk Index or CRC Handbook of Chemistry. If water is bound to the solute, the amount of water typically bound at laboratory conditions must be considered in weighing the molecular weight of the solute. A 1 molar solution is the molecular weight in grams of the solute dissolved in 1 liter (1000 ml) of the solvent. A 1 molar solution of sodium chloride (molecular weight = 58.5 g) is prepared by dissolving 58.5 grams of sodium chloride in 1 liter of water. A 0.1 molar solution of sodium chloride is 5.85 grams dissolved in 1 liter.

NORMAL SOLUTIONS

The preparation of a normal solution is based upon dissolving an equivalent weight of an equivalent single positive ionic species. Sometimes this is called the equivalent (molecular) weight. For example, if only one positive ion is present in a molecule, such as sodium chloride (NaCl), then the equivalent weight is the same as the molecular weight and a 1 normal solution is the same as a 1 molar solution; thus one molecular weight of sodium ions is present in the 1 N solution. In contrast, potassium sulfate (K_2SO_4) has two positive ions per molecule; thus the equivalent weight is the molecular weight divided by 2. In the case of calcium chloride [$Ca(Cl)_2$], the calcium with a positive charge (valence) of 2 is equivalent to two positive ions, so the normal (equivalent) weight is half the molecular weight. Thus the equivalent weight used to prepare normal solutions depends on the molecular weight **and** the ionic form of the molecule. The preparation of normal solutions is described in Table Appendix 2.4.

Table Appendix 2.3 Preparation of molar solutions

Solution	Weight of solute	Final volume of solution
1 molar	Molecular weight in grams	1000 ml
0.1 molar	0.1 × molecular weight	1000 ml
0.01 molar	10 ml of 0.1 molar	100 ml (90 ml solvent)
0.001 molar	10 ml of 0.01 molar	100 ml (90 ml solvent)

Table Appendix 2.4 Preparation of normal solutions

Normality	Species	Equivalent weight
1 N	$X^{+1}Y^{-1}$	Molecular weight
1 N	$X^{+2}Y^{-2}$	$1/2$ the molecular weight
1 N	$X^{+3}(Y^{-1})_3$	$1/3$ the molecular weight
0.5 N	$X^{+1}Y^{-1}$	$1/2$ the molecular weight
0.5 N	$X^{+2}Y^{-2}$	$1/4$ the molecular weight
0.1 N	Any species	1 part 1 N and 9 parts water
0.01 N	Any species	1 part 0.1 N and 9 parts water
0.001 N	Any species	1 part 0.1 N and 99 parts water

PREPARATION OF USEFUL SOLUTIONS

Acid alcohol

70% alcohol	99 ml
Concentrated hydrochloric acid	1 ml

Acid permanganate

0.5% aqueous potassium permanganate	50 ml
3% sulfuric acid	2.5 ml

Alcian blue (varying pH of solution)

pH 0.2	1 g in 100 ml of 10% sulfuric acid
pH 0.5	1 g in 100 ml of 0.2 M hydrochloric acid
pH 1.0	1 g in 100 ml of 0.1 M hydrochloric acid
pH 2.5	1 g in 100 ml of 3% acetic acid
pH 3.2	1 g in 100 ml of 0.5% acetic acid

Celestine blue

Celestine blue B	2.5 g
Ferric ammonium sulfate	25 g
Glycerin	70 ml
Distilled water	500 ml

Dissolve the ferric ammonium sulfate in cold distilled water and stir well. Add the Celestine blue to this solution, then boil the mixture for a few minutes. After cooling, filter the stain and add the glycerin.

Formalin ammonium bromide

Formalin	15 ml
Ammonium bromide	2 g
Distilled water	85 ml

Formal calcium

40% formaldehyde	100 ml
Distilled water	900 ml
10% calcium chloride	100 ml

Gram's iodine

Iodine	3 g
Potassium iodide	6 g
Distilled water	900 ml

Lugol's iodine

Iodine	1 g
Potassium iodide	2 g
Distilled water	100 ml

Magnesium chloride

(for alcian blue at different electrolyte concentrations)

0.05 M	1.01 g in 100 ml of distilled water
0.06 M	1.22 g in 100 ml of distilled water
0.3 M	6.09 g in 100 ml of distilled water
0.5 M	10.15 g in 100 ml of distilled water
0.7 M	14.21 g in 100 ml of distilled water
0.9 M	18.27 g in 100 ml of distilled water

Mayer's carmalum

Ammonium or potassium alum	10 g
Carminic acid	1 g
Distilled water	200 ml
Salicylic acid as preservative	0.2 g

Dissolve the alum and the carminic acid in the distilled water with the aid of gentle heat. Cool, filter, and then add the salicylic acid.

2% methyl green (chloroform washed)

Methyl green	2 g
Distilled water	100 ml

Dissolve the methyl green in the distilled water. Pour the solution into a separating funnel. Add 100 ml of chloroform and shake well. Run off the contaminated chloroform and repeat until no more violet is extracted (6–8 washes).

Picric acid (saturated)

The solubility of picric acid is 1.2 g/100 ml or 1.2%. Due to the hazards of dry picric acid, it is typically sold in a form containing 30–35% water.

Picric acid (hydrated)	1.6 g
Distilled water	100 ml

Note

Solutions of picric acid should not be allowed to evaporate, as dry picric acid is potentially explosive.

Scott's tap water

Potassium bicarbonate	2 g
Magnesium sulfate	20 g
Distilled water	1000 ml

Tincture of iodine

Potassium	2 g
Iodine	2 g
Distilled water	2 ml
90% alcohol	75 ml

TRIS–HCl buffered saline pH 7.6 (for immunoperoxidase wash)

Sodium chloride	8.1 g
TRIS (TRIS hydroxymethyl-aminomethane)	0.6 g
1 M HCl	3.8 ml
Distilled water	to 1000 ml

Van Gieson stain

Picric acid, saturated aqueous solution	50 ml
1.0% acid fuchsin, aqueous solution	9 ml
Distilled water	50 ml

Weigert's borax ferricyanide solution

Borax	2 g
Potassium ferricyanide	2.2 g
Distilled water	200 ml

Appendix III   Buffers

INTRODUCTION

The pH of a solution is defined as the logarithm to base 10 of 1 divided by the concentration of the free hydrogen ions in solution (i.e. $pH = \log_{10} 1/[A^+] = -\log_{10}[H^+]$). A neutral solution is defined as $pH = -\log_{10}[10^{-7}] = 7$. The pH may greatly affect may chemical and immunohistochemical reactions; thus it is frequently important to minimize large changes in free hydrogen ion content (i.e. in pH).

Buffers are typically solutions in which additions of small quantities of acids or bases cause little or no change in the pH of the solution. Thus the solution 'buffers' against a change in pH. This is accomplished by solutions of inorganic and organic acids or bases plus salts which together absorb free hydrogen or free hydroxyl ions to prevent major changes in pH. Several major buffer systems are used in histochemical and/or immunohistochemical staining. Buffer systems include citric acid, sodium citrate, acetic acid–sodium acetate, and mixtures of sodium or potassium phosphates. One frequently used system is based on the use of tri(hydroxyl methyl) aminomethane, called 'Tris'. Tris buffer systems include Tris–maleic acid. Tris buffers are susceptible to temperature changes, so pH values specified at multiple temperatures are shown. The following tables of buffers are prepared so that the material added is within parenthesis. Usually it is milliliters (ml) or cubic centimeters (ml) but may be in grams. The buffer tables given below are the primary buffers referred to in this edition. For any buffers required and not listed here, the reader is referred to Pearse (1980) and Lillie and Fullmer (1976), or to suitable biochemical texts.

General notes regarding buffer solutions

The salts and acids used in the preparation of buffers should be of at least laboratory reagent grade. When preparing buffers the molecular weight given on the reagent bottle should be checked, as many chemicals are available in a number of states of hydration.

Acetate buffer

Preparation of stock solutions
Stock A: 0.2 M acetic acid (MW 60.05)
1.2 ml of glacial acetic acid in 100 ml of distilled water.

Stock B: 0.2 M sodium acetate
1.64 g of sodium acetate trihydrate (MW 136) in 100 ml of distilled water.

0.2 M acetate buffer or Walpole buffer; 0.1 M acetate buffer

pH 0.2 M	pH 0.1 M	0.2 M acetic acid (ml)	0.2 M sodium acetate (ml)	0.1 M acetic acid (ml)	0.1 M sodium acetate (ml)
2.696	—	20	0	—	—
2.804	—	19.9	0.1	—	—
2.913	—	19.8	0.2	—	—
2.994	—	19.7	0.3	—	—
3.081	—	19.6	0.4	—	—
3.147	—	19.5	0.5	—	—
3.202	—	19.4	0.6	—	—
3.315	—	19.2	0.8	—	—
3.416	—	19.0	1.0	—	—
3.592	—	18.5	1.5	—	—
—	3.6	—	—	18.5	1.5
3.723	—	18	2	—	—
—	3.8	—	—	17.6	2.4
3.9	—	17	3	—	—
—	4.0	—	—	16.4	3.6
4.047	—	16	4	—	—
4.160	—	15	5	—	—
—	4.2	—	—	14.7	5.3
4.270	—	14	6	—	—
4.360	—	13	7	—	—
—	4.4	—	—	12.6	7.4
4.454	—	12	8	—	—
4.530	—	11	9	—	—
—	4.6	—	—	10.2	9.8
4.62	—	10	10	—	—
4.71	—	11	9	—	—
4.802	—	8	12	—	—
4.900	—	7	13	—	—
4.990	—	6	14	—	—
—	5.0	—	—	8.0	12
5.110	—	5	15	—	—
—	5.2	—	—	5.9	14.1
5.227	—	4	16	—	—
—	5.3	—	—	4.2	15.8
5.380	—	3	17	—	—
—	5.4	—	—	2.9	17.1
5.574	—	2	18	—	—
—	5.6	—	—	1.9	18.1
5.894	—	1	19	—	—
6.211	—	0.5	19.5	—	—
6.518	—	0	20	—	—

Cacodylate buffer

Preparation of stock solutions

Stock A: 0.2 M sodium cacodylate (MW 214)
4.28 g of sodium cacodylate in 100 ml of distilled water.

Stock B: 0.2 M HCl (MW 36.46)
1.7 ml of hydrochloric acid in 100 ml of distilled water.

Cacodylate buffer			
0.2 M sodium cacodylate (ml)	0.2 M HCl (ml)	pH	Distilled water (ml)
50	2.7	7.4	147.3
50	4.2	7.2	145.8
50	6.3	7.0	143.7
50	9.3	6.8	140.7
50	13.3	6.6	136.7
50	18.3	6.4	131.7
50	23.8	6.2	126.2
50	29.6	6.0	120.4
50	34.8	5.8	114.2
50	39.2	5.6	110.8
50	43.0	5.4	107.0
50	45.0	5.2	105.0
50	47.0	5.0	103.0

Source: Plumel M (1949) Bulletin de la Société de Chimie Biologique 30:129.

Phosphate buffer

Preparation of stock solutions

Stock A: 0.1 M sodium dihydrogen orthophosphate (MW 156)

1.56 g of sodium dihydrogen orthophosphate in 100 ml of distilled water.

Stock B: 0.1 M disodium hydrogen orthophosphate (MW 142)

1.415 g of disodium hydrogen orthophosphate in 100 ml of distilled water.

Phosphate buffer (Sorensen's buffer) (25°C)		
pH	0.1 M NaH$_2$PO$_4$ (ml)	0.1 M Na$_2$HPO$_4$ (ml)
4.41	50	0
5.31	48	2
5.53	47	3
5.67	46	4
5.78	45	5
5.86	44	6
5.94	43	7
6.02	42	8
6.08	41	9
6.12	40	10
6.17	39	11
6.23	38	12
6.28	37	13
6.33	36	14
6.37	35	15
6.41	34	16
6.45	33	17
6.49	32	18
6.53	31	19
6.55	30	20
6.58	29	21
6.61	28	22
6.65	27	23
6.70	26	24
6.76	25	25

Phosphate buffer (Sorensen's buffer) (25°C)		
pH	0.1 M NaH$_2$PO$_4$ (ml)	0.1 M Na$_2$HPO$_4$ (ml)
6.81	24	26
6.84	23	27
6.87	22	28
6.89	21	29
6.91	20	30
6.94	19	31
6.97	18	32
7.00	17	33
7.02	16	34
7.06	15	35
7.10	14	36
7.14	13	37
7.19	12	38
7.24	11	39
7.30	10	40
7.36	9	41
7.42	8	42
7.49	7	43
7.57	6	44
7.65	5	45
7.73	4	46
7.81	3	47
7.92	2	48
8.98	0	50
8.98	0	50

Phosphate–citrate buffer (McIlvaine's)

Preparation of solutions

Stock A: 0.2 M disodium hydrogen orthophosphate (MW 142.0)
2.83 g of disodium hydrogen orthophosphate in 100 ml of distilled water.

Stock B: 0.1 M citric acid (MW 210.0)
2.1 g of citric acid in 100 ml of distilled water.

Stock C: 0.2 M sodium dihydrogen phosphate (MW 156.01)
3.12 g sodium dihydrogen phosphate in 100 ml of distilled water.

Basic phosphate–citric acid buffer (McIlvaine's)				
pH	0.2 M Na$_2$HPO$_4$ (ml)	0.1 M Citric acid (ml)	0.2 M NaH$_2$PO$_4$ (ml)	Distilled water (ml)
2.2	0.4	19.6	—	—
2.4	1.24	18.76	—	—
2.6	2.18	17.82	—	—
2.8	3.17	16.83	—	—
3.0	4.11	15.89	—	—
3.2	4.94	15.06	—	—
3.4	5.70	14.30	—	—
3.6	6.44	13.56	—	—
3.8	7.10	12.90	—	—
4.0	7.71	12.29	—	—
4.2	8.28	11.72	—	—
4.4	8.82	11.18	—	—
4.6	9.35	10.65	—	—
4.8	9.86	10.14	—	—
5.0	10.30	9.70	—	—
5.2	10.72	9.28	—	—
5.4	11.15	8.85	—	—
5.6	11.60	8.40	—	—
5.8	12.09	7.91	—	—
5.8	8.0	—	92	100
6.2	13.22	6.78	—	—
6.2	18.5	—	81.5	100
6.4	13.05	6.15	—	—
6.4	26.5	—	73.5	100
6.6	14.85	5.45	—	—
6.6	37.5	—	62.5	100
6.8	15.45	4.55	—	—
6.8	49.0	—	51	100
7.0	16.47	3.53	—	—
7.0	61.0	—	39	100
7.2	17.39	2.61	—	—
7.2	72.0	—	28	100
7.4	18.17	1.83	—	—
7.4	81.0	—	19.0	100
7.6	18.73	1.27	—	—
7.6	87.0	—	13.0	100
7.8	19.15	0.85	—	—
7.8	91.5	—	8.5	100
8.0	19.45	0.55	—	—
8.0	94.7	—	5.3	100

Tris-HCl buffer

Preparation of stock solutions

Stock A: 0.2 M Tris (MW 121.0)
2.42 g of Tris (hydroxymethyl) aminomethane in 100 ml of distilled water.

Stock B: 0.1 M HCl (MW 36.46)
0.85 ml of hydrochloric acid in 100 ml of distilled water. Do not add water to acid.

Tris–HCl buffer and commercial Tris buffer						
pH at			25 ml 0.2 M Tris plus 0.1 M HCl in volumes indicated	TRIZMA® 0.05 M	TRIZMA®— base 0.05 M	Water
23°C	25°C	37°C	(ml)	(grams)	(grams)	(ml)
9.10		8.95	5.0	—	—	95
	9.0	8.7	—	0.76	5.47	994
8.92		8.78	7.5	—	—	92.5
	8.9	8.62	—	0.96	5.32	994
8.74		8.60	10	—	—	90
	8.8	8.51	—	1.23	5.13	993
8.62		8.48	12.5	—	—	87.5
	8.7	8.42	—	1.5	4.9	993
8.50		8.37	17.5	—	—	82.5
	8.6	8.31	—	1.83	4.65	993
8.40		8.27	20	—	—	80
	8.5	8.22	—	2.21	4.36	993
8.32		8.10	22.5	—	—	79.5
	8.4	8.1	—	2.64	4.03	993
8.14		8.0	25	—	—	75
	8.3	8.01	—	3.07	3.70	993
8.05		7.9	27.5	—	—	72.5
	8.2	7.91	—	3.54	3.34	993
7.96		7.82	30	—	—	70
	8.1	7.8	—	4.02	2.97	993
7.87		7.73	32.5	—	—	67.5
	8.0	7.71	—	4.44	2.65	993
7.77		7.63	35	—	—	65
	7.9	7.62	—	4.88	2.30	993
7.66		7.52	37.5	—	—	62.5
	7.8	7.52	—	5.32	1.97	993
7.54		7.40	40	—	—	60
	7.7	7.40	—	5.72	1.66	993
7.36		7.22	42.5	—	—	57.5
	7.6	7.30	—	6.06	1.39	993
7.20		7.05	45	—	—	55
	7.5	7.22	—	6.35	1.18	993
	7.4	7.12	—	6.61	0.97	992
	7.3	7.02	—	6.85	0.80	992
	7.2	6.91	—	7.02	0.67	992

REFERENCES

Bancroft J.D. (1975) Histochemical techniques, 2nd edn. London: Butterworths.

Gomori G. (1948) Histochemical demonstration of sites of choline esterase activity. Proceedings of the Society for Experimental Biology and Medicine 68:354.

Gomori G. (1955) Preparation of buffers for use in enzyme studies. Methods in Enzymology 1:138–146.

Lillie R.D., Fullmer H.M. (1976) Histopathologic technic and practical histochemistry, 4th edn. New York: McGraw-Hill.

McIlvaine T.C. (1921) A buffer solution for colorimetric comparison. Journal of Biological Chemistry 49:183.

Pearse A.G.E. (1980) Histochemistry: theoretical and applied, 3rd edn. Edinburgh: Churchill Livingstone, Vol. 1.

Appendix IV Solubility of some common Reagents and Dyes

In the following table, the weight of solute (in the third column), dissolved in the volume of distilled water (in the right-hand column) will produce 100 ml of a saturated solution at the temperature given in the left-hand column.

Solubility of useful reagents			
	Temp °C	Weight of solute (g)	Volume of distilled water (ml)
Aluminum ammonium sulfate	25	13	92.0
Aluminum potassium sulfate	25	7.02	99.1
Aluminum sulfate	25	63	66.0
Ammonium molybdate	25	39	88.0
Ammonium nitrate	25	90.2	41.8
Ammonium oxalate	25	5.06	97.0
Calcium chloride	25	67.8	79.2
Chloral hydrate	25	120	31.0
Citric acid	25	88.6	42.7
Cobalt nitrate	18	78.2	79.1
Cupric sulfate	25	22.3	98.7
Dextrose	25	59	60.0
Ferric ammonium sulfate	16.5	22.4	94.3
Ferric chloride	25	131.1	48.3
Ferric nitrate	25	70.2	79.2
Glycine	25	21.7	86.8
L-Glutamic acid	25	0.86	99.15
Hydroquinone	20	6.78	94.4
Lead nitrate	25	53.6	91.0
Lithium carbonate	15	1.38	100.0
Magnesium chloride	25	79	47.5
Magnesium nitrate	25	58.6	80.5
Magnesium sulfate	25	72	58.5
Oxalic acid	25	10.3	94.2
Phenol crystals	20	6.14	94.5
Phosphomolybdic acid	25	135	46.0
Phosphotungstic acid	25	160	64.0
Potassium acetate	25	97.1	44.3
Potassium bicarbonate	25	31.6	87.5

	Temp °C	Weight of solute (g)	Volume of distilled water (ml)
Potassium bromide	25	56	82.0
Potassium carbonate	25	82.2	73.5
Potassium chloride	25	31.2	86.8
Potassium dichromate	25	14.2	95.0
Potassium ferricyanide	22	38.1	80.8
Potassium ferrocyanide	25	28.2	89.2
Potassium hydroxide	15	79.2	74.2
Potassium iodide	25	103.2	69.1
Potassium nitrate	25	33.4	86.0
Potassium permanganate	25	7.43	97.3
Resorcin	25	67.2	47.2
Silver nitrate	25	164	65.5
Sodium acetate	25	40.5	80.0
Sodium bicarbonate	15	8.8	97.6
Sodium carbonate	25	28.1	96.5
Sodium chloride	25	31.7	88.1
Disodium hydrogen orthophosphate	17	4.4	99.9
Sodium hydroxide	25	77	74.0
Sodium hypophosphite	16	72.4	66.6
Sodium iodate	25	9.21	98.5
Sodium nitrite	20	62.3	73.8
Sodium periodate	25	13.9	96.2
Sodium sulfate	25	28.5	95.5
Sodium sulfite	25	26.4	94.5
Sodium thiosulfate	25	93	46.0
Sucrose	25	90.0	43.0
Trichloroacetic acid	25	149.6	12.41

Solubility of some dyes

Dye name	Generic name	Colour Index no.*	Approx. solubility (g/100 ml)	
			Water	Alcohol
Acridine Orange	Basic Orange 14	46005	Sol	Sol
Alcian Blue 8GX	Ingrain Blue 1	74240	5	1.6
Alizarin Red S	Mordant Red 3	58005	7.5	0.15
Aniline Blue (H_2O sol)	Acid Blue 22	42755	Sol	Slight
(Soluble blue 3 M or 2R, water blue)				
Auramine O	Basic Yellow 2	41000	0.7	4.5
Azophloxine	Acid Red 1	18050	3	Slight
Azur A (McNeal)		52005	Sol	Sol
Biebrich Scarlet	Acid Red 66	26905	Sol	0.05
Bismark Brown Y (Vesuvian Brown)	Basic Brown 1	21000	1.3	1.1
Carmine	Natural Red 4	75470	Sol	Slight

Solubility of some dyes

Dye name	Generic name	Colour Index no.*	Approx. solubility (g/100 ml)	
			Water	Alcohol
Carminic Acid	Natural Red 4	75470	8.3	–
Chromotrope 2R	Acid Red 29	16570	19	0.15
Congo Red	Direct Red 28	22120	Sol	0.2
Cresyl Fast Violet	–	–	Sol	Slight
Crystal Ponceau 6R (brilliant Crystal Scarlet 6R, Ponceau 6R)	Acid Red 44	16250	3	0.5
Crystal Violet	Basic Violet 3	42555	1.7	13
Eosin Yellowish (H$_2$O & alcohol sol, Eosin Y)	Acid Red 87	45380	44	2
Eosin Bluish (Eosin B, Erythrosin B)	Acid Red 51	45430	11	2
Fast Garner GBC salt	Azoic Diazo component 4	37210	5	–
Fast Green FCF	Food Green 3	42053	16	0.35
Fast Red B salt	Azoic Diazo component 5	37125	20	–
Fast Red TR salt	Azoic Diazo component 11	37085	20	–
Fluorescein	Acid Yellow 73	45350	–	2.1
Fuchsin acid	Acid Violet 19	42685	20	0.25
Fuchsin basic	Basic Violet 14	42510	0.4	8
Fuchsin new	Basic Violet 2	42520	1.13	0.41
Gallocyanine	Mordant Blue 10	51030	Insol	Slight
Hematoxylin	Natural Black 1	75290	1.5	>30
Indigo carmine	Food Blue 1	73015	1.1	–
Janus Green B	–	11050	5.3	1.1
Light Green SF	Acid Gren 5	42095	20	0.8
Luxol Fast Blue	Solvent Blue 38	–	V. Sol	Sol
Malachite Green	Basic Green 4	42000	7.60	7.52
Martius Yellow	Acid Yellow 24	10315	4.5	0.15
Metanil Yellow	Acid Yellow 36	13065	5.36	1.45
Methyl Blue	Acid Blue 93	42780	Sol	Slight
Methyl Green	Basic Blue 20	42585	Sol	Insol
Methyl Violet 2B	Basic Violet 1	42535	3	15
Methylene Blue	Basic Blue 9	52015	3.5	1.5
Neutral Red	Basic Red 5	50040	5.5	2.5
Nile Blue Sulfate	Basic Blue 12	51180	1.0	1.0
Oil Red O	Solvent Red 27	26125	Insol	0.5
Orange G	Acid Orange 10	16230	10	0.2
Patent Blue	Acid Blue 1	42045	8.4	5.23
Phloxine	Acid Red 92	45410	50	9
Phosphine	Basic Orange 15	46045	Sol	Sol
Picric Acid	–	10305	1.2	8
Ponceau 2R (Ponceau de xylidene)	Acid Red 26	16150	6	0.1
Pyronin Y (Pyronin G)		45005	9	0.6
Rhodamine B	Basic Violet 10	45170	0.8	1.5
Safranin O	Basic Red 2	50240	5.5	3.5

Solubility of some dyes

Dye name	Generic name	Colour Index no.*	Approx. solubility (g/100 ml)	
			Water	Alcohol
Solochrome cyanine RS (Eriochrome cyanine R)	Mordant Blue 3	43820	Sol	Sol
Scarlet R (Sudan IV)	Solvent Red 24	26105	Insol	0.2
Sudan Black B	Solvent Black 3	26150	Insol	1.13
Tartrazine	Food Yellow 4	19140	11	0.1
Thioflavine T	Basic Yellow 1	49005	Sol	Sol
Thionin	–	52000	0.25	0.25
Toluidine Blue	Basic Blue 17	52040	3.8	0.5
Victoria Blue B	Basic Blue 26	44045	0.5	4

*From Colour Index International, 3rd edn. Bradford, UK: Society of Dyers and Colourists and American Association of Textile Chemists and Colorists. Sol = soluble, Insol = insoluble, V. Sol = very soluble.

Appendix V Mounting Media and Slide Coatings

In order to provide the maximum degree of transparency to stained tissue sections, the refractive index of the mounting medium must approximate to that of dried protein, i.e. between 1.53 and 1.54. This is especially important for photographing slides. To visualize detail in unstained tissues, it may be desirable to employ a medium of lower or higher refractive index. The refractive index of a mounting medium may change on drying due to evaporation of solvents. Air bubbles should not be permitted to remain under coverslips since these air bubbles tend to expand.

AQUEOUS MOUNTANTS

Few aqueous mountants have a refractive index higher than 1.5, most being in the range 1.40 to 1.45. Higher refractives are usually achieved by the use of high concentrations of sugars.

Potassium acetate may be added to mountants, almost to the point of saturation, in order to reduce the 'bleeding' of cationic dyes, at the same time giving a pH of approximately 7.0.

Most pathology laboratories currently utilize commercial mounting media, usually non-aqueous. From the standpoint of safety and costs, this may be a laboratory's best approach to mounting. Aqueous mounting media are still important for special stains requiring aqueous media and for mounting immunohistochemical stains, for example with 3-amino-9-ethylcarbazole (AEC).

If a laboratory cannot afford to purchase commercially available mountant, the best choice might be polystyrene mountant. This can be made from polystyrene granules or recycled polystyrene (cups, packing crickets):

Polystyrene mountant (refractive index 1.54)

Polystyrene	25 g
Xylene	70 ml

If available, add 5 ml of dibutyl phthalate which keeps the mounting media from shrinking upon drying.

For other specialized mountants, see the appendices for the fifth edition of this text.

Apathy's mountant (modified by Lillie & Ashburn 1943), refractive index 1.41

Gum Arabic crystals	50 g
Cane sugar	50 g
Distilled water	100 ml
Thymol	100 mg

Dissolve with moderate heating.

Apathy's mountant (Highman's modification, 1946), refractive index 1.436

Gum Arabic crystals	50 g
Cane sugar	50 g
Potassium acetate	50 g
Distilled water	100 ml

Gentle heat may be used to dissolve the solids. 0.05 g of thymol or merthiolate may be added as a preservative.

FLUORESCENCE-FREE MOUNTING MEDIA

Some mounting media fluoresce in short wavelength light; this interferes with the examination of material under the fluorescence microscope. Fluorescence-free mountants are available commercially in both resinous and aqueous forms.

COMBINED COVERSLIP AND MOUNTANT

Several manufacturers supply a medium of a varnish-like nature which may be used to coat the section surface, by dipping, pouring, or spraying. This type of medium obviates the use of a coverslip.

For low-power microscopy, combined mountant and coverslip may prove quite satisfactory although little protection of the section to abrasion is given. High-power microscopy demands the use of optically flat slide surfaces with a coverslip of known thickness.

COATING OF SLIDES

Microscopic slides may be coated for several reasons:

1. To act as an adhesive to keep difficult tissue specimens attached. For example, fatty tissues such as breast; hard tissues such as bone, synovium, and cartilage; or cellular preparations.
2. To aid in cellular attachment when cells are to be grown on slides or coverslips.
3. To make staining more consistent when staining small structures (e.g. cultured cells) spread across microscope slides.

Multiple materials may be used to aid in the attachment of tissue to slides. Most of these can be obtained from specialty chemical supply sources. Methods to improve the attachment of tissues to microscope slides include the use of special commercial slides (silanized) or the preparation and use of silanized slides.

Silanized slides are prepared by cleaning the slides by washing, followed with a rinse in 95% ethanol. Some 4 ml of 3-aminopropyltriethoxy silane is added to 200 ml of acetone and slides are dipped for 30–60 seconds, followed by 60 seconds in agitated distilled water. The coated slides are then dried for 1 hour, and can be boxed for future use.

Polylysine slides are prepared similarly to silanized slides. First wash the slides followed by a rinse in 95% ethanol. Immerse the non-frosted portion of slides in a 5% solution of polylysine for more than 1 minute. Dry for over 1 hour. The slides can be boxed for future use.

Albumen-coated slides—wash slides followed by a 95% ethanol wash. Make a 5% solution of crude egg albumen Grade II and immerse non-frosted portion of slides for over 1 minute. Permit to dry for 1 hour and then fix in a solution of 10% neutral buffered formalin for over 1 hour. Dry and box slides for future use.

Chrome alum gelatin slides—'subbed slides'—wash slides followed by a rinse in 95% ethanol. Dissolve 1.0 gram of Type A powdered gelatin (300 bloom) in 80 ml of warm distilled water. Dissolve 0.1 g of chromic potassium sulfate ($CrK(SO_4)_2 \cdot 12H_2O$) in 20 ml of distilled water. Mix the gelatin and chromic potassium sulfate solutions together to form a working solution. Spread evenly over slides and dry for at least 1 hour. Box slides for future use.

REFERENCES

Highman B. (1946) Improved methods for demonstrating amyloid in paraffin sections. Archives of Pathology 41:559–562.

Lillie R.D., Ashburn L.L. (1943) A modification of Apathy's mounting medium. Archives of Pathology 36:432.

Staining Methods Index

Subject Index